MANIC-DEPRESSIVE ILLNESS

COLLABORATORS

S. NASSIR GHAEMI, M.D., M.P.H.
Associate Professor of Psychiatry and Public Health
Emory University

CONSTANCE HAMMEN, PH.D.
Professor of Psychology and Psychiatry
University of California, Los Angeles

TERENCE A. KETTER, M.D.
Professor of Psychiatry
Stanford University School of Medicine

HUSSEINI K. MANJI, M.D., FRCPC
Director, Mood and Anxiety Disorders Program
National Institute of Mental Health

FRANCIS M. MONDIMORE, M.D.
Assistant Professor of Psychiatry
The Johns Hopkins University School of Medicine

JAMES B. POTASH, M.D., M.P.H.
Associate Professor of Psychiatry
The Johns Hopkins University School of Medicine

HAROLD A. SACKEIM, PH.D.
Professor of Psychiatry and Radiology
College of Physicians and Surgeons of Columbia University

MYRNA M. WEISSMAN, PH.D.
Professor of Epidemiology in Psychiatry
College of Physicians and Surgeons of Columbia University

AND

Hagop S. Akiskal, M.D.
Professor of Psychiatry
University of California, San Diego

Gabrielle A. Carlson, M.D.
Professor of Psychiatry and Pediatrics
Stony Brook University School of Medicine

Miriam Davis, Ph.D.
Adjunct Assistant Professor of Epidemiology
 and Biostatistics (as of 2006)
The George Washington University School of Public Health
 and Health Services

J. Raymond DePaulo, Jr., M.D.
Professor of Psychiatry
The Johns Hopkins University School of Medicine

Jan Fawcett, M.D.
Professor of Psychiatry
University of New Mexico School of Medicine

Daniel Z. Lieberman, M.D.
Associate Professor of Psychiatry
The George Washington University Medical Center

Teodor T. Postolache, M.D.
Associate Professor of Psychiatry
University of Maryland School of Medicine

SECOND EDITION

MANIC-DEPRESSIVE ILLNESS
Bipolar Disorders and Recurrent Depression

FREDERICK K. GOODWIN, M.D.
Professor of Psychiatry
The George Washington University Medical Center

KAY REDFIELD JAMISON, PH.D.
Professor of Psychiatry
The Johns Hopkins University School of Medicine

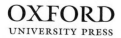
OXFORD
UNIVERSITY PRESS

2007

OXFORD
UNIVERSITY PRESS

Oxford University Press, Inc., publishes works that further
Oxford University's objective of excellence
in research, scholarship, and education.

Oxford   New York
Auckland   Cape Town   Dar es Salaam   Hong Kong   Karachi
Kuala Lumpur   Madrid   Melbourne   Mexico City   Nairobi
New Delhi   Shanghai   Taipei   Toronto

With offices in
Argentina   Austria   Brazil   Chile   Czech Republic   France   Greece
Guatemala   Hungary   Italy   Japan   Poland   Portugal   Singapore
South Korea   Switzerland   Thailand   Turkey   Ukraine   Vietnam

Published by Oxford University Press, Inc.
198 Madison Avenue, New York, New York 10016

www.oup.com

Oxford is a registered trademark of Oxford University Press

Please visit this volume's companion Web site at
www.oup.com/us/manicdepressiveillness2e

Citation to this volume should be given in the following way: Goodwin, F. K., and Jamison,
K.R. (2007). *Manic-Depressive Illness: Bipolar Disorders and Recurrent Depression,*
2nd edition. New York: Oxford University Press.

9 8 7 6 5 4 3 2 1

Printed in the United States of America
on acid-free paper

This book is dedicated to the memory of
John Cade and Mogens Schou,
whose pioneering work saved
the lives of hundreds of thousands of patients
and to our colleagues,
whose work will save the lives of countless more.

—F.K.G. and K.R.J.

AND

Also dedicated to my wife and colleague
Rosemary P. Goodwin, M.S.W.

—F.K.G.

In memory of
Richard Wyatt, M.D.,
husband and colleague

—K.R.J.

The original version of this book, published in 1990, was a unique contribution to the literature on manic-depressive illness. For a long time, certainly since Bleuler and Schneider developed broad criteria for schizophrenia, manic-depressive illness had been neglected both as a clinical diagnosis and as a topic for research. The influence of psychoanalysis and Meyer's psychobiology exacerbated this neglect. Meaningful attention to the illness began to increase with the discovery of lithium as a surprisingly effective treatment for mania (this book is very appropriately dedicated to John Cade and Mogens Schou). But it was Goodwin and Jamison's work, coming at a time when manic-depressive illness remained curiously marginalized in the scientific literature, that gave the subject the treatment it deserved. Remarkably, their text was lengthy enough to allow detailed accounts and comprehensive summaries of all the available literature while at the same time being accessible in style and presentation, with an authentic continuity in the voice of its two authors.

Kay Jamison and Fred Goodwin are, of course, giants in this field, and their contribution seemed even then a remarkable one: Jamison for her profound clinical and psychological understanding, and Goodwin for his immense pharmacological and biological knowledge. To attempt a repeat of their efforts in a new edition was an enormous challenge, especially since the rapid expansion of scientific and clinical information that has occurred in the last 20 years has made the single- or dual-author textbook an increasingly endangered species. The authors' solution for this new edition of *Manic-Depressive Illness* is an innovative one that works exceedingly well: by enlisting the help of close colleagues with various specialized interests and producing an interpretive synthesis of those views through the filter of their own unparalleled expertise, they have avoided creating a compilation of chapters written by individual authors and preserved the unity and structure of the original work.

The book is divided into five parts covering the diagnosis, clinical characteristics, psychology, pathophysiology, and treatment of manic-depressive illness. It is an exceptional record of the current state of the art, and we are confident that it will satisfy the most discriminating readers, from those who simply want to acquaint themselves with a single aspect of the illness and its many manifestations to those who wish to use this text as the basis for a comprehensive understanding of the subject.

A number of key differences between this and the first edition of the book deserve to be highlighted. The discussion of the spectrum diagnoses has been greatly expanded and informed by an increase in empirical work on the topic: diagnoses such as bipolar-II were not as commonly accepted prior to the publication of the *Diagnostic and Statistical Manual*, 4th edition (DSM-IV) in 1994, and the previously underappreciated topic of mixed states, especially depressive mixed states, is now properly included. Phenomenological studies of manic-depressive illness in children, women, and the elderly are now examined. The chapter on course of illness incorporates some major new outcome studies that began in the 1990s and have since expanded. The treatment chapters are, inevitably, greatly expanded to review the literature on benchmark therapies such as electroconvulsive therapy and lithium, as well as to accommodate the new literature on atypical antipsychotics, novel anticonvulsants, antidepressants, and structured psychosocial interventions. These chapters are also preceded by a discussion of the research methods now needed to evaluate increasingly complex clinical trials. Studies of molecular genetics, second messenger and intracellular mechanisms, and functional imaging were just starting two decades ago, but are quite central now. Even the historical assessment of how the illness was understood in previous eras is being revised on the basis of new evidence discussed in this edition.

The title of the second edition remains *Manic-Depressive Illness*, with the addition of a subtitle, *Bipolar Disorders and Recurrent Depression*. As in the first edition, the main emphasis is on the inclusive Kraepelinian concept of manic-depressive illness, a perspective too easily lost within the post–DSM-III nosology of mood disorders. This second edition underlines how Kraepelin's "central insight—that all of the recurrent major mood disorders (in today's terms) belonged together under the rubric of *manic-depressive illness*—still provides the best model for what we know to date, as well as for understanding emerging clinical, pharmacological, and genetic data."

We have no doubt that this second edition of *Manic-Depressive Illness*, like the first, will have an immense impact on the field; it will be a great resource for research, and it will help improve diagnosis and treatment of those who suffer from the illness. While the volume of new work it describes is encouraging, however, manic-depressive illness remains a much lower public health priority than schizophrenia and depression, not to mention many physical conditions, as evidenced by the relative paucity of research funds devoted to its study. Hence this second edition

can help us all in an important additional task: to promote awareness and investment of both time and money in this major illness by the best and brightest around the world. As Kraepelin said, "What goal could be more sacred than that of caring for a brother in distress, especially when the affliction stems from his very humanity . . . and when it cannot be halted by reason, rank or riches?"[1]

GUY GOODWIN, M.D.
Oxford

ATHANASIOS KOUKOPOULOS, M.D.
Rome

[1] Emil Kraepelin, quoting Anton Mueller, in *Hundert Jahre Psychiatrie* (Berlin: Verlag von Julius Springer, 1918), p. 112.

ACKNOWLEDGMENTS

Without the sustained commitment and clinical and scientific expertise of our collaborators, whose names appear opposite the title page, there would be no second edition of *Manic-Depressive Illness*. We are immensely indebted to them for their time and scholarship. The collaborators' individual contributions ranged from a slight to substantial updating of a first-edition chapter (retaining the original organization and most of the original material) to, in a few instances, the drafting of an entirely new chapter; most contributions fell somewhere in between. They followed general guidelines formulated by us, including our specifications about the conceptualization and usage of the terms *manic-depressive illness* and *bipolar disorder*, the critical need for rigorous and impartial review, and the shared goal of contributing to a book that would maintain the unified authorship voice of the first edition. There was extensive interaction between us and our collaborators throughout, with many drafts of each chapter going back and forth.

In each case the last draft provided to us by a collaborator was revised and updated, usually extensively, by one or both of us. When our judgment about a specific clinical or scientific point differed from that of a collaborator, which was not infrequently the case, we carefully considered the collaborator's point of view before making a final decision. In the end, the two authors take responsibility for the contents of the book.

The collaborators would like to acknowledge the contributions of Po Wang and John Brooks (Dr. Ketter); Susan Bachus, Lisa Catapano, Guang Chen, Jing Du, Holly A. Giesen, Fatemi Hosein, Libby Jolkovsky, Celia Knobelsdorf, Phillip Kronstein, Rodrigo Machado-Vieira, Andrew Newberg, Jennifer Payne, Jorge Quiroz, Giacomo Salvadore, Peter J. Schmidt, Jaskaran Singh, and Carlos A. Zarate, Jr. (Dr. Manji); Al Lewy, Joseph Soriano, John Stiller, Leonardo Tonelli, and Thomas Wehr (Dr. Postolache); Gregory Fuller (Dr. Potash); Rice Fuller (Dr. Sackeim); and Helena Verdeli (Dr. Weissman). Drs. Goodwin and Jamison would like to acknowledge additional colleagues who reviewed chapters or otherwise provided input: Jules Angst, Ross Baldessarini, Robert Belmaker, Charles Bowden, Joseph Calabrese, Kiki Chang, Guy Goodwin, Heinz Grunze, Dean Jamison, Athanasios Koukopoulos, Andreas Marneros, Roger Meyer, Gary Sachs, Mauricio Tohen, Eduardo Vieta, Jeremy Waletzky, and Peter Whybrow.

Dr. Goodwin's two research assistants, Mark Goldstein and Jaclyn Saggese Fleming, worked full time on this book and were essential to its production, Mr. Goldstein during the critical first two years of the project and Mrs. Fleming during the final three. Not only were they responsible for many of the literature searches and the preparation of tables and figures, they also often went beyond that, preparing summaries of critical areas of research. During the final two years in particular, Mrs. Fleming was the indispensable hub of the whole operation, coordinating the work of both the authors, the input from all of our collaborators, the work of our chief medical editor, and the editorial and production staff at Oxford University Press. She did this with a rare combination of intelligence, care and thoroughness, organization, blinding speed, and good humor. The ability of Mr. Goldstein and Mrs. Fleming to perform at such a high level is consistent with their career trajectories—Mr. Goldstein is already in medical school and Mrs. Fleming is in a post-baccalaureate biology program.

Dr. Goodwin is further indebted to his executive assistant, Joanne Davis, for facilitating his work on this book by skillfully keeping other aspects of his professional life on track. Dr. Goodwin would also like to acknowledge his first mentor, William E. Bunney, Jr., M.D., and his long-term colleague Dennis Murphy, M.D., who together contributed so much to the emergence of manic-depressive illness as a major focus of research at the National Institute of Mental Health. He would also like to thank the George Washington University Medical Center's Department of Psychiatry and Behavioral Sciences and its chairman, Jeffrey Akman, M.D., for support. Finally, the unceasing encouragement and support of Rosemary Goodwin, M.S.W., has been, as always, a mainstay.

Dr. Jamison would like to acknowledge the invaluable contributions of Silas Jones, William Collins, and Ioline Henter. It has been a delight to work with them and it would have been impossible to complete this book without their help. She would also like to acknowledge the support of her colleagues in the Department of Psychiatry at the Johns Hopkins School of Medicine. Adam Kaplin, M.D., Ph.D., has been particularly helpful and generous with his time. Most deeply she would like to extend her heartfelt appreciation to her psychiatrist, Daniel Auerbach, M.D., who not only taught her how to live with manic-depressive illness but also encouraged her to study and write about it. His profound clinical understanding of the medical and psychological aspects of bipolar disorder were life saving; they have also strongly influenced her research, clinical practice, and writing. She owes a deep debt as well to her late husband, Richard Wyatt, M.D. He too encouraged her to write about manic-depressive illness, from both a clinical and personal perspective, and provided the kind of love and support that made it possible. He was a wonderful husband, colleague, and friend.

It is impossible to overstate the contribution of our medical editor, Rona Briere. Her consummate editing abilities, coupled with an extraordinary level of professionalism and intellectual integrity, made working with her both an education and a pleasure. Alisa Decatur meticulously prepared the manuscript of each chapter, tracked and reconciled the text citations and reference lists, edited the references, and performed numerous additional tasks that were invaluable in finalizing the book. Deb Uffelman and Gerald Briere assisted with proofreading and preparation of the reference lists. We are also grateful to Marion Osmun, Nancy Wolitzer, and Sarah Harrington at Oxford University Press for their dedication, skill, and impressive ability to implement and meet near-impossible deadlines.

During the time that this book was in preparation, Dr. Goodwin received research support from George Washington University Medical Center, the Foundation for Education and Research on Mental Illness, the Dalio Family Foundation, GlaxoSmithKline, Pfizer, Eli Lilly, and Solvay. He has received honoraria from GlaxoSmithKline, Pfizer, Solvay, and Eli Lilly and unrestricted educational grants to support the production of this book from Abbott, AstraZeneca, Bristol Meyers Squibb, Forest, GlaxoSmithKline, Janssen, Eli Lilly, Pfizer, and Sanofi. Dr. Goodwin has been a consultant and/or advisor for Eli Lilly, GlaxoSmithKline, Pfizer, Janssen, Novartis, and Solvay. He is not a shareholder in any pharmaceutical or biotechnology company. He is a partner in Best Practice Project Management, Inc.

Dr. Jamison, as a MacArthur fellow, received generous financial support from the John D. and Catherine T. MacArthur Foundation, as well as funding from the Dana Foundation. She has received occasional lecture honoraria from AstraZeneca, GlaxoSmithKline, and Eli Lilly. She has received no research support from any pharmaceutical or biotechnology company, nor is she a consultant to, or shareholder in, any pharmaceutical or biotechnology company. As with the first edition of this text, all of her royalties go directly to a not-for-profit foundation that supports public education about manic-depressive illness.

F.K.G. AND K.R.J.

Contents

Melancholia is the beginning and a part of mania . . . . The development of a mania is really a worsening of the disease (melancholia) rather than a change into another disease.

—Aretaeus of Cappadocia, ca. 100 AD[1]

It has been 17 years since the publication of the first edition of this text; they have been the most explosively productive years in the history of medical science. In every field relevant to our understanding of manic-depressive illness—genetics, neurobiology, psychology and neuropsychology, neuroanatomy, diagnosis, and treatment—we have gained a staggering amount of knowledge. Scientists and clinicians have gone an impressive distance toward fulfilling the hopes articulated by Emil Kraepelin in the introduction to his 1899 textbook on psychiatry. Those who treat and study mental illness, he wrote, must first, from bedside observation, delineate the clinical forms of illness; they must define and predict its course, determine its causes, and discover how best to treat and then ultimately prevent insanity. Psychiatry, he argued, was a "young, still developing science," and it must, "against sharp opposition, gradually achieve the position it deserves according to its scientific and practical importance. There is no doubt that it will achieve the position—for it has at its disposal the same weapons which have served the other branches of medicine so well: clinical observation, the microscope and experimentation."[2] Kraepelin was right, as usual. And he was remarkably astute in his observations and predictions about the immensely complex group of disorders collectively known as manic-depressive illness.

Manic-depressive illness magnifies common human experiences to larger-than-life proportions. Among its symptoms are exaggerations of normal sadness and joy, profoundly altered thinking, irritability and rage, psychosis and violence, and deeply disrupted patterns of energy and sleep. In its diverse forms, manic-depressive illness afflicts a large number of people—the exact number depending on how the illness is defined and how accurately it is ascertained. First described thousands of years ago, found in widely diverse cultures, manic-depressive illness always has fascinated medical observers, even as it has baffled and frightened

most others. To those afflicted, it can be so painful that suicide seems the only means of escape; indeed, manic-depressive illness is the most common cause of suicide.

We view manic-depressive illness as a medical condition, an illness to be diagnosed, treated, studied, and understood within a medical context. This position is the prevailing one now, as it has been throughout history. Less universal is our diagnostic conception of manic-depressive illness, which evolved as we were writing both editions of this book. Derived from the work of Kraepelin, the "great classifier," our conception encompasses roughly the same group of disorders as the term *manic–depressive illness* in European usage. It differs, however, from contemporary concepts of bipolar disorder. Kraepelin built his observations on the work of a small group of nineteenth-century European psychiatrists who, in their passion for ever finer distinctions, had cataloged abnormal human behavior into hundreds of classes of disorder. More than any other single individual, Kraepelin brought order and sense to this categorical profusion. He constructed a nosology based on careful description, reducing the categories of psychoses to two: manic-depressive illness and dementia praecox, later renamed *schizophrenia*.

It is to Kraepelin, born in the same year as Freud, that we owe much of our conceptualization of manic-depressive illness. It is to him that we owe our emphasis on documenting the longitudinal course of the illness and the careful delineation of mixed states and the stages of mania, as well as the observations that cycle length shortens with succeeding episodes; that poor clinical outcome is associated with rapid cycles, mixed states, and coexisting substance abuse; that genetics is central to the pathophysiology of the disease; and that manic-depressive illness is a spectrum of conditions and related temperaments.

Kraepelin's model consolidated most of the major affective disorders into one category because of their similarity in core symptoms; presence of a family history of illness; and, especially, the pattern of recurrence over the course of the patient's lifetime, with periods of remission and exacerbation and a comparatively benign outcome without significant deterioration. Kraepelin viewed mania as one manifestation of the illness, not as the distinguishing sign of a separate bipolar disorder as it is regarded in today's American (and increasingly worldwide) diagnostic practice.

The European and American concepts of manic-depressive illness began to diverge almost immediately after Kraepelin's ideas became widespread in the early years of the twentieth century. Europeans, adhering to a traditional medical disease model, emphasized the longitudinal course of the illness in both research and clinical work. Ever pragmatic, Americans wanted to treat the illness with the techniques at hand, which at that time were derived from the "moral treatment" movement in mental hospitals and the emerging dynamic therapies based on psychoanalytic theory. Research and clinical efforts in the United States thus slighted clinical description and genetics and turned instead to the psychological and social contexts in which the symptoms of the illness occurred.

Exploration of the linkages between clinical typology and family history led to the formulation of the bipolar–unipolar distinction, by which manic-depressive patients were grouped according to the presence or absence of a prior history of mania or hypomania. First proposed by a German, Karl Leonhard, the distinction was elaborated by other Europeans, such as Jules Angst and Carlo Perris, and by the Washington University group in St. Louis, Missouri, the neo-Kraepelinians who gave impetus to the new concern for an etiology-free, description-based diagnostic system in the United States.

The bipolar–unipolar distinction represented a logical refinement of the already well-defined Kraepelinian model, with its emphasis on recurrence and endogeneity. As useful as the distinction is in both research and clinical contexts, it proved to be problematic when applied to the much broader American conception of affective disorders. The bipolar subgroup was clearly defined, but the other component of Kraepelinian manic-depressive illness—endogenous, recurrent unipolar depression—was obscured by its confusion with other affective disorders. In American usage, *unipolar* disorder came to mean any mood disorder that was not bipolar, regardless of its severity or course. Although the third edition of the *Diagnostic and Statistical Manual* (DSM-III) clarified the situation somewhat by requiring that criteria for major affective disorder be met before the bipolar–unipolar distinction is drawn, a diagnosis of unipolar disorder was still broader than the Kraepelinian concept since it did not require a prior course of illness. Even the DSM-III/IV category of recurrent depression is overly broad, requiring only two episodes in a lifetime.

Our own struggle to confine and limit the focus of the first edition of this text followed a course similar to the larger historical one. We started with a framework of Kraepelinian manic-depressive illness, that is, recurrent major affective illness with and without mania. Later, we focused more exclusively on bipolar disorder as a way of imposing workable boundaries on the scope of our efforts. Once thoroughly immersed in the subject, however, we became increasingly convinced that isolating bipolar disorder from other major depressive disorders and unduly emphasizing polarity over cyclicity (as do DSM-III and DSM-IV) prejudges the relationships between bipolar and unipolar illness and diminishes appreciation of the fundamental importance of recurrence. By the end, we had returned to a position close to where we began, convinced of the value of the original unified concept of manic-depressive illness, albeit with a special emphasis on the bipolar form. Scientific and clinical advances of the past two decades have only added to the strength of our belief that, as important as polarity is, cyclicity or recurrence is fundamental to understanding manic-depressive illness. This conviction is made clear in the second edition's new title: *Manic Depressive Illness: Bipolar Disorders and Recurrent Depression.* Genetic findings will have the ultimate etiologic and diagnostic say, of course, but in the interim we think a broader rather than narrower concept of the illness is warranted by the data; we also think it is heuristically most valuable.

DIMENSIONS OF THE ILLNESS

It bears repeating that the presence or absence of mania in addition to depression is but one critical aspect of manic-depressive illness. The other is cyclicity, which may ultimately prove to be as useful as polarity in differentiating forms of affective illness. The classic European focus on longitudinal studies has provided an ample database for redirecting the emphasis of pathophysiology to mechanisms of cyclicity—that is, the biology of recurrence. To conduct such research, an investigator must analyze each patient's biological functioning over time and relate it to the natural course of illness. The priority that American clinicians are beginning to assign to recurrence is a tribute to the persuasiveness of our European colleagues' meticulous longitudinal clinical observations. Kraepelin's descriptions have been enduring: again and again during our study of the contemporary literature, we returned to his original writings to rediscover modern ideas. To a remarkable degree, his work anticipated, explicitly and implicitly, contemporary theoretical developments. One example is the spectrum concept—the continuity of manic-depressive symptoms with normal fluctuations in mood, energy patterns, and behavior—a concept whose database has greatly expanded since the publication of the first edition.

The longitudinal view provided by Kraepelin and many others both before and since persuaded us to survey the literature on recurrent unipolar illness along with that on bipolar illness, our primary focus. If we had confined ourselves to the bipolar literature, we would have excluded many potentially relevant data and insights. This recognition of the essential unity of major recurrent affective illness is evident throughout the book. When discussing lithium prophylaxis in Chapter 20, for example, we point out that similarities between recurrent unipolar and bipolar illness constitute firm ground for speculating about common neurobiological substrates.

The issue of cyclicity opens up many new areas of inquiry. Manic and depressive episodes can be predicted to revert to normal at some finite time, either spontaneously or in response to effective treatment. The opportunity to compare biological measures during the illness with the same measures in the recovered state is essential in psychobiological research, since it permits longitudinal studies that can circumvent the problem of variability among individuals. The recurrent pattern of the illness—that of recovery to normal or change to an opposite state—makes it an unsurpassed paradigm for separating state and trait variables in mental illness. The regularity of recurrence in some patients permits the clinical investigator to anticipate the onset of an episode and thus to schedule data collection at critical points. The frequent rapidity of the switch from one state to another, especially the switch into mania, allows for intensive efforts to understand the relationships between stress and biological changes in the onset of illness by looking at the temporal sequence of events—one approach to the ultimate question of causality.

The bipolar form of the illness also is an interesting study in the coexistence of opposites or, more precisely, deviations from normal in opposite directions. Even lay observers may recognize that bipolar disorder is at times accompanied by periods of euphoric mood, productivity, and high energy, but at other times by despair and profound lassitude. Clinicians see a more subtle manifestation of this Janus-like illness in lithium's effects in preventing its apparently opposite expressions. Lithium's dual action, perhaps diminishing some of the silver lining along with the cloud, challenges the clinician's psychotherapeutic skills in managing the issue of treatment acceptance, especially medication adherence.

THE SCIENCE OF THE ILLNESS

Over the past six decades, research has yielded effective treatments that have radically altered clinical work in manic-depressive illness. Principally, it was the discovery of lithium that galvanized the treatment community, instilling new hope among clinicians, their patients, and the public. Also important, the emergence of lithium, the antidepressants, the antipsychotics, and the anticonvulsants gave birth to whole new fields of scientific investigation. Studies of the illness have dominated biological psychiatry, which itself has begun to lead the profession. Manic-depressive illness has been an increasingly important focus of work in other disciplines as well. Insights gained from the study of an illness that is biological in origin yet psychological in expression have underscored the urgency and inevitability of paradigms of mental illness that give balanced attention to biology, psychology, and the environment. Methodologies developed expressly for studies of manic-depressive illness have been incorporated as standard tools of clinical investigation in other areas of biomedical and behavioral research in psychopathology. Because symptoms of the illness shade over into normal human experience, it provides a model for the study of normal states as well.

Nearly 60 years have passed since the initial clinical observation of lithium's effectiveness in treating manic-depressive illness and 50 years since early clinical trials—most important, those completed by Mogens Schou, Poul Christian Baastrup, G. P. Hartigan, and Alec Coppen—were conducted so that lithium could be approved for general clinical use throughout the world. More recently, research on manic-depressive illness has played a central role in efforts to apply new and emerging techniques, such as molecular genetics, to the study of psychiatric conditions. The application of these techniques depends on the use of sensitive and reliable epidemiological and diagnostic case-finding methodologies to identify family pedigrees with a high incidence of the illness. Preliminary results suggest that several genotypes underlie different forms of manic-depressive illness. It is also possible that, as with the multiple genetic forms of diabetes, several genotypes are expressed in clinical phenomena commonly associated with the illness.

Research on manic-depressive illness also has contributed new, empirically based theories about the pathophysiology of psychiatric disorders, including the influence of the physical environment—light and temperature in particular—on their course and expression. Of equal interest are efforts to describe mechanisms by which the psychosocial environment interacts with the individual's biology to produce symptoms. One of the most promising lines of inquiry grew out of longitudinal observations: external stress appeared to activate or precipitate some initial episodes of illness, but eventually the illness seemed to take on a life of its own, since later episodes began without obvious precipitating stress.

OVERVIEW OF THIS TEXT

In a text of this size and scope, a certain amount of redundancy is inevitable. Issues pertaining to the dimensional aspects of manic-depressive illness, such as severity, polarity, and cyclicity, are introduced in the first two chapters and then discussed further throughout the book. Where an issue could logically be discussed in more than one chapter, our decisions on placement occasionally were somewhat arbitrary.

Clinical Description and Diagnosis

The text is divided into five parts, the first of which focuses on clinical phenomenology and diagnosis. Chapter 1 traces the evolution of the concept of the illness, which has remained remarkably consistent since the time of Hippocrates, and describes the spectrum of the illness in detail. We highlight the fact that diagnostic and subgroup boundaries represent somewhat arbitrary distinctions, with individual patients often falling in a gray area. Also emphasized is the spectrum of manic states, which, unlike the well-described depressive spectrum, is often overlooked. We stress that while the spectrum concept has validity and utility, there are risks in subclassifying the bipolar forms of the illness to such an extent that they are confusing, on occasion to the detriment of both clinical and research purposes.

We begin the chapter on clinical description (Chapter 2) with classic descriptions of the illness by early clinical observers who worked in the era before effective medications altered the natural expression of the illness; these are followed by patients' descriptions of their experiences of the illness. We also review data-based studies of mania, mixed states, and bipolar depression, with a particular emphasis on new research findings pertaining to mixed states and bipolar depression.

Chapter 3 guides the clinician through the problems of diagnosis. Most important is the differential diagnosis of bipolar disorder and unipolar depression, schizophrenia, organic brain disorders, substance abuse, and borderline personality disorders. The shortcomings of our current diagnostic systems, including their emphasis on polarity rather than cyclicity, the absence of a category for highly recurrent depression, the underrecognition of bipolar-II disorder, and the inadequacy of the diagnostic criteria for mixed states, are discussed in detail.

Clinical Studies

The second part covers various clinical aspects of manic-depressive illness. Appropriately, we begin in Chapter 4 with a discussion of course and outcome, fundamental characteristics of the illness that provide the basis for differentiating it from schizophrenia. In addition to its obvious importance for clinicians who are assessing prognosis and planning treatment, natural course is important to scientists since it offers many useful clues as to pathological processes. We consider historical observations on course and outcome together with data gathered from the large-scale studies conducted since the first edition of this text.

Chapter 5, on epidemiology, argues that manic-depressive illness, especially its bipolar form, is more common than is usually thought. Among the most important recent observations are the early age at onset documented in careful community surveys; determinations of the rates of bipolar-II and bipolar spectrum disorders; and the results of several important international studies, including those of death and disability, that document the high toll exacted by manic-depressive illness worldwide.

The next three chapters highlight special clinical aspects of manic-depressive illness. Chapter 6 addresses aspects of the illness in children and adolescents. Because there are essentially no data on highly recurrent depression in these populations, the chapter focuses exclusively on bipolar disorder, which all too often goes unrecognized in youth. Although relatively rare in prepubertal children, classic bipolar disorder often begins in adolescence; indeed, well over one-third of all cases begin before the age of 20. Were the kindling hypothesis substantiated, early recognition and immediate, vigorous treatment would be expected to reduce subsequent pathology. Early treatment would reduce the psychological scarring caused by untreated illness, as well as the high mortality rate from suicide, which is disproportionately likely to occur early in the course of bipolar disorder. All too typical is the individual, initially treated in his or her mid- to late twenties, who has already lived with the disorder for more than a decade, a period critical for life's major beginnings in relationships, education, and career. The research findings on childhood bipolar disorder published since the first edition of this text have been prodigious, but continue to be marked by confusion and controversy. Even so, many more young children with severe mood lability and behavioral dyscontrol are now being identified and treated with mood stabilizers, antipsychotics, and antidepressants.

A focus on the young highlights the frequent coexistence of drug and alcohol abuse among young manic-depressive patients. Growing recognition of the frequent coexistence of the illness with substance abuse prompted us to devote an entire chapter (Chapter 7) to describing these problems and another (Chapter 24) to reviewing their treatment. In these two chapters, we also discuss other important comorbid conditions, such as anxiety disorders, eating disorders, cardiovascular disease, thyroid dysfunction, overweight and obesity, and migraine, as well as their treatment. The presence of a depressive or anxiety disorder can double the chances of subsequent substance abuse. Conversely, illicit drugs and alcohol can adversely affect the course and treatment of manic-depressive illness by altering the same brain mechanisms that regulate mood, including the potential for kindling.

As with substance abuse and other comorbid conditions, the importance of suicide in manic-depressive illness is reflected in our devoting two chapters to the subject—one describing rates, putative causes, and clinical correlates (Chapter 8), and another detailing preventive measures (Chapter 25). The high mortality associated with this illness cannot be overemphasized. Fortunately, considerable progress has been made in understanding the causes of suicide in manic-depressive patients, in addition to the accumulating evidence that lithium exerts a strong protective influence.

The reader may note that there is no chapter on gender differences in manic-depressive illness, reflecting the relative scarcity of literature on this subject. However, reports of male–female differences are noted throughout the book; here we summarize those for which there is general agreement: the first episode is more likely to be mania in males and depression in females, while women have more mixed episodes (consistent with a predominance of depression) and are overrepresented among rapid cyclers; consistent with the general population, men are more likely to have comorbid substance abuse and histories of pathological gambling and conduct disorder, while women are more likely to have comorbid eating disorders as well as changes in appetite and weight during depressive episodes; and, in contrast to the general population, the completed suicide rate for bipolar women is higher than that for bipolar men. It may be that the risk of suicide associated with manic-depressive illness is so powerful that it overrides the usual male–female patterns. Bipolar women generally are more likely than their male counterparts to seek treatment, but there is as yet no consensus regarding gender differences in response to mood stabilizers.[3]

Psychological Studies

Manic-depressive illness has been a rich source of theory and data for investigators interested in psychological mechanisms. The third part of the book considers these developments. Manic-depressive illness has contributed to the general study of psychology by serving as a paradigm for explorations of state and trait differences. It also has been a model for the general psychological assessment of cognition and for the more specific differentiation of cognition in manic and depressive states from that in schizophrenia. We begin with a survey of what is known about neuropsychological deficits in mood disorders, including recent research documenting significant impairments in intellec-

tual functioning, attention, learning and memory, and executive functioning (Chapter 9).

The psychological manifestations of manic-depressive illness, observable in personality and behavior as well as cognitive patterns, can result in profound discord in family life and other social relationships; this is especially true for those with the bipolar form of the illness. In Chapter 10 we review studies of personality functioning in manic and depressed states and how it compares with that in normal states in patients themselves and in the general population. We also discuss personality disorders that commonly co-exist with manic-depressive illness, as well as the effects of medication on personality. The chapter then addresses interpersonal aspects of the illness, with emphasis on the bipolar subgroup.

Chapter 11 is devoted to the wide array of methods that now exists for assessing manic, mixed, and depressive states; these assessment measures add the perspective of formal psychological evaluation to the discussion of differential diagnosis in Chapter 3.

Widespread interest in creativity, the subject of Chapter 12, has lent visibility to this aspect of the study of manic-depressive illness. The age-old link between "madness" and creativity has been studied with increasingly sophisticated methods in recent years. Research has demonstrated that it is not schizophrenia but manic-depressive illness, especially its bipolar forms, that is more often associated with creative accomplishment. Among the most interesting developments in this field is the hypothesis that the genetic predisposition for manic-depressive illness also confers a creative edge on affected individuals and their close relatives. Explorations of the characteristics that help make some individuals more creative than others should have implications for the general population. Among the positive features of the bipolar form of the illness being examined in relation to creativity are the heightened energy level and speed of cognition of hypomania, linked to a global, inclusive associative process, and certain temperamental factors; positive (and painful) experiences derived from having affective illness are salient as well. In addition to raising important psychological, social, and ethical issues, these and related positive features of the bipolar form of the illness can play a key role in reducing the burden of stigma borne by patients. Understanding these features is, of course, necessary in dealing with one of the most sensitive and difficult issues in treatment—medication adherence.

Pathophysiology

The size of the fourth part of the book, the largest, testifies to the wealth of biological knowledge that has accrued through research on manic-depressive illness. The illness has come to represent an extraordinarily rich source of information about the interrelationships between behavioral and biological phenomena; certainly it has stimulated fascinating and productive theories about brain–behavior relationships.

We begin with a survey of the salient literature on genetics (Chapter 13). In this chapter we review genetic epidemiology, results of studies using the linkage method, alternative phenotypic definition, association methods, gene expression and pathogenesis, pharmacogenetics, and genetic counseling. We then look at the future of the field, including new technologies and what we can expect to learn from each.

Chapter 14, on neurobiology, provides the conceptual base necessary for an appreciation of the biochemical and pharmacological studies whose review follows. Much of modern neurobiology and neuropharmacology has been driven by efforts to understand the effects of mood-altering drugs. Indeed, attempts to understand why certain drugs affect mood have inspired major hypotheses about the neurobiology of behavior. The chapter also describes animal models designed to simulate affective illness and reviews the formidable literature on the major neurotransmitter, neuroendocrine, and neuropeptide systems involved in manic-depressive illness, along with extensive new findings related to postsynaptic signal transduction networks and gene expression.

With the emergence of highly sophisticated brain-imaging technologies, it has become important to review the anatomical correlates of mania and depression critically, if only to help guide the application of imaging approaches; we do so in Chapter 15. Functional neuroimaging work has advanced rapidly in recent years. We review research findings on cerebral activity in normal, depressed, and manic states, as well as summarize what is known about baseline cerebral activity markers of treatment response.

Chapter 16 covers sleep and biological rhythms, reflecting our judgment that these two fields, which developed independently of one another, have found a natural point of convergence in the pathophysiology of manic-depressive illness. It is increasingly clear that sleep physiology is important to circadian physiology and that sleep disturbances seen in affective illness reflect disturbances in circadian rhythms. This area of study has, in our estimation, yielded some of the most interesting developments in understanding manic-depressive illness. The identification of seasonal affective disorder, for example, represents a systematic, quantitative rediscovery of ancient observations of seasonality in mood disorders and suicide. The speed with which the initial observation of seasonal mood disorder was incorporated into the DSM nosology testifies to the responsiveness of our current diagnostic system. Research

on biological rhythms has spawned the development of three novel physiological but nonpharmacological treatments for mood disorders—sleep deprivation, phase advance, and high-intensity light—that are described in Chapter 19 on the treatment of acute depression, especially in bipolar patients. At a more general level, the contemporary focus on biological rhythms has given rise to environmental psychiatry, and thus the discussion of the subject in Chapter 16 emphasizes the subtle environmental influences on manic-depressive illness and offers relevant clinical suggestions.

Treatment

The final part of the book covers all aspects of the treatment of manic-depressive illness. It is traditional in its organization, separating acute from prophylactic treatment and medical from psychological treatment. Despite this division, we wish to emphasize the profound importance of integrating medical and psychological approaches. Although the structure of this part of the book is traditional, the organization of each chapter is not. Each begins with practical recommendations for clinical management and then reviews the treatment literature, highlighting areas inadequately explored in existing reviews, including the efficacy of lithium in treating depression as well as mania and the quality of the prophylactic response. We discuss treatment controversies such as antidepressant-induced mania, mixed states, and rapid cycling; the use of adjunctive treatments for breakthrough episodes during prophylactic treatment with mood stabilizers; the important but often overlooked distinction between prevention of relapse and prevention of recurrence (new episodes); the relative efficacy and side-effect profiles of the mood stabilizers and the antipsychotics; and the use of alternative or adjunctive approaches for patients who do not respond to initial treatment. It has been of great, often life-saving clinical importance to now have anticonvulsant and antipsychotic medications that provide an alternative for those patients who do not respond to or will not take lithium. We make clear our belief that lithium remains the gold standard of treatment, however, despite an increasing tendency to use less-proven medications.

The two chapters on adherence and psychotherapy (Chapters 21 and 22, respectively) should be read together. Our purpose here is not to provide a general psychotherapy primer but to focus on issues of special importance to the psychotherapy of manic-depressive illness, especially the bipolar form. These issues include fears of recurrence, the psychological scars left by the illness, and concerns about genetic vulnerability. The central issue in the psychological management of bipolar patients is medication adherence. Recent studies suggest that outcomes of medical treatment are substantially enhanced by adjunctive psychotherapy, no doubt reflecting the contribution of improved adherence. In our discussion of adherence, we return to the core issue of the paradox of drugs that are often very effective, yet can have an impact on some aspects of the illness that may be valued by the patient. Given clinicians' all-too-common tendency to be unaware of subtle adherence problems, we believe this issue warrants a separate chapter.

Chapter 23 is devoted to the special issues that arise in treating children and adolescents with bipolar illness. Chapter 24 deals with the treatment of comorbid conditions such as anxiety disorders, substance abuse, and medical conditions that frequently accompany manic-depressive illness.

The fact that manic-depressive illness is often lethal bears repeated mention. We have underscored this fact by summarizing what is known about rates and clinical correlates of suicide in Chapter 8; in Chapter 25, we emphasize clinical methods we believe to be most useful in reducing the risk of suicide among acutely ill patients. We emphasize again the fundamental premise that the best approach to the prevention of suicide is the effective and aggressive treatment of the underlying illness.

THE DEVELOPMENT OF THIS BOOK

The overwhelming size of the literature on manic-depressive illness makes it all but impossible for clinicians and researchers to keep pace with the latest findings and to see the broader clinical, human, and scientific picture. The National Library of Medicine's Medline file on bipolar disorder alone has grown from 16 citations in 1950; to approximately 600 citations in 1990, the year the first edition of this book was published; to more than 1,100 citations in 2006. We were aware of the problem before we began writing the first edition of this book. As we struggled through the scientific literature that had grown exponentially since 1990, we once again were concerned that the very magnitude of the new, scattered evidence threatens the ability to form a coherent overall view of the illness. In recent decades, research on manic-depressive illness has contributed to an extraordinary expansion of the knowledge base in increasingly specialized fields. The productivity of the research enterprise has generated diverse points of focus, which are often appreciated only by individuals in a given subfield. An unfortunate outgrowth of such specialization is that the wealth of new information typically has been made available only in the form of individual research reports or reviews of selected areas; at best, these occasionally are published in edited volumes.

Working during this period of extraordinary productivity and ferment in the study of manic-depressive illness, we saw the need for a comprehensive book that would attempt to impose order on a rich but vast and disparate literature. We were convinced that this goal could be accomplished only by seeing the subject through from beginning to end—in other words, by writing a book rather than editing a collection. We were able to accomplish this by jointly authoring the first edition. As indicated in our acknowledgments and in the list of collaborators for this edition, however, we found it imperative to seek the help of colleagues; we could not have completed this book without them. Our intent was to go beyond a review of the literature—to assess the nodal points in knowledge of the illness, to integrate them in a way that would enhance the quality of clinical care available, and to suggest opportunities for future research. In the early twenty-first century, manic-depressive illness continues to present new challenges and questions that extend from the realm of basic neurobiological science to those of clinical practice and social ethics. The skill the field brings to identifying these questions will determine the strategies formulated to answer them, and in turn will bear directly on future advances in treatment and prevention.

Throughout the writing of this edition of the book, as during the first, we have been impressed time and again by the excellent science, imaginative clinical research, and profoundly important treatment advances generated by our colleagues. We are delighted to acknowledge our debt to them, both for their science and for the lives they have saved. As before, our debt to our students and patients is immeasurable.

NOTES

1. Cited in Marneros, A., and Angst, J. Bipolar disorders: Roots and evolution (p. 6). Translated from the Greek by A. Marneros. In Marneros, A., and Angst, J. (2000). *Bipolar Disorders: 100 Years After Manic-Depressive Insanity.* Dordrecht, The Netherlands: Kluwer.
2. Kraepelin, E. (1990). *Psychiatry: A Textbook for Students and Physicians*, Sixth Edition. Translated by Helga Metoui. Canton, MA: Science History Publications, p. 8. Originally published as *Psychiatrie. Ein Lehrbuch fur Studierende und Arzte.* Leipzig: Johann Ambrosius Barth, 1899.
3. For reviews of gender differences in bipolar disorder, see Taylor and Abrams, 1981; Leibenluft, 1996; Blehar et al., 1998; Robb et al., 1998; Hendrick et al., 2000; and Kawa et al., 2005.

REFERENCES

Blehar, M.C., and Oren, D.A. (1997). Gender differences in depression. *Medscape Womens Health*, 2(2), 3.

Blehar, M.C., and Rudorfer, M.V. (1998). Women's mental health research—what is the need? *Psychopharmacol Bull*, 34(3), 237–238.

Blehar, M.C., DePaulo, J.R., Gershon, E.S., Reich, T., Simpson, S.G., and Nurnberger, J.I. (1998). Women with bipolar disorder: Findings from the NIMH Genetics Initiative sample. *Psychopharmacol Bull*, 34(3), 239–243.

Dorr, D.A., Rice, J.P., Armstrong, C., Reich, T., and Blehar, M. (1997). A meta-analysis of chromosome 18 linkage data for bipolar illness. *Genet Epidemiol*, 14(6), 617–622.

Hendrick, V., Altshuler, L.L., Gitlin, M.J., Delrahim, S., and Hammen, C. (2000). Gender and bipolar illness. *J Clin Psychiatry*, 61(5), 393–396, quiz 397.

Kawa, I., Carter, J.D., Joyce, P.R., Doughty, C.J., Frampton, C.M., Wells, J.E., Walsh, A.E., and Olds, R.J. 2005. Gender differences in bipolar disorder: Age of onset, course, comorbidity, and symptom presentation. *Bipolar Disord*, 7(2), 119–125.

Leibenluft, E. (1996). Women with bipolar illness: Clinical and research issues. *Am J Psychiatry*, 153(2), 163–173.

Robb, J.C., Young, L.T., Cooke, R.G., and Joffe, R.T. (1998). Gender differences in patients with bipolar disorder influence outcome in the medical outcomes survey (SF-20) subscale scores. *J Affect Disord*, 49(3), 189–193.

Stuart, S., O'Hara, M.W., and Blehar, M.C. (1998). Mental disorders associated with childbearing: Report of the Biennial Meeting of the Marce Society. *Psychopharmacol Bull*, 34(3), 333–338.

Taylor, M.A., and Abrams, R. (1981). Gender differences in bipolar affective disorder. *J Affect Disord*, 3(3), 261–271.

PART I

CLINICAL DESCRIPTION AND DIAGNOSIS

1 Conceptualizing Manic-Depressive Illness: The Bipolar–Unipolar Distinction and the Development of the Manic-Depressive Spectrum

Manic-depressive insanity . . . includes on the one hand the whole domain of the so-called periodic and circular insanity, on the other hand simple mania, the greater part of the morbid states termed melancholia and also a not inconsiderable number of cases of amentia [confusional insanity].

—*Emil Kraepelin*[1] *(1921, p. 1)*

It was the work of Angst and Perris that helped spread my theory that unipolar and bipolar diseases . . . have different clinical pictures. The bipolar form displays a considerably more colorful appearance; it varies not only between the two poles, but in each phase offers different pictures. The unipolar forms . . . return, in a periodic course, with the same symptomatology.

—*Karl Leonhard (1979, pp. 3–4)*

Medical conceptions of mania and depression are as old as medicine itself. From ancient times to the present, an extraordinary consistency characterizes descriptions of these conditions. Few maladies have been represented with such unvarying language. Yet while the essential features are recognizable in the medical literature through the centuries, the boundaries that define mania and depression and the relationship between them have changed during that time. In this chapter, we begin by reviewing the historical roots of our current concepts. We then discuss the two different but overlapping conceptualizations of manic-depressive illness: the bipolar–unipolar distinction and the manic-depressive spectrum.

HISTORICAL ROOTS

Pre–Nineteenth-Century Ideas

The medical writers of ancient Greece conceived of mental disorders in terms that sound remarkably modern.[2] They believed that melancholia was a psychological manifestation of an underlying biological disturbance, specifically, a perturbation in brain function. In documents dating back to the fifth and fourth centuries BC, Hippocrates and his school[3] described melancholia as a condition "associated with 'aversion to food, despondency, sleeplessness, irritability, restlessness,' and they stated that fear or depression that is prolonged means melancholia" (Jackson, 1986, p. 30). Early conceptions of melancholia and mania were, however, broader than those of today. The two terms, together with phrenitis, which corresponds roughly to an acute organic delirium, made up all mental illness throughout

most of the ancient period. As Jackson (1986, p. 249) pointed out, "disorders similar to our mania and our melancholia constituted significant portions of the larger groupings of mental disorders that were subsumed under those rubrics in ancient times."

As they did with other illnesses, the Hippocratic writers argued forcefully that mental disorders were not due to supernatural or magical forces, beliefs that characterized most primitive societies and that have resurfaced from time to time throughout history. In Greece, "Hippocrates did not encounter excessive resistance in the magical sphere because these diseases had long been interpreted as phenomena deriving from an underlying humoural disturbance" (Roccatagliata, 1986, p. 170). This essentially biological explanation for the cause of melancholia, which survived until the Renaissance, was part of the prevailing understanding of all health as an equilibrium of the four humors—blood, yellow bile, black bile, and phlegm—and all illness as a disturbance of this equilibrium. First fully developed in the Hippocratic work *Nature of Man* (ca. 400 BC), the humoral theory linked the humors with the seasons and with relative moistness. An excess of black bile was seen as the cause of melancholia, a term that literally means "black bile." Mania, by contrast, was usually attributed to an excess of yellow bile.

Aristotle, who differed with the Hippocratic writers by seeing the heart rather than the brain as the dysfunctional organ in melancholy, introduced the notion of a "predisposition" to melancholy. The "marker" of that predisposition was a relative excess of black bile, which he thought was common in small amounts in all people. As Whitwell[4] (1936, p. 59) pointed out, Aristotle thought those with the excess had melancholic temperaments that were associated with being gifted:

> Aristotle appears to have been the first to draw attention to the problem of the frequent occurrence of melancholia, or at least a degree of mental depression in the case of philosophers, statesmen, artists and poets, and he gives as examples Plato, Socrates and Empedocles. This is a question which is constantly recurring in later literature, the explanation of which is attempted by Marsilius Ficinus.[5]

Deliberations on the relationship between melancholia and mania date back at least to the first century BC, as noted by Soranus of Ephesus: "The followers of Themison, as well as many others, considered melancholy a form of the disease of mania" (Jackson, 1986, p. 250). Soranus himself (fl. 100 AD) believed that melancholia and mania were two distinct diseases, but with similar prodromal symptoms and requiring similar treatments (Jackson, 1986, p. 250):

> For Soranus, mania involved an impairment of reason with delusions; fluctuating states of anger and merriment, although sometimes of sadness and futility and sometimes "an overpowering fear of things which are quite harmless"; "continual wakefulness, the veins are distended, cheeks flushed, and body hard and abnormally strong"; and a tendency for there to be "attacks alternating with periods of remission." Melancholia involved being "downcast and prone to anger and . . . practically never cheerful and relaxed"; "signs . . . as follows: mental anguish and distress, dejection, silence, animosity toward members of the household, sometimes a desire to live and at other times a longing for death, suspicion . . . that a plot is being hatched against him, weeping without reason, meaningless muttering, and again, occasional joviality"; and various somatic symptoms, many of them gastrointestinal.

Aretaeus of Cappadocia, who lived in the second century AD, appears to have been the first (whose work has survived to modern times) to bring together the syndromes described in Greek medicine and propose that mania was an end stage of melancholia, a view that was to prevail for centuries to come. Roccatagliata (1986, p. 229), who referred to Aretaeus as "the clinician of mania," noted that he "isolated . . . a form of mental disease presenting phases of depression alternating with phases of mania," and reported Aretaeus's characterization of the illness:

> "Some patients after being melancholic have fits of mania . . . so that mania is like a variety of being

melancholy." He described a kind of cyclothymia which presented only intermittent stages of mania: "It arises in subjects whose personality is characterised by gayness, activity, superficiality and childishness." The mania was expressed in "furor, excitement and cheerfulness." Other types of mania, he said, had delirious manifestations of an expansive type, so that the patient "has deliriums, he studies astronomy, philosophy . . . he feels great and inspired." So he identified a bipolar cyclothymia, a monopolar one consisting only of manic phases, and a paranoid psychosis which he considered akin to schizophrenic mania.

Although Aretaeus included syndromes that today might be classified as psychoses beyond mania, his clear descriptions of the variety of manic conditions influenced medicine for many centuries, and have a modern ring to them (Roccatagliata, 1986, pp. 230–231):

> According to Aretaeus, the classical form of mania was the type that was associated with melancholia: the patient who previously was gay, euphoric, and hyperactive suddenly "has a tendency to melancholy; he becomes, at the end of the attack, languid, sad, taciturn, he complains that he is worried about his future, he feels ashamed." When the depressive phase is over, such patients go back to being gay, they laugh, they joke, they sing, "they show off in public with crowned heads as if they were returning victorious from the games; sometimes they laugh and dance all day and all night." In serious forms of mania, called furor, the patient "sometimes kills and slaughters the servants"; in less severe forms, he often exalts himself: "without being cultivated he says he is a philosopher . . . and the incompetent [say they are] good artisans . . . others yet are suspicious and they feel that they are being persecuted, for which reasons they are irascible."

Aretaeus believed that mania was a brain dysfunction that "deprived its imaginative functions" (Roccatagliata, 1986, p. 229). Melancholy, similarly, had an endogenous etiology; melancholic delirium arose (Roccatagliata, 1986, p. 231):

> "without motive, like the loss of reason, insomnia, and despair." The vital tone was subject to typical circadian variations, which in melancholy were inverted with respect to the normal person, so that the patients "wake up suddenly and are seized by a great tiredness."

The next important medical writer, Galen of Pergamon (131–201 AD), firmly established melancholia as a chronic and recurrent condition. His few comments on mania included the observation that it can be either a primary disease of the brain or secondary to other diseases. Galen's "contribution" was, in the opinion of most medical historians, his brilliant, all-encompassing elaboration of the humoral theory, a system so compelling that it dominated—and stifled—medical thought for more than a millennium.

Medical observations in succeeding centuries continued to reflect these conceptions of depression and mania laid down in classical Greece and Rome. As Jackson (1986) observed, most authors wrote of the two conditions as separate illnesses, but usually in adjoining chapters and ascribing them to humoral causes that suggested a close connection between them. Yet where mania and depression are considered in the historical medical literature, a link is almost always made, as can be seen in the time line in Box 1–1.

As we have seen, from classical Greece until the Middle Ages, mental and physical afflictions were primarily the concern of medical doctors. As illness gradually became the responsibility of the priests, the above early insights were submerged. The period that followed was, in retrospect, a dark age, when mental illness was generally attributed to either magic or sin or possession by the devil.

By the late Middle Ages, empirical science had attracted interest and the beginnings of acceptance, engendered by the ascendancy of Baconian philosophy. At that point, however, in the clinical realm now encompassed by psychiatry, scientific interpretations were limited to anatomical, physiological, and pathological studies of the brain.

Empirical clinical observations without religious overtones did not reappear until the beginning of the seventeenth century. A key figure in this descriptive renaissance was Felix Platter, who in 1602 published his systematic observations and classifications of mental disorders. Although his descriptions of mania and melancholia were extensive and methodical, there was little to suggest the longitudinal or recurrent nature of the illness, or the distinctions between manic-depressive illness[6] and what is now known as schizophrenia.

A unique eighteenth-century discussion of manic-depressive illness can be found in a 1759 monograph by Andres Piquer ("the Spanish Hippocrates"), physician to King Ferdinand VI of Spain ("Discurso sobre la Enfermedad del Rey nuestro Senor Fernando VI"), recently republished with an introduction by Eduard Vieta and Demetrio Barcia. Piquer diagnosed the king with "melancholic-manic affect" (p. 17), clearly anticipating later French and German authors in viewing this condition as a single illness: "Melancholy and mania, although treated in many medical books separately, are one and the same illness, and only differ according to the various grades of activity and diversity of affective states that occur in both." (pp. 57–58; translated

segments by Nassir Ghaemi) Piquer went on to quote Hippocrates and Arateus in support of his view.

As noted previously, the subsequent literature of the seventeenth and eighteenth centuries is replete with clinical observations of manic and depressive symptomatology. As pointed out by Pichot (1995), the disciples of Esquirol played a critical role as they paved the way for recognition of the mental disease that ultimately came to be known as manic-depressive insanity through the work of Kraepelin (1899). For instance, Jules Baillarger[7] wrote in 1854:

> There exists a special type of insanity characterized by two regular periods, the one of depression and the other of excitement. . . . This type of insanity presents itself in the form of isolated attacks; or, it recurs in an intermittent manner; or, the attacks might follow one another without interruption.

This theme is echoed in subsequent French psychiatric writing:

> By circular insanity, or *folie à double forme*, we understand a special form of mental derangement, the attacks of which are characterised by a regular sequence of two periods—one of depression, and another of excitement, or inversely. (Ritti, 1892)[8]

There are literally thousands of such observations, for the most part disconnected from one another. Many are accompanied by hastily erected classification systems and etiological speculations, which sometimes anticipate contemporary theory to a striking extent. As Jelliffe (1931) wrote, the "epidemic of classification" was further spread by the powerful influence of Linnaeus's work on the classification of plants. Even more new empirical observations were added when the advent of autopsies opened the door for neuropathologic observations and their attendant speculations. This evidence was gathering in a conceptual climate still dominated by the traditional separation of the mind ("soul") from the body. The era was not yet ready for a new synthesis or unifying insights, despite its increasing need of them.

Nineteenth-Century Ideas

The explicit conception of manic-depressive illness as a single disease entity dates from the mid-nineteenth century. As noted above, the French "alienists," Falret and Baillarger, independently and almost simultaneously formulated the idea that mania[9] and depression could represent different manifestations of a single illness. Students of Esquirol and, therefore, intellectual descendants of Pinel, they had been strongly influenced by Pinel's sharp disdain for the "classification epidemic," as well as by contemporary arguments for a unitary concept of general paresis.

BOX **1–1.** Linking of Mania and Depression throughout History[a]

ca. 400 BC An excess of black bile was seen as the cause of melancholia, a term that literally means "black bile." Mania, by contrast was usually attributed to yellow bile. (Hippocrates)

ca. 150 AD "Some patients after being melancholic have fits of mania . . . so that mania is like a variety of being melancholy." (Aretaeus of Cappadocia[b])

ca. 575 "Those affected with such a condition are not suffering from melancholia only, for they tend to become maniacal periodically and in a cycle. Mania is nothing else but melancholia in a more intense form." (Alexander of Tralles[c])

ca. 1000 "Undoubtedly the material which is the effective producer of mania is of the same nature as that which produces melancholia." (Avicenna[d])

ca. 1300 "Mania and melancholia are different forms of the same thing." (Joh. Gaddesden[e])

ca. 1500 "[Melancholia] manifestly differs from what is properly called mania; there is no doubt, however, that at some time or other, authorities agree that it replaces melancholia." (Joh. Manardus[f])

ca. 1549 "Perturbation of the spirit of the brain when mixed with and kindled by other matter can produce melancholia, or if more ardent, mania." (Felix Platter[g])

ca. 1672 "[Manics and melancholics] are so much akin, that these Distempers often change, and pass from one into the other; for the Melancholick disposition growing worse, brings on Fury; and Fury or Madness [mania] growing less hot, oftentimes ends in a Melancholick disposition. These two, like smoke and flame, mutually receive and give place to one another." (Thomas Willis[h])

ca. 1735 "If Melancholy increases so far, that from the great Motion of the Liquid of the Brain, the Patient be thrown into a wild Fury, it is call'd Madness [mania]. Which differs only in Degree from the sorrowful kind of Melancholy, is its Offspring, produced from the same Causes, and cured almost by the same Remedies." (Herman Boerhaave[i])

ca. 1759 "Melancholy and mania, although treated in many medical books separately, are one and the same illness, and only differ according to the various grades of activity and diversity of affective states that occur in both."—Andres, Piquer (quoted in "El trastorno bipolar en el siglo XVIII," by Eduard Vieta and Demetrio Barcia, 2000, Burdeos, Spain: Mra ediciones, pp. 57–58, segment translated by Nassir Ghaemi).

ca. 1806 "[Mania is] often no other than a higher degree of melancholia. . . . [I]t does not appear to me any wise difficult to suppose, that the same state of the brain may in a moderate degree give melancholia; and in a higher, that mania which melancholia so often passes into." (William Cullen[j])

ca. 1845 "Several distinguished masters, Alexander de Tralles, and Boerhaave himself, were of the opinion, that melancholy . . . was only the first degree of mania. This is in some cases true. There are in fact, some persons who, before becoming maniacs, are sad, morose, uneasy, diffident and suspicious." (Jean-Etienne-Dominique Esquirol[k])

---

[a]Although the idea for this time line was ours, locating the quotations would have been next to impossible without the excellent historical sources cited for each. We are especially indebted to Whitwell (1936), Jackson (1986), and Roccatagliata (1986). The quotations, particularly those from the Middle Ages, do not always represent prevailing thought, but they do illustrate the thread of this theme throughout history. Also, when the conditions we would characterize as manic-depressive illness were interpreted as medical rather than philosophical or religious problems, a relationship between mania and depression was almost always suggested, explicitly or implicitly.

[b]Cited by Whitwell (1936, pp. 163–164). From *De acut, et diut, morborum, causis, signis, et curatione* (Paris), 1554. Transl. R. Moffatt.

[c]Quoted by Whitwell (1936, p. 175), who gave Trallianus's birth and death dates as 525–605, from Trallianus Alexander: *Medici libri duodecim*, interpret, Guintherius (Basil), 1556.

[d]Quoted by Whitwell (1936, p. 181), who gave Avicenna's birth and death dates as 980–1037. Whitwell cited as a source Opera, ed.: *Alpagus et Benedictus* (Venet.), 1582, and *Morb. Ment.* (Paris) 1659. Italics in original.

[e]Quoted by Whitwell (1936, p. 196), who gave Gaddesden's birth and death dates as 1280–1361. Source cited is Gaddesden Joh.: *Practica Johanni Anglica—Rosa medicina nuncupata* (Papiae), 1492. Transl. Wolffe.

[f]Cited by Whitwell (1936, p. 205), who gave Manardus's birth and death dates as 1462–1536. Citation given is Manardus Joh: *Epist. Med.* (Venet.), 1542. Italics in original.

[g]Quoted by Whitwell (1936, p. 98), who gave Platter's birth and death dates as 1536–1614. Although it is not clear which of Platter's works is the source of this quotation, Whitwell later quoted from *Praxeos medicae Tomi tres* (Basil), 1656, and *Histories and Observations* (London: Culpeper and Cole), 1664.

[h]Quoted by Jackson (1986, p. 255) from Willis, T.: *Two Discourses Concerning the Soul of Brutes.* Transl. S. Pordage (London: Thomas Dring), Ch. Harper and John Leigh,[A] 1683, pp. 201, 205.

[i]Quoted by Jackson (1986, p. 256) from Boerhaave, H.: *Boerhaave's Aphorisms: Concerning the Knowledge and Cure of Diseases, Which Is That of a Vital and Sensitive Man. The First Is Physiological Shewing the Nature, Parts, Powers, and Affections of the Same. The Other Is Pathological, Which Unfolds the Diseases Which Affect It and Its Primary Seat; to Wit, the Brain and Nervous Stock, and Treats of Their Cures: with Copper Cuts* (London: W and J Innys), 1735, pp. 323–324.

[j]Quoted by Jackson (1986, p. 259) from Cullen, W.: *First Lines of the Practice of Physic.* 2 vols., in 1. ed. J. Rotheram (New York: E. Duyckinck), 1806, p. 497.

[k]Quoted by Jackson (1986, p. 262) from Esquirol, E.: *Mental Maladies: A Treatise on Insanity.* Transl. E. K. Hunt (Philadelphia: Lea and Blanchard), 1845, pp. 381–382.

In 1854, Falret described a circular disorder (*la folie circulaire*), which for the first time expressly defined an illness in which "this succession of mania and melancholia manifests itself with continuity and in a manner almost regular" (perhaps a foreshadowing of the modern concept of rapid cycling). In the same year, Baillarger (1854) described "double insanity" (*la folie à double forme*), emphasizing that the manic and depressive episodes were not two different attacks but rather two different stages of the same attack. Thus, cyclicity with or without clear-cut remission was already being described in these pioneering French contributions. Although clearly anticipating Kraepelin's later synthesis, these descriptions nonetheless focused on chronic illness with poor prognosis; the relationship of these "forms" to other varieties of mania or melancholia was not delineated. Other valuable contributions were made by Griesinger (1867), who provided rich clinical descriptions of melancholia and mania, although he described primarily chronic states with poor prognosis. As Aretaeus had centuries before, Griesinger conceived of mania as an end stage of a gradually worsening melancholia and of both as different stages of a single, unitary disease (Jackson, 1986).

Although mild cases of mania had been described by the ancients, as well as by Falret, Esquirol, and other observers, Mendel (1881) was the first to define *hypo*mania as "that form of mania which typically shows itself only in the mild stages abortively, so to speak." Kahlbaum (1882) described circular disorders (cyclothymia), which were characterized by episodes of both depression and excitement but did not end in dementia, as chronic mania or melancholia could. Despite these contributions, most clinical observers continued to regard mania and melancholia as separate entities, chronic in nature, and following a deteriorating course. Nonetheless, some German authors during this period, such as Hecker (see the translation by Koukopoulos, 2003), reserved cyclothymia for the milder, nondeteriorating, forms observed in private clinical practice. Hecker's work is actually quite consistent with what today we have come to recognize as bipolar-II disorder:

> Virtually all of the [patients with cyclothymia] presented with a depressive state. The state of excitation—and I should like to emphasize this—had escaped the attention, in the majority of milder cases, of the patient's doctor, his family and friends, and the patient himself. The patients only became aware of it when I described the characteristics of this state to them. Even more often, however, it was the patients themselves who, having up until that moment considered them as their 'healthiest' periods, were forced to recognize that they were ill in these periods also.

The Kraepelinian Synthesis

It was left to Kraepelin to segregate the two major psychotic illnesses—manic-depressive insanity and dementia praecox—from one another and clearly draw the perimeter around manic-depressive illness. The early editions of his textbook of psychiatry contained the seeds of his later synthesis, particularly his special emphasis on careful diagnosis based on both longitudinal history and the pattern of current symptoms. Nevertheless, these early editions still reflected a struggle with the then-traditional categories of melancholia and circular psychosis. In the sixth edition, published in 1899, the term *manic-depressive* encompassed the circular psychoses and simple manias. Kraepelin expressed doubt that melancholia and the circular psychoses (a category that includes today's bipolar and schizoaffective disorders) were really separate illnesses, but he was still reluctant to take a definite stand.

By 1913, in the eighth edition of Kraepelin's text, virtually all of the major clinical forms of melancholia had been subsumed under "manic-depressive illness." Under his unitary concept, much of what had once been considered involutional melancholia was reclassified as mixed states,[10] based on a follow-up study by his pupil, Dreyfus.[11] Kraepelin placed special emphasis on the features of the illness that differentiated it most clearly from dementia praecox (schizophrenia): the periodic or episodic course, the more benign prognosis, and a family history of manic-depressive illness.

Within a relatively short time, Kraepelin's views were widely accepted, thus bringing some unity to European psychiatry. His was the first fully developed disease model in psychiatry to be backed by extensive and carefully organized observations and descriptions. This model did not exclude psychological or social factors, and in fact, Kraepelin was one of the first to point out that psychological stresses could precipitate individual episodes. By including "slight colourings of mood," which "pass over without sharp boundary into the domain of personal predisposition," he also provided the basis for the development of spectrum concepts, described later in this chapter.

Wide acceptance of Kraepelin's broad divisions led to further exploration of the boundaries between manic-depressive illness and dementia praecox, the delineation of similarities across the two, and the possibility that subgroups could be identified within each. Kraepelin's extraordinary synthesis is important not because it drew the ultimately "correct" picture of nature, but because it built a solid and empirically anchored base for future work. This was his major accomplishment. Indeed, as we will see later, his central insight—that all of the recurrent major mood disorders (using current nomenclature) belonged together under the rubric of *manic-depressive illness*—still provides the best model for what we know to date, as well as for understanding emerging clinical, pharmacological, and genetic data.

Post-Kraepelinian Developments

After Kraepelin, the evolution of the concept of manic-depressive illness proceeded differently in Europe and the United States (Pichot, 1988). Europeans continued to place primary emphasis on the traditional medical disease model of mental illness, whereas psychiatrists in the United States were profoundly influenced by the new perspectives of psychoanalysis and other theories emphasizing psychological and social factors. During the first half of the twentieth century, the views of Meyer (1866–1950) gradually assumed a dominant position in American psychiatry, a position maintained for several decades. Meyer believed that psychopathology emerged from interactions between an individual's biological and psychological characteristics and his social environment.[12]

The disease model, by contrast, is based on the premise that clinical phenomena in a given patient are understandable (and therefore potentially predictable) in terms of a given disease with a specific natural history and pathophysiology. European psychiatry in the nineteenth and early twentieth centuries had successfully employed this traditional medical disease model in the definition and treatment of general paresis secondary to syphilis of the central nervous system and organic syndromes associated with vitamin deficiencies (especially pellagra).[13] Failure to identify mechanisms of pathophysiology in the major so-called functional psychoses, including manic-depressive illness, stimulated doubts about the continued usefulness of the model, particularly since the prevailing biological hypotheses emphasized infectious agents and neuropathological lesions. Consistent with this pessimism was the failure of the biologically based treatments of the time. In this climate, it is not surprising that American psychiatrists, manifesting the national penchant for pragmatism, were drawn to treatment approaches that emphasized psychological and social factors. When the Meyerian focus, considerably influenced by psychoanalysis, turned to manic-depressive illness, the individual and his environment were the natural focus, and clinical descriptions of symptoms and the longitudinal course of the illness were given less emphasis.[14]

Until the latter part of the twentieth century, the American nosological systems for affective disorders reflected these competing sets of etiological assumptions. Depression was divided into several dichotomies: reactive–endogenous, neurotic–psychotic, and, more recently,

primary[15]–secondary. Forgotten in these conceptions is the fact that a single parameter cannot differentiate aspects of illness that are at least partially independent of one another: severity, "neurotic features," thought disorder, precipitating events, physiological symptoms, and genetic vulnerability. Dichotomous systems thus foundered on their a priori assumptions about etiology. Even the primary–secondary distinction, although free of assumptions about severity, quality of symptoms, and precipitating events, is based on another supposition: it assumes that depression or mania associated with other illnesses is relatively free of genetic influence, an assumption that has not been supported by the data (Andreasen et al., 1988).[16]

In Europe, the post-Kraepelinian evolution of the concept of manic-depressive illness took a different turn. The European psychosocial and psychoanalytical traditions continued to develop in relative isolation from the mainstream of psychiatry, which largely retained its medical or disease orientation; psychoanalytic thinking per se did not have as important an influence on the European concept of manic-depressive illness as it did on the American concept. Although Kraepelin's fundamental distinction between manic-depressive illness and dementia praecox endured (Mayer-Gross et al., 1955), nosological disputes soon arose.

In his classic contributions to descriptive psychiatry, Bleuler (1924) departed from Kraepelin by conceptualizing the relationship between manic-depressive (affective) illness and dementia praecox (schizophrenia) as a continuum without a sharp line of demarcation.[17] Bleuler believed that a patient's location on the spectrum depended on the number of schizophrenic features he demonstrated. In that sense, Bleuler considered the affective symptoms to be nonspecific. These issues are explored more fully in Chapter 3.

Bleuler also broadened Kraepelin's concept of manic-depressive illness by designating several subcategories and using the term *affective illness*. The influence of his modifications of Kraepelin's taxonomy could be seen in the *International Classification of Diseases* (ICD) (8th and 9th editions) and the closely related early versions of the *Diagnostic and Statistical Manual,* the first and second editions (DSM-I and -II). Bleuler's subcategories of affective illness anticipated the principal contemporary subdivision of the classic manic-depressive diagnostic group—the bipolar–unipolar distinction.

THE BIPOLAR–UNIPOLAR DISTINCTION

From its inception, Kraepelin's unitary concept of manic-depressive illness was criticized for being too inclusive, but it was not until 1957 that Leonhard proposed a classification system that went beyond clinical description alone. Leonhard observed that, within the broad category of manic-depressive illness (i.e., recurrent affective illness), some patients had histories of both depression and mania, whereas others had depressions only. He then noted that patients with a history of mania (whom he termed *bipolar*) had a higher incidence of mania in their families as compared with those with recurrent depressions only (whom he termed *monopolar*). In 1966, Angst and Perris independently provided the first systematic family history data to support Leonhard's distinction, validating it by an independent criterion—family history. As discussed in Chapter 13, some of the subsequent family history studies are consistent with a model in which bipolar and the more highly recurrent forms of unipolar depression are variants of the same fundamental disorder (Kraepelin's manic-depressive illness), with bipolar illness representing the more severe end of the spectrum.

The bipolar–unipolar distinction was formally incorporated into the American diagnostic system, DSM, the third edition (DSM-III), in 1980; was subsequently carried forward into DSM, the fourth edition (DSM-IV); and became explicit in the international classification system in ICD-10. Unfortunately the structure of DSM-IV (see Fig. 3–1 in Chapter 3), which breaks out bipolar disorder as a separate illness distinct from all other mood disorders (i.e., from the depressive disorders) obscures the fact that originally, the bipolar–unipolar distinction was conceived of as a way to distinguish two forms of a *recurrent* illness. In other words, the DSM structure gives precedence to polarity over cyclicity, obscuring the reality that one rather common variant of unipolar illness is as recurrent or cyclic as bipolar illness. Further, DSM-IV really has no language for the unipolar patient with frequent recurrences, since its "recurrent" category is so broad as to include patients with only two depressions in a lifetime (see Chapter 3 for a more extensive discussion of this point).

Before the mid-1970s, the scientific literature on manic-depressive illness typically did not include information on the number of patients with or without a history of mania. During the past three decades, however, the bipolar–unipolar distinction has been examined in numerous studies encompassing family history, natural course, clinical symptoms, personality factors, biological measures, and response to various pharmacological treatments. The question of bipolar–unipolar differences in clinical features of depression is reviewed in this chapter; these as well as other reported bipolar–unipolar differences (e.g., biological, pharmacological, psychological) are summarized in Table 1–1 and further detailed in the relevant chapters (including this one—see also Table 1–3 on clinical differences later in the chapter). Our purpose in outlining these

reported differences here is to introduce a framework helpful in understanding them.

An Overview of Differentiating Features

The criteria that distinguish bipolar from unipolar illness have changed over the years, at least among American investigators. As noted above, in the original descriptions of Leonhard and the subsequent studies of Angst and colleagues (1998), Perris and colleagues (1971), and Winokur and colleagues (1981), both *bipolar*[18] and *unipolar* were used to describe patients with a phasic or cyclic course of recurrent episodes, characterized by autonomous "endogenous" features and clear functional impairment. It is worth repeating that in DSM-III and -IV, *unipolar* has come to mean all depressed patients without a history of hypomania or mania (i.e., to mean simply nonbipolar)—a heterogeneous population that includes both highly recurrent and nonrecurrent depressions, not to mention patients who might have been classified as "neurotic," "reactive," "characterological," or "atypical" in other diagnostic systems. As Roth (1983, pp. 47–48) observed about DSM-III:

> The significant point in this context is that Leonhard intended that bipolar–unipolar dichotomy for endogenous states alone. . . . When the endogenous syndrome is discarded, unipolar disorders become a large and compendious bag to be commingled with a wide variety of disorders of affect, including neuroses of different kinds.

The critical issue of recurrence is further obscured by DSM-IV, which does not include an item concerning prior history or course, despite evidence suggesting a clear distinction between family history and course in different illness subtypes (Winokur, 1979).[19] We believe that the next revision of the DSM and ICD systems should include a category (and operational definition) for the more recurrent forms of unipolar depression, which might be designated as "highly recurrent," or "cyclic." A related contributor to unipolar heterogeneity is the subgroup of unipolar patients with certain bipolar-like characteristics, as discussed below.

Bipolar groups are also heterogeneous. Most studies, particularly those first to use the distinction, did not specify criteria for bipolar beyond indicating a "history of mania." In many studies, bipolar included only those patients with a history of frank mania requiring hospitalization; in others, the bipolar group included patients with milder symptoms (hypomania). Then, Goodwin and colleagues at the National Institute of Mental Health (NIMH) suggested that bipolar patients could be classified more meaningfully as either bipolar-I or bipolar-II (Dunner et al., 1976b). They based this recommendation on their studies of hospitalized depressed patients who met criteria for primary

TABLE 1–1. Overview of Reported Differences between Bipolar and Unipolar Depression

Phenomenology of Depression	Bipolar (I and/or II)	Unipolar
Depressive Symptoms	See Table 1–3	See Table 1–3
Natural Course		
Age at onset	Younger	Older
	Narrower range	Broader range
Number of episodes	More	Fewer
Length of depressive episode[a]	Shorter	Longer
Cycle length	Shorter	Longer
Precipitants of episodes	More important at illness onset than for later episodes	Relation to illness onset not clear
Interepisode mood shifts	More	Fewer
Marital Status	Single status not a risk factor for episodes	Single status a risk factor
Epidemiology		
Lifetime risk	1.2–1.5%	5–10%
Proportion of major affective illness	20–50%	50–80%
Gender ratio	F = M	F > M
Substance abuse	More frequent	Less frequent
Suicide	Unclear	Unclear
Personality		
Depression/introversion	Less	More
Impulse control	Less	More
Stimulus seeking	More	Less
Personality profile	More normal	Less normal
Hyperthymic temperament	More	Less
Cyclothymia	More	Less
Family History/Genetics		
Monozygotic twin concordance rates	Higher	Lower
Mania among first-degree relatives	More	Less
Biological/Physiological		
Monoaminergic function (metabolites, receptors, neuroendocrine response, electrolytes, etc.)	Some studies report UP–BP differences (see Chapter 15)	
Pain sensitivity	Less	More
Hemispheric function dysfunction	More nondominant	?
Brain imaging parameters	? (see Chapter 15)	?

(continued)

TABLE 1–1. **Overview of Reported Differences between Bipolar and Unipolar Depression** *(continued)*

Phenomenology of Depression	Bipolar (I and/or II)	Unipolar
Sleep/Rhythms		
Sleep duration	Longer	Shorter
Phase advance	Less frequent (?)	More frequent (?)
Seasonal patterns	Fall/winter depression Spring/summer mania	Spring depression (?)
Pharmacological Response		
Response to antidepressants	Less (?)	More (?)
Speed of response to antidepressants	More rapid (?)	Less rapid (?)
Tolerance to antidepressants	More frequent	Less frequent
Antidepressant response to mood stabilizers	More frequent	Less frequent
Manic/hypomanic response to antidepressants	More frequent	Less frequent
Prophylactic response to lithium	Equivalent when bipolar and unipolar cycle length are comparable	
Prophylactic response to antidepressants	Poor	Good

[a]Studies demonstrating longer duration of episodes with unipolar versus bipolar depression are generally not corrected for number of episodes. See text.

Note: See individual chapters for details. Some of the bipolar–unipolar comparisons included both bipolar-I and -II, while others focused on either one or the other, an obvious source of heterogeneity. Not all of the reported differences have been replicated uniformly, which is not surprising given the heterogeneity of both the bipolar and "unipolar" groups (for example, early-onset, highly recurrent unipolar depression will be closer to bipolar depression in clinical characteristics). The sequence of the table follows that of the chapters in this volume.

F = female; M = male; UP–BP = unipolar–bipolar.

major affective disorders; that is, they had no prior history of another psychiatric diagnosis. Bipolar-I patients were defined as those with a history of mania severe enough to have resulted in treatment, usually hospitalization. Such full-blown mania was often accompanied by psychotic features. Bipolar-II patients, by contrast, had, in addition to major depression requiring hospitalization, a history of hypomania—that is, specific symptoms of sufficient magnitude to be designated as abnormal by the patient or the family and to result in interference with normal role functioning, but not severe enough to result in hospitalization.

This original distinction between bipolar-I and -II is different from that made in subsequent studies that also employed the bipolar-II terminology.[20] Whereas the work of Dunner and colleagues (1976b) and the NIMH Collaborative Program on the Psychobiology of Depression-Clinical Studies, as well as that of Angst and colleagues (2005) in

their long-term follow-up study, emerged from observations of hospitalized depressed patients without other psychiatric diagnoses, many of the more recent studies were conducted in patients in whom neither the depressed nor the hypomanic phase was severe enough to require hospitalization and in whom concomitant diagnoses (principally borderline personality disorder and substance abuse disorder) were not uncommon (Coryell et al., 1985, 1995; Endicott et al., 1985). Such definitional broadening is not universally accepted (Ghaemi et al., 2002). Thus, Baldessarini (2000) pointed out that mood fluctuations can be found in many if not most psychiatric disorders and expressed concern that the continued broadening of the bipolar diagnosis risks weakening the core concept of bipolar disorder. Similar concerns were expressed by van Praag (1993), and we agree.

Angst (1978), having earlier recognized the problem of the range of meanings that could confuse application of the bipolar-II category, proposed a nomenclature that would account for milder forms of both depression and mania. He divided bipolar patients into Md and mD, with *M* and *D* indicating episodes of mania and depression requiring hospitalization, and *m* and *d* episodes clearly different from normal but not of sufficient severity to necessitate hospitalization. Although Angst's mD group is analogous to the original definition of bipolar-II of Dunner and colleagues (1976b), other systems have no subcategory analogous to his Md group. This is unfortunate, since Angst reported interesting differences among these subgroups. For instance, the ratio of females to males is substantially higher in the predominantly depressed subgroups (unipolar and Dm), whereas males are a higher proportion of the predominantly manic subgroups (MD and Md); these data are consistent with the higher female-to-male ratio in bipolar-II compared with bipolar-I disorder (Weissman et al., 1996; Cassano et al., 1999). More recently, Angst completed a long-term follow-up study of his original 1959–1963 cohort. He concluded that the Md group, compared with their MD counterparts, have a more favorable course and are less likely to require long-term maintenance medication, while their first-degree relatives have a lower affective morbidity risk (Angst et al., 2004).

The extent of overlap between Angst's dm category and the bipolar-II outpatients in subsequent studies (by Akiskal, Benazzi, and others) cannot be assessed because Angst's system defines d episodes by an absence of hospitalization for depression, whereas a bipolar-II diagnosis is based on meeting DSM-IV criteria for major depression. Angst's dm grouping is inherently broader than bipolar-II and includes patients who would be classified as cyclothymic in DSM-III and -IV (see Chapter 3). Whatever the level of depressive severity,[21] however, bipolar-II patients represent a very important group. Moreover, as discussed below, both family history and pharmacological response data indicate that, while in some respects bipolar-II should be considered an intermediate form between bipolar-I and unipolar,[22] some of the data are consistent with its being a distinct subgroup.

As noted in the first edition of this text, one problem complicating research on bipolar-II disorder has been the poor reliability of the diagnosis, which results principally from the difficulty of establishing a history of hypomania (Andreasen et al., 1981; Dunner and Tay, 1993). Depressed patients are especially poor at recalling prior episodes of hypomania. Fortunately, family members generally do better. Moreover, the sensitivity to hypomania can be increased by multiple interviews over time (Rice et al., 1986). And current data indicate excellent reliability when clinicians trained in recognizing bipolar-II make the diagnosis (Dunner and Tay, 1993; Simpson et al., 2002). Other issues

involved in making a DSM diagnosis of hypomania include the not-always-warranted primacy accorded to elated mood over dysphoric mood and the durational requirement of 4 or more consecutive days, both of which have been widely criticized by clinical researchers (see the discussion in Chapter 3).

Most significant, contemporary data necessitate revision of the more traditional view of bipolar as substantially less common than unipolar illness. In Egeland and Hotstetter's (1983) study, using sensitive methods of ascertainment and considering cyclothymia, bipolar-II, and bipolar-I together, the incidence of bipolar disorder was approximately equal to that of unipolar illness—that is, it accounted for 50 percent of major affective illness.[23] Angst and colleagues (1978) also found that the ratio of bipolar to unipolar illness was about 1:1 in patients followed for up to 16 years, a ratio very close to that noted in the subsequent follow-up of that cohort, in which only 46 percent of the patients were still unipolar (Angst et al., 2002, 2004). Other recent studies using this broader definition of bipolar have found a similarly high bipolar/unipolar ratio.[24]

Unfortunately, many studies of recurrent affective illness employ relatively insensitive methods of ascertainment and correspondingly rigid criteria for an episode. Although such inflexible criteria are useful for certain research purposes, they exclude many patients from consideration. Egeland and Hotstetter (1983) referred to the bipolar illness typically cited in the literature (i.e., bipolar-I) as the "tip of the iceberg" of bipolarity. Current data indicate that manic-depressive spectrum conditions (see below), many of them below the threshold of mania, may be found in 5–8 percent of the population (Angst, 1978) (see Chapter 5). However, the validity of the diagnoses in most of these surveys (obtained by trained lay interviewers) has been questioned, primarily because estimates based on diagnoses by experienced clinicians tend to be substantially lower (see Chapters 4 and 5).

A broad range of bipolar–unipolar differences have been reported (see Table 1–1). They include four separate spheres of data—genetic, clinical, biological, and pharmacological. Considerable caution is warranted in interpreting these differences, however, given the heterogeneity in both groups. While most of these studies have focused on bipolar-I patients (reducing heterogeneity on that side),[25] the unipolar groups have been highly heterogeneous with respect to the critical variable of recurrence or cycle length; clearly the unipolar groups represented in Table 1–1 have generally not been selected for frequent recurrences (Cassano et al., 1992; Winokur et al., 1993, 1994, 1995; Judd et al., 2003a). Indeed, to our knowledge, there have been no studies comparing bipolar and unipolar illness in which the groups have actually been matched for episode frequency. This is a serious limitation in light of the increasing evidence that more highly recurrent unipolar patients appear to be quite similar to bipolar patients in some important respects (e.g., early age at onset, family history of mania, "atypical" features, and prophylactic response to lithium).

Implicit in the foregoing discussion of bipolar–unipolar distinctions is the need for a more explicit focus on the relationship between cyclicity and polarity. To what extent do differences in cyclicity contribute to or obscure reported bipolar–unipolar differences? In other words, how are we to know whether a given bipolar–unipolar difference is a function of the presence or absence of a history of mania/hypomania, or occurs because the bipolar group is more cyclic or recurrent than the unipolar group? These important questions are discussed later in the chapter. The relationship between polarity per se and other dimensions of affective illness—family history, age at onset, severity, psychotic features, response to treatment, and biological markers—generally has been studied one dimension at a time. A more comprehensive understanding of these interrelationships awaits studies that employ simultaneous weighing of multiple dimensions.

Unipolar Mania

The classic studies of Leonhard (1957), Perris (1966), Angst (1966), and Winokur and colleagues (1969) noted the relatively rare occurrence of manic patients with no apparent history of depression. In Leonhard's series, "pure mania" represented 9 percent of the bipolar group, whereas in the other studies it made up less than 5 percent. Although Leonhard initially considered patients with pure mania a separate group, subsequent studies indicated that they could not be distinguished from bipolar patients by either family history, course, treatment, or clinical features of mania. Thus, pure mania has generally been considered a variant of bipolar illness. Present knowledge suggests the likelihood that patients so identified either have had unreported depressions or have not been followed long enough to rule out future depressions. For some unipolar manic patients, depressive episodes are subsyndromal: they fail to be diagnosed because they lack a prominent or reported mood component; that is, the depressions manifest themselves primarily as episodes of increased sleep, decreased energy, and slowed thinking.

Abrams and colleagues[26] (Abrams and Taylor, 1974; Abrams et al., 1979) prompted a reevaluation of this question by reporting a 28 percent and an 18 percent incidence of unipolar mania among two relatively large independent samples of manic patients (N=127 for the two samples). Among the problems with these two studies, however, is the method used to ascertain a history of depression.[27] Like previous authors, Abrams and Taylor found that their "unipolar manics" did not differ fundamentally from the bipolar patients in demographic characteristics, family history variables, symptoms, or response to "doctor's choice" treatment.

Nurnberger and colleagues (1979) surveyed 241 bipolar-I patients in a lithium clinic and found that 16 percent had not been medically treated for depression, although most of them did show depressive features on a systematic interview. These authors, like other investigators, concluded from their review of phenomenological and family history data that unipolar mania is a variant of bipolar illness, not a separate entity. The NIMH Collaborative Program on the Psychobiology of Depression-Clinical Studies followed 27 patients (from a pool of 163 bipolar-I patients) initially admitted with a diagnosis of unipolar mania (Solomon et al., 2003) and found that 7 of them suffered no episodes of major depression during the 15- to 20-year follow-up; that is, unipolar mania represented 4 percent of the total bipolar sample. Yazici and colleagues (2002), by contrast, found that unipolar mania accounted for 16 percent of patients in their lithium clinic in Turkey, the higher rate perhaps reflecting cultural differences; that study also revealed a significantly higher rate of psychotic features associated with unipolar mania. Shulman and Tohen (1994) found the rate of unipolar mania to be 12 percent in a group of 50 elderly manic patients.

Perugi and colleagues (1998a) reported that hyperthymic temperament was the baseline in many unipolar manic patients, whose course appeared to be more chronic than that of the typical bipolar patient. Unlike the work of Angst and colleagues (2004), who reported a relatively favorable course among their pure M and Md patients, the findings of the two aforementioned studies suggest that unipolar mania represents a prognostically unfavorable variant of bipolar-I disorder. Yet this discrepancy may reflect differences in the populations designated as unipolar manics. For example, a late-onset bipolar disorder with predominantly manic course has been described, and is associated with evidence of organic contributions and negative family history for bipolarity (Shulman and Post, 1980; Moorhead and Young, 2003). The condition of these patients is best considered a phenocopy of mania, and should probably be excluded from the manic-depressive spectrum.

Future studies attempting to evaluate the validity of the concept of unipolar mania will have to employ careful diagnostic criteria, sensitive methods of ascertainment (especially family informants), and extensive follow-up periods. As the evidence now stands, we would agree with most authorities in the field that the existence of true unipolar mania as a separate entity is questionable. In our discussions here, it is included in the bipolar group.

False Unipolar Patients

As reviewed in the first edition of this volume, patients classified as unipolar who subsequently experience a manic or hypomanic episode—so-called *false unipolars*—confound studies of bipolar–unipolar differences (unipolar patients with some bipolar characteristics—sometimes called *pseudounipolar*—represent a different issue and are discussed below). Obviously, substantial numbers of false unipolar patients in a sample could distort or conceal bipolar–unipolar differences.

Table 1–2 presents data from three longitudinal studies (Perris, 1968; Angst et al., 1978; Grof, unpublished). The number of false unipolar patients is expressed as a percentage of the total unipolar group and as a function of numbers of depressive episodes without a mania. One might have expected the percentage of false unipolar patients to decrease as the group was "purified" by requiring more episodes of depression, that is, allowing more and more opportunity for latent bipolarity to express itself. In fact, however, the denominator (i.e., the number of true unipolar patients) also decreases as patients with more episodes are selected, since the unipolar patients who have only one, two, or three episodes are dropped. Thus, the actual percentage of false unipolar patients in the apparent unipolar population is relatively stable beyond the second episode, so that the convention of requiring more than two episodes of depression before diagnosing unipolar illness is ineffective in reducing the percentage of false unipolar patients. However, this convention does reduce the heterogeneity among unipolar groups

with respect to recurrence, increasing the chances that bipolar–unipolar comparisons will really be about polarity, as noted above. Perris's (1966) bipolar–unipolar studies come closest to this in that his unipolar patients had all experienced at least three depressions. But the median number of episodes experienced by his unipolar patients was still substantially below that of his bipolar group.

A number of important studies of the unipolar-to-bipolar conversion conducted since 1990 are not included in Table 1–2 because they do not provide this type of analysis. They generally found rates of conversion from an initial unipolar to a subsequent bipolar diagnosis that range up to 50 percent;[28] the highest rate was found in the study of the Angst group, which had the longest follow-up period. Generally, the younger the age at onset of depression, the higher was the rate of subsequent conversion to bipolar (see, for example, Rao et al., 1995; Geller et al., 2001). These issues are detailed in Chapter 4.

We have already noted that some unipolar patients have bipolar-like courses—namely early age at onset and frequent recurrences. Akiskal and Mallya (1987) pursued this observation by examining unipolar patients for depressive symptoms that might be considered analogous to mania/hypomania. Koukopoulos and Koukopoulos (1999) described these agitated depressions as "depressive mixed states," a concept that overlaps considerably with "agitated depression" (see Chapter 2). Depressive mixed states were studied more systematically in the Ravenna–San Diego Collaborative Study.[29] In that research, only three "manic-hypomanic" symptoms were required, the most frequent being psychomotor agitation (which was not goal directed), distractibility, and racing–crowded (predominantly

TABLE 1–2. **Estimates of Percent False Unipolar Using Different Cutoff Points for "Unipolar Depression"**

Required Number of Depressive Episodes	FALSE UNIPOLAR %		
	Grof (Unpublished)	Perris (1968)	Angst et al.[a] (1978)
1	18.5	—	28.4
2	15.3	13.1	26.2
3	11.9	11.4	22.5
4	13.2	12.5	22.9
5	7.8	10.7	25.0

[a]The larger percentages from the Angst et al. data may reflect a sampling bias toward more recurrent forms of the illness.

negative) thoughts, all symptoms traditionally associated with agitated depression.

The examination of depressive "mixed states" has accelerated since the first edition of this text was produced. For example, Benazzi (2001) found that 49 percent of his bipolar-II patients had three or more concurrent manic-like symptoms, versus only 3 percent of his unipolar patients. Likewise, Sato and colleagues (2003) found significantly more manic-like symptoms in their bipolar depressed patients—especially irritability, racing thoughts, and distractibility—than in their unipolar patients. In their study of 441 bipolar patients, Bauer and colleagues (2005) found that 70 percent had "clinically significant" manic-like symptoms while in a depressive episode. Maj and colleagues (2003) compared bipolar-I patients who became agitated when depressed with those who did not and found that one in four of the former had other manic-like symptoms, such as racing thoughts and pressured speech. In a more recent study of major depressive disorder, Maj and colleagues (2006) compared agitated patients with the same number of nonagitated patients, and found more bipolar relatives among the former. Serretti and Olgiati (2005) analyzed the patterns of "manic" symptoms in 372 patients diagnosed with major depressive disorder and identified agitated activity as the most frequent (18 percent), followed by irritable mood (7 percent), distractibility (3 percent), reduced need for sleep (2 percent), and reckless activity (2 percent). Note that in these studies, the most frequent "manic" symptom identified was psychomotor agitation, which recalls our speculation in the first edition of this text that agitation in unipolar depression may be analogous to mania in bipolar illness. However, we noted that manic hyperactivity and depressive agitation generally connote different phenomena, the former being more variable and goal directed, and the latter more repetitive, stereotyped, and purposeless.

The contention that these conditions should be called "mixed states" (and therefore bipolar) rather than "agitated depression" can complicate the interpretation of bipolar–unipolar differences because it broadens the concept of bipolarity to include patients *without* a history of mania or hypomania. While the finding of an elevated risk for bipolarity in first-degree relatives of agitated unipolar patients reinforces the conclusion that activation/agitation in a subgroup of unipolar patients may be a marker of a bipolar diathesis, it falls short of being an adequate basis for designating such unipolar patients as bipolar per se (Goodwin and Ghaemi, 2000). The contemporary delineation of depressive mixed states harkens back to Kraepelin (1899), who cited the existence of certain manic-like signs and symptoms during recurrent depression in some patients as he developed his argument for the essential unity of the recurrent affective disorders as manic-depressive

illness. Clearly this is a critical issue and one that is central to the discussion of mood disorders. The centrality of mixed affective states, along with the belief that recurrence/cyclicity is as or more defining a feature than polarity per se, underscores our use of the more inclusive diagnostic term manic-depressive illness. Future research on depressive mixed states and their relationship to bipolar disorder will in time clarify which characteristics of depression and mania are most important to differentiating among and understanding the affective illnesses.

The Primacy of Mania

Koukopoulos (2006) has made a novel suggestion about the relationship between mania and depression that may explain the occurrence and frequency of mixed states, as well as the connection between manic and depressive episodes in the course of this illness. According to his hypothesis, mania is primary, with depression being the consequence of a preceding mania. Thus according to this perspective, the recurrent unipolar subgroup of manic-depressive illness does not really exist since all depressive presentations are preceded by a manic presentation. Obviously, this hypothesis would require a much broader notion of mania than occurs in DSM-IV, one corresponding to concepts used 100 years ago and into ancient times. In this model, mania represents any kind of "excitement" or agitation. Thus in mania's most severe forms, we have type I bipolar disorder, while in its less severe forms, hypomania or hyperthymic personality precedes depressive episodes. Even with respect to nonrecurrent major depression, other manifestations of excitation (e.g., stress-induced anxiety conditions) could be seen as precursors of a later major depressive episode. As with any bold hypothesis, numerous objections can be made to the thesis of Koukopoulos; however, it is testable, and considering it in examining the spectrum of mood conditions may be heuristically useful.

Clinical Differences between Bipolar and Unipolar Depression

In his early observations, Leonhard noted that his bipolar patients (proportion of bipolar-I versus -II not specified) showed more symptomatic variability from episode to episode than did his recurrent unipolar patients, whose depressive symptoms he characterized as "stereotyped" (Leonhard, 1957). This differential brings to mind more recent comparisons in which bipolar-II depressed patients have been noted to have less stability and uniformity of symptoms across episodes than unipolar patients (Hantouche and Akiskal, 2005). Many studies over several decades, the results of which are summarized in Table 1–3, have found unipolar and bipolar-I differences over a wide

TABLE 1–3. Clinical Differences between Bipolar (Primarily Bipolar-I) and Unipolar Depressions

Symptom	Clinical Comparisons	Studies
Anxiety	UP>BP	Greenhouse and Geisser, 1959; Beigel and Murphy, 1971a; Brockington et al., 1982; Mitchell et al., 2001; Sato et al., 2005; Vahip et al., 2005
Tension/fearfulness	BP>UP	Perlis et al., 2006
Somatic complaints	UP>BP	Greenhouse and Geisser, 1959; Beigel and Murphy, 1971a; Vahip et al., 2002
Psychomotor retardation	BP>UP	Beigel and Murphy, 1971a; Himmelhoch et al., 1972; Kotin and Goodwin, 1972; Dunner et al., 1976a; Katz et al., 1982; Mitchell et al., 2001
	UP>BP	Popescu et al., 1991; Mitchell et al., 1992
Psychomotor agitation	UP>BP	Greenhouse and Geisser, 1959; Beigel and Murphy, 1971a; Katz et al., 1982; Kupfer et al., 1974
Atypical features	BP-II>UP	Ebert et al., 1993; Perugi et al., 1998c; Agosti and Stewart, 2001; Benazzi and Akiskal, 2001; Mitchell et al., 2001; Angst et al., 2002; Ghaemi et al., 2004; Akiskal and Benazzi, 2005; Hantouche and Akiskal, 2005
	BP-II=UP	Horwath et al., 1992; Robertson et al., 1995; Posternak and Zimmerman, 2002; Sullivan et al., 2002
Appetite loss	UP>BP	Papadimitriou et al., 2002
Depressive mixed states	BP>UP	Benazzi, 2001; Perugi et al., 2001; Maj et al., 2003; Sato et al., 2003; Akiskal and Benazzi, 2005; Bauer et al., 2005
Symptomatic variability across episodes	BP-I/-II>UP	Leonhard, 1957; Hantouche and Akiskal, 2005
Mood lability within episode	BP>UP	Brockington et al., 1982a; Hantouche and Akiskal, 2005
Irritability	BP-II>UP	Fava and Rosenbaum, 1999; Deckersbach et al., 2004; Perlis et al., 2004; Perugi et al., 2004; Benazzi and Akiskal, 2005
Insomnia (initial)	UP>BP	Mitchell et al., 2001; Hantouche and Akiskal, 2005
Insomnia (late)	BP>UP	Vahip et al., 2002
Hypersomnia	BP>UP	Mitchell et al., 2001
Postpartum episodes	BP>UP	Reich and Winokur, 1970; Kadrmas et al., 1979
Pain sensitivity	UP>BP	Davis and Buchsbaum, 1981
Fragmented REM sleep	BP>UP	Duncan et al., 1979; Mendelson et al., 1987; Rao et al., 2002

(continued)

TABLE 1–3. **Clinical Differences between Bipolar (Primarily Bipolar-I) and Unipolar Depressions** (continued)

Symptoms	Clinical Comparisons	Studies
Weight loss	UP>BP	Abrams and Taylor, 1980
Psychotic features	BP>UP	Guze et al., 1975; Akiskal, 1983c ; Coryell et al., 1985; Endicott et al., 1985; Parker et al., 2000; Mitchell et al., 2001
Comorbid substance abuse	BP>UP	Regier et al., 1990; Judd et al., 2003a; Marneros and Goodwin, 2006

BP = bipolar; UP = unipolar.

range of clinical features. We have already noted the heterogeneity in both the bipolar and unipolar groups (especially the latter), which makes any generalizations difficult to say the least. In addition to the unknown variability in extent of recurrence (cycle lengths), most of these studies did not control for differences in severity of depression or age at onset.[30]

It is worth noting that the comparisons in Table 1–3 are predominantly between unipolar and bipolar-I patients (although several of the studies refer only to "bipolar" without specifying subtype). Indeed, it has been suggested that bipolar–unipolar differences become clearer when the bipolar-II group is excluded. The most widely replicated studies point to a picture of the bipolar-I depressed patient as having more mood lability, psychotic features, psychomotor retardation, and comorbid substance abuse. In contrast, the typical unipolar patient in these studies had more anxiety, agitation, insomnia, physical complaints, anorexia, and weight loss. As noted in the table, there are a number of other features for which there is only one study or conflicting studies; certainly some of the apparent disagreement may be related simply to inadequate description of the bipolar or unipolar samples.

There is a much smaller body of data on unipolar–bipolar-II comparisons, and most of these data focus on depressive "mixed states" (more frequent in bipolar-II, as discussed above and in Chapter 2) and on so-called atypical features. Atypical depression was originally described in unipolar patients on the basis of a group of symptoms including hypersomnia, increased weight and appetite, leaden paralysis, interpersonal rejection sensitivity, and preferential response to monoamine oxidase inhibitors (MAOIs) (reviewed by Raskin and Crook, 1976). Given the suggestion of earlier studies that MAOIs are preferentially effective in bipolar depression (Himmelhoch et al., 1991), an interest in the relationship between atypical features and bipolar illness has developed. Following up on studies of atypical features reviewed in the first edition, a number of more recent

studies have reported more atypical symptoms in bipolar-II than in unipolar depressed patients.[31] On the other hand, not all investigators have found such differences.[32,33] Some of these latter studies, however, did not systematically assess bipolar-II as recommended by Dunner and Tay (1993) and Ghaemi and colleagues (2002), among others. As noted above, heterogeneity among samples of unipolar patients is another potential source of divergent findings. For example, Benazzi (2003) found that some bipolar–unipolar differences depended on the age at onset in the unipolar sample: only those unipolar patients with later age at onset were significantly different from the bipolar-II group with respect to bipolar family history, atypical features, number of episodes, and depressive mixed states.

Another approach to examining the relationship between atypical depression and bipolar disorder was pursued by Akiskal and Benazzi (2005). They examined 602 consecutively evaluated outpatients with DSM-IV major depression (58 percent were bipolar-II,[34] 42 percent unipolar), 43 percent of whom met DSM-IV criteria for atypical features, in agreement with the data of Perugi and colleagues (1998a) and Angst and colleagues (2002). They found a robust association between atypical features (especially leaden paralysis and hypersomnia) and a bipolar family history.[35] In a recent analysis of this same cohort, Akiskal and Benazzi (2006) found that hypomania scores (using The Hypomania Interview Guide) were distributed normally, not bimodally and there was a "dose response" relationship between these scores and the extent of bipolar family history, both findings suggesting that highly recurrent unipolar and bipolar II are on the same spectrum rather than representing seperate categories. On this basis, Akiskal and Benazzi suggested that atypical depression may represent a bridge between unipolar and bipolar-II disorder.

Heun and Maier (1993) interviewed 80 bipolar and 108 unipolar patients and 80 controls, along with their first-degree relatives, and found that while the morbid risk for bipolar-I was equivalent in relatives of the bipolar-I and -II groups (and was higher for both than for the unipolar group), the morbid risk for bipolar-II distinguished the relatives of this group (6.1 percent) from those of the bipolar-I group (1.8 percent). Like the findings of earlier studies (Dunner et al., 1976b; Gershon et al., 1982), these data suggest that bipolar-II may be genetically heterogeneous, some evidence being consistent with categorical integrity (Simpson et al., 1993) and some with a bipolar-I–bipolar-II spectrum. (These genetic issues are discussed more thoroughly in Chapter 13.)

Clinical Differences between Bipolar-I and -II Depressions

In the first edition, we reported on a series of NIMH clinical, genetic, pharmacological, and biological studies of bipolar–unipolar differences in which bipolar-I and -II patients were analyzed separately (Dunner et al., 1976a; Dunner, 1980). On some measures (for example, a family history of mania), the bipolar-I and -II groups were similar to one another and dissimilar to the unipolar patients. On other measures (for example, age at onset), the bipolar-II group appeared to be intermediate between the bipolar-I and unipolar groups. Finally, on some measures (for example, "atypical" features of depression), the bipolar-II patients were more similar to the unipolar than to the bipolar-I patients. One problem limiting interpretation of this interesting series of studies is the fact that the initial diagnosis of depressive illness was made prior to the availability of formal diagnostic criteria; thus, even though all of the patients had depressions severe enough to require hospitalization, the unipolar groups were undoubtedly heterogeneous.

Endicott and colleagues (1985) advanced the field by applying the formal Research Diagnostic Criteria (RDC) to 122 bipolar-I, 66 bipolar-II, and 104 recurrent unipolar depressed patients (two or more episodes of major depressive disorder). In the earlier study of Dunner and colleagues (1976) of patients hospitalized for depression, the age at onset of the bipolar-II group was intermediate (consistent with a spectrum based on severity of mania), whereas in the study of Endicott and colleagues (1985), the age at onset of the two bipolar groups was similar and different (younger) from that of the unipolar group. On the other hand, bipolar-II and unipolar patients were similar (and different from bipolar-I patients) in that both had higher proportions of time spent depressed, a finding that was confirmed and extended by the longitudinal NIMH Collaborative Program on the Psychobiology of Depression-Clinical Studies (Judd et al., 2003c) (see Chapter 4). Bipolar-II females had higher rates of alcoholism than unipolar or bipolar-I females, consistent with the earlier findings of Dunner and colleagues (1979), and they

were more likely to suffer from premenstrual dysphoria. Most important, Coryell and colleagues (1984) and Endicott and colleagues (1985) found that bipolar-I and -II patients tended to breed true. That is, bipolar-I patients tended to have bipolar-I relatives and bipolar-II patients to have bipolar-II relatives, a finding that is in agreement with the data of Fieve and colleagues (1984)[36] and Simpson and colleagues (1993) and partly with those of Gershon and colleagues (1982).

Table 1–4 updates those findings with studies published since the first edition. One important question is how these reported bipolar-I–bipolar-II differences may affect our understanding of the relationship between unipolar and bipolar depression and the concept of the manic-depressive spectrum. Focusing on the most replicated findings, a picture emerges of the bipolar-II patient as more likely to be female, with less severe but more frequent and more chronic depressions, shorter interepisode intervals, and more comorbid anxiety and alcohol abuse (the latter among females). By contrast, the bipolar-I patient has more severe and prolonged depressions with more psychosis and hospitalizations. With regard to age at onset, agitation, irritability, and frequency of rapid cycling, there is no consensus on bipolar-I–bipolar-II differences.

Examining Tables 1–3 and 1–4 together, one notes that bipolar-II is closer to unipolar in some respects (e.g., percent female and time spent depressed), but closer to bipolar-I in others (e.g., number of episodes and substance abuse).

As noted earlier, the DSM-IV construct of bipolar-II requires a threshold of 4 or more days. However, findings of more recent studies suggest that 2 days may be a more appropriate threshold (judged on the basis of external validating strategies, such as age at onset, depressive recurrence, and familial bipolarity). These are mainly cross-sectional studies from different clinics in the United States (Akiskal and Mallya, 1987; Manning et al., 1997) and Italy (Cassano et al., 1992; Benazzi, 2001). Epidemiologic data reveal that most hypomanias are of 1–3 days' duration (Wicki and Angst, 1991). It is interesting to note that if one takes a dimensional view of hypomania in manic-depressive illness (symptoms rather than syndrome), bipolar–recurrent unipolar differences are attenuated (Cassano et al., 2004);[37] these clinical observations require independent validation by external markers, such as family history and prospective course.

Few long-term studies have been conducted with lower thresholds for hypomania. The two exceptions are derived from the prospective NIMH Collaborative Program on the Psychobiology of Depression-Clinical Studies, which showed, first, longitudinal stability of bipolar-II over time (Coryell et al., 1995) and, second, no significant differences in clinical and course parameters when either 2- or 7-day

TABLE 1–4. **Clinical Differences between Bipolar-I and Bipolar-II**

Symptom	Clinical Comparisons	Studies
Anxiety	BP-II >BP-I	Dunner et al., 1976b; Hantouche et al., 1998; Judd et al., 2003c
Time spent in depression (major and minor)	BP-II >BP-I	Endicott et al., 1985; Vieta et al., 1997; Judd et al., 2003
Interepisode intervals	BP-II <BP-I	Judd et al., 2003b
Number of episodes	BP-II >BP-I	Vieta et al., 1997; Judd et al., 2003c; Akiskal and Benazzi, 2005
Rapid cycling	BP-II >BP-I	Coryell et al., 1992; Maj et al., 1999; Baldessarini et al., 2000
	BP-II = BP-I	Vieta et al., 1997; Coryell et al., 2003
Psychotic features	BP-I >BP-II	Vieta et al., 1997; Mitchell et al., 2001
Suicide/suicide attempt	BP-II >BP-I	Dunner et al., 1976; Goldring and Fieve, 1984; Arato et al., 1988; Rihmer and Pestality, 1999
	BP-I = BP-II	Coryell et al., 1989; Vieta et al., 1997
Premenstrual dysphoria	BP-II >BP-I	Endicott et al., 1985
Hospitalizations	BP-I >BP-II	Vieta et al., 1997
Agitation; irritability	BP-I >BP-II	Dunner et al., 1976b; Hantouche et al., 1998; Serretti and Olgiati, 2005
Alcohol abuse (females)	BP-II >BP-I	Dunner et al. 1976b; Endicott et al., 1985; Ferrier et al., 2001
Percent female	BP-II >BP-I	Weissman et al., 1996; Cassano et al., 1999
Severity of depressive episodes	BP-I >BP-II	Coryell et al., 1985; Vieta et al., 1997; Benazzi, 1999
Length of depressive episode	BP-I >BP-II	Coryell et al., 1985
Percent medicated	BP-I >BP-II	Coryell et al., 1985

BP = bipolar.

thresholds were applied to RDC-defined bipolar-II patients (Judd et al., 2003b). Akiskal and Pinto (1999) suggested that those with the shortest duration of hypomania are more unstable and have a highly recurrent course, typically arising from a cyclothymic temperamental base, which they designate bipolar-II ½.[38] It remains to be seen whether such continued splitting of diagnostic groups is productive or is simply confusing to the field. This is an empirical question, one that will be resolved ultimately by genetic studies. It is noteworthy that Angst and Gamma (2002), in defining subthreshold bipolarity, set no thresholds for the duration of hypomania as long as the hypomania is recurrent.

EMERGENCE OF THE MANIC-DEPRESSIVE SPECTRUM

The concept of a spectrum is used in two different ways in the description of affective disorders, both clearly delineated by Kraepelin. On the one hand, spectrum conceptualizes a continuum between bipolar and unipolar illness—historically, this is the manic-depressive spectrum. On the other hand, a spectrum is a way to conceptualize the relationship between full-blown affective illness, either bipolar or unipolar, and milder states or characteristics that might be construed as temperament. When we refer to the manic-depressive spectrum here, we are using it in this latter way.

Kraepelin (1921, p. 1) was the first to formally posit a continuum between the psychotic and less severe of affective disorders, merging imperceptibly with normality (although this concept was implicit among many of the ancient physicians):

Manic-depressive insanity . . . [includes] certain slight and slightest colourings of mood, some of them periodic, some of them continuously morbid, which on the one hand are to be regarded as the rudiment of more severe disorders, on the other hand pass without sharp boundary into the domain of personal predisposition. In the course of the years I have become more and more convinced that all the above-mentioned states only represent manifestations of a single morbid process.

As we noted in the first edition, the classic descriptions cited in Chapter 2, systematic observations reported in the literature, and our own research and clinical experience and that of our colleagues all convince us that the cardinal features of manic-depressive illness are dimensional, that is, distributed along a spectrum. Indeed, to give emphasis to the spectrum concept in the first edition, we devoted a separate chapter to it. Our 1990 conclusion was echoed by an international panel of experts that summarized the increasingly rich and sophisticated database supporting such a spectrum (Akiskal et al., 2000). More recently, Ghaemi and colleagues (2004) proposed a definition of bipolar spectrum disorder (or as we would prefer for clarity, the manic-depressive spectrum), which is outlined in Box 1–2.

We further explore the spectrum model here because it introduces concepts that shaped the formal diagnostic systems reviewed in Chapter 3, and it clarifies our own conceptions of manic-depressive illness, implicit in discussions throughout this volume.

Although diagnosis is central to all of medicine, the assumptions underlying its various meanings are seldom examined. The most common medical classification model—the categorical approach—posits discrete diagnostic entities or discrete subtypes within a larger diagnostic group. Dimensional approaches, the most common competing model, characterize the individual patient according to where he or she falls on a number of separate dimensions. In this model, each individual represents the point of intersection of multiple parameters. Both models have gained support from studies using discriminate function analysis and other statistical techniques. Clearly, the categorical approaches tend to prevail, not because they are supported more compellingly by the empirical evidence, but because they are much easier to grasp conceptually and to deal with statistically. Indeed, multidimensional approaches, however eloquently descriptive of an individual patient, will remain essentially unhelpful if they cannot test generalizations—that is, be applied to prediction.

Contrary to the common assumption, the categorical approach does not preclude the concept of a continuum (Grayson, 1987; Kraemer et al., 2004). A diagnostic category need not have absolutely discrete and discontinuous boundaries. Let us suppose for the moment that individuals with depressive disorders are distributed more or less evenly along a continuum with self-limiting grief reactions on one end and severe, disabling major depressive illness on the other (Kendell, 1968; Goodwin, 1977). Even if discontinuity (i.e., clustering at discrete points along the spectrum) is not

---

BOX 1–2. A Proposed Definition of Bipolar Spectrum Disorder

A. At least one major depressive episode
B. No spontaneous hypomanic or manic episodes
C. Either one of the following, plus at least two items from criterion D, or both of the following plus one item from criterion D:
  1. A family history of bipolar disorder in a first-degree relative
  2. Antidepressant-induced mania or hypomania
D. If no items from criterion C are present, six of the following nine criteria are needed:
  1. Hyperthymic personality (at baseline, nondepressed state)
  2. Recurrent major depressive episode (>3)
  3. Brief major depressive episodes (on average, <3 months)
  4. Atypical depressive features (increased sleep or appetite)
  5. Psychotic major depressive episode
  6. Early age at onset of major depressive episode (before age 25)
  7. Postpartum depression
  8. Antidepressant tolerance ("wear-off," acute but not prophylactic response)
  9. Lack of response to >3 antidepressant treatment trials

Source: Ghaemi et al., 2004.

---

demonstrable, a useful category can still be defined by establishing a minimum (or maximum) threshold of symptoms for inclusion in the category; consider, for example, hypertension and hypothyroidism. And the pattern of illness characteristics—symptoms, course, family history, and treatment response, for example—reflects a convergence of several dimensional variables. Such a model should be acceptable to those who are comfortable with large, internally variable categories—the "lumpers"—as well as to those who want to create a new category for every variant—the "splitters." This conception is simply for the sake of narrative convenience, not to reflect a conviction that any particular group has discrete, discontinuous boundaries. On the contrary, and as we emphasized in the first edition of this book, we are impressed with the subtlety of the shadings.[39] How these issues bear on diagnosis is discussed in Chapter 3.

Exploration of spectrum models is important for several reasons. The reliable characterization and validation of subsyndromal states similar to bipolar illness would enhance research on genetic markers and modes of genetic transmission, as discussed in Chapter 13, as well as provide an approach for identifying individuals at risk for the development of full-blown bipolar illness (Alda, 2004). Additionally, a spectrum model would permit the evaluation of treatments for attenuated variants, including the question of whether early intervention could lessen the chance of progression to bipolar illness. Existing prospective and retrospective data indicate that approximately one-third of individuals with subthreshold conditions phenomenologically related to bipolar illness (i.e., cyclothymia) will go on to develop the full bipolar syndrome (Akiskal et al., 1979a, 1995; Depue et al., 1981, 1989; Cassano et al., 2002, 2004). The possibility that this progression may be hastened by treatment with antidepressant drugs (see Chapter 19) lends further urgency to identifying subsyndromal precursors of bipolar disorder. Indeed, the term *bipolar spectrum*, which conveys the continuum of cyclothymia with bipolar-II and with hypomanias associated with antidepressants, is a logical extension of concepts laid out long ago by Kraepelin and his predecessors.

The concepts of secondary depression and secondary mania have received considerable attention because they are important to differential diagnosis (see Chapter 3) and because they may shed light on the pathophysiology of mood states (see Chapter 14). Reexamined in light of spectrum models, secondary mania and depression, like their primary counterparts, also appear to be expressions of an underlying diathesis, but a weaker one, which therefore requires a greater perturbation to be expressed clinically. This possibility is most credible in the case of pharmacologically induced hypomanias.

Bearing on the concept of a manic-depressive spectrum (i.e., the relationship between unipolar and bipolar illness), recent data from the French national EPIDEP (Epidemiology of Depression) study (Akiskal et al., 2003a) suggest a familial vulnerability for hypomania associated with antidepressant pharmacotherapy, which is similar to that for spontaneous bipolar-II disorder (see Table 1–1), but one that is probably less severe than that associated with spontaneous hypomanic episodes. For this reason, Akiskal and colleagues (2003a) have suggested the term *bipolar-III* for this group of patients. A prospective study by Kovacs and colleagues (1994) showed that many dysthymic children followed up beyond puberty do switch to hypomania and/or mania even without pharmacological treatment. These data suggest a threshold of vulnerability among subjects with early-onset dysthymia that may not routinely require external triggers, such as antidepressants.

Along the same lines, Akiskal and colleagues (1979b) reported that familial affective "loading" (defined as more than three affected members in a pedigree) predicted those "neurotic depressives" who progressed to hypomania and/or mania during prospective follow-up. In another study, Akiskal and colleagues (1978) followed 100 outpatients with mild depressive states—variously referred to as "neurotic," "reactive," or "situational"—for 3 to 4 years. They found that 40 percent developed a major affective disorder, and nearly half of these were bipolar.

The terminology applied to the "soft bipolar spectrum" includes overlapping conditions in the less-than-manic range. The soft spectrum includes Dunner and colleagues' (1980) "bipolar, not otherwise specified," as well as conditions described by Akiskal and Akiskal (1988) as depressions arising from cyclothymic and hyperthymic temperament. In addition, it includes hypomanic reactions occurring during antidepressant and other somatotherapies for depression.

An elevated risk for familial bipolarity (Cassano et al., 1992; Akiskal, 2001) represents the main external validation of the bipolar nature of these "soft" phenotypes. Akiskal and colleagues (2003a) and Hantouche and colleagues (2003a) have suggested that within the broadly conceived cyclothymic temperamental domain there are "dark" and "sunny" types. Although family history for bipolar disorder is equally high in both groups, in clinical practice bipolar-II associated with the darker core cyclothymic temperament is more likely to be diagnosed as a personality disorder. There is little justification for this practice, because as in the case of full-blown bipolar patients, those with spectrum diagnoses in the broad cyclothymic–bipolar-II realm are equally likely to engage in dramatic and socially inappropriate behaviors (Akiskal, 1994; Deltito et al., 2001). In the end, it may not be easy to distinguish among clinical, subclinical, subthreshold, and personality expressions of bipolarity (Akiskal et al., 1979a; Sass et al., 1993; Akiskal, 2001). Again, it is important to stress that although the spectrum concept is essential, there must be concern that the spectrum of bipolarity can become so far extended that it becomes theoretically and clinically meaningless (if not actually damaging, as would be the case with a diagnostic overinclusiveness resulting in the inappropriate diagnosis and treatment of individuals with intense normal variants of temperament).

The Akiskal and Pinto (1999) formulation acknowledging more subtle intermediary forms, a formulation indebted to the observations of many earlier clinicians and investigators, captures the dilemmas of the clinician and the researcher working within a spectrum model of bipolar illness from the most severe (mood-incongruent mania) to the least severe (hyperthymic temperament). Similar dilemmas are encountered when exploring the manic-depressive spectrum between bipolar disorder and unipolar depression.

Using both clinical and nonclinical populations of college students, Depue and colleagues developed a systematic approach to the evaluation of subsyndromal affective states, focusing particularly on bipolar forms. The touchstone of this series of studies was the development of the General Behavioral Inventory (GBI), a self-report measure of traits that can assess the pattern of cyclothymia over time (Depue et al., 1981; Depue and Klein, 1988). Each of its

73 items, drawn from clinical descriptions of hypomania and depression and focused on lability, incorporates the dimensions of intensity, duration, and frequency. (The GBI is described in more detail in Chapter 11.) GBI scores for depression are distributed across normal, cyclothymic, and bipolar-II populations; each group merges imperceptibly into the other, consistent with the concept of a spectrum.[40] These studies imply that the concept of a depressive spectrum applies equally to bipolar and unipolar depression, challenging the conventional wisdom that neurotic depression should be subsumed entirely in the unipolar spectrum.

Unfortunately, the cyclothymic scale introduced by Depue and colleagues did not command sufficient interest in the literature, conceivably because its system for assessing mood lability, intensity, and cyclicity was quite elaborate. A new instrument was subsequently developed to measure the broader temperamental domain of bipolarity (Akiskal et al., 1998b): the temperament scale of Memphis, Pisa, Paris, and San Diego (TEMPS), which, while lacking the psychometric sophistication and strong validating research base of the GBI, appears to be somewhat less unwieldy from a psychometric standpoint and represents the dominant tendency for each of the cyclothymic, hyperthymic, irritable, and depressive types.[41]

As noted earlier, and as elaborated in Chapter 2 on clinical description, Kraepelin described a "manic temperament," which he originally termed "constitutional excitement." The antithesis of the "depressive temperament," the manic temperament, at its most severe, was defined as a handicapping condition marked by desultory, incoherent, and aimless thought; hasty and shallow judgment; restlessness; and exalted, careless, and confident mood. Kraepelin viewed the manic temperament as a "link in the long chain of manic-depressive dispositions," which in its least severe form could still be considered normal.

Akiskal and colleagues (1979a) characterized—and psychometrically validated (Akiskal et al., 1998b)—the most discriminatory features of what they termed the "hyperthymic temperament," representing the softest expression of Kraepelin's manic type. Like cyclothymia, hyperthymia represents a trait and possibly a lifelong disposition, with a familial excess of bipolar disorder as compared with depressive states without bipolar temperaments (Cassano et al., 1992; Akiskal, 2001; Akiskal et al., 2005). Unlike the studies of Kagan and colleagues (see Chapter 10), however, these studies of temperament have not been carried out across the lifetime or in a prospective context, which limits our understanding of the relationship among measured "hyperthymia," subsyndromal illness, and actual illness.

In his discussion of the manic spectrum based on cross-sectional observations, Klerman (1981) described a continuum from normal happiness or joy through cyclothymic personality, nonpsychotic hypomania, and psychotic mania. It is clear, however, that this string of states does not reflect a spectrum of ever-increasing happiness and joy, since these pleasant emotions are replaced by qualitatively very different moods and sensations as one crosses the line from hypomania into mania. Klerman's recommendation that the term "elations" be used to encompass the spectrum of mania emphasizes mood over other important features, such as energy level, activity, behavior, and cognition. As noted earlier, the terminology can be confusing. In Klerman's spectrum, cyclothymic personality falls between normal happiness and hypomania. In DSM-IV, a diagnosis of cyclothymia requires hypomanic episodes. In this diagnostic system, cyclothymia is differentiated from bipolar-II major affective disorder on the basis of its less severe depressions, which do not meet criteria for major depressive disorder. Using elation as the criterion for the manic spectrum also is reminiscent of older formulations in which depression and mania were at opposite ends of a continuum, with normal in the middle. Such a continuum is quite limited as a model, primarily because it cannot account for mixed states, which, as discussed in Chapter 2, are quite common. Some believe it preferable to consider the depressive and manic spectra as independent and capable of interacting in a variety of combinations and permutations.[42] It is interesting that in both the Endicott (1989) and the Angst and Gamma (2002) schema, the manic-depressive spectrum is dominated by depressive recurrences, with very mild and short hypomanias. This conception is in line with our view that recurrence and cyclicity are more fundamental than polarity, which in turn accords with Kraepelin's nosologic position. We remain concerned, however, that relatively little research has been conducted on the continuum of manic states (Jamison, 2004), a concern we expressed in the first edition of this text.

As reviewed in Chapter 2, severe psychotic features, including mood incongruence, are extensively documented for bipolar patients in both the classical and the recent literature. The boundary between severe mania and schizobipolar disorder is not clear (see Chapter 3). Suffice it to say that new data appear to be consistent with the view that schizobipolar patients lie on a continuum with severe mania, whether one examines family history (Van Eerdewegh et al., 1987; Toni et al., 2001) or course (Cutting, 1990).

If we integrate the depressive and manic spectra, we can construct an overall spectrum of bipolar illness. At one end is cyclothymic personality; then cyclothymic disorder (bipolar, other in Dunner's terms or md in Angst's terms[43]); followed by bipolar-II disorder (mD or bipolar disorder, not otherwise specified, in DSM-IV); then Md (often misdiagnosed as unipolar mania); and finally MD (i.e., bipolar-I), which is the core critical bipolar disorder.[44] Figure 1–1 illustrates this spectrum by displaying the mood variation characteristic of each subgroup. Note that in this spectrum, we implicitly consider mania to be more severe than depression, since the Md form is closer than mD (bipolar-II) to the severe end of the spectrum. Current international data indicate that much of the bipolar spectrum is in the midrealm (type II) and beyond.[45]

As presented here, the spectra are only descriptive. They do not necessarily imply a progression, nor do they require that all these states share some unitary relationship. Individuals fitting the description of cyclothymic personality, for example, may have a family history or response to treatment unrelated to bipolar-I disorder. The data reviewed in this chapter suggest, however, that a large percentage of individuals with soft or subsyndromal states apparently analogous to bipolar disorder do indeed belong in the bipolar spectrum by virtue of their positive family history and their tendency to progress to full clinical disorder. While those on the soft end of the spectrum may not be bipolar in the formal sense of having a history of diagnosable mania or hypomania, many of them no doubt have a bipolar diathesis.

Once we move beyond the temperaments into cyclothymic disorder (described more fully in Chapter 2), the evidence argues compellingly for the inclusion of cyclothymic disorder in the bipolar spectrum. Cycles of mood and energy can continue indefinitely, constituting a mild form of bipolar illness, or they can progress to a more severe expression of the disorder, sometimes after years.

As noted in Chapter 2, Kraepelin assumed that cyclothymia is part of the bipolar spectrum, and modern investigators[46] have argued persuasively for its inclusion on the basis of (1) family history data linking cyclothymia with the more severe forms of bipolar illness, (2) overlap and similarity of symptom patterns between cyclothymia and bipolar disorder, (3) comparability of rates for pharmacologically induced hypomania, and (4) the subsequent development of full syndromal illness in many patients initially diagnosed as cyclothymic. In some instances, cyclothymia can be regarded as a milder expression of bipolar illness and in others as a precursor to the full syndrome.

Some bipolar-II patients show considerable erratic "character" pathology (often referred to as "cluster B" or borderline—see Chapters 2 and 10), interepisode lability, and related problems of substance abuse. Conventional wisdom (e.g., DSM-IV) would suggest that an intrinsic association of these features with bipolar disorder is less convincing, on the assumption that such features are simply a consequence of the fact that bipolar-II patients often lead chaotic lives, have poor or unpredictable social support systems, and fail to adhere to medications.[47] Nonetheless, new findings from the French EPIDEP study, as described in Chapter 2, suggest that from a familial standpoint, these patients may be as bipolar as those with bipolar-II. Perugi and colleagues (1999, 2003) have proposed a common link among these cyclothymic traits, borderline personality, and atypical depression.

Criticism notwithstanding, the concept of a manic-depressive spectrum appears to be shaping a new paradigm, much of it extending into the domain of traditional depressive disorders. Indeed, whether one examines bipolar pedigrees (Gershon et al., 1982; Tsuang et al., 1985), offspring of bipolars (Akiskal et al., 1985), epidemiologic samples (Angst et al., 2003), or the microstructure of the course of bipolar-I and -II disorders (Judd et al., 2002, 2003b), bipolar illness is

Figure 1–1. Range of total mood variation by subgroup.

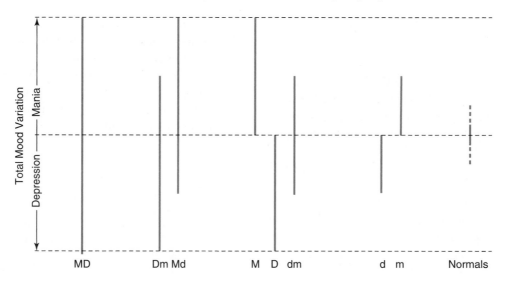

dominated by depressive symptomotology.[48] In this respect, bipolar-I and -II appear to be quite similar (Judd et al., 2003a). This is where a great deal of the disability associated with the illness appears to reside—in the subdepressive symptomotology between episodes (Altshuler et al., 2002). Given that the depressive dominance is found in epidemiologic samples and in pedigree and family studies, one cannot criticize the foregoing clinical studies on the basis of tertiary referral bias, by which the more depression-prone bipolar patients are retained in follow-up studies. As detailed in Chapter 2, the depressive phase of bipolar disorder and depressive presentations in clinical practice represent a highly important aspect of bipolarity.

The spectrum concept is not just a recent peculiarity of the clinical and research focus on soft bipolarity. As reviewed here and in Chapter 2, these concepts are ancient. Indeed, it has been suggested that all major mental disorders can perhaps best be characterized in spectrum models (Maser and Akiskal, 2002). As noted earlier, Baldessarini (2000) criticized the concept of a broad bipolar spectrum on methodological grounds, arguing that it risks diluting the concept of bipolar disorder, thereby reducing the rigor of contemporary research. We agree. It is true that most authors cited by Baldessarini as having made major contributions to the field (from Aretaeus on) endorsed a broad conceptualization of manic-depressive illness; as we noted earlier, however, "manic-depressive spectrum" denotes something different from "bipolar spectrum."

While the more recently proposed soft forms of bipolarity make some clinical and intuitive sense to us, they still require considerably more research from a wider range of independent research groups focused on external validators, especially family history, treatment response, and long-term outcome. For the clinician dealing with individuals, deciding whether one is encountering one end of a normal range of behavior, a personality disorder, or manic-depressive illness requiring treatment remains a challenge.

CONCLUSIONS

The existence of the "softer" phenotypes on the fringes of classic or "hard" bipolar phenotypes that encroach into the territory of unipolar depression indicates the need for at least a partial return to the unitary Kraepelinian concept of manic-depressive illness. While some view the bipolar spectrum as the modern heir of this classic broader position, subsuming all conditions under the rubric of "bipolar" is a less than totally satisfactory way to emphasize the close relationship between bipolar illness and highly recurrent unipolar depression (many patients with the latter condition, after all, remain nonbipolar in the usual sense).

If our diagnostic systems were to return to the Kraepelinian position of taking recurrence as the first principle for organizing the affective disorders (as we propose in Chapter 3), one would not have to posit that all early-onset recurrent depressions are part of the bipolar spectrum. On the other hand, contemporary studies[49] of "depressive mixed states" appear to provide some empirical support for Kraepelin's descriptions of "excited depression" and "depression with flight of ideas," apparently representing those highly recurrent unipolar patients who, despite not having a history of manic or hypomanic episodes, may have enough manic-like features when depressed, as well as sufficient bipolarity in their family histories, to be considered part of the bipolar spectrum in the sense of having some bipolar diathesis. For conceptualizing the relationship between bipolar disorder per se and recurrent depressive disorders, however, we still prefer the Kraepelinian concept of manic-depressive illness because it is unitary; all recurrent affective illness is encompassed, although Kraepelin anticipated the later bipolar–unipolar subdivision. Indeed, while much future research needs to be conducted to fully validate the concept of a manic-depressive spectrum, the pendulum appears to have shifted distinctly in favor of the Kraepelinian position, which includes much of the domain of frequently recurrent depression under the broad manic-depressive rubric.

Finally, we should reiterate why the exploration of spectrum models of manic-depressive illness is so important. First, for the bipolar subgroup, validation of subsyndromal states will enhance research on genetic markers and modes of genetic transmission. Second, it will allow the identification of individuals potentially at risk for the development of full bipolar illness, opening up the possibility of trials of early interventions that could reduce the likelihood of progression. Lastly, the model of a manic-depressive spectrum increases clinicians' awareness of the close relationship between bipolar illness and some forms of unipolar depression (an understanding that has been undermined by the structure of DSM-IV). It is only this awareness that can help the clinician avoid the all-too-common misdiagnosis of bipolar patients as unipolar, a mistake that can lead to the almost always ill-advised treatment decision, discussed in Chapter 19, of administering an antidepressant in the absence of a mood stabilizer.

NOTES

1. The authors acknowledge a deep intellectual debt to the great German psychiatrist Emil Kraepelin. Kraepelin, the son of an actor, was born in 1856 in Neustrelitz, near the Baltic Sea. His older brother Karl, a biology teacher, influenced Emil's decision to become a doctor and an academician. Interested in

psychiatry while still at the Würzburg Medical School, Kraepelin, upon graduation in 1878, studied with the neuroanatomists Bernard von Gudden and P. E. Flechsig. He then turned to experimental psychophysiological research, under the tutelage of Wilhelm Wundt. He held psychiatric hospital appointments in Munich, Leubus, and Dresden. In 1886, he became professor of psychiatry in Dorpat, then moved to the same position in Heidelberg in 1890 and to Munich in 1904 [or 1903?]. In 1922, he retired from teaching and became head of the Research Institute of Psychiatry in Munich.

According to Alexander and Selesnick (1966), Kraepelin's training, personality, and dedication were well suited to the task of classifying and generalizing the myriad clinical observations made during the nineteenth century: "He learned early to respect authority, order, and organization.... "Imperial German psychiatry" was said to have gained its prominence under the "chancellorship" of Kraepelin, one of Bismarck's admirers" (pp. 162–163). As Bismarck unified Germany, Kraepelin brought order to the balkanized psychiatry of the turn of the century. The first edition of his textbook, which he continued to revise throughout his life, was published in 1883. In succeeding editions, he refined and expanded the textbook from the brief outline of the first edition to the 2,425 pages of the ninth edition, published in 1927, a year after his death. The textbook was notable for its division of major psychiatric illness into two categories and for its emphasis on prognosis. The third and fourth parts of the eighth edition, covering manic-depressive "insanity" and paranoia, were published separately in 1921, and it is that monograph that is cited throughout this book.

Zilboorg (1941), from his psychoanalytical perspective, summarized the personal observations of Kraepelin from those who knew him personally:

[They] tell of his rather pleasant, responsive personality, of his tactful ability in bringing people together to work as an organized group, and of his great gifts as a teacher; yet it is curious that his scientific personality was so very detached, almost distant from the inner life of the patient. To Kraepelin a mentally sick person seems to have been a collection of symptoms. He was a true son of the great, energetic, and creative age that was interested greatly in humanity but comparatively little in man. Perhaps this trait in Kraepelin as a psychiatrist, which today would be considered a defect, was the very characteristic which helped rather than hindered him in the creation of his great system and school. He was able to collect and to study thousands of case histories, covering not only the story of each illness, but the history of each patient's life before the illness and a follow-up history of his life after he left the hospital. Dealing with such large masses of data, Kraepelin was able to sort out everything these many individuals had in common, leaving out of consideration the purely individual data. He thus arrived at an excellent general picture, at a unique perspective of a mental illness as a whole. But he seems to have been almost unaware that in his careful study he lost the individual. (p. 452)

Berrios and Hauser (1988) took issue with this assessment, noting the "great depth and beauty" of Kraepelin's late conceptual writing. They quoted from a 1920 work: "If these observations approximate the truth we will have to look for the key to the understanding of the clinical picture primarily in characteristics of the individual patient ... his expectations play a decisive role."

2. For the material in this section we are indebted to the historians in our field, especially to Jackson (1986) and Roccatagliata (1986) for their extensive scholarship. Whitwell (1936), in his modestly titled *Historical Notes on Psychiatry*, provided translations of ancient manuscripts and insights into the apparent manic-depressive symptoms of literary and historical figures, such as Orestes, Saul, and Herod the Great. Although not as sharply focused on affective illness, other sources have proved valuable in understanding the historical context in general medicine and psychiatry; they include Ackerknecht (1959, 1982), Zilboorg (1941), Alexander and Selesnick (1966), and Wightman (1971).

3. Medical historians believe that the works attributed to Hippocrates probably represent the work of his school. According to Ackerknecht (1982, p. 55), for example:

From fifty to seventy books were later attributed to Hippocrates, and in the third century B.C. they were collected in Alexandria into the Corpus Hippocraticum. It is not known which of these books, if any, were actually written by the great physician. As a matter of fact, none of them contains the ideas attributed to him in the writings of Plato and Menon.

4. Quoted by Whitwell (1936, p. 212) from Pratensis Jason: *De cerebri morbis* (Basil), 1549.

5. According to Jackson (1986, p. 100), Marsilius Ficinus (Marsilio Ficino) was a fifteenth-century philosopher, physician, and priest who revitalized Aristotle's views "with far-reaching effects on his own and later times."

6. Despite the presence of schizophrenic-like symptoms during the manic episodes, the diagnosis of manic-depressive illness was confirmed on follow-up. Demographic data suggested that the patients in this study were like manic-depressive patients in other studies in relapse frequency, duration of illness, and other features.

7. Quoted by Jackson (1986, p. 263) from Baillarger, 1854, p. 352.

8. Quoted by Jackson (1986, p. 268) from Ritti, A.: "Circular insanity." In *A Dictionary of Psychological Medicine Giving the Definition, Etymology and Synonyms of Terms Used in Medical Psychology, with the Symptoms, Treatment and Pathology of Insanity and the Law of Lunacy in Great Britain and Ireland*, edited by D. Hack Tuke, 2 vols. (Philadelphia: P. Blakiston), 1892, p. 214.

9. Some psychoanalytic writers implied that different phases of manic-depressive illness were linked through some underlying mechanism. Prominent here is the conception of mania as a defense against depression (see Chapter 11). This analytical formulation, reminiscent of the earliest observations that mania grew out of melancholia, could be said to have anticipated the current continuum model.

10. Some investigators (e.g., Koukopoulos et al., 1983; Akiskal and Akiskal, 1988; Cassano et al., 1988) focused on the opposite temperaments—depressive and hyperthymic—and proposed that a fundamental characteristic of bipolarity is the shift from one temperamental state into the opposite

extreme in the form of an episode. Thus, depressive temperaments are vulnerable to a swing into hypomania or mania, whereas those with hyperthymic temperaments are likely to swing into depressions. According to Akiskal and colleagues (1998b), such propensities may serve as the basis for mixed states (see Chapter 2).

11. The very existence of depressive mixed states (isolated intradepressive "manic" symptoms) argued for a continuum, which is consistent with the contemporary work of Benazzi and Akiskal (2001) and Sato and colleagues (2003).

12. Although not incompatible with Kraepelin's descriptions of manic-depressive illness, Meyer's approach implied a different conceptual framework. The Meyerians, although allowing for the operation of biological and genetic factors, understood them as part of an individual's vulnerability to specific psychological and social influences. This perspective was symbolized by the rubric "manic-depressive reaction" in the first official diagnostic manual of the American Psychiatric Association, published in 1952.

13. This would apply most clearly to German and British psychiatry, perhaps less so to French psychiatry (Leff, 1977).

14. This emphasis on presenting episode rather than course was somewhat ironic, because Meyer's own writings emphasized a longitudinal perspective.

15. *Primary* is defined as depression in the absence of any preexisting or antecedent psychiatric or medical disorder.

16. At any rate, from a clinical and epidemiologic standpoint, current data indicate that the foregoing depressive dichotomies are best regarded as part of a depressive spectrum (Judd and Akiskal, 2000).

17. To Bleuler, a patient was predominantly schizophrenic or predominantly manic-depressive. Patients were distributed all along this spectrum, and an individual patient could be at different points on the spectrum at different times.

18. Compared with unipolar patients, bipolar depressed patients were reported to have lower ratings of anxiety, anger, and physical complaints (Beigel and Murphy, 1971b); more psychomotor retardation (Beigel and Murphy, 1971b; Himmelhoch et al., 1972; Kotin and Goodwin, 1972; Dunner et al., 1976a; Katz et al., 1982); lower levels of measured physical activity (Kupfer et al., 1974); and more total sleep time (Hartmann, 1968; Kupfer et al., 1972; Duncan et al., 1979).

19. Winokur divided his primary unipolar patients (none of whom had a family history of mania) into familial pure depressive disease (FPDD), sporadic pure depressive disease (SPDD), and depression spectrum disease (DSD). (*Primary* was defined as depression in the absence of any preexisting or antecedent psychiatric or medical disorder.) The two pure types had no other preceding psychiatric diagnoses and no alcoholism among first-degree relatives. The distinction between them was that FPDD patients had a first-degree relative with primary depression, whereas SPDD patients did not. DSD patients were those with alcoholism or antisocial personality among first-degree (male) relatives; they were predominantly female patients with early onset. Winokur (1980) suggested that genetically, the FPDD subtype was closely related to bipolar illness.

20. Akiskal, 1981, 1983a, 1998; Benazzi, 1997, 2001, 2003; Akiskal and Pinto, 1999; Angst and Marneros, 2001; Benazzi and Akiskal, 2001, 2003; Marneros, 2001; Hantouche et al., 2003b.

21. Some of the differences among individual manic-depressive patients reflect differences in the illness per se, whereas others reflect the interaction of the illness with individual characteristics, some of which certainly involve genetic differences unrelated to manic-depressive illness. The reactive–endogenous and neurotic–psychotic dichotomies (or spectra) should not be taken simply as a reflection of differential severity, that is, from mild to severe in consequences for the patient. As observed by Lewis (1936, p. 998):

> It may be said, simply, that severe emotional upsets ordinarily tend to subside, but that mild emotional states, when often provoked or long maintained, tend to persist, as it were, autonomously. Hence the paradox that a gross blatant psychosis may do less damage in the long run than some meager neurotic incubus: a dramatic attack of mania or melancholia, with delusions, wasting, hallucinations, wild excitement and other alarms, may have far less effect on the course of a man's life than some deceptively mild affective illness which goes on so long that it becomes inveterate. The former comes as a catastrophe, and when it has passed the patient takes up his life again, active, cheerful, normal in every way, while with the latter he may never get rid of his burden.

22. Akiskal et al., 1977, 1979a; Depue et al., 1981; Egeland and Hotstetter, 1983; Akiskal and Pinto, 1999; Angst and Marneros, 2001; Marneros, 2001; Ghaemi et al., 2002.

23. It is possible that the high bipolar/unipolar ratio in Egeland's Amish data reflects special genetic factors limited to that population. As noted below, however, Angst's (1978) group also found a 1:1 ratio of bipolar to unipolar illness when the sample was followed for many years and hypomania was ascertained.

24. Ghaemi et al., 1999; Goldberg et al., 2001; Dilsaver and Akiskal, 2005; Hantouche and Akiskal, 2005; Rybakowski et al., 2005; Sharma et al., 2005; Smith et al., 2005.

25. Some bipolar–unipolar differences become more clear when bipolar-II is deleted from the comparison.

26. In their second study, however, Abrams and Taylor (1979) found a higher morbid risk for unipolar depression in unipolar manic patients compared with bipolar patients.

27. The method relied on reports of the manic patients themselves at or near admission, presumably while they were still ill. Davenport and colleagues (1979) at NIMH showed (as common sense would suggest) that manic patients report substantially fewer past depressive episodes than their families remember.

28. Akiskal et al., 1995, 2005; Coryell et al., 1995; Goldberg et al., 2001; Angst et al., 2005.

29. Benazzi and Akiskal, 2001; Maj et al., 2003; Akiskal and Benazzi, 2004; Biondi et al., 2005; Sato et al., 2005; Serretti and Olgiati, 2005.

30. Even in the study by Katz and colleagues (1982), which employed prior screening by the Research Diagnostic Criteria (RDC) (see Chapter 3), greater heterogeneity in the unipolar group is plausible since the research criteria allowed for sleep and appetite changes in either direction. In fact, Kupfer and colleagues (1975), examining unipolar depressed patients with a variety of clinical and personality measures, described a subgroup with symptoms similar to those of

bipolar depression. Like bipolar patients, these unipolar depressed patients were more retarded, had lower levels of anxiety, and ate and slept more. They, like the bipolar patients, had been hospitalized more often in the past than the unipolar patients, although the incidence of past depressive episodes, suicide attempts, and substance abuse was similar for all the patients. Kupfer suggested that this subgroup of unipolar patients may share some common biological and pharmacological response characteristics with bipolar patients. Overlapping with this grouping are the unipolar patients described by Winokur and Clayton (1967) as having familial pure depressive disease and by Mendels (1976) as "pseudounipolar." In a similar vein, Benazzi (2003) described a group of early-onset unipolar patients who, unlike later-onset patients, were very similar to his bipolar-II group.

31. Ebert et al., 1993; Perugi et al., 1998a; Serretti et al., 1998; Akiskal et al., 2000; Agosti and Stewart, 2001; Mitchell et al., 2001; Angst et al., 2002; Benazzi, 2003; Ghaemi et al., 2004; Akiskal and Benazzi, 2005; Hantouche and Akiskal, 2005.
32. Horwath et al., 1992; Robertson et al., 1996; Levitan 1997; Posternak and Zimmerman, 2002; Sullivan et al., 2002.
33. The negative studies generally involved small and/or unbalanced samples.
34. The DSM IV criteria were modified to require only 2 days for hypomania.
35. Other features that have been reported to differentiate unipolar from bipolar-II patients are irritability and agitation, symptoms that overlap with the concept of depressive "mixed states."
36. Unpublished data cited by Dunner (1987).
37. In the Cassano et al. study (2004), recurrent unipolar patients endorsed a substantial number of manic/hypomanic symptoms over their lifetimes.
38. Hantouche and colleagues (2003b) and Akiskal and colleagues (2003b) have argued for the existence of such a bipolar-II variant on the basis of clinical, psychometric, and temperamental characteristics; further, the bipolar nature of the more unstable bipolar-II ½ patients is suggested by the observation that the rates of familial bipolarity in bipolar-II and bipolar-II ½ groups are highly similar.
39. Even within categories, variation always occurs. Cantor and Genero (1986, p. 236) pointed out that the "natural" categories into which human beings organize their perceptual experiences do not have "obvious necessary and sufficient criterial properties, so that boundaries between closely related categories are ill-defined." People find it extraordinarily difficult or impossible to specify criteria for common object categories, such as furniture, birds, fruit, or clothing. Instead, they identify correlated features that imply a continuum of category membership, ranging from a prototype (an apple is a very typical fruit, for example) to a more atypical member (a tomato is a fruit often thought to be a vegetable). Assigning such atypical members to one category or another can be difficult, and the overlap of characteristic features from one category to another also "runs counter to the intuitive notion of well-defined, orthogonal categories with clearly demarcated boundaries."
40. With appropriate cut-off scores, the GBI can be used for case identification in either nonclinical or clinical populations. It may be particularly useful in family studies. For example, evaluated against clinically determined DSM-III diagnoses, the GBI was found to have a sensitivity of 90 percent and a specificity of 98 percent when used with adolescent offspring of bipolar-I parents and parents with nonaffective major psychiatric diagnoses (Klein et al., 1986b). Originally structured to identify only bipolar affective states, the GBI has been broadened to apply to the separation of bipolar from unipolar subjects with considerable success (Depue et al., 1989).
41. TEMPS exists in an interview format (TEMPS-I) (Akiskal et al., 1998a; Placidi et al., 1998) and a self-rated autoquestionnaire version (TEMPS-A) (Akiskal and Akiskal, 2005). The cutoffs, determined by extreme distributions based on z-scores (corresponding to +2 standard deviations), represent individuals at putative risk for clinical bipolar disorder. Akiskal (1995) actually proposes that temperaments can both provoke and react to life events, thereby leading to complex life situations, emotional arousal, and, eventually, affective episodes. This viewpoint is supported by data on juvenile subjects indicating that cyclothymic reactivity is associated with stress, anxiety, and behavioral disturbances (Signoretta et al., 2005). Only new research will reveal the extent to which the promise of TEMPS-A will be justified. Such research is in progress.
42. Joffe et al., 1999; Angst and Marneros, 2001; Angst et al., 2003.
43. The DSM-III-R category bipolar disorder–not otherwise specified, was originally meant to apply to bipolar-II patients; however, many such patients meet DSM-III-R criteria for bipolar major affective disorder, given that the criteria for major depression are broad enough to encompass a wide range of severity. On the other hand, cyclothymia in DSM-III-R reflects a milder state, referred to by Dunner as "cyclothymic personality," that is also milder than the cyclothymia described by Akiskal.
44. More recently, using nonclinical community samples, Angst (1991) identified recurrent brief depression (RBD) or recurrent brief hypomania (RBM), each with a minimum of 12 episodes a year. He suggested that these are part of the bipolar spectrum.
45. Akiskal and Mallya, 1987; Cassano et al., 1992; Simpson et al., 1993; Benazzi, 1997; Manning et al., 1997; Hantouche et al., 1998; Angst and Gamma, 2002; Mainia et al., 2002.
46. Akiskal et al., 1977, 1978, 1979a, 1983: Depue et al., 1978; Waters, 1979; Akiskal, 1981, 1983a,b.
47. As detailed in Chapter 21, nonadherence is a major problem for both bipolar-I and bipolar-II patients, although the factors that contribute to it may be different in each group.
48. This predominance of depression in bipolar disorder might be reconciled with the proposal of Koukopoulos and others that mania represents the underlying state in bipolar disorder by noting that many depressions in the bipolar spectrum involve activation and other manic-like symptoms.
49. The widespread use of effective pharmacological treatments, along with earlier recognition, probably accounts for the fact that contemporary studies of manic-depressive illness are more dependent on outpatient samples, whereas earlier studies were predominantly of inpatients.

2 Clinical Description

[N]otwithstanding manifold external differences certain *common fundamental features* yet recur in all the morbid states mentioned. Along with changing symptoms, which may appear temporarily or may be completely absent, we meet in all forms of manic-depressive insanity a quite definite, narrow group of disorders, though certainly of very varied character and composition. Without any one of them being absolutely characteristic of the malady, still in association they impress a uniform stamp on all the multiform clinical states.

—*Emil Kraepelin (1921, p. 2)*

To understand manic-depressive illness—to diagnose it accurately and to treat it effectively—requires close familiarity with what Kraepelin calls "the common fundamental features" of the disease. This chapter gives a general clinical description of hypomania and mania, bipolar depression and recurrent unipolar depression, and mixed states, as well as the cyclothymic and other temperamental traits that often underlie these states. Clinical description is approached from three perspectives: that of uniquely experienced classic clinical observers, such as Kraepelin; that of manic-depressive patients themselves (especially the bipolar subgroup); and that of contemporary investigators who have conducted data-based clinical studies. By combining these perspectives (at the unavoidable cost of some redundancy), we hope to capitalize on the descriptive and heuristic strengths of each while avoiding the limitations of any one alone.

We have chosen to cite extensively the classic clinical literature, most of which predates the modern treatment era. We have done this for several reasons. First, descriptions found in these sources are powerful and have not been surpassed; Kraepelin, particularly, remains without peer. Second, the lack of effective treatments and the provision of residential care for patients over many years, often lifetimes, allowed prepharmacotherapy clinicians to observe the natural course of the illness in all its severity. Third, modern diagnostic systems, although vital in advancing treatment and research, have resulted in less emphasis on clinical description and proportionately more emphasis on quantifications susceptible to stastistical analysis, employing symptom checklists, rating scales, and diagnostic algorithms. Regrettably, few psychiatric residents, graduate students, scientists, and clinicians now read Kraepelin and Bleuler. Fewer still have read Aretaeus,

Griesinger, Weygandt, Falret, Jaspers, Baillarger, Campbell, or Henderson and Gillespie. We believe the clinical writings of these classic authors provide both historical perspective and a singular understanding of the nature of manic-depressive illness.

The accounts of manic-depressive (predominantly bipolar) patients presented in this chapter provide the personal dimension missing from clinicians' and researchers' reports, however astute their observations. These descriptions, which vary widely, reflect both the nature of the illness and the nature of the people suffering from it. In the scientific literature, relatively scant attention is paid to firsthand accounts of manic-depressive illness; rather, the emphasis is on the use of objective observer ratings as a basis for studying and describing major affective disorders, including their psychotic variants. One reason for this virtual exclusion of experiential information is that firsthand accounts are subjective and necessarily biased. Thus, patients may remember with clarity some aspects of their disorder and forget or ignore others; they may verbalize what is easiest to describe and say little about aspects less readily articulated. They may relate only those experiences most novel to them, thus giving disproportionate weight to out-of-the-ordinary events, or they may describe what they think the observer wishes to hear. In addition, moods can radically alter memory and perception, resulting in state-dependent distortions. Finally, those individuals most capable of discussing their experiences in an articulate manner may belong, by virtue of this fact, to a more introspective and less representative group.

These are legitimate concerns for anyone desiring systematic, clear-cut, and reducible data. Clinicians have long been aware, however, that experiential accounts are vital to an understanding of individuals and their illnesses.

Likewise, the heuristic value of hypotheses generated from patients' descriptions of their feelings, thoughts, and behaviors is well established. Good clinical management of manic-depressive illness, both pharmacological and psychotherapeutic, depends upon recognizing the concerns of patients and the consequences (both negative and positive) the illness has for them. Descriptive information gathered from patients also has been important in clinical research, such as that describing the switch process (Bunney et al., 1972a,b,c), unraveling the paradoxical effects of lithium as both antidepressant and antimanic agent (Goodwin et al., 1969), and elucidating the occasional positive qualities of manic states (Jamison, 1993, 2004; Jamison et al., 1980), as well as the clinically related difficulties some patients have in adhering to a treatment regimen (see Chapter 21).

There are strong limitations on the effective use of language to describe unusual events, such as extreme moods, gross cognitive and perceptual distortions, and both subtle and profound changes in sensory experience. Despite the shortcomings of language and the highly personalized vocabulary often used by patients in describing their manic-depressive illness, certain words, phrases, and metaphors are chosen time and again, forming a common matrix of experiences. Often these images center on nature, weather, the day–night cycle, and the seasons; often, too, they convey unpredictability, periodicity, violence, tempestuousness, or a bleak dearth of feelings. Religious themes and mystical experiences pervade the language, conveying an extraordinary degree and type of experience—beyond control, comprehension, or adequate description.

At a narrower conceptual level, certain individual words and phrases are heard repeatedly by clinicians treating patients with manic-depressive illness. Depression is associated with common language fragments. The patient is "slowed down," "in a fog," or "exhausted" and describes life as having "lost its color," "dull, flat, and dreary." Everything is "hopeless," "heavy," "too much of an effort," "drab, colorless, pointless." Life is a "burden"; there is no point to living; all is meaningless. Hypomania and mania elicit descriptions of a more vivacious and energetic kind. Life is "effortless," "charged with intensity," and filled with special meaning. The patient is "upbeat," "racing," "full of energy," "speeded up," "wired," "hyper," "high as a kite," "moving in the fast lane," "ecstatic," "flying." Other people are described as "too slow" and unable to "keep up."

Clinical descriptions derived from data-based studies compensate, in part, for the selective attention of both clinicians and patients. They provide a more objective view of the frequency and character of symptoms in manic-depressive illness. In selecting such studies for review in this chapter, we have to some extent emphasized manic states, partly because differential diagnosis can be problematic in mania (see Chapter 3), and partly because more systematic studies of symptoms and their syndromic profiles have been carried out on mania than on bipolar depression, recurrent unipolar depression, mixed states, or cyclothymia. Moreover, we agree with Koukopoulos (2005) and those before him (Pinel, 1801; Heinroth, 1818; Griesinger, 1845) that mania is the fundamental clinical state in bipolar disorder.

In the first edition of this volume, we noted the relative scarcity of data-based studies of bipolar depression and mixed states as a cause for both surprise and concern. This was in contrast to an exceedingly large general literature on depression, one that seldom differentiated bipolar depression from the many nonbipolar forms. Fortunately, there has been a proliferation of studies of both bipolar depression and mixed states in recent years, and their inclusion here is an important addition to the first edition. Older data-based clinical studies, although using standardized diagnostic criteria and making the necessary distinctions between bipolar and unipolar depression, tended not to focus on clinical patterns of bipolar depression but on such issues as psychotic versus nonpsychotic status. Typically, bipolar patients were excluded from these samples. There is next to no research on the nature of depressions in unipolar patients with highly recurrent illness, which were included in Kraepelin's concept of manic-depressive illness, and how they may differ from that of depressions in patients with the less recurrent unipolar forms.

The same caveats about methodology that apply to earlier research findings on manic-depressive illness in general, particularly the bipolar form, apply as well to the older studies discussed in this chapter. First, diagnostic criteria, especially for mixed states, varied greatly across studies. Second, investigators often failed to specify the stage, severity, or duration of the affective state. Third, measurement techniques lacked sophistication; there was a tendency, for example, to measure only the presence or absence of a symptom rather than its intensity, constancy, and duration. Other methodological problems were widespread. The pioneering clinical study of mania, bipolar depression, and mixed states conducted by Winokur and colleagues (1969), for example, although an invaluable contribution to the literature, involved the analysis of data based on multiple episodes (e.g., 100 episodes of mania in 61 patients). To the extent that a given individual showed a similar symptom pattern from one affective episode to another, a contaminating element was introduced. Early clinical studies, while often methodologically flawed, were nonetheless important for the questions they raised and the patients they studied, individuals whose illnesses were generally uncomplicated by changes in clinical presentation due to treatment, especially antidepressant use. We have included the findings of many of these pre-1990 studies because of their historical as well as clinical and scientific interest.

With greater attention to clinical research on bipolar disorder since 1990, the limitations of the older literature have to some extent been addressed. For instance, the twin French collaborative studies of the clinical epidemiology of mania (EPIMAN) and bipolar depression (EPIDEP) have focused on carefully measured clinical nuances of manic, mixed, and bipolar-II disorders, as well as their temperamental foundations (e.g., Hantouche et al., 1998). *Bipolarity beyond Classic Mania*, an extensive examination of soft bipolar variants (Akiskal, 1999), and a European monograph entitled *Bipolar Disorder One Hundred Years after Manic Depressive Illness* (Marneros and Angst, 2000) were published to pay tribute to—and extend—Kraepelin's clinical vision and methodology. Another trans-Atlantic monograph, *Bipolar Disorders*, focuses on mixed, atypical, and rapid-cycling bipolar disorder (Marneros and Goodwin, 2003). Finally, an entire issue of the *Journal of Affective Disorders* devoted to "soft" and "hard" phenotypes within the bipolar spectrum was published in 2003. The data-based contributions of this monograph came from the United States, France, Italy, Switzerland, and Germany, countries where clinical research is currently being conducted on the phenomenology of the broadly conceived manic-depressive spectrum.

In this chapter we address only those aspects of symptom presentation relevant to clinical description. These include the observable patterns of mood, energy, sleep, thought, and behavior typically used in clinical diagnosis. (Detailed discussion of related topics is found in Chapters 1, 3, 9, 10, and 15.) Before proceeding, we emphasize that while many generalizations can be drawn from clinical descriptions of manic-depressive illness, individuals are bound to differ widely with regard to an illness that is at once genetically based, environmentally influenced, and psychologically expressed. Kraepelin (1921), although committed to the idea and practice of classification, also was sensitive to the infinite capacity for individual expression in the illness. Referring to the subclassifications proposed by earlier writers, he concluded (p. 139): "I am convinced that that kind of effort . . . must of necessity wreck on the irregularity of the disease." The clinical differences seen across individuals can be striking (as are, more often, the similarities), but it remains unclear to what extent one episode resembles another in a given individual. Anecdotal accounts, along with several studies discussed later, support some constancy of clinical presentation, including the presence or absence of melancholic and psychotic features, in the same patient across time.[1]

Finally, although much of the clinical description presented here emphasizes differences among clinical states, we stress from the outset that the coexistence of affective states is fundamental to bipolar disorder and that oscillation into, out of, and within the various forms and states of manic-depressive illness is, in its own right, a hallmark of the disease. As we shall see, "pure" affective states are rare: mania is often complicated by depressive symptoms, and conversely, depression, especially the bipolar form, usually is accompanied by at least one or more symptoms of mania. Bauer and colleagues (2005), for example, found in their study of 441 bipolar patients that clinically significant depressive symptoms occurred in 94 percent of those with mania or hypomania, while 70 percent of patients in a depressive episode had clinically significant manic symptomatology. Thus, far from being a "bipolar" disorder, with the assumption of clinically opposite states, the illness is characterized by co-occurrence of manic and depressive symptoms more often than not. Bauer and colleagues (2005) also found that depressive and manic symptoms were positively, not inversely, correlated, suggesting that "a dimensional conceptualization of mood state in this disorder is more valid than the categorical conceptualization presumed by both the DSM [*Diagnostic and Statistical Manual*] and ICD [*International Classification of Diseases*]" (p. 88).

Patterns of manic and depressive symptoms clearly have a cyclic quality, but their overlapping, transitional, and fluctuating aspects are enormously important in describing and understanding the illness overall. Thus, Kraepelin (1921, p. 54) wrote:

> The delimitation of the individual clinical forms of the malady is in many respects wholly artificial and arbitrary. Observation not only reveals the occurrence of gradual transitions between all the various states, but it also shows that within the shortest space of time the same morbid case may pass through most manifold transformations.

Campbell (1953, pp. 112–113) emphasized this fundamentally dynamic nature of bipolar illness by comparing the illness to a film:

> The fluidity, change, and movement of the emotions, as they occur in the ever-changing cyclothymic process, may be compared to the pictures of a cinema, as contrasted with a "still" photograph. Indeed, the psychiatrist, observing a manic-depressive patient for the first time, or as he undergoes one of the many undulations in mood, from melancholia to euphoria or from hypomania to a depression, is reminded of the experience of entering a movie during the middle of the story. No matter where one takes up the plot, the story tends to swing around again to the

point where it started. The examiner may observe the manic-depressive patient first in a manic reaction, later in a depression, but eventually, if followed long enough, in another manic reaction. Like the movie, which is a continuous but constantly changing process, the cyclothymic process is also continuous even though for the moment the observer is attracted by the immediate cross-section view. This conception of change, or constant undulation of the emotions, is much more accurate than a static appraisal.

In the following sections, we address in turn manic, depressive, and mixed states and cyclothymia. For each we present clinical description in three general areas of functioning: mood, cognition and perception, and activity and behavior.

MANIC STATES

Classic Clinical Descriptions

Manic states are typically characterized by heightened mood, more and faster speech, quicker thought, brisker physical and mental activity levels, greater energy (with a corresponding decreased need for sleep), irritability, perceptual acuity, paranoia, heightened sexuality, and impulsivity. The degree, type, and chronicity of these cognitive, perceptual, and behavioral changes determine the major subclassification of mania, namely hypomania or mania. In hypomania, the above changes are generally moderate and may or may not result in serious problems for the individual experiencing them. In more intense episodes, however, they profoundly disrupt the lives of patients, their families, and society.

Mood

Mood in hypomania is usually ebullient, self-confident, and exalted, but with an irritable underpinning. Most early clinical descriptions emphasized the elevated, volatile, and fluctuating nature of hypomanic mood. Campbell (1953, pp. 151, 153) described its euphoric aspect:

> Associated with the euphoria there is a genuine feeling of well-being, mentally and physically, a feeling of happiness and exhilaration which transports the individual into a new world of unlimited ideas and possibilities. . . . When a 19-year-old [hypo]manic was advised that he was indeed ill, he replied, "if I'm ill, this is the most wonderful illness I ever had."

Kraepelin (1921, p. 56) likewise described the euphoric aspect of hypomanic mood, but also emphasized the integral quick changes, irritability, and extreme volatility:

Mood is predominantly exalted and cheerful, influenced by the feeling of heightened capacity for work. The patient is in imperturbable good temper, sure of success, "courageous," feels happy and merry, not rarely overflowingly so. . . . On the other hand there often exists a great emotional irritability. The patient is dissatisfied, intolerant, fault-finding . . . he becomes pretentious, positive, regardless, impertinent and even rough, when he comes up against opposition to his wishes and inclinations; trifling external occasions may bring about extremely violent outbursts of rage.

Mood in acute mania is not well described by the classic writers, perhaps because extreme changes in cognition and behavior are more clearly observable than subjective mood states. Two thousand years ago, however, Aretaeus of Cappadocia noted that those who are manic are gay, active, and expansive. They are naturally joyous; they laugh and they joke: "they show off in public with crowned heads as if they were returning victorious from the games; sometimes they laugh and dance all day and all night" (quoted in Roccatagliata, 1986, pp. 230–231). Kraepelin (1921, p. 63), writing centuries later, agreed, but stressed the instability of the manic mood:

> Mood is unrestrained, merry, exultant, occasionally visionary or pompous, but always subject to frequent variation, easily changing to irritability and irascibility or even to lamentation and weeping.

Jaspers (1997, p. 596; first published in 1913) emphasized the essential liveliness of mood and behavior in *pure mania*, making the distinction, as Kraepelin had, between pure and mixed manic states:

> The feeling of delight in life is accompanied by an increase in instinctual activities: increased sexuality, increased desire to move about; pressure of talk and pressure of activity which will mount from mere vividness of gesture to states of agitated excitement. The psychic activity characterized by flight of ideas lends an initial liveliness to everything undertaken but it lacks staying-power and is changeable. All intruding stimuli and any new possibility will distract the patient's attention. The massive associations at his disposal come spontaneously and uncalled for. They make him witty and sparkling; they also make it impossible for him to maintain any determining tendency and render him at the same time superficial and confused.

Cognition and Perception

Cognition and perception, especially the former, are strongly altered in hypomania. Falret (1854, cited in Sedler, 1983) wrote that "profusion of ideas [in manic states] is prodigious," and most early clinicians emphasized that, to a point, associational fluency is furthered by mild hypomania. Bleuler (1924, pp. 466, 468), for example, commented that thought remains relatively intact in the less severe forms of mania:

> The *thinking* of the manic is flighty. He jumps by by-paths from one subject to another, and cannot adhere to anything. With this the ideas run along very easily and involuntarily, even so freely that it may be felt as unpleasant by the patient. . . . Because of the more rapid flow of ideas, and especially because of the falling off of inhibitions, artistic activities are facilitated even though something worth while is produced only in very mild cases and when the patient is otherwise talented in this direction. The heightened sensibilities naturally have the effect of furthering this.

Tuke (1892, p. 765), in his *Dictionary of Psychological Medicine*, described the quickened senses so many manic patients appear to have:

> Increased acuity in the perception of sense impressions certainly exists. Attention is lively and sharp though entirely unstable. The acute maniac appears to see and hear better than a sane person because every impression tells upon him. . . . Everything attracts his notice.
>
> The filling of the mind with an enormous number of sense impressions, the blurring as it were of the mental canvas by the superposition of a crowd of details . . . account in a great degree for the confusion of memory which is one of the ordinary phenomena of mania. . . . Objects seen appear to serve chiefly as the starting-point of trains of ideas which change rapidly with slight changes in the visual surroundings.

Thinking becomes fragmented and often psychotic in acute mania. Coherence gives way to incoherence; rapid thinking proceeds to racing and disjointed thinking; distractibility becomes all-pervasive. Paranoid and grandiose delusions are common, as are illusions and hallucinations. In Kraepelin's (1921, p. 62) description, patients

> show themselves sensible and approximately oriented, but extraordinarily distractible in perception and train of thought. Sometimes it is quite impossible to get into communication with them; as a rule, however, they understand emphatic speech, and even give isolated suitable replies, but they are influenced by every new impression; they digress, they go into endless details.

Kraepelin (pp. 68–69) went on to describe the progressively worsening clinical state of *delusional mania*:

> The Delusions and Hallucinations, which in the morbid states hitherto described are fugitive or merely indicated, acquire in a series of cases an elaboration which calls to

mind paranoid attacks. His surroundings appear to the patient to be changed; he sees St. Augustine, Joseph with the shepherd's crook, the angel Gabriel, apostles, the Kaiser, spirits, God, the Virgin Mary.[2] . . . The delusions, which forthwith emerge, move very frequently on religious territory. . . . He preaches in the name of the holy God, will reveal great things to the world, gives commands according to the divine will.

Benjamin Rush (1812, pp. 244–245), author of the first major psychiatric treatise published in the United States, gave a particularly graphic account of the grandiose and "disjointed or debilitated faculties of the mind" in an acutely delusional manic patient:

> The following short extract, taken down by Mr. Coats, from the constant conversation of a young man of a good education, and respectable connections, now deranged in the Pennsylvania Hospital, will exhibit an affecting specimen of this disjointed state of the mind, and of the incoherence of its operations. "No man can serve two masters. I am king Philip of Macedonia, lawful son of Mary queen of Scots, born in Philadelphia. I have been happy enough ever since I have seen general Washington with a silk handkerchief in High-street. Money commands sublunary things, and makes the mare go; it will buy salt mackerel, made of tenpenny nails. Enjoyment is the happiness of virtue. Yesterday cannot be recalled. I can only walk in the night-time, when I can eat pudding enough. I shall be eight years old tomorrow. They say R. W. is in partnership with J. W. I believe they are about as good as people in common—not better, only on certain occasions, when, for instance, a man wants to buy chincopins, and to import salt to feed pigs. Tanned leather was imported first by layers. Morality with virtue is like vice not corrected. L. B. came into your house and stole a coffee-pot in the twenty-fourth year of his majesty's reign. Plumb-pudding and Irish potatoes make a very good dinner. Nothing in man is comprehensible to it. Born in Philadelphia. Our forefathers were better to us than our children, because they were chosen for their honesty, truth, virtue and innocence. The queen's broad R originated from a British forty-two pounder, which makes two [sic] large a report for me. I have no more to say. I am thankful I am no worse this season, and that I am sound in mind and memory, and could steer a ship to sea, but am afraid of the thriller. ****** ****** son of Mary queen of Scots. Born in Philadelphia. Born in Philadelphia. King of Macedonia."

Activity and Behavior

Activity and behavior are greatly increased and diversified in mania. Patients appear to be indefatigable; they are rash, virulently opinionated, and interpersonally aggressive. Additionally, as Campbell (1953, pp. 152, 154–155) wrote:

> The manic patient may expend a considerable amount of his energy and pressure of ideas in writing. His writing is demonstrative, flashy, rhetorical and bombastic. He insists that the physician must read every word, even though the content is biased, full of repetition, rambling and circumstantial. Capital letters are used unnecessarily, sentences are underscored and flight of ideas and distractibility destroy the coherence of the theme. The subject of the manic's writing often pertains to the correction of wrongs, religious tangents, gaining his freedom, institution of lawsuits. . . . One patient made three visits to Washington to obtain a patent on a cotton-chopping machine; another attempted to speak to the President by long-distance telephone to warn him that the Russians might land on the coast of Florida. Urged on by the pressure of ideas as well as an excess of physical energy the manic patient has an inner drive which will not allow him to rest.

For many patients, excessive energy translates directly into pressured writing and an inordinate production of written declarations, poetry, and artwork. Kraepelin (1921, pp. 34–36) gave a concise description of this phenomenon, along with a specimen of handwriting produced during mania (see Fig. 2–1):

Figure 2–1. Specimen of handwriting produced during mania. (*Source*: Kraepelin, 1921, p. 35. Reproduced with permission.)

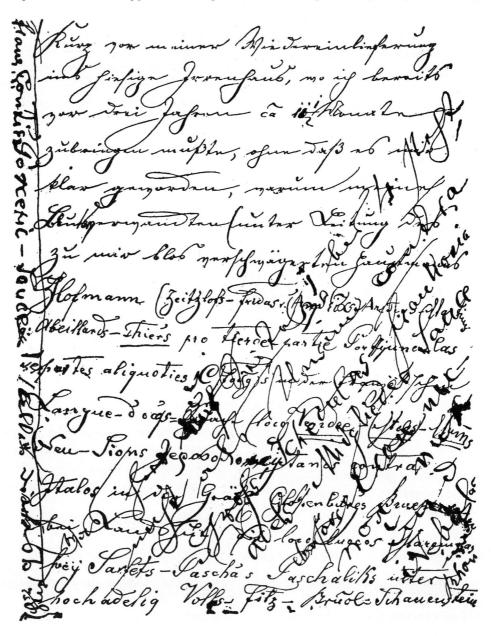

The handwriting of the patients may at first be quite regular and correct. In consequence of the excitability, however, it usually becomes gradually always larger, more pretentious and more irregular. There is no more consideration for the reader; the letters run through one another, are scribbled; more words are underlined; there are more marks of exclamation; the flourishes become bolder. . . . The number of documents produced by manic patients is sometimes astonishing, though certainly they themselves do not count on their being read; the pleasure of writing itself is the only motive.

The progression from hypomania to acute mania is usually accompanied not only by instability of mood and a sense of impending doom or premonitions of madness, but also by increasingly erratic behavior. Rush (1812, p. 142) made this clear in his monograph *Medical Inquiries and Observations upon the Diseases of the Mind*:

Its premonitory signs are, watchfulness, high or low spirits, great rapidity of thought, and eccentricity in conversation, and conduct; sometimes pathetic expressions of horror, excited by the apprehension of approaching madness; terrifying or distressing dreams; great irritability of temper; jealousy, instability in all pursuits; unusual acts of extravagance, manifested by the purchases of houses, and certain expensive and unnecessary articles of furniture, and hostility to relations and friends.

Sexual or erotic excitement is common in mania. Aretaeus of Cappadocia (150 AD) (quoted in Jelliffe, 1931, p. 20), for example, wrote that "a period of lewdness and shamelessness" exists in mania. Likewise, Kraepelin (1921, p. 22) noted that sexual excitability "is increased and leads to hasty engagements, marriages by the newspaper, improper love-adventures, conspicuous behaviour, fondness for dress, on the other hand to jealousy and matrimonial discord." Tuke (1892, pp. 764–765) described this as well:

A very common symptom in maniacal conditions is erotic excitement. This varies from a mere coquetry, a somewhat extended application of the command "love one another," an undue attention to the opposite sex, and so forth, up to the extreme of salacity, when the mind is wholly occupied by the urgent sexual appetite, and all restraint is abandoned.

Particularly dramatic and extreme among the clinical features of acute mania are the frenetic, seemingly aimless, and occasionally violent activities of manic patients. Bizarre, driven, paranoid, impulsive, and grossly inappropriate behavior patterns are typical. Kraepelin (1921, pp. 64–65) provided a graphic overview of these behaviors:

The patient cannot sit or lie still for long, jumps out of bed, runs about, hops, dances, mounts on tables and benches, takes down pictures. He forces his way out, takes off his clothes, teases his fellow patients, dives, splashes, spits, chirps and clicks. . . . [There are] discharges of inner restlessness, shaking of the upper part of the body, waltzing about, waving and flourishing the arms, distorting the limbs, rubbing the head, bouncing up and down, stroking, wiping, twitching, clapping and drumming. . . . [Death may be caused] by simple exhaustion with heart failure (collapse) in long continuing, violent excitement with disturbance of sleep and insufficient nourishment, by injuries with subsequent blood-poisoning.

Delirious mania, or Bell's mania, is a relatively rare, grave form of mania characterized by severe clouding of consciousness. When Bell (1849) described the syndrome in the mid-nineteenth century, he noted its sudden onset and symptoms of severe insomnia, loss of appetite, disorientation, paranoia, and extremely bizarre hallucinations and delusions.[3] Kraepelin (1921, pp. 70, 71) also remarked upon the syndrome's acute onset and noted that patients were "stupefied, confused, bewildered," in addition to being completely disoriented as to time and place. At the core of the illness he found a "dreamy and profound clouding of consciousness, and extraordinary and confused hallucinations and delusions." Griesinger (1867) also emphasized the acute onset of the syndrome and observed that the primary emotion experienced by patients is anxiety. Bond (1980) noted that acute delirious mania can be distinguished by its precipitous onset, with or without premonitory signs of irritability, insomnia, or emotional withdrawal; the presence of the hypomanic or manic syndrome at some point during the illness; development of the signs and symptoms of delirium; a personal and/or family history of either mania or depression; and responsiveness to standard treatments for mania. (Patients with delirious mania often respond to electroconvulsive therapy, despite the delirium [Mann et al., 1986; Fink 1999].)

Mayer-Gross and colleagues (1960, pp. 213–214) gave a general overview of extreme manic confusion, emphasizing the medical gravity of the untreated clinical situation:

These states are seriously debilitating and may endanger life. *Sleep* is severely disturbed in these graver psychoses, but it is also shortened in the milder forms. Another bodily symptom is the exhaustion which supervenes on months of hyper-activity and reduced sleep. The intake of food may be seriously interfered with, for the manic may never take an uninterrupted meal, being constantly diverted to something else. *Body-weight*, which increases in the milder stages, rapidly drops, and very careful nursing is required. . . . The possibility that the atypical features in manic confusion or delirium are due to nutritional deficiencies of the same kind as those sometimes causing delirium in infective illness, cannot be excluded.

Mood during delirious mania may shift rapidly between extreme melancholia and mania, suggesting a clinical link to mixed states. In Kraepelin's (1921, p. 71) words, mood is "very changing, sometimes anxiously despairing ('thoughts of death'), timid and lachrymose, distracted, sometimes unrestrainedly merry, erotic or ecstatic, sometimes irritable or unsympathetic and indifferent." The extreme cognitive and perceptual changes during delirious mania are manifested primarily through clouding of consciousness, hallucinations, and delusions. The profoundly disturbed and psychotic behavior of delirious mania underscores the origin of the phrase "raving maniac." Kraepelin (1921, pp. 71–72) graphically described this behavior:

> At the beginning the patients frequently display the signs of senseless raving mania, dance about, perform peculiar movements, shake their head, throw the bedclothes pell-mell, are destructive, pass their motions under them, smear everything, make impulsive attempts at suicide, take off their clothes. A patient was found completely naked in a public park. Another ran half-clothed into the corridor and then into the street, in one hand a revolver in the other a crucifix. . . . Their linguistic utterances alternate between inarticulate sounds, praying, abusing, entreating, stammering, disconnected talk, in which clang-associations, senseless rhyming, diversion by external impressions, persistence of individual phrases, are recognised. . . . Waxy flexibility, echolalia, or echopraxis can be demonstrated frequently.

More recently, Fink (1999, pp. 57–58) described a series of modern cases of delirious mania:

> Patients with delirious mania are excited, restless, fearful, paranoid, and delusional. They sleep poorly, are often confused and disoriented, and they confabulate. The onset develops within a few hours or a few days. Fever, rapid heart rate, tachycardia, hypertension, and rapid breathing are common. Patients hide in small spaces, close the doors and blinds on the windows, remove their clothes, and run nude from their home. Garrulous, incoherent, and rambling speech alternates with mutism. Negativism, stereotypy, grimacing, posturing, echolalia, and echopraxia occur. When examined, they are poorly oriented for place, date and time, are unable to recall their recent experiences, or numbers given them.

Fink argued that we do not know the true incidence of delirious mania, nor do we have adequate diagnostic criteria to distinguish it reliably from malignant catatonia, excited catatonia, rapid-cycling mania, or mania with psychotic features.

Chronic mania was observed and described by many early clinicians, including Pinel (1801), Esquirol (1838), Griesinger (1865), Schott (1904), Kraepelin (1921), and Wertham (1929). According to Schott, only the lack of recovery distinguished the chronic from the acute form of the illness (see also Chapter 4). A first manic episode after the age of 40 was thought to put the patient at much higher risk for chronicity than one occurring earlier (Henderson and Gillespie, 1956), an observation consistent with the results of subsequent research (see Chapter 4). Wertham (1929) outlined the central features of chronic mania: reduced intellectual productivity and general activity levels, increased behavioral stereotypy, and an overall intellectual weakening. Hare (1981), in an excellent historical review of the concept of mania, discussed the declining interest in the subject of chronic mania after the nineteenth century. He attributed this in part to the decreasing morbidity of manic illness, and maintained that improvements in general health and hygiene had resulted in significant changes in the manifestation, severity, and consequences of mania. He acknowledged, however, that there still existed "the ghost as it were, of a process of mental enfeeblement which can occur in affective psychosis and which generally *did* occur, to a more severe degree, until towards the end of the nineteenth century" (p. 97).

Kraepelin (1921, pp. 161–162) provided an overview of the intellectual and emotional blunting in chronic mania; he also drew a distinction between chronic mania and extreme, continuous, rapid cycling and discussed possible contributory factors:

> Here manic features dominate the picture. The patients are in general sensible and reasonable, and perceive fairly well; memory and retention are also fairly well preserved. On the other hand there exist increased distractibility, wandering and desultoriness of thought, a tendency to silly plays on words, poverty of thought. The patients have no understanding of their state, consider themselves perfectly well and capable of work.
>
> Mood is exalted, but no longer exultant, enjoying activity, but silly and boastful; occasionally it comes to flaring up without strength or durability. The finer emotions are considerably injured. . . . Only the coarser enjoyments, eating, drinking, smoking, snuffing, still arouse in them vivid feelings, further the satisfaction of their personal wishes and wants; everything else has become to them more or less indifferent. . . .
>
> At this point we have to mention in a few words another group of cases, in which the psychic decline

reveals itself in continual, abrupt fluctuation between lachrymose anxiety, irritability, and childish merriment. States of this kind sometimes appear to be developed from a continuous accumulation of short circular attacks.

Subjective Experiences of Patients

Mood

In his memoir *Wisdom, Madness, and Folly: The Philosophy of a Lunatic*, John Custance (1952, p. 30), a writer and former Royal Navy intelligence officer who suffered from bipolar illness, described the sense of well-being at the beginning of his manic episodes:

> First and foremost comes a general sense of intense well-being. I know of course that this sense is illusory and transient. . . . Although, however, the restrictions of confinement are apt at times to produce extreme irritation and even paroxysms of anger, the general sense of well-being, the pleasurable and sometimes ecstatic feeling-tone, remains as a sort of permanent background of all experience during the manic period.

As it progresses, this feeling of well-being often is accompanied by a sense of benevolence and communion with nature; frequently it is associated with what Henderson and Gillespie (1956) and others have called a "heightened sense of reality." These feelings, analogous to the beatific and mystical experiences of saints and other religious leaders, share certain features with contemporary experiences of "universal communion" induced by mescaline, LSD, and other hallucinogenic substances. The interaction among emotional, cognitive, and sensory–perceptual changes is complex, as we see in the following passages by Custance (1952, pp. 37, 40):

> It is actually a sense of communion, in the first place with God, and in the second place with all mankind, indeed with all creation. It is obviously related to the mystic sense of unity with the All. . . .
>
> A feeling of intimate personal relationship with God is perhaps its paramount feature. . . .
>
> The sense of communion extends to all fellow-creatures with whom I come into contact; it is not merely ideal or imaginative but has a practical effect on my conduct. Thus when in the manic state I have no objection to being more or less herded together—as is inevitable in public Mental Hospitals—with men of all classes and conditions. Class barriers cease to have any existence or meaning.

Likewise, poet Theodore Roethke (quoted in Seager, 1991, p. 101) captured the mystical merging of identity in his description of the early, euphoric stage of one of his manic episodes:

> For no reason I started to feel very good. Suddenly I knew how to enter into the life of everything around me. I knew how it felt to be a tree, a blade of grass, even a rabbit. I didn't sleep much. I just walked around with this wonderful feeling. One day I was passing a diner and all of a sudden I knew what it felt like to be a lion. I went into the diner and said to the counter-man, "Bring me a steak. Don't cook it. Just bring it." . . . I went to the Dean [at the university where Roethke taught] and said, "I feel too good. Get me down off this." So they put me into the tubs.

Cognition and Perception

During hypomanic and manic states, thinking becomes very fluid and productive—to the point of loosening of normal patterns of association, as well as racing thoughts and flight of ideas. The dendritic, branching-out quality of manic thinking was described by nineteenth-century art critic and writer John Ruskin (quoted in Rosenberg, 1986, p. 151):

> I roll on like a ball, with this exception, that contrary to the usual laws of motion I have no friction to contend with in my mind. . . . I am almost sick and giddy with the quantity of things in my head—trains of thought beginning and branching to infinity, crossing each other, and all tempting and wanting to be worked out.

Perhaps most pathognomonic of hypomanic and manic cognitive patterns are flight of ideas and the subjective experience of racing thoughts. The overwhelming and often terrfying nature of racing thoughts is expressed below in one patient's account of manic illness. Grandiosity of delusional proportions and a compelling sense of moral and social awareness also are described (Reiss, 1910):

> The condition of my mind for many months is beyond all description. My thoughts ran with lightning-like rapidity from one subject to another. I had an exaggerated feeling of self importance. All the problems of the universe came crowding into my mind, demanding instant discussion and solution—mental telepathy, hypnotism, wireless telegraphy, Christian science, women's rights, and all the problems of medical science, religion and politics. I even devised means of discovering the weight of a human soul, and had an apparatus constructed in my room for the purpose of weighing my own soul the minute it departed from my body. . . .
>
> Thoughts chased one another through my mind with lightning rapidity. I felt like a person driving a wild horse with a weak rein, who dares not use force, but lets him run his course, following the line of least resistance. Mad

impulses would rush through my brain, carrying me first in one direction then in another. To destroy myself or to escape often occurred to me, but my mind could not hold on to one subject long enough to formulate any definite plan. My reasoning was weak and fallacious, and I knew it.

Russian poet Velimir Khlebnikov (quoted in Markov, 1975, pp. 362–363), hospitalized for his erratic behavior and wild mood swings, described a euphoric grandiosity that ratcheted upwards into a delusional system of cosmic proportions. He was convinced that he possessed equations "for the stars, equations for voices, equations for thoughts, equations of birth and death." The artist of numbers, he believed, could draw the universe:

> Working with number as his charcoal, he unites all previous human knowledge in his art. A single one of his lines provides an immediate lightninglike connection between a red corpuscle and Earth, a second precipitates into helium, a third shatters upon the unbending heavens and discovers the satellites of Jupiter. Velocity is infused with a new speed, the speed of thought, while the boundaries that separate different areas of knowledge will disappear before the procession of liberated numbers cast like orders into print throughout the whole of Planet Earth.
>
> Here they are then, these ways of looking at the new form of creativity, which we think is perfectly workable.
>
> The surface of Planet Earth is 510,051,300 square kilometers; the surface of a red corpuscle—that citizen and star of man's Milky Way—0.000, 128 square millimeters. These citizens of the sky and the body have concluded a treaty, whose provision is this: the surface of the star Earth divided by the surface of the tiny corpuscular star equals 365 times 10 to the tenth power (365×10^{10}). A beautiful concordance of two worlds, one that establishes man's right to first place on Earth. This is the first article of the treaty between the government of blood cells and the government of heavenly bodies. A living walking Milky Way and his tiny star have concluded a 365-point agreement with the Milky Way in the sky and its great Earth Star. The dead Milky Way and the living one have affixed their signatures to it as two equal and legal entities.

The perceptual and somatic changes that almost always accompany hypomania and mania reflect the close and subtle links among elevated mood, a physical sense of well-being, expansive and grandiose thoughts, and heightened perceptual awareness. Custance (1952, p. 16) described the temporal ordering of somatic, mood, and cognitive symptoms during the initial phases of his manic episodes:

> Thus at the onset of phases of manic excitement I have sometimes noticed the typical symptoms, the pleasurable tingling of the spinal chord [sic] and warm sense of well-being in the solar plexus, long before any reaction in the mental sphere occurred. The same thing happens with the sinking feeling of fear and horror which accompanies extreme depression.

Clearly, as with virtually all signs and symptoms of bipolar illness, perceptual and somatic changes vary in degree and kind—from mild increases in awareness of objects and events actually present in the individual's environment to total chaotic disarray of the senses, resulting in visual, auditory, and olfactory experiences unrelated to existing physical phenomena. At the milder end of perceptual change, one patient described the relationship of heightened awareness, strongly charged but normal emotional reactions, and psychotic perceptions (Coate, 1964, p. 1):

> In normal life at times of strong emotion, and especially at moments of great fear, we find that we are more keenly aware than usual of the external details of our world. The sunshine on wet roofs across the way, the faded edge to the blue window curtain, a scent of pipe tobacco in the room, the way the man in the armchair clasps and unclasps his hands—all is more clearly etched in consciousness because of the feeling aroused by the nearness of enemy bombers, or the gravity of an operation taking place next door, or the tenseness of waiting until an expected person, acutely loved or deeply hated, will walk in. In psychotic states, where the fate of the whole universe may be at stake, awareness of material objects and of trivial events can be heightened to an extent that is outside the range of sane experience.

Custance wrote of his sensory experiences while in the preliminary stage of a manic episode (1952, pp. 31–32):

> The first thing I note is the peculiar appearances of the lights—the ordinary electric lights in the ward. They are not exactly brighter, but deeper, more intense, perhaps a trifle more ruddy than usual. Moreover, if I relax the focusing of my eyes, which I can do very much more easily than in normal circumstances, a bright star-like phenomenon emanates from the lights, ultimately forming a maze of iridescent patterns of all colours of the rainbow, which remind me vaguely of the Aurora Borealis. . . . Connected with these vivid impressions is a rather curious feeling behind the eyeballs, rather as though a vast electric motor were pulsing away there.
>
> All my other senses seem more acute than usual. Certainly my sense of touch is heightened; my fingers are much more sensitive and neat. . . .
>
> My hearing appears to be more sensitive, and I am able to take in without disturbance or distraction many different sound-impressions at the same time.

Custance (1952, p. 59) also described specific physical sensations he experienced during his manic episodes. His perceived imperviousness to pain and cold, as well as his delusional beliefs about electrical and other influences, occur in many manic patients:

> Metabolism is rapid. I can stand cold without difficulty or discomfort; an inner warmth seems to pervade me. I can, for example, walk about naked out of doors on quite cold nights—to throw off my clothes is incidentally a strong impulse and presumably symbolises the freedom from restraint which is a feature of the whole condition. My skin seems peculiarly resistant; I have walked barefooted on stony and thorny ground, squeezed myself naked through furze fences and so on without suffering discomfort. Perhaps this is akin to the strange feats of fire walkers or dancing Dervishes. It certainly seems to show the influence of mind over matter. I fear nothing—freedom from fear is another notable symptom—so nothing seems to hurt me.

Activity and Behavior

Behavioral changes during mania include increases in psychomotor activity and in the pressure and rate of speech; heightened irritability and aggressive behaviors; increases in spending and other impulsive behaviors; hypersexuality; and frenzied, bizarre, often aimless activity. Detailed clinical descriptions of these behavioral changes—especially those by Kraepelin—were given earlier in this chapter, and specific discussions of hypomanic and manic behavior can be found elsewhere in the volume. We present here first-person accounts of only a few common or especially interesting behavioral changes in manic states. Two passages describe increased enthusiasm for and involvement in a wide variety of creative interests and activities. The first, from Coate (1964, pp. 84–85), reflects the clear influence of mood and grandiosity on thinking and behavior. The sense of time urgency and the special significance of events and objects also are evident:

> I must record everything and later I would write a book on mental hospitals. I would write books on psychiatric theory too, and on theology. I would write novels. I had the libretto of an opera in mind. Nothing was beyond me. My creative impulse had found full outlet and I had enough now to write to last me for the rest of my life.
>
> I made notes of everything that happened, day and night. I made symbolic scrap-books whose meaning only I could decipher. I wrote a fairy tale; I wrote the diary of a white witch; and again I noted down cryptically all that was said or done around me at the time, with special reference to relevant news bulletins and to jokes which were broadcast in radio programmes. The time, correct to the

nearest minute, was recorded in the margin. It was all vitally important. The major work which would be based on this material would be accurate, original, provocative, and of profound significance. All that had ever happened to me was now worthwhile.

Because her thinking was not yet psychotically fragmented or delusional, Coate was able to concentrate intensely and to keep in order a broad diversity of ideas and sensations. This ability is not uncommon in hypomania, although many bipolar patients who experience scattered thinking early in their episodes never go through this hyperalert but concentrated phase. Those who do and who also possess creative ability find this stage can be an exceptionally productive one (see Chapter 12). For Custance (1952, pp. 244–245), both creativity and learning were heightened:

> In some forms of insanity, including especially mania, this ripening of the instinct, this eager readiness to absorb and learn new things, to become interested in fresh games, sports and forms of work, seems to recur. It certainly does in my own case. I have, in actual fact, learnt more while confined in Mental Hospitals than anywhere else, including my School and University. I have learnt drawing, shorthand, some languages, studied philosophy and psychology as deeply as I was able, collected and systematically written down and filed innumerable scraps of information on all sorts of subjects, and, above all, read in the book of human nature, which is as it were exposed in the raw. I know the history, background and medical diagnosis of many of the patients in the wards I have been in. Finally I have written this book.

A common aspect of the manic state is impulsive and irrational financial behavior. The psychological and interpersonal consequences, as well as the economic ones, can be devastating. The return of postmanic reason and subsequent awareness of financial extravagances and other painfully embarrassing actions often occur in the harsh context of severe postmanic depression. The humorous aspects of many manic purchases often obscure the acute shame and dire financial consequences experienced by patients with bipolar illness:

> When I am high I couldn't worry about money if I tried. So I don't. The money will come from somewhere; I am entitled; God will provide. Credit cards are disastrous, personal checks worse. Unfortunately, for manics anyway, mania is a natural extension of the economy. What with credit cards and bank accounts there is little beyond reach. So I bought twelve snake bite kits, with a sense of urgency and importance. I bought precious stones, elegant and unnecessary furniture, three watches within an hour of one another (in the Rolex rather than Timex

class: champagne tastes bubble to the surface, are the surface, in mania), and totally inappropriate siren-like clothes. During one spree in London I spent several hundred pounds on books having titles or covers that somehow caught my fancy: books on the natural history of the mole, twenty sundry Penguin books because I thought it could be nice if the penguins could form a colony, five Puffin books for a similar reason, on and on and on it went. Once, I think, I shoplifted a blouse because I could not wait a minute longer for the woman-with-molasses feet in front of me in line. Or maybe I just thought about shoplifting, I don't remember, I was totally confused. I imagine I must have spent far more than $30,000 during my two major manic episodes, and God only knows how much more during my frequent milder manias.

But then back on lithium and rotating on the planet at the same pace as everyone else, you find your credit is decimated, your mortification complete: mania is not a luxury one can easily afford. It is devastating to have the illness and aggravating to have to pay for medications, blood tests, and psychotherapy. They, at least, are partially [tax] deductible. But money spent while manic doesn't fit into the Internal Revenue Service concept of medical expense or business loss. So, after mania, when most depressed, you're given excellent reason to be even more so. (Jamison, 1995, pp. 74–75)

Clinical Studies

Mania is a complex, volatile, and fluctuating cauldron of symptoms. "The form and ways which mania manifests are manifold," said Aretaeus (translated by Jelliffe, 1931, p. 20) nearly 2000 years ago. "Some are cheerful and like to play . . . others passionate and of destructive type, who seek to kill others as well as themselves." Although classically described as a state of extraordinary energy and activity, mania can also present clinically as manic stupor and "catatonia." Manic mood, frequently characterized as elated and grandiose, as often as not is riddled with depression, panic, and extreme irritability; mania without significant mixed features is what is known as "classic" mania. For years, mania was differentiated mistakenly from schizophrenia because it reputedly lacked a thought disorder. It now is recognized as an often floridly psychotic condition, as we shall see below.

Manic episodes differ from person to person and in the same individual from time to time, although Falret (1854, cited in Sedler, 1983) and Kraepelin (1921) noted a tendency for constancy in symptom patterns across episodes in the same individual. While few systematic data are available on this latter point, Wellner and Marstal (1964, p. 176), reporting on a study of 279 manic episodes in 221 patients, concluded that "atypical attacks are followed by atypical, and typical by typical significantly more often than not

($p=0.002$), indicating the patients' inclination to reproduce the type of their psychoses." Beigel and Murphy (1971a) found that patients with multiple manic attacks tended to exhibit similar behavior and mood patterns during subsequent episodes. Two more recent studies (Cassidy et al., 2001a; Woods et al., 2001) demonstrated that manic and mixed episodes show diagnostic stability over time; the interepisode stability of depressive mixed states, while significant, is considerably less pronounced than is the case for manic states (Sato et al., 2004). Francis and colleagues (1997) found that the symptom profile of catatonia is highly consistent across episodes, while Cassidy and colleagues (2002), who evaluated 77 bipolar patients during two distinct manic episodes separated, on average, by 2 years, concluded that manic symptomatology remains generally consistent from episode to episode. Specifically, they found that severity of mania, dysphoria, hedonic activation, psychosis, and irritable aggression tends to correlate across episodes; psychomotor symptoms do not.

Regardless of the degree of constancy of the clinical picture across attacks, it is clear that symptoms vary widely during any given manic episode as it progresses through various stages. These stages, characterized by Carlson and Goodwin (1973) and discussed more fully below, begin with elation or irritability, evolve into a more severe form as arousal and hyperactivity escalate, and culminate in floridly psychotic disorganization.

Mood

Research on mood symptoms in mania, summarized in Table 2–1, demonstrates that most patients, on average, are depressed (46 percent) or labile (49 percent) nearly as often as they are euphoric (63 percent) or expansive (60 percent); they are irritable (71 percent) even more often. The depression, irritability, and mood lability are generally seen less often in early stages of an episode, although few studies have specified the stage, level, or severity of mania at the time of observation.

Winokur and colleagues (1969) observed depressed mood in 68 percent of their manic patients, as well as more severe depressive symptoms (including depressive delusions and psychomotor retardation) in a significant subgroup. They found that "short depressive contaminations in the manic episode" were significantly more common in women (79 percent) than in men (49 percent) (p. 64). Like many investigators, they were particularly impressed by the volatility of mood during manic episodes:

In our series of patients, the degree of mood elevation varied from patient to patient and from time to time during the same episode. The changes in mood were capricious, responding to internal as well as external stimuli

TABLE 2–1. **Mood Symptoms during Mania: Percent Displaying Symptoms**

Study	Patients (N)	Irritability (%)	Euphoria (%)	Depression (%)	Lability (%)	Expansiveness (%)
Clayton et al., 1965	31		97			
Winokur et al., 1969	100[a]	85	98	68[b]	95	
Beigel and Murphy, 1971a	12		67	92		
Kotin and Goodwin, 1972	20			100		
Carlson and Goodwin, 1973	20	100	90	55	90	
Taylor and Abrams, 1973	52	81	31			66
Murphy and Beigel, 1974	30			90		
Winokur and Tsuang, 1975	94	70	92[c]			
Abrams and Taylor, 1976	78	76	44		59	
Leff et al., 1976	63		97			
Loudon et al., 1977	16	75	81[d]	63[e]	56	44
Taylor and Abrams, 1977	119	81	39		52	60
Carlson and Strober, 1979	9[f]	100	89			
Prien et al., 1988	103			67[g]		
Cassidy et al., 1998[h]	316	51	59	29[i]	42	
Serretti and Olgiati, 2005	158	91				
Total n[j]	1121					
Weighted Mean[j]		71	63	46	49	60

[a]100 episodes, 61 patients.
[b]Depressive delusions in 24%, suicidal ideation in 7%.
[c]Irritable only (8%), euphoric only (30%), irritable and euphoric (62%).
[d]Hypomanic affect.
[e]Suicidal ideation in 25%.
[f]Adolescents.
[g]Mild depression (45%), moderate to severe depression (22%).
[h]High threshold value used for signs and symptoms.
[i]Dysphoria.
[j]Winokur et al. not included in calculation because units are in episodes, not in patients.

and so very changeable that they defied measurement. . . . In only 5% was the mood unchanging over a period of hours or days. (p. 62)

As noted earlier, Carlson and Goodwin (1973) described progressive stages of mania, from mild hypomania to delirious psychotic mania. The principal features of the three stages are outlined in Table 2–2; the relationship of these stages to daily behavioral ratings is illustrated in Figure 2–2. The stages were inferred from a study of 20 hospitalized, unmedicated bipolar patients who had experienced a manic episode at some time during their hospitalization.

TABLE 2–2. **Clinical Features of the Stages of Mania**

	Stage I	Stage II	Stage III
Mood	Lability of affect; euphoria predominates; irritability if demands not satisfied	Increased dysphoria and depression; open hostility and anger	Clearly dysphoric; panic-stricken; hopeless
Cognition	Expansivity, grandiosity, overconfidence; thoughts coherent but occasionally tangential; sexual and religious preoccupation; racing thoughts	Flight of ideas; disorganization of cognitive state; delusions	Incoherent, definite loosening of associations; bizarre and idiosyncratic delusions; hallucinations in one-third of patients; disorientation as to time and place; occasional ideas of reference
Behavior	Increased psychomotor activity; increased initiation and rate of speech; increased spending, smoking, telephone use	Continued increased psychomotor acceleration; increased pressured speech; occasional assaultive behavior	Frenzied and frequently bizarre psychomotor activity

Source: Adapted from Carlson and Goodwin, 1973.

Figure 2–2. Relationship between states of a manic episode and daily behavior ratings. (*Source*: Carlson and Goodwin, 1973.)

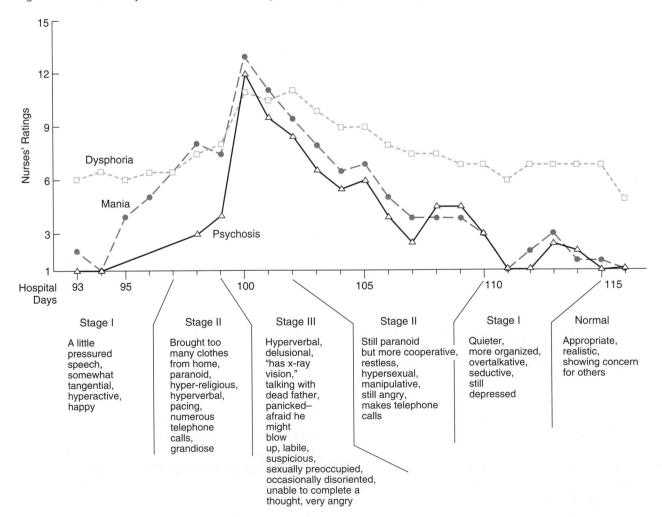

Manic episodes were identified by means of global mania ratings determined twice a day by consensus of the nursing research team, and were corroborated by the psychiatrists' and nurses' written descriptions of patients' affect, psychomotor activity, and cognitive state. The sequence of mood, cognitive, and behavioral symptoms over the course of the episode was recorded. Based on analysis of this information, the patients' longitudinal course was divided into three stages, with predominant mood as the primary criterion—from the euphoria of stage I, to the anger and irritability of stage II, to the severe panic of stage III. In some of the patients, the onset of mania (the switch) was gradual, clearly unfolding in a sequence until the full syndrome had developed. In others, the onset was sudden and dramatic; even in these cases, however, the earlier stages were present, if transient.

As Carlson and Goodwin elaborated, the initial phase of mania (stage I) typically is characterized by increased activity; by a labile mood that can be euphoric, irritable, or both; and by expansive, grandiose, and overconfident thoughts. Thinking remains coherent but is often tangential. Patients describe this change as "going high" and frequently report racing thoughts. In some instances, the "high" does not go beyond stage I, which corresponds to hypomania.

Many episodes progress to the next stage, however. Psychomotor activity increases—evident in the even more rapid speech—and the mood state becomes more labile, characterized by a mix of euphoria and dysphoria. Irritability turns into open hostility and anger, and the accompanying behavior often is explosive and assaultive. As racing thoughts progress to a definite flight of ideas, cognition becomes increasingly disorganized. Preoccupations intensify, with grandiose and paranoid trends that are apparent as frank delusions. This level, which corresponds to acute mania, is designated as stage II.

In some patients, the manic episode progresses further to an undifferentiated psychotic state (stage III), experienced by the patient as clearly dysphoric, usually terrifying, and accompanied by frenzied movement. Thought processes that earlier had been only difficult to follow become incoherent, and definite loosening of associations often is seen. Delusions commonly are bizarre and idiosyncratic, and some patients experience ideas of reference, disorientation, and a delirium-like state. This phase of the syndrome is difficult to distinguish from other acute psychoses, at least superficially. In general, as the manic episode unfolds, stage I is dominated by elation (or irritability) and grandiosity, stage II by increasing hyperactivity and arousal, and stage III by florid psychotic disorganization.

In the Carlson and Goodwin study, many of the rated items showed graded continuous distributions, whereas others evidenced definite thresholds involving apparently qualitative shifts. The level of psychomotor activity escalated continuously through all three stages, and ratings for manic mood increased in like manner through stages I and II. Ratings of psychosis, by contrast, were not clearly distributed along a continuum. This point is illustrated by the case example presented in Figure 2–2. As can be seen, stage III mania was characterized by the relatively abrupt and initial appearance of hallucinations, formal thought disorder in the Schneiderian sense, and organic delirium.

In their study of mania, Kotin and Goodwin (1972) found depressive affect to be pervasive. Indeed, in 10 of their 20 manic patients the mean depression rating was significantly higher during the manic episode than during nonmanic, depressed periods in the hospital. The authors noted that mania and depression ratings were correlated positively in a majority of patients both during manic periods and for the entire hospital stay. These findings, observed the authors, "are contrary to the common view that a patient is either manic or depressed" (p. 683). Recent studies of mania, discussed later, bear out its mixed nature.

Cognition and Perception

Nonpsychotic cognitive symptoms are common during mania. Grandiosity and flight of ideas—experienced subjectively as racing thoughts—were observed in approximately three-quarters of the manic patients described in the clinical studies summarized in Table 2–3. Less clearly and more variably defined were distractibility, poor concentration, and confusion, a fact that may account in part for the broader range of results on these variables—16 to 100 percent for distractibility, for example, and 8 to 58 percent for confusion. Definitions were especially wide-ranging for confusion—from "somewhat confused and unable to follow the gist of a conversation" to the more severe clinical usage of the term to denote disorientation and serious memory disturbance.

Thought Disorder. There is no single or comprehensive definition of formal thought disorder. Instead, thought disorder has been used as a general phrase to describe problems with the ability to attend to, abstract, conceptualize, express, or continue coherent thought. Deficits in thought and language were at one time described in general terms; today these deficits are defined by specific measures (e.g., the Thought Disorder Index or the Scale for the Assessment of Thought, Language and Communication). This increased specificity makes it possible to disentangle, at least in part, disorders of thought from those of language or speech (accordingly, we discuss the

TABLE 2–3. Cognitive Symptoms during Mania (Excluding Psychotic Features)

Study	Patients (N)	Grandiosity (%)	Flight of Ideas/ Racing Thoughts (%)	Distractibility/ Poor Concentration (%)	Confusion[a] (%)
Lundquist, 1945	95				23
Clayton et al., 1965	31	79	100	97	58
Winokur et al., 1969	100[b]	86	93	100	8
Carlson and Goodwin, 1973	20	100	75	70	35
Taylor and Abrams, 1973	52		77		33
Abrams and Taylor, 1976	78	71	41		26
Leff et al., 1976	63		49	16	
Loudon et al., 1977	16	50	58[c]	75	
Taylor and Abrams, 1977	119				27
Carlson and Strober, 1979	9	67	56	67	
Braden and Ho, 1981	11		91[d]	55	
Cassidy et al., 1998	316	72	78		
Serretti and Olgiati, 2005	158		95	97	
Total n[e]	968				
Weighted mean[e]		73	76	75	29

[a]Disorientation and memory lapses; unclear criteria in some studies.
[b]100 episodes, 61 patients.
[c]Flight of ideas = 25%.
[d]Persistent = 55%.
[e]Winokur et al. not included in calculation because units are in episodes, not in patients.

latter separately below). Although difficult, this distinction is important, since it is possible to have either disorder without the other (Holzman et al., 1985). Much of thought is nonverbal, and individuals often say one thing while thinking another. Here we use as a working definition of thought disorder one provided by Solovay and colleagues (1987, p. 13): thought disorder "is not intended to denote a unitary dimension or process; rather, it refers to any disruption, deficit, or slippage in various aspects of thinking, such as concentration, attention, reasoning, or abstraction."

Certain psychotic features of mania and bipolar depression—delusions and hallucinations—are relevant but not central to the concept of thought disorder. The specificity of thought disorder to the major psychoses—mania and schizophrenia—represents an important conceptual issue and is a major focus here. Results of recent genetic studies indicate that psychosis may be an overlapping feature of bipolar illness and schizophrenia (see Chapter 13); therefore, studies that address the similarities and dissimilarities in the psychotic presentation of the two illnesses are of particular interest. Holzman and colleagues (1985, p. 228) asked: "Is thought disorder a nonspecific accompaniment of psychotic behavior, whatever the etiology of that psychosis, just as fever is nonspecific for a variety of systemic conditions; or is there a set of specific disorders of thinking that accompanies specific psychotic conditions?"

Several methods have evolved for studying thought and communication disorders in schizophrenia and affective illness. These methods were categorized by Harvey (1983) as (1) clinical (the examination of speech patterns on the basis of clinical interactions, e.g., in the manner of Kraepelin and Bleuler); (2) laboratory (the study of underlying cognitive processes that result in or contribute to disordered speech); and (3) natural-language (the examination of speech samples from a variety of sources in an attempt to "identify the discourse processes that lead to the problems listeners have in understanding the speech of psychotics" [p. 368]). Several specific measures have been developed, three of which, summarized below, form the basis for most of the research relevant to the study of thought disorder in bipolar illness. Taken together, these three measures can provide a reasonably comprehensive assessment of formal thought disorder.

Holzman and colleagues (1985) developed the Thought Disorder Index using verbal protocols (most typically verbatim responses to the Rorschach test). Based on earlier indices (Watkins and Stauffacher, 1952; Rapaport et al., 1968), the Thought Disorder Index comprises 23 categories of thinking disturbances evaluated at four levels of severity (Johnston and Holzman, 1979; Shenton et al., 1987; Solovay et al., 1987). The least severe level includes vagueness and peculiar verbalizations; the most severe includes thought contamination and neologisms.

Andreasen (1979a,b) characterized different language behaviors that she considered to be subtypes of thought disorder and developed them into another measure, the Scale for the Assessment of Thought, Language and Communication. Some subtypes occur frequently in psychotic speech (e.g., poverty of content of speech, pressure of speech, tangentiality, derailment, loss of goal, and perseveration), whereas others are relatively uncommon and, correspondingly, less useful (e.g., clanging, blocking, echolalia, neologisms, and word approximations).

Finally, Harrow and colleagues[4] have used a battery of measures taken from the Wechsler Adult Intelligence Scale (WAIS) (Social Comprehension Subtest), the Goldstein-Scheerer Object-Sorting Test, and the Gorham Proverbs Test to assess bizarre and idiosyncratic thinking and behavior, as well as conceptual style. Detailed discussions of the development, reliability, and validity of their test battery are provided elsewhere.[5]

Virtually all studies of formal thought disorder in mania and schizophrenia, the results of which are summarized in Table 2–4, have found comparably high levels in both diagnostic groups.[6] In fact, although Resnick and Oltmanns (1984) observed more thought disorder in schizophrenic patients, Harrow and colleagues (1982) found a trend toward greater levels in manic patients.[7] There is,

therefore, no indication that thought disorder per se is in any way specific to schizophrenia. This observation is consistent with the evidence for the strong presence in mania, as well as in schizophrenia, of psychotic features, such as hallucinations and delusions. (See Chapter 13 for discussion of potential genetic factors underlying psychosis in both bipolar disorder and schizophrenia.) Findings of qualitative comparisons of manic and schizophrenic thought disorder are less consistent, although increased pressure of speech appears to be more characteristic of mania,[8] as are increased derailment, loss of goal, and tangentiality (Andreasen, 1984; Simpson and Davis, 1985). Poverty of speech and other negative symptoms were reported by Andreasen (1984) to be more characteristic of schizophrenic thought, although Ragin and Oltmanns (1987), using the same scale, did not confirm this finding. More recent studies have found greater poverty of thought, less complexity of speech, and less overall quantity of speech in schizophrenic than in manic patients.[9]

Studies of differences between manic and schizophrenic patients on measures of idiosyncratic and/or bizarre thinking have yielded mixed results, with some authors finding higher levels in manic patients (Andreasen and Powers, 1975; Harrow et al., 1982) and others higher levels in schizophrenic patients (Simpson and Davis, 1985; Shenton et al., 1987; Docherty et al., 1996). In general, investigators have found that those with mania have more complex speech than those with schizophrenia (Thomas et al., 1996; Lott et al., 2002). Simpson and Davis (1985) made the useful distinction that manic patients appear to be more disordered in *thought structure*, whereas schizophrenic patients appear to be more disordered in *thought content*. Jampala and colleagues (1989, p. 462) argued that manic patients with formal thought disorder may "have a more severe rather than a different condition than manic patients without formal thought disorder. The fact that more manic patients with formal thought disorder had a first-degree relative with affective illness supports this interpretation."

Qualitative differences in thought disorder between mania and schizophrenia are more distinct in the use of combinatory thinking, the "tendency to merge percepts, ideas, or images in an incongruous fashion" (Shenton et al., 1987, p. 23). In a study of 20 manic patients, 43 schizophrenic patients, and 22 normal subjects, Solovay and colleagues (1987), using the Thought Disorder Index, found no significant difference in the quantity of thought disorder in manic and schizophrenic patients, but did note that manic thought disorder was "extravagantly combinatory, usually with humor, flippancy, and playfulness." Schizophrenic thought disorder, by contrast, was "disorganized, confused, and idealistically fluid, with many peculiar words and

TABLE 2–4. Thought Pathology in Mania and Schizophrenia: Similarities and Differences

Study	Thought Disorder Measure	Similarities	Differences
Breakey and Goodell, 1972	Bannister Grid Text	Same frequency of thought disorder	
Andreasen and Powers, 1975	Goldstein-Scheerer Object Sorting Test		**Manic patients:** ↑behavioral overinclusion; ↑conceptual overinclusion, ↑idiosyncratic thinking **Schizophrenic patients:** ↑underinclusiveness
Grossman et al., 1981	Gorham Proverbs Test Goldstein–Scheerer Object Sorting Test Wechsler Adult Intelligence Scale (WAIS), Social Comprehension Subtest	Similar in overall level of severity, course of disturbance, and loose association of ideas; intermingling of inappropriate personal ideas or concerns into responses to neutral stimuli; gaps in communication of ideas, odd outlooks, and other manifestations of bizarre thinking	**Manic patients:** ↑behavioral activity and responsiveness, ↓response time on word association test, ↓deficits in behavioral activity or impoverished activity, ↑grandiose ideas
Harrow et al., 1982	Gorham Proverbs Test Goldstein–Scheerer Object Sorting Test WAIS, Social Comprehension Subtest		**Manic patients:** may be more thought disordered than schizophrenics, "although the results are not conclusive"; ↑bizarre–idiosyncratic thinking
Andreasen, 1984	Scale for the Assessment of Thought, Language and Communication	Similar in number of abnormalities	**Manic patients:** more positive thought disorder; ↑tangentiality, ↑derailment, ↑incoherence, ↑illogicality, ↑pressure of speech **Schizophrenic patients:** more negative thought disorder, ↑poverty of speech, ↑poverty of content **Schizoaffective patients:** thought disorder is midway between that of manic and schizophrenic patients
Resnick and Oltmanns, 1984	Global ratings of thought disorder		**Manic patients:** less overall thought disorder; ↑pressure of speech

Reference	Measure	Findings
Simpson and Davis, 1985	Scale for the Assessment of Thought, Language and Communication Brief Psychiatric Rating Scale	**Manic patients:** more disordered thought structure; ↑loss of goal, ↑tangentiality, ↑derailment, ↑circumstantiality, ↑illogicality, ↑pressure of speech, ↑incoherence **Schizophrenic patients:** more disordered thought content; ↑hallucinatory statements, ↑hallucinatory behavior, ↑unusual thought content
Ragin and Oltmanns, 1987	Scale for the Assessment of Thought, Language and Communication	Similar levels of poverty of speech, derailment, loss of goal
Shenton et al., 1987	Thought Disorder Index	High level of thought disorder in both manic and schizophrenic patients **Manic patients:** ↑combinatory thinking **Schizophrenic patients:** overall higher level of thought disorder; ↑idiosyncratic and autistic thinking, ↑absurdity, ↑confusion **Schizoaffective patients:** thinking disorders more similar to those of schizophrenic patients than to those of manic patients
Solovay et al., 1987	Thought Disorder Index	Equal amount of thought disorder **Manic patients:** Thought disorder "extravagantly combinative, usually with humor, flippancy and playfulness" **Schizophrenic patients:** "disorganized, confused, and ideationally fluid, with many peculiar words and phrases"
Jampala et al., 1989	Authors' measures of thought disorder	**Manic patients:** ↑flight of ideas **Schizophrenic patients:** ↑non sequiturs, ↑tangentiality, ↑driveling, ↑neologisms, ↑private use of words, ↑paraphasias

(continued)

47

TABLE 2–4. **Thought Pathology in Mania and Schizophrenia: Similarities and Differences** (*continued*)

Study	Thought Disorder Measure	Similarities	Differences
Docherty et al., 1996	Communication Disturbance Index	Structural unclarities; confused, wrong words and vague references	**Manic patients:** ↑ amount of speech; ↑ ambiguous word meanings
			Schizophrenic patients: ↑ references to information unknown to listener
Thomas et al., 1996	Brief Syntactic Analysis		**Schizophrenic patients:** ↓ complexity of speech
Lott et al., 2002	Authors' measures of thought, language, and communication	Most measures of deviant speech	**Manic patients:** ↑ complexity of speech
			Schizophrenic patients: ↑ poverty of speech

phrases." The authors elaborated further on these differences (pp. 19–20):

[M]anic thought disorder manifests itself as ideas loosely strung together and extravagantly combined and elaborated . . . appearance of irrelevant intrusions into social discourse that may at times appear inappropriately flippant and playful. . . . Schizophrenic thought disorder, on the other hand, seems devoid of the playful, compulsively elaborative, and ideationally loose constructions of the manic patients. Characteristic of the schizophrenic patients in this study were fluid thinking, interpenetrations of one idea by another, unstable verbal referents, and fragmented and elliptical communications.

These differences are portrayed in Figure 2–3, which shows standardized Thought Disorder Index scores (on factors derived from a principal components analysis) for 12 schizoaffective (manic) and 10 schizoaffective (depressed) patients, as well as for the manic, schizophrenic, and normal subjects discussed earlier (Shenton et al., 1987). Of note, on the one "manic" factor (combinatory thinking), schizoaffective manic patients were most similar to the manic group, but on the five "schizophrenic" factors (idiosyncratic thinking, autistic thinking, fluid thinking, absurdity, and confusion), they performed more like the schizophrenic patients. The schizoaffective depressed patients more strongly resembled the normal subjects. Andreasen (1984) found that her schizoaffective patients were midway in thought disorder between the manic and schizophrenic patients. Jampala and colleagues (1989) observed a greatly increased rate of flight of ideas in their manic patients (72 percent) compared with schizophrenic patients (10 percent).

In summary, although the overall amount of thought disorder does not differentiate manic from schizophrenic patients, qualitative differences do exist. Manic patients are more likely than schizophrenics to exhibit more pressured and complex speech; grandiosity; flight of ideas; combinatory and overinclusive thinking; and a strong affective component to thought that is characterized by humor, playfulness, and flippancy. The causal relationships among affect, psychomotor acceleration, and the often strikingly different manifestations of the underlying thought disorders in mania and schizophrenia remain unclear.

A few studies have followed the course of manic thought disorder over time. Andreasen (1984) observed that most manic patients, unlike schizophrenic patients, demonstrated a reversible thought disorder. Other than a continuing pressure of speech, they showed nearly complete recovery over time. Schizoaffective patients, to a lesser

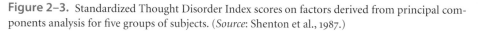

Figure 2–3. Standardized Thought Disorder Index scores on factors derived from principal components analysis for five groups of subjects. (*Source*: Shenton et al., 1987.)

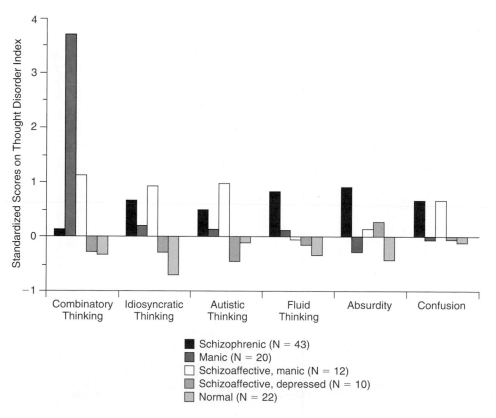

extent than the manic patients, also recovered. Ragin and Oltmanns (1987), on the other hand, found that manic patients displayed moderate levels of derailment and loss of goal at initial testing and, unlike other thought-disordered subjects, did not show significant decreases in either of these features at follow-up. The most extensive longitudinal studies of manic thought disorder were conducted by Harrow and colleagues (Harrow et al., 1982, 1986; Grossman et al., 1986). Using a battery of cognitive tests designed to assess bizarre–idiosyncratic thinking (Goldstein-Scheerer Object Sorting Test, Gorham Proverbs Test, and WAIS Social Comprehension Subtest), the investigators tested manic thought disorder in the acute phase (Harrow et al., 1982), 1 year after hospitalization (Harrow et al., 1986), and 2 to 4 years after hospitalization (Grossman et al., 1986). Initial levels of manic thought pathology and changes over time were compared with those obtained for schizophrenic and nonpsychotic psychiatric patients and normal subjects. The results of these comparisons are summarized in Figure 2–4 and presented in further detail below.

In the acute phase, manic patients were extremely thought disordered; 94 percent showed some definite evidence of abnormal thinking, and 73 percent of hospitalized manic patients demonstrated severe levels of bizarre–idiosyncratic thinking. There were no significant differences in levels of thought disorder between medicated and unmedicated manic patients. Manic patients were at least as thought disordered as, if not more so than, schizophrenic patients (Harrow et al., 1986).

In the short-term follow-up phase (7 weeks), manic thought disorder in medicated patients improved, although some patients continued to show severe thought disorder. Manic patients did not show a more rapid reduction in thought pathology relative to the schizophrenic patients (Harrow et al., 1982).

One year after hospital discharge, a "surprisingly large number" of manic patients showed relatively severe bizarre–idiosyncratic thinking or positive thought disorder (Fig. 2–4). There was also a significant reduction in severity of thought pathology for both manic and schizophrenic patients at follow-up. Manic patients showed a greater reduction in pathology (from 73 to 27 percent rated as severe or very severe) relative to the schizophrenic patients (from 50 to 27 percent) (Harrow et al., 1986).

Two- to 4-year follow-up data revealed that of the manic patients, 30 percent had severe or very severe thought disorder, and another 30 percent had definite signs of abnormal thinking. Of the 14 formerly hospitalized manic patients who showed severe or very severe thought disorder, only 4 were rehospitalized at the time of the follow-up assessment.

Figure 2–4. Composite level of thought disorder during and after hospitalization in manic, schizophrenic, and nonpsychotic psychiatric patients and normal subjects. (*Source*: Grossman et al., 1986; Harrow et al., 1982, 1986.)

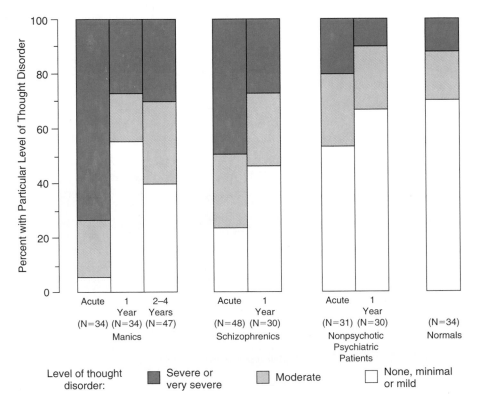

TABLE 2–5. Relationship of Manic Behavior and Psychosis to Thought Disorder in 47 Formerly
Hospitalized Manic Patients at 2- to 4-Year Follow-Up

	No or Mild Thought Disorder (%) (n=19)	Signs of Abnormal Thought Disorder (%) (n=14)	Severe or Very Severe Thought Disorder (%) (n=14)
Ratings of Manic Behavior			
None	58	71	29
Equivocal	42	7	36
Definite	0	21	36
Ratings of Psychosis			
None	74	29	43
Equivocal	26	36	29
Definite	0	36	29

Source: Grossman et al., 1986. Reprinted with permission from the *American Journal of Psychiatry*, Copyright 1986, American Psychiatric Association.

Positive thought disorder was associated with manic behavior; that is, those patients who showed more manic behaviors had more severe thought disorder (see Table 2–5). There was a significant correlation between thought disorder and psychosis, but psychotic symptoms alone did not account for all of the variance associated with thought disorder at follow-up. Manic patients with more than one previous hospitalization or with a more chronic manic course had significantly more thought disorder than patients with only one or no previous hospitalizations (Grossman et al., 1986).

These findings of Harrow's group are indicative of the fact that manic thought disorder can prevail long past an acute episode, a point suggesting the need for caution in accepting assumptions of a relatively benign course of illness or of a return to normality for all patients with bipolar illness (see Chapter 4 for further discussion of the problematic course of bipolar disorder). The findings must be tempered, however, by certain methodological constraints, especially one relevant to recent investigations. In the current era, manic-depressive patients seen and treated in university teaching hospitals represent a disproportionately ill and treatment-refractory group. Bipolar patients with a more typical (i.e., salutary) course are now treated, for the most part, by the general psychiatric community. Those patients less responsive to standard medical interventions are more frequently referred to research centers for evaluation and treatment. Further confounding interpretation of the above findings are issues of patient nonadherence to medication regimens (see Chapter 21), medication side effects, and seasonal biases (e.g., annual assessments, if completed 1, 2, or 4 years after an acute episode, may increase the likelihood of testing during a periodic recurrence rather than a remission). The continuance of significant thought pathology in many manic patients is of both clinical and theoretical relevance and is an important area for further research (see Perugi et al., 1998a, for a discussion of cognitive decline in chronic mania).

Linguistic and Communication Patterns. Investigators have found differences in linguistic patterns between manic and schizophrenic patients (Kagan and Oltmanns, 1981; Harvey, 1983; Ragin and Oltmanns, 1987). Hoffman and colleagues (1986) found that total speech deviance and utterance length were greater in manic than in schizophrenic patients. The authors concluded that "manic speech difficulties were due to shifts from one discourse structure to another, while schizophrenic speech difficulties reflected a basic deficiency in elaborating any discourse structure" (p. 836). In a related study, Fraser and colleagues (1986) found that schizophrenic patients had less syntactically complex speech than manic patients. This finding is consistent with those of the more recent work of Thomas and colleagues

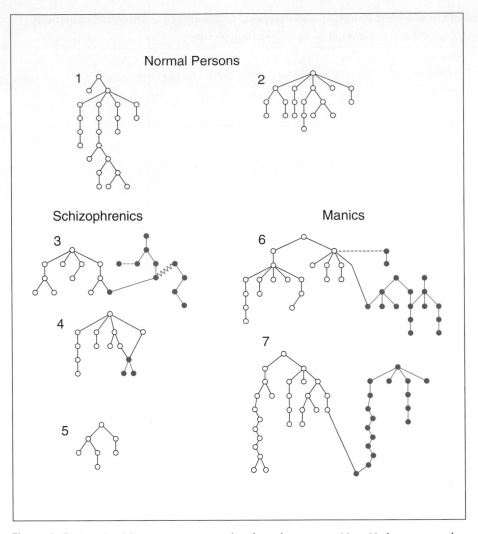

Figure 2–5. Sample of discourse structures taken from three groups. Note: Nodes correspond to statements generated by text. Linkages are formed from dependency relations. Substructures identified by open circles correspond to largest subtree embedded in segment. Jagged line indicates nontransitive dependency; broken lines represent nondependent associations. Upward branching nodes can be seen to receive more than one chain of superordinate statements. Two manic patients have larger subtrees compared with three schizophrenic patients. 1, 2, and 5 are well-formed trees. (*Source*: Hoffman et al., 1986.)

(1996) and Lott and colleagues (2002), who also found that manic speech was more complex. The structural differences in language are schematized in Figure 2–5. Hoffman and colleagues (1986) speculated that the shift from one discourse structure to another is related to the manic patient's increased distractibility and general level of overactivation, each of which involves both verbal and nonverbal behavior. Distractibility in bipolar illness, which is pervasive and often severe, is discussed in detail in Chapter 9.

Predictability of verbal communication has been studied through close analysis, a measure of the ability of normal subjects to guess words deleted from transcripts of speech samples. Using this technique, Ragin and Oltmanns (1983) found that depressed speech was the most predictable,

schizophrenic the least, and manic somewhere in between. Andreasen and Pfohl (1976) analyzed the frequency of syntactical elements in speech samples taken from 16 manic and 15 depressed patients. Their results are summarized in Table 2–6 and as follows by the authors (p. 1366):

The analysis of syntactical elements was particularly useful in distinguishing between the two groups . . . [D]epressive speech tends to be more vague, qualified, and personalized, while manic speech is more colorful and concrete . . . [D]epressed patients tend to qualify more, to talk more in terms of a "state of being," and to talk more both about themselves and other people. Manics, on the other hand, tend to talk more about things

TABLE 2–6. Frequency of Syntactical Elements in Manic and Depressed Patients

Manic = Depressed	Manic > Depressed	Depressed > Manic
• Lexical diversity (number of words, number of different words) • Syntactical complexity	• Colorfulness • Action verbs • Adjectives • Concreteness • Words reflecting power and achievement	• Vagueness • Qualifying adverbs • First-person pronouns • Overstatement

Note: Sample = 16 manic patients, 15 depressed patients.
Source: Adapted from data in Andreasen and Pfohl, 1976.

than about people, to discuss them in terms of action, and to use more adjectives to describe them.

Delusions and Hallucinations. Problems in the assessment of delusions and hallucinations are many and troublesome. Orvaschel and colleagues (1982) found that family reports of affective delusions identified only 18 percent of probands who admitted such symptoms on direct interview with the Schedule for Affective Disorders-Lifetime (SADS-L). In a study of psychosis in 89 bipolar patients, Rosen and colleagues (1983a) found that 49 (55 percent) emerged as psychotic on the basis of interviews (SADS) alone. After a review of all interviews and prior records, however, 63 were identified as psychotic. Price and colleagues (1984), like Orvaschel and colleagues (1982), found a lack of reliability in reports from family members. Yet as Pope and Lipinski (1978) observed in their early review of the literature, the general findings of all these studies, despite wide differences in time, setting, and sample selection, are reasonably consistent.

Table 2–7 summarizes findings from 33 studies of psychotic features in mania. Approximately two-thirds of the bipolar patients in these studies were found to have a lifetime history of at least one psychotic symptom (phase of illness usually unspecified, but when specified, more often manic). The range of rates was 47 to 90 percent. These results are consistent with Carlson and Goodwin's (1973) finding that 30 percent of their bipolar-I patients (i.e., those with a history of mania) did not progress to stage III mania. Rosenthal and colleagues (1979) also observed that 33 percent of their bipolar-I patients never became formally psychotic during mania. The high prevalence of psychotic features in these studies is consistent with the presence of a psychosis factor in most factorial studies of mania and with Koukopoulos's (2005) assertion that the manic syndrome is basically a psychotic condition.

Some evidence suggests that early age at onset of bipolar illness is likely to be associated with an increased rate of psychotic symptoms. Carlson and Strober (1979) found that bipolar illness first appearing during adolescence was characterized by especially florid psychotic symptoms. Rosenthal and colleagues (1980) observed that those bipolar-I patients who also met Research Diagnostic Criteria (RDC) for schizoaffective illness had a younger age at onset and more non-Schneiderian delusions and hallucinations. Rosen and colleagues (1983b) found a negative correlation of 0.4 between age at onset and psychotic symptom score. The authors also suggested that their findings raise the possibility that RDC schizoaffective disorders are really a form of bipolar-I disorder. More recent, larger studies have not found a significant correlation between early age at onset and psychotic symptoms, however (Perugi et al., 2000; Toni et al., 2001; Baethge et al., 2005). Age-specific issues relevant to delusions and hallucinations are discussed more fully in Chapter 6.

Akiskal and colleagues (1983) reported that in patients who switched from depression to mania during a prospective observation period of 3–4 years, the index depressive episode was often psychotic. Findings of a new study (Othmer et al., in press) based on more than 1,000 outpatients confirm the strong association between early-onset psychotic depression and eventual manic switch.

Some evidence relates the presence of psychotic symptoms to severity of illness. Abrams and Taylor (1981) found "only a trend" toward an association between severity of manic syndrome and "schizophrenic features," including delusions and hallucinations. Carlson and Goodwin (1973), however, reported covariance between ratings of psychosis and ratings of manic severity. Likewise, Young and colleagues (1983) found a positive relationship between total score on the Mania Rating Scale and the presence of psychotic symptoms. More recently, Baethge and colleagues (2005) found that hospitalizations for bipolar patients who had hallucinations averaged 17 percent longer than those for bipolar patients who did not.

TABLE 2–7. Psychotic Symptoms during Mania

Study	Patients N	DELUSIONS				HALLUCINATIONS				Presence or History of Psychotic Symptoms[a] (%)	Thought Disorder (%)	First-Rank Schneiderian Symptoms (%)
		Any (%)	Grandiose (%)	Persecutory/ Paranoid (%)	Passivity (%)	Any (%)	Auditory (%)	Visual (%)	Olfactory (%)			
Lange, 1922	700						7				8	
Bowman and Raymond, 1931–1932a,b	1009			20			17	9				
Rennie, 1942	66	24				22						
Lundquist, 1945	95					13						
Astrup et al., 1959	96			18	9		24					9
Clayton et al., 1965	31	73			47							
Winokur et al., 1969	100[b]	48		19	22		21	9				
Beigel and Murphy, 1971a	12			33								
Carlson and Goodwin, 1973	20	75		65	20	40						
Carpenter et al., 1973	66											23
Taylor and Abrams, 1973b	52		60	42			48	27	15			12
Murphy and Beigel, 1974	30			23								
Guze et al., 1975	19									53[b]		
Abrams and Taylor, 1976	78			55			44					
Leff et al., 1976	63	67										
Loudon et al., 1977	16		43	25								

54

Study	n											
Taylor and Abrams, 1977	119	52	65	47						84		11
Carlson and Strober, 1979	9	56	33							44		
Rosenthal et al., 1979	66	35[c]	35[c]	30[c]	21[c]					67[c]		
Brockington et al., 1980[a]	32	53		34						9	34	
Rosenthal et al., 1980	71	41	30	25						74[c]	34	
Rosen et al., 1983a	89									55 (71)[e,f]		
Rosen et al., 1983b	71									75[c]		
Winokur, 1984	122	54	14						9	64[c]		4
Endicott et al., 1986	298[d]									47[c]		
Black and Nasrallah, 1989	467	44				13	6	14				
Vieta et al., 1997	34[g]									90		
Cassidy et al., 1998	316									78–90[h]		
Coryell et al., 2001	139									65		
Suppes et al., 2001	214[g]									67		
Serretti et al., 2002	863[g]	61	31			31				50		
Keck et al., 2003	352[c]	42	34	25						68	22	17
Baethge et al., 2005	196(48)[i]				11 (23)[i]							
Total n	5973											
Weighted means[j] (individual episode data[a])		53	31	39	12	23	18	14	15	61	19	17

(continued)

TABLE 2–7. Psychotic Symptoms during Mania (*continued*)

Study	Patients N	DELUSIONS				HALLUCINATIONS				Presence or History of Psychotic Symptoms[a] (%)	Thought Disorder (%)	First-Rank Schneiderian Symptoms %
		Any (%)	Grandiose (%)	Persecutory/ Paranoid (%)	Passivity (%)	Any (%)	Auditory (%)	Visual (%)	Olfactory (%)			
Weighted means[j] lifetime data[a]		—	35	22	—	—	18	10	—	60	9	34
Weighted means[j] (all)		53	31	29	12	23	18	12	15	61	19	18

[a]Lifetime or course of illness.
[b]100 episodes, 61 patients.
[c]Phase of illness not specified.
[d]Bipolar fraction unclear.
[e]38 reported psychotic symptoms during manic phase only, 6 during both manic and depressed phases, and 5 during depressed phase only.
[f](71) refers to total % psychotic (only 55% were considered psychotic on the basis of interview alone).
[g]Bipolar I patients only.
[h]Low and high symptom threshold values.
[i]Mixed mania figures are in parentheses.
[j]Winokur et al. not included in calculation because units are in episodes, not in patients.

The relationship between the presence or a history of psychotic features and the long-term course of illness is unclear. While several studies have not found a correlation between psychosis and poorer outcome,[10] many more have.[11] There is even more agreement that mood-incongruent psychotic features predict a less positive course.[12] Only one early investigation (Abrams and Taylor, 1983) and a single recent study (Keck et al., 2003) found otherwise. Keck and colleagues hypothesized that their findings, which are at variance with most others, may reflect the high morbidity and poor functional outcome in the great majority of the patients they studied. There does not appear to be a significant correlation between psychosis and an increased likelihood of attempting suicide (Grunebaum et al., 2001; Black et al., 2003; Keck et al., 2003; see Chapter 8).

Young and colleagues (1983) examined the relationship between psychotic features and other manic symptoms. They found no association of psychotic features with insight, disruptive–aggressive behavior, appearance, and rate and amount of speech, or with demographic variables, such as age, gender, and race. They did find, however, that psychotic patients were significantly more likely than nonpsychotic patients to have grandiose and expansive mood, increased psychomotor activity and energy, and increased sexual interest, and were also more likely to report sleep-disturbance symptoms. Baethge and colleagues (2005), who studied hospitalized bipolar patients, found that those who reported hallucinations were less well educated and had higher anxiety scores, longer hospitalizations, and less insight into their illness. Comparisons of bipolar-I and -II patients have found, as one would expect, a greatly elevated rate (nearly three-fold) of psychotic symptoms in those with bipolar-I (Vieta et al., 1997; Suppes et al., 2001; Serretti et al., 2002).

Finally, Endicott and colleagues (1986) studied 1,084 first-degree relatives of 298 probands with schizoaffective, psychotic, and nonpsychotic unipolar and bipolar major depressive disorders. They found that over the course of a lifetime, bipolar disorder and psychosis were positively associated in both probands and relatives. Bipolar illness in a proband did not predict psychosis in relatives, however, whereas psychosis in a proband was related to increased risk of psychosis (but not to bipolarity) in relatives. According to Endicott and colleagues, these findings suggest that, although bipolarity and psychosis often occur in the same individuals, they may not reflect the same genetic influence. The authors speculated that "the risk for the 'expression' of psychotic symptoms is increased in individuals who also have had a bipolar disorder" (p. 11). Interestingly, Winokur and colleagues (1986; Winokur and Kadrmas, 1989) showed that the risk for psychosis, as well as polyepisodic course in bipolar

patients, is predicted by a history of mania and polyepisodic course in the family.

Delusions, like thought disorder, vary widely in severity, fixedness, content, and effect on overt behavior (Jaspers, 1913; Kraepelin, 1921; Garety, 1985). The degree to which they are contingent upon fluctuating affect also varies.

Manic delusions are usually grandiose and expansive in nature, often religious, and not infrequently paranoid. They generally can be differentiated from schizophrenic delusions by their tendency to be wish-fulfilling in nature and oriented more toward communion than segregation (Lerner, 1980). Winokur and colleagues (1969, p. 70) distinguished the presentations of delusions in the two illnesses as follows:

> The delusions that are seen in schizophrenia usually last for months or years and are often primary; that is, they do not explain a real or disordered perception. They fulfill the definition of a delusion as a fixed, false belief. In mania the delusions are quite different. They are often evanescent, appearing or disappearing during the course of a day, or even during an interview. They also vary with the patient's total state, being more frequent when he is more active; and his flights of ideas become more pronounced and fading as he becomes more quiet. Frequently they are extensions of the patient's grandiosity.
>
> At times the patient can be talked out of his delusion, and at other times he gives the impression that he is only being playful rather than really being deluded. In our group the delusions were often secondary to the patient's exalted affect. This was especially true of those patients who felt their mood could be described only as a religious experience.
>
> The most subtle and earliest distortions of reality are manifest in the frequent extravagance and grandiose self-image expressed by the patients.

Kraepelin (1921, pp. 68–69) also emphasized the changing nature of manic delusions (especially when contrasted with those expressed during the depressive phase, which he thought were for the most part "uniformly adhered to"): manic delusions "change frequently, emerge as creations of the moment and again disappear"; they "move very frequently on religious territory," tending to be grandiose; and "patients often narrate all sorts of journeys and adventures, secret experiences." He also reported that the same delusional ideas often appeared again in subsequent attacks. Winokur and colleagues (1969, p. 72), like Kraepelin, suggested that delusions of mania are "not well systematized and, apart from grandiose optimism, tend not to be acted upon." They attributed the fact that manic patients seldom act on their delusions (a point perhaps worth disputing) to the brief duration of the delusions and the patient's "inability to make any sort of concerted action." They noted further that both manic and depressive delusions, which occur primarily in the most disturbed patients, tend to be appropriate to the patient's mood and not to be systematized. The same investigators found that religious themes were the most common manic delusions in both men (27.0 percent) and women (30.1 percent). Political themes were more common in men (18.9 percent) than in women (3.2 percent), and sexual and financial themes were about equally common (13.5 and 9.5 percent, respectively, in men; 5.4 and 7.9 percent, respectively, in women).

Hallucinations, or perceptions of sensory impressions without the existence of external physical stimuli, represent a fascinating, not uncommon, and yet relatively unstudied part of the clinical phenomenology of affective illness. They occupy a portion of the continuum of dream-state–illusory–hallucinatory phenomena, which ranges from distortions and misperceptions on the one hand to the total conjuring of fully developed images on the other. Hallucinations can vary in a wide range of aspects, such as their extent (frequency and duration), location, constancy, intensity, effect on overt behavior, affect produced, content, and causal attributions (Lowe, 1973). Yet despite these complexities, hallucinations are most commonly presented in the psychiatric research literature as simply present or absent in a given sensory modality (e.g., auditory or visual).

Hallucinations generally occur less frequently than delusions in both the manic and depressed phases of bipolar illness, although Carlson and Strober (1979) reported a significantly higher rate of hallucinations in bipolar depression. Baethge and colleagues (2005) found comparable rates of hallucinations in mania and depression, but twice as high a rate in bipolar mixed patients (see Table 2–8). The lifetime history data presented earlier in Table 2-7 suggest that at least half of all patients report a history of delusions, but only about a fifth report the experience of hallucinating while depressed or manic. Auditory hallucinations, averaged across the data-based studies, are more common than visual ones.

Kraepelin (1921, pp. 5–6) found that in mania, the perception of external impressions was "invariably encroached upon" and that defective perceptions often were related to "extraordinary distractibility of attention." He described not only the blurring of illusions, hypnagogic phenomena, and hallucinations, but also their overlap with mood and thinking in the bipolar form of manic-depressive illness (pp. 8, 11):

> Isolated hallucinations are observed frequently and in the most different states, although they do not very often

appear conspicuously in the foreground. It is generally a case of illusionary occurrences, the appearance of which is favoured by the incompleteness and slightness of perception, but especially by the lively emotions peculiar to the disease. The substance of the illusions therefore is invariably in close connection with the trains of thought and the moods of the patients. . . .

> Auditory hallucinations frequently appear only in the night-time, or at least much more then. They seem, as a rule, not to possess complete sensory distinctness. They are voices "as in a dream". . . . Their origin is relatively seldom referred to the external world. . . . Much more frequently the hallucinations have their seat in the patient's own body.

In an early study, Bowman and Raymond (1931–1932b) compared hallucinations in 1,009 patients with manic-depressive psychoses, 1,408 with schizophrenia, and 496 with general paresis. They found an overall tendency for more women than men to have a history of hallucinations (especially of a visual nature), and observed that women with "seclusive personalities" were at particularly high risk for auditory and visual hallucinations. A recent study of hallucinations in bipolar patients also found that women were more likely than men to report hallucinations (Baethge et al., 2005). Bowman and Raymond found no significant relationship between the presence of hallucinations and religion, age at admission, or level of intelligence. They did observe a close relationship between the clinical nature of the hallucinations in bipolar illness and those present in patients with general paresis. This latter finding is consistent with Lowe's (1973) conclusion that bipolar hallucinations resemble more those of the organic psychoses than those of schizophrenia or paranoia. (This similarity to organic psychosis [toxic versus defect] is also discussed in Chapters 3, 9, and 15.)

Winokur and colleagues (1969) found that manic hallucinations tended to be brief, grandiose, often part of a delusional idea, usually religious ("the face of God," "Heaven in all its glory"), and frequently in the form of a command from God. Manic and depressive hallucinations shared a fragmented and fleeting quality and usually occurred in the most severely disturbed patients. The authors stressed the theoretical importance of a severity profile in bipolar illness, after noting that hallucinations—the least common of symptoms—were also the first symptoms to disappear during recovery from a manic episode, followed in turn by delusions, flight of ideas, push of speech, and distractibility (a general pattern later confirmed by Carlson and Goodwin, 1973).

Although finding hallucinations of generally limited use in differential diagnosis, D.W. Goodwin and colleagues

TABLE 2–8. Comparison of Psychotic Features during Mania and Bipolar Depression

Category of Symptoms	PERCENTAGE OF PATIENTS					
	Winokur et al., 1969[a]	Carlson and Strober, 1979	Rosenthal et al., 1980	Black and Nasrallah, 1989	Mantere et al., 2004	Baethge et al., 2005
Delusions						
Mania	48	56	96[c]	44		
Depression	33	66	28	12		
Hallucinations						
Mania	21[b]	33	66	14		11 (23[d])
Depression	6[b]	50	24	8		11
Psychotic Symptoms[e]						
Mania					44	
Depression					9	
Mixed					40	

[a]100 episodes, 61 patients.
[b]Episodes of auditory hallucinations only.
[c]Includes delusions during euthymic states.
[d]Mixed state.
[e]Delusions or hallucinations not specified. Bipolar-I patients.

(1971), in one of the few (albeit small) phenomenological studies, were able to draw several conclusions about the nature of hallucinations in their 28 patients (7 bipolar) with affective illness: (1) the modality of hallucinations (e.g., auditory or visual) was not consistent from one affective episode to another; (2) patients with affective illness were far more likely than those with schizophrenia to hallucinate only when no other person was there; (3) color was usually normal; (4) the people who appeared in the hallucination were usually of normal size and appearance; (5) the hallucinations were intermittent; (6) they were often in several sensory modalities; and (7) accusatory voices were not specific to affective illness—indeed, they were more common in schizophrenia.

Lowe (1973) studied 22 bipolar patients in a particularly intensive and interesting investigation of hallucinations. In comparing these patients with others who had organic, paranoid, or schizophrenic psychoses, he found that they reported mainly auditory and visual hallucinations when manic; that these hallucinations were less frequent and briefer than those occurring in other neuropsychiatric conditions; that in retrospect, the hallucinations were believed by patients to be "less real" but were also perceived to be less controllable; that women were more likely to report rarer types of hallucinations; and finally, that the patients always believed the hallucinations to be experienced only by themselves. Consistent with other investigators, Lowe concluded that manic hallucinations were more similar in nature to those reported by patients with organic psychoses than to those reported by patients with schizophrenia or paranoia.

Lerner (1980), who also investigated qualitative differences between the psychotic experiences of mania and schizophrenia, concluded that mania was more characterized by enhanced sensory awareness and ecstatic or beatific experiences. Manic hallucinations tended to be more of the visual type; strikingly vivid and associated with bright, colorful sensations; and often coupled with intensely pleasurable or ecstatic feelings (similar to psychedelic experiences). Silberman and colleagues (1985) compared histories of transient sensory phenomena akin to hallucinations in 44 euthymic affective patients (34 bipolar), 37 patients with a history of complex partial seizures, and 30 hypertensive controls. Affective and epileptic patients were similar in their reports of sensory changes, including visual and auditory hallucinations and altered perceptual intensities. Epileptic patients, however, were far more likely to have experienced epigastric, vestibular, and gustatory hallucinations.

In summary, hallucinations occur less frequently than delusions in both the manic and depressed phases of bipolar illness. Hallucinatory phenomena appear to represent the extreme end of the symptomatic picture, being nonexistent in milder forms of depression and mania and most pronounced in the gravest, most delirious states. Hallucinations during mania are frequently ecstatic and religious in nature, brief and fleeting in duration, and inconstant in their modality of expression. They appear qualitatively, at least in the few studies in which they have been addressed, to be more similar to organic than to schizophrenic psychoses. Gender differences in the experience of hallucinatory phenomena are unclear, although there is some evidence that women are more likely to report having had hallucinations.

Activity and Behavior

The results of studies of activity and behavior during manic states, summarized in Table 2–9, show that disturbed sleep and speech, as well as hyperactivity, are common in mania. About 80 percent of manic patients have either insomnia or a decreased need for sleep. Virtually all, 80–90 percent, exhibit hyperverbosity and rapid or pressured speech. An overwhelming majority are hyperactive, more than half are hypersexual, and one in four exhibits catatonia. There are few studies of gender differences in manic activity and behavior, although a recent New Zealand investigation of 90 bipolar males and 121 bipolar females found that men were significantly more likely to report the presence of "problem behaviors" (the nature of which was not specified) and "excitement or inability to hold a conversation" (Kawa et al., 2005, p. 122). Gender differences in manic sexual behavior are discussed in Chapter 10.

Factorial Studies of Mania

Although a great deal of research has been done on the factorial structure of nonbipolar depressive disorders, the literature on the structure of bipolar depressive states is relatively sparse (reviewed in Azorin, 2000). Until recently, this was also the case for mania. Initially, Beigel and colleagues (1971) concluded, on the basis of a relatively small National Institute of Mental Health (NIMH) sample, that pure manic and dysphoric subtypes could be delineated. Subsequently, new data derived from large clinical samples have confirmed this conclusion, but also painted a much more complex clinical portrait of mania.[13] The French EPIMAN study (Akiskal et al., 2003a) is multicentered, with patient information being collected by means of a standardized

protocol in at least four regions of France. The main findings of this study are generally consistent with those of earlier research in indicating that further phenomenological understanding of mania requires a multidimensional perspective. The authors of this study went beyond the euphoric–dysphoric dichotomy and proposed the existence of independent euphoric, depressive, hostile, psychotic, and deficit factors, each of which was correlated with a core activation (disinhibition–instability) factor of mania.

Like Bauer and colleagues (1994), Akiskal and colleagues (2001) concluded that, rather than euphoria/irritability, the central definitional focus of mania should be psychomotor activation. This conclusion is consistent with the emphasis of Heinroth (1818) and Koukopoulos (2005), which posits that excitement is the fundamental state of the bipolar subgroup of manic-depressive illness. By incorporating new features of mania derived from the EPIMAN study (e.g., pathological gregariousness and overfamiliarity) and using clinical expertise, different groups of investigators have developed a factorial structure of mania that incorporates psychomotor activation as the major criterion, along with mood disturbance, other signs and symptoms, and a lack of insight and judgment; this work, in conjunction with that of other investigators, has led to proposed changes in the DSM-IV criteria for mania. Ghaemi and colleagues (1995) also underscored the cognitive dysfunction in the areas of insight and judgment in mania; similar findings were reported by Dell'Osso and colleagues (2000). Interestingly, insight appears to be less impaired during mixed mania (Cassidy et al., 2001a; see Chapters 21 and 22).

Table 2–10 summarizes the findings of factorial studies of the structure of mania. It is clear that current diagnostic systems fail to reflect the actual complexity of the state. Nor do most diagnostic formulations adequately capture the essential relationship, indeed the often total overlap, between major subtypes of mania and mixed states. Virtually all investigations of the structure of mania have noted common underlying dimensions: a mood component, characterized by either predominantly euphoric or dysphoric qualities; psychomotor activation; psychotic features; and irritability and/or aggression.

There are fewer data on the structure of hypomania, but as with mania, cardinal manifestations are irritability, coupled with heightened activation and behavioral excess. Serretti and Olgiati (2005) compared patterns of manic symptoms in 158 bipolar-I and 122 bipolar-II patients (see Table 2–11). The bipolar-I patients had a higher prevalence of reckless activity, distractibility, psychomotor agitation, irritable mood, and increased self-esteem. Juruena and colleagues (2006) compared 27 bipolar-I patients with

Table 2–9. Activity and Behavior Symptoms during Mania

Study	Patients (N)	Hyper-activity (%)	Decreased Sleep[a] (%)	Violent/ Assaultive Behavior (%)	Rapid/ Pressured Speech (%)	Hyper-verbosity (%)	Nudity/ Sexual Exposure (%)	Hyper-sexuality (%)	Extrav-agance (%)	Religiosity (%)	Head Decoration (%)	Regression (Pronounced) (%)	Catatonia (%)	Fecal Inconti-nence/ Smearing (%)
Lange, 1922	700											27		
Allison and Wilson, 1960	24							70						
Clayton et al., 1965	31		94		100			74						
Winokur et al., 1969	100[b]	76	90		99			65	69					
Carlson and Goodwin, 1973	20	100		75	100	100		80		50		45		
Taylor and Abrams, 1973	52	100		48	100		23				33		14	19
Abrams and Taylor, 1976	78	100		46	100		33				38			14
Leff et al., 1976	63	81	63			86		27	32					
Loudon et al., 1977	16	56	69		75			25		25				
Taylor and Abrams, 1977[c]	123			46			29				32		28	10
Carlson and Strober, 1979	9	100	78		89			78				56		

(continued)

TABLE 2–9. **Activity and Behavior Symptoms during Mania** (continued)

Study	Patients (N)	Hyper-activity (%)	Decreased Sleep[a] (%)	Violent/ Assaultive Behavior (%)	Rapid/ Pressured Speech (%)	Hyper-verbosity (%)	Nudity/ Sexual Exposure (%)	Hyper-sexuality (%)	Extrav-agance (%)	Religiosity (%)	Head Decoration (%)	Regression (Pronounced) (%)	Catatonia (%)	Fecal Inconti-nence/ Smearing (%)
Abrams and Taylor, 1981	111												19	
Bräunig et al., 1998	61												31	
Cassidy et al., 1998	316[d]	85	79	46	80									
Krüger et al., 2003	99												27[c]	
Serretti and Olgiati, 2005	158	98	99		93									
Total n[f]	1857													
Weighted mean[f]		90	83	47	88	89	29	51	32	39	34	28	24	13

[a]Includes decreased need for sleep and insomnia.
[b]100 episodes, 61 patients.
[c]Calculations based on a sample of 119 patients (except for catatonia rating).
[d]Based on high-threshold scores.
[e]Of mixed manic patients, 62% displayed catatonia; of pure manic patients, only 5%.
[f]Winokur et al. not included in calculation because units are in episodes, not in patients.

Table 2–10. Findings of Factorial Studies of the Structure of Mania

Study	Sample Size	Assessment Tool	Primary Factors	Core Dimensions/ Clusters
Murphy and Beigel, 1974	30	MSRS		I. Euphoria–grandiosity II. Paranoia–destructiveness
Double, 1991	81	RDC MRS CPRS	10 nondelineated factors	I. (Mild) excitation II. Elation–pressured speech–flight of ideas III. Psychosis–severity IV. Psychomotor activation–aggressive overactivity
Cassidy et al., 1998	237	DSM-III-R MSRS Clinical assessment	1. Dysphoric mood 2. Psychomotor pressure 3. Psychosis 4. Euphoric mood 5. Irritability, aggression	
Dilsaver et al., 1999	105	RDC DSM-III-R	1. Manic activation 2. Depressed state 3. Sleep disturbance 4. Irritability/paranoia	I. Mania with depressed mood II. Mania without depressed mood
Cassidy et al., 2001a	327	DSM-III-R SMS	1. Hypomania; low psychosis; mild, classic mania 2. Severe, classic "pure" mania; devoid of dysphoric features 3. Grandiosity and psychosis, but without marked psychomotor pressure, sleep disturbance, hypersexuality, humor, and irritable paranoia 4. Dysphoria; complete absence of euphoric mood or humor; little grandiosity or hypersexuality 5. Dysphoria, but less than factor 4. Higher levels of grandiosity, humor, psychomotor activation, hypersexuality	Hypomania Acute mania Delusional mania Depressive or anxious mania Mixed state

(continued)

TABLE 2–10. Findings of Factorial Studies of the Structure of Mania (continued)

Study	Sample Size	Assessment Tool	Primary Factors	Core Dimensions/ Clusters
Swann et al., 2001	162	DSM-III-R SADS ADRS	1. Impulsivity 2. Hyperactivity 3. Anxious pessimism 4. Distressed appearance 5. Hostility 6. Psychosis	I. Depressive II. Delusional III. Classic IV. Irritable
Sato et al., 2002	576	DSM-IV GAF AMDPS	1. Depressive mood 2. Irritable aggression 3. Insomnia 4. Depressive inhibition 5. Pure mania 6. Emotional liability/agitation 7. Psychosis	I. Pure mania II. Aggressive mania III. Psychotic mania IV. Depressive (mixed) mania
Akiskal et al., 2003a	104	DSM-IV MSRS GAF HDRS	1. Disinhibition 2. Hostility 3. Deficit 4. Psychosis 5. Elation 6. Depression 7. Sexuality	
González-Pinto et al., 2003	103	DSM-IV MRS HDRS	1. Depression 2. Dysphoria 3. Hedonism 4. Psychosis 5. Activation	I. Hedonism II. Dysphoria III. Activation

ADRS = Affective Disorders Rating Scale; AMDPS = Association for Methodology in Psychiatry System; CPRS = Comprehensive Psychopathology Rating Scale; DSM-III-R = *Diagnostic and Statistical Manual*, 3rd edition, revised; DSM-IV = *Diagnostic and Statistical Manual*, 4th edition; GAF = Global Assessment of Functioning; HDRS = Hamilton Depression Rating Scale; MRS = Mania Rating Scale (Young); MSRS = Manic State Rating Scale; MVAS-BP = Multiple Visual Analogue Scales of Bipolarity; RDC = Research Diagnostic Criteria; SADS = Schedule for Affective Disorders; SMS = Scale for Manic States.

25 bipolar-II patients. Those with bipolar-I reported a higher frequency of racing thoughts, grandiosity, impaired judgment, and decreased total sleep time. Patients with bipolar-II disorder experienced 3.5 times more depressive episodes and four times the rate of lifetime substance abuse disorders. Benazzi (2005) emphasized that there are no clear boundaries between mania and hypomania and that overactive behavior during hypomania is at least as important as hypomanic mood. To date, fewer factors have been derived for hypomania: energy–activity; irritability–racing thoughts, which, as noted earlier, is putatively a

dysphoric expression of hypomania (Benazzi and Akiskal, 2003); and, more recently, an "elevated mood" factor that includes elevated mood and increased self-esteem (Benazzi, 2006). Hantouche and colleagues (2003) also found a dual structure of hypomania, although the factors were slightly different: one factor was defined by positive (driven–euphoric) features, and the other by greater irritability and risk taking.

The factorial structure of mania and hypomania is a relatively new area of clinical investigation, and future studies are needed to follow up on this preliminary work.

TABLE 2–11. **Occurrence of Manic Symptoms in Bipolar-I and -II**

Symptom	BP-I (n = 158) (%)	BP-II (n = 122) (%)	Probability	Risk Ratio	95% Confidence Interval
Excessive activity	98.1	96.7	0.47	1.32	0.56–3.13
Reckless activity	72.1	41.8	<0.01	1.81	1.40–2.33
Distractibility	96.8	79.5	<0.01	3.67	1.64–8.22
Reduced need for sleep	98.7	96.7	0.41	1.71	0.55–5.32
Agitated activity	87.9	52.4	<0.01	3.13	2.08–4.71
Pressured speech	93.0	86.0	0.07	1.48	0.93–2.38
Racing thoughts	94.9	89.3	0.11	1.52	0.87–2.67
Elevated mood	90.5	94.2	0.27	0.82	0.60–1.10
Irritable mood	91.1	68.8	<0.01	2.34	1.48–3.71
Increased self-esteem	86.7	63.9	<0.01	1.97	1.37–2.84

Source: Adapted from Serretti and Olgiati, 2005.

In particular, little is known about the longitudinal stability of these factors, although the findings of one short-term follow-up study suggest such a possibility for the manic and mixed subtypes (Cassidy et al., 2002).

DEPRESSIVE STATES

Classic Clinical Descriptions

The bipolar depressive states, in sharp contrast to the manias, are usually characterized by a slowing or decrease in almost all aspects of emotion and behavior: rate of thought and speech, energy, sexuality, and the ability to experience pleasure. As with the manic states, severity varies widely. Symptoms can range from mild physical and mental slowing, with very little distortion in cognition and perception, to profound depressive stupors, delusions, hallucinations, and clouding of consciousness. Of the three major symptomatic groups we have been examining—mood, cognition and perception, and activity and behavior—mood is perhaps the least variable across the continuum of depressive states, although, as we shall see, irritability and anger often accompany the more usual melancholic picture. Cognition and perception, on the other hand, change profoundly, as do activity and behavior. We begin with extensive classic descriptions of depressive mood, then discuss

changes in cognition and perception and activity and behavior in various depressive states (i.e., nonpsychotic, psychotic, and stuporous depressions). Cognition and perception are treated most extensively in the discussion of psychotic depression, whereas activity and behavior figure more prominently in the discussion of stuporous depression. First, however, we present an ancient description of melancholia from Aretaeus (*Extant Works*, pp. 299–300):

> The patients are dull or stern, dejected or unreasonably torpid, without any manifest cause: such is the commencement of melancholy. And they also become peevish, dispirited, sleepless, and start up from a disturbed sleep.
>
> Unreasonable fear also seizes them, if the disease tend to increase, when their dreams are true, terrifying, and clear: for whatever, when awake, they have an aversion to, as being an evil, rushes upon their visions in sleep. They are prone to change their mind readily; to become base, mean-spirited, illiberal, and in a little time, perhaps, simple, extravagant, munificent, not from any virtue of the soul, but from the changeableness of the disease. But if the illness become more urgent, hatred, avoidance of the haunts of men, vain lamentations; they complain of life, and desire to die. In many, the understanding so leads to insensibility and fatuousness, that they become ignorant

of all things, or forgetful of themselves, and live the life of the inferior animals. . . . They are voracious, indeed, yet emaciated; for in them sleep does not brace their limbs either by what they have eaten or drunk, but watchfulness diffuses and determines them outwardly.

Mood

Mood in all of the depressive states is bleak, pessimistic, and despairing. A deep sense of futility is often accompanied, if not preceded, by the belief that the ability to experience pleasure is permanently gone. The physical and mental worlds are experienced as monochromatic, as shades of gray and black. Heightened irritability, anger, paranoia, emotional turbulence, and anxiety are common. The frightening lack of color and the inability to experience meaningful emotional responses were described by Campbell (1953, p. 106):

> General impairment in emotional feeling is another symptom often described by the manic-depressive patient in a depressive episode. In addition to distortions in sensing impressions, such as a queer, odd or unreal feeling, the patient may complain of a universal dulling of the emotional tone. This symptom, like the feeling of unreality, frightens the patient because it tends to alienate him from his environment. Indeed, it is an important constituent of the patient's fear of insanity. It is bad enough not to speak the same language as other people—it is worse not to feel the same emotions.

Mayer-Gross and colleagues (1960, p. 209) emphasized the negative cognitive and affective tone of depressed patients:

> There is a diminished capacity for normal affective response to sad as well as happy events, a phenomenon which is merely one aspect of a *generalized insufficiency of all mental activities.* . . . Whatever is experienced seems to be painful. Even enjoyable experiences have this effect, partly by making the patient more acutely aware of his incapacity for normal appreciation, partly because he is at once sensible of any unfortunate aspect they may have; he may in fact show considerable ingenuity in seeing the bad side of everything. Past, present, and future are alike seen through the same dark and gloomy veil; the whole of life seems miserable and agonizing. The depth of the affect cannot easily be measured from its *outward expression.* The silent shedding of tears may be seen in an otherwise expressionless face; another patient will mock at himself and at his complaints with a grim and sardonic but surprising humour or call himself a fraud or a fool: in another a sudden smile or expression of gaiety will deceive the physician about the severity of the underlying emotion.

Cognition and Perception

Most mental activity is markedly slowed during depression. By definition, patients with nonpsychotic depression do not manifest clouding of consciousness, nor do they experience delusions or hallucinations. Suicidal thinking, however, is often of dangerous proportions, and morbidly ruminative and hypochondriacal thinking is common. The profoundly slowed but nonpsychotic nature of this type of depressive thought and its indecisive and ruminative quality are portrayed in the following passage from Kraepelin (1921, p. 75)[14]:

> Thinking is difficult to the patient, a disorder, which he describes in the most varied phrases. He cannot collect his thoughts or pull himself together; his thoughts are as if paralyzed, they are immobile. . . . He is no longer able to perceive, or to follow the train of thought of a book or a conversation, he feels weary, enervated, inattentive, inwardly empty; he has no memory, he has no longer command of knowledge formerly familiar to him, he must consider a long time about simple things, he calculates wrongly, makes contradictory statements, does not find words, cannot construct sentences correctly.

Jaspers (1997, p. 597; first published in 1913) described the profound impairment of will, pervasive gloom, and dearth of ideas in depression. The central core of pure depression, he wrote, is formed from

> an equally unmotivated and profound sadness to which is added a retardation of psychic events, which is as subjectively painful as it is objectively visible. All instinctual activities are subjected to it. The patient does not want to do anything. The reduced impulse to move and do things turns into complete immobility. No decision can be made and no activity begun. Associations are not available. Patients have no ideas. They complain of a complete disruption of memory. They feel their poverty of performance and complain of their inefficiency, lack of emotion and emptiness. They feel profound gloom as a sensation in the chest or body as if it could be laid hold of there. The depth of their melancholy makes them see the world as grim and grey. They look for the unfavourable and unhappy elements in everything. They accuse themselves of much past guilt (self-accusations, notions of having sinned). The present has nothing for them (notions of worthlessness) and the future lies horrifyingly before them (notions of poverty, etc.).

Activity and Behavior

Like thought and verbal expression, activity and behavior are slowed in bipolar depression. Fatigue, lack of activity, withdrawal from the company of others, impairment in the volition of will, and profoundly altered sleep and eating patterns are hallmarks of this type of depression (see Chapter 16 for detailed discussion of altered sleep and activity patterns). Campbell (1953, p. 85) described the fatigued, psychomotorically retarded appearance of depressed patients:

Depressed mood is often suggested by the bearing, gait or general appearance of the patient. The depressed individual usually walks slowly and reacts sluggishly. He appears to push himself along, as if he were being held back, rather than propelling himself with normal agility. There are no unnecessary movements with the hands or feet, the patient sitting in a languorous but not restful posture. The shoulders sag, the head is lowered and the entire body seems to droop; loosely hanging clothes sometimes suggest the weight loss often present in the melancholic individual. Everyone is acquainted with the tendency of the angles of the mouth to turn down in the saddened person; a smile, when it occurs, must be forced, and even then there is something sickly or distorted in its expression. The facial musculature of the depressed individual lacks tone, giving the face an inert, myasthenic appearance. The upper eyelids also manifest this careworn expression. . . .

The eyes, which normally portray the spark, vitality and curiosity of the personality, are dull and lustreless. In some individuals the eyes have a faraway, unnatural stare, which even the layman recognizes as a mark of extreme pre-occupation or mental illness.

Disturbances in both the quality and quantity of sleep during depression can be profound but variable. Jaspers (1997, p. 234) noted that depressive sleep is

sometimes abnormally deep, so that patients sometimes feel as if they had been dead. It may however be abnormally light and the patients never feel refreshed, but have vivid, restless and anxious dreams, and feel as if only half of their being had been asleep, the other half had stayed awake and watched. *Duration of Sleep* may be very lengthy . . . in some depressed states. The patients are always wanting to sleep and sometimes sleep twelve hours uninterruptedly. On the other hand we find sleep abnormally curtailed. The patients go to sleep but are awake again soon after and then lie awake all night long. Or they only manage to get off to sleep towards morning.

Suicide is an all-too-frequent outcome of bipolar depression (see Chapter 8). In the words of Kraepelin (1921, pp. 25, 87–88):

The torment of the states of depression, which is nearly unbearable, according to the perpetually recurring state-

ments by the patients, engenders almost in all, at least from time to time, weariness of life, only too frequently also a great desire to put an end to life at any price. . . .

The extraordinarily strong tendency to suicide is of the greatest practical significance. Sometimes it continually accompanies the whole course of the disease, without coming to a serious attempt owing to the incapacity of the patients to arrive at a decision. . . . Sometimes the impulse to suicide emerges very suddenly without the patients being able to explain the motives to themselves. . . .

Occasionally after indefinite prodromata the first distinct morbid symptom is a suicidal attempt. Only too often the patients know how to conceal their suicidal intentions behind an apparently cheerful behaviour, and then carefully prepare for the execution of their intention at a suitable moment.

Psychotic depression (Kraepelin's *melancholia gravis*) is characterized by the same signs and symptoms as those present in nonpsychotic depression, usually in worsened form, with the addition of delusions and/or hallucinations. The following is Bleuler's (1924, pp. 475–476) description of the nature and extent of depressive delusions, hallucinations, and paranoia, as well as their primary content areas of expression (somatic, religious, and financial):

In the severer cases delusions are invariably present and may stand in the foreground. At the same time the hallucinations usually but not always increase. . . . The devil appears at the window, makes faces at the patients. They hear themselves condemned, they hear the scaffold erected on which they are to be executed, and their relatives crying who must suffer on their account, or starve or otherwise perish miserably.

But the *delusions* especially are never absent in a pronounced case and always as delusions of economic, bodily, and spiritual ruin. The patients think that they became poor, and it does no good to show them their valuables or their balance in the bank; that has no significance for them. Debts are there anyway, or demands are to be expected that will wipe out everything.

A more severe form of psychotic depression, although still less severe than delirious depression, was termed by Kraepelin *fantastic melancholia* (equivalent to Griesinger's *melancholia with delusions*, or what other clinicians have called *depressive insanity*). Delusions and hallucinations are more pronounced, some clouding of consciousness usually occurs, and violent excitement can alternate with mild stuporous states. As described by Kraepelin (1921, pp. 89–95):

[a] further, fairly comprehensive group of cases is distinguished by a still greater development of *delusions*. We

may perhaps call it "fantastic melancholia." Abundant *hallucinations* appear. . . . [T]here are also multifarious delusional interpretations of real perceptions. The patient hears murderers come; some one is slinking about the bed; a man is lying under the bed with a loaded gun; an electro-magnet crackles. . . . The trees in the forest, the rocks, appear unnatural, as if they were artificial, as if they had been built up specially for the patient, in fact, even the sun, the moon, the weather, are not as they used to be. . . .

Hypochondriacal delusions usually reach a considerable development; they often completely resemble those of the paralytic. . . .

Consciousness is in this form frequently somewhat clouded. The patients perceive badly, do not understand what goes on, are not able to form clear ideas. They complain that they cannot lay hold of any proper thought, that they are beastly "stupid," confused in their head, do not find their way, also perhaps that they have so many thoughts in their head, that everything goes pell-mell. . . .

The Volitional Disorders are also not quite uniform. The activity of the patients is frequently dominated by volitional inhibition; they are taciturn, even mute, cataleptic; they lie with vacant or strained expression of countenance in bed. . . .

At times more violent states of excitement may be interpolated. The patients scream, throw themselves on the floor, force their way senselessly out, beat their heads, hide away under the bed, make desperate attacks on the surroundings. . . . Serious attempts at suicide are in these states extremely frequent.

Delirious melancholia represents the most severe stage of cognitive and perceptual distortion and disorientation. Delusional thought becomes progressively unclear and fragmented, and hallucinations are particularly vivid, bizarre, and frightening. It is a depressive state characterized predominantly by clouding of consciousness. Kraepelin (1921, pp. 95–97) wrote more than anyone since about the mental and physical aspects of this stage of depression:

Gradual transitions lead to a last, delirious group of states of depression, which is characterized by *profound visionary clouding of conscience*. Here also numerous, terrifying hallucinations, changing variously, and confused delusions are developed. . . .

During these changing visionary experiences the patients are outwardly for the most part strongly inhibited; they are scarcely capable of saying a word. They feel confused and perplexed; they cannot collect their thoughts, know absolutely nothing any longer, give contradictory, incomprehensible, unconnected answers, weave in words which they have heard into their detached,

slow utterances which they produce as though astonished. . . . For the most part the patients lie in bed taking no interest in anything.

Depressive stupor, the most severe form of psychomotor retardation, often constitutes an acute medical emergency. Although it is rarely seen today, it is an important clinical presentation and one that provides insight into the severity of the illness prior to the modern treatment era. The state was described by Henderson and Gillespie (1956, p. 258):

This condition may be defined as a state of intense psychic inhibition during which regression may occur to an infantile, if not more primitive level. The patient, usually, is confined to bed, is mute, inactive and unco-operative. His bodily needs require attention in every way; he has to be fed, washed and bathed. Precautions have to be taken to prevent the retention of faeces, urine and saliva. In some cases all attempts at movement are strongly resisted. In other cases the muscles are more flaccid, and the body and limbs can be moulded into any position. On the surface it may seem as if there was a total absence of feeling or emotion, but that is often more apparent than real, for, after recovery, many patients give a vivid account of the distress which they have experienced. The idea of death is believed by some to be almost universal in stupor reactions, and may be regarded as a form of expiation for the wickedness for which they hold themselves responsible. Some patients may have a clear appreciation of their position and surroundings throughout the whole period of the stupor, but in the majority a considerable dulling of consciousness occurs.

During all these stages of depression the *physical health* suffers greatly. The patient becomes weak, loses weight, has a poor appetite, a coated tongue, and constipation. The circulation is enfeebled, and there is cyanosis, especially of the extremities.

Subjective Experiences of Patients

Mood

Mood in bipolar depression tends to be dominated by a dull, flat, and colorless sense of experience; by despair, hopelessness, and pessimism, often fueled by marked physical and mental lethargy; and by a sharp decrease in the pleasure obtained from ordinarily gratifying events, interests, and people.

Depression is paralyzing and suffocating to those in its grasp. Five years before she killed herself, Sylvia Plath (1982, p. 240) wrote of this in her journal: "I have been and am battling depression. I am now flooded with despair, almost hysteria, as if I were smothering. As if a great muscular owl were sitting on my chest, its talons clenching and constricting my heart." British writer Alan Garner (1997, pp. 208–209) portrayed the deadening and the horror of the beginning of his manic-depressive breakdown:

> The next thing I remember is that I was standing in the kitchen, the sunlit kitchen, looking over a green valley with brook and trees; and the light was going out. I could see, but as if through a dark filter. And my solar plexus was numb.
>
> Some contraption, a piece of mechanical junk left by one of the children, told me to pick it up. It was cylindrical and spiky, and had a small crank handle. I turned the handle. It was the guts of a cheap musical box, and it tinkled its few notes over and over and over again, and I could not stop. With each turn, the light dimmed and the feelings in my solar plexus spread through my body. When it reached my head, I began to cry with terror at the blankness of me, and the blankness of the world.
>
> A scene from Eisenstein's "Alexander Nevsky" swamped my brain: the dreadful passage in which Nevsky dupes the Teutonic Knights onto the frozen lake, and the ice breaks, and their faceless armour takes them under. The cloaks float on the water before being pulled down, and the hands clutch at the ice floes, which flip over and seal in the knights.
>
> All that helplessness, cold and horror comprised me. I was alone in the house, and throughout the afternoon I turned the tinkle tinkle tinkle of the broken toy, which became the sound of the ice. My body was as heavy as the armour and the waterlogged cloaks as I slid beneath the ice.
>
> When the family came home, I was lying on the kitchen settle, in a foetal position, without moving or speaking, until I went to bed at midnight. Sleep was unconsciousness without rest. . . .
>
> I was incapable of emotion except that of being incapable of emotion. I had no worth. I poisoned the planet.

Composer Hugo Wolf's account of his depression (quoted in Walker, 1968, p. 322) focused, as have many descriptions written by depressed or formerly depressed individuals, on the painful contrast between the subjective experience of an arid, sterile reality and a perception of the external world as an unobtainable, visible but not habitable world of light, warmth, and creation:

> What I suffer from this continuous idleness I am quite unable to describe. I would like most to hang myself on the nearest branch of the cherry trees standing now in full bloom. This wonderful spring with its secret life and movement troubles me unspeakably. These eternal blue skies, lasting for weeks, this continuous sprouting and budding in nature, these coaxing breezes impregnated with spring sunlight and fragrance of flowers . . . make me frantic. Everywhere this bewildering urge for life, fruitfulness, creation—and only I, although like the humblest grass of the fields one of God's creatures, may not take part in this festival of resurrection, at any rate not except as a spectator with grief and envy.

The sense of lost energy is of singular importance in understanding the subjective experience of depression. The ebb and flow of life's force or vitality and its painful absence in depression were described by F. Scott Fitzgerald in *The Crack-Up* (1956, p. 74; first published in 1936), a harrowing account of his nervous breakdowns:

> [O]f all natural forces, vitality is the incommunicable one. In days when juice came into one as an article without duty, one tried to distribute it—but always without success; to further mix metaphors, vitality never "takes." You have it or you haven't it, like health or brown eyes or honor or a baritone voice. "*Ye are the salt of the earth. But if the salt hath lost its savour, wherewith shall it be salted?*"—Matthew 5:13[15]

Cognition and Perception

Cognitive changes during depression can be subtle or profound and often are a combination of both. Depressed patients frequently complain that their process of thinking has slowed down. They are confused and ruminative, cannot concentrate, and feel inadequate and useless. John Custance (1952, p. 62) wrote:

> I seem to be in perpetual fog and darkness. I cannot get my mind to work; instead of associations "clicking into place" everything is inextricable jumble; instead of seeming to grasp a whole, it seems to remain tied to the actual consciousness of the moment. The whole world of my thought is hopelessly divided into incomprehensible watertight compartments. I could not feel more ignorant, undecided, or inefficient. It is appallingly difficult to concentrate, and writing is pain and grief to me.

Irrational fears, which can range from fear and panic to obsession and delusion, are common in depression. Fitzgerald (1956, p. 75) summed up the experience as "the dark night of the soul":

> Now the standard cure for one who is sunk is to consider those in actual destitution or physical suffering—this is an all-weather beatitude for gloom in general and fairly salutary day-time advice for everyone. But at three o'clock in the morning, a forgotten package has the same tragic importance as a death sentence, and the cure doesn't work—and in a real dark night of the soul it is always three o'clock in the morning, day after day.

Robert Schumann (quoted in Niecks, 1925, p. 142) was even more explicit about his terror:

> I was little more than a statue, neither cold nor warm; by dint of forced work life returned gradually. But I am still so timid and fearful that I cannot sleep alone. . . . Do you believe that I have not courage to travel alone to Zwickan for fear that something might befall me? Violent rushes of blood, unspeakable fear, breathlessness, momentary unconsciousness, alternate quickly.

Preoccupation with sin and perceived religious transgressions are not uncommon in severe depression, and many deeply depressed patients would empathize with Cowper's "strong sense of God's wrath, and a deep despair of escaping it." William James wrote definitively of this preoccupation, as well as of religious ecstasies, in *The Varieties of Religious Experience* (1902).

Finally, as noted above, thoughts of suicide often accompany the despair, apathy, guilt, and feelings of inadequacy associated with depression. Extensive discussion of suicidal thoughts and behaviors is given in Chapter 8; here we present one woman's description of the depression leading up to a nearly lethal suicide attempt (Jamison, 1995; pp. 110–111, 113):

> A floridly psychotic mania was followed, inevitably, by a long and lacerating, black, suicidal depression; it lasted more than a year and a half. From the time I woke up in the morning until the time I went to bed at night, I was unbearably miserable and seemingly incapable of any kind of joy or enthusiasm. Everything—every thought, word, movement—was an effort. Everything that once was sparkling now was flat. I seemed to myself to be dull, boring, inadequate, thick brained, unlit, unresponsive, chill skinned, bloodless, and sparrow drab. I doubted, completely, my ability to do anything well. It seemed as though my mind had slowed down and burned out to the point of being virtually useless. The wretched, convoluted, and pathetically confused mass of gray worked only well enough to torment me with a dreary litany of my inadequacies and shortcomings in character, and to taunt me with the total, the desperate, hopelessness of it all. What is the point in going on like this? I would ask myself. Others would say to me, "It is only temporary, it will pass, you will get over it," but of course they had no idea how I felt, although they were certain that they did. Over and over and over I would say to myself, If I can't feel, if I can't move, if I can't think, and I can't care, then what conceivable point is there in living?
>
> The morbidity of my mind was astonishing: Death and its kin were constant companions. I saw death everywhere, and I saw winding sheets and toe tags and body bags in my mind's eye. Everything was a reminder that everything ended at the charnel house. My memory always took the black line of the mind's underground system; thoughts would go from one tormented moment of my past to the next. Each stop along the way was worse than the preceding one. . . .
>
> At the time, nothing seemed to be working, despite excellent medical care, and I simply wanted to die and be done with it. I resolved to kill myself. I was coldbloodedly determined not to give any indication of my plans or the state of my mind; I was successful.

Activity and Behavior

Although social isolation, psychomotor retardation or agitation, and other behavioral changes accompany depression, changes in sleep patterns are among the most pervasive, quantifiable, and pathognomonic symptoms. They are also highly distressing for patients. (Research on sleep disturbances is discussed in detail in Chapter 16.) Sylvia Plath—probably bipolar, certainly hospitalized and treated for severe depression—described her experience thus in her autobiographical novel *The Bell Jar* (1971, pp. 142–143):

> I hadn't washed my hair for three weeks. . . .
>
> I hadn't slept for seven nights.
>
> My mother told me I must have slept, it was impossible not to sleep in all that time, but if I slept, it was with my eyes wide open, for I had followed the green, luminous course of the second hand and the minute hand and the hour hand of the bedside clock through their circles and semicircles, every night for seven nights, without missing a second, or a minute, or an hour.
>
> The reason I hadn't washed my clothes or my hair was because it seemed so silly.
>
> I saw the days of the year stretching ahead like a series of bright, white boxes, and separating one box from another was sleep, like a black shade. Only for me, the long perspective of shades that set off one box from the next had suddenly snapped up, and I could see day after day after day glaring ahead of me like a white, broad, infinitely desolate avenue.
>
> It seemed silly to wash one day when I would only have to wash again the next.
>
> It made me tired just to think of it.
>
> I wanted to do everything once and for all and be through with it.

Likewise for Scott Fitzgerald (1956, pp. 72–73; first published in 1936), sleep and hating to face the night became sources of terror:

> [E]very act of life from the morning toothbrush to the friend at dinner had become an effort . . . hating the night

when I couldn't sleep and hating the day because it went towards night. I slept on the heart side now because I knew that the sooner I could tire that out, even a little, the sooner would come that blessed hour of nightmare which, like a catharsis, would enable me to better meet the new day.

Clinical Studies

There has been much less quantitative study of the clinical features of bipolar depression than is the case for either mania or nonbipolar depression. In fact, the substantial literature on depression seldom differentiates bipolar from unipolar depression,[16] and until recently, bipolar depression was usually excluded from study and discussion. Further complicating matters, bipolar depression has frequently been misdiagnosed as unipolar depression, or not discussed in the context of its often mixed forms. For our data-based clinical description of bipolar depression, we have relied primarily upon the early monograph of Winokur and colleagues (1969), Benazzi's series of outpatient studies,[17] and the work of several other researchers (Perugi et al., 1998a; Koukopoulos and Koukopoulos, 1999; Mitchell et al., 2001). Specific comparisons of bipolar and unipolar depression are presented in Chapter 1.[18] In this section we present the findings of data-based studies with regard to symptom presentation in bipolar depression, psychotic features, depressive mixed states, and bipolar–unipolar differences in depressive symptomatology.

Mood

Winokur and colleagues (1969) studied the symptomatology and clinical course of 21 treated bipolar depressed patients (5 men and 16 women, with a combined total of 33 separate depressive episodes). They described the onset of depression as abrupt in 5 episodes (15 percent) and gradual in 28 (85 percent). Mood was observed to be melancholic or tearful in virtually all patients (100 and 94 percent, respectfully), with approximately half (52 percent) displaying hopelessness. Fully three-fourths of bipolar depressed patients were described as irritable, almost as high a percentage (85) as was found by the same authors in manic patients (see Table 2–1). Irritability, which is pervasive during bipolar depression (Deckersbach et al., 2004; Benazzi and Akiskal, 2005), is considered more extensively later in this section, as well as in the subsequent discussion of mixed depressive states.

Cognition and Perception

Winokur and colleagues (1969) found widespread cognitive and perceptual changes during bipolar depression. Self-deprecatory and self-accusatory thoughts were present in almost all patients (97 and 91 percent, respectively).

With few exceptions, patients also reported substantially impaired cognitive ability: 91 percent reported poor concentration, diminished clarity of thought, and/or diminished speed of thought. Half complained of poor memory. Suicidal thoughts were common (82 percent), a figure in close agreement with the rate (83 percent) found in a later study of bipolar depressed adolescents (Carlson and Strober, 1979).

Frequencies of thought disorder in manic, depressed, and normal subjects (as measured by the Scale for the Assessment of Thought, Language and Communication) were analyzed in three early studies (Ianzito et al., 1974; Andreasen 1979a, 1984). Manic patients were more likely than depressive patients to exhibit pressured speech, distractibility, derailment, illogicality, loss of goal, perseveration, and a higher overall global rating of thought disorder. Depressed patients, by contrast, were more likely than manic patients to demonstrate poverty of speech. There were no differences between manic and depressed patients in ratings of poverty of content of speech, tangentiality, clanging, neologisms, word approximations, circumstantiality, echolalia, blocking, or stilted speech. When compared with normal subjects, depressed patients displayed greater poverty of content of speech, as well as increased tangentiality, circumstantiality, and self-reference. Normal subjects were more likely than depressed patients to exhibit derailment. Andreasen (1979a,b, 1984) found less evidence of thought disorder in her depressed patients than in schizophrenic patients, perhaps reflecting either true differences or differences in illness severity, assessment techniques, and diagnostic criteria (bipolar–unipolar differences were not specified).

Delusions and hallucinations often occur in severe bipolar depression, but they are less frequent than psychotic symptomatology in mania. Depressive delusions tend to focus on fixed ideas of guilt and sinfulness, poverty, hypochondriacal and somatic concerns, and feelings of persecution.[19] As shown in Table 2–8 (presented earlier), delusions were present in 12 to 66 percent of bipolar depressive episodes versus 44 to 96 percent of manic episodes. Hallucinations, less common in both mania and depression, were relatively more frequent in manic episodes. Several investigators have found a constancy in the presence or absence of psychotic symptoms across major depressive episodes,[20] although generalizability from unipolar to bipolar depression has not been demonstrated. Charney and Nelson (1981) found that 95 percent of their delusional patients but only 8 percent of their nondelusional patients had experienced prior delusional episodes. Among patients whose index admission was psychotic, 89 percent of all previous episodes had been psychotic as well. Helms and Smith (1983) reported that 92 percent of their psychotic depressive patients with recurrent illness had experienced another admission for psychotic depression, while Lykouras and colleagues (1985) found that 92 percent of their delusional depressive patients had experienced previous episodes with delusional ideation, compared with 36 percent of their nonpsychotic depressive patients. Nelson and colleagues (1984, p. 298) observed:

> It would appear that the presence of delusions during an index episode of depression may be not merely an indicator of severity of that episode, but additionally a distinct stable trait which would be expressed in the biologically vulnerable individual during prior and subsequent episodes.

Aronson and colleagues (1988), studying bipolar as well as unipolar delusional depressive patients, also found a consistency of psychotic expression across episodes, as well as an association with a marked rate of relapse. They noted that psychoticism may be an independent variable that can present in either bipolar or nonbipolar depression. The question of whether psychoticism is to some extent independent of polarity and diagnosis (for example, schizophrenia and bipolar illness) is discussed in Chapter 13, as are family-history studies of bipolar and unipolar delusional depression; additional reviews of clinical correlates of unipolar delusional depression are presented elsewhere.[21] A recent large-scale analysis (N = 4,274) of three family studies found that the diagnosis of bipolar-I was far more predictive of psychotic symptoms during depression than was the diagnosis of recurrent major depression (odds ratio [OR] = 5.13) (Goes et al., in press).

Bipolar patients who experience psychotic depressions tend to have a more severe and more chronic course than those who do not. They also have fewer atypical features and less Axis I comorbidity (Benazzi, 1999c).

Activity and Behavior

Activity, behavior, and somatic symptoms during bipolar depression as noted by Winokur and colleagues (1969) are summarized in Table 2–12; comparison figures from Carlson and Strober (1979) and Casper and colleagues (1985) also are given. Sleep difficulties are pronounced and pervasive. Fatigue and psychomotor retardation are seen in approximately three-fourths of bipolar depressed patients; loss of appetite and sexual drive are common as well. Women are more likely than men to report weight and appetite changes during periods of bipolar depression (Benazzi, 1999; Kawa et al., 2005). Most patients have somatic complaints, and the majority report a diurnal mood variation (most feel worse in the morning and better in the evening).

MIXED STATES

Mixed states, in which symptoms of depression and mania combine, represent a complex and often confusing aspect of the clinical presentation of bipolar illness. They can be conceived of as transitional states from one phase of illness to another or as independent clinical states combining various mixes of mood, thought, and activity components. To a considerable extent, mixed states are even more vulnerable to the inadequacies of modern diagnostic systems than other types or stages of affective illness. Indeed, systematic diagnostic criteria, impressively standardized for most other types and phases of affective disorders, are least validated for mixed states. Differential diagnosis—especially among mixed states, agitated depressions, and borderline pathologies—can be a difficult clinical problem (see Chapter 3).

Mixed states are broadly defined as the simultaneous presence of depressive and manic symptoms. Yet we know, for example, as noted earlier, that mania frequently is accompanied by moderate to severe depression. Should depression during mania be conceptualized as a mixed state, a typical mania, an atypical mania, or a severe (stage-related) form of mania? Should a mixed depressive episode be defined by the presence of four manic symptoms or only two? Are the diagnostic criteria of DSM-IV prohibitively strict, as most researchers think? (According to DSM-IV, a diagnosis of mixed states requires that all of the criteria, except duration, for both a manic and a depressive episode be met "nearly every day" during at least a 1-week period, and that the symptoms be severe enough to cause "marked impairment" or necessitate hospitalization, or that there be psychotic features.) Until more systematic and discriminating definitions and criteria are developed, the pragmatism of the immediate clinical or research issue will determine the answers to such questions.

Classic Clinical Descriptions

Mixed states are important for both theoretical and clinical reasons. (Their implications for pathophysiology are discussed in Chapter 17 and for treatment in Chapters 18 and 19.) Despite the diagnostic difficulties noted above, their existence has been recognized for centuries. A seventeenth-century physician (Brouchier, 1679; cited in Dewhurst, 1962, p. 122) described the alternating and combining qualities of mania and melancholy in one of his patients, a Lady Grenville. Characterizing the illness as "her Ladyship's annual raving," he wrote to her husband:

> For there are twin symptoms, which are her constant companions, Mania and Melancholy, and they succeed each other in a double and alternate act; or take each other's place like the smoke and flame of a fire; so that the

TABLE 2–12. **Activity, Behavior, and Somatic Symptoms in Bipolar Depression**

Category of Symptoms	PERCENTAGE OF PATIENTS		
	Winokur et al., 1969[a]	Carlson and Strober, 1979	Casper et al., 1985
Sleep Disorder			
Insomnia	100		
Global sleep disturbance			85
Difficulty falling asleep	58		
Early-morning awakening	27		77
Hypersomnia	23		
Activity			
Fatigue	76		
Psychomotor retardation	76	83	
Social withdrawal	100		
Weight and Appetite			
Loss of appetite	97	50	45
Increase in appetite			23
Loss of weight			26
Libido			
Loss of sexual interest	73		77
Somatic Complaints	67		
Diurnal Mood Variation	64		72

[a]100 episodes, 61 patients.

noble patient is first melancholy, while her animal spirits are unable to disentangle themselves from the dense cloud of fumes which surround them; and then maniacal, when the saline and sulphureous atoms of the blood are stirred up and loosened by the immoderate heat of their surroundings.

Heinroth (1818) delineated, in detail, mixed states of exaltation and depression (see Marneros, 2001). Later in the mid-nineteenth century, Falret (cited in Sedler, 1983) noted the strong depressive quality often observed before, during, and after manic episodes, as well as *melancolie anxieuse*. The latter state, he wrote, is "characterized by constant pacing and inner turmoil, which incapacitates these patients

so they cannot concentrate, and this state sometimes ends up as manic agitation." Kraepelin (1921, pp. 4, 191–192) described mixed states and their similarities and dissimilarities to manic and depressive states as follows:

We observe also clinical "*mixed forms,*" in which the phenomena of mania and melancholia are combined with each other, so that states arise, which indeed are composed of the same morbid symptoms as these, but cannot without coercion be classified either with the one or with the other. . . . The mixed states frequently fall outside the limits of the ordinary states in a very conspicuous way. . . . Our customary grouping into manic and melancholic attacks does not fit the facts, but requires substantial enlargement, if it is to reproduce nature. At the same time it turned out that this enlargement ran out in the direction not of the fitting in of fresh morbid symptoms, but only of the different combination of morbid symptoms known for long. Further, it was seen that the mixed states, even when they appeared not as interpolations but as independent attacks, behaved with regard to their course and issue quite similarly to the usual forms, and lastly, that they might in the same morbid course simply take the place of the other attacks especially after a somewhat long duration of the malady.

Kraepelin conceptualized mixed states as primarily transitional phenomena, but recognized their existence as individual attacks that frequently occur in later stages of the illness, often associated with poor outcome. Table 2–13 summarizes Kraepelin's classification and description of mixed states, which he conceptualized as different combinations of the manic and depressive symptoms of mood, activity, and thought. Below is Kraepelin's (1921, pp. 103–104) description of two of the most important kinds of these mixed states, *depressive* or *anxious mania* and *excited depression*:

> Depressive or Anxious Mania—If in the picture depression takes the place of cheerful mood, a morbid state arises, which is composed of flight of ideas, excitement, and anxiety. The patients are distractible, absent-minded, enter into whatever goes on round them, take themselves up with everything, catch up words and continue spinning out the ideas stirred up by these; they do not acquire a clear picture of their position, because they are incapable of systematic observation, and their attention is claimed by every new impression. They complain that they must think so much, their thoughts come of themselves, they have a great need of communicating their thoughts, but easily lose the thread, they can be brought out of the connection by every interpolated question, suddenly break off and pass to quite other trains of thought. Many patients display a veritable passion for writing, and scrawl over sheets and sheets of paper with disorderly effusions. At the same time ideas of sin and persecution are usually present, frequently also hypochondriacal delusions, as we have formerly described them.
>
> Mood is anxiously despairing; it gives itself vent in great restlessness, which partly assumes the form of movements of expression and practical activity, but partly also passes over into a wholly senseless pressure of activity. The patients run about, hide away, force their way out, make movements of defense or attack; they lament, scream, screech, wring or fold their hands, beat them together above their head, tear out their hair, cross themselves, slide about kneeling on the floor. With these are associated rhythmical, rubbing, flourishing, snatching,

turning, twitching movements, snapping with the jaw, blowing, barking, growling. If one will, one might here speak of a "depressive" or "anxious" mania.

> Excited Depression—If in the state described the flight of ideas is replaced by inhibition of thought, there arises the picture of excited depression. It is here a case of patients who display, on the one hand, extraordinary poverty of thought but, on the other hand, great restlessness. They are communicative, need the doctor, have a great store of words, but are extraordinarily monotonous in their utterances. To questions they give short answers to the point, and then immediately return to their complaints again, which are brought forth in endless repetition, mostly in the same phrases. About their position in general they are clear; they perceive fairly well, understand what goes on, apart from delusional interpretation. Nevertheless they trouble themselves little about their surroundings, they are only occupied with themselves.
>
> Mood is anxious, despondent, lachrymose, irritable, occasionally mixed with a certain self-irony. Sometimes one hears from the patients witty or snappish remarks. Delusions are frequently present, but they are usually scantier and less extraordinarily spun out than in the form just described. The excitement of the patients also is usually not so stormy or protean. They run hither and thither, up and down, wring their hands, pluck at things, speak loud out straight in front of them, give utterance to rhythmic cries and torment themselves as well as their surroundings often to the uttermost by continuous, monotonous lamenting.

Jaspers, while noting occasional ambiguity in Kraepelin's nosology of mixed states, acknowledged its clinical utility. The many possible combinations of components—euphoria, flight of ideas, and pressure of movement on the one hand, and sadness and retardation of thought and of movement on the other—made possible a better understanding of the wide variety of affective states seen in clinical practice. Thus, Jaspers (1997, p. 598; first published in 1913) described a mixed melancholia, one that he suggested might be characterized as a "querulant mania" or "nagging depression" in some, and as a "wailing melancholia" in others:

> In this state the over-valued or compulsive depressive ideas become delusionlike. They are fantastically elaborated (the patients are the cause of all the misfortune in the world; they are thought to be beheaded by the devil, etc.). The ideas are believed even though the patient seems relatively sensible. Underlying the experiences there are a host of *body sensations* (which soon lead to hypochondriacal delusions: the patients are filled up to the neck with excreta; the food falls through the empty body right to the bottom); then there are the most severe

TABLE 2–13. Kraepelin's Classification of Mixed States

	I. Depressive or Anxious Mania	II. Excited or Agitated Depression	III. Mania with Poverty of Thought
Mood	*Anxiety* Anxiously despairing.	*Anxiety* Anxious, despondent, lachrymose, irritable, occasional self-irony.	*Elation* Cheerful, pleased, unrestrained; somewhat irritated, repellent, or afterwards breaking into a merry laugh.
Activity	*Overactivity* Great restlessness; wholly senseless pressure of activity.	*Overactivity* They run hither and thither, wring their hands, pluck at things; loud rhythmic cries; monotonous lamenting.	*Overactivity* Excitement is often limited to making faces, dancing about, throwing things, changes in dress; many conduct themselves so quietly and methodically that superficial excitement does not appear at all; incapable of regular occupation, very abrupt, short-lived, impulsive outbursts of violence.
Thought	*Flight of Ideas* Distractible, absent-minded; incapable of systematic observation; veritable passion for writing with disorderly effusions; thoughts come of themselves.	*Inhibition of Thought* Delusions are frequently present; extraordinary poverty of thought; extraordinarily monotonous in utterances; perceive well, understand what goes on, apart from delusional interpretation.	*Inhibition of Thought* Perceive slowly and inaccurately; cannot immediately call things to mind. Their conversation is monotonous, not infrequently making an impression of weak-mindedness; state is subject to great fluctuation.
Summary Mood Activity Thought	Depressed Manic Manic	Depressed Manic Depressed	Manic Manic Depressed

(continued)

TABLE 2–13. Kraepelin's Classification of Mixed States *(continued)*

	IV. Manic Stupor	V. Depression with Flight of Ideas	VI. Inhibited Mania
Mood	*Elation*	*Depression*	*Elation*
	Cheerful; smile without recognizable cause; supportive, erotic.	Cast-down and hopeless; anxiety; sad and moody.	More exultant, occasionally irritable, distractible, inclined to jokes.
Activity	*Gross Motor Retardation*	*Motor Retardation*	*Motor Retardation*
	Usually inaccessible; lie quiet in bed; decorate themselves, without sign of restlessness or excitement. Not infrequently catalepsy can be demonstrated. Unexpectedly give utterance to loud and violent abuse, throw their food, suddenly take off their clothes, and immediately sink back into inaccessibility.	They read much, show interest in, and have understanding of their surroundings, although almost mute, and rigid in their whole conduct.	In outward behaviors, conspicuously quiet; it appears, however, as if a great inward tension existed, as patients may suddenly become very violent.
Thought	*Inhibition of Thought*	*Flight of Ideas*	*Flight of Ideas*
	Occasionally isolated delusions of changing content find utterance; for the most part they prove themselves fairly sensible and well oriented.	Incited by delusions; occasionally patients who cannot give utterance in speech are capable of writing; often desultory, full of ideas of sin and delusional fears; heaping up of synonymous phrases, jumping off to side thoughts, show flight of ideas, recognizable only in writings.	They easily fall into chattering talk with flight of ideas and numerous clang associations.
Summary			
Mood	Manic	Depressed	Manic
Activity	Depressed	Depressed	Depressed
Thought	Depressed	Manic	Manic

Source: Kraepelin, 1921. Reproduced with permission.

forms of *depersonalization* and *derealisation*: the world is no more, they themselves no longer exist, but still since they seem to exist they will have to live for ever (nihilistic delusions); finally there is extreme *anxiety*: the patients seek relief from this by keeping constantly on the move and indulging in a monotonous pressure of talk which almost becomes verbigeration: 'God, God, what will come of it, all, everything is gone, everything is gone, everything is gone, what will come of it?' etc. Even when the anxiety and melancholy have lifted, the patterns of movement, the facial expression and pressure of talk seem to maintain an *ossified* state until—often after a considerable time—the phase finally abates and recovery commences.

Manic stupor, according to Kraepelin's student and colleague Weygandt (1899, translated into English in the *Harvard Review*, 2002, p. 276), is the most important of the mixed states:

> Manic stupor as a phase of manic-depressive insanity is characterized by psychomotor inhibition and manic, elevated mood, with inhibition of thought (which usually occurs in a depressive state) instead of flight-of-ideas. This condition can occur transiently during a manic or depressive episode, particularly during switching from the manic phase to the depressive, when a shift has already taken place in psychomotor activity but not in affect . . . .
>
> The psychopathological condition is usually characterized by psychomotor manifestations (specifically stupor) as the prominent feature: some patients lie [in bed] showing very severe inhibition for a long time. Their limbs are cold; they refuse food, and every attempt to feed them is vain due to their opposition; for months they are mute. Only the facial expression, which shows no trace of depression and often shows a slight smile, reveals that a case is not typical circular [manic-depressive] stupor with depressed mood. In other cases, the [psychomotor] block is less intense: such patients may answer if asked questions, but they speak in a soft voice and hesitate before replying. They prefer not to speak spontaneously at all. Furthermore, these patients want to stay in bed all the time and refuse to work. Considerable retardation in their movements can be observed immediately: the gait is heavy and leaden; they hesitate to shake hands; and their writing is clearly slowed down. In less severe cases, the [psychomotor] block is occasionally interrupted by a fast, goal-directed movement.

Campbell (1953, pp. 144, 146), with his characteristic and important emphasis on the ever-fluctuating nature of moods, reiterated the mixed nature of most of the emotional and physical states associated with bipolar illness:

> There are more mixed reactions of this disease than is generally realized. It could truly be stated that, to some extent, all manic-depressive reactions are "mixed" types, in that the symptomatology is anything but static.
>
> The mixed type of manic-depressive psychosis epitomizes the entire cyclothymic process, in that it contains the symptoms characteristic of the various phases. Whether it is a sustained reaction or represents a phase of metamorphosis between the major forms, the mixed type emphasizes the underlying similarities between the depressive and hypomanic, the fact that the manic and depressive reactions may be superimposed, and that the same individual possesses the potentialities for either form. . . . Manic-depressive is a dynamic, constantly changing process which, at times, may manifest symptoms of both phases simultaneously. It is in the mixed form that the observer graphically realizes the homogeneity of the entire process.

Subjective Experiences of Patients

The extreme mental anguish often experienced during mixed states, including the terrifying thoughts and feelings associated with racing thoughts, delusions, and auditory hallucinations, was described by one bipolar patient whose mixed state was experienced at the height of a manic episode that, prior to that point, had been purely euphoric (as had countless hypomanias). Despite the strong and prolonged preponderance of classic euphoric mania in each of her episodes, the occasional transition into a mixed state was a potent feature of her illness. The simultaneous existence of suicidal thinking and mania is clearly portrayed in this description (Jamison, 1995, pp. 82–83):

> I felt infinitely worse, more dangerously depressed, during this first manic episode than when in the midst of my worst depressions. In fact, the most dreadful I have ever felt in my entire life—one characterized by chaotic ups and downs—was the first time I was psychotically manic. I had been mildly manic many times before, but they had never been frightening experiences—ecstatic at best, confusing at worst. I had learned to accommodate quite well to them. I had developed mechanisms of self-control, to keep down the peals of singularly inappropriate laughter, and had set rigid limits on my irritability. I avoided situations that might otherwise trip or jangle my hypersensitive wiring, and I learned to pretend I was paying attention or following a logical point when my mind was off chasing rabbits in a thousand directions. My work and professional life flowed. But nowhere did this, or my upbringing, or my intellect, or my character, prepare me for insanity.
>
> Although I had been building up to it for weeks, and certainly knew something was seriously wrong, there was

a definite point when I knew I was insane. My thoughts were so fast that I couldn't remember the beginning of a sentence halfway through. Fragments of ideas, images, sentences raced around and around in my mind like the tigers in a children's story. Finally, like those tigers, they became meaningless melted pools. Nothing once familiar to me was familiar. I wanted desperately to slow down but could not. Nothing helped—not running around a parking lot for hours on end or swimming for miles. My energy level was untouched by anything I did. Sex became too intense for pleasure, and during it I would feel my mind encased by black lines of light that were terrifying to me. My delusions centered on the slow painful deaths of all the green plants in the world—vine by vine, stem by stem, leaf by leaf they died and I could do nothing to save them. Their screams were cacophonous. Increasingly, all of my images were black and decaying.

At one point I was determined that if my mind—by which I made my living and whose stability I had assumed for so many years—did not stop racing and begin working normally again, I would kill myself by jumping from a nearby twelve-story building. I gave it twenty-four hours. But, of course, I had no notion of time, and a million other thoughts—magnificent and morbid—wove in and raced by. Endless and terrifying days of endlessly terrifying drugs—Thorazine, lithium, valium, and barbiturates—finally took effect. I could feel my mind being reined in, slowed down, and put on hold. But it was a very long time until I recognized my mind again, and much longer until I trusted it.

In the nineteenth century, composer Hector Berlioz (1966, translated by Cairn, 1970, pp. 226–228), described his episodes of "spleen," or depression, one type of which he characterized as an agitated and deeply "malignant" state:

The fit fell upon me with appalling force. I suffered agonies and lay groaning on the ground, stretching out abandoned arms, convulsively tearing up handfuls of grass and wide-eyed innocent daisies, struggling against the crushing sense of absence, against a mortal isolation.

Yet such an attack is not to be compared with the tortures that I have known since then in ever-increasing measure. What can I say that will give some idea of this abominable disease? . . .

There are . . . two kinds of spleen; one mocking, active, passionate, malignant; the other morose and wholly passive, when one's only wish is for silence and solitude and the oblivion of sleep.

George Gordon, Lord Byron (in a letter dated August 1819) described his agitated and fluctuating moods during one of his many mixed depressive episodes:

I am so bilious—that I nearly lose my head—and so nervous that I cry for nothing—at least today I burst into tears all alone by myself over a cistern of Gold fishes—which are not pathetic animals. . . . I have been excited—and agitated and exhausted mentally and bodily all this summer—till I really sometimes begin to think not only "that I shall die at top first"—but that the moment is not very remote—I have had no particular cause of grief—except the usual accompaniments of all unlawful passions.

In a letter to a friend (written in December 1793), Scottish poet Robert Burns, who was also afflicted with a vexacious melancholia on and off throughout his life, provided a particularly graphic description of the terrible agitation that can accompany depression (*The Letters of Robert Burns*, ed. G.R. Roy, 1985):

Here I sit, altogether Novemberish, a damn'd mélange of Fretfulness & melancholy; not enough of the one to rouse me to passion; nor of the other to repose me in torpor; my soul flouncing & fluttering round her tenement, like a wild Finch caught amid the horrors of winter newly thrust into a cage.

Clinical Studies

To date, the best historical discussions of mixed states are those of Weygandt (1899), Kraepelin (1921), Campbell (1953), Winokur and colleagues (1969), Himmelhoch (1979), and Koukopoulos (Koukopoulos et al., 1992; Koukopoulos and Koukopoulos, 1999). These authors described the clinical course, presentation, and correlates of mixed states, as well as hypotheses regarding their etiology and nature (including their relationship to the continuum hypothesis of affective illness, kindling and rapid cycling, and mixed-heredity hypotheses).

Reported rates of mixed states vary as a function of the inclusion criteria—that is, whether the diagnostic criteria are narrow or broad—and the nature of the rating scales employed,[22] as reflected in the wide range of rates reported by the 18 studies summarized in Table 2–14. An average of 28 percent of affectively ill patients experienced mixed states across these studies. By any standard, mixed states are not as rare as they once were reputed to be. (Kraepelin and Weygandt, of course, were fully aware of how common mixed states are. In a study of 150 manic-depressive patients at the Heidelberg Psychiatric Clinic, 36 percent were diagnosed with a form of mixed states: 15 percent with sustained mixed episodes, 8 percent with agitated depression, 7 percent with manic stupor, and 6 percent with unproductive mania [Weygandt, 1899].)

Symptomatic presentations of mixed states range from a single opposite-state symptom found in the midst of an

TABLE 2–14. **Rates of Mixed Manic States in Representative Studies**

Study	Patients (N)	%
Winokur et al., 1969	61	16
Kotin and Goodwin, 1972	20	65
Himmelhoch et al., 1976	84	31
Akiskal and Puzantian, 1979	60	25
Nunn, 1979	112	36
Prien et al., 1988	103	67
Secunda et al., 1988	18	44
Post et al., 1989	48	46
Dell'Osso et al., 1991	108	45
McElroy et al., 1995	71	40
Perugi et al., 1997	261	>50[a]
Akiskal et al., 1998a	104	37
Cassidy et al., 1998	237	14
Dilsaver et al., 1999	105	54
Cassidy et al., 2001	327	13
Sato et al., 2002	576	10
Gonzalez-Pinto et al., 2003	103	24
Krüger et al., 2003	99	39
Total no. of patients	2,497	
Weighted mean		28[b]

[a]Because of the sampling methods, the use of enriched criteria from European concepts of mixed states (Berner et al., 1992) and various thresholds for diagnosing mixed states beyond the strict DSM-IV guidelines, the rate of mixed states in this study cannot be given as a single round figure. If excluded, weighted mean becomes 26%.

[b]Assuming the minimum 50% for Perugi et al.

otherwise "pure" manic or depressive syndrome (such as depressive mood during mania or racing thoughts during depression) to more complex mixes of mood, thought, and behavior. Documentation of the frequent occurrence of depressive mood during mania was presented earlier in Table 2–1. Kotin and Goodwin (1972) systematically inves-

tigated the relationship of depression to mania in 20 hospitalized patients. Through an analysis of nurses' and physicians' behavioral ratings and notes, they found a statistically significant positive association between mania and depression in the majority of cases.

Racing thoughts during depression can be considered another type of mixed state, one observed by earlier clinicians (Kraepelin, 1921; Lewis, 1934). More recently, this state was examined by Ianzito and colleagues (1974) and Braden and Qualls (1979). Ianzito's group found a relatively low rate of racing thoughts in their 89 depressed inpatients (5 percent), but they used the Present State Exam, which emphasizes the pleasurable and exciting quality as well as the rapidity of thought. Braden and Qualls, by contrast, found that one-third to one-half of their depressed inpatients reported racing thoughts, with a definite diurnal variation (worsening in the evening, greatest severity at bedtime). They drew the following conclusion (pp. 17–18):

> In bipolar patients and cyclothymics, the racing thoughts may occur in both "high" and "low" states. The symptom may thus be related more to the underlying pathology of the affective illness than to the characteristics of either "pole."

Other authors (Akiskal and Mallya, 1987; Koukopoulos and Koukopoulos, 1999; Benazzi and Akiskal, 2001) have favored the interpretation that racing—especially "crowded"—thoughts are indicative of mixed depressive states, and have invoked a significant excess of bipolar family history as validation of the bipolar nature of the phenomenon.

The symptomatic presentation of severe mixed states has been characterized in a variety of studies as dysphoric mood alternating with elevated mood, racing thoughts, grandiosity, suicidal ideation, persecutory delusions, auditory hallucinations, severe insomnia, psychomotor agitation, and hypersexuality (Cassidy et al., 1998; Perugi et al., 2001a; Brieger et al., 2003). Kotin and Goodwin (1972, p. 60) summarized their clinical impressions of mixed states as follows:

> Mania was nevertheless clearly identifiable by pressure of speech, increased motor activity, anger, intrusiveness, grandiosity, and mood instability. Depression during mania was frequently evidenced by expressed feelings of helplessness and hopelessness and thoughts of suicide. Sleep disturbance, irritability, anorexia, and many other symptoms are common to both conditions.

In their early study, Winokur and colleagues (1969) documented the course and symptoms of mixed states; the quantitative results of their work are given in Table 2–15. They concluded that the single most striking feature of

TABLE 2–15. Symptoms of Mixed Manic-Depressive Psychosis

Category of Symptoms	Percentage of Patients
Mood	
Depressed	100
Euphoric	100
Irritable	100
Labile	100
Hostile	79
Cognition and Perception	
Distractibility	100
Grandiosity	57
Flight of ideas	43
Delusions (depressive)	36
Delusions (nondepressive)	21
Auditory hallucinations	14
Visual hallucinations	7
Disorientation	7
Activity and Behavior	
Increased psychomotor activity	100
Insomnia	93
Pressure of speech	93
Decreased sexual interest	63
Suicidal threats or attempts	43
Increased alcohol intake	43
Anxiety attacks	43
Extravagance	14

Note: Based on 14 episodes of mixed manic-depressive psychosis in 10 patients.
Source: Adapted from Winokur et al., 1969.

mixed states was variability and lability of mood: "It is this panoply of varying and contrasting emotions which makes these patients difficult to diagnose" (p. 81). Winokur's group observed that mixed states tended to resemble mania in push of speech, physical activity, and hyperactivity. Delusions, on the other hand, tended to be depressive in nature, as did mood and vegetative signs and symptoms. The authors found that in 79 percent of cases, mixed states were gradual; that there was prior depression of appreciable clinical proportions in 71 percent of patients; that diurnal variation occurred in 64 percent; that the average period from onset to euthymia was 24 days; and that more than half (57 percent) of mixed episodes were followed by a depression.

Women made up 60 percent of Nunn's (1979) sample of patients with mixed states, consistent with the finding of Himmelhoch and colleagues (1976a) that 55 percent of their sample were women. Winokur and colleagues (1969) found a far more striking gender difference: 9 of their 10 patients with mixed episodes were women, and 13 of the 14 episodes they analyzed were experienced by women. The degree of this discrepancy almost certainly is due to the more stringent criteria used by these authors in defining mixed states. In the most comprehensive study to date, 908 bipolar patients were followed over a period of 7 years to assess mixed and euphoric hypomanias (Suppes et al., 2005). Mixed hypomania was more common than euphoric hypomania, and women were significantly more likely to experience a mixed symptomatic picture ($p < .001$).

Himmelhoch and colleagues (1976a) found no correlation between mixed states and severity of illness or rapidity of mood swings. They did find, however, that patients with mixed states were far more likely to have a history of substance abuse, especially alcoholism. This has been confirmed in some studies (Sonne et al., 1994; McElroy et al., 1995; Goldberg et al., 1999) but not in subsequent, larger investigations (Brieger, 2000; Cassidy et al., 2001). Current data indicate that mixed mania, unlike pure mania, which peaks in the spring, is more likely to peak in the late summer (Cassidy and Carroll, 2002), and both types of episodes tend to remain consistent over a prospective course (Cassidy et al., 2001b; Woods et al., 2001; Suppes et al., 2005). A recent study (Sato et al., 2006) found significant seasonal differences between 95 bipolar depressive patients and 77 unipolar patients with depressive mixed states when compared with 786 unipolar depressive patients without mixed states. Depressive episodes peaked in the spring in those without mixed states, but in those with mixed states (whether bipolar or unipolar), there was a significant autumn peak in depressive episodes. (It is not clear why unipolar patients with mixed states were not diagnosed as bipolar by the researchers.)

Winokur and colleagues (1969) examined the nature of delusions during mixed states and found, not surprisingly, that the type of delusion fluctuated with the patient's mood. Although depressive delusions were more frequent, manic-like delusions (nondepressed, grandiose, all religious) also occurred. Himmelhoch (1979, p. 453) emphasized the importance of manic delusions in differentiating unipolar agitated depression from mixed states:

> The clue to recognizing it [a mixed state] is the presence of distinct maniacal coloration of the psychotic material in the midst of all the severe depressive symptomatology . . . [for example] . . . grandiose, radiant, beatific religious delusions . . . out of tune with the patient's misery.

Recent studies have found a significant rate of delusions (23 percent) or delusions and/or hallucinations (40 percent) in mixed states (Mantere et al., 2004; Baethge et al., 2005). As some overlap exists between depressive and manic signs and symptoms (insomnia, anorexia, psychomotor agitation), the question arises of what constitutes the depressive manifestations "uncontaminated" by mania that would be suitable for the diagnostic assessment of mixed states. On the basis of a comprehensive review of the data (McElroy et al., 1992; Bauer et al., 1994, Cassidy et al., 1998), Akiskal and colleagues (2000) proposed the following depressive symptoms to support a diagnosis of dysphoric mania: depressed and/or labile mood, irritability, anhedonia, hopelessness/helplessness, suicidal thinking or behavior, guilt, and fatigue. Nonspecific symptoms, according to these authors, include agitation, changes in weight, and insominia.

Akiskal (1992b) proposed that mixed states arise when temperament and episodes are opposite in polarity—that is, mania arising from a depressive temperament and depression arising from a hyperthymic temperament. There has now been some preliminary validation of this view in several Italian, French, and German studies (Dell'Osso et al., 1991; Perugi et al., 1997; Brieger et al., 2003), but the diverse presentation of mixed states makes any single explanation necessarily incomplete and premature. Temperament may be decisive in determining the manifestation of mixed states in some individuals but ultimately is far less important than other factors—for example, comorbidity, chronicity of illness, medication effects—in many or even most patients.

While much of the research on mixed states has been in dysphoric or depressive mania, depressive mixed states (hypomanic behavior and/or symptoms intruding into depressive episodes) have been described since Kraepelin's (1899) and Weygandt's (1899) original contributions in this area. The most common manifestations of the excitatory pole in depressive mixed states are psychomotor activation and/or agitation, irritability and mood lability, racing or crowded thoughts, and sexual arousal, as well as severe insomnia, panic attacks, and suicidal crises in severely complicated variants.[23] Indeed, increased suicidality and the risk of suicide are particularly associated with mixed states (Hantouche et al., 2003; Strakowski et al., 1996; Marneros et al., 2004; see Chapter 8). A recent study of bipolar adolescents found that mixed states contributed independently to the risk of suicidal behavior, but the increased risk was among the girls only (Dilsaver et al., 2005). In a meta-analysis of risk factors for suicide and attempted suicide, Hawton and colleagues (2005) at the University of Oxford also found mixed states to be a significant risk factor.

Consistent with Aretaeus, who had observed that melancholics could be "angry without reason," Mammen and colleagues (2004) found that 39 percent of their bipolar patients reported anger attacks during depression. Such attacks may well represent a form of depressive mixed state.

As discussed in Chapter 1, Benazzi and Akiskal (2005) compared the relationship between irritability and other clinical features in a large number of bipolar-II and unipolar major depressive subjects. Major depressive episodes with irritability were present in 60 percent of their bipolar-II patients and in 37 percent of their depressive patients. In the bipolar-II patients, those who presented with irritability had a significantly younger age at index episode, higher rates of atypical depressive features, and more significant Axis I comorbidity relative to those who did not. They also were more likely to meet the study criteria for depressive mixed states, defined by the investigators as a major depressive episode plus three or more concurrent intradepressive hypomanic symptoms (whether occurring in the bipolar-II or major depressive patients). In the unipolar patients, those who presented with irritability had a significantly younger age at onset and higher rates of atypical depression; they were also more likely to meet criteria for a depressive mixed state and to have a family history of bipolar illness. According to the authors, their data demonstrate that irritability may be a good marker of depressive mixed states, a view consistent with that of others who have found high rates of irritability and anger attacks associated with these states (e.g., Fava and Rosenbaum, 1999; Deckersbach et al., 2004; Perlis et al., 2004). The relationship between age at onset and mixed states is unclear. Some investigators have found that earlier age at onset is associated with mixed states (Nunn, 1979; Post et al., 1989; McElroy et al., 1997), but others have not (Marneros et al., 1991a,b; Strakowski et al., 1996; Perugi et al., 1997).

In their discussion of depression with manic features, Koukopoulos and Koukopoulos (1999) suggested that all types of agitated depressions should be called "mixed depression." They proposed that the following diagnostic criteria be used: (1) major depressive episode and (2) at least two of the three symptoms of motor agitation, psychic agitation or intense inner tension, and racing or crowded thoughts. Perugi and colleagues (2001) have distinguished between depressive mixed states and non-mixed bipolar depression on the basis of depressive mixed states being characterized by fewer episodes of longer duration; less cyclicity; greater likelihood of mixed state at first episode; more previous mixed episodes; less interepisode remission; more incongruent psychotic features; and more agitation, irritability, pressured speech, and flight of ideas.

CYCLOTHYMIA AND MANIC-DEPRESSIVE TEMPERAMENTS

Classic Clinical Descriptions

Cyclothymia and related temperamental types represent a significant portion of the manic-depressive spectrum. The relationship of predisposing personalities (or temperaments) and cyclothymia to the subsequent development of manic-depressive illness is a fundamental one (as discussed further below, as well as in Chapters 1, 5, 6, and 10). *Cycloid temperament*, a generic term for the spectrum of manic-depressive personality types, is generally manifested as predominantly depressive, manic or hypomanic, irritable, or cyclothymic.[24] Campbell (1953, pp. 25–26) described these personality types and their relationship to manic-depressive illness and to one another:

> The term *cycloid personality* is an overall or general appellation, indicating all forms of the prepsychotic manic-depressive personality. The cycloid personality may occur in one of three forms, with innumerable gradations and mixtures between the three. First, is the hypomanic personality, the overactive, jovial, friendly, talkative and confident individual who, if he becomes psychotic, *usually* develops the manic form of manic-depressive psychosis. . . . Second, is the depressive type, the worried, anxious, thoughtful, sorrowful, individual who, if he becomes psychotic, *usually* develops the depressive form of manic-depressive psychosis. The third form of the cycloid personality is the cyclothymic personality who may have mixed traits, or be euphoric and friendly at one time, and depressed and pessimistic at another, and who may develop either a manic or depressive reaction, or swing from one into the other. It is important to realize

that the manic reaction, melancholia, hypomanic reaction, cyclothymic personality, cycloid personality, depressive personality and periodic insanity, are all a part of the same disease process, and that any one of these may change into any other.

The generic term *cycloid personality* used by Kretschmer encompasses all types of prepsychotic personality in manic-depressive patients. Kretschmer, too, stressed the overlap among these personality types (1936; cited in Campbell, 1953, pp. 26–27):

> Men of this kind have a soft temperament which can swing to great extremes. The path over which it swings is a wide one, namely between cheerfulness and unhappiness. . . . Not only is the hypomanic disposition well known to be a peculiarly labile one, which also has leanings in the depressive direction, but many of these cheerful natures have, when we get to know them better, a permanent melancholic element somewhere in the background of their being. . . . The hypomanic and melancholic halves of the cycloid temperament relieve one another, they form layers or patterns in individual cases, arranged in the most varied combinations.

Clearly, not all cyclothymic or cycloid personalities go on to develop the full manic-depressive syndrome, and here we concern ourselves primarily with clinical descriptions of the range of cycloid temperaments and cyclothymic disorders. Kraepelin (1921, pp. 119–120) described a *depressive temperament*, which is characterized by a "permanent gloomy emotional stress in all the experience of life":

> Patients, as a rule, have to struggle with all sorts of internal obstructions, which they only overcome with effort; . . . they lack the right joy in work. . . . From youth up there exists in the patients a special susceptibility for the cares, the difficulties, the disappointments of life . . . in every occurrence feel the small disagreeables much more strongly than the elevating and satisfying aspects. . . . Frequently . . . a capricious, irritable, unfriendly, repellent behaviour is developed. The patients are occupied only with themselves, do not trouble themselves about their surroundings. . . .
>
> Every task stands in front of them like a mountain; life with its activity is a burden which they habitually bear . . . without being compensated by the pleasure of existence.

In manic temperament, Kraepelin went on to say, the patients' "understanding of life and the world remains superficial"; their "train of thought is desultory, incoherent, aimless"; and their mood is "permanently exalted, careless, confident." (Centuries earlier, Aretaeus [cited in

Roccatagliata, 1986, p. 229] had described a predominantly manic form of illness that arose in those "whose personality is characterized by gayness, activity, superficiality and childishness." The mania itself was manifest in "furor, excitement and cheerfulness") Kraepelin (1921, pp. 126–128) said that such patients are

> convinced of their *superiority* to their surroundings. . . . Towards others they are haughty, positive, irritable, impertinent, stubborn. . . . *unsteadiness and restlessness* appear before everything. They are accessible, communicative, adapt themselves readily to new conditions, but soon they again long for change and variety. Many have belletristic inclinations, compose poems, paint, go in for music. . . . Their mode of expression is clever and lively; they speak readily and much, are quick at repartee, never at a loss for an answer or an excuse. . . . With their surroundings the patients often live in constant *feud.*

Kraepelin also discussed a milder form of manic temperament within the "domain of the normal," but still a "link in the long chain of manic-depressive dispositions," a form that progresses to what he termed the *irritable temperament.* In Kraepelin's (1921, pp. 129–131) words:

> It concerns here brilliant, but unevenly gifted personalities with artistic inclinations. They charm us by their intellectual mobility, their versatility, their wealth of ideas, their ready accessibility and their delight in adventure, their artistic capability, their good nature, their cheery, sunny mood. But at the same time they put us in an uncomfortable state of surprise by a certain restlessness, talkativeness, desultoriness in conversation, excessive need for social life, capricious temper and suggestibility, lack of reliability, steadiness, and perseverance in work, a tendency to building castles in the air . . . periods of causeless depression or anxiety. . . .
>
> The *irritable temperament,* a further form of manic-depressive disposition, is perhaps best conceived as a *mixture of the fundamental states* . . . in as much as in it manic and depressive features are associated. . . . The patients display from youth up extraordinarily great fluctuations in emotional equilibrium and are greatly moved by all experiences, frequently in an unpleasant way. While on the one hand they appear sensitive and inclined to sentimentality and exuberance, they display on the other hand great irritability and sensitiveness. They are easily offended and hot-tempered; they flare up, and on the most trivial occasions fall into outbursts of boundless fury. "She had states in which she was nearly delirious," was said of one patient; "Her rage is beyond all bounds," of another. It then comes to violent scenes with abuse, screaming and a tendency to rough behaviour. . . . The patients are positive, always in a mood for a fight, endure no contradiction, and, therefore, easily fall into disputes with the people round them, which they carry on with great passion. . . . The colouring of mood is subject to frequent change. . . .
>
> Their power of imagination is usually very much influenced by moods and feelings. It, therefore, comes easily to delusional interpretations of the events of life. The patients think that they are tricked by the people round them, irritated on purpose and taken advantage of.

Cyclothymic temperament is characterized, according to Kraepelin (1921, p. 131), by "frequent, more or less regular fluctuations of the psychic state to the manic or to the depressive side." He described cyclothymic individuals as follows (p. 132):

> These are the people who constantly oscillate hither and thither between the two opposite poles of mood, sometimes "rejoicing to the skies," sometimes "sad as death." To-day lively, sparkling, beaming, full of the joy of life, the pleasure of enterprise, and pressure of activity, after some time they meet us depressed, enervated, ill-humoured, in need of rest, and again a few months later they display the old freshness and elasticity.

Kretschmer (1936, p. 132) pointed out a tendency of these individuals to drift toward either mania or depression:

> The temperament of the cycloids alternates between cheerfulness and sadness, in deep, smooth, rounded waves, only more quickly and transitorily with some, more fully and enduring with others. But the mid-point of these oscillations lies with some nearer the hypomanic, and with others nearer the depressive pole.

Slater and Roth (1969, pp. 206–207) provided a general description of the "constitutional cyclothymic," emphasizing the natural remissions and seasonal patterns often inherent in the temperament. The alternating mood states, each lasting for months at a time, are continuous in some individuals but subside, leaving periods of normality, in others. In Slater and Roth's words, the cyclothymic constitution

> is perhaps less frequent than the other two "basic states," but its existence in artists and writers has attracted some attention, especially as novelists like Björnsen and H. Hesse have given characteristic descriptions of the condition. Besides those whose swings of mood never intermit, there are others with more or less prolonged *intervals of normality.* In the hypomanic state the patient feels well, but the existence of such states accentuates his feeling of insufficiency and even illness in the depressive phases. At such times he will often seek the advice of his practitioner,

complaining of such vague symptoms as headache, insomnia, lassitude, and indigestion. . . . In typical cases such alternative cycles will last a lifetime. In cyclothymic artists, musicians, and other creative workers the rhythm of the cycles can be read from the dates of the beginning and cessation of productive work. Some cyclothymics have a *seasonal rhythm* and have learned to adapt their lives and occupations so well to it that they do not need medical attention.

According to Koukopoulos (2003, p. 202), observing a cyclothymic patient who is depressed, "one is spontaneously reminded of a machine in which the oil has run dry and the gears grind on in laborious suffering, rasping against one another until they seize up in pain." When hypomanic, on the other hand, the patient is entirely different (p. 203):

> Instead of the inhibition that was previously felt, the course of thoughts is now faster, the perception of external impressions easier and more immediate, so the patient appears to be more intelligent, full of wit and more entertaining than in the healthy days. As for the increased capacity for criticizing, which as already mentioned may present itself also in the depressive state, this may now become so strong as to be considered vexing by the patient himself. It often betokens itself by an arrogant, mocking smirk. The elevated mental capacity leads in the majority of cases to a restless, non-stop activity and dynamism which develops in the widest variety of directions. It is not only the stamina of the patient, which appears greater than that of the healthy days, but the level of skill and ability that is increased in various ways. Many, for instance, who had a rather mediocre voice and in their depressive intervals—were without much musical talent—now sing not only with great eagerness, but also with a better tone of voice and a livelier expressiveness. Others display, in manual tasks and their mode of dress, a skill and taste which they did not formerly possess. And others manifest a literary bent that was quite alien to them before.
>
> All these characteristics are, as I observed above, due to the expression of the expansive mood, which as a rule sweeps over the patient suddenly. All at once he sees the rosy side of life and at the same time feels a desire to have others partake in his joy, to help his fellow men and carry out activities that frequently bear fruit in the fields of charity and humanitarian interests.

Clinical Studies

Compelling evidence argues for including cyclothymia as an integral part of the spectrum of manic-depressive illness. The data presented here describe several aspects of cyclothymia: its clinical presentation; symptomatic patterns of mood, cognition, and behavior; and subsequent development of full affective episodes in cyclothymic patients.[25] (Related issues are discussed in Chapters 1, 10, and 11.)

In his early review of the literature, Waters (1979) cited widespread agreement that mood and energy swings often precede clinical illness by years. In a study of 33 patients with definite bipolar illness, he found that one-third reported bipolar mood swings or hypomania predating the actual onset of their illness. These subsyndromal mood swings were characterized by (1) onset in early adulthood; (2) occurrence most often in spring or fall; (3) occurrence on an annual or biennial basis; (4) onset unrelated to current life events (with the exception of the first episode); (5) persistence of symptoms for 3 to 10 weeks; (6) a change in energy level, rather than the experience of dysphoria; and (7) sensitivity to lithium treatment (comparable to that for manifest bipolar illness). More recently, Kochman and colleagues (2005) assessed 80 depressed children and adolescents with the Kiddie-SADS semistructured interview and a newly developed questionnaire to measure cyclothymic–hypersensitive temperament. At the end of the 2- to 4-year follow-up period, 43 percent of the sample had been diagnosed as bipolar. Of the children and adolescents who had been categorized as cyclothymic–hypersensitive, 64 percent developed bipolar disorder; of those who had not been so categorized, only 15 percent experienced a hypomanic or manic episode ($p < .001$).

In a study of the natural course or progression of cyclothymia, that is, the relationship of cyclothymic states to the subsequent development of bipolar affective episodes, approximately one-third (36 percent) of 50 cyclothymic patients, in contrast to only 4 percent of 50 nonaffective controls, developed full syndromal depression, hypomania, or mania (Akiskal et al., 1979b). Of the 25 cyclothymic patients requiring antidepressant medication for their depressive illness, 11 (44 percent) became hypomanic. This rate was comparable to the switch rate in bipolar controls (35 percent).

Akiskal and colleagues further described and quantified these "subsyndromal" mood swings. Box 2–1 presents revised operational criteria for cyclothymia based on a population study that tested the authors' clinically derived criteria (Akiskal et al., 1979a, 1998b). Their original sample of 50 cyclothymic patients was characterized by the following: a female/male ratio of 3:2; young age at onset, which is consistent with other data suggesting an onset of first symptoms between ages 12 and 14 (Akiskal et al., 1977; Depue et al., 1981); and a tendency for the first clinical presentation to be perceived as a personality rather than a mood disorder, with family members and friends describing the

Biphasic subclinical mood swings with abrupt and labile shifts, and with variability in duration, measured from hours to a few days. At least four of the following constitute the habitual long-term baseline of the subject:

- Lethargy alternating with eutonia
- Shaky self-esteem alternating between low self-confidence and overconfidence
- Decreased verbal output alternating with talkativeness
- Mental confusion alternating with sharpened and creative thinking
- Unexplained tearfulness alternating with excessive punning and jocularity
- Introverted self-absorption alternating with uninhibited people seeking

Source: Akiskal et al., 1998b. Reprinted with permission from Elsevier.

patient as "high-strung," "explosive," "moody," "hyperactive," or "sensitive."

Mood, cognitive, and behavioral patterns in 46 patients with cyclothymia were studied by Akiskal and colleagues (1977); although based on a small sample, their findings are useful in providing an overall view of cyclothymic states. As might be expected, the mood and cognitive aspects parallel, in milder form, those for mania and depression. Three-fourths of Akiskal and colleagues' patients met criteria for alternating patterns of sleep disorder, fluctuating levels in the quality and quantity of work or school productivity, and financial disinhibition. One-half of the patients reported periods of irritability or aggressiveness, patterns of frequent shifts in interests or plans, drug or alcohol abuse, or fluctuating levels of social interaction. Episodic promiscuity or extramarital affairs were reported by 40 percent of the sample, and joining new movements with zeal, followed by disillusionment, by 25 percent. Although frequencies of specific behavior patterns are of interest, replicated and comparison population figures are necessary. Thus we await more detailed studies of cognitive and perceptual changes across mood states, much larger sample sizes, and replications utilizing more standardized measures.

Cyclothymia is a common temperamental variant, occurring in 0.4 to 6.3 percent of the population (Depue et al., 1981; Placidi et al., 1998; Chiaroni et al., 2005). According to Akiskal (1998), the most frequent subtypes of cyclothymia are *pure cyclothymia* (equal proportion of depressive and hypomanic swings, alternating in an irregular fashion), *predominantly depressed cyclothymia* (depressive periods dominating the clinical picture,

interspersed with "even," "irritable," and occasional hypomanic periods), and *hyperthymia* (hypomanic traits—decreased need for sleep, expansive behavior, "wild lifestyle"—dominating, with occasional depressive and irritable episodes). Systematic qualitative data to verify this taxonomy do not exist, however.

Discriminatory criteria for the irritable temperament have remained elusive (Akiskal, 1992a; Akiskal et al., 1998b). The hyperthymic type, by contrast, is probably distinct from the cyclothymic (Akiskal, 1992a). Indeed, in a factor analytic study of temperaments in an Italian student population, the cyclothymic and hyperthymic types emerged as separate superfactors (Akiskal et al., 1998b). The hyperthymic type is best described as adaptive-trait hypomania (which distinguishes it from hypomanic episodes), consisting of the triad of high energy, overconfidence, and cheerfulness, with virtually no depressive dips (which distinguishes this type from the cyclothymic type proper). Again, while such speculations are interesting, they need greater validation and replication.

The validated criteria for the cyclothymic type summarized in Box 2–1 portray a temperament with greater instability than the hyperthymic type, and for that reason one perhaps more proximal to bipolar disorder; indeed, cyclothymia often precedes or underlies bipolar-II disorder (Hantouche et al., 1998; Perugi and Akiskal, 2002). Of the affective temperaments, cyclothymia is the most correlated with emotional and behavioral problems (Signoretta et al., 2005).

On the other hand, the hyperthymic type represents a more adaptive set of traits. The criteria for hyperthymic temperament, as validated by Akiskal and colleagues (1998a), require that four of the following traits (which constitute the habitual long-term functioning of the individual) be present: (1) warm, people seeking, or extraverted; (2) cheerful, overoptimistic, or exuberant; (3) uninhibited, stimulus seeking, or risk taking; (4) overinvolved and meddlesome; (5) vigorous, overenergetic, and full of plans; (6) self-assured, overconfident, or boastful; and (7) overtalkative or articulate. Researchers in Italy (Maremmani et al., 2005) compared responses from 1,010 students aged 14 to 26 on Cloninger's revised Tridimensional Personality Questionnaire (TPQ) (Cloninger, 1987) and on the semi-structured affective temperament interview (TEMPS-I) (Placidi et al., 1998). The TPQ constructs of gregariousness, exploratory excitability, uninhibited optimism, attachment, confidence, extravagance, independence, vigor, and impulsiveness correlated highly with the temperamental construct of hyperthymia. Jamison (2004) has discussed at length the relationship among exuberant, hyperthymic, and extraverted temperaments, as well as the relationship between such temperaments and psychological resilience (see also Chapter 10).

Psychiatric studies of temperament would benefit enormously from the addition of the perspectives and methodologies used by developmental psychologists who have studied early manifestations of temperament and the development of temperament over time, from infancy to adulthood. Particularly relevant here is the paradigm used by Jerome Kagan and colleagues in their important studies of inhibited and uninhibited temperaments.[26] At present, we lack the sophisticated developmental and genetic approaches that ultimately will provide the kind of information needed to adequately understand the manic-depressive spectrum of temperaments.

CONCLUSIONS

This chapter has presented a clinical description of manic-depressive illness (with emphasis on the bipolar form) that combines three methods of observation: descriptions of both ancient and modern clinical observers, first-person accounts from patients with manic-depressive illness, and results obtained from clinical studies. Each method is unique, invaluable, but incomplete. Good clinical description is beholden to all three perspectives.

Pathognomonic cycles of mood and activity serve as a background for ongoing fluctuations in thinking, perception, and behavior. The bipolar form of manic-depressive illness encompasses the extremes of human experience. Moods swing between euphoria and despair, irritability and panic. Cognition can range from psychosis or delirium to a pattern of fast, clear, and sometimes creative associations; it can also manifest as retardation so profound that consciousness is clouded. Behavior can be seductive, hyperactive–expansive, and dangerous; or it can be reclusive, sluggish, and suicidal.

The rapid undulations and combinations of such extremes result in an intricately textured clinical picture. It is important to note that the designation "mixed states" is often arbitrary. Indeed, manic patients are depressed and irritable at least as often as they are elated, and bipolar depressed patients are frequently agitated and may have racing thoughts.

NOTES

1. Falret, 1854 (translated by Sedler, 1983); Kraepelin, 1921; Campbell, 1953; Wellner and Marstal, 1964; Beigel and Murphy, 1971a; Cassidy et al., 2001a, 2002; Woods et al., 2001; Sato et al., 2004.

2. Kraepelin continued:

> Statues salute him by nodding; the moon falls down from the sky; the trumpets of the Day of Judgment are sounding. He hears the voice of Jesus, speaks with God and the poor souls, is called by God dear son. There are voices in his ears; the creaking of the floor, the sound of the bells take on the form of words. The patient has telepathic connection with an aristocratic fiancée, feels the electric current in the walls, feels himself hypnotized; transference of thought takes place.

3. As discussed later in this chapter, Carlson and Goodwin (1973), in their systematic study of the stages of mania, found that mania usually evolves gradually. In their hospitalized patients, the early stages of mania could be discerned in nurses' recordings of mood and behavior reviewed after the apparently sudden onset of manic episodes.

4. Harrow et al., 1972a,b, 1982, 1983, 1986; Harrow and Quinlan, 1977; Harrow and Prosen, 1978.

5. Harrow et al., 1972a,b, 1986; Himmelhoch et al., 1973; Adler and Harrow, 1974; Harrow and Quinlan, 1977; Grossman et al., 1981.

6. Breakey and Goodell, 1972; Grossman et al., 1981; Andreasen, 1984; Shenton et al., 1987; Solovay et al., 1987.

7. The discrepancy between the results of these two groups may be due in part to differences in the assessment of thought disorder. Resnick and Oltmanns (1984) used a global rating, whereas Harrow and colleagues (1982) used specific tests.

8. Andreasen, 1984; Resnick and Oltmanns, 1984; Simpson and Davis, 1985; Ragin and Oltmanns, 1987.

9. Morice and Ingram, 1983; Morice and McNicol, 1986; Docherty et al., 1996; Thomas et al., 1996; Lott et al., 2002.

10. Pease, 1912; Rosenthal et al., 1979; Harrow et al., 1990; Goldberg et al., 1995; Keck et al., 2003.

11. Beigel and Murphy, 1971b; Murphy and Beigel, 1974; Taylor and Abrams, 1975; Rosen et al., 1983b; Young et al., 1983, Winokur et al., 1985; Coryell et al., 1990, 2001; Tohen et al., 1990; Young and Klerman, 1992; Toni et al., 2001.

12. Brockington et al., 1983; Winokur, 1984; Coryell et al., 1990; Miklowitz, 1992; Tohen et al., 1992; Fennig et al., 1996; Perugi et al., 1999; Strakowski et al., 2000.

13. Double, 1990; Bauer et al., 1994; Cassidy et al., 1998; Dilsaver et al., 1999; Perugi et al., 2001b; Swann et al., 2001; Sato et al., 2002.

14. Suicidal behavior, discussed in the next section, is covered more fully in Chapter 8.

15. All quotations from this source are from F. Scott Fitzgerald, *The Crack-up*, copyright © 1945 by New Directions Publishing Corp. Reprinted by permission of New Directions Publishing Corp.

16. It is even more rare for a clinical study of unipolar depression to differentiate the highly recurrent form (part of Kraepelin's manic-depressive illness) from the nonrecurrent form.

17. Benazzi, 1999b, 2000a,b, 2001, 2003, 2004.

18. More specialized reviews of related clinical topics can be found in Chapters 1, 8, 9, 10, 11, and 16.

19. Kraepelin, 1921; Bowman and Raymond, 1931–1932a; Schneider, 1959; Beck, 1967; Winokur et al., 1969.

20. Charney and Nelson, 1981; Frangos et al., 1983; Helms and Smith, 1983; Winokur, 1984. Baethge et al., 2005.

21. Charney and Nelson, 1981; Frances et al., 1981; Glassman and Roose, 1981; Coryell and Tsuang, 1982; Nelson et al., 1984; Spiker et al., 1985; Roose and Glassman, 1988.

22. McElroy et al., 1992, 1995; Cassidy and Carroll, 1998; Cassidy et al., 1998; Sato et al., 2002.

23. Akiskal and Mallya, 1987; Koukopoulos and Koukopoulos, 1999; Benazzi, 2000b; Benazzi and Akiskal, 2001; Sato et al., 2003; Biondi et al., 2005; Benazzi, 2006; Oedegaard et al., 2006.

24. Reiss, 1910; Kraepelin, 1921; Bleuler, 1924; Kretschmer, 1936; Campbell, 1953; Slater and Roth, 1969.

25. *Cyclothymia* in the German literature refers to the temperament as well as the full range of bipolar disorders. In the English literature, it is restricted to a subthreshold disorder.

26. Kagan et al., 1988, 1992; Kagan, 1989; Kagan and Snidman, 1991; Fox et al., 2001; Schwartz et al., 2003.

Diagnosis

The symptom-complexes of pure mania and depression seem extraordinarily "natural" to us because of the thread of meaningful connection which runs through their individual features, but very many of these patients do not correspond at all to these "natural" complexes which are only ideal types of construct.

—*Karl Jaspers (1913, p. 597)*

The history of psychiatric diagnosis has been notable for its confusion, reflected in the myriad overlapping systems for classifying and subdividing depressive disorders. As discussed in Chapter 1, however, Kraepelin brought order to the diagnosis of depression by grouping all of the recurrent affective disorders under the rubric of manic-depressive illness, a broad category later divided into unipolar and bipolar subgroups. Although the original meaning of *unipolar* as a form of recurrent affective disorder has been obscured in our current diagnostic system, bipolar illness has remained a relatively consistent and stable diagnostic category; characterizing patients as bipolar leads to valid predictions about family history, course, prognosis, and treatment response. In this chapter, we review the formal criteria for the diagnosis of manic-depressive illness, focusing on the bipolar form. With the category thus defined, we then reexamine the boundaries it shares with other major diagnostic categories, some of which were introduced in our earlier discussion of the manic-depressive spectrum (see Chapter 1). Here the focus is on clinical decision making.

A reading of the relevant literature makes clear that reliable diagnosis of manic-depressive illness requires a longitudinal as well as a cross-sectional view of the patient.[1] This literature also charts a course for clinicians, underscoring the need to meet repeatedly with the patient and to seek out other people, particularly family members, who can help in forming an accurate picture of the patient's history, symptoms, and behavior. Such practices decrease the clinician's dependence on cross-sectional data and increase the reliability of diagnoses. Clinicians will need to remain careful and skilled diagnosticians even if future genetic and biological studies provide more clues as to the etiology of manic-depressive illness. This is so because both the bipolar and highly recurrent unipolar forms of manic-depressive illness undoubtedly involve complex interactions among genetic and environmental factors that do not allow for the kinds of direct cause-and-effect relationships seen, for example, with inborn errors of metabolism.

The first section of this chapter summarizes the development of contemporary diagnostic systems. This is followed by a review of the diagnostic criteria for those disorders salient to diagnosis of manic-depressive illness. We then examine findings of recent studies addressing the key issue of whether psychotic conditions should be classified as separate conditions or as falling along a continuous spectrum. Finally, we look at the problem of differential diagnosis of bipolar disorder and other disorders with which it shares overlapping features.

DEVELOPMENT OF CONTEMPORARY DIAGNOSTIC SYSTEMS

Successive versions of the *International Classification of Diseases* (ICD), now in its tenth revision (Sato et al., 2002), represent the official diagnostic system used by clinicians throughout most of the world. The major exception, of course, is the United States, where clinicians use the American Psychiatric Association's (APA) *Diagnostic and Statistical Manual*, the fourth edition of which (DSM-IV) was published in 1994. The different diagnostic systems are illustrated in Boxes 3–1a and 3–1b. Two European systems of classification are also important—the Present State Examination (PSE)-Catego (Wing and Nixon, 1975) and the system developed by the Association for Methodology and Documentation in Psychiatry (Guy and Ban, 1982).

BOX 3–1a.   DSM-IV Mood Disorders

Depressive Disorders

2.96	Major depressive disorder
	.2x single episode
	.3x recurrent
300.4	Dysthymic disorder
	—specify if: early onset/late onset
	—specify: with atypical features
311	Depressive disorder not otherwise specified

Bipolar Disorders

296	Bipolar I disorder
	.0x single manic episode
	—specify if mixed
	.40 most recent episode hypomanic
	.4x most recent episode manic
	.6x most recent episode mixed
	.5x most recent episode depressed
	.7 most recent episode unspecified
296.89	Bipolar II disorder
	—specify (current or most recent episode) hypomanic/depressed
301.13	Cyclothymic disorder
296.8	Bipolar disorder not otherwise specified
293.83	Mood disorder due to (indicate the general medical condition)
	—specify type: with depressive/manic/mixed features
	—specify if: with onset during intoxication/withdrawal
	—see substance-related disorders for codes
	for specific drugs of abuse
	for other agents (including antidepressants)
292.84	Code as other substance–induced mood disorder
296.90	Mood disorder not otherwise specified
295.70	Schizoaffective disorder
	—specify: bipolar type/depressive type
295.40	Schizophreniform disorder
	—specify: with or without good prognostic features
298.8	Brief psychotic disorder
	—specify: with or without marked stressor, with postpartum onset
298.9	Psychotic disorder not otherwise specified

Source: Reprinted with permission from the *Diagnostic and Statistical Manual of Mental Disorders*, Fourth Edition, Text Revision (Copyright 2000). American Psychiatric Association.

BOX 3–1b.   ICD-10 Mood Disorders (Affective Disorder)

F 32	Depressive episode
F 33	Recurrent depressive disorder
F 34	Persistent mood (affective) disorders
F 34.1	Dysthymia
F 34.8	Other persistent mood (affective) disorders
F 34.9	Persistent mood (affective) disorders, unspecified
F 38	Other mood (affective) disorders
F 38.0	Single mixed affective episode
F 38.1	Recurrent brief depressive episode
F 31	Bipolar affective disorder (BAD)
F 30	Manic episode
	—specify if hypomania, mania with or without psychosis
F 31.0	BAD, current episode hypomania
F 31.1, 31.2	BAD, current episode manic with or without psychosis
F 31.6	BAD, current episode mixed
F 31.3, 31.4, 31.5	BAD, current episode depressed with or without psychotic symptoms
F 31.8	Other bipolar affective disorders
	—specify if bipolar-II disorder or recurrent manic episodes
F 34.0	Cyclothymia
F 31.9	BAD, unspecified
F 10-19	Mental and behavioral disorders due to psychoactive substance abuse
F 25.0	Schizoaffective disorder, manic type
F 25.1	Schizoaffective disorder, depressive type
F 25.2	Schizoaffective disorder, mixed type
F 25.9	Schizoaffective disorder, unspecified
F 23	Acute and transient psychotic disorder
F 23.2	Acute schizophrenic-like psychotic disorder

Source: From *International Classification of Diseases*, 10th edition. Reprinted with permission from WHO.

Classification of Causes of Death. The ICD was designed as a system that could be applied throughout the world; thus its developers attempted to encompass a great variety of conceptual backgrounds, which in turn resulted in overlap among many of its categories. The 16 different subtypes of affective disorder in ICD-9, grouped under eight different main headings, cannot readily be compared with the descriptive diagnostic systems that have recently evolved from systematic research on these disorders.

The APA's first diagnostic manual (DSM-I) was published in 1952. Although developed independently of the ICD, the American system likewise was not derived from

ICD-6 through ICD-9 and DSM-I and DSM-II

The first effort to establish a universal diagnostic system for psychiatric illnesses was made by the World Health Organization (WHO) in its 1948 ICD-6, formerly the International systematic research. In DSM-I, manic-depressive reaction appeared along with psychotic depressive reaction as sub-categories of affective reactions, which in turn formed one of four categories of psychosis.

In 1968, the eighth revision of the ICD appeared, as did the revised APA manual (DSM-II); the two generally paralleled each other. Manic-depressive reaction became manic-depressive illness and, with involutional melancholia, was classified under major affective disorders. Psychotic depressive reaction was removed from the affective disorders category and became a separate class. As was true of prior versions, the categories in ICD-9, which appeared in 1978, overlapped conceptually.

Empirically Based Systems: Research Diagnostic Criteria, DSM-III-R, and ICD-10

The transition from DSM-II to DSM-III and more recent systems has been characterized by a movement from psychiatric dogmas to greater reliance on empirical research. ICD-9 and DSM-II were fundamentally flawed, despite their greater use of descriptive material and implicit recognition of the bipolar–unipolar distinction, because they were essentially compromises constructed around isolated, mutually exclusive belief systems about etiology. In DSM-II, each school of psychiatric thought appeared to be assigned its own category, which reflected its own etiologic assumptions. For example, a presumed psychosocial etiology was the defining characteristic for depressions not associated with physiological disturbances or major functional impairment. Depressions associated with these latter features were presumed to be endogenous, that is, biological in origin. In both ICD-9 and DSM-II, manic-depressive illness stayed in the "endogenous" column. Neurotic (reactive) depression and psychotic depressive reaction (or reactive depressive psychoses) were excluded from the manic-depressive illness category, implying that the presence of precipitating factors was incompatible with such a diagnosis.

Clearly, what was desperately needed was a nosological system that was etiologically neutral, a system that would allow independent assessment of the types and severity of symptoms, the presence of precipitating events, the extent of functional impairment, personality characteristics, and the presence of other psychiatric diagnoses. Without such a system, the long-standing debate pitting biological predispositions against psychological causes and social influences would remain an exercise in polemics. Likewise, attempts to foster understanding of manic-depressive illness by bridging these insular schools of thought would continue to flounder, as would efforts to clarify the relationship between affective illness and schizophrenia.

The evolution of psychiatric nosology toward DSM-III was propelled by the rise in influence of the "neo-Kraepelinian" school, based in the United States at Washington University at St. Louis. The shift was toward descriptive criteria, based to the extent possible on empirical evidence, with no etiologic commitments. Since diagnostic validity was and remains elusive, the framers of DSM-III sought to at least establish diagnostic reliability—agreed-upon empirically testable definitions—which is a prerequisite to validity. A precursor to DSM-III was the Research Diagnostic Criteria (RDC)[2] (Spitzer et al., 1978).

The systems as they have evolved thus far are by no means ideal. For example, as illustrated in Figure 3–1, the organization of both DSM-III and DSM-IV implies that bipolar disorder is distinct from all forms of major depression. This division discourages consideration of underlying unifying relationships between bipolar and the more highly recurrent forms of unipolar disorder, including the possibility that they fall along a continuum (Angst et al., 2003; Smith et al., 2005; see also Chapter 1). It appears that

Figure 3–1. DSM-IV classification of mood disorders. NOS = not otherwise specified.

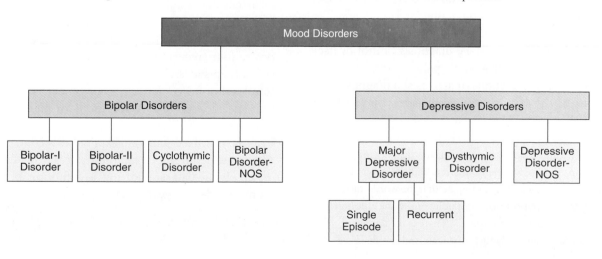

the designers of DSM-III and -IV arbitrarily chose polarity over cyclicity or recurrence as the primary principle for organizing a diagnostic system. This approach left the depressive disorder category as hopelessly heterogeneous, defined only by not being bipolar (see Chapter 1). Another drawback of DSM-III, DSM-III-R, and DSM-IV is that they lack the rich clinical descriptiveness of ICD-9.

Other criticisms can be made of the DSM-IV system in general, not just of the bipolar category. First, natural course, longitudinal patterns, and family history in recurrent affective illness are not included in the DSM-IV criteria, despite their clear importance. The lack of attention to course means that the DSM-IV schema often results in defining an episode more reliably than the disorder. For example, in longitudinal studies of patients with mixed affective and schizophrenic symptoms, numerous investigators[3] have noted a significant proportion who undergo syndrome shifts; that is, at one point in their history they can be diagnosed as schizophrenic, and at another as having an affective disorder.

Other studies of diagnostic stability—defined as the degree to which a diagnosis is confirmed at subsequent assessment points (Fennig et al., 1994)—have shown a similar propensity to diagnostic shifting, with an original diagnosis of unipolar depression later changing to one of bipolar disorder.[4] In a 20-year follow-up of 406 hospitalized depressed patients initially diagnosed as unipolar (Angst et al., 2005), the diagnoses were changed to bipolar at a rate of approximately 1.5 percent per year (1 percent to bipolar-I, 0.5 percent to bipolar-II), cumulatively 39.2 percent over the 20-year follow-up period; those with six or more depressive episodes were especially likely to be rediagnosed as bipolar. In an interesting study of the relationship of diagnostic criteria to the stability of the bipolar diagnosis, Amin and colleagues (1999) found that 91 percent of those diagnosed as bipolar according to ICD-10 maintained that diagnosis at a 3-year follow-up, compared with only 78 percent of those so diagnosed using DSM-IV (see also Chapter 3).

Another problem with DSM-IV is that since all criteria are weighted equally, a DSM-IV diagnosis cannot by itself replicate the complex process of pattern recognition by which the experienced clinician arrives at a diagnosis. The limitations of the system were emphasized by van Praag (1993, p. 97):

> One can witness a standardized interview degenerating into a question-and-answer game: answers being taken on face value, not caring for the meaning behind the words, disregarding the as-yet-unspoken and oblivious to the emotional content of the communication. . . . There is the danger of the desk researcher studying rating scale and standardized

interview results rather than actual patients. These may be data collected not by himself, but by a research assistant with little psychiatric experience and training.

ICD-10 became official in 1993. Heavily influenced by the development of DSM-IV, it groups all mood disorders together by replacing manic-depressive psychosis with bipolar affective disorder and recurrent depressive disorders. ICD-10 does stay more true to the original Kraepelinian vision by linking the two recurrent forms of major affective disorder.[5] Neurotic depression, reactive depressive psychosis, and affective (cyclothymic) personality disorder are relocated to the major groups of affective disorders. The classification scheme for ICD-10 is reviewed in Box 3–1b, presented earlier.

Transition from DSM-III-R to DSM-IV

DSM-III-R was criticized for its definitions of mood disorders on a number of grounds. First, bipolar-II disorder was only a residual category and not recognized as a distinct presentation. Second, there was no operational definition of rapid cycling or mixed states. Third, there was no duration requirement for manic, mixed, or depressive episodes in bipolar disorder, leading to some confusion in distinguishing among rapid cycling, mixed episodes, and cyclothymic disorder. Fourth, certain system-level flaws from prior DSM criteria persisted, such as an absence of clinical description and no information regarding age at onset, course, or family history.

DSM-IV was introduced in 1994. Major revisions are as follows:

- Bipolar-II is designated as a diagnostic entity in its own right.
- Antidepressant-induced mood states are excluded from the diagnosis of bipolar disorder.
- Episodes are descriptive but not formally categorized with codes; instead, mood disorders are coded as either recurrent or single episode. This simple distinction between recurrent and single episode is still too broad since it includes everyone with more than one episode; more useful would be a further distinction between those with two to four (recurrent) and more than four (highly recurrent) episodes.
- Information on course, age, and gender is included. A time specification of 1 week is given for manic or mixed episodes.
- Criteria for mixed states are explicitly stated.
- A separate definition of rapid cycling is provided, based on empirical data supporting a definition of four or more episodes per year (see Chapter 4).

DSM-IV makes no change in the overall diagnostic schema for major depressive disorder.

Of the above changes, perhaps the most important clinically are the introduction of bipolar-II disorder, the definition of rapid cycling, the definition of mixed episodes, and the exclusion of antidepressant-induced mood states from the diagnosis of bipolar disorder. In general, it would appear that the DSM-IV task force attempted to balance the expansion of the bipolar diagnosis to include type II and a clearly defined rapid-cycling course with more restrictive definitions of mixed states and antidepressant-induced mania.

On the latter point, there is indeed significant evidence that antidepressant-induced mania is a predictive marker for bipolar disorder (Akiskal and Benazzi, 2003; Akiskal et al., 2003). The exclusion of this diagnostic group is not supported clinically or empirically by most of the available evidence. To quote Dunner (1998) (a member of the DSM-IV task force):

> There was a sense from the Task Force that bipolar conditions should not be overdiagnosed in the community; if they are, lithium might be too broadly applied to patients with mood disorders. . . . The criteria for bipolar II were defined in a way that is somewhat restrictive. . . . Hypomanic episodes occurring in response to treatment with antidepressant pharmacotherapy would not count toward the diagnosis of bipolar II but would instead be termed substance-induced hypomania. Frankly, this latter option makes little sense to me and is inconsistent with the natural course of bipolar disorder. . . . It is difficult to induce mania or hypomania in a true unipolar patient; there is a likelihood that patients who develop hypomania in response to treatment are actually bipolar.

Given the (probably unfortunate) reality that the majority of patients with bipolar disorder take antidepressants most of the time, it can be difficult to be sure about the identification of true spontaneous manic or hypomanic episodes.

The definition of mixed episodes (discussed further below) in DSM-IV requires that complete criteria for a major depressive episode and a manic episode be met simultaneously for 1 week. This strict definition can exclude many classic descriptions of dysphoric mania and agitated depression that have historically been referred to as mixed states and appear to share characteristics distinct from pure depression or pure mania (see Chapter 2). As discussed below, these more broadly defined mixed states may be valid categories that are, unfortunately, excluded from DSM-IV.

Finally as noted above, DSM-IV continues to leave unaddressed Kraepelin's original observation of the essential unity of the recurrent affective disorders, both bipolar and unipolar, and the possibility that these two recurrent subgroups exist along a spectrum with intermediate forms.

Thus, while DSM-IV incorporates some useful new features, it leaves considerable room for improvement. It may be hoped that this will be accomplished. The APA and the National Institute of Mental Health (NIMH) have commissioned a series of white papers on various diagnostic issues as a way to launch the process of the development of DSM-V. Also, the APA and WHO are jointly sponsoring a series of conferences to stimulate and coordinate the empirical research necessary to fill key information gaps relevant to improving current diagnostic systems; the promotion of international collaborations is a key goal of the APA–WHO effort (American Psychiatric Association, 2005). Figure 3–2 presents our proposal for the organization of mood disorders in DSM-V.

We now turn to the specific diagnostic criteria set forth in DSM-IV. For mania, depression, and mixed states, the criteria define episodes; for bipolar-II disorder, cyclothymia, and schizoaffective disorder, they include a definition of the disorder. The role of biological correlates of diagnosis is reviewed in Chapters 9, 13, 14, and 15.

DIAGNOSTIC CRITERIA

When making a diagnosis, the clinician should assess presenting signs and symptoms, and weigh them together with the patient's history and prior response to treatment, as well as the family's history. Individual symptoms—even clusters of symptoms—examined at one point in time often lack diagnostic specificity, although such cross-sectional views are sometimes the only ones available. In the following sections, we use the relevant DSM-IV categories as a framework for discussing diagnostic criteria for mania and hypomania, depression, mixed states, cyclothymia, and schizoaffective disorder. We also review problems involved in applying the DSM-IV criteria.

Mania and Hypomania

The DSM-IV definition of a manic episode is given in Box 3–2. Among the criteria for mania, perhaps the most objective is decreased need for sleep. In more subtle cases of hypomania in particular, this feature—decreased need for sleep—appears to be the most reliable single indicator of the diagnosis (Rice et al., 1992) and can alert the clinician to explore for other manic features.

As detailed in Chapter 2, the structure of mania has been examined in recent phenomenological studies using factor analytic and other methods. These studies have revealed that the most common signs of mania are motor activation, flight of ideas, pressured speech, and decreased sleep, while elated mood and increased sexuality are decidedly less common. These studies have also identified four types of mania that coincide with Kraepelin's observations:

BOX 3–2.   DSM-IV Definition of a Manic Episode

DSM-IV (p. 328) defines a manic episode as follows:

Criterion A: A *manic episode* is a distinct period during which there is an abnormally and persistently elevated, expansive, or irritable mood. This period of abnormal mood must last at least 1 week (or less if hospitalization is required).

Criterion B: The mood disturbance must be accompanied by at least three additional symptoms from a list that includes inflated self-esteem or grandiosity, decreased need for sleep, pressure of speech, flight of ideas, distractibility, increased involvement in goal-directed activity or psychomotor agitation, and excessive involvement in pleasurable activities with a high potential for painful consequences. If the mood is irritable (rather than elevated or expansive), at least four of the above symptoms must be present.

Criterion C: The symptoms do not meet criteria for a mixed episode.

Criterion D: The disturbance must be sufficiently severe to cause marked impairment in social or occupational functioning or to require hospitalization, or it is characterized by the presence of psychotic features.

Source: Reprinted with permission from the *Diagnostic and Statistical Manual of Mental Disorders*, Fourth Edition, Text Revision (Copyright 2000). American Psychiatric Association.

hypomania, acute mania, delusional mania, and depressive or anxious mania.

As in DSM-III-R, diagnostic criteria for manic episodes in DSM-IV include psychotic features—even the Schneiderian first-rank symptoms that some investigators have thought to be pathognomonic of schizophrenia. The framers of DSM-IV (and its DSM-III-R precursor) departed from earlier diagnostic systems because evidence had accumulated to confirm the presence of considerable thought disorder and gross psychotic content in patients clearly defined as manic by all other indicators, corresponding to Kraepelinian delusional mania. Specific exclusionary criteria are used to rule out other psychotic or secondary mental disorders, a point developed later in the section on differential diagnosis.

The diagnostic distinction between pure mania and mixed states is supported by the identification in these studies of a factor linking dysphoria in mania with depressed mood, lability, guilt, anxiety, suicidality, and the absence of elation. This finding supports the idea of frequent mixed states in manic presentations, as well as the validity of the distinction between pure mania and mixed states (see Chapter 2).

Impulsivity as a prime phenomenological feature of mania has also been underscored by the recent studies reviewed in Chapter 2. Using the Barratt Impulsiveness Scale, Swann and colleagues (2003) found that impulsivity appears to persist even outside of the acute mood state in

Figure 3–2. Mood disorders in DSM-V: a proposal. BP=bipolar; NOS=not otherwise specified.

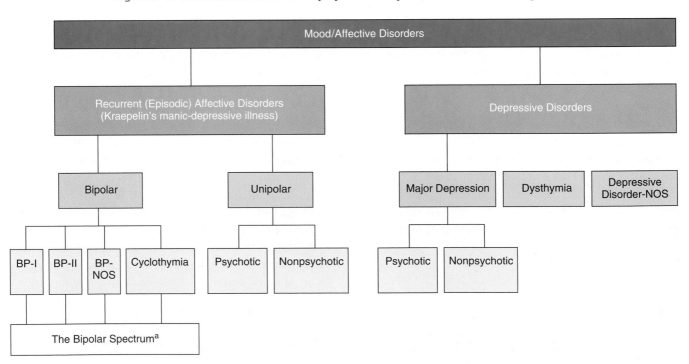

DSM-IV (p. 335) defines a hypomanic episode as follows:

Criterion A: *Hypomanic episode* is defined as a distinct period during which there is an abnormally and persistently elevated, expansive, or irritable mood that lasts at least 4 days.

Criterion B: Normal mood must be accompanied by at least three additional symptoms from a list that includes inflated self-esteem or grandiosity (nondelusional), decreased need for sleep, pressure of speech, flight of ideas, distractibility, increased involvement in goal-directed activities or psychomotor agitation, and excessive involvement in pleasurable activities that have a high potential for painful consequences.

Criterion C: If the mood is irritable rather than elevated or expansive, at least four additional symptoms must be present (from a list identical to that provided for a "manic episode"). . . . Hypomanic episodes must be clearly different from the individual's usual nondepressed mood, and there must be a clear change in functioning that is not characteristic of the individual's usual functioning.

Criterion D: These changes in mood and functioning must be observable by others.

Criterion E: In contrast to a manic episode, a hypomanic episode is not severe enough to cause marked impairment in social or occupational functioning or to require hospitalization, and there are no psychotic features.

Source: Reprinted with permission from the *Diagnostic and Statistical Manual of Mental Disorders*, Fourth Edition, Text Revision (Copyright 2000). American Psychiatric Association.

bipolar disorder, suggesting that it may represent both a state and a trait feature of the illness.

Research on the structure of manic episodes indicates that they are stable, appearing with similar presentations if and when they recur. The symptom factors reviewed in Chapter 2 have been found to be highly correlated in separate episodes.

The inclusion of hypomanic episodes in DSM-IV was based on accumulating empirical evidence that hypomania could be diagnosed reliably by experienced clinicians using semistructured interviews (Dunner and Tay, 1993; Simpson et al., 2002; Benazzi, 2003); that it was stable; and that it could be distinguished from bipolar-I disorder or unipolar depression on the basis of symptoms, course, family history, and treatment response (Coryell et al., 1989; Dunner and Tay, 1993).[6] The diagnostic criteria for a hypomanic episode in DSM-IV, which are much more specific than those in DSM-III-R, are listed in Box 3–3.

The key differentiating feature between a manic and hypomanic episode in DSM-IV is not in the manic symptoms themselves, as they are largely the same for both diagnoses. Rather, the key difference is in the impact of those symptoms on social or occupational functioning. In a manic episode, social or occupational functioning must be characterized by "marked" impairment. In a hypomanic episode, "the episode is not severe enough to cause marked impairment in social or occupational functioning, or to necessitate hospitalization, and there are no psychotic features." In simple terms, there should be no such thing as a hypomanic hospitalized patient; if manic-like symptoms lead to hospitalization, the diagnosis must be mania, not hypomania. The same holds true if psychosis is present. With regard to functional impairment, much hinges on one's definition of the word "marked," which DSM-IV has left deliberately vague, perhaps reflecting the limited literature on the subject. Indeed, the main reason for the low reliability of a bipolar-II diagnosis in many routine clinical settings is that clinicians disagree on the limits of marked functional impairment. Hypomanic episode is one of the few if not the only major Axis I primary psychiatric diagnosis in DSM-IV in which marked impairment of social or occupational functioning is not part of the definition of the syndrome; indeed as noted, the clinician must rule out such impairment before making the diagnosis. Almost all the impairment in bipolar-II is due to the depressive phase. As Vieta and colleagues (1997, p. 100) observed:

It is worth emphasizing that although bipolar-II disorder is milder than bipolar-I disorder in terms of manic symptoms, it is not less severe in terms of depressive morbidity. In fact, bipolar-II disorder is more severe in terms of an increased propensity for rapid-cycling and a greater number of mood episodes than bipolar-I disorder.

Another important difference between the DSM-IV definitions of mania and hypomania has to do with the duration of the syndrome, defined as 1 week for the former and a minimum of 4 days for the latter. Clinical and research experience suggests that 2 to 3 days of hypomania appears to identify a cohort of patients with a variant of bipolar illness that is milder in manic symptomatology than the classic form (Angst, 1998). Duration of 1 day or less of hypomania is more controversial, often making it difficult to distinguish the state from the rapid mood alternations of borderline personality disorder or normal variants in temperament. The following is Dunner's (1992, p. 13) account of how the 4-day minimum criterion came to be set:

The initial definition proposed by Dunner et al. had posited a 3-day or longer duration of hypomania. This definition was based on a study of "normal" women who were being assessed for a premenstrual mood disturbance and who on interview were sometimes found to have 1–2 days of hypomanic symptoms. Because 1–2 days of hypomania could occur in "normal" women, the proposed minimal criteria for the duration of hypomania for bipolar II patients became 3 days or more. There were no data to support the minimal duration criteria [*sic*] for hypomania, and the ICD-10 group had arbitrarily chosen 4 days or more as the minimal criterion. The [DSM-IV] Work Group opted for that definition in order to be consistent.[7]

Just as with mania, an exclusive focus on euphoria can miss patients in whom irritability is the primary manifestation, with hypomania, overactivity can be a more sensitive (but less specific) indicator of hypomania than euphoria (Akiskal, 2005). Angst and Cassano (2005) have argued for broadening this concept so that overactivity and/or euphoria and/or irritability are used together.

Bipolar-II disorder is defined as at least one hypomanic episode along with at least one major depressive episode. The diagnostic criteria for this condition are listed in Box 3–4. If a patient meets criteria for hypomania and has a history of depressions not severe enough to be designated as major depression, the appropriate DSM-IV diagnosis is

---

BOX **3–4.   DSM-IV Definition of Bipolar-II**

DSM-IV (p. 359) defines bipolar-II as follows:

Criterion A: The essential feature of bipolar-II disorder is a clinical course that is characterized by the occurrence of one or more major depressive episodes.

Criterion B: Accompanied by at least one hypomanic episode.

Criterion C: The individual experiences rapidly alternating moods (sadness, irritability, euphoria) accompanied by symptoms of a manic episode and a major depressive episode. The presence of a manic or mixed episode precludes the diagnosis of bipolar-II disorder.

Criterion D: Episodes of substance-induced mood disorder (due to the direct physiological effects of a medication, other somatic treatments for depression, drugs of abuse, or toxin exposure) or of mood disorder due to a general medical condition do not count toward a diagnosis of bipolar-II disorder. In addition, the episodes must not be better accounted for by schizoaffective disorder and are not superimposed on schizophrenia, schizophreniform disorder, delusional disorder, or psychotic disorder not otherwise specified.

Criterion E: The symptoms must cause clinically significant distress or impairment in social, occupational, or other important areas of functioning.

Source: Reprinted with permission from the *Diagnostic and Statistical Manual of Mental Disorders*, Fourth Edition, Text Revision (Copyright 2000). American Psychiatric Association.

---

cyclothymia (discussed below), which is not easily distinguishable from bipolar-not otherwise specified (NOS).

Additional discussion relevant to the bipolar-II diagnosis is included in Chapters 1 and 2. For example, Benazzi and Akiskal (2005) have offered a definition of trait mood lability and suggested that it can be used as a screening tool for bipolar-II.

Depression

DSM-IV criteria for a major depressive episode are presented in Box 3–5. As with the criteria for mania, the boundaries of major depressive disorder were considerably broadened in DSM-III-R through the incorporation of additional psychotic features, including mood-incongruent delusions, and this broadened definition carries over into DSM-IV. We return to this issue later in the section on differential diagnosis. The required minimum 2 weeks' duration is regarded as too short by many clinicians, who prefer the 1 month originally given in the criteria of Feighner and colleagues (1972).

As noted earlier in this chapter and in Chapter 1, one of the major, and in our opinion unfortunate, changes in the transition to ICD-10 and DSM-IV is that both of these nosologies, as a first principle, separate bipolar disorder from major depression (single or recurrent), thereby reinforcing the bipolar–unipolar dichotomy. Within the DSM-IV framework, there is no attempt to differentiate bipolar from unipolar depression on any grounds other than the presence or absence of a history of mania. Clinical features reported to differentiate bipolar from unipolar depression as described in Chapter 1 are not incorporated into the DSM-IV system. In contrast, ICD-9, under the rubric of manic-depressive psychoses–depressed type, properly emphasized the recurrent nature of endogenous forms of depression, implying that such depressions are closely related to bipolar illness (i.e., Kraepelin's manic-depressive illness).

Mixed States

The factor analytic studies referred to earlier (and reviewed in Chapter 2) reported two types of mixed states with marked lability of mood: one displayed depression with labile periods of pressured, irritable hostility and paranoia; the other displayed an incongruous mix of elated mood and psychosis, which would switch frequently to anxiety, depression, and irritability.

Kraepelin originally viewed mixed states as the most common form of manic-depressive illness. In fact, in the 1899 edition of his textbook, he placed a great deal of emphasis on six types of mixed states, including forms that clinicians today may label as mania (dysphoric mania) or depression (agitated depression, depression with racing

BOX 3–5. DSM-IV Definition of a Major Depressive Episode

DSM-IV (p. 320) defines a major depressive episode as follows:

Criterion A1: The essential feature of a major depressive episode is a period of at least 2 weeks during which there is either depressed mood or the loss of interest or pleasure in nearly all activities. In children and adolescents, the mood may be irritable rather than sad. The individual must also experience at least four additional symptoms drawn from a list that includes changes in appetite or weight, sleep, and psychomotor activity; decreased energy; feelings of worthlessness or guilt; difficulty thinking, concentrating, or making decisions; or recurrent thoughts of death or suicidal ideation, plans, or attempts. To count toward a major depressive episode, a symptom must either be newly present or must have clearly worsened compared with the person's pre-episode status. The symptoms must persist for most of the day, nearly every day, for at least 2 consecutive weeks. The episode must be accompanied by clinically significant distress or impairment in social, occupational, or other important areas of functioning. For some individuals with milder episodes, functioning may appear to be normal, but requires markedly increased effort. The mood in a major depressive episode is often described by the person as depressed, sad, hopeless, discouraged, or "down in the dumps."

Criterion A2: Loss of interest or pleasure is nearly always present, at least to some degree.

Criterion A3: When appetite changes are severe (in either direction), there may be a significant loss or gain in weight, or, in children, a failure to make expected weight gains may be noted.

Criterion A4: The most common sleep disturbance associated with a major depressive episode is insomnia.

Criterion A5: Psychomotor changes include agitation (e.g., the inability to sit still, pacing, hand-wringing; or pulling or rubbing of the skin, clothing, or other objects) or retardation (e.g., slowed speech, thinking, and body movements; increased pauses before answering; speech that is decreased in volume, inflection, amount, or variety of content, or muteness).

Source: Reprinted with permission from the *Diagnostic and Statistical Manual of Mental Disorders,* Fourth Edition, Text Revision (Copyright 2000). American Psychiatric Association.

---

thoughts) (Marneros, 2001; Salvatore et al., 2002).[8] Recent work has confirmed that agitated depression and dysphoric mania are distinguishable syndromes—the differences lying primarily in manic-like symptoms, with depressive and anxiety features being rather similar (Swann et al., 1993). Koukopoulos (1999) considers agitated depression to be a mixed depressive state, as did Kraepelin (1921) and Waygandt (1899). This category can include cases without motor agitation but with intense psychic agitation or inner tension. To clarify the differential diagnosis between anxiety and inner agitation, Koukopoulos has proposed certain criteria[9] (Koukopoulos et al., 2005).

A third kind of mixed state, unique to bipolar-II disorder, has also recently been proposed: the "depressive mixed state" (Benazzi, 2000b). This condition, described more fully in Chapters 1 and 2, reflects the occurrence of a major depressive episode and *at least three* hypomanic symptoms in an individual with bipolar-II disorder (past pure depressive and spontaneous "hypomanic" episodes).

Compared with DSM-III-R and ICD-10, DSM-IV provides a more definitive treatment of mixed episodes. DSM-IV still does not, however, provide separate empirically derived criteria for mixed states, but instead refers to the criteria for mania and depression. DSM-IV also avoids addressing criteria for the diagnosis of agitated depression or dysphoric mania. The main DSM-IV and ICD-10 criteria for bipolar-I disorder, most recent episode mixed, are provided in Box 3–6. DSM-IV's description is more extensive than in the past, whereas the ICD-10 definition is somewhat vague and spotty.

Despite the advance toward a clear definition of mixed episodes, the DSM-IV criteria remain unlinked to empirical

BOX 3–6. DSM-IV and ICD-10 Definitions of a Mixed Episode

DSM-IV (p. 333) defines a mixed episode as follows:

Criterion A: A *mixed episode* is characterized by a period of time (lasting at least 1 week) in which the criteria are met both for a manic episode and for a major depressive episode nearly every day.

The individual experiences rapidly alternating moods (sadness, irritability, euphoria) accompanied by symptoms of a manic episode and a major depressive episode. The symptom presentation frequently includes agitation, insomnia, appetite dysregulation, psychotic features, and suicidal thinking.

The ICD-10 definition is as follows (p. 58)[a]:

Bipolar affective disorder, current episode mixed: The patient has had at least one authenticated hypomanic, manic, depressive, or mixed affective episode in the past, and currently exhibits either a mixture or a rapid alternation of manic and depressive symptoms.

---

[a]In the first edition, we also referred to the Vienna Research Criteria for Mixed States, which before DSM-IV provided the clearest definition. Unlike DSM-IV, the Vienna Research Criteria were derived more directly from empirical studies of mixed states. It appears the DSM-IV task force felt the need to provide a clear definition of mixed states in light of the burgeoning literature on the topic. Yet it chose to use the most restrictive definition possible, contrary to the empirical evidence supporting somewhat broader definition of mixed states (see discussion in the text).

Source: Reprinted with permission from the *Diagnostic and Statistical Manual of Mental Disorders,* Fourth Edition, Text Revision (Copyright 2000). American Psychiatric Association.

studies of such episodes—specifically those studies that support the validity of definitions in which criteria for mixed episodes are met by mania accompanied by as few as two or more depressive symptoms (dysphoric mania) (McElroy et al., 1992). Using this definition, for instance, one study (reviewed in Chapter 18) suggested greater treatment response with valproate than with lithium.

Some research suggests that, under the narrow DSM-IV criteria, fewer than 10 percent of episodes in patients with bipolar disorder meet criteria for a mixed episode. One study reviewed in Chapter 2 found that only 54 percent of 143 broadly defined mixed states (using Kraepelinian definitions) met DSM-III-R (or DSM-IV) criteria for a mixed episode (Perugi et al., 1997). Data suggest that using broader criteria for mixed states, incorporating the clinical concept of dysphoric mania and perhaps also agitated depression, in patients with bipolar disorder would result in more than 50 percent of episodes in bipolar disorder being diagnosable as mixed states.

Further work is needed to demonstrate empirically the appropriate boundaries for mixed states. Findings of other studies reviewed in Chapter 2 suggest that the DSM-IV criteria will need to be broadened. For instance, when dysphoric mania was defined as two or more depressive criteria plus a manic episode (McElroy et al., 1992), 36 percent of manic episodes were identified as dysphoric (Hantouche et al., 2001). In a study of the "depressive mixed state," Perugi and colleagues (1997) found that 32 patients with depressive mixed states could be distinguished from 36 patients with pure bipolar depression by the presence of increased cyclicity with greater frequency of episodes in the latter group, as opposed to longer episodes with less interepisode recovery in the depressive mixed state group (Perugi et al., 2001).

There is also some evidence, reviewed in Chapter 19, that patients with depressive "mixed states" (analogous or perhaps identical to agitated depression), unlike those with pure depression, may not respond well to antidepressants and may even worsen with their use. Thus it would appear that depressive mixed states are distinct from pure major depression in phenomenology, course, treatment response, and family history, a supposition that may justify a broadening of DSM-IV criteria for mixed episodes. It is also important to recall the point made in Chapters 1 and 2 that, while irritability often occurs in mixed states, irritability is nonspecific, occurring also in pure mania as well as in pure depression.

Cyclothymia

Consistent with our discussion of cyclothymia in Chapter 2, DSM-IV notes that the boundaries between this disorder, bipolar disorder, and bipolar-NOS are not well defined, and that many investigators believe cyclothymia to be simply a mild form of bipolar illness. The DSM-IV definition of cyclothymia is presented in Box 3–7.

Note that DSM-IV allows for a dual diagnosis of a major depressive, manic, or mixed episode and cyclothymia if such episodes occur after the described 2-year period. The clinical relevance of this provision is not clear. DSM-IV also allows for a dual diagnosis of borderline personality disorder, noting that the two disorders are sometimes difficult to distinguish. We find the notion of combining two diagnoses because they are difficult to differentiate questionable at best; we discuss problems involving borderline personality disorder comorbidity in Chapter 2 and in the section on differential diagnosis below.

It should be noted that the DSM-IV residual category of bipolar-NOS allows for the inclusion of many suspected

---

BOX 3–7.   DSM-IV Definition of Cyclothymia

DSM-IV (p. 363) defines cyclothymia as follows:

Criterion A: *Cyclothymic disorder* is a chronic, fluctuating mood disturbance involving numerous periods of hypomanic symptoms and numerous periods of depressive symptoms.

Criterion B: The hypomanic symptoms are of insufficient number, severity, pervasiveness, or duration to meet full criteria for a manic episode, and the depressive symptoms are of insufficient number, severity, pervasiveness, or duration to meet full criteria for a major depressive episode. During the 2-year period (1 year for children or adolescents), any symptom-free intervals last no longer than 2 months.

Criterion C: The 2-year period of cyclothymic symptoms must be free of major depressive, manic, and mixed episodes.

Criterion D: After the initial 2 years of the cyclothymic disorder, manic or mixed episodes may be superimposed on the cyclothymic disorder, in which case both cyclothymic disorder and bipolar-I disorder are diagnosed. Similarly, after the initial 2 years of cyclothymic disorder, major depressive episodes may be superimposed on the cyclothymic disorder, in which case both cyclothymic disorder and bipolar-II disorder are diagnosed. The diagnosis is not made if the pattern of mood swings is better accounted for by schizoaffective disorder or is superimposed on a psychotic disorder, such as schizophrenia, schizophreniform disorder, delusional disorder, or psychotic disorder not otherwise specified.

Criterion E: The mood disturbance must also not be due to the direct physiological effects of a substance (e.g., a drug of abuse, a medication) nor a general medical condition (e.g., hyperthyroidism).

Source: Reprinted with permission from the *Diagnostic and Statistical Manual of Mental Disorders*, Fourth Edition, Text Revision (Copyright 2000). American Psychiatric Association.

cases of bipolar disorder that are excluded by the manual's rather strict definitions of hypomania and mixed episodes. Thus, bipolar-NOS

> includes disorders with bipolar features that do not meet criteria for any specific Bipolar Disorder. Examples include 1. Very rapid alternation (over days) between manic symptoms and depressive symptoms that do not meet minimal duration criteria for a Manic Episode or a Major Depressive Episode; 2. Recurrent Hypomanic Episodes without intercurrent depressive symptoms; 3. A Manic or Mixed Episode superimposed on Delusion Disorder, residual Schizophrenia, or Psychotic Disorder not otherwise specified; 4. Situations in which the clinician has concluded that a Bipolar Disorder is present but is unable to determine whether it is primary, due to a general medical condition, or substance induced. (p. 366)

In effect, most cases of bipolar spectrum illness that are more atypical than bipolar-II disorder or cyclothymia fall under the nonspecific rubric of bipolar-NOS. We should note here that, although DSM-IV does not address bipolar spectrum disorder (which is covered in Chapter 1), there is an emerging literature proposing criteria for its diagnosis.[10]

Schizoaffective Disorder

In DSM-I and -II, schizoaffective illness was included as a subtype of schizophrenia, reflecting the broad Bleulerian concept of schizophrenia as discussed later in this chapter. Subsequent research (reviewed in Chapter 2) documented the frequent occurrence of Schneiderian first-rank[11] and related schizophrenic symptoms (e.g., catatonic features, paranoia, bizarre behavior, formal thought disorder) in individuals whose family history, natural course, other symptoms, and treatment outcome clearly placed them in the manic spectrum. American psychiatry departed significantly from the Bleulerian tradition when, in DSM-III, the scope of affective illnesses was substantially broadened to include nonaffective psychotic symptoms. Schizoaffective illness was moved from schizophrenia to an intermediate category labeled "psychotic disorders not elsewhere classified." With DSM-III-R and ICD-9, schizoaffective disorder was given its own criteria. Those criteria essentially restated the acute symptoms required for a diagnosis of schizophrenia, but without continuous signs of illness for 6 months or more. The schizoaffective category was thus reserved for patients who met the acute symptomatic criteria for mania (or depression) and for schizophrenia and who had delusions or hallucinations in the absence of prominent mood symptoms for more than 2 weeks. (If the delusions or hallucinations were present for less than 2 weeks, the patient met criteria for a primary affective disorder.)

In DSM-IV, the main change is in criterion C. This criterion had previously been worded as follows: "Schizophrenia has been ruled out, [when] the duration of all episodes of a mood syndrome has not been brief relative to the total duration of the psychotic disturbance." In DSM-IV, this wording is somewhat clearer: "Symptoms that meet criteria for a mood episode are present for a substantial portion of the total duration of the active and residual periods of the illness." By still using the somewhat deliberately vague phrase "substantial portion," the DSM-IV definition seeks to increase the relevance of mood symptoms to the definition of schizoaffective disorder. In other words, one might diagnose DSM-IV schizoaffective disorder in a person with prominent mood syndromes and only a relative excess of psychotic symptoms (e.g., 2 weeks of psychosis outside of a mood syndrome). Yet one would not diagnose the disorder in a person with prominent chronic psychosis and only brief mood episodes (e.g., 2 weeks of a major depressive episode). Mood episodes must be relatively frequent and lengthy in the DSM-IV definition of schizoaffective disorder. Otherwise, the appropriate diagnosis would appear to be schizophrenia with comorbid major depressive episodes (in the case of depression). This tendency of the DSM-IV definition of schizoaffective disorder to be weighted toward the presence of mood symptoms is intended to focus this diagnosis on persons whose illness is closely related to mood disorders.

Some controversy persists over whether this newly delineated category is closer to affective illness or to schizophrenia, or whether it is a valid diagnosis in its own right. There are at least five major schools of thought on the matter, among them that schizoaffective illness represents

- A separate illness.
- An intermediate form on the continuum of psychosis.
- Comorbidity of schizophrenia and affective disorders.
- A more severe variant of bipolar disorder.
- A less severe variant of schizophrenia.

Some investigators believe that since patients with mood-incongruent symptoms are now included under mood disorders in DSM-IV, the remaining individuals with a mix of schizophrenic and affective symptoms (particularly depressive symptoms) are closer to the schizophrenic end of the schizoaffective spectrum (Kendler et al., 1986). As outlined in Chapter 13, family history studies support an association between DSM-III-R (or RDC) schizoaffective disorder and manic-depressive illness, as well as schizophrenia. Yet most studies have not found that schizoaffective disorder runs in families, as would be expected if it were a separate disease entity (Kendler et al., 1993). The genetic finding of co-occurrence of schizophrenia and bipolar disorder in at least some genealogies of schizoaffective disorder supports most strongly two of the above five models—either the continuum (described below) or comorbidity perspective. The latter perspective, perhaps the newest, holds that schizoaffective disorder results when schizophrenia and bipolar disorder (two relatively common medical conditions) happen to occur in the same individual.

The position that schizoaffective illness will ultimately occupy on the spectrum of schizophrenia and affective illness may depend on whether one is referring to schizomanic or schizodepressive conditions. The schizomanic condition clearly appears to be associated more closely with affective illness, with a somewhat worse course than bipolar disorder (Gershon et al., 1982; Coryell et al., 1990). Schizoaffective depressed patients, by contrast, often demonstrate outcomes or neuropsychological profiles similar to those of the schizophrenic pole (Brockington et al., 1980; Tsuang and Coryell, 1993; Evans et al., 1999).[12]

An integrative perspective on these models and the associated data may be similar to that proposed by Tsuang and Simpson (1984). According to this perspective, in some individuals with predominantly manic symptoms and less pronounced psychosis, the diagnosable schizoaffective condition may represent a more severe variant of bipolar disorder. In individuals with predominantly psychotic symptoms and less pronounced mood symptoms (which are solely depressive), the diagnosable schizoaffective condition may represent a less severe variant of schizophrenia. And in others with a nearly equal mix of psychosis and mood symptoms (both mania and depression), the diagnosable schizoaffective disorder may represent a true comorbidity of schizophrenia and bipolar disorder, a condition not likely to be very common. Indeed, recent epidemiological studies have found the community prevalence of schizoaffective disorder to be a fraction of a percent, as might be expected if the comorbidity model is correct (Kendler et al., 1993, 1996). In contrast, clinical samples often show quite high diagnostic rates for schizoaffective disorder, perhaps reflecting the fact that those with more than one condition are more likely to come to clinical attention. In addition, higher rates of schizoaffective diagnosis could reflect the clinical tendency at times to overdiagnose schizoaffective disorder rather than engage in the arduous task of identifying psychotic and mood syndromes.

Problems in Applying the DSM-IV Criteria

We have discussed conceptual problems inherent in the DSM-IV system, including those engendered by the separation of bipolar disorder from depressive disorders. Here we note the practical problems that arise when applying this system in the clinical context.

As noted above, DSM-IV lists bipolar disorder first and then assigns depressive disorders to a totally separate category. This separation of categories at the outset is incompatible with the reality of clinical practice, where assessing patients with depressive symptoms is the most common diagnostic decision faced. The clinician's first task is to determine whether the patient meets criteria for major depressive disorder or dysthymia, and then to review the individual's history for evidence of bipolar or unipolar illness (if at all possible with the assistance of a family member). Compounding the problems caused by separating bipolar and depressive disorders "from the top," milder depressive states are listed only under the depressive disorders—that is, the nonbipolar disorders. A patient who is mildly or moderately depressed and also has a history of mania finds a niche in this system only by some awkward fitting. The system implies more homogeneity and separateness for the bipolar category than is justified by the data.

Clinical Summary

The nosological systems that evolved during the latter part of the 20th century are in many respects superior to those used earlier. They are, for the most part, etiologically neutral, allowing for independent assessment of the types and severity of symptoms, the presence of precipitating events, the extent of functional impairment, personality characteristics, and the presence of other psychiatric diagnoses. Problems remain in the classification of manic-depressive illness, however. For example, DSM-IV implies that bipolar disorder is a separate illness and fundamentally different from all forms of unipolar depression; this supposition goes beyond the data, especially with respect to the more recurrent forms of unipolar depression. Also troubling is the absence from all categories of affective illness of criteria concerning long-term course and family history and the failure to provide for a mild form of depression in bipolar illness. These and other features of the system are problematic for clinical as well as conceptual reasons.

THE PSYCHOSES: SEPARATE OR CONTINUOUS?

In the first edition of this volume, we emphasized the controversial and important topic of whether psychotic conditions should be classified as a few major conditions or as one continuous spectrum. The ensuing decade and a half has not resolved this debate, though overall, perhaps, the available evidence is accumulating more in support of than against the Kraepelinian dichotomy. Readers interested in the history of this topic may refer to Tables 3–1a and 3–1b.

TABLE 3–1a. The Two-Entities Tradition

Author	Schizophrenia	Manic-Depressive Illness
Kraepelin, 1896	Characterized by a steady downhill course into chronic dementia	Characterized by an episodic course with intermittent recovery.
Bleuler, 1911	Certain symptoms are specific and pathognomonic—namely, those symptoms that define splitting of thought from feeling and behavior.	Symptoms are nonspecific; diagnosis is made only after schizophrenia is excluded.
Kraepelin, 1919	Some patients appeared to recover.	Some patients followed a progressive chronic course.

TABLE 3–1b. A Schizophrenia–Affective Continuum

Study	Findings
Kasanin, 1933	Coined the term "schizoaffective psychosis" to describe a group of relatively young patients with good premorbid adjustment who in response to stress developed the rapid onset of a psychosis characterized by "marked emotional turmoil" and "false sense impressions," but without "passivity."
Langfeldt, 1937	Coined the term "schizophreniform" to describe patients who today would probably be referred to as schizoaffective.
Slater and Roth, 1969	Contended that the patient with a mix of affective and schizophrenic symptoms who is observed long enough can usually be confidently diagnosed as having either an affective illness or schizophrenia.
Brockington and Leff, 1979	Applied eight different published definitions of schizoaffective illness to a sample of patients, and found virtually no agreement among the various definitions.

The Two-Entities Tradition

Kraepelin's (1913) lucid discrimination of pattern in a mass of confusing clinical phenomena led him to propose a dichotomy of fundamentally different classes of psychotic illness. Lacking knowledge of etiology or pathophysiology, he based the distinction on family history, age at onset, course, and outcome. In his original formulation, dementia praecox was marked by a steady downhill course into chronic dementia, and manic-depressive illness followed an episodic course with intermittent recovery.

Kraepelin's original contribution was followed rapidly by the revision of Bleuler (1968), who changed the term "dementia praecox" to "schizophrenia," extended the condition's boundaries, and focused on intrapsychic symptoms. The concept of manic-depressive illness, in contrast, grew increasingly narrow with time, especially in the United States, where it attracted little interest on the part of psychoanalytic groups. A U.S.–U.K. study (Copper et al., 1972) highlighted how far American clinicians had likely gone in overdiagnosing schizophrenia and underdiagnosing manic-depressive illness. With the introduction of DSM-III, this situation gradually began shifting back to one of greater balance, though there is some evidence that bipolar disorder is still misdiagnosed as schizophrenia, particularly, perhaps, in state hospitals in the United States or in developing nations (Vieta and Salva, 1997; Ghaemi et al., 1999).

A Schizophrenia–Affective Disorder Continuum

As noted previously, the complex concept of schizoaffective disorder could be seen as a rejection of the Kraepelinian dichotomy, as suggested by Crow (1998); on the other hand, the available evidence does not support the validity of schizoaffective disorder as a unique disease entity. This view was well expressed as early as 1969, in the revision of Mayer-Gross' *Clinical Psychiatry*, in which Slater and Roth contended that the patient with a mix of affective and schizophrenic symptoms who is observed long enough can usually be confidently diagnosed as having either affective illness or schizophrenia. This assertion implies that, by and large, the schizoaffective category has reflected incomplete or imperfect diagnoses rather than a meaningful diagnostic entity.

This observation is supported in part by epidemiologic studies of schizoaffective disorder conducted since the first edition of this book was published in 1990. In both the Roscommon study (2003) and the National Comorbidity Survey, schizoaffective disorder appeared to represent a small fraction of 1 percent of the population (Kendler et al., 1993, 1996). This finding contrasts with what one might expect from the unitary psychosis model, in which schizoaffective presentations, occurring in the middle of the psychotic continuum, would be presumed to be quite frequent. The Roscommon family study in particular also appeared to provide a new explanation for schizoaffective disorder—the idea of comorbidity. It could be that if families with propensities to develop schizophrenia and bipolar disorder were to merge, some offspring would develop both types of symptoms, presenting phenotypically as schizoaffective disorder. The genetic data from that study strongly support this interpretation.

Some support for a continuum model is provided by the observation that neurobiological studies have not clearly distinguished between affective disorders and schizophrenia (Crow, 1990). This observation, if accurate in the long run, does not necessarily entail the continuum model, however. Two diseases can be different phenomenologically, as well as in their etiologies, but share many pathophysiological mechanisms. In the case of the brain, the presence of many shared "final common pathways" is a well-known feature of brain function. In any case, the neurobiological or neuropsychological findings of some studies do suggest differences between patients with schizophrenia and those with affective disorders (Keri et al., 2001), although there are enough conflicting reports to leave this question open (see Chapters 9, 14, and 15). Ketter and colleagues (2004) have proposed a mixed dimensional/categorical model that they believe allows for a more flexible approach to considering pathophysiological findings and treatment options. It is their view that a dimensional construct may be best when evaluating relationships between biological or other variables and symptoms such as psychosis in bipolar disorder or schizophrenia, while a categorical construct allows evaluation of diagnostic reliability.

Findings of a carefully conducted nosological study by Kendler and colleagues (1998) argue against the concept of a nosologic continuum. That study assessed diagnostic groupings based on family data, as well as symptom groupings. It found that most patients appeared to fall into different diagnostic categories rather than one (as suggested by Crow). Similarly, based on a factor analysis of a group of 191 psychotic patients whose diagnoses included schizophrenia and mood disorders with psychosis, Dikeos and colleagues (2006) concluded that diagnosis by itself explained the large majority of the clinical characteristics examined, although dimensional measures were more useful than diagnosis as predictors of clinical course. Others who have explored the predictive value of diagnostic versus dimensional measures in psychotic patients across both schizophrenic and affective disorder patients include van Os and colleagues (1996, 1998), Toomey and colleagues (1998), Ventura and colleagues (2000) and Serretti and colleagues (2001). Finally, another view, closer to that of Crow, is expressed by Craddock and Owen (2005, p. 364) who pointed to the emerging evidence for shared and overlapping susceptibility genes as "the beginning of the end for the Kraepelinian dichotomy," a topic that is explored in Chapter 13.

DIFFERENTIAL DIAGNOSIS

Until the 1980s, the most commonly encountered problems in making differential diagnoses of bipolar illness involved its overlapping boundaries with schizophrenia and schizoaffective illness, as well as with personality disorders, especially borderline disorders. These two major differential diagnoses remain highly important, but to them must be added the most clinically significant problem—the differential diagnosis of bipolar disorder and unipolar depression. Bipolar illness also must be distinguished from schizophreniform disorder, brief reactive psychosis, cycloid psychosis, atypical psychosis, organic brain disorders, and epilepsy. The overlap between primary affective diagnoses and substance abuse is of such importance that we address it in a separate chapter (see Chapter 7).

Schizophrenia and Schizoaffective Disorder

As discussed previously, the clinician should be able to assign the great majority of patients a diagnosis of either affective illness or schizophrenia by carefully applying the diagnostic criteria shown in Box 3–8. Schizoaffective

---

BOX 3–8.   DSM-IV Definition of Schizoaffective Disorder

DSM-IV (p. 309) defines schizoaffective disorder as follows:

Criterion A: The essential feature of schizoaffective disorder is an uninterrupted period of illness during which, at some time, there is a major depressive, manic, or mixed episode concurrent with symptoms that meet Criterion A for schizophrenia.

Criterion B: In addition, during the same period of illness, there have been delusions or hallucinations for at least 2 weeks in the absence of prominent mood symptoms.

Criterion C: Finally, the mood symptoms are present for a substantial portion of the total duration of the illness.

Source: Reprinted with permission from the *Diagnostic and Statistical Manual of Mental Disorders*, Fourth Edition, Text Revision (Copyright 2000). American Psychiatric Association.

---

disorder can sometimes be excluded by considering previous episodes; a history of either clear affective illness or clear schizophrenia cautions against diagnosing a present episode as schizoaffective.

Mania versus Schizophrenia or Schizoaffective Disorder

Differentiating mania from schizophrenia or schizoaffective illness is a diagnostic challenge often faced by clinicians. Viewed cross-sectionally, acute symptoms of irritability, anger, paranoia, thought disorder, and catatonic-like excitement cannot distinguish mania from schizophrenia. Because presenting symptoms can be similar in mania and schizophrenia, the clinician must give equal attention to the level of premorbid functioning, family history, natural course, and the character of any prior episodes. This differential diagnosis has been made more rational and straightforward by the previously discussed broadening of the criteria for mania to include a range of psychotic features.

A key DSM-IV criterion for diagnosing psychotic mania or depression in the presence of schizophrenic symptoms is the more or less continuous prominence of the affective symptoms. Thus, bizarre mood-congruent delusions or hallucinations (including Schneiderian first-rank symptoms) are not inconsistent with a diagnosis of mania as long as they have been accompanied substantially by affective symptoms most of the time (the DSM-IV criteria for mania allow for up to 2 weeks of delusions or hallucinations free of other prominent manic symptoms, whereas the RDC allow for 1 week).

If the period of quiet (i.e., affect-free) delusions or hallucinations is substantial (by criterion, exceeding 2 weeks), a diagnosis of either schizophrenia or schizoaffective illness should be considered. Schizophrenia would be diagnosed if, in addition, the patient continuously manifested overt signs of a psychotic illness for at least 6 months, and the manic symptoms were brief relative to the duration of the schizophrenic symptoms. On the other hand, schizoaffective illness, manic type, would be diagnosed if the criterion of 6 months of continuous psychotic illness were not met, but there had been more than 2 weeks of quiet delusions or hallucinations.

It is now well recognized that strict application of the Bleulerian concept of thought disorder as pathognomonic of schizophrenia can result in misdiagnosis of manic-depressive patients (see Chapters 1 and 10). More than a quarter of patients with mania have "classic" Bleulerian symptoms of schizophrenia (Pope and Lipinski, 1978).[13] See Chapter 2 for further discussion of psychosis and thought disorder in mania and schizophrenia.

Bipolar Depression versus Schizophrenia or Schizoaffective Disorder

As with mania, the DSM-IV criteria for differentiating bipolar depression from schizophrenia and schizoaffective disorder focus on the prominence of the affective symptoms, their temporal relationship to the psychotic or schizophrenic symptoms, and the length of time the patient has been continuously delusional or hallucinatory. (As for mania, the DSM-IV criteria for major depression allow for up to 2 weeks of "mood-free" delusions or hallucinations, whereas the RDC allow for 1 week.) These criteria reemphasize classic descriptions that include considerable psychosis among the affective disorders.

Studies emerging since the first edition of this book was published have emphasized other clues to psychosis in the depressive syndrome, which are especially relevant to many bipolar patients with psychotic depression (Schatzberg and Rothschild, 1992). Those clues include relatively intact insight, marked guilt, and marked psychomotor changes. Intact insight in particular can lead to an increased effort on the part of the patient to mask psychotic symptoms.

Mixed Bipolar States versus Schizophrenia or Schizoaffective Disorder

Mixed bipolar states can pose special problems of differential diagnosis because of their instability, the often confusing mix of manic and depressive symptoms, and the fact that these states occur most characteristically in association with the most severe stage of mania (stage III) (Carlson and Goodwin, 1973). Frequently associated with mixed states is the presence of alcohol or drug intoxication, which can further mask pure affective symptoms and confuse differential diagnosis.

Clinical Summary

The clinician can distinguish manic-depressive illness from schizophrenia or schizoaffective disorder in most cases by careful attention to the patient's personal and family history, premorbid functioning, age at onset, and sequence and patterning of symptoms. In manic-depressive illness, delusions or hallucinations generally follow a period of either manic or depressive symptoms, and affective symptoms are prominent almost continuously.

Unipolar Depression

As noted in Chapter 1, evidence has begun to accumulate over the last decade that the misdiagnosis of bipolar disorder as unipolar depression is a major clinical problem. There are likely five primary causes for this development: (1) patients' lack of insight with regard to manic as opposed to depressive symptoms; (2) clinicians' neglect of information available from family members or other third parties; (3) clinicians' relative focus on euphoric rather than dysphoric or irritable mood as a criterion for hypomania; (4) the structure of DSM-IV, which by separating out bipolar from all depressive disorders has obscured the close relationship between early-onset recurrent depression and bipolar disorder; and (5) widespread interest in and use of "second-generation" antidepressants.

In some clinical studies, between 40 and 60 percent of patients with bipolar disorder appear to have been misdiagnosed with unipolar depression in both inpatient and outpatient psychiatric settings (Benazzi, 1999; Ghaemi et al., 1999, 2000). Data that are not widely known because they were collected as part of a family history study (Tsuang et al., 1980) illustrate the extent of the problem. When patients who had previously been hospitalized for mania were evaluated by an extensive research diagnostic interview several years later (but without input from a family member), about 60 percent had forgotten or denied that they had ever been manic. These findings, reported in the United States, appear to hold true in other countries as well; similar results were found in Spain, for example, although the latter study also noted a high rate of misdiagnosis as schizophrenia and personality disorder (Vieta and Salva, 1997). In another study, careful evaluation of the history of 108 patients in primary care revealed that 48 (44 percent) had hypomanic symptoms, thus indicating an apparent misdiagnosis rate of about 40 percent in the primary care setting as well (Manning et al., 1997). Hence careful attention to the differential diagnosis of bipolar disorder and unipolar depression is essential.

As we note throughout this text, much of the problem of the misdiagnosis of bipolar disorder as unipolar depression has to do with the structure of DSM-IV itself (recall

Fig. 3–1). Since DSM-III, the diagnostic system used in the United States has separated bipolar disorder from all depressive disorders "from the top," as does ICD-10. Major depressive episodes are always identified initially as unipolar (not bipolar), and a diagnosis of bipolar disorder relies entirely on diagnosis of a spontaneous manic or hypomanic episode. By excluding antidepressant-related mania or hypomania and by providing a very strict definition of mixed episodes, DSM-IV makes it likely that unipolar depression will be diagnosed more and bipolar disorder less frequently.

Unfortunately, in the case of the depressed patient, a diagnosis of bipolar disorder becomes entirely dependent on obtaining a history of past spontaneous mania or hypomania. A number of factors—related to both patient and clinician—mitigate against a complete and accurate diagnosis in such circumstances (see Box 3–9).

Among patient factors, lack of insight is perhaps most important. Researchers have demonstrated that about half of patients with acute mania lack insight into their symptoms (Amador et al., 1994; Ghaemi et al., 1995). Thus among depressed patients, that proportion or more would be unable to provide an accurate history of mania simply because they had never recognized having its symptoms. For example, in one study, patients reported prodromal

---

BOX 3–9.   Patient, Clinician, and Illness Factors Leading to Misdiagnosis of Bipolar Disorder as Unipolar Depression

Patient Factors

- Lack of insight with regard to mania
- Impaired memory during the depressive state and/or memory selective for past depressions (state-dependent memory)
- Experiencing of hypomania as normal "good times"
- Cultural positive feedback for manic/hypomanic symptoms

Clinician Factors

- Failure to include a family member in the diagnostic evaluation
- Structure of DSM-IV, which, "from the top," separates bipolar from all depressions
- Inadequate knowledge of manic criteria
- Intuitive "prototype" approach to diagnosis
- Practical desire to make a diagnosis (e.g., unipolar depression) for which many effective treatments exist
- Lack of awareness of the high population rate of bipolar illness

Illness Factors

- First episode of illness is often depression, not mania
- Dysphoric depression is not conceptualized as a mixed state
- Depressive episodes last longer than the often fleeting hypomanic states

behavioral symptoms of mania only half as frequently as did family members (Keitner et al., 1996). These data strongly support the need to obtain family or other third-party reports (e.g., teachers, halfway-house staff, social workers, psychotherapists, friends) in assessing the bipolar diagnosis. In fact, one might reasonably say that it is virtually impossible to rule out bipolar disorder with any degree of confidence in the absence of third-party reports.

Depressed patients' self-reports are also impaired by the depressive state. As is well known, depression not only impairs memory but also makes it more likely that memories will focus on past depressions—that is, memory can be state dependent. Thus, even if patients had previously possessed some insight into their manic symptoms, they might have difficulty recalling those symptoms clearly and accurately enough for the clinician to make a definitive diagnosis. Also, patients are often in such psychic pain during a depressive episode that they may be unmotivated to search their memory carefully for times when they may have felt better (albeit pathologically). Even then the mania may be remembered simply as "good periods."

Even more challenging is the ascertainment of prior hypomania, given the ill-defined boundary between hypomania and normal good mood (Gershon et al., 1982). Indeed, patients often cannot distinguish the hypomanic state, since they may not view it as behaviorally different from their usual personality—a phenomenon recognized by DSM-IV in requiring third-party reports for the diagnosis of hypomania. Cultural factors are also relevant: in the United States, hypomanic traits are often prized and socially promoted, making it difficult for some patients, as well as some observers, to recognize them as "abnormal."

Clinician-related factors are important as well. First and foremost, clinicians are often not aware of manic symptoms. In one study, clinicians could not describe accurately more than three of the seven manic criteria when asked to write them down, as compared with their ability to describe seven of the eight major depressive criteria (Sprock, 1988). This apparent ignorance of the features of mania may be due in part to the "prototype" phenomenon (Cantor et al., 1980), which relates to diagnosis by clinical intuition alone. Clinicians often practice with prototypes of the common syndromes in mind—the "typical" patient with depression, schizophrenia, or mania. Experience over the years has taught, however, that such prototypes need to be augmented by careful attention to empirically based diagnostic criteria. Furthermore, prototypes usually represent cross-sectional symptomatic presentations (e.g., the manic patient is agitated and grandiose); we know that such observations need to be augmented with longitudinal data regarding age at onset and course, as well as family history and prior medication responses.

In the past, such intuitive diagnostic techniques tended to lead to overdiagnosis of schizophrenia and probably to underdiagnosis of major depression as well. In the last decade or so—in part as a result of major continuing medical education programs often underwritten by the pharmaceutical industry (with interests in the multitude of new antidepressants)—much greater attention has been paid to major depression, and clinicians now routinely apply DSM-IV diagnostic criteria to that disorder. The evidence suggests, in contrast, that many if not most clinicians fail to apply the diagnostic criteria for mania routinely, and instead rely on a largely intuitive approach to diagnosis of the condition. With this approach, it is likely that only patients with pure euphoric mania at the time of the evaluation will be diagnosed; mixed episodes, rapid-cycling episodes, and bipolar depressed patients will tend to be missed.

Clinicians are practitioners first and foremost. The recent tendency to diagnose bipolar disorder less frequently may relate to the relative paucity of mood-stabilizing options. The advent of new mood stabilizers appears to be generating increased interest in bipolar disorder. Unfortunately, a recent survey of the members of the National Depressive and Manic-Depressive Association (now renamed the Depression and Bipolar Support Alliance) in the United States failed to find improvement in diagnosis of bipolar disorder in 2000 (Lewis, 2001) relative to 1994 (Lish et al., 1994). About half of patients had initially been misdiagnosed with unipolar depression, and the accurate diagnosis of bipolar disorder had usually been delayed by about a decade after initial evaluations with mental health professionals. On average, more than three mental health professionals had been seen before the accurate diagnosis of bipolar disorder had been made.[14] Relatively recent clinical studies have confirmed these findings. Thus, despite increasing attention to affective disorders in recent years, follow-up of treatment experience in a U.S. advocacy group population (which admittedly is probably not representative of bipolar illness generally) revealed little improvement during the last decade in the ability of U.S. practitioners to diagnose bipolar disorder (Hirschfeld et al., 2003). In one study, the mean time to a bipolar-I diagnosis from the first visit to a mental health professional (6 years) was twice that for unipolar depression (3.3 years), and the mean time to the correct diagnosis of bipolar-II disorder was even longer (nearly 12 years) (Ghaemi et al., 2000).

Of relevance to bipolar diagnosis is a self-report questionnaire, the Mood Disorder Questionnaire (MDQ), developed as a screening instrument for bipolar disorder (Hirschfeld et al., 2000).[15] This questionnaire reflects DSM-IV criteria. Patients are asked to report whether they have experienced those symptoms, whether the symptoms occurred simultaneously, and whether they led to significant social and occupational dysfunction. The sensitivity or true positive rate (the proportion of those actually ill thus identified) and specificity or true negative rate (the proportion of those not ill thus identified) of this self-report questionnaire depend on the population it is used to evaluate. Thus, as discussed more thoroughly in Chapter 11, relatively high sensitivity was achieved among patients from a university affective disorders clinic with a high proportion of bipolar-I patients who, moreover, were likely to have been educated about their illness. By contrast, in a community-based sample (where a screening instrument is presumably most useful), sensitivity was only 28 percent; that is, the MDQ missed more than 70 percent of those diagnosed as bipolar by a clinician using the Structured Clinical Interview for DSM (SCID) (Zimmerman et al., 2004). Similarly, in an independent validation study with a clinical sample, the MDQ was found to be more diagnostically sensitive for 26 patients with bipolar-I disorder (69 percent) than for 8 patients with bipolar-II disorder (30 percent) (Miller et al., 2002). Further, patients with impaired insight would be expected to deny their symptoms on the MDQ.[16] These studies suggest that the MDQ may be more useful in a clinical than in a community setting (Hirschfeld et al., 2003). Modifications to the MDQ that might increase its utility as a screening tool in community samples have been discussed by Miller and colleagues (2004) (see Chapter 11).

Besides the issue of differential sensitivity in community versus clinical settings, the larger question is whether it is appropriate to use the MDQ as a diagnostic tool without further clinical assessment. Here the concept of predictive value is relevant (Phelps and Ghaemi, 2006). Sensitivity and specificity are characteristics of a scale; predictive values are characteristics of a sample to which the scaled is applied. If the underlying prevalence of an illness is low, then even a highly sensitive scale can have a low positive predictive value, just as a highly specific scale can have a weak negative predictive value. For instance, if the MDQ, based on its two main validation studies, is applied in a community setting where the baseline rate of bipolar illness is 10 percent, a positive predictive value of less than 45–51 percent is obtained. In other words, only about half of the MDQ-positive subjects actually have bipolar disorder. In contrast, the negative predictive value of the MDQ in such settings would be quite high, over 92–97 percent. Thus in the community setting, the MDQ can help rule out but not rule in bipolar disorder. This limitation again highlights the importance of combining the MDQ or any self-report diagnostic scale with clinician-based interview evaluations. Further, this limitation should be taken into account in some quite large research studies that assume that MDQ-positive scores are equivalent to a valid bipolar diagnosis.

In addition to clinician and patient factors, an important natural history factor can make it likely for bipolar disorder to be misdiagnosed as unipolar depression: the occurrence of depressive episodes before manic episodes in the onset of the illness (false unipolar depression). As noted in Chapters 1 and 4, this is a frequent presentation in bipolar illness, especially in females. Again, it is important to recognize that there is a relationship between false unipolar depression and age at onset. As detailed in Chapter 4, the risk of switching from false unipolar depression to bipolar disorder is highest in childhood and young adulthood, occurring at a rate of about 3 to 5 percent per year; it then decreases by the late 30s, at which point it flattens out to about 1 percent per year. Thus in any depressed child or young adult, the index of suspicion for bipolar disorder should be high, as opposed to depressed individuals in their 30s or older.

In addition to identifying past hypomanic or manic symptoms, clinicians should seek to assess clinical data in three areas that can better delineate the distinction between unipolar and bipolar depression: natural course (especially age at onset and episode frequency), family history, and treatment response.[17] (For a more detailed analysis of the distinction between unipolar and bipolar depression, see Chapter 1.)

Attention-Deficit Hyperactivity Disorder (ADHD)

In children, a major differential for the diagnosis of bipolar disorder is ADHD, a topic discussed in more detail in Chapter 6. A principal overlap in symptomatology is distractibility, which is one of the criteria for mania. Child psychiatrists report that co-occurrence of marked irritability and aggression, often with major depressive episodes, should raise suspicion of bipolar disorder, at least comorbid with ADHD (Danielson et al., 2003; Fergus et al., 2003; Scheffer and Niskala Apps, 2004; Citrome and Goldberg, 2005). Retrospective data in adults suggest that in patients with bipolar disorder, symptoms of ADHD or anxiety disorder may predominate in childhood, and mood symptoms in adolescence and early adulthood (Sachs et al., 2000). Thus in some patients, ADHD may represent an early manifestation of an overall illness that later presents as a mood disorder. Another particularly informative feature is family history of bipolar disorder, which markedly increases the likelihood of bipolar disorder as opposed to ADHD. Also, if stimulant medications are ineffective or cause worsened aggression and irritability or even manic symptoms, the likelihood of bipolar disorder increases.

Finally, further research is required to establish the validity of adult ADHD. This is especially urgent now, given that adult ADHD is becoming an increasingly common diagnosis (some of this increase in diagnosis is, no doubt, in response to a new agent being marketed with this condition as an indication).

In the National Comorbidity Survey, adult ADHD was diagnosable in about 4.4 percent of the adult population (Kessler et al., 2006). However, 86 percent of these individuals were also diagnosable with mood or anxiety disorders. The authors, and many ADHD experts view these data as simply representing comorbidity; thus the importance of diagnosing and treating adult ADHD is emphasized. An equally possible if not more logical conclusion would be that since adult ADHD is hardly diagnosable without concomitant other mood or anxiety disorder diagnoses, those other diagnoses may account for most if not all of the cognitive symptoms that are labeled ADHD. This perspective flows from an appreciation of the concept of diagnostic hierarchy, whereby mood disorders in particular can cause other kinds of symptoms (whether psychotic, anxiety, or cognitive); thus those other diagnoses should not be made in the presence of an active mood disorder (Surtees and Kendell, 1979). In other words, if those mood or anxiety disorders are adequately treated, the cognitive symptoms will improve, suggesting that no separate ADHD diagnosis is necessary. Such extensive overlap between diagnoses should raise the possibility of a single diagnosis with multiple manifestations, not simply the concept of multiple diagnoses. Further, advocates for the diagnosis of adult ADHD often point to retrospective data in adults with bipolar disorder, in which 9.5 percent of such patients are retrospectively diagnosable with ADHD in childhood (Nierenberg et al., 2005). Yet such data do not necessarily support the common presence of ADHD in adulthood, but rather are compatible with the alternative view that many children with purported ADHD develop bipolar disorder in adulthood, raising the possibility that the ADHD-like presentation in childhood may have represented an early manifestation of the bipolar illness. In other words, instead of thinking that such persons had one illness in childhood and have another in adulthood, it may be more plausible that the same illness manifested itself differentially at different ages, with ADHD-like symptoms in childhood and more classic bipolar symptoms in adulthood.

In sum, given these possibilities, we would urge caution in the diagnosis and treatment of adult ADHD, always giving preference to initially diagnosing and treating mood disorders until euthymia is achieved before making the ADHD diagnosis or seeking to treat it with stimulants. Most experts would agree (given the abuse potential of stimulants) that prescribing such agents for cognitive symptoms of distractibility without first trying to treat concurrent mood or anxiety conditions is not scientifically or clinically well informed.

Brief Psychotic Disorder

Brief psychotic disorder is a DSM-IV category (see Box 3–10) reserved for individuals who experience a psychotic episode lasting from a day to a month with "eventual full return to premorbid level of functioning." The psychotic symptoms may or may not follow immediately after a major psychological or social stress, or they may occur postpartum. If the criteria for mania or major depressive episode are met, the affective diagnosis takes precedence. Often, individuals initially placed in the category of brief psychotic disorder eventually show symptoms that permit a diagnosis of either bipolar illness or schizophrenia. In particular, postpartum psychosis (often with depressive features) is highly associated with bipolar illness and may represent the first episode of the disorder (with manic episodes to follow) (Viguera and Cohen, 1998).

Cycloid Psychosis

The concept of cycloid psychosis, first described by Leonhard (1957), like that of schizoaffective disorder, a hybrid rooted in the overlapping symptoms of schizophrenia and recurrent (predominantly bipolar) affective illness, was discussed in more detail in the first edition of this volume. The condition occurs predominantly among females and

---

BOX **3–10.** **DSM-IV Definition of a Brief Psychotic Episode**

DSM-IV (p. 139) defines a brief psychotic episode as follows:

Criterion A: The essential feature of brief psychotic disorder is a disturbance that involves the sudden onset of at least one of the following positive psychotic symptoms: delusions, hallucinations, disorganized speech (e.g., frequent derailment or incoherence), or grossly disorganized or catatonic behavior.

Criterion B: An episode of the disturbance lasts at least 1 day but less than 1 month, and the individual eventually has a full return to the premorbid level of functioning.

Criterion C: The disturbance is not better accounted for by a mood disorder with psychotic features, by schizoaffective disorder, or by schizophrenia and is not due to the direct physiological effects of a substance (e.g., a hallucinogen) or a general medical condition (e.g., subdural hematoma).

Source: Reprinted with permission from the *Diagnostic and Statistical Manual of Mental Disorders*, Fourth Edition, Text Revision (Copyright 2000). American Psychiatric Association.

has a good prognosis. One study of 73 inpatients who met Perris's (1988) criteria for cycloid psychosis concluded that it is best regarded as an atypical variety of affective psychosis (Cutting, 1990). However, a more recent controlled family study of cycloid psychosis found a significantly lower morbidity risk for bipolar illness in first-degree relatives compared with relatives of patients with bipolar illness (Pfuhlmann et al., 2004). The authors concluded, therefore, that cycloid psychosis cannot be integrated into either the bipolar or the schizophrenic spectrum, but exists as an independent entity. Because of these conflicting results, further research is needed. Given the genetic vulnerability to psychosis that may cross the schizophrenia–affective boundary, it will be interesting to see what genetic studies of cycloid psychosis ultimately reveal.

Psychotic Disorder-Not Otherwise Specified

Classically, atypical psychosis was diagnosed in patients who had schizophrenic symptoms but showed rapid fluctuations in emotional states, an episodic course, and a generally favorable outcome. Mitsuda (1965) concluded from his study of monozygotic twins that atypical psychosis could be distinguished genetically from schizophrenia and, to a lesser extent, from manic-depressive illness. However, the relationship between this disorder and the cycloid psychosis delineated by Leonhard (1957) and Perris (1990) is not clear.

In DSM-IV, psychotic disorders-NOS is a residual category for patients with psychotic symptoms who do not meet criteria for any other DSM-IV disorder. For purposes of differential diagnosis, such patients would appear to fall in the schizoaffective spectrum.

Borderline Personality Disorder

The overlap between bipolar disorder and borderline personality disorder is quite controversial, and is discussed in more detail in Chapters 10 and 11. As a clinical rule of thumb, however, it may be good practice to use great caution in diagnosing borderline personality disorder in the midst of an active affective disorder (Parker et al., 2004). In other words, during a major depressive or hypomanic/manic episode, patients often may meet criteria for borderline personality disorder, whereas once the episode has ended, borderline features are no longer evident. Thus if possible, it is best to evaluate borderline personality disorder during periods of euthymia.

Making a differential diagnosis between bipolar depression and the depressive affect associated with borderline personality disorder involves attention to issues of lability, reactivity, and the overall symptom cluster. The depressive affect associated with borderline personality disorder is marked by considerable day-to-day or even hour-to-hour variability, whereas the depressive mood associated with a bipolar episode is generally experienced as a discrete episode with a clear onset and termination and a relatively stable course during the episode. The mood of the borderline patient is more likely to remain reactive to the environment and, although intensely dysphoric, to change quickly with an appropriate stimulation or intervention. As noted earlier, the symptom cluster of bipolar depression generally involves pervasive changes in the regulation of sleep and appetite (usually hyperphagia and hypersomnia). These features are not associated as prominently with depressive mood in the borderline patient unless bipolar disorder also is present.

In evaluating elevated mood, duration is important as well. Given the extreme lability of mood in borderline personality disorder, mood elevation probably does not last long enough to meet the criteria for mania. On duration alone, the mood elevation in borderline personality disorder could overlap with that in hypomania or cyclothymia. The usual associated symptoms of hypomania, however, such as racing thoughts and decreased need for sleep, are generally not part of the mood lability of the borderline patient. The absence of events either precipitating or terminating the hypomanic mood would also suggest a true case of bipolar disorder, as would a positive family history of the disorder, although the latter would not be conclusive. In practical terms, emphasis on the linkage between borderline and bipolar diagnoses is important because all too often, the diagnosis of bipolar disorder is missed when borderline features are also present, especially in adolescents. As discussed in Chapter 6, bipolar disorder can be especially difficult to diagnose in this age group, since a wide range of apparently nonspecific symptoms is common. Not infrequently, moreover, individuals rediagnosed as bipolar on follow-up experienced their first manic or hypomanic episode after exposure to an antidepressant drug. The possibility of this outcome argues for considerable care in ruling out a bipolar diathesis before treating depressive syndromes in adolescents with presumed borderline features.

It is our impression that many patients who may have bipolar disorder, particularly the rapid-cycling type II variety, receive a diagnosis of borderline personality disorder because of an overreliance on the intuitive prototype approach described above. The clinical picture of the rapid-cycling bipolar patient can approximate that of borderline personality cross-sectionally. However, careful application of the criteria for mania or hypomania often distinguishes rather clearly between patients with bipolar disorder and characterological illness (Akiskal, 2005; Benazzi, 2000a).[18] In some settings, moreover, patients with borderline personality disorder may be mistakenly diagnosed as bipolar when the clinician relies overly on mood lability alone for a bipolar diagnosis, rather than assessing both the full criteria for a mood episode and the unique course features associated with bipolar disorder (Berns et al., 2003).

Organic Brain Disorders

Since manic-depressive illness has its own underlying biological foundation, differentiating it from secondary brain disorders can be semantically and diagnostically confusing. DSM-IV represents an advance over DSM-III-R in this regard. Whereas DSM-III-R applied the term "organic" to disorders in which psychological and behavioral abnormalities are "associated with transient or permanent dysfunction of the brain," DSM-IV refers to "secondary" psychiatric disorders, in which symptoms are secondary to a specific medical condition, a specific medication or other substance, or identifiable conditions such as delirium or dementia of the Alzheimer's type. With DSM-IV, the designations "functional" and "organic" were replaced by "primary," meaning no definitive established etiology, and "secondary," with reference to the specific established etiology. This terminology is more precise and accurate, and allows for the fact that many primary psychiatric disorders, such as manic-depressive illness, may have biological etiologies that are not yet identifiable. The catch-all DSM-III-R diagnoses of "organic mood syndrome" and "organic personality syndrome," which often overlapped with manic-depressive illness, do not appear in DSM-IV.

The absence of specific pathognomonic neuropsychiatric manifestations of secondary brain disorders means that differentiating these disorders from bipolar illness requires an understanding of the variety of potentially associated conditions. Some behavioral features—principally changes in cognitive function, including impairment of orientation, memory, general intellectual function, and judgment—are more prominent in most of these disorders than in bipolar illness (see Chapter 9). Of comparable importance in making a differential diagnosis is a history of bipolar illness. However, the absence of such a history does not rule out primary bipolar illness, especially when the patient is still within the age of risk for onset of the disorder; here a positive family history of bipolar disorder can be helpful.

A standard neurological examination usually does not aid in differential diagnosis, since in most organic psychiatric syndromes, the results of such an examination remain normal until the disease is far advanced. The so-called soft neurological signs often thought to mark secondary brain disease have not proven to be specific.

Neuropsychological testing can be helpful in quantifying the extent of impairment but is not particularly useful in the initial differential diagnosis. This is so because, as detailed in Chapter 9, both depression and mania can be associated with substantial disturbances in responses on a wide variety of neuropsychological tests designed to measure cognitive changes. Procedures such as magnetic resonance imaging (MRI), computed tomography (CT) scans, and electroencephalograms (EEGs) may be helpful, but unless they can identify a localized lesion, they have not yet proven reliable in differentiating secondary brain disorder from bipolar illness. Newer methods, such as functional MRI (fMRI), positron emission tomography (PET), and single photon electromagnetic transmission (SPECT), provide enhanced functional assessments of anatomic function, which can be particularly useful in assessing changes during varying mood states. However, their utility remains limited primarily to research.

The Concept of Secondary Affective Episodes

Krauthammer and Klerman (1978) made an important conceptual contribution by reviewing the literature for reports of manic syndromes occurring shortly after medical, pharmacological, or other somatic dysfunctions. As described previously, DSM-IV places a great deal of emphasis on secondary causes of mania or hypomania. Box 3–11 lists conditions that have been associated with secondary manic or hypomanic symptoms.

Studies of secondary mania are uncommon. One study found that EEG abnormalities in patients with bipolar disorder predicted better valproate than lithium response (Stoll et al., 1994). Studies of secondary depression are more common. Its occurrence is frequently related to stroke or other neurological disorders (Whyte and Mulsant, 2002).

In general, while the primary–secondary distinction in psychiatry has not been carefully validated, it appears to have clinical utility and theoretical attraction.[19] As discussed in Chapter 1, however, an alternative to dividing mania and depression into primary and secondary categories is a spectrum model reflecting varying levels of vulnerability. The greatest vulnerability would be expressed as a *primary* case, in which little or no external stress was required; lower levels of vulnerability might show up only as *secondary* cases, that is, requiring the operation of external factors for the episode to appear. (For a more complete discussion of secondary affective presentations, see Chapter 17.)

We now review three specific secondary conditions: two related but nonaffective states—delirium and dementia—and epilepsy.

Delirium

The DSM-IV diagnostic criteria for delirium are given in Box 3–12. Severe (stage III) mania (Carlson and Goodwin, 1973) can involve clouding of consciousness, occasionally rendering it difficult to differentiate from delirium

BOX 3–11.   DSM-IV Features Associated with Secondary Mania or Hypomania

DSM-IV (p. 328) defines features associated with a manic episode as follows:

Individuals with a manic episode frequently do not recognize that they are ill and resist efforts to be treated. Ethical concerns may be disregarded even by those who are typically very conscientious. The person may be hostile and physically threatening to others. Some individuals, especially those with psychotic features, may become physically assaultive or suicidal. Adverse consequences of a manic episode (e.g., involuntary hospitalization, difficulties with the law, or serious financial difficulties) often result from poor judgment and hyperactivity. Some individuals describe having a much sharper sense of smell, hearing, or when catatonic symptoms (e.g., stupor, mutism, negativism, and posturing) are present, the specifier with catatonic features may be indicated (see p. 382). Mood may shift rapidly to anger or depression. Depressive symptoms may last moments, hours, or, more rarely, days. Not uncommonly, the depressive symptoms and manic symptoms occur simultaneously. No laboratory findings that are diagnostic of a manic episode have been identified. However, a variety of laboratory findings have been noted to be abnormal in groups of individuals with manic episodes compared with control subjects. Laboratory findings in manic episodes include polysomnographic abnormalities, increased cortisol secretion, and absence of dexamethasone nonsuppression. There may be abnormalities involving the norepinephrine, serotonin, acetylcholine, dopamine, or gamma-aminobutyric acid neurotransmitter systems, as demonstrated by studies of neurotransmitter metabolites, receptor functioning, pharmacological provocation, and neuroendocrine function.

DSM-IV (p. 335) defines features associated with a hypomanic episode as follows:

Associated features of a mixed episode are similar to those for manic episodes and major depressive episodes. Individuals may be disorganized in their thinking or behavior. Because individuals in mixed episodes experience more dysphoria than do those in manic episodes, they may be more likely to seek help. Laboratory findings for mixed episode are not well studied, although evidence to date suggests physiological and endocrine findings that are similar to those found in severe major depressive episodes.

Source: Reprinted with permission from the *Diagnostic and Statistical Manual of Mental Disorders*, Fourth Edition, Text Revision (Copyright 2000). American Psychiatric Association.

BOX 3–12.   DSM-IV Definition of Delirium

DSM-IV (p. 127) defines delirium as follows:

Criterion A: The essential feature of a delirium is a disturbance of consciousness that is accompanied by a change in cognition that cannot be better accounted for by a preexisting or evolving dementia. The disturbance develops over a short period of time, usually hours to days, and tends to fluctuate during the course of the day. The disturbance in consciousness is manifested by a reduced clarity of awareness of the environment. The ability to focus, sustain, or shift attention is impaired.

Criterion B: There is an accompanying change in cognition (which may include memory impairment, disorientation, or language disturbance) or development of a perceptual disturbance.

Criterion C: In mild delirium, disorientation to time may be the first symptom to appear. Disorientation to self is less common. Language disturbance may be evident as dysnomia (i.e., the impaired ability to name objects) or dysgraphia (i.e., the impaired ability to write). In some cases, speech is rambling and irrelevant, in others pressured and incoherent, with unpredictable switching from subject to subject. The disturbance develops over a short period of time and tends to fluctuate during the course of the day.

Source: Reprinted with permission from the *Diagnostic and Statistical Manual of Mental Disorders*, Fourth Edition, Text Revision (Copyright 2000). American Psychiatric Association.

in delirium than in stage III mania. The sustained euphoria (or irritability) characteristic of mania, by contrast, is not likely in delirium.

As with all diagnoses of organic brain disorders, indications (from the patient's history, physical examination, or laboratory data) of a specific organic etiological factor are important to the diagnosis. As noted in Chapter 7, manic episodes are commonly associated with substance abuse, particularly in young patients, and here the challenge is to differentiate a pure organic delirium from a manic episode precipitated and colored by alcohol or drugs.

Dementia

The DSM-IV criteria for dementia, given in Box 3–13, overlap somewhat with those for delirium. The considerable attention that has been paid to differentiating between true dementia and depressive pseudodementia is often justified since the pseudodementia associated with depression is highly treatable. Recent data suggest, however, that depression in the elderly can often herald dementia, making the distinction less exclusive than may earlier have been assumed (Jorm, 2000). As discussed in Chapter 9, bipolar patients in particular often experience profound deficits in

(see Chapter 2) (Fink, 1999). Indeed, delirious mania was well described by Kraepelin (1921) and others. The absence of the preceding stages of mania or of a history of mania is sometimes helpful in making this differential diagnosis. Perceptual disturbances usually have a more sudden onset

BOX 3–13.   DSM-IV Definition of Dementia

DSM-IV (p. 139) defines dementia as follows:

Criterion A1: The essential feature of a dementia is the development of multiple cognitive deficits that include memory impairment and at least one of the following cognitive disturbances: aphasia, apraxia, agnosia, or a disturbance in executive functioning. Memory impairment is required to make the diagnosis of a dementia and is a prominent early symptom.

Criterion A2a: Deterioration of language function (aphasia) may be manifested by difficulty producing the names of individuals and objects.

Criterion A2b: Individuals with dementia may exhibit apraxia (i.e., impaired ability to execute motor activities despite intact motor abilities, sensory function, and comprehension of the required task).

Criterion A2c: Individuals with dementia may exhibit agnosia (i.e., failure to recognize or identify objects despite intact sensory function).

Criterion A2d: Disturbances in executive functioning are a common manifestation of dementia and may be related especially to disorders of the frontal lobe or associated subcortical pathways.

Criterion B: The items in both Criterion A1 (memory impairment) and Criterion A2 (aphasia, apraxia, agnosia, or disturbance in executive functioning) must be severe enough to cause significant impairment in social or occupational functioning (e.g., going to school, working, shopping, dressing, bathing, handling finances, and other activities of daily living) and must represent a decline from a previous level of functioning. The nature and degree of impairment are variable and often depend on the particular social setting of the individual.

Source: Reprinted with permission from the *Diagnostic and Statistical Manual of Mental Disorders*, Fourth Edition, Text Revision (Copyright 2000). American Psychiatric Association.

cognition and memory, and consequently are sometimes misdiagnosed as having primary dementia. This misdiagnosis occurs most frequently with elderly patients, in whom clinicians tend to neglect affective symptoms and focus instead on somatic and cognitive symptoms. Although a history of manic or depressive episodes is quite helpful in making this differential diagnosis, it cannot be used absolutely: on the one hand, a small percentage of bipolar patients do not have their first episode until they are in their 50s or 60s; on the other hand, bipolar patients may independently develop dementia later in life. Since a high proportion of late-onset bipolar patients have frequent cycles (see Chapter 4), the clinical picture may convey chronicity and therefore appear to be associated with an organic etiology.

Other aspects of the depressive syndrome, such as sleep and appetite dysregulation, are not especially helpful in differentiating bipolar illness from dementia. Neuropsychiatric testing can be useful, especially if a focal lesion is involved, but it cannot be relied upon to establish a clear differential because bipolar depression can also be associated with profound cognitive impairment. As with other differential diagnostic questions, it is important to look for atypical forms of mania in the patient's history, particularly episodic irritability or agitation in the absence of euphoria. The periods of secondary affective lability sometimes associated with primary dementing illnesses do not appear as discrete episodes. Obviously, a definitive diagnosis can be made if an organic cause for the dementia can be uncovered. Box 3–14 lists diseases or conditions that have been associated with dementia.

Because of its enormous public health importance, the issue of acquired immunodeficiency syndrome (AIDS) dementia deserves special attention (Melton et al., 1997). The human immunodeficiency virus (HIV) belongs to a class of retroviruses that are neurotrophic; that is, they have a special affinity for the nervous system. By the time AIDS has reached its peak, involvement of the central nervous system is almost universal. More important to the issue of

BOX 3–14.   DSM-IV Definition of Diseases Associated with Dementia

DSM-IV (pp. 133–134) defines the physical examination findings and general medical conditions associated with dementia as follows:

The associated physical examination findings of dementia depend on the nature, location, and stage of progression of the underlying pathology. The most common cause of dementia is Alzheimer's disease, followed by vascular disease, and then by multiple etiologies. Other causes of dementia include Pick's disease, normal-pressure hydrocephalus, Parkinson's disease, Huntington's disease, traumatic brain injury, brain tumors, anoxia, infectious disorders (e.g., human immunodeficiency virus [HIV], syphilis), prion diseases (e.g., Creutzfeldt-Jakob disease), endocrine conditions (e.g., hypothyroidism, hypercalcemia, hypoglycemia), vitamin deficiencies (e.g., deficiencies of thiamine, niacin, vitamin B), immune disorders (e.g., polymyalgia rheumatica, systemic lupus erythematosus), hepatic conditions, metabolic conditions (e.g., Kufs' disease, adrenoleukodystrophy, metachromatic leukodystrophy, and other storage diseases of adulthood and childhood), and other neurological conditions (e.g., multiple sclerosis).

Source: Reprinted with permission from the *Diagnostic and Statistical Manual of Mental Disorders*, Fourth Edition, Text Revision (Copyright 2000). American Psychiatric Association.

differential diagnosis, however, is the finding that among 20–25 percent of AIDS patients, the presenting symptoms originate in the central nervous system. These early AIDS symptoms may be difficult to distinguish from depression (Price et al., 1986; Bridge et al., 1988). Mania has also been reported as an early symptom (Gabel et al., 1986; Lyketsos et al., 1997; Yang et al., 2005). As the condition progresses, memory, concentration, and rapid alternating movements are impaired. Other indications include pyramidal tract signs, ataxia, leg weakness, and tremor. AIDS dementia becomes the presumptive diagnosis when the antibody test is positive. In addition, neuropsychological tests and MRI scans may be helpful in making the differential diagnosis. Of course it must be remembered that bipolar patients may also have AIDS, perhaps at a higher rate than comparable populations, given the prominence of reckless sexual behavior during mania.

Epilepsy

Epilepsy comprises a group of disorders of the central nervous system that, like other organic disorders, must be differentiated from bipolar illness. The condition is commonly associated with psychiatric symptoms, which can be divided into those occurring during actual seizure activity and those manifested only during interictal periods.

Findings of epidemiologic surveys of large numbers of patients with epilepsy (see, e.g., Gibbs and Gibbs, 1952) indicate that psychotic symptoms are about 10 times more likely to occur in association with temporal lobe than with generalized epilepsy (reviewed by McKenna et al., 1985; Kanner, 2004). The psychoses associated with temporal lobe epilepsy were initially described at a time when the broad Bleulerian concept of schizophrenia was prevalent. It is thus not surprising that patients with these psychoses tended to be described as schizophrenic, and less frequently as affectively ill. Clinically, these psychoses are generally mixed syndromes with a prominence of visual and olfactory hallucinations, rapid fluctuations of mood, catatonic features, and dreamlike states—all of which occur in an episodic course.

In his studies of patients with temporal lobe epilepsy, Flor-Henry (1969) found that 40 percent had either manic-depressive or schizoaffective features, and 42 percent had predominantly schizophrenic symptoms. Further frustrating attempts to understand the association between psychosis and temporal lobe epilepsy is the fact that patients can at times manifest predominantly affective symptoms and at other times predominantly schizophrenic symptoms. Flor-Henry also found an association between ictal laterality and type of mood syndrome: left-side epileptic foci in temporal lobe epilepsy were associated with depressive syndromes, whereas right-side epileptic foci were associated

with manic syndromes. While intriguing, this observation has not been well replicated. Conversely, Post and Weiss (2004) at the NIMH observed a relatively high frequency of epileptic-like phenomena in bipolar patients, particularly those with rapid cycles.

The specific relationship between epilepsy per se and bipolar disorder is relatively understudied. The most recent study of the topic compared 13 patients with generalized epilepsy and interictal manic episodes and 13 patients with primary bipolar disorder (Kudo et al., 2001). In that study, patients with epilepsy and mania tended to experience somewhat less severe manic episodes than did patients with primary bipolar disorder. The epileptic patients also tended to have substance-induced episodes somewhat more frequently than the primary bipolar disorder group. The epileptic foci were frontal or temporal in location.

Clinical Summary

Given the possibility that the pathophysiology of manic-depressive illness may overlap with that of some identifiable brain disorders, differential diagnosis cannot easily be reduced to simple formulas. For practical purposes, however, a differential diagnosis is critical to making an accurate treatment selection and prognosis. Thus, the clinician's first task when presented with manic or depressive symptoms is to consider other (possibly correctable) factors that might explain the symptoms. The absence of a personal or family history of affective illness and poor response to traditional treatments for manic-depressive illness are important clues suggesting the possibility of an organic etiology (McElroy et al., 1992). Although no single medical screening test is definitive, certainly a neurological examination, formal neuropsychiatric testing, an MRI, an EEG, a CT scan, and a chemical screen for metabolic and toxic disturbances should supplement the careful taking of the patient's history. Where the evidence points to a possible commingling of manic-depressive illness and a seizure disorder diathesis, anticonvulsants with a primary effect on temporal lobe disorders (e.g., carbamazepine, valproate, or lamotrigine) should be the treatment of choice.

CONCLUSIONS

To make an accurate diagnosis of bipolar disorder, the patient's history should be reviewed carefully with the patient *and* a family member; this focus on history is at least as important as a full description of the presenting episode. Whenever possible, the onset, duration, and treatment response of all past episodes should be recorded on a life chart, along with important life events. Much of this information can be obtained before the initial appointment by having the patient and family members fill out a life chart form. The most important differential diagnostic issue in evaluating depression is determining whether the patient has a unipolar or bipolar form of the illness. Obviously, this distinction must rest on knowledge of the patient's history, especially any prior episodes of mania or hypomania. Once again we must emphasize the importance of obtaining information from the family, especially given that impairment of insight is a major problem in about half of patients with bipolar disorder. Without family input, more than half of patients with a prior history of mania will deny or forget it, and the resulting overdiagnosis of unipolar depression is even more likely when the bipolar history involves hypomania only.

If the patient has had two or more previous depressions without evidence of mania or hypomania, an age at onset above 25 or 30, and a family history negative for bipolar disorder, it is reasonably safe to assume a unipolar diagnosis, even though about 10 percent of such patients will later develop a manic episode and be reclassified as bipolar. In children and adolescents presenting with depression, the likelihood of an eventual bipolar course is much higher. As noted above, a family history of mania can provide an important clue to a possible bipolar diathesis, and may be helpful in choosing a mood stabilizer over an antidepressant for the treatment of highly recurrent depression. When manic-like symptoms characterize the presenting picture, the clinician may face difficult questions of differential diagnosis. If a patient is in the hyperactive psychotic state described as stage III mania (see Chapter 2) and a complete patient or family history is not available, the clinician must rely on an analysis of the presenting symptoms. (If there is a history of manic or depressive episodes, especially with well intervals, bipolar illness is the presumptive diagnosis, despite the atypical presenting symptoms.)

The principal alternative diagnoses that should be ruled out in diagnosing the manic phase of bipolar illness are acute schizophrenia and psychoses secondary to substance abuse or a general medical condition, although the latter can, and often do, occur in an individual with bipolar illness. The presence of delusions (including paranoid delusions), hallucinations, and thought disorder does not support a diagnosis of schizophrenia over that of mania. Schizophrenia should be suspected, however, if the delusions are organized into a formal and stable system that has continued for a considerable time in the absence of prominent mood symptoms. As a practical matter, differentiating acute stage III mania from schizoaffective illness and schizophrenia is not absolutely critical, since the initial treatment—antipsychotic medication (especially an atypical agent)—often is essentially the same for all three. If an affective component is suspected, the addition of a mood stabilizer, such as lithium or an anticonvulsant, should be considered. When the acute psychotic episode is under control, differential diagnosis often becomes clearer, even if information on the patient's personal or family history is still missing. If delusions or hallucinations persist in the absence of manic mood or hyperactivity (i.e., the patient is quietly delusional), schizophrenia or schizoaffective disorder is the more appropriate diagnosis. If the patient meets criteria for both schizophrenia and affective illness in the present episode or by history, schizoaffective illness is the appropriate diagnosis. Care should be taken to avoid overuse of the schizoaffective diagnosis simply because the patient's past history is unavailable. Distinguishing between bipolar disorder and schizophrenia can be particularly difficult in an adolescent because at that age, psychotic features are especially common in manic syndromes.

When vivid hallucinations (especially visual ones) or delusions dominate the clinical picture, particularly in a young person, a drug-induced state should be suspected, and a urine screen becomes especially important. Indeed, for most adolescent patients, it is sensible to employ a urine screen routinely. True mania may be present even if these suspicions are borne out, because it is not at all uncommon for initial manic episodes to be precipitated by drugs of abuse. In such cases, differential diagnosis can be difficult during the acute phase.

When presented with milder manic-like symptoms (or a history of such symptoms), the clinician must differentiate between clinical hypomania and normal elevated mood. Here it is important to recall the spectrum concepts outlined in Chapter 1. The threshold for a DSM-IV diagnosis of hypomanic episode is reached when (1) elation, excitement, and/or irritability cluster in discrete episodes lasting at least 4 days; (2) the symptomatic criteria outlined previously are met; (3) symptoms are out of proportion to any environmental precipitant; (4) symptoms represent a clear change in the individual's normal functioning; and/or (5) the episodes have a high potential to result in negative social, professional, and/or financial consequences. While the criteria for hypomania can be met without (4) or (5), the latter are prominent in the DSM-IV definition of a hypomanic episode. Again, we cannot overstate the importance of obtaining corroborating information from a spouse or other family member in evaluating the presence (or history) of hypomanic symptoms.

When presented with psychotic depressive symptoms, the clinician faces a somewhat different diagnostic challenge. Again, assuming that no history is available, one must rule out schizophrenia and schizoaffective illness, drug-induced states, and dementia. If delusions are present, they should be depressive in content to support an affective diagnosis. Among the depressive disorders, delusions are more likely to be associated with the bipolar form. Differentiating the bipolar form of manic-depressive illness from personality disorders or post-traumatic stress disorder (PTSD) is complex. Frequently, the conditions can co-occur. If any acute episodes meet the criteria for mania or hypomania, bipolar disorder should be diagnosed, regardless of the extent of concomitant PTSD or personality disorder features. If the course is almost completely characterized by physical or sexual trauma, along with the typical features of borderline personality (interpersonal conflict and rage, repeated self-injury, manipulative relationships), then the occurrence of mood lability *by itself* likely will not justify the bipolar diagnosis. Again, attention should be paid to family history, and more emphasis placed on course of illness rather than acute presentation.

NOTES

1. Andreasen et al., 1981; Tsuang et al., 1981; Andreasen and Grove, 1982; Keller and Baker, 1991; Blacker and Tsuang, 1992; Dunner, 1992; DeBattista et al., 1998; Goodwin and Ghaemi, 1998.
2. The RDC, together with the Schedule for Affective Disorders and Schizophrenia, proved to be reliable diagnostic instruments when used by interviewers from different centers around the country to rate past psychiatric symptoms and lifetime diagnoses in patients who were mentally ill at the time of assessment. However, the lifetime diagnoses of hypomania and recurrent unipolar depression were not as reliable as other categories (Keller et al., 1981).
3. Angst, 1980; Marneros et al., 1988, 1989, 1991, 2000; Maj et al., 1989.
4. Akiskal et al., 1995; Goldberg et al., 1995, 2001, Kessing, 2005.
5. Outside the United States, most of the rest of the world is characterized by geographically stable populations, making it easier to recognize the recurrent nature of the affective disorders.
6. Not all studies are consistent. For instance, one study found that bipolar-II disorder was much less stable (33 percent unchanged diagnostically 6 years later) than bipolar-I disorder (60 percent unchanged); it also found that decreased need for sleep was the best predictor among diagnostic criteria for bipolar-II disorder (Rice et al., 1992). Dunner also found that the reliability of the bipolar-II diagnosis was much greater when made by clinicians with expertise in mood disorders than when based solely on research diagnostic instruments such as the Structured Clinical Interview for DSM (SCID) (Dunner and Tay, 1993).
7. Testing the DSM-IV definition, Benazzi (2001) reported that almost all patients who met the DSM-IV definition of bipolar-II disorder also experienced 2 to 3 days of hypomania.
8. A recent excellent historical review demonstrated that Kraepelin's original conception of mixed states was derived largely from Weygandt, and that Kraepelin and Weygandt viewed mixed states not as uncommon, but as being the most common form of manic-depressive illness (Salvatore et al., 2002).
9. Along with major depression and inner agitation, at least three of the following symptoms must be present: (1) racing or crowded thoughts, (2) irritability or unprovoked feelings of rage, (3) absence of signs of retardation, (4) talkativeness, (5) dramatic descriptions of suffering or frequent spells of weeping, (6) mood lability and marked emotional reactivity, and (7) early insomnia (which is often associated with racing or crowded thoughts).
10. See Chapter 2; also, especially, Akiskal, 1996, 2002; Ghaemi et al., 2002.
11. The Schneiderian first-rank symptoms that overlap most commonly between schizophrenia and manic-depressive illness include thought broadcasting, thought insertion, experiences of influence, delusional perceptions, and incomplete auditory hallucinations (Schneider, 1959). Descriptive data suggest that manic patients with first-rank and/or catatonic symptoms cannot be distinguished from those without such symptoms on the basis of family history or treatment response (Jampala et al., 1989). Jampala and colleagues (1985) reported that manic patients with so-called emotional blunting—"a constricted, inappropriate, unrelated affect of diminished intensity, with indifference or unconcern for loved ones, lack of emotional responsivity, and a loss of social graces"—had family histories suggestive of schizophrenia, but with a pattern of treatment response related more closely to mania without emotional blunting.
12. Schizoaffective depressed patients do not have a history of mania; that is, they are unipolar.
13. The following case history reported by Pope (1983, pp. 326–327) illustrates the devastation that can follow the misdiagnosis of manic-depressive illness as schizophrenia:

> Ms. B, a 28-year-old woman, had been a psychiatric inpatient in a state hospital for the greater part of nine years. She had first been admitted at the age of 19 when she developed psychotic symptoms. . . . A history taken at that time by the admitting psychiatrist elaborately described her delusions and hallucinations but gave no information about whether Ms. B displayed mood change, activity change, an increase or decrease in energy level, or other affective symptomatology. No family history data were elicited. . . . Ms. B had been treated with virtually every antipsychotic drug available but had never been treated with lithium or ECT [electroconvulsive therapy]. . . . [Her] hospital records revealed that she had had periods of unusual irritability, coupled with increased activity and talkativeness . . . [and] had also displayed distractibility, grandiosity, and interpersonal intrusiveness. However, during most of her hospitalization, she was described as apathetic, with hypersomnia of 10 to 11 hours a night, lacking in energy and concentration, eating poorly, and displaying little interest in social contact. She was also markedly self-deprecating and was described as having long guilty ruminations on religious themes. She had made two suicide attempts during these periods.
>
> During Ms. B's ninth year in the hospital, her 21-year-old brother was admitted to a private psychiatric hospital. He was suffering from a relatively typical manic episode . . . [and] responded relatively well to lithium carbonate. When the brother's psychiatrist learned of Ms. B's illness, he elicited more information about the family and discovered that a maternal aunt and the

maternal grandmother had had major depressive episodes. This evidence seemed to support his theory that Ms. B was suffering from a chronic form of bipolar disorder.... [T]he brother's psychiatrist made further inquiries about the possibility of the sister's being given a trial of lithium carbonate. The doctors at the state hospital refused, saying that the patient was "clearly schizophrenic." ... However, after a great deal of pressure from Ms. B's mother, [they] reluctantly agreed to start Ms. B on lithium.

Within about three weeks Ms. B became markedly less agitated, less irritable, and more cooperative with staff. Shortly thereafter she was discharged to the quarterway house. Within two months, she transferred to a halfway house setting and was able to engage in a productive job with only a modest degree of supervision. However, she then became somewhat more depressed, and shortly thereafter stopped both her lithium and her antipsychotic drugs. Within a week, she had become sleepless, hyperactive, irritable, distractible, and grandiose. She was readmitted to the state hospital where she was treated with antipsychotic drugs but not with lithium. In spite of the clear temporal association between use of lithium and clinical response, the doctors claimed that the patient's "schizophrenic" symptoms ruled out a diagnosis of manic-depressive illness, and were unwilling to resume lithium therapy. At last report Ms. B's mother was still battling with the state hospital to reinstitute lithium.

14. Although the association's samples are not likely to be representative of patients with bipolar disorder in general, the point is that in this sample, early ascertainment of bipolarity had not improved recently.

15. The MDQ is a five-part questionnaire. The first part comprises 13 brief yes-or-no statements related to manic symptoms, all of which begin with the precursor "Has there ever been a period of time when you were not your usual self and. . . ." These questions assess various bipolar symptoms, such as hypersexuality ("you were much more interested in sex than usual?") and racing thoughts ("thoughts raced through your head or you couldn't slow your mind down?"). The second part is one yes-or-no question, which asks whether those manic symptoms occurred simultaneously. The third part has the subject evaluate the problems caused by those manic behaviors along a four-point scale, ranging from "no problem" to "serious problem." The fourth and fifth parts assess bipolar disorder in the subject's relatives and previous bipolar diagnoses, respectively.

16. One study found that 93 percent of patients who joined a voluntary bipolar disorder case registry accurately reported having bipolar disorder in agreement with a research diagnostic interview (Cluss et al., 1999). However, 94 percent of these patients had previously been diagnosed by professionals with bipolar disorder. It would appear likely that they would be influenced by such professional interactions. What is of concern for a screening instrument is how well it accurately diagnoses individuals who have never been correctly diagnosed with bipolar disorder despite having the condition, and in those circumstances, impairment of insight would appear to predict low accuracy of self-report.

17. Mitchell et al., 1992; Akiskal et al., 1995; Akiskal, 1996; Benazzi, 2000b; Benazzi and Rihmer, 2000; Ghaemi et al., 2004; Akiskal and Benazzi, 2005.

18. It also has been suggested that personality inventories, such as Cloninger's Temperament Character Inventory, may be used to distinguish between bipolar disorder and borderline personality disorder (Atre-Vaidya and Hussain, 1999).

19. In their review of reported reserpine-induced depressions, Goodwin and Bunney (1971) found that the great majority of reserpine "depressions" were, in fact, pseudodepressions that did not mimic the full natural syndrome. Those with full endogenous or melancholic symptoms generally had a personal or family history of affective illness. These authors inferred that reserpine merely uncovered a vulnerability rather than inducing depression de novo (see Chapter 19).

PART II

CLINICAL STUDIES

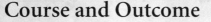

4 Course and Outcome

The universal experience is striking, that the attacks of manic-depressive insanity . . . never lead
to profound dementia, not even when they continue throughout life almost without interrup-
tion. . . . As a rule the disease runs its course in isolated attacks more or less sharply defined
from each other or from health, which are either like or unlike, or even very frequently are
[the] perfect antithesis.

—Emil Kraepelin (1921, p. 3)

Emil Kraepelin's central insight, one that continues as an organizing principle in modern descriptive psychiatry, was his division of the major psychoses into two groups based largely on course and outcome. He observed that whereas dementia praecox (schizophrenia) tends to be chronic and to follow a deteriorating course, manic-depressive illness is episodic and ultimately exacts a less devastating toll from those affected. Today we face a paradox: whereas the discovery of the prophylactic potential of lithium and, subsequently, some of the anticonvulsants and atypical antipsychotics has revived interest in the natural course of manic-depressive illness, widespread use of these prophylactic agents, as well as antidepressants, has substantially altered that course. Investigators must confront the fact that "natural" course now includes the largely unquantified effects of routine, acute, and prophylactic treatment.

In this chapter, after briefly reviewing salient methodological issues, we examine findings of the literature on the following aspects of the course and outcome of manic-depressive illness: premorbid functioning, age at onset, number of episodes, frequency of episodes (cycle length), onset and duration of episodes, polarity, pattern, precipitants of episodes, long-term outcome, mortality, the course of bipolar-II disorder, and mechanisms of recurrence. Studies assessing the impact of prophylactic treatment are reviewed in Chapter 20, and biological correlates of natural course are covered in Chapter 14.

METHODOLOGICAL ISSUES

As with most fields of inquiry, studies of the course and outcome of manic-depressive illness involve methodological complexities that should be kept in mind when interpreting the study results. Two issues are especially important.

The first relates to patient selection. The index hospitalization required in many older outcome studies can produce either underestimates or overestimates of recurrence. Underestimates can result when, during a single hospitalization, a patient has multiple rapid cycles that are counted as a single episode. On the other hand, overestimates can result from basing recurrence rates on hospital admission data, because those data exclude patients who experience a single episode, recover without hospitalization, and never have a recurrence. While some recent studies (virtually all of which focused on the bipolar subgroup) have avoided these problems by recruiting patients from the general community, other samples (e.g., those of the Stanley Foundation Bipolar Network) have been drawn from clinics in which sicker, treatment-resistant patients tend to be overrepresented. Indeed, clinical samples are, by definition, not representative, because a substantial portion of the bipolar population is not receiving treatment at any given time.

The second issue has to do with diagnosis. Many of the classic studies of natural course do not distinguish between the bipolar and recurrent unipolar subgroups. Numerous interpretive problems result, particularly in studies from the United States, where diagnostic criteria for unipolar illness (i.e., depressions that are not bipolar) allow for considerable heterogeneity (see the discussions of this issue in Chapters 1 and 3). For this reason, we emphasize the literature on bipolar patients, although some conclusions may be relevant to the more recurrent forms of unipolar illness as well. Furthermore, most classic studies of bipolar patients have involved patients hospitalized for mania and thus have not included the bipolar-II subgroup. The extent to which patients with schizoaffective features are included in the sample is another diagnostic issue (see the later discussion).

In addition to these issues, a traditional methodological problem is the lack of a generally accepted convention for collecting data on the course of manic-depressive illness or for defining recovery and relapse. Standardized methods for charting the course of the illness, proposed for both retrospectively derived data (Post et al., 1988; Honig et al., 2001) and prospectively derived data (Keller et al., 1987; Leverich et al., 2001), have improved this situation but are still far from universally applied. These methods have clinical as well as research uses. For example, detailed description of the prior course of the illness may reveal that medications, such as lithium, given to the patient in the past were mistakenly judged ineffective when they actually led to improvement. Conversely, charting may uncover instances in which certain drugs, such as antidepressants, exacerbated the course of the illness. In addition, previously unrecognized associations of episode onsets with anniversaries, life events, or other stressors may aid in psychotherapeutic understanding and behavioral management. These standardized charting methods are all the more important in industrialized countries, where population mobility is exacerbating a situation in which there are increasingly fewer opportunities for a single clinic or clinician to follow a cohort of patients over a lifetime.

A final methodological consideration in reviewing this literature is its largely retrospective nature, a troublesome aspect given the problems inherent in recalling the past, especially for depressed patients. Future studies need to be prospective and to focus on patients in naturalistic treatment settings.

PREMORBID FUNCTIONING

The distinction between "premorbid" functioning in children and childhood manifestations of full-blown manic-depressive illness can be somewhat arbitrary, because the disorder may present a different clinical picture in childhood than in adolescence or adulthood. We discuss clinical manifestations of possible childhood variants of the illness, as well as premorbid functioning in its early-onset forms, in Chapter 6, issues of premorbid/underlying personality in Chapter 10, and issues of neurocognitive development in Chapter 9. Here we focus on other measures of premorbid functioning (e.g., social, academic) in samples that do not include childhood-onset recurrent mood disorder.

In the original Kraepelinian definition, patients with manic-depressive illness were free of any morbid symptoms before the onset of their illness. Some modern data are consistent with this impression. In an elegant prospective study, Reichenberg and colleagues (2002) examined results from an extensive array of tests designed to measure level of functioning in persons who later developed schizoaffective, schizophrenic, or nonpsychotic bipolar disorder. Patients were matched with normal controls on age and education level. The nonpsychotic bipolar group showed no significant impairment on intellectual tests, reading/writing, or various behavioral measures.[1] Schizophrenic patients displayed premorbid impairment across most measures of intellectual and behavioral functioning, whereas schizoaffective patients showed less consistent impairment, suggesting a psychotic continuum of premorbid impairment.[2]

Some studies of premorbid functioning in psychotic bipolar patients paint a picture slightly different from the Kraepelinian model. For example, in their retrospective analysis comparing a large sample of bipolar and unipolar patients, Stephens and McHugh (1991) found significantly greater premorbid impairment on descriptive measures of social and work functioning in the bipolar group, which also had significantly higher rates of mood-congruent psychosis; however, the unipolar group was not selected for the more recurrent form. In a retrospective study using maternal interviews, Cannon and colleagues (1997) compared hospitalized schizophrenic patients with hospitalized psychotic bipolar patients and healthy controls on measures of premorbid social functioning and school performance. The psychotic bipolar group scored significantly worse than healthy controls on premorbid social adjustment measures, but significantly better than schizophrenic patients. Other studies have corroborated the finding that patients with psychotic and/or severe forms of bipolar disorder displayed significantly less premorbid impairment than did schizophrenic patients, lending weight to the notion that degree of premorbid impairment is an important distinction between bipolar disorder and schizophrenia.[3] Nevertheless, it appears that subtle premorbid dysfunction (especially cognitive dysfunction) may exist in some patients with bipolar disorder, particularly those with psychotic forms of the illness. More prospective data from epidemiologic samples, employing *Diagnostic and Statistical Manual* (DSM)-IV diagnoses and incorporating both psychotic and nonpsychotic forms of the disorder, are needed to further elucidate the premorbid phenomenology of bipolar disorder.

AGE AT ONSET

The age when manic-depressive illness most often begins (in both its bipolar and recurrent unipolar forms) is intrinsically important to genetically vulnerable individuals and their clinicians and may offer clues to future course. In this section, we examine the literature on this issue in general; Chapter 6 focuses on studies of early onset in prepuberty and adolescence, and Chapter 13 examines how differences in age at onset relate to estimates of the degree of genetic vulnerability.

We pooled data from 15 studies published after 1990 (i.e., since the first edition of this text appeared) reporting average age at onset in samples of patients with bipolar illness (summarized in Table 4–1) and derived a weighted mean of 22.2 years.[4] When gender was specified, the difference for males and females was not significant (Fogarty et al., 1994; Hendrick et al., 2000; Suppes et al., 2001). Studies reporting separate figures for bipolar-I and -II disorder showed similar averages for the two groups (McMahon et al., 1994; Judd et al., 2003).

It is interesting that the post-1990 mean is 6 years younger than the weighted mean taken from the 22 pre-1990 studies examined in the first edition, which used the same basic inclusion criteria. Because the data are not normally distributed, however, these figures may be misleading. Averages can be raised by a relatively small number of patients with late onset, for example. When median age at onset is reported, it is usually in the early twenties. Here again, these medians are several years younger than those found in the literature before 1990.

As noted earlier, some of the variance across individual studies in Table 4–1 is related to differing criteria for onset. In general, the age when symptoms first appear is younger than the age when patients meet diagnostic criteria, and the age of first clinical contact is later still. (Studies of first hospitalization are not included in Table 4–1 because this measure says very little about age at onset.) Some studies have used age at first clinical contact on the assumption that dating of initial symptoms would be too imprecise. Egeland and colleagues (1987a), however, using information gleaned from patient charts and interview records to compare six clinical indices of onset for bipolar disorder, obtained high interrater reliability ($r = .89$) using the measure of first achievement of Research Diagnostic Criteria (RDC) for a major affective disorder.[5] As might be expected, the ages obtained with this measure are significantly younger than those derived from first treatment or first hospitalization.

Indeed, the literature is consistent in finding a significant time gap between onset of the illness and first treatment. Meeks (1999) found that mean age at first symptoms in a bipolar and unipolar population was almost 6 years younger than age at first treatment. A demographic study of the first 261 patients in the Stanley Foundation Bipolar Network (which may represent patients on the more severe end of the spectrum) revealed an 8-year difference between age at first diagnosis and age at first medical treatment (22.9 and 30.4 years, respectively), whereas age at first symptoms was only 2 years before age at diagnostic onset (Suppes et al., 2001). In a Stanley Foundation recruitment survey administered by Kupfer and colleagues (2002), more than 50 percent of a large bipolar sample indicated that they had received no treatment for their first affective episode. Thus it is to be expected that age at first treatment is a poor indicator of onset. Although retrospective self-reporting has its own pitfalls—which should be controlled for whenever possible with corroborating family reports and medical/academic records—using "first episode" as an onset measure with standardized (*International Classification of Diseases* [ICD]-10 or DSM-IV) criteria appears to be the most accurate indicator.

The lower age at onset in more recent studies reflects, in part, a cohort effect that is supported in the literature. For example, Chengappa and colleagues (2003) examined two separate cohorts of patients with bipolar disorder in a large patient sample and found that the more recent cohort had a mean age at onset 3 years younger than that of the older cohort. When the investigators examined a third, still more recent cohort in a post hoc analysis, they found that onset occurred at an even younger age, with a statistically significant different mean among the three cohorts. Kupfer and colleagues (2002) made similar findings in their examination of separate birth cohorts in a patient population from the Stanley Center's Bipolar Disorder Registry: the earliest birth cohort (1900–1939) was 3.5 years older at onset than the later two cohorts.

Researchers have advanced several hypotheses to explain this reduction in age at onset. Changes in nosology and illness definition could be a partial explanation. With the exception of the retrospective studies, the data in Table 4–1 were taken largely from samples of patients diagnosed in the past three decades (Stephens and McHugh, 1991). Many of these patients might have been classified as "schizophrenic" 50 years ago. The diagnostic inclusion of more psychotically ill subgroups could lower the age at onset, particularly in light of the earlier impairment observed in these groups (as discussed earlier). Genetic anticipation could play a role in the heightened predisposition to development of the disorder with each subsequent generation (see Chapter 13). Some investigators have proposed that the increasing use of antidepressants and stimulants in adolescents and children may help induce the onset of bipolar disorder at an earlier age in those already susceptible (Goodwin and Ghaemi, 1998; Cicero et al., 2003; Reichart, 2004).[6] This phenomenon would be consistent with what we know about the effect of antidepressants on mania induction and cycle acceleration, but more research is necessary to draw a solid conclusion. Similar to the antidepressant association is the hypothesis that the increased use of recreational drugs and alcohol among young people contributes to earlier onset. Here again, sound evidence is lacking, and it is difficult to establish a unidirectional association between onset of affective symptoms and onset of drug use.[7]

To gauge more accurately the distribution of the published ages at onset in the bipolar patient population, we

TABLE 4–1. Average Age at Onset in Studies Since 1990

Study	Sample	Average Age at Onset (Years)	Purpose/Design	Other Findings
Stephens and McHugh, 1991	235 bipolar	26.7	Retrospective analysis of notes on patients treated and monitored at a large institution, 1913–1940	Average age at onset lower in bipolar than in unipolar patients by approximately 6 years; average of 6 years between average age at onset and age at first admission
Kessler et al., 1993; Weissman et al., 1996	116 bipolar	23.3	Data from national comorbidity survey	—
Fogarty et al., 1994	22 bipolar	20.3: 20.5 male, 20.0 female	Determined clinical characteristics of mania by survey of randomly selected households	Age at onset: 5th percentile, ~9.0; 50th percentile, ~18.5; 95th percentile, ~25.5
Benazzi, 1999	186: 45 bipolar-I, 141 bipolar-II	26.7: 28.5 bipolar-I, 26.0 bipolar-II	Determined first episode using retrospective Structured Clinical Interview for DSM (SCID)/patient interview	No significant difference in age at onset ($p = .53$) in bipolar-I vs. bipolar-II
Meeks, 1999	86 bipolar	24.9	Determined factors of functioning in late-life bipolar disorder through patient interviews conducted three times over 8 months	Early onset related to poor functioning, increase in episode number and severity
Hendrick et al., 2000	37 bipolar-II	20.5: 21.8 male, 19.6 female	Gender comparison for average age at onset and a number of other clinical variables; first episode determined by retrospective questionnaire	—
Johnson et al., 2000	190 bipolar	31.4 (range 14.0–78.0)	Examined relationship between average age at onset and family history, early life events; average age at onset = first episode as determined by retrospective questionnaire	
Bellivier et al., 2001	211 bipolar-I	25.9 (standard deviation 4.5)	Used admixture analysis (a clustering method) to determine average age-at-onset distribution patterns/first diagnosis	Three subgroups of bipolar patients based on average age-at-onset distribution with distinct clinical profiles; findings support average age-at-onset subtypes

Citation	Sample	Age at onset	Method	Findings
McElroy et al., 2001	288 bipolar (I or II)	22.3: 26.0 noncomorbid diagnosis, 20.3 comorbid diagnosis	Compared attributes of bipolar patients with comorbid Axis I diagnosis and purely bipolar patients through retrospective interviews	Comorbidity related to earlier average age at onset
Suppes et al., 2001	261: 211 bipolar-I, 42 bipolar-II, 5 bipolar-not otherwise specified (NOS), 3 schizoaffective-bipolar type	22.9: 23.4 (±11.0) male, 22.5 (±10.0) female	Descriptive analysis of demographic features and course for 261 recruits in Stanley Foundation Bipolar Network; average age at onset ascertained by first full syndrome development using SCID	Early average age at onset associated with increased mood switching, worsening course of illness, history of early abuse
Carlson et al., 2002	123 bipolar	25.66 (standard deviation 9.9)	Outcome as a function of early vs. late average age at onset, first-episode SCID history, records, third-party interviews	22% <19.0, 78% >19.0. Early average age at onset an independent influence on poor functioning
Dittmann et al., 2002	152 bipolar	24.4 (standard deviation 10.9)	Follow-up of 152 patients entered in Stanley registry clinical sample, mostly hospitalized	No associations with age at onset included in this report
Judd et al., 2002, 2003	232 bipolar	22.2	Combined data reported in two studies on bipolar-I and -II patients from National Institute of Mental Health's Collaborative Depression Study. Average age at onset based on Research Diagnostic Criteria for first episode	Average age at onset did not correspond with measures of chronicity in either bipolar-I or bipolar-II group. Median age: bipolar-I=21.0; bipolar-II=19.0 (nonsignificant)
Kupfer et al., 2002	2,308 bipolar	19.8	Analysis of clinical and demographic characteristics of respondents to a Stanley recruitment survey; average age at onset determined by self-report using DSM-IV criteria for first manic or depressive episode	Median age = 17.5; younger cohort (1950–1959) had higher median average age at onset (22.5) than two older cohorts (1940–1949=19.0; 1900–1939=19.0); more than 50% of participants received no treatment for first episode

Note: Weighted means; 15 studies since 1990 (N=4,494) = **22.2**; studies before 1990 (N=4,210) = **28.1**; studies 1907–present (N=8,704) = **25.1**.

pooled data from seven studies specifying the number of patients with first episodes beginning in each decade of life (a total of 2,968 patients). This finer-grained analysis resulted in a peak in the age range of 15 to 19, followed closely by the 20–24 and 10–14 ranges, which were almost equal (Fig. 4–1). Note that the age-at-onset distribution is similar for men and women. Note also that this distribution provides only a rough picture and is heavily influenced by the large cohort of bipolar survey participants recruited by the Stanley Center Bipolar Registry, in which the largest subset (approximately 26 percent) of a sample of 2,308 participants were aged 15 to 19 (Kupfer et al., 2002).[8] Still, the rising concentration of bipolar diagnosis before age 20 is a clear trend in the recent literature and is consistent with Epidemiological Catchment Area (ECA) data showing hazard rates for the development of mania to be at their highest in the 15–19 age range (Burke et al., 1990).

Some investigators have defined two primary groups by age at onset—early and late (Carlson et al., 2000; Schurhoff et al., 2000; Suppes et al., 2001; Patel et al., 2006), with bimodal cutoff points ranging from the late teens (Goldstein and Levitt, 2006) to the mid-twenties (Grigoroiu-Serbanescu et al., 2001). Others have proposed three subgroups of onset—early (child or early adolescent), intermediate or typical (late adolescent, young adult), and later life (after age 35) (Sax et al., 1997; Bellivier et al., 2001; Mick et al., 2003; Lin et al., 2006). These hypotheses can be difficult to verify because "early," "late," and varying degrees of intermediate categories have tended to be defined inconsistently and arbitrarily.[9] However, Bellivier's group (2001)

used "admixture analyses" to determine the subgrouping model of best fit in a sample of 211 patients. Their findings correspond to an early–intermediate–late model (that is, a trimodal distribution), with mean onset at ages 16.9, 26.9, and 46.2, respectively. In a subsequent study (Bellivier et al., 2003), this group tested the fitness of this model on a different patient population (N=368). The model fit within the bounds of statistical sameness, further validating the trimodel distribution of onset age. Also, Bellivier and colleagues (2001) reported that bipolar siblings of a patient in a particular subgroup were statistically more likely to be part of the same age subset (p=.0001), a finding that supports a genetic etiological component to age-at-onset subgroups. A similar familial aggregation by age at onset was recently reported by Lin and colleagues (see Chapter 13).

Very late onset (i.e., after age 60) generally has been considered rare (Carlson et al., 1974; Loranger and Levine, 1978), although some data suggest that it may be more common than previously thought (Spicer et al., 1973; Shulman and Post, 1980; Stone, 1989; Wylie et al., 1999; Almeida and Fenner, 2002; Kessing, 2006). Angst and colleagues (1978) reported a secondary peak of late onset among women in the 40–50 age range (see Fig. 4–1). Patients with very late onset are less likely to have a family history of the disorder and more likely to be organically impaired. For example, Tohen and colleagues (1994) compared two groups of elderly patients, one with late-onset mania (first episode after age 65) and one with multiple manic episodes before age 65. The former group was significantly more likely to

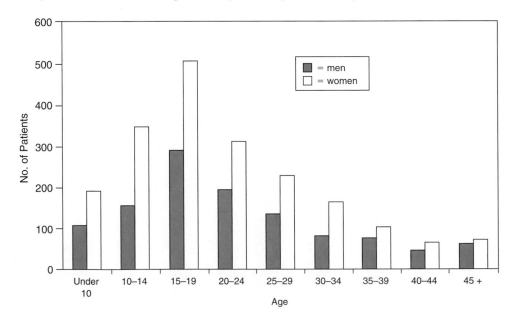

Figure 4–1. Distribution of age at onset (years) in bipolar-I and -II patients across seven studies.

experience neurological abnormalities.[10] These observations highlight the importance of differential diagnosis of primary mood disorders and mood disorders that occur secondary to specific neuropathology (see Chapter 3).

It is not yet clear to what extent grouping patients by age at onset really identifies distinct subgroups with differential phenomenology, pathophysiology, family history, outcome, and/or treatment response. Studies examining family history in early- versus late-onset groups have generally shown more genetic loading for recurrent mood disorder associated with early onset (see below).[11] But age at onset did not differ significantly in several studies comparing patients with mixed and pure mania (McElroy et al., 1995[12]; Akiskal et al., 1998; Brieger et al., 2003), and it does not appear to be a distinguishing feature of bipolar-I versus bipolar-II disorder (Benazzi, 1999). On the other hand, early onset has shown rather consistent correlations with certain clinical features, including rapid cycling, presence of comorbid anxiety disorder, suicidal behavior, psychotic features, and treatment resistance.

Carlson and colleagues (2002) reported that patients with an early onset (before age 19) had significantly worse outcomes on a variety of measures than those with later onset (after age 19).[13] Likewise, a French study of 58 early-onset (before age 18) versus 39 late-onset (after age 40) bipolar patients found that the former group experienced more psychosis (in agreement with the data of McGlashan [1988] and Schulze et al. [2002]), mixed episodes, panic disorder comorbidity, and lithium resistance and were more likely to have first-degree relatives with bipolar disorder (Schurhoff et al., 2000).[14] Among 320 bipolar-I and -II patients, those with onset younger than age 18 had more comorbid anxiety, rapid cycling, suicidality, and substance abuse compared with those with an onset above age 18 (Carter et al., 2003). An examination of a large cohort of Stanley Foundation Bipolar Network patients showed significant correlations between early onset (up to age 17) and greater incidence of learning disabilities, rapid-cycling course, and family history of bipolar disorder (Suppes et al., 2001),[15] while Ernst and Goldberg (2004) found that onset below age 19 was associated with more rapid cycling and comorbid substance abuse.[16] Engstrom and colleagues (2003) reported lower levels of treatment response and significantly greater numbers of suicide attempts in early-versus late-onset patients in a Swedish population.

Although the evidence for a connection between early onset and the complicating illness features described is compelling, one must exercise caution when using cross-sectional studies to distinguish damaging effects of the illness from so-called "clinical subtype" features. That is, worse outcomes in early-onset patients could be a factor of longer duration of illness rather than a phenotypic characteristic.

The issue of duration of illness is discussed later in this chapter.

The genetic literature is discussed in detail in Chapter 13, but it is worth noting here that newer linkage/mapping studies, coupled with older family studies, support the proposition that different age-at-onset subsets represent genetically heterogeneous groups of bipolar patients. Several studies cited in the first edition of this text reported that earlier onset was linked to higher familial bipolar morbidity and to early onset in bipolar relatives (Baron et al., 1981; Smeraldi et al., 1982–1983). Grigoroiu-Serbanescu and colleagues (2001), using segregation analysis of a large sample of 177 bipolar-I probands and 2,407 relatives, found that early-onset bipolar-I disorder was transmitted with a different pattern of heritability (non-mendelian major gene model) than late-onset bipolar-I. Recently, polymorphisms in serotonin transporter (5-HTTLPR) and a glycogen synthase kinase (GSK3-β) were associated with age at onset within bipolar populations (Bellivier et al., 2002; Benedetti et al., 2002). A recent chromosomal linkage study also confirmed the heritability of onset age, linking it to three chromosomal regions (Faraone et al., 2004). Taken as a whole, the evidence for age at onset as a possible marker for genetic subtypes of bipolar disorder is robust (see the review by Leboyer and colleagues [2005]).

The association between psychotic features and early onset among bipolar patients has considerable support in the literature. In an extensive review, Angst (1986c) cited 10 studies reporting this relationship, a conclusion supported by Blumenthal and colleagues (1987) in their study of the Amish and confirmed by subsequent research (Dell'Osso et al., 1993; Verdoux and Bourgeois, 1993; Schulze et al., 2002). Yet adolescent-onset mania is not always associated with psychotic features, as evidenced by cross-sectional comparison studies (Coryell and Norten, 1980; McElroy et al., 1997). A more recent cross-sectional study comparing early with non-early onset groups likewise failed to find a significantly higher presence of psychotic features in the former (Perlis et al., 2004). However, cross-sectional studies cannot determine subsequent development of psychosis and may easily miss prior psychotic features, especially if the investigators rely on patient recall. Taken as a whole, the evidence for a connection between psychotic features and younger age at onset is strong. Coupled with the association between premorbid impairment and level of psychosis discussed earlier, this evidence supports the hypothesis that pervasive psychotic features mark a more severe form of the disorder that sometimes entails earlier syndromal manifestation and is more often characterized by premorbid impairment. The relationship between age at onset and episode frequency is discussed later in this chapter.

NUMBER OF EPISODES

In his classic 1921 monograph, Kraepelin noted that of 459 manic-depressive patients he had studied (which included unipolar patients), only 55 percent had experienced more than one episode and only 28 percent more than three. A careful reading of Kraepelin's clinical descriptions suggests, however, that many of his ostensibly single-episode patients were in fact severely and chronically ill and had experienced multiple episodes, which at that time required continuous hospitalization (the single hospitalization being counted as single episode).

Considered together, findings of longitudinal studies of manic-depressive patients not taking prophylactic medication (Table 4–2), which included those with both bipolar and unipolar forms of the illness, indicate that most patients—particularly those studied in the past 35 years—had more than one episode.[17] Table 4–2 also indicates that most patients with major affective disorder (i.e., Kraepelinian manic-depressive illness) have a recurrent course. Many textbooks, apparently relying on older data, fail to emphasize this point sufficiently.

The near-total likelihood of recurrence is supported by recent research. In a 4-year naturalistic follow-up study of 75 bipolar patients, only 28 percent remained in remission (Tohen et al., 1990). If relapse were to continue at this rate over the long term (18 percent per year), fewer than 1 percent of patients would remain in remission at about 10 years' follow-up. In the National Institute of Mental Health's (NIMH) Collaborative Program on the Psychobiology of Depression-Clinical Studies (CDS), relapse into a new episode within 5 years was observed in 81 to 91 percent of patients, the variability in percentage being related to the polarity of the index episode (i.e., depressive, mixed, or manic states) (Keller et al., 1993).

In contrast, relapse in unipolar depression is not as frequent and is more dependent on the number of previous episodes, with a much higher risk of relapse after the third major depressive episode. In a separate analysis of the data from the NIMH Collaborative Program on the Psychobiology of Depression-Clinical Studies, the 5-year recurrence rate was 64 percent among 380 patients with unipolar depression, rising to 80 percent at 10 years and 85 percent at 15 years (Mueller et al., 1999). In a Japanese collaborative study (Kanai et al., 2003), 95 previously untreated unipolar depressed subjects (70.5 percent first episode, 29.5 percent recurrent; mean age 44.3) were followed for 6 years. In this cohort, lower rates of relapse were seen, with only 45 percent experiencing a new episode at 6 years. This lower relapse rate may reflect the fact that, unlike the CDS cohort, most of these patients had not already experienced recurrent major depressive episodes. The lower rate of episode

recurrence in unipolar compared with bipolar disorder does not address the issue of subsyndromal chronicity, however (see later discussion).

Angst (1980) subdivided his patients into three categories according to their pattern of recurrence: MD, Md, and Dm. As described in Chapter 2, MD represents the core illness, with both major manic and major depressive episodes; Md patients have full manic episodes, but their depressive episodes do not require hospitalization; and Dm patients have been hospitalized for depression, but their manic episodes are not severe enough for hospitalization (i.e., they have a history of hypomania).[18] Angst's MD patients showed a tendency toward having the most episodes. In the larger cohort described in the CDS, however, Dm (bipolar-II) patients had the most prior episodes, although this number was not significantly different from that for bipolar-I patients (Coryell et al., 1989).[19]

As noted earlier in our discussion of methodological issues, some differences among studies relate to varying definitions of what counts as an episode. Some studies underestimate recurrence because they rely solely on hospitalization as a marker of episodes.[20] Other studies may be prone to overestimate recurrence because of treatment factors, such as use of antidepressants and selection of lithium clinic patients for study.

On the question of the contribution of antidepressant drugs, it is important to note that the highest relapse rates generally are the most recent. Thus it is conceivable, as suggested in the first edition of this text and by Koukopoulos and colleagues (1980) and Wehr and Goodwin (1987), that the increased use of antidepressants may have influenced the results. Indeed, in his analysis of the incidence of manic switches in one hospital studied over six decades, Angst (1985) noted a four-fold increase when the pretreatment decades were compared with the decades after electroconvulsive therapy (ECT) and antidepressant drugs became widely used. Some more recent studies (Altshuler et al., 1995; Ghaemi et al., 1999, 2000), but not all (Altshuler et al., 2001), support the possible impact of anti-depressants. Although other explanations, such as better diagnostic detection of mania, are plausible, these explanations also are consistent with the hypothesis that effective antidepressant treatments altered the course in some manic-depressive patients (perhaps particularly those with the bipolar form) toward more frequent recurrences. The evidence for and against this hypothesis is reviewed extensively in Chapter 19.

Another possibility is that a bias toward higher relapse rates is likely when an outcome study draws all of its subjects from patients referred to a lithium maintenance clinic. The studies of Angst and of Grof cited elsewhere in this chapter, however, included all patients who came to

TABLE 4–2. **Total Number of Episodes**

Study	Sample Size	Years of Observation	TOTAL EPISODES (%)				Comments
			1	2–3	4–6	7+	
Kraepelin, 1921	459	Variable, up to a lifetime R	45	27	—	28	Many "single-episode" patients were chronically hospitalized with continuous cycling
Pollock, 1931	5,739	11 R	55	35	8	2	Excluded episodes occurring before index admission
Rennie, 1942	66	26 R	8	29	26	37	"Several" had 20 or more episodes
Lundquist, 1945	103	20% <10 R 38%, 10–20 R 42%, 20–30 R	50	25	—	25	28% were chronic and were included in the "single-episode" category; excluded episodes occurring before index admission
Stenstedt, 1952	62	1.2–20+ R	26	42	—	32	Included nonrecovered patients as single-episode
Bratfos and Haug, 1968	42	1–12 P	13	42	—	45	"Not free of symptoms for any length of time"; half of these were "chronic"
Perris, 1968	131	19.6 R	0	17	40	43	Average number of episodes: bipolar=7, unipolar=4
Carlson et al., 1974[a]	53	10 P	4	17	32	47	One third of these were rapid cyclers (4 or more episodes/year).
Angst, 1978, 1979b[a]	95	26 P, R	0	8	22	69	16% had >20 episodes. "New episode" required >4 weeks asymptomatic interval
Zis et al., 1980	105	P, R	6	13	33	48	—
Fukuda et al., 1983	96	18–28 R	15	40	20	25	Hospitalized; questionnaire and chart review; no treatment with lithium, but other drugs used
Total	**6,951**		0–55	13–42	8–40	2–69	

Note: Studies reported here included both bipolar and unipolar patients.
P = prospective; R = retrospective.
[a]These studies included some patients treated prophylactically; most of the other studies included patients treated acutely.
Source: Update of Goodwin and Jamison (1984).

the clinic for treatment of an episode without regard to previous episodes (i.e., not just those deemed eligible for maintenance treatment). Other studies appear to have focused primarily on those judged eligible for lithium maintenance (Baldessarini et al., 1999, 2000). As noted earlier, both underestimations and overestimations of true natural recurrence rates have occurred in the literature. It appears that some recent studies may be prone to overestimation of recurrence rates as a result of the uncontrolled effects of treatment and to potential selection bias, although underestimation also occurs.[21]

FREQUENCY OF EPISODES (CYCLE LENGTH)

Cycle length is defined as the time from the onset of one episode to the onset of the next. Variation in cycle length reflects primarily variation in the length of the symptom-free interval, because the duration of episodes tends to be relatively constant in a given individual. Onset is used to calculate cycle length because it is generally easier to pinpoint than termination of an episode. In addition, treatment can easily obscure an episode's natural length. Most investigators agree that cycle length tends to grow shorter with subsequent recurrences; that is, episodes become more frequent. What is not as clear is the proportion of bipolar patients whose illness accelerates. After three to five episodes, however, the extent of shortening slows considerably and approaches a leveling off, or maximum frequency of episodes.

In the first edition of this text, we speculated that episode frequency might represent a familial trait, as suggested by Gershon and colleagues (1982). Subsequently, Fisfalen and colleagues (2005), examining 86 families with at least three members with a major affective disorder, found that episode frequency (evenly distributed over a wide range) was correlated among relatives (r = 0.56, p < .004). They also noted that, compared with the lowest quartile of episode frequency, the highest quartile was significantly (and independently) associated with bipolar-II, early age at onset, psychotic features, alcoholism, and suicidal behavior.

Decrease in Well Intervals with Increasing Number of Episodes

Kraepelin was the first to report that intervals of euthymia appear to decrease in duration in manic-depressive illness with increasing numbers of affective episodes. This observation later became a central impetus for the kindling model, with its prediction that episodes become more frequent over time, and that euthymic intervals between episodes become increasingly shorter. This observation was subsequently confirmed in a number of clinical studies. Recently, however, some methodological flaws underlying those

studies have been identified, and not all of the study findings have been consistent.

Figure 4–2 illustrates the relationship between average cycle length and episode number. This graph is based on six studies involving a total of 20,660 patients. Despite substantial individual variability, the averages show a remarkably consistent pattern across the studies. For example, note the pattern in the 105 bipolar patients of Zis and colleagues (1979): the average cycle length between the first and second episodes was 36 months, diminishing to about 24 months, then to 12 months. In 46 bipolar patients studied by Roy-Byrne and colleagues (1985a), the mean cycle lengths for the first seven episodes were 53, 28, 25, 20, 12, 15, and 9 months. In 95 bipolar patients from Angst's Zurich clinic, the median first cycle length was 48 months, compared with 22 months for the second cycle, 24 for the third, 14 for the fourth, and 12 for the fifth (Angst, 1981b). The longer average cycle length in the Kraepelin data reflects the inclusion of unipolar patients, whose cycles are longer than those of bipolar patients (Angst, 1981b; Fukuda et al., 1983).

The findings of the six studies illustrated in Figure 4–2 are consistent with the retrospective data of Taschev (1974), who found the average second cycle to be as long as the first, but the fourth cycle to be half as long as the second. A prospective study of patients in the 1980s (Keller et al., 1982) also documented the increasing probability of an

Figure 4–2. Episode number versus cycle length. BP = bipolar, UP = unipolar. (*Source*: Update of Goodwin and Jamison, 1984.)

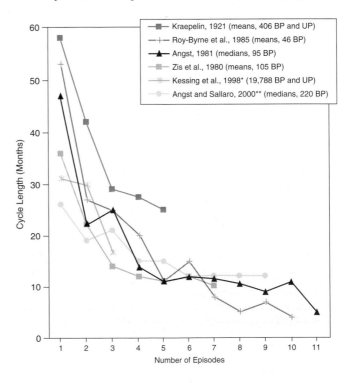

earlier relapse with each episode, a finding suggesting that some fundamental characteristics of the illness course may persist despite treatment. The methodological consideration of "Slater's fallacy"—the impact of the number of episodes on cycle length—needs to be taken into account when assessing these studies, however (see later discussion).

Recent studies have not been consistent with regard to the progressive shortening of cycle length. In a reanalysis of his Zurich cohort (identified 1959–1963, followed to 1997; N=220 bipolar patients), Angst and Selloro (2000) found shortening of cycle length in the first few but not in later episodes. In the studies of Winokur and colleagues (1993) and Turvey and colleagues (1999), who analyzed data from the same large NIMH cohort, bipolar patients did not appear to have more frequent and shorter episodes with time, nor was there a correlation between poor outcome and such a course. Rather, poor outcome was associated with "polyphasic" mood episodes; that is, immediate switching from mania to depression to mania without intervening euthymia.

Findings of other contemporary studies suggest that at least a subgroup of patients with bipolar disorder do experience a progressive shortening of cycle length. For instance, Goldberg and Harrow (1994) reported that 50 percent of 20 bipolar patients with two or more previous hospitalizations had experienced intervals between episodes of less than 1 year (defined as "kindlers"), whereas 19 other patients with fewer than two hospitalizations had experienced intervals between episodes of more than 1 year ("nonkindlers"). At 4.5-year follow-up, the kindlers were more likely to have had a recurrence than the nonkindlers. In a hospital-based case register study, Kessing and colleagues (1998a) found that 40 percent of a large sample (N=1,712) had shortening between first and second intervals, and 25 percent of this sample showed progressive shortening across two consecutive intervals.

The considerable individual variability in patterns of relapse was pointed out by Kraepelin (1921, p. 149):

> If we give no more examples that is not because those already given represent adequately the multiplicity of the courses taken by manic-depressive insanity; it is absolutely inexhaustible.

The complexity of this topic increases when we pay attention to the above-noted methodological problem first raised by Eliot Slater in 1938 but ignored by most researchers until recently. Slater's fallacy, as revived by Oepen and colleagues (2004), posits that patients with more episodes tend also to have shorter cycle lengths, and those with fewer episodes to have longer cycle lengths.[23] Thus if the two groups are pooled, as in Kraepelin's original data, it will ap-

pear as if cycle length decreases with more episodes in the sample as a whole, whereas this apparent effect may be an artifact of pooling the two distinct subgroups of patients, those with few and those with many episodes. To truly demonstrate shortening of cycle length, then, one would need to correct for number of episodes.

Because this important methodological point went underrecognized for decades, we reanalyzed the studies described in the first edition of this text with regard to cycle length, as well as newer studies conducted since 1990. We found that the majority of studies either did not correct for number of episodes or did not address the subject. A number of investigators, however, without directly referring to Slater's finding, appear to have been cognizant of this issue.[23] In two of these studies (Bratfos and Haug, 1968; Angst et al., 1973), correction for number of episodes led to results similar to those reported by Slater; that is, no consistent evidence of progressive shortening of well intervals. In two other studies (Roy-Byrne et al., 1985a; Goldberg and Harrow, 1994), however, a "sensitization" or "kindling" pattern was identified in about half of patients with refractory bipolar disorder and not in the others (see Fig. 4–2). In a large Norwegian community-based study of hospitalized bipolar patients, half of those with three or fewer episodes also appeared to have progressive shortening of intervals of wellness, but a similar pattern was seen in only 25 percent of patients with four or more episodes (Kessing et al., 1998a). Slater's fallacy was also avoided in a contemporary Italian study of 426 hospitalized research patients with mood disorders (182 unipolar, 244 bipolar) (Cusin et al., 2000). In that study, in which all patients had experienced periods of euthymic recovery (continuous and rapid-cycling courses were excluded), progressive shortening of cycle length was observed (based on retrospective evaluation) after correction for total number of episodes, up to a plateau of about one episode per year. In a recent 40-year follow-up of Angst's Zurich cohort (N=406, 186 with recurrent unipolar depression, 220 with bipolar disorder), Kessing and colleagues (2004) specifically conducted their analysis to control for Slater's fallacy by using a Cox regression model in which one of the variables was episode number, thus adjusting the overall hazard ratio for number of previous episodes. They found an increased likelihood (hazard ratio) of more episodes with increasing number of episodes (e.g., the hazard ratio for 1 episode was 1.0 as the reference point, while for 4 episodes it was 1.52 and for 10 episodes 2.19).

In these studies, then, correction for episode frequency revealed decreasing length of well intervals mainly in the first three episodes, with unchanging well intervals of about one per year for further episodes, which in fact was what the Goodwin group found earlier (Zis et al., 1980). These findings suggest that studies of well intervals that fail to capture the first three episodes of illness are unlikely to observe any kindling-like effect. This point may be relevant to some studies that fail to find this effect, such as that of Turvey and colleagues (1999), in which the first episode was captured in only 15 percent of subjects recovered from the index episode. On the other hand, the recent data from the McLean-Harvard First-Episode Mania Study do not show evidence of shortened intervals of wellness, although the period of follow-up was brief (2 to 4 years) (Tohen et al., 2003).[24]

As alluded to earlier, if the finding of shortening of well intervals cannot be applied to an entire sample of patients with manic-depressive illness, the question arises of whether it may be a subgroup effect. It is important to note that Post and colleagues (Post et al., 1986a; Post, 1990) proposed the kindling hypothesis as relevant to only a subset of patients with bipolar illness, particularly those who are unresponsive to lithium, more responsive to anticonvulsants, and with other "nonclassical" features of the illness. Granting Slater's critique, such a proposal would not be inconsistent with the available literature.

Clearly, the kindling model does not depend solely on the prediction of shortening of euthymic intervals of wellness. As discussed previously, the model makes other predictions as well, such as increasing frequency of episodes, increasing episode duration with time, decreasing importance of psychosocial triggers with time, and increasing treatment resistance with greater numbers of episodes (or differential efficacy in early versus later phases of illness). An important issue bearing on the generalizability of the kindling model is the proportion of patients with bipolar disorder whose course is consistent with these predictions.

Research on psychosocial triggers of episodes has revealed interesting data regarding this issue. Kendler and Karkowski-Shuman (1997) analyzed their sample of patients with recurrent unipolar depression so as to account for "within-person analyses." They reported on a sample of 2,395 female twin pairs followed for 9 years, in whom later mood episodes were associated less and less frequently with psychosocial triggers, as predicted by the kindling model.[25] They concluded (p. 542):

> These results indicate the observed decline in the association between stressful life events and depressive onsets with increasing numbers of previous depressive episodes is a true within-individual phenomenon and cannot be explained by systematic differences between the kind of individuals who have a low versus high number of previous depressive episodes.

Is there any evidence that episodes increase in frequency over time? Kessing and Andersen (1999) reported that such was the case for both unipolar depression (15 percent increased risk of recurrence with each episode)

and bipolar disorder (9 percent) in a case register study of all hospitalized admissions in Denmark (7,925 unipolar, 2,011 bipolar; 1971–1993 time frame). A similar conclusion was reached by Bockting and colleagues (2006) on the basis of a study of 172 patients meeting DSM-IV criteria for recurrent unipolar depression.

Increasing treatment resistance with number of episodes has been reported in some studies (e.g., Koukopoulos et al., 2000) but not in others (e.g., Baldessarini et al., 1999). Kessing and colleagues (1998b) failed to find other evidence of worsened outcome, such as increased mortality, associated with a sensitization pattern of progressive shortening of cycle length, although there was an interesting association between that kindling-like pattern and an increased risk of dementia.[26]

Recall that the kindling model predicts that outcome will be worse after more episodes. The outcome of both untreated and treated courses could be expected to reflect this pattern. This prediction is supported by some but not all studies. For instance, Gitlin and colleagues (1995) found that more previous episodes predicted earlier relapse at 4.3-year follow-up (2.2 versus 3.5 years; $p = .007$), a finding similar to that of Goldberg and Harrow (1994) noted earlier. On the other hand, in a 4.6-year study of outcome among 360 bipolar-I (n = 220) and bipolar-II (n = 140) patients on lithium maintenance therapy, Baldessarini and colleagues (1999) did not confirm the kindling-based prediction of worsening outcome with each successive episode. These investigators assessed delay in beginning lithium treatment after onset of bipolar illness and compared response to lithium treatment in subgroups of patients with few (0 to 4), some (4 to 9), or many (more than 10) mood episodes before treatment began. They reported no difference in lithium treatment response among these conditions; that is, lithium response was neither better nor worse if patients had experienced few or many previous mood episodes, or if they had begun lithium treatment soon after the onset of their illness as opposed to later. It is worth noting that lithium treatment had not been started until an average of 8 years after the onset of illness in this sample, which suggests that a significant delay occurred in most patients. Also, because this study was naturalistic, information about previous episodes and onset of illness was retrospective and subject to recall bias. It is notable that the average age at onset of bipolar illness in this sample (29.6 years)[27] was much older than the age in most other studies, a fact that may suggest the effects of recall bias or a difference in patient selection. It is also relevant that the kindling model may not be pertinent to the long-term outcome of lithium treatment. In the early work of Post and colleagues (Post and Weiss, 1989; Post, 1990), kindling was invoked to explain the treatment-refractory course of illness in those patients who failed to respond to lithium and who appeared to respond to anticonvulsant agents.

Taken as a whole, the findings reviewed here, although not decisively confirming the validity or generalizability of the kindling model, appear to suggest its relevance to at least some patients with manic-depressive illness, including both bipolar and recurrent unipolar forms.[28]

Other Cycle-Length Patterns

The relationship between frequency of episodes and age at onset remains somewhat unclear. Several older studies[29] found an increasing frequency of relapse with increased age at onset, but two studies failed to show this association (Dunner et al., 1980; Roy-Byrne et al., 1985a), and two found the opposite (Okuma and Shimoyama, 1972; Winokur and Kadrmas, 1989).[30] A multiple-regression analysis of the 105 bipolar patients studied by Grof and colleagues (1995) showed that the patient's age and age at onset each contributed independently to the prediction of relapse (Zis et al., 1979). Onset in the 20s was associated with a 20 percent probability of recurrence within 24 months, onset in the 30s with a 50 percent probability, and late onset (age 50 years or older) with a very high (80 percent) probability. Only the first cycle length (the time between the first and second episodes) was related to age at onset, however.[31]

A final question about the pattern of cycles in bipolar illness is whether burnout occurs. Kraepelin observed that the illness tends to decline after the fourth decade, although he did not elaborate on his observation. In a prospective follow-up study of 215 bipolar patients (150 bipolar-I, 65 bipolar-II) over a period of 17 to 21 years, Angst (1986d) found no age-related decrease in frequency of episodes; 26 percent of the bipolar patients (versus 42 percent of the unipolar patients) were free of relapses over 5 or more years, although most patients were still actively ill through their 60s, when the follow-up usually ended. Likewise, findings of recent studies do not generally support the concept of burnout (Goldberg and Harrow, 1999), although long-term follow-up from adulthood into the elderly years is rare.

Rapid Cycling

The inclusion of rapid cycling in DSM-IV was based to a large extent on a study by Bauer and colleagues (1994), who compared 120 patients with rapid-cycling bipolar disorder and 119 non–rapid-cycling patients. They found that 45 percent of the rapid cyclers had bipolar-II disorder, compared with 38 percent of the non–rapid cyclers, a difference that did not achieve statistical significance. Those with rapid cycling, not surprisingly, had more episodes in a 12-month prospective follow-up period; there were also more females in the rapid-cycling group. Based on these

differences in course and demographics, the investigators supported the differentiation of rapid-cycling bipolar disorder as a valid course specifier for inclusion in DSM-IV. They also supported the cutoff definition of four episodes per year, because of an increase in the number of patients who experienced four to eight episodes per year, versus two to three episodes, during the prospective follow-up (although this was observed only among the females). It is notable that this was an observational study, in which adjustments were not made for potential confounding variables or effect modifiers. Therefore, similarities or differences between the two groups in this study may or may not be related to rapid cycling per se. This limitation holds for most of the research on rapid cycling.

Rapid cycling is thought to be equally common in type I and type II bipolar illness, but there is no firm consensus on this point.[32] Indeed, rapid-cycling unipolar depression (although uncommon) has been reported. It has generally been thought that rapid cycling develops later in the course of the illness and may reflect underlying pathophysiological mechanisms, such as the progressive kindling, or sensitization, discussed earlier (Fig. 4–3.). Late rapid cycling may also reflect the impact of certain treatments, especially antidepressants, in accelerating the natural course of the illness (see Chapter 19). The concept of rapid cycling as a later manifestation of bipolar illness has been proposed but is not supported by all investigators (see the later discussion) (Coryell et al., 1992). There may also be a predominance of rapid cycling in females (Koukopoulos et al., 1980; Coryell et al., 1992; Bauer et al., 1994), although Kupka and colleagues (2005) examined 539 outpatients in the Stanley Network and found that female preponderance was limited to those with eight or more episodes per year.

Box 4–1 highlights what is known about the relationship between rapid-cycling and non-rapid-cycling bipolar disorder. A study of the frequency distribution of cycle lengths could answer the question of whether rapid cycling represents a distinct subgroup or is simply one end of a continuum. Cycle-length data presented by Coryell and colleagues (1992) do not support a separate short-cycle-length group. The existing family history data also are more consistent with the continuum notion, in that the families of rapid-cycling patients have the same frequency of non-rapid-cycling affective disorders as families of non-rapid-cycling patients (Nurnberger et al., 1988b; Wehr et al., 1988; Coryell et al., 1992). The largest single prospective study of rapid cycling (Coryell et al., 1992) found that it is transient and not associated with the end stage of severe bipolar illness. The data in this study are based on the CDS, conducted in five tertiary-care academic health centers, in which 243 bipolar and 674 unipolar patients were

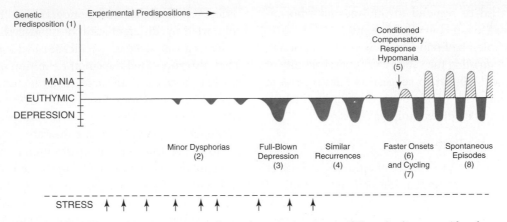

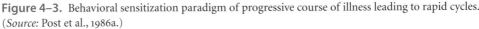

Figure 4–3. Behavioral sensitization paradigm of progressive course of illness leading to rapid cycles. (*Source:* Post et al., 1986a.)

BOX **4–1.**   **Relationship between Rapid-Cycling and Non–Rapid-Cycling Bipolar Disorder**

- Data are insufficient to determine whether cycle length is distributed normally.
- In general, rapid-cycling patients appear to be related genetically and phenotypically to non-rapid-cycling patients (Nurnberger et al., 1988b; Wehr et al., 1988; Coryell et al., 1992).
- Illness in rapid-cycling patients can include a non-rapid-cycling course.
- Rapid cycling may be viewed as an extreme development of tendencies inherent in a non-rapid-cycling course:
  — Increasing frequency of episodes[*] (Grof et al., 1974)
  — Switches into new episodes with no normal interval between[*] (Winokur et al., 1969)
  — Circularity of episodes (Koukopoulos and Reginaldi, 1973)
- Rapid cycling may exhibit a somewhat different pharmacological response profile.
- Relative frequency in bipolar-I versus -II is unsettled.

---

   [*]Potentiated by antidepressants, which are also capable of inducing rapid cycling (Wehr and Goodwin, 1979, 1987).

---

followed for 1 to 5 years, with interviews conducted every 6 months. The investigators found that 45 patients, all but one of them bipolar, developed a rapid-cycling course in the first year of follow-up; however, this group did not experience a lower rate of recovery at 5-year follow-up. Only 1 of the 39 rapid cyclers followed for the full 5 years continued to have four or more episodes in each year. In years 3 to 5, rapid cyclers did not differ from non–rapid cyclers in recovery from their index episode at the beginning of the study. However, there was a statistical trend for rapid cyclers to be less likely to experience a final follow-up year

with no affective symptoms (only 10 percent of rapid cyclers, versus 49.5 percent of non–rapid cyclers; $p = .09$).

Although the CDS has the major advantage of being the kind of careful prospective, naturalistic study needed by the field, it is limited by those same study methods. Patients who remained in the study after having been recruited into one of the five tertiary-care centers in which it was conducted may not have been representative of the larger population of patients with rapid-cycling bipolar disorder—individuals whose chaotic lives often do not allow for long-term prospective follow-up in a systematic research study. Nonetheless, one cannot ignore the findings of this study, especially given the fact that, in a separate cohort, Maj and colleagues (1994) also found that only 18.9 percent of 37 individuals with rapid cycling continued to experience four or more episodes per year during 5-year follow-up. Future prospective research on more community-based samples may clarify these questions that are so important to the estimation of prognosis in individual patients.

Rapid cycling appears to represent a generally treatment-refractory state compared with non–rapid cycling. Most of the studies on this issue have involved lithium, which has led to the common belief that rapid-cycling patients do not respond well to lithium and respond better to anticonvulsants. In fact, as discussed in Chapters 18, 19, and 20, it appears that most rapid-cycling patients do not respond particularly well to any medication—lithium or anticonvulsants. Alternatively, as suggested by a number of investigators (Koukopoulos et al., 1983; Wehr et al., 1988; Baldessarini et al., 2000), the responsiveness of rapid-cycling patients to mood stabilizers may be greatly enhanced when concomitant antidepressant use is avoided.

Recent genetic studies on rapid cycling have yielded instructive, if inconclusive, results. Associations have been reported with the serotonin transporter gene polymorphism (Rousseva et al., 2003) and with a low-activity allele for the catechol-O-methyltransferase (COMT) gene (Kirov et al., 1998; Papolos et al., 1998), although the COMT allele association was not seen in a study of 52 children (mean age 10.9 years) (Geller and Cook, 2000). A family history study in 165 patients with rapid-cycling bipolar disorder did not identify major differences in familial mental illness compared with non-rapid-cycling bipolar disorder, with the exception of a suggestion of more substance abuse among relatives of rapid-cycling bipolar probands (Lish et al., 1993).

Taken together, the data tend to favor the concept that rapid cycling represents one extreme of a bipolar spectrum of cyclicity, but it is generally not a stable characteristic in an individual patient.

ONSET AND DURATION OF EPISODES

Often, the onset of manic episodes is abrupt, developing over a few days. Depressive episodes develop more gradually, over weeks, although bipolar depressive episodes are more abrupt in onset than unipolar depressive episodes (Winokur, 1976; Molnar et al., 1988; Keitner et al., 1996).

As we noted in the first edition, some patients experience a "hypomanic alert" (Jacobsen, 1965), a period of days or even weeks of hypomanic symptoms before the switch into mania. The most common prodrome is sleep disturbance, which had a prevalence of 77 percent in one study (Jackson et al., 2003). Family members are twice as likely as patients to observe early behavioral symptoms of mania (Keitner et al., 1996) (see Chapter 22).

Older estimates of the average duration of episodes in manic-depressive illness were derived from studies conducted before medications were available. In the CDS 5-year follow-up of a largely treated sample, the mean time to recovery was 6 weeks with pure mania, 11 weeks with pure depression, and 17 weeks with mixed states (Coryell et al., 1990). In a follow-up study conducted by Angst and Preisig (1995), the mean episode length was 4.3 months. Pure manic and pure depressive episodes lasted the same amount of time—approximately 3 months. Mixed episodes also lasted about 3 months, but "cyclic" episodes were longer (mean 4.2 months). The Baltimore site of the ECA community-based study of psychiatric disorders found that episodes lasted a median of 8 to 12 weeks (Eaton et al., 1997), with depressions lasting longer than manias. Maj and colleagues (2003) found longer duration of agitated depressive episodes compared with nonagitated depression in bipolar-I disorder (mean time to 50 percent recovery, 12 versus 9 weeks; N = 120) (Maj et al., 2003).

POLARITY

Estimates of the proportion of bipolar patients who begin the illness with a manic episode range from 34 to 79 percent, averaging just over 50 percent. It is important to recognize that the other half of patients with the bipolar form of manic-depressive illness will go undiagnosed as bipolar at the onset of their condition, because they initially experience only major depressive episodes[33]; this condition is sometimes called "false" unipolar depression. This dilemma arises from the current DSM nosology (see Chapters 1 and 3), which places primary emphasis on polarity at the expense of cyclicity or recurrence. This approach guarantees an initial misdiagnosis in many patients who have bipolar disorder but have not yet experienced their first manic episode. The problem was less acute with the classic construct of manic-depressive illness, which took into account other course factors, such as recurrence of episodes, as well as family history.

One study of false unipolar depression examined 17,447 patients with mood disorders who were hospitalized in Denmark over a 22-year period (1971–1993) (Kessing, 1999). Among those whose first episodes were depressive, if a manic episode was to develop, it usually did so within 5 years. Patients with false unipolar depression experienced more recurrent depressive episodes than did patients with true unipolar depression.[34]

It is also important to recognize that there is a relationship between false unipolar depression and age at onset (see Chapter 1). An often-cited figure is that 1 to 2 percent of patients with depression may experience a hypomanic/manic episode in every year of follow-up. This figure is based on the CDS cohort (Coryell et al., 1995), in which 10.2 percent of a depressed subgroup (mean age 36.8 years) had a manic or hypomanic episode during 10 years of follow-up. A younger age at onset within this cohort was associated with increased risk of manic/hypomanic switch, however. Other younger cohorts have confirmed higher natural switch rates to mania (see Chapter 6). For example, in a group of 72 depressed children (mean age 10.3 years), Geller and colleagues (2001) found that 49 percent had experienced a manic or hypomanic episode at 10-year follow-up. In a group of 74 depressed young adults (mean age 23.0 years), Goldberg and colleagues (2001) observed that 46 percent had experienced a manic or hypomanic episode at 15-year follow-up. Thus the risk of switching from false unipolar depression to bipolar disorder is highest in childhood and young adulthood, occurring at a rate of about 3 to 5 percent per year; it then decreases by the late 30s, at which point it flattens out to about 1 percent per year.

Studies showing the highest estimates of manic onset utilize first hospitalization as the onset criterion. It is possible that these high estimates result from underestimation of depressive onsets, because many depressions do not require hospitalization. On the other hand, hypomanic onsets are probably underestimated compared with depressive onsets, because patients are more likely to experience (and report) depressive symptoms as illness. Angst (1978) reported manic onset of illness in the majority of his bipolar sample (N = 95), where onset was defined as the first occurrence of symptoms requiring treatment. On the other hand, Roy-Byrne and colleagues (1985a), who defined onset as the first symptoms meeting the RDC for an affective episode, found that 60 percent of 71 bipolar patients had a depressive first episode.

Onset may influence the later pattern of illness. Perris and d'Elia (1966) reported that among patients with a manic first episode, 62 percent went on to have a predominantly manic course, and only 25 percent a predominantly depressive course. It is interesting that a predominantly manic course may herald a better outcome. In a hospital chart review study based on the premedication treatment era, Stephens and McHugh (1991) reported on outcomes in 297 bipolar and 945 unipolar patients admitted to the Johns Hopkins Hospital from 1913 to 1940. Only 2 percent of all patients with mood disorder experienced unipolar manic episodes, and their outcome was best (75 percent recovered or improved), followed by that of those with unipolar depression (69 percent) and bipolar disorder (57 percent) (Stephens and McHugh, 1991). This report is supported by another study of 320 patients with bipolar-I disorder (Perugi et al., 2000), in whom depressive episode onset was associated with higher levels of later rapid-cycling course, as well as suicide attempts. Later psychotic features were more likely to be associated with manic onset, however. In light of these findings of a relationship between polarity at onset and subsequent course, a recent report that the polarity of onset appears to be familial (Kassen et al., 2006) is especially interesting.

It has generally been observed that women tend to be more likely to have a predominantly depressive pattern to their bipolar illness, and men a predominantly manic pattern.[35] More recent data have not uniformly supported these findings, however. In one chart review of 131 patients (63 women and 68 men) (Hendrick et al., 2000), there were no statistically significant gender differences in age at onset, number of depressive or manic episodes, and number of hospitalizations for depression. However, women had been hospitalized for mania significantly more often than men, whereas substance abuse, although high in both groups, was more prevalent among men. Also, in a cross-sectional analysis of 500 subjects in the NIMH Systematic Treatment Enhancement Program for Bipolar Disorder (STEP-BD) study cohort, there were no gender differences in number of past depressive versus manic episodes (87.4 percent of women and 86.8 percent of men had experienced three or more manic episodes; 92.1 percent of women and 92.3 percent of men had experienced three or more depressive episodes) (Baldassano et al., 2002).[36] As noted earlier in relation to age at onset of depression and false unipolar depression, polarity distinctions are not stable until approximately age 40.[37] Before that age, depressed individuals remain at a relatively elevated risk of eventual occurrence of manic or hypomanic episodes.

Some investigators have noted that polyphasic polarity patterns are associated with poor outcomes (Turvey et al., 1999; Maj et al., 2002). For instance, Maj and colleagues (2002) compared 10-year outcome in 97 patients with bipolar disorder whose index episode included switching from one mood phase to another and 97 patients whose index episode was monophasic. Overall, they found that a subgroup of those who switched had experienced multiple polarity switches (n = 23) and had worse outcomes (ill 56 percent of the time during the follow-up period), compared with those who had one polarity switch (ill 26 percent of the time; n = 74) or those with a monophasic index episode (ill 20 percent of the time; n = 97).

A related question (discussed further in Chapter 19) is whether depression that occurs alone (preceded and followed by euthymia) is different in duration or risk of an antidepressant-related manic switch from depression that occurs immediately following mania. This pattern of differential risk was noted in a post hoc analysis of a small randomized clinical trial comparing the addition of paroxetine to a mood stabilizer (lithium or valproate) with a combination of the two mood stabilizers (Goldberg, 2001). Another study (Gitlin et al., 2003) examined 72 prospectively observed depressive episodes in 28 patients with bipolar-I disorder. It was found that 65 percent of depressive episodes were monophasic, and 35 percent were postmanic. Duration of episodes was somewhat longer in the monophasic group (82 ± 65 days) than in the postmanic group (62 ± 48 days). Antidepressant-induced manic switching was also higher in the postmanic group (36 percent, 4 of 11 patients) than in the monophasic group (26 percent, 9 of 34 patients). Although the authors interpreted these differences as unimportant because of a lack of statistical significance, there is a large risk of type II false-negative error due to the small sample size. Whether future research will confirm this suggestion of higher susceptibility to antidepressant-induced mania and perhaps an increased cycling rate in those with polyphasic as compared to monophasic depressive episodes remains an open question.

The features of a manic episode may also be related to the course of illness. In a retrospective assessment, Swann and colleagues (2001) found that mania with depressive features (mixed states) was associated with an earlier onset of illness and more prior episodes than mania with irritable features (but no concomitant depressive affect).

PATTERN

The topic of episode pattern is of historical importance. Early investigators demonstrated that three basic patterns were apparent: mania followed by depression and then a well interval (MDI), depression followed by mania and then a well interval (DMI), and continuous cycling (MDMD).[38] There is some evidence from these studies that the MDI pattern may have the best outcome (Koukopoulos et al., 1980) and the MDMD pattern the worst. As we suggested in the first edition, the DMI pattern appears to be associated with mania occurring after treatment of the depressive phase with antidepressants (Maj et al., 1989).

Contemporary studies of episode pattern are not entirely consistent with this older literature. In a study of all hospitalized cases of bipolar and unipolar disorders in Denmark over a 22-year period (1971–1993; N = 17,447), the DMI and MDI courses were associated with a similar number of recurrences (Kessing, 1999). On the other hand, in a recent reanalysis of data from the CDS in which 165 bipolar-I patients were followed for 15 years, Turvey and colleagues (1999) reported that mood episodes beginning with depression (depression only or depression followed by mania) were associated with worse 15-year outcomes than those beginning with mania. Also, polarity sequences tended to remain stable over time: 75 to 80 percent of individuals whose first observed mood episode began with mania continued to have mood episodes beginning with mania, and 55 to 60 percent of those whose mood episodes began with depression also maintained that pattern. This study is the longest outcome study assessing polarity. Its findings suggest that patterns of mood episodes are sustained over time and that the poorer prognosis of depressive as opposed to manic episodes persists in the long run.

Finally, it should be noted that some confusion regarding the patterning of episodes has been introduced by recent treatment guidelines asserting that the polarity of the index episode predicts the polarity of a relapse following the episode. As discussed in detail in Chapters 17 and 20, this conclusion should apply only to those relapses that occur shortly after remission is achieved, and these generally occur as a result of an effective treatment's being withdrawn before the continuation phase of treatment is completed. In an analysis of the course of patients on placebo participating in an 18-month study of maintenance treatment with lithium or lamotrigine when the time frame beyond the continuation phase of treatment was examined the next new episode was almost always (85 percent of the time) of opposite polarity confirming classic observations (F. Goodwin and Calebrese [in preparation]).

PRECIPITANTS OF EPISODES

Findings of most studies of diagnostically heterogeneous groups of depressed patients suggest that stressful life events, such as losing a loved one, changing jobs, or moving, are more frequent during the 3 to 12 months preceding the onset of a depressive episode. Although the literature on events precipitating depression is extensive, that pertaining specifically to bipolar patients is more modest. It comprises primarily interesting but ultimately inconclusive case reports (reviewed by Ellicott, 1988), an intriguing report on increased relapses among bipolar patients after a hurricane,[39] and 14 systematic studies, all but 3 of which were retrospective. These studies are outlined in Table 4–3; their conclusions are summarized in Box 4–2. Taken together, they provide considerable support for the importance of stressful events in the onset of episodes in bipolar patients.

Although some theories assign primary causal importance to psychosocial environmental forces, it is now generally accepted that environmental conditions—psychosocial or physical—contribute more to the timing of an episode than to underlying vulnerability, which is largely genetic (see Chapter 13). Thus modern biological theory reaffirms the classic position of Kraepelin (1921, pp. 180–181):

> We must regard all alleged injuries as possibly sparks for the discharge of individual attacks, but that the real cause of the malady must be sought in permanent internal changes, which at least very often, perhaps always, are innate. . . . Unfortunately, the powerlessness of our efforts to cure must only too often convince us that the attacks of manic-depressive insanity may be to an astonishing degree independent of external influences.

Early precipitating events, rather than merely influencing the timing of an episode, may actually activate the preexisting vulnerability, thereby making the individual more vulnerable to subsequent episodes, as recently demonstrated by Dienes and colleagues (2006). The theoretical significance of this possibility, proposed by Post and colleagues (1986a), is elaborated in Chapters 14 and 17.

More recent evidence supports the conclusion that the influence of life events in triggering mood episodes is more prominent in earlier than in later phases of bipolar disorder. The studies summarized in Table 4–3 (total of 688 patients) generally support this observation.

TABLE 4–3. Life Events, Kindling, and Mood Episodes in Bipolar Disorder

Study	Sample Size	Life Event (LE) Method	Findings	Supports Kindling	Comments
Ambelas, 1979	67	Paykel LE scale	First-episode patients were overrepresented in LE-associated mania.	Yes	Retrospective only; hospitalized manic episodes assessed
Dunner et al., 1979b	79	Own LE questionnaire	52% reported LEs before first episode, compared with 15% before subsequent episodes.	Yes	Retrospective study of outpatients; not limited to hospitalized episodes
Glassner and Haldipur, 1983	53	Own interview with patients and families	23% of early-onset bipolar patients (age <20) had LEs before episodes, compared with 63% of late-onset bipolar patients (age >20). However, early-onset patients had the same percentage LEs before first and subsequent episodes (23%), as did late-onset patients (64% and 61%, respectively).	Indeterminate	Retrospective; included inpatients and outpatients
Perris et al., 1984	149	Own LE interview	More patients with later episodes than first episode of depression reported no preceding negative LEs (50% vs. 38%; $p < .02$) or conflict events (81% vs. 57%; $p < .001$).	Yes	Prospective; combined bipolar and recurrent unipolar disorders in sample
Bidzinska, 1984	36	Puzynski LE questionnaire	LEs preceded more of first three episodes (2.6) than fourth through sixth episodes (1.9; $p < .05$).	Yes	Retrospective; compared findings with those of studies of unipolar patients, in which results did not support kindling; criteria for episodes unclear

Study	N	Measure	Findings		Comments
Swann et al., 1990	66	Two Schedule for Affective Disorders and Schizophrenia (SADS) scale items asking clinicians and patients to give impressions of stressful LEs and current episode	Perceived roles of stressful LEs (combined clinician and patient scores) were greater in patients with fewer previous episodes (3.7) than in those with more previous episodes (13.4; $p < 0.05$).	Yes	Retrospective; careful rating scale and diagnostic assessments; data for bipolar and unipolar patients not separate
Winokur et al., 1993	148	None	Patients with one or more previous episodes were more likely than first-episode patients to have a recurrence in 2-year follow-up (0.64 episodes vs. 0.46; $p = .18$), but not statistically significant.	Indeterminate	Prospective; episodes based on Research Diagnostic Criteria and not just hospitalization, up to 5-year follow-up
Palao et al., 1997	26	Scale of Assessment of LE and Social Support of the California Department of Mental Health	Fewer LEs were found before the first episode of bipolar disorder compared with the following two episodes ($p < .02$).	No	Outpatients; complete data not available, presented as abstract; method for assessing episodes not clear (apparently retrospective)
Hlastala et al., 2000	64	SADS-Lifetime (SADS-L) or Structured Clinical Interview for DSM (SCID)	Number of episodes experienced did not appear to have a significant effect on reactivity of bipolar-I patients to external stressors.	No	Prospective

Note: Total sample = 688 (limited to patients identified as having bipolar disorder, with exception of Perris et al., 1984).

Recently, Kendler and colleagues (2000) conducted a large twin study involving 2,395 individuals with unipolar depression, interviewed four times over a period of 9 years, and found that stressful life events were increasingly less associated with triggering a major depressive episode over time. This pattern held for the first nine episodes, then tapered off. Although this study investigated unipolar disorder, its findings on precipitation of episodes appear to be highly relevant to mood disorders in general. A major strength of this study is that it employed a twin research paradigm and therefore could control for the effects of the environment, as opposed to genetics, in a way that clinical studies cannot. Employing this paradigm and mathematical models that can be used to predict genetic versus environmental causation, the investigators were able to suggest that the relationship between life events and major depressive episodes was causal and not simply correlational. Similar findings have reported from non-twin studies of recurrent unipolar depression (Brown et al., 1994; Hammen et al., 2000; Bockting et al., 2006.)

The older literature on an association between life events and relapse is supported by a study of 62 patients with bipolar disorder (Hunt et al., 1992), in which a more frequent rate of severe life events (19 percent) was found in the month before relapse, compared with the background monthly rate of such events (5 percent), during the 2-year follow-up period. In another study, recovery from mood episodes in 67 hospitalized patients with bipolar-I disorder was delayed three-fold in the presence of a precipitating negative life event (Johnson and Miller, 1997).

Because external life events have been established as associated with mood episodes, recent research has focused on other aspects of the psychosocial circumstances of individuals with bipolar disorder. For instance, Staner and colleagues (1997) reported that, among 27 patients with bipolar disorder in remission for 1 year, social support, self-esteem, and attributional styles were not associated with increased risk of subsequent episodes of bipolar illness, but social maladjustment was.

Specific life events that deserve separate mention are pregnancy and childbirth. The earlier literature suggested a significant risk of postpartum (puerperal) depression or mania.[40] More recent data indicate a high risk of depression during pregnancy or the postpartum period in bipolar women (30 to 50 percent), as well as some risk of mood instability during pregnancy itself.[41,42] The treatment implications of pregnancy and the postpartum period of treatment are discussed in Chapter 20.

Comorbidity of personality disorders may be another factor that interacts with psychosocial stressors in increasing the risk of relapse in bipolar disorder (see Chapter 10). In one study of 52 euthymic U.S. military veterans with bipolar disorder, 38 percent met DSM-III-R criteria for personality disorder, which, in an unadjusted analysis, was associated with lower employment status and increased substance abuse (Kay et al., 2002). In another study, 72 bipolar-I patients were assessed dimensionally for the presence of hyperthymic versus depressive temperaments. Adjusted for age, sex, and occupational level in a multiple-regression analysis, higher depressive temperament trait scores were associated with greater number of mood episodes, especially of depressive polarity, and more suicide attempts (Henry et al., 1999). The interaction between personality and psychosocial stressors is an important clinical and research topic for further evaluation.

Drugs and physical illness, unlike life events, are sometimes not recognized as significant precipitating factors for manic or depressive episodes, but they should be (Table 4–4). Both drugs and alcohol can, in their own right, precipitate manic episodes, and they also can impair both the quantity and quality of sleep, thereby increasing the probability of mania. The special situation of mania precipitated by antidepressant treatment is discussed in detail in Chapter 19; we review some of that literature here as it relates to precipitation of mood episodes.

In his cohort study, Angst (1981a) found no association between long-term administration of antidepressants and recurrence, although he did not report the raw data. Turvey

TABLE 4–4. Conditions and Drugs Reported to Precipitate Manic Episodes

General Category	Specific Factor	Study
Endocrine States or Substances	Cushings (increased steroids)	Glaser, 1953; Goolker and Schein, 1953
	Hyperthyroidism	Corn and Checkley, 1983
	Androgens	Freinhar and Alvarez, 1985b
	Steroid and steroid withdrawal	Goldstein and Preskom, 1989; Pope and Katz, 1988; Venkatarangam et al., 1988; Viswanathan and Glickman, 1989
Drugs	Isoniazid[a]	Chaturvedi and Upadhyaya, 1988; Jackson, 1957; Kane and Taylor, 1963
	Procarbazine	Mann and Hutchinson, 1967
	Levodopa	O'Brien et al., 1971; Ryback and Schwab, 1971; Van Woert et al., 1971; Chase et al., 1973
	Methyldopa withdrawal	Labbate and Holzgang, 1989
	Hallucinogens (e.g., LSD, PCP and mescaline)	
	Cocaine[b]	
	Alcohol[b]	
	Bromide	Sayed, 1976
	Sympathomimetic amines	Waters and Lapierre, 1981
	Cimetidine; amantadine	Hubain et al., 1982; Lazare, 1979; Rego and Giller, 1989
	Tolmetin	Sotsky and Tossell, 1984
	Iproniazid	Crane, 1956
	Methylphenidate	Koehler-Troy et al., 1986
	Triazolam	Weilburg et al., 1987
	Zidovudine[c]	Maxwell et al., 1988; O'Dowd and McKegney, 1988; Schaerf et al., 1988;
	Busipirone	Wright et al., 1989; Liegghio and Yeragani, 1988; Price and Bielefeld, 1989
	Alprazolam	France and Krishnan, 1984
	Lorazepam	Rigby et al., 1989
	Guanfacine[d]	Horrigan and Barnhill, 1999
	Lisinopril[d]	Skop and Masterson, 1995
Metabolic Conditions	Postoperative state	Muncie, 1934
	Hemodialysis	Cooper, 1967
Infections	Influenza	Maurizi, 1985; Steinberg et al., 1972
	Q Fever	Schwartz, 1974
	Post–St. Louis type A encephalitis	Weisert and Hendrie, 1977
	Cryptococcal meningitis	Johnson and Naraqi, 1993
Central Nervous System (CNS) Pathology Neoplasms[a]	Suprasellar diencephalic tumor	Guttman and Hermann, 1932; Greenberg and Brown, 1985
	Head trauma	Stern and Dancey, 1942; McKeown and Jani, 1987; Jorge et al., 1993

(continued)

TABLE 4–4. **Conditions and Drugs Reported to Precipitate Manic Episodes** (continued)

General Category	Specific Factor	Study
	Parasagittal meningioma	Oppler, 1950
	Benign pheno-occipital tumor	Bourgeois and Campagne, 1967
	AIDS	Dauncey, 1988; Gabel et al., 1986; Kermani et al., 1985; Mijch et al., 1999
	Creutzfeld-Jakob Disease	Lendvai et al., 1999
	Syndenham's chorea	Black and Perlmutter, 1997
	Multiple sclerosis	Casanova et al., 1996; Heila et al., 1995
	Chondroma	Salazar-Calderon et al., 1993
Vascular Lesions[e]	Aneurysm	Jampala and Abrams, 1983
	Infarction	Cummings and Mendez, 1984; Fujikawa et al., 1995; Kulisevsky et al., 1993; Vuilleumier et al., 1998
Other	Epilepsy—right temporal focus	Rosenbaum and Barry, 1975
	Vitamin B_{12} deficiency	Goggans, 1984
	L-glutamine	Mebane, 1984
	Aspartame	Walton, 1986
	Metrizamide as a contrast agent in myelography	Kwentus et al., 1984

Note: This table is based on the definition of secondary mania provided by Krauthammer and Klerman (1978); the data have been updated by our own review and those of Lazare (1979), Yassa and colleagues (1988a), and Sultzer and Cummings (1989).

[a]Mania induced by antidepressants (tricyclic monoamine oxidase inhibitors [MAOIs] and selective serotonin reuptake inhibitors [SSRIs]) is thoroughly discussed in Chapter 20. Reports of antipsychotic-induced mania are discussed in Chapter 18.

[b]The impact of alcohol and illicit drug abuse on manic-depressive illness is detailed in Chapters 7 and 21.

[c]Used for treatment of acquired immunodeficiency syndrome (AIDS).

[d]Antihypertensive medications.

[e]A comprehensive review of secondary mania in association with central nervous system (CNS) pathology can be found in Chapter 17.

and colleagues (1999), analyzing the CDS data, reported that polyphasic as opposed to monophasic mood episodes were not associated with antidepressant use. Although polyphasic mood episodes were associated with poor outcome and initial depression was correlated with polyphasic mood episodes, antidepressant use could not be shown to be a factor in the poor outcome later observed. This study was a longer-term reanalysis of the same sample previously discussed (with similar findings) by Coryell and colleagues (1992). Because treatments were not randomized, one cannot know what influenced clinicians to use or not use antidepressants.

Other investigators, using other samples, have reported different results. As detailed earlier, Altshuler and colleagues (1995) found that about 25 percent of bipolar patients appeared to show an association between antidepressant use and rapid cycling. This figure was confirmed by Ghaemi and colleagues (2000), who reported that 24 percent of individuals treated in a university-affiliated health maintenance organization demonstrated such an association. Although

these latter reports are retrospective, rather than prospective like the CDS, the inability to replicate the findings of the CDS in other samples raises questions about the generalizability of the CDS sample.

Wehr and colleagues (1987a) proposed that sleep reduction may be the common denominator of several disparate events and stressors that reportedly precipitate mania. Indeed, this suggestion is well supported by our clinical experience. Sleep loss is common to reports of manic episodes following (1) various stressful events, such as bereavement (e.g., Krishnan et al., 1984); (2) the postpartum state; and (3) jet lag associated with flying across time zones. Selective serotonin reuptake inhibitor (SSRI) antidepressants are capable of destabilizing sleep patterns. Because of the importance of this issue, we outline in Chapter 19 specific approaches designed to minimize sleep loss in bipolar patients.

Another important potential trigger for mood episodes is the season of the year. Issues regarding light and seasonality were addressed extensively in the first edition and are further discussed in Chapter 16 of this volume. In the context of course of illness, patients with bipolar and recurrent unipolar conditions often experience seasonal patterns. In one study published since the first edition of this text, 49 percent of 146 patients who met DSM-III-R criteria for seasonal affective disorder (Faedda et al., 1993) were diagnosable with bipolar disorder, mainly type I (30 percent of the total sample; 19 percent were type II), meaning that these patients tended to experience full manic episodes in spring or summer. While winter depression is often the focus in the diagnosis and treatment of seasonal affective disorder, the high likelihood of summer mania should also be noted.[43]

LONG-TERM OUTCOME

The literature on long-term outcome in bipolar disorder can be quite confusing. We have already noted some problems that can contribute to this confusion, such as effects of treatment in studies done in the modern era, selection bias in studies from academic health centers, and lack of adjustment through appropriate statistical techniques (e.g., multivariate regression) for other potential predictors of outcome (such as socioeconomic status and antidepressant use). Another problem is multiple publications over time based on the same dataset, which can appear to readers to represent different datasets. For this reason, we have grouped studies of long-term outcome by their initial recruitment location, rather than by specific publications.

The literature from the 1970s and 1980s on long-term outcome in bipolar illness tended to find somewhat better outcomes than have more recent studies. For instance, in a report on a 35-year follow-up of the original 100 patients admitted for mania in the Iowa 500 study, Tsuang and colleagues (1979) found that when marital, residential, occupational, and psychiatric (symptomatic) status were combined, outcome was good in approximately 64 percent of patients, fair in 14 percent, and poor (i.e., chronic) in 22 percent. This study, while more than 25 years old, still encompasses the modern era in which pharmacological treatments were available.

Modern Prospective Cohort Studies

Since 1990, there have been reports on 11 prospective cohort studies of natural history in manic-depressive illness, all but one of which were limited to bipolar disorder (Table 4–5).[48] The two largest and most carefully examined are the CDS and McLean-Harvard first-episode cohorts, which are discussed at the end of this section. Two more recent cohorts are those of the Stanley Foundation Bipolar Network and STEP-BD. Longitudinal outcome data are beginning to become available from both of these studies.

The Zurich cohort consisted of 406 patients, 186 with unipolar depression and 220 with bipolar disorder, initially recruited on admission to a psychiatric hospital during 1959–1963 and then reinterviewed at 5-year intervals. In a follow-up period that lasted up to 20 years, Angst and colleagues (2005) reported that only 24 percent of the bipolar sample and only 30 percent of the unipolar sample had fully remitted (that is, had experienced no further episodes). Many patients, however, had experienced periods free of illness, comprising on average about 80 percent of the time; chronically ill outcomes were seen in only 16 percent of the bipolar and 13 percent of the unipolar sample. In a recent reanalysis involving a follow-up period of more than 40 years, only 16 percent of the total sample had fully recovered by age 68 (Global Assessment Scale score above 60, with no episodes in the past 5 years), and 52 percent still had recurrent episodes. A subgroup (16 percent) remained chronically ill, and 7.8 percent had committed suicide (Angst and Preisig, 1995).

The Chicago cohort consisted of 139 hospitalized patients, 73 with mania and 66 with unipolar depression, recruited from area hospitals in the late 1980s. Outcome was assessed with a scale that incorporated both symptomatic and functional assessments. In a follow-up period that lasted on average 1.7 years, 25 percent of unipolar and 19 percent of bipolar subjects had a good outcome, while 14 percent of unipolar versus 25 percent of bipolar subjects had a consistently poor outcome (Harrow et al., 1990). In a follow-up that extended up to 5 years (mean 4.5 years), outcomes looked somewhat better, with 41 percent of unipolar and bipolar subjects demonstrating a good outcome, versus 14 percent of unipolar and 22 percent of bipolar subjects having a consistently poor outcome (Goldberg et al., 1995).

The University of California-Los Angeles (UCLA) cohort consisted of 82 bipolar patients recruited to the university outpatient clinic from 1984 to 1990, followed for a minimum of 2 years (which led to the exclusion of 78 patients initially recruited) and then for up to 5 years (mean 4.3 years) (Gitlin et al., 1995). Among this sample, 37 percent had relapsed at 1-year follow-up and 73 percent at 5 years, with only 17 percent consistently euthymic. Most relapses (70 percent) involved multiple episodes.

The Cincinnati cohort consisted of two groups. The first comprised 134 hospitalized patients with DSM-III-R bipolar disorder recruited from their academic psychiatric units during 1992–1995. At 1-year follow-up (Keck et al., 1998), 48 percent had experienced syndromal recovery; 26 percent symptomatic recovery (full remission); and 24 percent functional recovery (defined as regaining premorbid occupational and residential status), which was associated with higher initial socioeconomic status and paralleled

TABLE 4–5. **Prospective Cohort Natural-History Studies in Manic-Depressive Illness Since 1990**

Study	Sample Size	Follow-up Period	Findings
Chicago cohort (Harrow et al., 1990; Goldberg et al., 1995)	139	Up to 4 years	22% poor overall outcome, 41% good overall outcome in bipolar subgroup
McLean/Harvard cohort I (Tohen et al., 1990)	75	Up to 4 years	Multiepisode cohort; 100% follow-up obtained. 28% poor functional outcome; only 28% episode-free
National Institute of Mental Health (NIMH) Collaborative Program on the Psychobiology of Depression-Clinical Studies cohort (Coryell et al., 1993, 1994, 1995; Akiskal et al., 1995, 1998; Judd et al., 1998; Turvey et al., 1999; Judd et al., 2002, 2003)	428	Up to 20 years	Mood symptoms presented in about one half of the follow-up period, primarily those associated with chronic subsyndromal depression
University of California-Los Angeles (UCLA) cohort (Gitlin et al., 1995)	82	Up to 5 years	Only 17% "consistently euthymic"
Cincinnati cohort I (Keck et al., 1998)	134	Up to 1 year	48% syndromal recovery; 28% symptomatic recovery; 24% functional recovery
Cincinnati cohort II (Strakowski et al., 1998)	50	Up to 1 year	First-episode mania cohort. 30% not improved; 30% with continued subsyndromal symptoms
McLean/Harvard cohort II (Tohen et al., 2000, 2003)	173	Up to 4 years	First-episode cohort; classic Kraepelinian features; almost complete syndromal recovery (98%), but less symptomatic (72%) and functional (43%) recovery
Stanley Foundation Bipolar Network cohort (Post et al., 2001, 2003; Suppes et al., 2001; Keck et al., 2003)	648	Up to 1 year	33% were substantially well, 67% mostly ill; 63% had a prospective rapid cycling course; cohort was depressed for 33% of the follow-up period and manic for 11%
Systematic Treatment Enhancement Program for Bipolar Disorder (STEP-BD) cohort (Kogan et al., 2004)	1000	Up to 5 years	Prospective data pending
Jorvi Bipolar Study cohort (Mantere et al., 2004)	191	N/A	A polyphasic episode was current in 51.3%, rapid cycling in 32.5%, and psychotic symptoms in 16.2%; mixed episodes occurred in 16.7% of bipolar-I and depressive mixed states in 25.7% of bipolar-II patients
Zurich cohort (Angst and Preiseg, 1995)	406	Up to 40 years	Only 16% fully recovered; only 16% had chronic outcome

symptomatic recovery. Incidentally, only 47 percent of patients were fully adherent to treatment at follow-up, which is consistent with the literature reviewed in Chapter 21. A second Cincinnati cohort project, initiated in 1996, recruited bipolar patients hospitalized with their first manic episode. The initial 50 subjects enrolled between 1996 and 1998 were characterized at about 6.8 months of follow-up (Strakowski et al., 2000). On average, the subjects remained in a full syndromal mood episode for about 30 percent of the follow-up period, spending an additional

30 percent of the time in subsyndromal mood states. Initial mood-incongruent psychosis predicted worse outcome than initial mood-congruent psychosis (after adjusting for some clinical factors with analysis of covariance).

The CDS and McLean-Harvard cohorts can be seen as complementary, because they represent different types of patients. Data on the CDS cohort were collected at five U.S. academic health centers. The cohort consisted of patients in their 30s and 40s initially, whose illness usually had begun a decade or more earlier with depression as its primary presenting feature (for which the patients had been treated primarily with antidepressants), and who tended to have comorbid diagnoses. This represents a "modern" manic-depressive illness cohort, with nonclassical features of illness. The McLean-Harvard cohort consisted completely of hospitalized bipolar patients, most of whom were psychotic and experiencing their first manic episode. Most were insured, of middle to high socioeconomic status, and with few psychiatric comorbidities. This cohort is close to a modern analogue of the classic patients of the pretreatment era, similar to those Kraepelin described from among psychotic patients hospitalized at the Munich asylum. As Grof and colleagues (1995) suggested, it could be that the natural history of the bipolar variant of classic Kraepelinian manic-depressive illness is quite different from that of the bipolar disorder identified in many cohorts today. At any rate, differences in findings among contemporary cohorts need to be assessed in light of the different samples they represent. Each cohort is discussed below in turn.[45]

The CDS has produced the most published data in recent years on the course of manic-depressive illness. The sample in that study consisted of roughly one-third outpatients and two-thirds inpatients initially recruited during the years 1978–1981 at five U.S. academic health centers. This cohort has now been followed for up to 25 years, with a retention rate in follow-up of more than 80 percent. As of 2003, about 80 percent of this cohort was reportedly in continued treatment with pharmacotherapy (R. Keller, personal communication, 2003). At 5-year follow-up, more previous episodes predicted more relapses but also quicker recovery (recovery at 6 months was 55 percent for a first episode, 73 percent for one or two previous episodes, and 90 percent for more than three previous episodes). Psychosis predicted only 37 percent recovery at 6 months, versus 65 percent in nonpsychotic patients. At 5-year follow-up, all of the patients initially treated for pure mania had recovered, compared with 89 percent of those with pure depression and 83 percent of those with mixed states. Despite ongoing "high-intensity somatotherapy" in the majority of subjects (75 percent), early relapse rates were relatively high: at 6 months, 20 percent of patients with pure mania had relapsed, compared with 33 percent of those with pure depression and 36 percent of those with mixed states. By 1 year, 48 percent of patients initially with pure mania had had a relapse, versus 57 percent of those with mixed states; at 5 years, these rates were up to 81 and 91 percent, respectively. Relapse rates among those initially treated for depression were similar to those among patients with mixed episodes (Keller and Boland, 1998). The question of antidepressant-induced worsening of the long-term course of bipolar illness also raises the possibility that these poor outcomes may have occurred in part because of (rather than despite) the high-intensity somatotherapy received by patients (although adherence to treatment was not reported).

Despite sustained syndromal recovery for 2 years, most of the sample of 148 bipolar and 240 unipolar patients experienced severe impairment of psychosocial functioning (Coryell et al., 1993). In the index episode, the co-occurrence of psychotic features with mixed states (depressive symptoms during acute mania) was associated with more long-term psychosis than was the co-occurrence of index psychotic features with pure mania (Coryell et al., 2001).

Other analyses of the CDS data were reviewed earlier in the discussion of kindling. More recent results from the CDS are presented later in the discussion of subsyndromal outcomes.

The McLean-Harvard First-Episode Mania Study consisted of two cohorts. The first (Tohen et al., 1990) included 75 bipolar patients who were recruited over a 1-year period (1983–1984) from the psychiatric units of McLean Hospital after admission for acute mania and followed for up to 4 years (100 percent of subjects were followed for the entire outcome period). This was primarily a multiple-episode cohort (68 percent). The second cohort (Tohen et al., 2000, 2003) started with bipolar patients in their first hospitalized episode; 173 such patients were recruited from 1989 to 1996 at the same hospital and followed for up to 4 years. The characteristics of this second cohort were as follows: 84.9 percent were Caucasian, with gender about equally distributed; 88.6 percent were psychotic; 75.3 percent were in a pure manic (not mixed) episode; only 18.7 percent had substance abuse comorbidity; and only 8.4 percent had another psychiatric comorbidity. As noted earlier, this second cohort can be viewed as representing close to the classic Kraepelinian description of what would now be referred to as the bipolar subgroup of manic-depressive illness.

In the first, multiple-episode cohort (Tohen et al., 1990), 28 percent were unable to work or study at 4-year follow-up, and 19 percent were unable to live independently. Only 28 percent were episode-free, and 28 percent had experienced three or more relapses, with a predominance of manic polarity. Poor occupational and residential status was correlated with subsyndromal interepisode illness (r = .42 to .46). After Cox proportional hazard regression to predict time to relapse, adjusted for 13 risk factors, the statistically significant main predictors were, in order of magnitude, past alcoholism (hazard ratio [HR] = 3.9), index psychosis (HR = 2.2), and index depressive symptoms during the manic episode (HR = 2.0). A reanalysis assessing psychotic features found that mood-incongruent psychosis in particular predicted a quicker relapse (adjusted HR = 2.6) (Tohen et al., 1992).

In the second McLean-Harvard cohort (patients initially hospitalized for mania/mixed states), those with past substance abuse were less likely than nonabusers to be recovered at 2-year follow-up (86 versus 98.5 percent). Among patients with initial mixed episodes, only 33 percent were living independently at 2 years, compared with 82 percent of those who had been admitted for pure mania. Further, although almost all patients had recovered syndromally at 2 years (98 percent), fewer (72 percent) had achieved full remission, and only 43 percent had recovered functionally (defined as regaining premorbid occupational and residential status). New episodes had been experienced by 59 percent of patients—20 percent mania, 20 percent depression, and 19 percent polyphasic switches (Tohen et al., 2000, 2003). These data suggest that functional recovery lags behind episode recovery and, further, that complete symptomatic remission does not ensure functional recovery, even in a classic Kraepelinian group of patients with relatively good prognosis. Predictors of earlier syndromal recovery (using Cox regression to adjust for other clinical factors) were as follows: short initial hospitalization (HR = 1.99; 95 percent confidence interval [CI] = 1.36 to 2.93), female gender (HR = 1.72; 95 percent CI = 1.16 to 2.56), and fewer index depressive symptoms (HR = 1.65; 95 percent CI = 1.14 to 2.39). For functional recovery (using multiple logistic regression), predictors were older than age 30 at index episode (odds ratio [OR] = 3.28; 95 percent CI = 1.58 to 6.82) and shorter initial hospitalization (OR = 2.82; 95 percent CI = 1.36 to 5.88). Further analyses suggest that initial pure mania and mood-congruent psychosis predicted manic relapse, whereas initial mixed episode predicted depressive relapse. Further, there appeared to be more manic relapse among those with lower baseline occupational status and more depressive relapse among those with higher status.

In the Stanley Foundation Bipolar Network cohort (N = 258) (Nolen et al., 2004), poor prognostic factors at 1 year of prospective follow-up (in an adjusted multivariate regression model) were comorbid substance abuse, more than 10 prior manic or depressive episodes, family history of substance abuse, past rapid-cycling course, and poor occupational functioning at study entry. In a German subgroup of this cohort (n = 152), predictors of poor outcome at 2.5 years of follow-up were bipolar-I disorder, comorbid Axis I disorders, and past rapid cycling (Dittmann et al., 2002).

In the first 1,000 subjects analyzed in the STEP-BD cohort, early age at onset (Perlis et al., 2004), past substance abuse (Weiss et al., 2005), and past comorbid attention-deficit disorder (Nierenberg et al., 2005) were associated with poor outcome (age-at-onset data only, based on an adjusted multivariate regression model).

Other Features of Long-Term Outcome

Another feature of long-term outcome that may be related to poor occupational functioning is cognitive impairment.[46] Findings of a number of studies indicate that cognitive impairment and neuroanatomical changes may be associated with the long-term effects of multiple mood episodes and/or duration of illness and/or treatment in both recurrent unipolar and bipolar patients (see Chapters 9 and 14). In one study using magnetic resonance imaging (MRI), lateral ventricles were larger in multiple-episode patients with bipolar disorder compared with 17 first-episode patients and 32 healthy subjects (Strakowski et al., 2002). In another study, duration of bipolar disorder (N = 43) was associated with impaired performance on general memory tasks (Donaldson et al., 2003). In neither of these studies, however, was the potential impact of pharmacological treatment evaluated. Neuropsychological test abnormalities were confirmed in another study of 26 euthymic patients with recurrent unipolar or bipolar illness, with an association being found between degree of neuropsychological impairment and number of past hospitalized episodes (Tham et al., 1997). This finding was confirmed in another study of 25 euthymic patients with bipolar disorder compared with 22 age-matched normal controls (van Gorp et al., 1998).

It has been suggested that neuropsychological dysfunction may be a consequence of increased activity of the hypothalamic–pituitary–adrenal axis during mood episodes, which has been shown to lead to excitotoxic damage to sensitive brain regions, particularly the hippocampus (Lee et al., 2002). Hippocampal atrophy is more likely to occur in patients with greater numbers of mood episodes than in those with fewer mood episodes or in normal controls (Altshuler et al., 1991), and pilot data (detailed in Chapter 14) suggest that patients taking lithium, compared with similar patients not taking lithium, do not suffer such atrophy (Moore et al., 2000).

It should be noted that studies in this area focus primarily on symptomatic outcome, although some recent studies have begun to focus on functional outcome. As previously noted, these two kinds of outcome are correlated, but not completely. In other words, while episode recurrence and subsyndromal chronicity are, not surprisingly, both associated with worse functional outcomes, about 40 percent of euthymic patients with minimal detectable symptoms still appear to be functionally impaired. Long-term state-independent cognitive impairment is one likely explanation for this asymptomatic functional impairment, but this link remains to be established.

Beyond functional recovery, moreover, the question of quality of life remains. Even if patients are working and living in normal circumstances, the quality of their work and level of satisfaction with life remain largely unexamined by standard functional outcome measures. In a study of 50 euthymic persons with bipolar disorder, Sierra and colleagues (2005) found that quality of life was lower than in normal controls, and Yatham and colleagues (2004) found that some aspects of quality of life may be worse in bipolar compared with unipolar depression. Findings of another study from Europe were more optimistic, noting some improvement in recent years in bipolar patients' reports of their quality of life as they learned more about the nature of their disorder and the need for treatment (Morselli et al., 2004). With regard to pharmacological treatment, our review of the quality-of-life literature revealed that, although mood-stabilizing treatments clearly improve symptomatic outcomes in the majority of patients with bipolar disorder, their effect on quality of life remains to be established (Revicki et al., 2005).

Finally, with regard to subsyndromal morbidity and interepisode symptoms, the most recent reanalysis of the CDS data (Judd et al., 2002) found chronic subsyndromal depression to be the main outcome of treated bipolar-I disorder. In a follow-up period ranging up to 20 years (mean 12.8 years; N=146), patients were symptomatic 47 percent of the time. During these symptomatic periods, patients were predominantly depressed (67 percent of symptomatic period, 32 percent of total follow-up period), rather than manic or hypomanic (19 and 9 percent, respectively) or in mixed states (13 and 6 percent, respectively). Depressive periods were almost three times more likely to be spent in subsyndromal states (25 percent of total period) than in major depressive states (9 percent of total follow-up period). In sum, these data reflect primarily subsyndromal or interepisode periods of chronicity. The fact that depressive rather than manic symptoms are responsible for the bulk of the morbidity and functional impairment associated with bipolar disorder has also been noted in a community survey using self-reports (Calabrese et al., 2004).

It should be noted that similar rates of subsyndromal chronicity were reported in the CDS cohort for patients with unipolar depression (N=431) (Judd, 1998). This cohort consisted of a first-episode group (28 percent; n=122), a recurrent-depression group (48 percent; n=205), and a "double-depression" group meeting criteria for recurrent

episodes and dysthymia (24 percent; n=104). In a follow-up of up to 20 years (mean 8.7 years), patients were symptomatic 59 percent of the time. During these symptomatic periods, depressive symptoms were again almost three times more likely to be associated with subsyndromal states (43 percent of total follow-up period) than with major depressive states (15 percent of total period).

As a result of these studies, Judd and colleagues (2002) and others (Kupka et al., 2005) have urged a shift in long-term studies to focus on chronicity and subsyndromal morbidity. One example of such work is a study that found subsyndromal depressive morbidity in bipolar disorder (N=25) to be associated with increased functional impairment (Altshuler et al., 2002).

It is also notable that subsyndromal manic morbidity was found to be most prominent in a 4-year follow up of children (N=86; mean age at baseline 10.8 years) (Geller et al., 2004). In this cohort, patients spent 57 percent of the follow-up time in manic or hypomanic states, versus 47 percent in depressive states and 37 percent in mixed states. (The total exceeds 100 percent because mixed states were included in all three categories.) These findings suggest that the chronic subsyndromal depressive course is a feature of adult bipolar disorder, whereas in children a more chronic manic/mixed course predominates (see Chapter 6).

A number of considerations arise in interpreting the results of outcome studies. The first is the extent to which these outcomes reflect natural history as opposed to being either attenuated or exacerbated by treatment effects. Most of the investigators cited earlier noted that their patients were treated primarily according to current standards, although information on specific treatments was not provided. When treatment effects were addressed, it was generally in the context of the assumption that continuing morbidity had to be occurring despite these effective treatments. Another possibility exists, however: that in some cases, treatment is only minimally beneficial or neutral, but capable of exacerbating the course of bipolar illness. As noted earlier and discussed in detail in Chapter 19, this possibility is especially salient for antidepressants, which may lead to subsyndromal cycling states that could in turn account for the outcomes described by Geller and colleagues (2004). The issue of how to treat subsyndromal chronic bipolar depression is a vexing problem for clinicians and an important unanswered question for researchers. If antidepressants are related to cycling, one option would be to decrease their use. On the other hand, if antidepressants were not being used, their possible benefits in some patients would be missed. The use of cognitive-behavioral and other psychotherapies would appear to be appropriate in this situation (see Chapter 22), although this approach has not been well studied. Other behavioral interventions, such as enhancement of sleep hygiene, have also been suggested (Morris, 2002; see also Chapter 16).

MORTALITY

Suicide is a frequent outcome of manic-depressive illness; in bipolar patients, it occurs more frequently early in the course of the illness (see Chapter 8). Although suicide is the single most important factor contributing to increased mortality in manic-depressive patients,[47] other causes, such as the increased risk of cardiovascular disease, contribute as well. Indirect consequences of psychotic behavior during untreated episodes—including malnutrition, exposure, and exhaustion—all compromise general health and presumably contribute to a higher mortality rate. So, too, do smoking and alcohol and drug abuse. As reviewed in Chapters 14 and 15, some of the biological dysfunction noted in manic-depressive patients involves systems other than the brain. These dysfunctions could also contribute to higher-than-normal mortality rates.

Recent studies of mortality in bipolar disorder are listed in Table 4–6, along with the weighted mean standardized mortality ratio (SMR) from studies reviewed in the first edition of this text.[47] Early studies of mortality rates in manic-depressive illness, which did not separate bipolar from unipolar forms, claimed substantially increased mortality—up to six times the rate expected for the same age group in a normal population. More recent studies have found a less striking but still considerable increase in mortality, averaging approximately 2.3 times the expected rate in the general population. This difference in results probably reflects improvements in psychiatric care, particularly the availability of specific treatments for the depressive and manic phases. Thus in Derby's (1933) study, 22 percent of hospitalized manic patients died, and 40 percent of these deaths were from "exhaustion," whereas in the Iowa 500 follow-up, Tsuang and colleagues (1980) found a significant increase only in "circulatory" deaths and only among women. Corroborating the earlier Iowa findings in a follow-up of 1,593 affective patients, Black and colleagues (1987a) noted that non-suicide-related deaths were excessive only among those patients with a concurrent medical disorder.

The largest recent prospective study of mortality in bipolar disorder involved up to 38 years of follow-up of depressed hospitalized patients in Zurich. Angst and colleagues (1999) reported that, overall, these patients demonstrated increased mortality compared with the general population, with a 61 percent higher risk of death (SMR = 1.6). The greatest risk was associated with suicide (SMR = 18), but statistically significant risks were also associated

with cardiovascular disease (SMR = 1.6) and accidents (SMR = 1.9). Those with bipolar depression were somewhat less likely to commit suicide than those with unipolar depression (SMR = 12.3 versus 26.7) but somewhat more likely to die from cardiovascular disease (SMR = 1.8 versus 1.4). Treated patients had lower suicide risks than untreated persons with bipolar disorder (SMR = 6.4 versus 29.2), but confounding factors were not controlled statistically in this observational study. It is also noteworthy that since cardiovascular disease is much more common than suicide, the absolute amount of improvement in mortality associated with suicide was the result primarily of decreased cardiovascular-related mortality. In concluding this discussion of mortality it is important to note that, with adequate lithium treatment, the mortality associated with bipolar illness can be reduced to a level indistinguishable from that of the general population, an effect no doubt related, at least in part, to the antisuicide effect of lithium (Muller-Oerlinghausen et al., 1996; Tondo et al., 2001). This point is discussed in greater detail in Chapters 8 and 25.

BIPOLAR-II DISORDER

The course of bipolar-II disorder has not been as well studied as that of bipolar-I illness; moreover, one of the issues in research on bipolar-II disorder is the relative lack of reliability for this diagnosis (see Chapter 3). The CDS in particular, however, has begun to shed light on the course of this condition. In 5-year follow-up, while bipolar-II subjects were less likely than bipolar-I subjects to be hospitalized, no other clinical differences in outcome (cycle length, number of mood episodes, suicide attempts) were found (Coryell et al., 1989b). Depressive episodes and symptom severity did not differ between the two groups, nor did frequency or duration of hypomanic versus manic episodes (in the bipolar-I group). Differences in psychosocial outcome between the two groups also were not evident. Manic episodes, by definition, occurred exclusively in the bipolar-I group. In a follow-up period of up to 10 years, only 7.5 percent (N = 64) of individuals with bipolar-II illness switched to type I. However, if one includes dropouts from follow-up in that study, which may reflect the disinclination of more severely ill patients to continue to participate in the biennial interviews, rates of switch from type II to type I approach 15 percent. In a follow-up of up to 20 years, the primary morbidity over time was chronic subsyndromal depression, and the prominence of depression was even more pronounced than in the bipolar-I cohort (Judd et al., 2003). During the follow-up period (mean 13.4 years; N = 86), patients were symptomatic 54 percent of the time. During these symptomatic periods, patients were predominantly depressed (93 percent of symptomatic period,

TABLE 4–6. Contemporary Studies of Mortality in Bipolar Disorder

Study	Sample Size	Duration of Observation (Years)	Deceased (%)	Standard Mortality Ratio[a]	Suicide % of all Deaths	Cardiovascular Disease % of all Deaths	Comments
Sharma and Markar, 1994	472	12–17	12.1	—	15.7	42.1	Population included psychiatric patients who had at least one episode of mania; SMR for CVD=3.0; and for suicide=23.4
Ahrens et al., 1995	473 F 354 M	6.75 (avg.)	4.9 5.9	1.23 1.07	21.7 9.5	30.4 33.3	Patient sample included BP, UP, and SZA patients attending outpatient lithium clinic; suicide mortality greater than expected, but overall mortality and CVD-caused mortality not different from general population
Broderson et al., 2000	133	16	30.1	2.50	27.5	17.5	All patients admitted to psychiatric hospital and given lithium prophylaxis; Dx=BP, UP, atypical affective disorders; SMR for CVD=1.23 and for suicide=20.5
Hoyer et al., 2000	34,465 F 19,638 M	1–20	26.8 32.4	1.8 2.2	17.9 23.1	26.5 28.5	Main analysis included hospitalized BP and UP patients; SMR for CVD=1.5, $p < .0001$ and SMR for suicide=17.12, $p < .0001$
Kallner et al., 2000	299 F 198 M	1–30	15.1 18.7	1.3	25.6	20.7	424 BP, 97 UP; all started on prophylactic lithium; SMR for suicide=14.0 ($p < .001$)
Ösby et al., 2001	8808 F 6578 M	11.5 (mean) 10.5 (mean)	19.8 26.1	27 2.5	18.7 20.1	29.9 32.1	Included only BP patients; all causes of death and diagnoses obtained from Swedish national registers; SMR for CVD=2.6 (F), 1.9 (M) and for suicide=22.4 (F), 22.9 (M)

(continued)

TABLE 4–6. Contemporary Studies of Mortality in Bipolar Disorder *(continued)*

Study	Sample Size	Duration of Observation (Years)	Deceased (%)	Standard Mortality Ratio[a]	Suicide % of all Deaths	Cardiovascular Disease % of all Deaths	Comments
Angst et al., 2002	291 F 115 M	34–38	72.2 82.6	1.59 1.64	13.8 15.8	35.2 26.3	186 UP and 220 BP; BP patients had SMR for CVD=1.84 vs. UP SMR for CVD=1.36; treated BP patients had lower SMR for CVD than untreated (1.68 vs. 2.23)
Weighted mean pre-1990s[b]				2.28			

BP=bipolar; CVD=cardiovascular disease; Dx=diagnosis; UP=unipolar; SMR=standard mortality ratio; SZA=schizoaffective.
[a]Ratio of observed mortality to expected mortality based on a normal demographically matched comparison population.
[b]Based on a total of 7,584 subjects from 11 pre-1990 studies in which excess mortality was determined.

50 percent of total follow-up period), and minimally hypomanic (2.4 and 1.3 percent, respectively) or mixed (4.3 and 2.3 percent, respectively). Depressive symptoms were almost three times more likely to be subsyndromal (37 percent of total follow-up period) compared with major depression (13 percent); again, then, these data reflect primarily subsyndromal or interepisode chronicity.

Vieta and colleagues (1997) reported that bipolar-II (n = 22) compared with bipolar-I patients (n = 38), had more past depressive episodes (5.6 versus 2.6), more hypomanic episodes (7.0 versus 3.2), and, of course, more total lifetime episodes (12.6 versus 6.3). Again, bipolar-I disorder was associated with more hospitalizations (3.0 versus 1.0).

The phenomenon of double-depression refers to the persistence of milder depressive states (dysthymia) following recovery from an episode of major depression (Keller et al., 1983). Klein and colleagues (1988) noted that, compared with other unipolar patients, those with double-depression had a higher incidence of hypomanic episodes during follow-up.

MECHANISMS OF RECURRENCE

Considering that recurrence is a major characteristic of manic-depressive illness, particularly in the bipolar form, it is surprising how little attention has been paid to its underlying mechanisms. None of the dominant neurotransmitter theories attempts to account for repeated episodes.

As noted earlier, the most widely cited explanation of the recurrent course of bipolar disorder is kindling, proposed by Post (1990) on the basis of experimental work on rodents (Weiss et al., 1990). The neurobiology of kindling is discussed extensively in Chapter 14, and earlier in this chapter we reviewed those aspects of the course of the illness that are relevant to evaluating this model. Those points bear repeating here.

Epileptic seizures are known to be generated by repeated subthreshold stimulation. The kindling model assumes that repeated stress and trauma can induce a similar progressive process in bipolar patients. Numerous studies have found fewer precipitants with increasing number of episodes in bipolar illness. Kindling may also be applicable in some cases to atypical DSM-IV bipolar disorder, with patients often reporting childhood traumas in retrospect. Unfortunately, none of the other predictions suggested by the kindling model appears to apply to classic bipolar disorder. For example, the kindling model would predict that patients treated later, after "a latency" and after more episodes, would have worse outcomes, but this hypothesis is not supported by the data (Baldessarini et al., 1999; Baethge et al., 2005). The kindling model would also predict that cycle length would shorten with more episodes,

but this is not a characteristic feature of later episodes of bipolar illness. Although regression analysis of cycles would create such an impression (Angst et al., 1970), progressive shortening is demonstrable only in a subgroup of patients, the MD type—patients who experience both major depressions and full manias (Angst, 1986c). Furthermore, 7 to 8 percent of patients actually show a gradual lengthening of cycle (Lat, 1973). Similarly, the kindling model might predict that patients fully stabilized after long-term lithium treatment would experience fewer episodes after gradual discontinuation than before the treatment, and this certainly is not the case.

Other proposed explanations of recurrence include those derived from biological rhythm models (see Chapter 16), especially catastrophe theory, based on a nonphysiological intersection of several endogenous rhythms. Other investigators have concluded that, in some cases, recurrent patterns of deterministic chaos may underlie the course of bipolar disorder (Bauer and Whybrow, 1988; Post et al., 1995).

CONCLUSIONS

The natural course and outcome of manic-depressive illness contribute to its definition and its differentiation from schizophrenia. For the clinician, understanding natural course can help answer a patient's questions about the most important estimate of all, the prognosis: Will it return, and when? Here we summarize the key points of this chapter that can help answer these questions.

Despite substantial methodological problems of both earlier and recent studies and limited data from prospective follow-up studies, the literature on the course and outcome of manic-depressive illness supports the following conclusions:

- The bipolar subtype has the earliest age at onset, followed by the more recurrent forms of unipolar depression, followed by the less recurrent forms. For the bipolar subgroup, the representative value varies with the definition of onset, ranging from the appearance of first symptoms (such as mood lability) before age 20 to the first hospitalization (in the 25–30 age range).
- Almost all bipolar patients experience relapse, given adequate observation time. Results of contemporary studies indicate higher relapse rates than those found in earlier studies; extended use of antidepressants may have contributed to this increase. Highly recurrent unipolar depression is a risk factor for developing bipolar illness.
- Cycle length does not change predictably with time, although it may shorten progressively in the initial stages of illness in a subgroup of individuals.

- An appreciable proportion of bipolar patients develop rapid cycling. Rapid cycling may represent one extreme of the bipolar spectrum rather than a completely autonomous group. The nosological status of rapid cycling remains unclear, however.
- The literature shows rather consistently that manic episodes are briefer than depressive or mixed episodes. The average episode duration remains stable throughout the illness.
- About 1–2% per year of unipolar patients experience a first manic or hypomanic episode, suggesting that over a long period of follow-up, a large minority of previously diagnosed unipolar patients will switch to diagnosable bipolar disorder. The pattern of initial depression followed later by mania is associated with poor long-term outcome. Antidepressants may have a role in hastening poor long-term outcome.
- Psychosocial and physical stresses continue to appear to be robust predictors of the timing of relapse, although these severe life events most likely interact with a patient's underlying vulnerability in a complex manner. Life events appear to be associated with relapse more in earlier than in later phases of bipolar illness.
- Long-term data suggest that up to one third of bipolar patients achieve complete remission, and a similar number achieve complete functional recovery. Although syndromal recovery is two or more times more frequent, fewer patients go on to recover premorbid levels of function. Chronic persistence of symptoms can be expected in about 20% of cases, and social incapacity in about 30%. Poor outcome in recent studies may be influenced by selection bias toward the inclusion of more severely ill patients in tertiary care centers. In the community setting, outcomes could be better than those cited here. Early age at onset, depression, mixed episodes, psychosis, substance abuse, medication noncompliance, and probably the long-term use of antidepressants are all associated with poor outcome. Mortality and suicide rates are increased in bipolar illness but can be substantially reduced by adequate lithium treatment.
- There are several interesting theories of the mechanisms of recurrence, including chronobiological explanations and kindling theory. Kindling may represent a subgroup effect, being relevant to a more severe or atypical subgroup of individuals with bipolar disorder.

NOTES

1. Behavioral, intellectual, and language tests were part of the standard examination battery administered by the Israeli Draft Board Registry. Anyone previously diagnosed with the aforementioned disorders by the time of the draft examinations or directly thereafter was excluded from the study. The experimental group was culled from those who developed the disorders at least 1 year after examination. To control for instability of diagnosis, the authors included only patients whose diagnosis after a 4-year follow-up was the same as the entry diagnosis.

2. Psychotic bipolar patients were excluded from this study because part of the cohort had been assessed using *International Classification of Diseases* (ICD)-9 criteria, before the bipolar definition had been broadened to include more psychotic features.

3. van Os et al., 1995; Bromet et al., 1996; Vocisano et al., 1996; McClellan et al., 2003.

4. While some of these data were taken from subanalyses of large epidemiological samples, most were gathered from clinical populations. We discuss age-at-onset results from epidemiological samples in Chapter 6. Although it is impossible to eliminate selection bias completely, we took care here to select only those patient samples that appeared to represent the general bipolar population.

5. Reliability measures were based on age-at-onset assessments made by two independent physician raters. Reliability coefficients for first treatment and first hospitalization were 0.94 and 0.97, respectively.

6. One must also consider the possible contributions of changes in maternal behavior (smoking and drinking during pregnancy), as well as changes in dietary factors, such as decreased intake of omega-3 fatty acids (since World War II) due to changes in infant formulas (see Chapter 5).

7. It is likely that the lower age at onset seen in more recent birth cohorts results from a confluence of these multiple factors.

8. Additional information about this survey was obtained from the study authors for the present review. Although subject to recall bias and not administered by a trained clinician, the survey used to determine age at onset did adhere to DSM-IV episodic criteria. Furthermore, to control for underreporting of later ages at onset, the authors did not include the youngest cohort of participants (born after 1959) in their analyses.

9. For example, Mick and colleagues (2003) compared measures of cognitive and global functioning, comorbidity, and clinical features across three groups arbitrarily designated as childhood, adolescent, and adult onset. They found significantly more comorbid anxiety disorders in the child and adolescent groups compared with the adult group, but no difference among groups in cognitive or global functioning. However, there was a trend for more rapid cycling and mixed episodes in the earlier-onset group, although the sample size lacked the power to permit evaluation of statistical significance for some of these measures.

10. Neurological abnormalities were descriptive and based on medical records. Among 14 patients in the elderly-onset mania group, 10 had neurological problems such as seizures, gait disturbance, recurrent cerebral contusions, and cerebral infarcts.

11. Winokur and colleagues (1993) found no association between a family history of bipolar disorder and age at onset. Lish (1994) and colleagues, however, found a significant correlation between childhood/adolescent onset and a family history of the disorder. This finding was replicated by Engstrom and colleagues (2003). Johnson and colleagues (2000) reported that patients with a family history of bipolar disorder had a significantly lower age at onset than those with no such family history.

12. However, a recent study from this group did find that mixed episodes were more common in a bipolar group with an early age at first hospitalization (younger than 18) compared with those first hospitalized in their twenties (Patel et al., 2006).

13. Although this study included patients with adolescent onset (minimum age=15), the authors confirmed the diagnosis at intake and at follow-up with clinician-administered Structured Clinical Interview for DSM (SCID) results and corroborating evidence from family reports, as well as school and medical records.

14. Here again, both early- and late-onset groups were adults at the time of assessment (mean age 33.6 and 60.2, respectively). Diagnosis was verified with DSM-IV criteria and corroborating medical records, as well as family interviews.

15. At the time of assessment, the sample included all adults (mean age 43.1) diagnosed with DSM-IV bipolar disorder. Age at onset was determined by clinician-administered questionnaire, medical records, and family interviews in some cases. Confirming other reports, Suppes and colleagues (2001) also found a highly significant relationship between incidence of childhood sexual abuse and early onset (p ≤ .001), a possible triggering phenomenon discussed in Chapter 7.

16. As in most studies of this kind, Ernst and Goldberg ascertained age at onset retrospectively, in this instance using life charts.

17. Perris (1968) found 83 percent with four or more episodes and 43 percent with seven or more. In a 1978 paper, Angst (1978) updated a careful longitudinal study of 95 bipolar patients who at that time had been followed for an average of 26 years (standard deviation ±11.9). The study included both retrospective and prospective phases, the latter involving direct patient and family contact at least every 5 years. Patients by and large did not receive prophylactic treatment, although most had individual episodes treated with medications. The number of episodes ranged from 2 to 54, with a median of 9; 84 percent had 5 or more episodes, 69 percent had 7 or more, and 42 percent had 11 or more. A naturalistic study of 51 bipolar patients who received unsystematic acute and prophylactic treatment showed that all but 2 of the patients had experienced 3 or more episodes, with a median of 15 (Roy-Byrne et al., 1985a). Although this finding is consistent with earlier data, it is important to remember that the patient groups are not comparable, because the research setting of the Roy-Byrne study tended to select treatment-resistant patients. In a chart review study of 236 bipolar patients from the prepharmacotherapy era (between 1920 and 1950), Winokur and Kadrmas (1989) found that, during a follow-up period averaging 2.4 years, 28 percent had 1 episode, 22 percent had 2, 14 percent had 3, 11 percent had 4, 4 percent had 5, 2 percent had 6, 0.8 percent had 7, 0.4 percent had 8, and 11 percent had 9 or more.

18. Angst's Dm group is roughly analogous to the bipolar-II subgroup in DSM-III-R, although hospitalization is not necessary for the diagnosis of either major depression or mania in DSM-III-R.

19. Today, given modern treatment, relatively few patients would actually meet this criterion (i.e., hospitalization).

20. In their 1979 review of the literature on the natural course of manic-depressive illness (both unipolar and bipolar, with the index episode usually a hospitalization), Zis and Goodwin (1979) divided studies that showed low rates of relapse from those that showed high rates. They found that those with low relapse rates were marred by methodological limitations, including short duration of observation, focus on episodes involving hospitalization, exclusion of episodes preceding index admission, inclusion of nonrecovered patients, combined episodes treated as single episodes, and high unipolar/bipolar patient ratio. For example, studies with low relapse rates tended to include only episodes requiring hospitalization, introducing a bias toward patients with longer and more severe episodes. Thus in Perris's 1968 study, only 40 percent of patients had had four or more episodes involving hospitalization, but when all episodes were included, more than 80 percent had had four or more. Obviously, excluding episodes preceding the index hospital admission also leads to underestimation. When, for instance, Bratfos and Haug (1968) included preadmission episodes, the proportion of patients with single episodes dropped to 13 percent.

As noted previously, early studies often found a high proportion of single-episode patients because they included in that single-episode count the many chronic patients who in fact had had multiple (but uncounted) episodes while hospitalized. Cutler and Post (1982a) traced the long-term course of illness in a group of bipolar patients who were chronically hospitalized in a state institution. Their detailed analysis indicated that each of these patients displayed a pattern similar to what Kraepelin had observed more than half a century earlier: multiple, discrete episodes embedded in a single long-term hospitalization. Estimates of relapse rates probably were lower than justified in the older studies, even when based on patients who were not chronically hospitalized. In those cases, combined episodes (e.g., a mania followed by a depression, perhaps interspersed with a brief well interval) may have been counted as a single episode. The presence of a continuously circular course (Koukopoulos et al., 1980) or rapid cycles (Dunner et al., 1976b) makes it more likely that multiple episodes will be counted as one.

21. It may also be that recurrence is related to other features of bipolar illness, such as age at onset and genetic risk. This interesting possibility has not been adequately explored since the time of a chart review conducted during the prepharmacology era (Winokur and Kadrmas, 1989), which suggested that certain clinical features may be associated with the illness's natural tendency to recur. Winokur and Kadrmas found that, compared with patients who had only one or two episodes during a follow-up period averaging 2.4 years, patients with a polyepisodic course (more than three episodes) were more likely to have had an early age at onset, a finding that replicates an earlier report by Okuma and Shimoyama (1972). Winokur and Kadrmas also found that a polyepisodic course was associated with a more insidious onset of the index episode and a greater frequency of bipolar illness in first-degree relatives. They speculated that this last finding could indicate that cyclicity more than polarity is genetically transmitted: the more total episodes, the greater the likelihood of manic episodes.

22. In 1938, Eliot Slater of the Maudsley Hospital in London published a paper ("On the Periodicity of Manic Depressive Insanity") (Slater, 1938a) in which he reexamined cases of patients who had been the source for Kraepelin's data regarding the shortening of cycle length. Unfortunately perhaps for later generations, Slater's paper, published in a German psychiatric

journal that was prominent before World War II, lapsed into obscurity in succeeding decades, especially in the non-German-speaking world. (This lack of attention in the Anglo-American setting is particularly ironic given that Slater was an Englishman.) In our review, we found the initial peer review and the most extensive discussion of "Slater's fallacy" in English in a 1996 paper by Haghighat (1996), who also noted earlier citations in book chapters by Angst (1988). In 2000, Angst and Sellaro (2000) again referred to Slater's report in English, and we recently obtained an English translation of the original paper.

In that study, Slater reviewed 116 charts of patients diagnosed by Kraepelin in Munich with manic-depressive illness. Among the features he assessed, Slater highlighted his reexamination of Kraepelin's report of decreasing intervals of wellness with an increase in the number of episodes, which became a central feature of what would later be called the kindling model. Slater confirmed that the duration of mood episodes appeared to increase to a small degree over time. However, his key finding was that the apparent decrease in euthymic intervals between episodes was a statistical artifact. Slater pointed out that "people who have longer intervals between episodes will not fall ill as often as those in whom the intervals are shorter." In other words, if all patients are included in the analysis, some will experience only two episodes and others six, for example. It may be that those with six episodes have short periods of wellness between episodes, whereas those with two episodes experience long periods of wellness. If those two types of patients are added together, as was done by Kraepelin, there will appear to be a progressive decrease in euthymic intervals. The actual state of affairs will not necessarily be so. One would have to demonstrate that intervals of wellness shortened over time *in the same patients*, whether they had two episodes or six. In sum, interepisode intervals of wellness need to be corrected for the number of episodes. When Slater made this correction, Kraepelin's finding vanished (except to a small degree for earlier episodes). In a recent outcome study of first-episode manic patients at McLean Hospital, Baldessarini and colleagues (2000) found the same effect. Taken as a group, the sample appeared to demonstrate progressive shortening of intervals of wellness, but when the data were corrected for number of episodes, there was no apparent shortening of well intervals.

We would like to acknowledge and thank Dr. Ross Baldessarini for bringing this long-neglected paper to our attention. We would also like to acknowledge and thank our colleague, Dr. Godehard Oepen, for assistance in translating and interpreting Slater's study.

23. Bratfos, 1968; Bratfos and Haug., 1968; Angst et al., 1973; Roy-Byrne et al., 1985a; Goldberg, 1993; Goldberg and Harrow, 1994; Kessing, 1998; Kessing et al., 1998a; Cusin et al., 2000.

24. Another study found that number of episodes did not predict recurrence at 1-year prospective follow-up (Staner et al., 1997). Such short-term studies are less useful in refuting kindling hypotheses, however, because the kindling model is a long-term model. The studies of the groups led by Coryell and colleagues (2001) and Baldessarini and colleagues (1999) were longer-term (up to 10 years).

25. Kendler and Karkowski-Shuman (1997) also assessed this finding within individuals by stratifying their dataset by individual

and assuming a separate hazard function for their Cox proportional hazards model for each person in the study.

26. In a study with the methodological limitation of including only hospitalized patients, there was no evidence of a difference in episode severity in individuals experiencing their first manic episode as opposed to one of multiple episodes (Keck et al., 1995). However, because all patients were hospitalized, differential severity may have been difficult to detect.

27. The sample was from the Mediterranean island of Sardinia.

28. Independent confirmation or refutation of the kindling model based on other lines of evidence may gradually develop. For instance, Huber and colleagues (2001) presented a mathematical nonlinear model of sensitization. This model has two components: a positive feedback loop (more episodes lead to more episodes) and a long time interval. The authors showed that this mathematical model can support autonomous disease progression as well as irregular rapid cycling as an end stage of disease, as predicted by the kindling hypothesis.

29. Swift, 1907; MacDonald, 1918; Pollock, 1931; Angst and Weis, 1967; Zis et al., 1979.

30. The 1989 study of Winokur and Kadrmas (1989), although limited by its chart review methodology, is nevertheless of interest because it is based on the prepharmacology era. The authors reported that patients with a polyepisodic course (more than three episodes per average follow-up of 2.4 years) were significantly more likely to have an early age at onset (before age 20) than those with one or two episodes.

31. Another question is whether episodes come in bursts or clusters, as originally described by Kraepelin in his studies of predominantly chronic patients with frequent relapses. As discussed in Chapter 20, this issue is important in assessing prophylactic treatment, and indeed in making treatment decisions. If episodes of manic-depressive illness characteristically occur in clusters, it may be difficult to interpret prophylactic trials in individual patients. The evidence on this issue is somewhat conflicting. Saran (1970) compared episode frequencies in six untreated bipolar patients for 2 years before and 3 years after an arbitrary point in time. Even in such a small number of patients, there was some suggestion of episode clustering. In a 2- to 20-year follow-up (mean 5.6 years) of patients admitted for manic episodes, Winokur (1975) found that 91 percent of first-episode patients had experienced another episode during follow-up, compared with only 53 percent of those with a history of previous episodes—a result interpreted as evidence of episode clustering. Angst and colleagues (1970) did not find different relapse rates before and after lithium treatment. It is also worth noting that there may be some methodological issues with extrapolating from such group findings to clustering in individual patients.

32. For example, Kupka and colleagues (2005) found more bipolar-I than bipolar-II patients among 539 outpatients in the Stanley Network.

33. In a study of 320 hospitalized patients with bipolar-I disorder, the polarity of the first episode was determined to be major depressive in 52 percent, mixed in 26 percent, and pure manic in 22 percent. Patients whose illness began with depression were more likely to develop a rapid-cycling course and experienced more suicide attempts but less psychosis than the other groups. The mixed group tended to be more

chronic and made frequent suicide attempts but generally did not experience a rapid-cycling course (Perugi et al., 2000).

34. In this study, the incidence of false unipolar (pseudounipolar) depression was strikingly low (4.4 percent) and out of line with the rest of the psychiatric literature. This observation may suggest that studies based on hospitalization will overreport the incidence of manic as opposed to depressive episodes, because the latter lead less frequently to hospitalization than the former.

35. Taschev, 1974; Angst, 1978; Koukopoulos et al., 1980; Roy-Byrne, 1985a; Coryell et al., 1989b.

36. The literature is inconsistent in the relationships reported between predominantly manic or predominantly depressive episodes and age at onset or family history of affective disorder. Three studies (Mendlewicz et al., 1972a; Taylor and Abrams, 1973a; Stone, 1989) found a positive family history of affective disorder to be associated with an earlier age at onset, but this finding was not replicated by Winokur (1975). An association between earlier age at onset and a higher proportion of manic episodes in the course of illness was reported by Mendlewicz and colleagues (1972a) and by Angst (1978), but not by others (Taylor and Abrams, 1973a; Carlson et al., 1977; Roy-Byrne et al., 1985a).

37. Other studies have tended to confirm the general observation of stability of polarity in the course of illness, but most have not addressed or corrected for age (Cassidy, Cassidy, Perugi, Woods). The one study (Perugi et al., 2000) with data on age at onset in the 20s found consistent polarity for manic and mixed episodes in the course of illness. Among those patients whose illness began with a depressive episode, however, future episodes were equally likely to be manic/mixed versus depressed.

38. Winokur et al., 1969; Angst, 1978; Koukopoulos et al., 1980; Roy-Byrne and colleagues, 1985a.

39. Sleep deprivation would appear to be a likely explanation for hurricane-induced manias; this recalls the earlier suggestion of Wehr and colleagues (1987a) that sleep loss is the final common pathway by which various stressors can trigger mania (Aronson and Shukla, 1987).

40. Bratfos and Haug, 1968; Reich and Winokur, 1970; Kendell et al., 1976, 1987; Kadrmas, 1979.

41. Viguera and Cohen, 1998; Viguera et al., 2002; Akdeniz et al., 2003.

42. The occurrence of sexual abuse as a precipitant or predictor of mood episodes has also been studied. In one study, the rate of self-reported childhood sexual abuse was high in 142 persons with DSM-III-R bipolar disorder (18 percent of women and 4 percent of men) and was similar to the rates found in a unipolar comparison group of 191 persons (16 percent in women, 3 percent in men) (Hyun, 2000).

43. An interesting suggestion has been made that part of the mechanism for seasonal instability in psychiatric conditions may be attributable not only to increased sunlight, but also to increased ambient light due to the cycles of the moon (Raison, 1998; also see Chapter 16).

44. Here we are excluding lithium prophylaxis studies (O'Connell et al., 1991; Maj et al., 1995), which are discussed in Chapter 22. We are also excluding retrospective cohort studies, of which there have been a number, including a Cologne cohort (Marneros et al., 1990; Deister and Marneros, 1993), a Johns Hopkins cohort (Stephens and McHugh, 1991), an Indian cohort (Khanna et al., 1992), a Danish cohort (Kessing, 1998, 1999), an Italian cohort (Cusin, 2000), and a Taiwanese cohort (Tsai, 2001).

The Cologne cohort consisted of 106 patients with DSM-III mood disorders, a subgroup of a total cohort of 402 patients (the rest with psychotic disorders). With a mean of 27.9 years of outcome data, 64 percent of the mood disorder sample was fully remitted (Marneros et al., 1990). Subclassification of bipolar and unipolar conditions was not performed. In multivariate analysis, male gender was a major predictor of poor functional outcome (Diester et al., 1993). Other apparent predictors were an "asthenic low self-confident" premorbid personality and a higher number of mood episodes.

The Johns Hopkins cohort, also mentioned in this chapter in the discussion of polarity, consisted of patients hospitalized between 1913 and 1940, and therefore represents a true pretreatment natural-history sample. The study group consisted of 914 patients with at least 5 years of medical record follow-up data. With a mean follow-up of 13.5 years, only 11 percent of the bipolar group (n=297) and 22 percent of the unipolar group (n=945) did not experience future mood episodes. About one third of the total sample had a chronic outcome, somewhat worse in the bipolar subgroup (43 percent), and 13 percent committed suicide.

The Indian cohort consisted of 95 patients with bipolar disorder hospitalized in an academic psychiatric hospital over a period of 3 months in 1989. Medical records were assessed for course of illness. The main findings were more manic than depressive episodes and worse outcomes in those with initial manic episodes (unadjusted for other clinical factors statistically). The sample was predominantly male (84 percent) and predominantly manic (83 percent of first episodes reported). Interestingly, not a single case of a rapid-cycling course or of polyphasic episodes was documented, a finding that one might speculate is related to lack of antidepressant exposure in a setting in which many patients remain untreated.

The Denmark cohort is described further in this chapter in the discussion of kindling.

The Italian cohort consisted of 244 patients with bipolar disorder with 14-year outcome data. The main finding was that an initial manic as opposed to depressive episode predicted a higher frequency of episodes in the outcome period.

In the Taiwanese cohort, 101 patients with bipolar disorder were identified by hospital records and agreed to follow-up after 15 years. The main predictor of poor psychosocial outcome was medication nonadherence, which was observed in 33 percent of the sample.

45. Although the second McLean-Harvard cohort is a proxy for a first-episode study, it is notable that 24.7 percent had experienced previous nonhospitalized major depressive episodes. Therefore, this subgroup did not really consist of first-episode bipolar subjects.

46. In Chapter 9, we review the evidence that some neurocognitive impairment may exist even prior to the onset of the illness.

47. In a postmortem study of 122 bipolar patients, for example, Taschev (1974) found that 27 percent had died by suicide. Among manic patients from the Iowa 500 series, Winokur and Tsuang (1975b) found that 8.5 percent of the deaths were

suicides. Perris and d'Elia (1966) found that 11 percent of the deaths in their patients had resulted from suicide, exactly the same proportion as in Tsuang's (1978) 40-year follow-up. Reviewing the literature, Guze and Robins (1970) noted that about 15 percent of all deaths among patients with major affective disorders can be traced to suicide. See Chapter 9 for a more comprehensive review.

48. The large epidemiologic study on the association between depression and its treatment and cardiovascular disease (known as the SAD HEARTS study) was not included. While it provides an invaluable amount of information on the relationship between depression and heart disease, the study focused exclusively on unipolar patients, and the majority were nonrecurrent, having fewer than two episodes.

5 Epidemiology

Seek the points of contact which may reveal the underlying law. Some things can be learned only by statistical comparison.

—Sir William Osler (in Thayer, 1920, p. 52)

Epidemiology, which has been called the basic science of public health, is the study of the distribution of disorders in human populations, the variation in rates that may provide clues to their cause, and the risk factors associated with their onset and course. Epidemiology focuses on populations rather than individuals. An observation that a disorder is considerably higher in one group than another can be used to identify an epidemic or determine protective factors. Studying the variation in rates by specific characteristics (risk factors) yields clues as to how altering those characteristics may interrupt the process that leads to a disorder. This information also provides a scientific basis for assessing the overall health status of a population and identifying who is or is not receiving treatment.

Epidemiologic methods are common to studies of all chronic noninfectious diseases, including psychiatric disorders. These methods fall into three categories (see the review by Rothman and Greenland, 1998): *descriptive* methods, used to study the rates of disorder in a population; *analytic* methods, used to explore variations among different groups in order to identify risk factors; and *experimental* methods, used to test the association between a risk factor and a disorder by controlling the risk factor to see whether a reduction in onset or reoccurrence results. In this chapter, we focus primarily on results of descriptive studies. We begin by reviewing the application of epidemiologic methods in studies of psychiatric disorders, and then examine the key methodological issues that arise in such studies. Next we summarize the methods and results of epidemiologic studies of manic-depressive illness, with an emphasis on the bipolar subgroup. (The term *manic-depressive illness* in the pre–*Diagnostic and Statistical Manual* [DSM]-III literature sometimes referred to patients

that would be called bipolar in today's nosology, while in other contexts, the term referred to all recurrent mood disorders.) The studies we review are of the bipolar subgroup and involve community surveys of adults and of children and adolescents, as well as studies conducted by the World Health Organization (WHO). Finally, we review what is known about correlates, or features associated with bipolar disorder.

APPLICATION OF EPIDEMIOLOGIC METHODS IN STUDIES OF PSYCHIATRIC DISORDERS

Population samples are utilized to understand the full magnitude of a disorder, as well as its spectrum, including mild and untreated forms. WHO's international projections of the disability associated with mood disorders in both developing and developed countries (discussed later in this chapter) have garnered the attention of mental health planners and have made international epidemiologic data on mood disorders the focus of considerable interest.[1] Yet epidemiologic methods utilizing large-scale studies of populations have been applied to psychiatric disorders relatively recently. The first large-scale epidemiologic studies of psychiatric disorders were reported in the 1980s. Since then, there has been a rapid increase in the number of such studies. Moreover, their quality has improved significantly.

Over the past decade, much more reliable data on the rates of psychiatric disorders have become available as concern regarding biases, inconsistencies, and inadequacies in the psychiatric epidemiology literature has led investigators to become increasingly more systematic and sophisticated in their methodologies. Yet although the newer epidemiologic data on bipolar disorder are the product of considerable advances in methodology, they are not without difficulties:

- The findings almost always are based on structured interviews conducted by nonclinicians; studies comparing such data with diagnoses by experienced clinicians tend to show only modest correspondence.
- The relatively low prevalence of bipolar disorder requires large population samples for accurate estimates.
- There is an absence of community-based data on highly recurrent major depression, which falls within the spectrum of bipolar disorder (see Chapter 1).
- The boundary between normal mood and mild hypomania that may also be part of the spectrum, or an early sign of the illness, is ambiguous.
- Controversy exists about the nature of the disorder's clinical presentation in children and adolescents, which may complicate the ascertainment of true age at onset.
- One of the most important risk factors for bipolar disorder, family history, has not been included in epidemiologic surveys.

These problems do not in general apply to the same extent for major depression, which has a considerably higher prevalence than bipolar disorder and for which there is a more extensive body of research on first presentation in children and adolescents, although, as noted above, there is virtually no information on the more recurrent forms of depression in these age groups.

In the late 1970s, the National Institute of Mental Health (NIMH) sponsored the development of a diagnostic instrument, the Diagnostic Interview Schedule (DIS), suitable for use in large-scale epidemiologic studies of psychiatric disorders (Robins et al., 1981). In 1980, the Epidemiologic Catchment Area (ECA) study was initiated (Robins and Regier, 1991). This study included more than 18,000 adults aged 18 and older living in five U.S. communities (New Haven, Connecticut; Baltimore, Maryland; Piedmont County, North Carolina; St. Louis, Missouri; and Los Angeles, California). Using the DIS as the diagnostic instrument, lay interviewers generated DSM-III diagnoses (American Psychiatric Association [APA], 1980). The study was longitudinal, with a 1-year follow-up to determine incidence (i.e., first onset). Oversampling of African Americans, the elderly, Hispanic Americans, and the rural poor ensured that accurate rates of disorders and treatment needs among these groups could be ascertained.

The ECA demonstrated that the use of comparable and reliable methods allows rates of psychiatric illness to be compared across geographic regions. Over the course of the 1980s, comparable epidemiologic studies were undertaken in Edmonton, Canada (Orn et al., 1988); Puerto Rico (Canino et al., 1987); the former Republic of West Germany (Wittchen et al., 1992); Florence, Italy (Faravelli et al., 1990); Paris, France (Lépine et al., 1989); Beirut, Lebanon (Karam, 1992); Christchurch, New Zealand (Wells et al., 1989); Taiwan (Hwu et al., 1989); and Korea (Lee et al., 1990a,b). A collaboration among the lead investigators—called the Cross-National Collaborative Group—was undertaken to conduct joint analyses (Weissman et al., 1996).

In the 1990s, the National Comorbidity Study (NCS) was initiated in the United States (Kessler et al., 1994). This study was unique in that it was a national probability sample, and it used a new diagnostic method, the Composite International Diagnostic Interview (CIDI) (WHO, 1990), which had the capacity to generate both *International Classification of Diseases* (ICD) (WHO, 1991) and DSM-III diagnoses (see Chapter 11). Thus, it was possible to use variable diagnostic criteria to make direct comparisons with cross-national studies.

The ECA, the Cross-National Collaborative Group, and the NCS, as well as other epidemiologic surveys in different parts of the world, demonstrated that the majority of psychiatric illnesses had their onset in childhood and adolescence.[2] The pressing need for a direct epidemiologic study of children became apparent, but such studies of children present even more methodological problems than those of adults. Many questions arise: Should the diagnostic criteria used with adults also be used with children (a question discussed below under methodological issues)? Who is the best informant? Should parents, children, or both be interviewed? What risk factors should be included? What is the youngest age at which psychiatric disorders can be meaningfully assessed? These questions have not yet been fully resolved. Nonetheless, the National Institute of Mental Health's (NIMH) Methods for the Epidemiology of Child and Adolescent Mental Disorder (MECA) study was initiated in the 1990s in New Haven, Connecticut; Westchester County, New York; Atlanta, Georgia; and Puerto Rico. Its purpose is to develop and test methods for a large national epidemiologic study (Lahey et al., 1996). Other studies of children are also under way, as described later.

Because of the relative lack of information on the epidemiology of childhood psychiatric disorders, NIMH has begun to capitalize on ongoing national physical health surveys of children by adding questions about mental health. These surveys include the National Health and Nutrition Examination Survey (U.S. Department of Health and Human Services [US DHHS], 1998) for children aged 8 to 18, the National Health Interview Survey (US DHHS, 1996) for those aged 4 to 17, and the National Household Survey on Drug Abuse (US DHHS, 1999) for those aged 12 to 17. The first two surveys are investigating the comorbidity of psychiatric with physical problems, and the third is examining comorbidity with drug abuse. The inclusion of questions on mental health in ongoing national surveys of physical health among young people in the United States provides much-needed monitoring data on both psychiatric disorders in children and the relationship of these disorders to physical health. It is not clear whether bipolar disorder will be examined separately from other mood disorders.

By 1995, the availability of epidemiologic information from community surveys had made possible the first textbook on psychiatric epidemiology (Tsuang et al., 1995). At the close of the twentieth century, WHO, in collaboration with The World Bank and Harvard University (Murray et al., 1994), turned to developing methods for assessing the global burden of disease. Given changing disease patterns, including a decrease in communicable diseases, as well as increasing longevity, investigators sought measures other than the traditional mortality used in international projections. They found that four psychiatric disorders, including bipolar disorder, appeared among the top 10 disabling illnesses in both developed and developing countries. This information drew worldwide attention and laid the groundwork for the future generation of epidemiologic studies, which are global in scope.

METHODOLOGICAL ISSUES

The chapter on epidemiology in the first edition of this text focused on methodological problems because at the time there were more problems than data. Although these problems cannot be ignored in interpreting the growing body of data now emerging, we need not dwell on them because they have been addressed in many of the more recent studies. Therefore, this section reviews only those methodological issues that are particularly relevant to current understanding of the epidemiology of bipolar disorder.

Variable Diagnostic Criteria

During the past decade, methods for obtaining diagnostic data have improved significantly. Reliability across interviewers has improved, and many new approaches to diagnostic interviews are available. Yet despite these improvements, different diagnostic interview formats yield different rates of psychiatric disorders. Even when the same methods are used, comparing published rates across studies can be difficult because of differences in data presentation. Some investigators confine the data to cases that show an episodic pattern of mania and major depression (bipolar-I), whereas others include cases with a pattern of hypomania and major depression (bipolar-II). Still others combine bipolar-I and -II rates or include cyclothymia. For major depression, most investigators do not separate out the more recurrent forms (which are part of the manic-depressive spectrum) from the less recurrent forms, and some older studies reporting rates of manic-depressive illness do not separate the bipolar from the recurrent unipolar groups. The Cross-National Collaborative Group, mentioned earlier, was formed to address these differences in the reported data by standardizing methods for analysis and data presentation. The results of the group's efforts are presented in Table 5–1.

As detailed in Chapter 3, DSM-III, DSM-III-R, and DSM-IV improved specification of the diagnostic criteria for bipolar disorder; however, slight changes in the criteria over time have made comparisons of studies conducted even less than a decade apart problematic. In DSM-III, hypomania was classified as a disturbance similar to but not as severe as a manic episode, but no specific criteria were given (APA, 1980, p. 209) (see Chapter 3). Hypomania first appeared as a specific diagnostic entity in DSM-III-R, where it was defined as a distinct period of elevated mood but not severe enough to warrant the diagnosis of mania (APA, 1986, p. 218). In the 1990s, DSM-IV operationalized the criteria for hypomania,

TABLE 5–1. One-Year Disorder Prevalence (Percent Standard Error), Before and After Applying Clinical Significance Criteria

Disorder	Survey	Before CS	After CS
Unipolar major depression	Epidemiologic Catchment Area	4.9 (0.3)	4.0 (0.3)
	National Comorbidity Study	8.9 (0.6)	5.4 (0.5)
Bipolar-I disorder	Epidemiologic Catchment Area	0.9 (0.1)	0.5 (0.1)
	National Comorbidity Study	1.3 (0.2)	1.3 (0.2)

Note: Encompasses ages 18–54 years.
CS = clinical significance.
Source: Narrow et al., 2002.

requiring a persistently elevated, expansive, or irritable mood for at least 4 days (APA, 1994, p. 338); these criteria are consistent with those of ICD-10.

Even when diagnostic criteria are clear, mild forms of mania (such as hypomania) can fail to be detected. Most hypomanic episodes go undiagnosed even by psychiatrists, who when asking about episodes of depression may not elicit information about periods of unusual activity before and after an episode. As we emphasized in the first edition of this book, unless the patient and a family member are both carefully questioned about past hypomania, the bipolar nature of a depression may be missed (Simpson et al., 1993; Angst and Gamma, 2002). Indeed, hypomania is not well defined in research instruments. In community surveys, as the data presented later in this chapter suggest, it is exceedingly difficult to distinguish mild states of euphoria due to positive changes in a subject's life from the abnormal highs of hypomania; many patients initially diagnosed as having agitated depressions subsequently turn out to have had dysphoric hypomanias. In short, misdiagnosing and overlooking hypomanic states often leads to an underestimate of the true rate of bipolar disorder.[3] (See Chapters 1 and 3 for a detailed discussion of these issues.) Higher incidence rates are obtained when a broader range of cases belonging to the presumed spectrum of bipolar disorder, such as cyclothymia or atypical bipolar illness, are included in the survey.

In the absence of a clear understanding of the pathophysiology involved, the distinctions among bipolar disorders, highly recurrent unipolar disorder, other mood disorders, and psychotic disorders remain unclear (see Chapters 1 and 3). These distinctions are especially difficult to make in community studies that include greater numbers of mild and untreated cases. At the psychotic end of the spectrum, a large number of patients have illnesses with features of both schizophrenia and bipolar disorder, termed schizoaffective disorder. The line between hypomania and mania is also difficult to draw, and DSM-IV offers differential diagnoses depending on the severity of symptoms and impairment. Patients with bipolar-II disorder are unlikely to present for treatment for hypomania, and even more unlikely to report it as pathology in community surveys (Akiskal, 1995, 1996; Coryell et al., 1995). Therefore, as shown later, the rates of bipolar-II are low in community surveys and are likely to be underestimated. (The reliability of diagnosis of bipolar-I and bipolar-II in community surveys is discussed further in the presentation of results of U.S. surveys.) Thus the distinction between bipolar-I and bipolar-II disorder is usually based on retrospective accounts, limiting reliability (Dunner and Tay, 1993). Moreover, applying criteria related to the clinical significance of a disorder based on impairment and the need for treatment

can markedly alter rates (Narrow et al., 2002) (see the later discussion).

Age-Specific Issues

The criteria for diagnosing bipolar disorder in children are even less clear than those used for adults (for example, see the discussion of problems in defining age at onset in children and adolescents later in this chapter and in Chapter 6). Indeed, since 1980 (DSM-III, DSM-III-R, and DSM-IV), adult criteria have been applied to diagnose mania and depression in children without taking into account differences in age and developmental stage (Sanchez et al., 1999). Bipolar disorder in young people may therefore be misdiagnosed or underdiagnosed. Moreover, although mania in youth can be a severe illness frequently associated with mixed features, psychosis, rapid cycling, and comorbid disruptive disorders, there is often a clinical bias against making a diagnosis of mania in children. And the relationship between bipolar disorder and other, more prevalent childhood psychiatric illnesses, such as attention-deficit hyperactivity disorder (ADHD), is problematic (see the later discussion of surveys of children and adolescents). Estimates of the age at onset of bipolar disorder must take into account this lack of clarity regarding first presentation of the disorder in youth. Eventually, longitudinal studies of children from families with a high risk of bipolar disorder may clarify issues of first presentation (see Chapter 6).

The effects of duration and severity on prevalence must also be considered when reviewing the literature on prevalence of childhood bipolar disorder (Sanchez et al., 1999). DSM-III-R removed the 7-day minimum duration criterion for mania required by DSM-III. Consequently, reports based on DSM-III-R criteria may overdiagnose mania, especially in childhood. In DSM-IV, the duration criterion was reinstated, and the severity requirement was added.

In April 2000, NIMH convened a group of experts for a Bipolar Child Roundtable to discuss possible approaches for addressing outstanding issues related to research on prepubertal bipolar disorder. The major issues of relevance to epidemiology addressed at the roundtable were the earliest age at which bipolar disorder can be diagnosed and the predictive value of the early manifestations of bipolar illness in children and adolescents. The experts generally agreed that a diagnosis of bipolar disorder using DSM criteria is possible in prepubertal children.

Discussion among the expert group resulted in agreement on two basic definitions: (1) a narrow phenotype that adheres strictly to bipolar-I and bipolar-II criteria, and (2) a broader phenotype that encompasses more heterogeneity—basically bipolar-not otherwise specified (NOS)—and includes children who do not quite meet the criteria (especially the durational criterion) for an episode but still are severely impaired by symptoms of mood instability. Consensus on the former phenotype was that it can be diagnosed with available psychiatric assessment instruments, such as the semistructured Kiddie Schedule for Affective Disorders and Schizophrenia (KSADS) (Chambers et al., 1985). For clear communication, however, the importance of establishing thresholds for the boundaries between bipolar disorder subtypes (bipolar-I, bipolar-II, and cyclothymia) was emphasized because homogeneity is essential for biological, genetic, and epidemiologic research.

Currently, children with severely impairing mood disturbance who do not meet full DSM-IV criteria for bipolar-I or -II are not included in research studies and are difficult to assess in epidemiologic studies because of the perceived uncertainty of diagnosis. The expert group agreed that bipolar-NOS could be used as a working diagnosis to advance research on this broader phenotype, as long as the children were well described (with particular attention to symptoms of ADHD). Because available diagnostic instruments may not generate a reliable and replicable diagnosis of bipolar-NOS, it was recommended that careful assessment include all of the behaviors that are impairing, giving consideration when relevant to the frequency with which they occur, as well as their severity. Examples of the behaviors to be included are aggressiveness, agitation, explosiveness, irritability, mood lability (fluctuation independent of input), thought disorder (paranoia, misinterpretation of social cues), communication disorder (pragmatic language disorder that can look like flight of ideas, receptive and expressive language disorder that can interfere with the accurate performance and interpretation of structured interviews), and cognitive ability/cognitive impairment (significantly low intelligence quotient [IQ], reading disabilities).

Once agreement has been reached on exclusion criteria (certain comorbidities, such as pervasive developmental disorder and/or physical disease) as well as inclusion criteria for the broader phenotype, it should be possible to address questions about relationships among the disorders—for example, whether bipolar-NOS or its subtypes are precursors of bipolar-I and/or bipolar-II or have a different course. The expert group noted, for instance, that whereas the course of classic bipolar illness includes well periods, these children tend not to have such periods. Moreover, it should be possible to identify and fully characterize children who have bipolar symptoms and are severely impaired and to follow them prospectively, with attention to developmental stages and transitions, in order to resolve whether they have a childhood-onset variant of bipolar disorder (see Chapter 6 for a more complete discussion).

Validation studies also need to take developmental manifestations into account. The expert group suggested that studies could encompass children as young as 4 years of age. Reconstruction of the history of adults with early-onset bipolar illness may be useful as well. For example, in studies of the offspring of bipolar parents, which should include all of their children, parents should be asked about their own age at onset. The group deemed it important also that children with possible bipolar disorder, as well as their parents, be interviewed with developmentally appropriate measures.

Information about instruments currently employed in NIMH-funded studies of childhood-onset bipolar disorder was assembled for use at the roundtable. The most commonly used diagnostic instrument is KSADS—in most cases, the Washington University (St. Louis) version (WASH-U-KSADS) or KSADS with the WASH-U-KSADS sections on mood disorders and rapid cycling added. Ancillary instruments being used include the Child Behavior Checklist (CBCL) (Achenbach, 1991a,b).

Efforts that might be undertaken to resolve the diagnostic issues raised above include the following: describing the course of bipolar-I, bipolar-II, cyclothymia, and bipolar-NOS, with attention to the impact of development on changing patterns of symptoms; establishing the predictive validity of bipolar disorder in prepubertal children; defining thresholds for and boundaries between bipolar-I, bipolar-II, and cyclothymia in prepubertal children; and identifying occasions on which combining versus separating bipolar-I and -II would be appropriate (in treatment studies of mania, for example, where severity is an issue, combining manic with hypomanic patients may be inappropriate). Although future epidemiologic studies will need to incorporate the clinical findings of studies conducted to date, the unresolved issues of diagnosis in children described here make the accuracy of estimates of rates of childhood bipolar disorder and determinants of age at onset uncertain. See Chapter 6 for a comprehensive discussion of these issues.

Epidemiologic findings for the elderly are also ambiguous. In geriatric inpatient units, the prevalence of treated bipolar disorder has been described as reaching 10 percent (Yassa et al., 1988). Yet there is a disparity between the prevalence of bipolar disorder among elderly patients in hospitals and elderly individuals living in the community. Moreover, the rates of bipolar disorder are dramatically lower among community-dwelling elderly people than among younger persons (Shulman and Hermann, 1999). One reason for this is the increased early mortality from medical causes, such as cardiovascular disease and suicide among those with the disorder (Snowdon, 1991).

Diagnostic Methods

Over the years, we have seen the development of a number of structured interview instruments that have improved the precision with which psychiatric disorders can be identified and their rates estimated (see Chapters 3 and 11). Yet different diagnostic criteria or revised versions of the same criteria can affect rates and their comparisons. Thus differences among diagnostic instruments used in community studies may explain some of the variation in the rates obtained.

The DIS (Robins et al., 1981a), mentioned earlier, is a highly structured interview designed for large-scale epidemiologic studies. It generates DSM-IV diagnoses in computer algorithm form for the major psychiatric disorders. The CIDI (WHO, 1990; Wittchen et al., 1998a), also noted previously, consists of state-of-the-art structured diagnostic interviews based on the DIS and generates DSM-IV and ICD diagnoses. Trained lay interviewers administer both the DIS and the CIDI. The two instruments differ in that the DIS includes impairment criteria when generating diagnoses, whereas the CIDI does not. Moreover, after an initial round of questions about symptoms, the CIDI returns to reassess those symptoms, while the DIS asks about symptoms only once. A modification of the CIDI made by the University of Michigan Institute for Social Research (UM-CIDI) (Kessler, 1995) simplified that instrument's complex questions. Qualifiers such as "a lot" (as in the question, "Did the symptom interfere with your life and activities a lot?") were clarified (as in the question, "How much did the symptom interfere with your life or activities—a lot, some, a little, not at all?").

Another semistructured interview instrument is the Schedule for Affective Disorders and Schizophrenia (SADS) (Endicott and Spitzer, 1978), which is tied to the Research Diagnostic Criteria (RDC) (Spitzer et al., 1978) and the DSM. This instrument has been used less often than the DIS or the CIDI in community surveys because it must be administered by trained mental health professionals.

The Structured Psychopathological Interview and Rating of the Social Consequences of Psychiatric Disturbances for Epidemiology (SPIKE for the original German) (Angst et al., 1984) is yet another semistructured clinical interview. It allows the assessment of 29 separate syndromes, including hypomania, in terms of symptoms, their length, their frequency of occurrence, subjective suffering, social consequences, treatment, and family history, and generates DSM-III diagnoses.

The Structured Clinical Interview for DSM (SCID) is a semistructured clinical interview used for making a major Axis I DSM-III-R or DSM-IV diagnosis. Through a decision-tree approach, the SCID guides the clinician in testing diagnostic hypotheses as the interview is conducted (see Chapter 11 for a discussion of issues involved in using decision trees). The output of the SCID is a record of the presence or absence of each of the disorders being considered for current episodes (past month) and for lifetime occurrence.

The Diagnostic Interview for Genetic Studies (DIGS) (Nurnberger et al., 1994) yields DSM-IV and RDC diagnoses and requires trained clinical interviewers. Questions on mania/hypomania in the mood disorder module are designed to assess current and most severe disorder, presence of psychotic features, impairment, organic factors, and treatment seeking. Mixed affective states and cycling are also assessed. The DIGS was designed for large-scale genetic studies and has not been used in community-based epidemiologic studies (see Chapter 13).

Finally, with few exceptions (Italy, Israel, Switzerland), the larger epidemiologic community surveys use trained nonclinical interviewers because it is costly and usually infeasible to send doctoral-level clinicians to conduct in-home interviews with thousands of subjects. Results of testing the congruence between findings obtained by nonclinical and clinical interviewers are described later in the presentation of the ECA findings.

Nonresponse or Refusal to Participate in the Survey

Another bias in community surveys that may affect the rates of bipolar disorder obtained is the failure of some subjects to participate, which may occur in the early phase of sample designation and again at measurement and interviewing. Because one cannot assume that nonresponse is randomly distributed across the intended sample, it can be a major source of bias. Nonresponse bias that occurs during the process of selecting and contacting the sample includes sample mortality, sample loss, and missing data (Badawi et al., 1999); also significant is refusal to respond in the middle stages of data collection.

The predictors of nonresponse bias were investigated in a 15-year follow-up of individuals in a probability sample from the household population of the Baltimore, Maryland, ECA. Mania was found to be associated with increased mortality, some of which may be related to the high rates of suicide, alcohol and drug abuse, and cardiovascular disease among this population (Badawi et al., 1999).

In the NCS, a special effort was made to estimate the rate of disorders among people who initially refused to participate in the survey. The results indicated that these individuals had higher rates of mental disorders, including bipolar disorder, than those who agreed to participate. Such data might be used to adjust prevalence estimates.

Other Issues

Sample Size

The relatively short duration of many manic and depressive episodes and the presence of mixed states cause difficulties in assessment. Short episodes are counted in some studies but overlooked in others that use diagnostic instruments with long-duration criteria. Short episodes also are responsible for large differences in rates of point and annual prevalence. Gagrat and Spiro (1980) explained this difficulty and underscored the problems created by studying a phenomenon with a low baseline rate. As they noted, point prevalence studies for a short-duration disorder with a yearly prevalence of 0.7 percent would require the screening of very large numbers of people. Even allowing for a mean duration of manic episodes of 2 months (a mean duration of 2 months assumes that many of the manic episodes in the community are shortened by treatment), the point prevalence rate would be on the order of 0.2 percent if the annual prevalence in the population at large were 1.0 percent. This means it would be necessary to screen 1,000 people to find 2 active cases. Epidemiologic studies of several hundred thousand people at a time would be required to determine the point prevalence in the population at large. Moreover, it is questionable whether current epidemiologic research instruments would be reliable in such studies.

Except for demographic characteristics such as age and gender, the relatively low prevalence of bipolar disorder makes estimates of variations in rates by risk factor difficult even in reasonably sized epidemiologic surveys. For example, in a sample of 5,000, which would be considered a reasonably sized community survey, a lifetime prevalence of 2 percent for a disorder would yield at most 100 cases. Few epidemiologic studies have 5,000 subjects. When the population is segmented by age, gender, and race, moreover, the sample size in each group dwindles rapidly. Finally, as discussed later, time constraints prevent any one study from including all the relevant risk factors, and multiple instruments are required.

Incidence and Prevalence Rates

Population measures of disease frequency include incidence and prevalence rates, the latter divided by different points in time (period prevalence). *Incidence* is defined as the number of new cases of disease in a *population at risk* for that disease per unit time. Incidence rates are used to determine differences in risk factors and are always difficult to obtain because they require a longitudinal study to identify new cases. Determining the incidence of bipolar disorder is yet more difficult because of the problems of determining subtle changes in mood and of knowing when a case of major depression converts to bipolar. The lack of clarity of presentation in children and the need for large samples, as discussed previously, can further compound the problem. Indeed, few of the epidemiologic studies published since the first edition of this text have provided incidence data. The 13-year follow-up of the Baltimore ECA (described later) excluded incidence data for bipolar disorder because of an insufficient sample size (Badawi et al., 1999). Likewise, a 40-year follow-up of the Stirling County study in Nova Scotia assessing the incidence of depression did not include bipolar disorder (Murphy et al., 2000).

Prevalence is defined as the number of existing cases of disease in a *total population* per period of time. Prevalence rates can help identify unmet need. The studies reviewed in this chapter provide data on period prevalence, usually annual and lifetime. The lifetime prevalence is the proportion of the population that has had a disease at some point during a lifetime (Kramer et al., 1980). It is the rate obtained in response to the question, "Have you ever had . . . ?" Lifetime prevalence as a measure has been criticized for numerous reasons, including problems of recall. However, it is still applied widely as one of the imperfect but useful tools available for counting cases.

Functional Impairment

The assessments used in recent epidemiologic studies require some evidence of functional impairment to determine the clinical significance of the case. Questions about impairment of major roles or treatment seeking are designed to elicit this information. Variations in these questions can seriously alter rates among studies, as revealed by the comparison of the rates in the ECA and the NCS, described later.

Age at Onset

Different methods may be used for computing the age at onset of bipolar disorder. One method is to use two measures of central tendency: the mean or average age at onset and the median, or the age that corresponds to the 50th percentile of the distribution. An advantage of using this method is that age at onset can be summarized as one estimate. The disadvantage is that both the mean and the median can be biased by extreme values at either the lower or higher end of the distribution of ages.

Another method for analyzing age at onset is to compute the incidence (or hazard) rate of bipolar disorder for each age of life. This is done by taking the number of new cases that appear at each age and dividing it by the population at risk for that age. The major advantage of this method is that trends in incidence rates can be compared across all ages, although the population at risk becomes smaller as age increases, inflating the incidence rate for older ages.

COMMUNITY SURVEYS AMONG ADULTS

In this section we review the methods and results of two surveys conducted among adults in the United States in the late 1970s, the two major epidemiologic studies conducted during the 1980s and 1990s, and comparable cross-national studies conducted throughout the world since the 1980s. Recent epidemiologic studies conducted among children and adolescents are discussed in the next section. Studies were included if they used standardized diagnostic assessments and defined sampling methods. When raw data were available, we undertook data analysis. In some cases, we used published results, so there is no standard presentation across sites; for example, bipolar-I and -II were sometimes combined in published results, and sometimes only annual, not lifetime, prevalence rates were given. The data presented are primarily annual and lifetime prevalence rates and incidence rates, where available.

New Haven Survey

The first community survey to use standardized diagnostic assessments and criteria was the New Haven survey, which was conducted in 1975 using the SADS-Lifetime (SADS-L) diagnostic instrument, based on the RDC (Weissman and Myers, 1978). This survey, considered a pilot study because it was a follow-up of a cohort identified 10 years earlier, included only 511 adults. A lifetime rate of 0.6 percent for bipolar-I was reported. The addition of bipolar-II raised the rate to 1.2 percent. Bipolar disorder was represented equally in males and females. These findings are comparable to those of subsequent large-scale community surveys.

The Amish Study

The Amish study of Egeland and colleagues (1983) is unusual in its assessment of the prevalence of affective disorders in a population that is culturally and genetically homogeneous. This subculture, a highly conservative Protestant religious sect in Pennsylvania, offered an "unheralded opportunity to study multigenerational pedigrees with large sibships" (Egeland and Hostetter, 1983, p. 70). Variables that confounded past research are not present in this population; for example, alcohol and drug abuse are virtually nonexistent, and criminal acts and violence are rare. Other obstacles had to be overcome, however. In applying specific diagnostic criteria to this group, the RDC definitions for mania and depression needed to be considered within the context of Amish culture. For example, manic behaviors to the Amish include racing one's horse

and carriage too fast, buying or using machinery or worldly items, using the public telephone excessively, and planning vacations during the wrong season (Egeland et al., 1983).

The Old Order Amish, 12,500 people who live primarily in Lancaster County, Pennsylvania, keep extensive genealogical and medical records of ancestors going back 30 generations (Egeland and Hostetter, 1983). The Amish study, which spanned the 5-year period from 1976 to 1980, attempted to identify all individuals who were actively ill, thus yielding incidence and period prevalence rates. As the authors noted, the close interactions among the Amish prevented even mild cases of emotional disturbance from being overlooked. Once an active case had been identified, medical records were abstracted and sent to a psychiatric board, which made a consensus diagnosis based on the RDC. If medical records did not exist, patients were interviewed directly using the SADS-L.

Reliability estimates were made based on the agreement between board consensus and a separate psychiatrist's diagnosis (Hostetter et al., 1983). Kappa statistics for reliability generally were high and consistent for any major affective disorder, for unipolar depression, and for bipolar-I disorder (0.87, 0.95, and 0.86, respectively). Only with bipolar-II disorder was the kappa coefficient much lower (0.68), suggesting a possible misrepresentation of this diagnosis among the Amish and less reliability in the diagnostic category. Indeed, the problem of unreliability in estimates of bipolar-II in community samples was found in subsequent studies described later.

During the survey period, 112 cases of mental illness were reported, 80 percent of which were affective disorders (71 percent major affective disorders), involving 1 percent of the Amish population (Egeland and Hostetter, 1983). A further breakdown of these rates revealed that 34 percent of the psychiatric cases were either bipolar-I or bipolar-II disorder, and 37 percent were unipolar depression. The remaining 9 percent comprised minor depression and hypomania (8 and 1 percent, respectively). As the authors pointed out, both the rate of major affective disorders and the rate of mental illness in general appeared to be below the general population average.

The most interesting finding is the apparent equivalence in rates of bipolar and unipolar illness. Other studies have shown a lopsided ratio. Weissman and Klerman (1978) and many subsequent investigators have found an almost 4:1 unipolar:bipolar diagnosis ratio across the United States, and some studies have shown a 10:1 ratio. In an attempt to explain these discrepant findings, Egeland and Hostetter (1983) noted that their sample of bipolar patients would have been greatly reduced had not community reports of behaviors suggestive of a "high" led to early SADS-L interviewing. In fact, the Amish data may more accurately reflect the actual bipolar:unipolar ratio. Recent clinical research indicates that many cases diagnosed as unipolar illness may be variants of bipolar disorder (see Chapters 1, 2, 13, and 19). Another explanation for the discrepancy is the finding of Egeland and colleagues (1983) that 79 percent of their bipolar-I patients had previously been diagnosed as schizophrenic. Cultural factors may be partly responsible for this incidence of misdiagnosis: earlier clinicians, unfamiliar with the customs of the Amish, may have viewed thought disorder, paranoia, and grandiosity as symptoms of schizophrenia rather than mania (Egeland and Hostetter, 1983; Egeland et al., 1983). Of particular note are grandiose symptoms with marked religious overtones, because religion is central to the Amish. If other manic symptoms are not noted or are overlooked (as is apparent in early medical records), these symptoms may easily be seen as schizophrenic. Likewise, it is probable that Amish individuals who are the most ill stay within the community, whereas the less ill may emigrate.

Among both bipolar and unipolar patients in the Amish study, gender was equally distributed. Although this finding is consistent with others for bipolar illness, the majority of subsequent studies have found a 2:1 female:male ratio for unipolar depression. The most obvious explanation for this discrepancy, according to Egeland and Hostetter (1983), is that alcoholism and sociopathy do not mask depression in Amish males as they do in males in the general population.

Although the findings of this study have been debated, they provide a view of major affective disorders relatively untainted by violence, alcohol and drug abuse, and other variables that might otherwise mask such a disorder's presence.

Epidemiologic Catchment Area Study

The ECA study, conducted during 1980–1984, was the first comprehensive epidemiologic study of mental illness in the United States. It was designed to obtain accurate and uniform epidemiologic data on mental disorders in the United States that would be comparable across sites, as well as to assess the adequacy of services to the mentally ill (Regier et al., 1984). The design required representative sampling of populations from both community and institutional settings at two different time points 1 year apart (waves 1 and 2). In wave 1, prevalence data were gathered for lifetime, annual, 6-month, 1-month, and 2-week periods. Wave 2 was a follow-up to ascertain rates of relapse and remission, as well as to determine incidence rates (Eaton et al., 1989).

More than 18,000 people were interviewed by lay interviewers, who used the DIS, together with criteria from the DSM-III, RDC, and Feighner diagnostic systems. (The latter two sets of diagnostic criteria are now used infrequently.) Subjects were first asked whether they had ever experienced a symptom at any time during their lives and whether they had experienced impairment in life activities from that symptom. For each symptom, the interviewer ascertained whether alcohol, drugs, medication, or physical illness was the underlying cause. Subjects were then asked whether they had experienced the symptom during the last 2 weeks, the last month, the last 6 months, and the last year, and this information was used to generate a diagnosis for period prevalence. The DIS determined the severity of a disorder in addition to its presence and duration.

The DIS appears to have relatively high reliability for diagnosing major depression but considerably less reliability for manic episodes. In comparing the agreement between the DIS administered to the same subjects by a lay interviewer and a physician, the kappa statistic for major depression was found to be 0.50 and for mania 0.21 (Helzer et al., 1985). Some questions remain about the continued use of the DIS and interpretation of the data it yields (see, e.g., Anthony et al., 1985). The accuracy of lifetime recall has been questioned, as has the lack of comparability of diagnoses made by lay interviewers and by experienced clinicians, whose pattern recognition and access to family history are likely to produce a more accurate diagnosis. Robbins and colleagues (1982) compared 1-month prevalence rates of depression and mania at two ECA sites (St. Louis and Baltimore) based on diagnoses by lay interviewers and psychiatrists using the DIS. Although the rates were not significantly different in Baltimore, both disorders were diagnosed three times more often by psychiatrists than by lay interviewers in St. Louis. A recent study of 41,838 individuals in the Swedish Twin Registry underscores the considerable problem in interpreting findings obtained by lay interviewers (Soldani et al., 2005). Telephone screening for mania, when compared with actual hospitalization and other medical records, resulted in spuriously high false-positive rates for mania in particular and for bipolar disorder in general. The investigators concluded that instead of the reported rate of 1.6 percent, a more accurate estimate would be 0.9 percent. These discrepancies suggest that some caution should be applied in interpreting ECA data, although the study is methodologically superior overall to past attempts at estimating the prevalence and incidence of bipolar illness.

The lifetime and annual prevalence and annual incidence for bipolar-I disorder for the total noninstitutionalized ECA sample and each of the five sites are presented in Table 5–2. The total sample size was 18,571 respondents aged 18 and older, 59 percent of whom were female. The overall response rate was 76 percent. The lifetime

TABLE 5–2. Lifetime and Annual Prevalence/100 (Standard Error) and Incidence Rate/100 of Bipolar-I Disorder in Five Epidemiologic Catchment Area Sites

Parameter	New Haven, CT	Baltimore, MD	St. Louis, MO	Durham, NC	Los Angeles, CA
Number in sample	5,034	3,481	3,004	3,921	3,131
Response rate (%)	77	78	79	79	68
% Female	59	62	60	60	53
Lifetime prevalence/100					
Total	1.2 (0.21)	0.6 (0.20)	1.0 (0.20)	0.3 (0.14)	0.6 (0.16)
Males	1.0 (0.27)	0.7 (0.22)	1.1 (0.30)	0.1 (0.11)	0.6 (0.23)
Females	1.3 (0.30)	0.5 (0.24)	1.0 (0.27)	0.6 (0.25)	0.5 (0.21)
M/F Ratio	0.8	1.4	1.1	0.2	1.2
Annual prevalence/100					
Total	1.0 (0.16)	0.5 (0.14)	1.0 (0.20)	0.2 (0.08)	0.4 (0.13)
Males	0.9 (0.22)	0.5 (0.21)	1.0 (0.30)	0.0	0.3 (0.15)
Females	1.1 (0.23)	0.5 (0.18)	1.0 (0.27)	0.4 (0.16)	0.5 (0.20)
M/F Ratio	0.8	1.0	1.0	0.0	0.1
Annual Incidence/100					
Total	0.6 (0.12)	0.2 (0.09)	0.1 (0.07)	0.3 (0.10)	0.5 (0.15)
Males	0.4 (0.15)	0.0	0.0	0.1 (0.09)	0.5 (0.21)
Females	0.7 (0.19)	0.4 (1.6)	0.2 (0.13)	0.5 (0.18)	0.5 (0.20)

Note: Encompasses ages 18 years and older.

prevalence of bipolar-I disorder was 0.8/100, ranging from 0.3/100 at Durham to 1.2/100 at New Haven. In general, the lifetime prevalence was the same for males and females, with slightly higher rates for males at Baltimore (M/F ratio = 1.4) and higher rates for females at Durham (M/F ratio = 0.2). The overall annual prevalence was 0.6/100, and the incidence was 0.4 per 100 cases per year. There was a tendency for females to have a higher incidence rate of bipolar-I than males, but this varied by site. The mean age at onset of bipolar-I disorder ranged from 14.6 years at St. Louis to 22.3 years at Baltimore (overall at the five sites, 18.6 years; overall median age, 18 years). (See the later discussion of the Cross-National

Collaborative Group for results and a discussion of rates for bipolar-II.)

The ECA also examined the use of mental health services by patients with bipolar disorder (Narrow et al., 1993; Regier et al., 1993). Overall, 61 percent of all individuals with bipolar disorder had been treated in the service sector within the past year—46 percent by specialty mental health providers and 29 percent by general medical providers. This was the highest rate of use of mental health services in the affective disorder group. It translates, on a population level, to approximately 1.1 million people with bipolar disorder making 16 million visits to outpatient mental health care facilities in the year before their wave 1 interview (Narrow et al., 1993).

One-third (33.4 percent) of bipolar patients receiving inpatient care did so at a general hospital facility, 19.5 percent at a private mental hospital, and 34.4 percent at a Veterans Affairs (VA) psychiatric hospital unit. The rest were treated at state and county facilities, community mental health centers, alcohol/drug units, or nursing home facilities.

National Comorbidity Survey

The NCS, administered by the staff of the Survey Research Center at the University of Michigan in Ann Arbor, was conducted between 1990 and 1992, or 10 years after the ECA. It was based on a probability sample of 8,098 individuals aged 15 to 54 from the noninstitutionalized populations of the 48 conterminous states; the response rate was 84 percent. Subjects were interviewed using the UM-CIDI, which made DSM-III-R diagnoses (Kessler et al., 1994). Unlike the ECA, which was based on five geographic sites, the NCS included a representative national sample from across the United States. Diagnoses known to have a low prevalence in population-based surveys (e.g., somatization disorder) or poor interrater reliability in the ECA (e.g., obsessive-compulsive disorder) were excluded. Respondents as young as age 15 were included because there was an interest in the comorbidity of substance abuse and other psychiatric disorders, and because the ECA had shown that the rates of psychiatric disorders were higher in younger than in older persons. Ten years after the NCS was completed, Kessler and colleagues (2005) conducted a replication (the NCS-R) of their initial study. Face-to-face diagnostic interviews were carried out on 9,282 English-speaking subjects by professional interviewers from the Institute for Social Research at the University of Michigan. DSM-IV diagnoses were generated based on the World Mental Health Survey initiative version of the CIDI (WMH-CIDI).

Table 5–3 shows the rates obtained for bipolar-I disorder in the NCS and NCS-R. Data on rates for bipolar-II were not reported in the NCS because of the unreliability of diagnosis of this disorder (see the later discussion); these rates were, however, ascertained in the replication study. The NCS and NCS-R rates shown in the table were adjusted for nonresponse and weighted to the sociodemographic characteristics of the target population from the 1989 U.S. National Interview Survey (US DHHS, 1992) and from the 2000 U.S. Census, respectively. In the NCS, the lifetime prevalence of bipolar-I disorder was 1.7 percent, with equal rates in males and females. The annual prevalence was 1.3 percent, also with equal rates by gender. The rates of bipolar-I were about twice as high in the NCS as in the ECA. The mean age at onset for bipolar-I disorder was 23.3 years (median 21 years). This onset age is about 3 years later than that found in the ECA.

The lifetime prevalence of bipolar-I disorder in the NCS-R was slightly lower, 1.0, than that reported in the NCS. The NCS-R found a lifetime prevalence of 1.1 in females and 0.8 in males. The annual prevalence for the total sample was 0.6. The mean age at onset for bipolar-I was 21.4 (median 19 years). For bipolar-II in the NCS-R, the lifetime prevalence was 1.1 (males, 0.9; females, 1.3); the annual prevalence was 0.8 (males, 0.7; females, 0.9); and the mean age at onset was 25.2 years (median 20 years).

There has been some debate about the reasons for the discrepancies in findings between the ECA and the NCS, and several attempts have been made to understand how differences between the two instruments (Table 5–4) might explain these discrepancies (Kessler et al., 1997; Regier et al., 1998; Narrow et al., 2002). The most obvious difference is the sampling frame. The ECA encompassed five selected sites, compared with a probability sample of all 48 conterminous states in the NCS. The ECA included persons living in institutions (prisons, boarding houses, nursing homes, and hospitals), while the NCS did not. The age structure of the two samples was also different, as mentioned earlier. Even when comparable age groups (18 to 54 years) are considered, however, the lifetime rate of bipolar disorder in the NCS remains at 1.7.

The controversy over which results are closer to the actual prevalence has not been resolved. However, there is agreement that any differences in rates are not true differences, but likely due to differences in sampling and methods between the studies (see note 2 for details). Moreover, although the rates of bipolar disorder are disparate between the ECA and NCS, the actual range of rates is not that large, and the demographic risk factors (discussed later) do not vary greatly between the two studies.

Table 5–5 compares the rates of bipolar-I disorder by demographic characteristics using an identical age group (18 to 54 years) to see whether the patterns of variation are similar. There are no significant differences in the rates of bipolar-I disorder by gender, educational level, or rural/urban domicile in either the ECA or the NCS. There is no difference in the rates by family income in the ECA. In the NCS, however, there is an inverse relationship between the rates of bipolar disorder and family income: the lower the income, the higher the rates ($p = .04$). Persons who are separated or divorced have higher rates in both the ECA ($p = .02$) and the NCS ($p = .002$). The age at onset is 5 years younger in the ECA compared with the NCS ($p = .001$).

Cross-National Collaborative Group

The success of the ECA in the United States led to the conduct of similar studies using the DIS in various parts of the world. Data from some countries began to appear in the late 1980s. However, it was difficult to make cross-national

TABLE 5–3. Lifetime and Annual Prevalence of Bipolar-I Disorder
in the U.S. National Comorbidity Survey (NCS)
and in the U.S. National Comorbidity
Survey Replication (NCS-R)

Parameter	NCS (1994)	NCS-R (2005)
Number in sample	8,098	9,282
Response rate (%)	84	71
Interview measure	UM-CIDI	CIDI
Diagnostic outcome	DSM-III-R	DSM-IV
Interviewers	Lay	Lay
% Female	52	52
Lifetime prevalence/100 (Standard Error)		
Total	1.7 (0.20)	1.0 (0.1)
Males	1.6 (0.28)	0.8 (0.1)
Females	1.7 (0.28)	1.1 (0.2)
Annual prevalence/100 (Standard Error)		
Total	1.3 (0.18)	0.6 (0.1)
Males	1.4 (0.25)	0.6 (0.1)
Females	1.3 (0.24)	0.7 (0.1)
Age at Onset (years)		
Mean	23.3 (0.9)	21.4 (1.2)
Median	21.0	19.0

CIDI = Composite International Diagnostic Interview; DSM = *Diagnostic and Statistical Manual*; UM-CIDI = University of Michigan Institute for Social Research's modification of the CIDI.
Sources: Kessler et al., 1994; National Comorbidity Study Replication (2005).

comparisons, even with studies using the same diagnostic assessment methods, because of variability in the data presentation. As noted earlier, the Cross-National Collaborative Group was formed in the 1990s to directly compare rates and risks for psychiatric disorders and to help overcome this problem of disparate presentation of data by standardizing analysis across sites. The hope was that real differences in rates by country, not due to differing analytic methods, might thereby emerge. Ten countries, including the United States, that had used Version III of the DIS and DSM-III formed the collaboration. Only 7 of these 10 provided data

on bipolar disorder; nonetheless, these 7 countries represent diverse geographic, political, and cultural areas in North America, the Caribbean, Europe, Asia, and the Pacific Rim. The investigators in each country translated the DIS; details on the translation and the methodology employed are included in the references for each study. In addition to the ECA, data were obtained from the following sources:

• The Edmonton Survey of Psychiatric Disorders (Orn et al., 1988) was conducted in the city of Edmonton, Alberta, Canada.

TABLE 5–4. Comparison of the Epidemiologic Catchment Area Study (ECA) and the National Comorbidity Survey (NCS)

Parameter	ECA	NCS
Date conducted	1980–1984	1990–1992
Sample size	18,571	8,089
Site	5 U.S. sites	48 U.S. states
Age range (years)	18–65	15–54
Instrument	DIS	CIDI
Diagnosis	DSM-III	DSM-III-R
Interviewers	Lay	Lay

CIDI = Composite International Diagnostic Interview; DIS = Diagnostic Interview Schedule; DSM = *Diagnostic and Statistical Manual.*

- The Puerto Rico Study of Psychiatric Disorders (Canino et al., 1987) included persons living in households throughout Puerto Rico, in addition to household members temporarily away and those in institutions.
- The Munich Follow-up Study (Wittchen et al., 1992) was a 7-year follow-up investigation of a stratified random general population sample drawn from the former West Germany.
- The Taiwan Psychiatric Epidemiology Project (Hwu et al., 1989) sampled three population areas representing metropolitan Taipei and township and rural areas.
- The Korean Epidemiologic Study of Mental Disorders (Lee et al., 1990a,b) sampled persons in urban Seoul and in scattered rural regions across South Korea.
- The Christchurch Psychiatric Epidemiology Study (Wells et al., 1989) included adults living in Christchurch on the South Island of New Zealand.

Table 5–6 shows the target population and sample size, response rate, and gender and age distributions for each study that collected data on bipolar disorder. Statistical analyses of these data standardized the rates at each site to the age and gender distribution of the ECA. Because of different age distributions at each site, analysis was restricted to the 18- to 64-year age group (26 to 64 years in West Germany). The standardization was performed according to methods described by Breslow and Day (1987). Weighted prevalence rates yielded estimates that would be derived if each site had the same age and gender distribution as the ECA. The ECA, Edmonton, Puerto Rico, Munich, Taiwan,

Korea, and Christchurch surveys collected data on both bipolar-I and bipolar-II disorder, which are the basis for the rates presented here; the NCS data are shown for comparison purposes. Note that both the ECA and NCS rates presented in the following tables may vary slightly from the rates presented earlier in Tables 5–2 and 5–3 because of the differing age ranges included.

The lifetime prevalence for bipolar-I range from 0.3 percent in Taiwan to 1.7 percent in the United States (NCS) (Weissman et al., 1996) (Table 5–7). The rates are moderately consistent cross-nationally. The male/female ratio is almost equal for the United States and Taiwan. Men have slightly higher rates than women in the Edmonton, Puerto Rico, and New Zealand surveys, and much higher rates in the Korea survey. Mean age at onset is on average 6 years younger for bipolar-I than for major depression, ranging from 17 in Edmonton to 27 in Puerto Rico (median 18 to 25). The West German rates are not stable because of the small sample size. The data on mean age at onset for bipolar-I may represent underestimates, because some of those surveyed had not yet passed through the age of risk, and no one older than age 64 was included.

The lifetime rates for bipolar-II are lower than those for bipolar-I, a result that probably reflects the difficulty of distinguishing mild highs from normal mood fluctuations in a community sample, as discussed previously. The rates are relatively consistent across sites (range 0.1 to 0.9 percent). There is no consistent gender ratio, although the rate of bipolar-II disorder is more often higher among females than males, a result suggested by clinical studies (Leibenluft, 1996). These rates, too, are probably underestimates. The lower rates of bipolar-II compared with bipolar-I reflect the uncertainty associated with diagnosis of bipolar-II in a nonpatient sample—a conclusion discussed previously and also reached by Kessler and colleagues (1997) in their validity study of the NCS.

Table 5–8 shows the very high rates of suicide attempts among persons with versus those without bipolar-I disorder in the United States and five other countries in the 1980s and 1990s (see Chapters 8 and 25). These figures were adjusted for age and gender at each site. Regardless of the variation in rates of bipolar disorder across countries, the association with suicide attempts is consistent and strong: the difference in prevalence of suicide attempts among those with and without bipolar disorder (odds ratio) ranges from 5.5 to 25.7/100.

Table 5–9 shows the significant association between panic disorder and bipolar disorder (see Chapter 7). Although the actual numbers of persons with this comorbidity were quite small in Puerto Rico, Taiwan, Korea, and Christchurch, the association is statistically significant across all sites. The association between the two disorders

TABLE 5–5. Lifetime Prevalence/100 (Standard Error) of Bipolar-I Disorder by Demographic Characteristics in the United States

Characteristic	ECA (1980)	NCS (1990)
Gender		
Male	1.0 (0.16)	1.6 (0.29)
Female	1.1 (0.17)	1.8 (0.30)
p Value	.43	.77
Mean age at onset, years	18.7 (6.1)	24.0 (7.5)
Median	18	22
Educational level		
Less than high school	1.3 (0.25)	2.2 (0.61)
High school graduate	1.1 (0.21)	2.0 (0.36)
College or higher	0.9 (0.16)	1.2 (0.27)
p Value	.33	.12
Total Family Income		
$0–$19,999	1.2 (0.22)	2.7 (0.53)
$20,000–$34,999	0.7 (0.21)	1.4 (0.38)
$35,000–$69,999	1.2 (0.33)	1.6 (0.34)
$70,000+	N/A	0.8 (0.39)
p Value	.34	.04
Marital status		
Married	0.8 (0.13)	1.3 (0.22)
Separated/divorced	1.6 (0.40)	3.8 (0.93)
Never married	1.3 (0.23)	1.8 (0.48)
p Value	.02	.002
Domicile		
Rural	0.9 (0.26)	1.3 (0.39)
Urban	1.1 (0.13)	1.8 (0.24)
p Value	.63	.31

Note: Encompasses ages 18–54 years.
ECA = Epidemiologic Catchment Area study; NCS = National Comorbidity Study.

TABLE 5–6. Target Population, Sample Size, Response Rate, and Gender and Age Distributions for the Cross-National Sites

Characteristic	ECA[a]	NCS[b]	Alberta, Edmonton	Puerto Rico	West Germany	Taiwan	Korea	New Zealand
Size of target population	1,198,000[c]	247,005,000[d]	397,965[e]	1,792,127[c]	29,240,900[f]	1,681,118[c]	13,520,908[c]	181,000[g]
Total number in study, age 18+ years	18,571	8,098	3,258	1,513	481	11,004	5,100	1,498
Response rate (%)	76	84	72	91	76	90	83	70
% Female	59	52	59	57	52	48	52	66
% Age at Interview (years)								
18–25	14	19	22	22	N/A	25	20	20
26–45	33	59	46	50	55	43	49	55
46–64	21	16	21	28	45	24	30	24
65+	31	N/A	11	N/A	N/A	7	0.5	N/A

Note: Figures shown are in raw percentages; percentages may not add to exactly 100 at certain sites because of missing values
N/A = not assessed.
[a]U.S. Epidemiologic Catchment Area Study, 1980.
[b]U.S. National Comorbidity Survey, 1990.
[c]Population figures according to 1980 census.
[d]Population figures drawn from 1990 U.S. Census of 48 conterminous states.
[e]Population figures according to 1981 census.
[f]Population figures according to 1974 census of West Germany, former Federal Republic of Germany.
[g]Population figures according to 1986 census.

TABLE 5–7. Lifetime Prevalence/100 (Standard Error) of Bipolar-I Disorder in Samples of the Cross-National Collaborative Group Study

Survey Site	Overall	Males	Females	M/F Ratio	Age at Onset (years)	Median Age at Onset (years)
United States						
ECA, 1980	0.9 (0.10)	0.8 (0.14)	1.0 (0.15)	0.7	18.1 (0.68)	18
NCS, 1990[a]	1.7 (0.21)	1.6 (0.29)	1.8 (0.30)	0.9	24.0 (0.92)	23
Edmonton	0.6 (0.16)	0.7 (0.25)	0.5 (0.21)	1.4	17.1 (1.12)	22
Puerto Rico	0.6 (0.23)	0.8 (0.38)	0.5 (0.27)	1.6	27.2 (3.40)	18
Munich[b]	0.5 (0.37)	N/A	1.0 (0.71)	N/A	29.0	25
Taiwan	0.3 (0.06)	0.3 (0.09)	0.3 (0.07)	1.0	22.5 (1.90)	22
Korea	0.4 (0.09)	0.6 (0.16)	0.2 (0.09)	3.0	23.0 (2.54)	18
Christchurch	1.5 (0.36)	1.7 (0.56)	1.2 (0.45)	1.4	18.2 (5.90)	N/A

Note: Encompasses ages 18–64 years unless otherwise noted.
N/A = not assessed.
[a]Ages 18–54 years.
[b]Ages 26–64 years. Only one case of bipolar disorder was reported.

TABLE 5–8. Lifetime Prevalence/100 (Standard Error)[a] of Suicide Attempts in Persons with and without Bipolar-I Disorder

Survey Site	Persons with Bipolar Disorder	Persons without Bipolar Disorder	Odds Ratio (95% CI)[b]	p Value
United States				
ECA, 1980	23.9 (4.70)	2.9 (0.18)	9.6 (5.6–16.6)	.0001
NCS, 1990[c,d]	40.5 (6.08)	4.2 (0.33)	15.8 (9.3–26.9)	.0001
Edmonton	44.5 (12.72)	3.6 (0.38)	25.7 (8.6–76.6)	.0001
Puerto Rico	24.5 (25.50)[e]	5.8 (0.67)	5.6 (1.0–29.8)	.04
Taiwan	11.8 (5.84)[e]	0.7 (0.08)	18.1 (5.8–57.0)	.0001
Korea	15.1 (8.40)[e]	3.1 (0.25)	5.5 (1.5–20.2)	.01
Christchurch	32.7 (11.69)	4.0 (0.59)	13.1 (4.2–41.1)	.0001

Note: Encompasses ages 18–64 years unless otherwise noted.
CI = confidence interval.
[a]Standardized to U.S. 1980 Census.
[b]Odds ratio adjusted by age and gender at each site.
[c]Ages 18–54 years.
[d]Weighted to 1989 National Health Interview Survey.
[e]Indicates cells with a frequency of 5 or less.

TABLE 5–9. Lifetime Prevalence/100 (Standard Error)[a] of Panic Disorder in Persons with and without Bipolar-I Disorder

Survey Site	Persons with Bipolar Disorder	Persons without Bipolar Disorder	Odds Ratio (95% CI)[b]	p Value
United States				
ECA, 1980	16.2 (4.09)	1.5 (0.13)	12.8 (6.8–24.1)	.0001
NCS, 1990[c,d]	27.0 (5.49)	3.1 (0.28)	12.5 (6.9–22.6)	.0001
Edmonton	16.7 (9.55)	1.3 (0.68)	16.5 (4.0–67.6)	.0001
Puerto Rico	49.6 (18.00)[e]	1.3 (0.33)	79.2 (17.3–323)	.0001
Taiwan	14.5 (6.36)[e]	0.3 (0.06)	53.5 (17.9–160)	.0001
Korea	9.0 (6.70)[e]	1.7 (0.19)	14.1 (2.6–77.3)	.002
Christchurch	20.6 (10.09)[e]	1.8 (0.40)	17.2 (4.3–69.1)	.0001

Note: Encompasses ages 18–64 years unless otherwise noted.
CI = confidence interval.
[a]Standardized to U.S. 1980 Census.
[b]Odds ratio adjusted by age and gender at each site.
[c]Ages 18–54 years.
[d]Weighted to 1989 National Health Interview Survey.
[e]Indicates cells with a frequency of 5 or less.

has also been noted in genetic studies showing an increased familial aggregation of panic disorder in probands with bipolar disorder (MacKinnon et al., 1998). The meaning of these results and whether they represent a specific genetic subtype are unclear (see Chapter 13).

Table 5–10 shows the significant association between substance abuse or dependence and bipolar disorder in all countries except Puerto Rico and New Zealand. These results suggest that cultural differences in substance abuse may explain some of the association (see Chapter 7).

Other International Studies

The data reported in the preceding section are from seven countries that used the DIS in their surveys and provided raw data for analyses. The NCS used the CIDI, not the DIS, but the raw data were available so that direct comparisons, with standardization for age and gender, could be made, thus reducing methodological differences as a source of variance in rates. Other well-designed epidemiologic studies have been conducted cross-nationally and published in the last decade; these studies have limitations for present purposes, however, in that they group all affective disorders together and do not present rates for bipolar disorder separately. Results of studies that do report on bipolar-I or bipolar-II disorder are presented sepa-

rately from the results of the Cross-National Collaborative Group study in Table 5–11, even if the former studies used the same diagnostic measures, as they employed somewhat different methods for either data collection or analysis that could explain differences in the results. Because the raw data were not available, standardization for age and gender differences could not be performed. Therefore, only published rates are presented. A uniform presentation across sites as shown in Tables 5–7 through 5–10 is not possible.

Iceland

The Icelandic study was drawn from a case register and represented a birth cohort born in 1931 and residing in Iceland on December 1, 1986; 2,396 persons met these criteria. Among 1,195 persons randomly selected, 862 interviews (79 percent) were completed. DSM-III diagnoses were derived from DIS interviews administered by trained lay interviewers. The lifetime prevalence rates for bipolar-I (0.2 percent) and bipolar-II (0.5 percent) were low, with equal gender ratios (Stefansson et al., 1991). The sample of bipolar subjects was too small to permit interpretation of associations with marital status. The lower rates obtained in this study could be explained by the age of the cohort (about 56) at the time of the interview.

TABLE 5–10. Lifetime Prevalence/100 (Standard Error)[a] of Any Substance Abuse or Dependence (Alcohol or Drug) in Persons with and without Bipolar-I Disorder

Survey Site	Persons with Bipolar Disorder	Persons without Bipolar Disorder	Odds Ratio (95% CI)[b]	p Value
United States				
ECA, 1980	57.2 (5.51)	17.5 (0.41)	7.6 (4.7–12.1)	.0001
NCS, 1990[c,d]	58.2 (6.11)	23.4 (0.69)	5.0 (3.0–8.4)	.0001
Edmonton	60.0 (12.53)	20.1 (0.82)	6.4 (2.1–19.5)	.001
Puerto Rico	0.0	12.8 (1.00)	—	—
Taiwan	19.3 (7.13)	6.7 (0.25)	3.3 (1.2–9.0)	.02
Korea	54.8 (11.68)	22.8 (0.61)	4.6 (1.3–12.5)	.02
Christchurch	23.7 (10.60)	20.9 (1.23)	0.8 (0.9–2.8)	.77

Note: Encompasses ages 18–64 years unless otherwise noted.
CI = confidence interval.
[a]Standardized to U.S. 1980 Census.
[b]Odds ratio adjusted by age and gender at each site.
[c]Ages 18–54 years.
[d]Weighted to 1989 National Health Interview Survey.

Shantin (Hong Kong)

A large-scale community survey was conducted in Shantin using the DIS and DSM-III (Chen et al., 1993). A two-phase design yielded 7,229 respondents. A flagged sample was given the Self-Reporting Questionnaire (SRQ) as a screen and the full DIS. The DIS was administered only to respondents among an unflagged sample who were positive on one of the screens of the SRQ. With this design, the lifetime prevalence of bipolar disorder was very low, and similar for males (0.15 percent) and females (0.16 percent). These rates are slightly lower than those reported for the two Asian countries (Taiwan and Korea) in the Cross-National Collaborative Group study (see Table 5–7). Chen and colleagues (1993) suggested that the difference could be due to the location of their study; because Shantin was a new town attracting healthy workers, people with serious mental illnesses would not have relocated there.

Hungary

A national community study was conducted in Hungary to estimate the prevalence of affective disorders in the adult population aged 18 to 64, sampled from the registries of 15 general practitioners in five different geographic areas

(Szadoczky et al., 1998). In this study, 2,953 respondents were interviewed using the DIS. The lifetime prevalence for bipolar-I was 1.5/100, similar to the U.S. rate; for bipolar-II, the lifetime rate was 2.0/100. There were few differences in the rates by gender. The first symptoms were reported slightly earlier for females (at 17.9 years) than for males (at 22 years), and the highest risk for first onset of bipolar-I was at ages 15 to 19. Persons with bipolar disorder had a higher level of education, a higher rate of unemployment in males, and a higher rate of marital disruption or never being married compared with those without the disorder.

Florence, Italy

This study included a community sample of 1,000 people in Florence, Italy, drawn from the registries of general physicians (Faravelli et al., 1990). In contrast to the majority of the other epidemiological surveys, the interviews were carried out by qualified psychiatrists or third-year trainees. The annual prevalence for bipolar-I was 1.9/100 for females and 0.6/100 for males, for an overall prevalence of 1.3/100. These rates are again in the same range as the U.S. rates, except for higher rates in females. For bipolar-II disorder, the overall prevalence was 0.2/100. The high annual rates of bipolar disorder are similar to lifetime rates

TABLE 5–11. Prevalence/100 of Bipolar Disorder from Other Cross-National Community Surveys

Study	Country/Year	Sample Size	Age Range (Years)	Diagnostic Method	Diagnosis	Time Period	Prevalence/100
Angst et al., 1984	Zurich, Switzerland, 1978–1982	4,547	19–20	SPIKE	BP-I	Annual	0.7
Faravelli et al., 1990	Florence, Italy, 1987	1,000	15–89	DIS	BP-I	Annual	1.3
					BP-II	Annual	0.2
Stefansson et al., 1991	Iceland, 1987	862	Cohort born in 1931	DIS	BP-I	Lifetime	0.2
					BP-II	Lifetime	0.5
Chen et al., 1993	Shantin, Hong Kong, 1984–1986	7,229	18–64	DIS	BP I or II	Lifetime	Males, 0.15; females, 0.16
Levav et al., 1993	Israel, 1987	2,741	24–33	SADS	BP-I	6 months	0.7
					BP-II		0.9
Brewin et al., 1997	Nottingham, England, 1992–1994	397,048[a]	16–64	SCAN, SANS	BP	2-year incidence	0.005
Szadoczky et al., 1998	Hungary, 1998	2,953	18–64	DIS	BP-I	Lifetime	1.5
					BP-II	Lifetime	2.0
Scully et al., 2000	Ireland, 1995–2000	29,542	Not stated	SCID-III-R	BP	Annual incidence	0.0022: males, 0.00037; females, 0.00060
Kringlen et al., 2001	Oslo, Norway, 1994–1997	2,066	18–65	CIDI	BP	Lifetime	1.6
						Annual	0.9
Andrade et al., 2002	São Paulo, Brazil, 1994–1996	1,464	18+	CIDI	BP	Lifetime	1.0
						Annual	0.5
Regeer et al., 2002	Netherlands, 1996–1999	7,067	18–64	CIDI	BP-I	Annual incidence	0.3
					BP-NOS	Lifetime	2.0
Mitchell et al., 2004	Australia	10,641	18+	CIDI	BP[b]	Annual	0.5
Negash et al., 2005	Butajira, Ethiopia	68,378	15–49	CIDI	BP-I	Lifetime	0.5: males, 0.6; females, 0.3
Vicente et al., 2006	Chile	2,978	15+	CIDI	BP-I	Lifetime	1.9: males, 1.5; females, 2.2

BP = bipolar; BP-NOS = bipolar disorder–not otherwise specified; CIDI = Composite International Diagnostic Interview; DIS = Diagnostic Interview Schedule; SANS = Schedule for Assessment of Negative Symptoms; SCAN = Schedules for Clinical Assessment in Neuropsychiatry; SCID = Structured Clinical Interview for DSM; SPIKE = Structured Psychopathological Interview and Rating of the Social Consequences of Psychiatric Disturbances for Epidemiology.

[a] Population at risk from 1991 Nottingham population census.

[b] Euphoric type.

reported in other studies, a result that may be attributable to having the interviews conducted by psychiatrists, who were better able to probe for symptoms of mania. Also, this study assessed only mood disorders; therefore, the results may include other disorders with mood disturbance. The low rate of bipolar-II disorder found in this study again suggests the difficulty of discriminating between mild mood disorders and normal mood in a community survey. This was also the only epidemiologic study to report rates of recurrent depression (annual prevalence 2.6 percent).

Israel

In an epidemiologic study of mental disorders among young adults in Israel, a 10-year birth cohort (1949–1958) was interviewed by psychiatrists using the Israeli version of SADS, based on RDC criteria. A two-stage screening process was used. Subjects scoring positive on the screen (about a fifth of the sample) received the full diagnostic interview by a psychiatrist. The screened positive sample included 2,741 Israeli-born offspring of Jewish immigrants. The 6-month prevalence was 0.7 percent for bipolar-I disorder and 0.9 percent for bipolar-II disorder. Annual or lifetime prevalence rates were not reported. The rates did not vary significantly by gender. The 6-month prevalence of *definite* bipolar-I disorder was higher among Israelis of European ethnicity (0.61) compared with Israelis of North African ethnicity (0.15, $p < .05$) (Levav et al., 1993). There were no significant differences by education.

Zurich, Switzerland

Subjects for the Zurich Cohort Study were drawn from the total population of the canton of Zurich. The sample was the result of a two-stage design that selected subjects at high risk for psychiatric disorders and applied random controls for 4,547 subjects at the ages of about 19 (males) and 20 (females). Reassessments were conducted when the subjects were about 22, 27, 29, and 34 years of age. Screening took place in 1978, the first and second interviews were conducted in 1979 and 1981, and the last (fifth) interview was conducted in 1993. Each interview covered the previous 12 months. Symptomatology was assessed using SPIKE (Angst et al., 1984), administered by trained clinical psychologists in the subjects' homes. SPIKE is a semistructured clinical interview, which, as noted earlier, allows the assessment of 29 separate syndromes, including hypomania, in terms of symptoms, their length, their frequency of occurrence, subjective suffering, social consequence, treatment, and family history.

The 1-year prevalence of bipolar-I disorder was 0.7 percent (Angst et al., 1984). The study identified brief hypomania (recurrent and sporadic), a condition characterized by short episodes of 1 to 3 days' duration and high recurrence, as a new diagnostic group with a 1-year prevalence rate (cumulative) of 2.8 percent (see later discussion).

The lifetime prevalence of bipolar spectrum disorder, which included a full range of manic symptoms (see the later discussion of bipolar spectrum) was 5.5 percent (Angst, 1995). Overall, the study demonstrated the high prevalence rates of DSM-IV hypomania and brief hypomania among the general population and the clinical and social relevance of these diagnoses. Because this was a prospective study with five waves of interviews focusing on rates from the previous year, it may have been more successful than other studies at identifying fluctuating hypomanic episodes. There have been no other epidemiologic studies of comparable design.

Ireland

A prospective study in rural Ireland of 29,542 subjects from 39 electoral districts was initiated in 1995–2000 to assess all *first episodes* of bipolar disorder. The SCID-III-R (Spitzer et al., 1992) and DSM-III-R were used. As of 2002, the annual incidence of bipolar-I for women was 0.0006 and for men was 0.00037; the overall incidence was 0.0022.[5]

Nottingham, England

This study estimated the incidence rate of ICD manic psychosis in first referrals to general adult psychiatric clinics over the 2-year period 1992–1994. It differs from the others reviewed here in that it was not community based. Therefore, patients who did not present for treatment—most likely milder cases—were not included (Brewin et al., 1997). New patients were evaluated with the Schedule for Clinical Assessment in Neuropsychiatry (SCAN) (WHO, 1994) and the Schedule for Assessment of Negative Symptoms (SANS) (Andreasen, 1982). Using the 1991 Nottingham population census as the population at risk (denominator) and new referrals meeting the ICD criteria for manic psychosis as the case (numerator), the incidence rate was 0.005, with a slightly higher rate among females (Brewin et al., 1997).

Norway

A sample of 2,066 subjects aged 18 to 65, randomly selected from the Norwegian National Population Registry, was interviewed with the CIDI between 1994 and 1997 (Kringlen et al., 2001). The overall annual prevalence of bipolar disorder was 0.9 percent (0.8 percent for males and 1.0 percent for females). The overall lifetime prevalence for bipolar disorder was 1.6 percent, with little difference by gender (1.7 percent for males and 1.4 percent for females). These rates are close to those found in the NCS, which also used the CIDI.

The Netherlands

A prospective survey of 7,067 subjects aged 18 to 64 years from the Dutch general population was conducted at three points in time between 1996 and 1999, using the CIDI (de Graaf et al., 2002; Regeer et al., 2002). Summing of the responses at the three points yielded a lifetime prevalence for bipolar-I or bipolar-NOS of 2.4 percent. A clinical reappraisal, blind to the original diagnosis, was conducted by trained clinicians using the SCID. The results led to a reduction of the rate to 2.0 percent. The annual incidence was 0.3 and was higher in females than in males, but these rates are based on small numbers (Bijl et al., 2002).

São Paulo, Brazil

A community survey of a sample of 1,464 adults living in one catchment area of a large hospital complex in São Paulo was conducted using the CIDI (Andrade et al., 2002). The lifetime and annual rates of bipolar disorder were 1.0 and 0.5, respectively. The rates among men and women were similar. Data on the association with other demographic characteristics were not presented for bipolar disorder separately from other mood disorders.

Chile

The CIDI was administered to a stratified random sample of 2,978 individuals from four provinces representative of Chile's population aged 15 and above (Vicente et al., 2006). The lifetime and annual rates of manic disorder were 1.9 and 1.4, respectively. Lifetime rates were higher in women (2.2) than in men (1.5).

Bipolar Spectrum

The rates of bipolar disorder reported above may be underestimates because many subjects who have brief recurrent hypomanic episodes may not be captured in surveys (see Chapters 2 and 3). Moreover, there is controversy about what symptoms should be included in the full spectrum of bipolar disorder. Some epidemiologic data on the spectrum that include hypomanic episodes are now available.

The relatively low reported rates of hypomania noted in previous surveys may be due to the fact that hypomania is frequently unrecognized by subjects themselves as a pathological condition. However, there may be a wide bipolar spectrum in clinical samples (Angst, 1998). The bipolar spectrum includes mania, hypomania, recurrent brief hypomania, sporadic brief hypomania, and cyclothymia. Modern concepts of bipolar disorder are still developing and can include bipolar-I and -II, hypomania, cyclothymia, mania with depression, and depression with hypomania, as well as highly recurrently major depression.[6] Six subtypes of bipolar disorder were described by Klerman (1981): (1)

mania, (2) hypomania, (3) hypomania or mania precipitated by drugs, (4) cyclothymic personality, (5) depression with a familial history of bipolar disorder, and (6) mania without depression. The concept of "soft" bipolar spectrum (Akiskal, 1996) includes Klerman's subtypes 3 through 6, as well as recurrent depression without spontaneous hypomania but with hyperthymic temperament (Angst, 1998). Epidemiologic studies have found lifetime prevalence rates for certain segments of the bipolar spectrum that range from 3.0 to 8.3 percent (Table 5–12). The further the spectrum is extended, however, the lower is the diagnostic reliability.

In this context, longitudinal epidemiologic studies of young adults to determine instances of subtle onset of symptoms could provide data for use in testing the hypothesis of a bipolar spectrum. However, almost all epidemiologic studies are cross-sectional. One attempt to study the spectrum was the longitudinal study of Angst (1998), discussed previously. In that study, the cumulative prevalence (based on four interviews over 12 years) for DSM-IV hypomania/mania was 5.5 percent. Brief (recurrent or sporadic) hypomania had a prevalence of 2.8 percent. Therefore, the inclusion of brief hypomania raised the Zurich rate for bipolar spectrum to 8.3 percent (Akiskal 2000). All of the subgroups in this study—those that met the DSM-IV criteria for hypomania and those with sporadic or brief recurrent hypomania—had similar symptom profiles and a family history of depression (Angst, 1998). Angst recommended that the bipolar spectrum be broadened to include brief hypomania in light of its high prevalence and clinical relevance.

The largest study of bipolar spectrum disorder included more than 85,000 adults in the United States and used the Mood Disorder Questionnaire (MDQ), a screening instrument of uncertain reliability. This study found a rate of bipolar spectrum of 3.7 percent. The relationship between data on bipolar spectrum obtained from a screening questionnaire and from a full diagnostic interview is unclear, however (Hirschfeld et al., 2001, 2003a,b; see Chapter 11).

The recent NCS-R found a lifetime prevalence of bipolar spectrum of 4.4 percent: 1.4 percent for bipolar-I, 1.6 percent for bipolar-II, and 1.4 percent for bipolar subthreshold (defined as those individuals who have euphoria or irritability plus two other symptoms for 4 days or longer with at least mild impairment and a history of major depression). Males were more likely to be diagnosed with subthreshold bipolar disorder than were females (1.7 and 1.0 percent, respectively) (Kessler et al., 2006).

Bipolar spectrum is an ambiguous classification and includes subtypes that are subtle and difficult to diagnose. There is general agreement, however, that bipolar disorder encompasses a broad spectrum and that clinically

TABLE 5–12. Lifetime Prevalence/100 of Bipolar Spectrum Disorder

Study	Country	Age Range (Years)	Diagnostic Method	Time Period	Prevalence/100
Oliver and Simmons, 1985	United States	15+	DIS	Lifetime	3.3
Faravelli and Incerpi, 1985	Italy	15–89	DIS	Annual	3.4
Szadoczky et al., 1998	Hungary	18–64	CIDI	Lifetime	5.1
Weissman and Meyers, 1978	United States	18–64	SADS-L	Lifetime	3.0
Heun and Maier, 1993	Germany	20–60	SADS-L	Lifetime	6.5
Levav et al., 1993	Israel	24–33	SADS-L	6-month	2.6
Angst, 1998	Switzerland	19–35	SPIKE	Lifetime	5.5[a]
Hirschfeld et al., 2002	United States	18+	MDQ	Lifetime	3.7
Judd and Akiskal, 2003	United States	18+	DIS	Lifetime	6.4
Moreno and Andrade, 2005	Brazil	18+	CIDI	Lifetime	8.3
Kessler et al., 2006	United States	18+	CIDI	Lifetime	4.4
Faravelli et al., 2006	Italy	14+	MINI	Lifetime	5.5

CIDI = Composite International Diagnostic Interview; DIS = Diagnostic Interview Schedule; MDQ = Mood Disorder Questionnaire; MINI = Mini International Neuropsychiatric Interview; SADS-L = Schedule for Affective Disorders and Schizophrenia-Lifetime; SPIKE = Structured Psychopathological Interview and Rating of the Social Consequences of Psychiatric Disturbances for Epidemiology.

[a]8.3 if brief hypomania is included.

significant cases within that spectrum are not captured in epidemiologic or even clinical studies.

COMMUNITY SURVEYS WITH CHILDREN AND ADOLESCENTS

As discussed earlier, the onset and clinical presentation of bipolar disorder in children and adolescents are less clear than in adults (see also Chapter 6). Moreover, there is considerable controversy about clinical presentation in children (Geller et al., 2002; Lewinsohn et al., 2003; Biederman et al., 2004). In particular, there is controversy as to whether hyperactive, inattentive children with emotional lability represent early presentations of mania or ADHD. Biederman (1995), Farone and colleagues (1997), Geller and colleagues (1998), and Wozniak and colleagues (1995) examined ADHD uncomplicated by any other psychiatric disorder in an effort to understand the possible symptomatology of childhood mania. Biederman and colleagues (1995) found that 96 percent of children referred with symptoms of mania fulfilled criteria for a diagnosis of ADHD; however, only 16 percent of the children referred with symptoms of ADHD met the criteria for mania. The diagnosis of bipolar disorder in pediatric populations is complicated by insufficient information on the clinical development of childhood symptomatology into adulthood; a clinical bias against a diagnosis of mania in childhood (Carlson, 1996), similar to the bias seen 20 years ago against the diagnosis of depression in children (Angold, 1988); and overlap of symptomatology between bipolar

disorder and other, more prevalent childhood psychiatric illnesses (ADHD and conduct disorder) (see Chapter 6).

Compared with the gender distribution in adulthood, reports of mania in childhood based on clinical and epidemiologic studies suggest that prepubertal onset of mania may be more frequent in boys than in girls (Varanka et al., 1988; Geller et al., 1998). The incidence of mania appears to increase after the onset of puberty, and the prevalence of mania during late adolescence is estimated to approximate that in adulthood.[7]

Table 5–13 presents the prevalence rates of bipolar disorder from community-based epidemiologic studies of adolescents. Only the MECA study included children; all of the other studies included only adolescent samples. The table demonstrates the paucity of data in this area. Note that the considerable variation in age ranges included in the different studies affects the rates derived and accounts for discrepancies shown in the table.

Results of both the NCS and the MECA study are on public-use tapes, making it possible to undertake the analyses presented here. The NCS, as described previously, included subjects aged 15 to 54. In that study, the lifetime rate for bipolar-I was 1.3/100 among 468 adolescents aged 15 to 17.

The MECA study was conducted among a population-based sample of children and adolescents (see Table 5–13). As noted, this is the only published epidemiologic study to include children; however, the sample was too small to be divided by age, and pubertal status was not obtained. Probability household samples of 1,285 youths aged 9 to 17 were selected at four sites (Atlanta, Georgia; New Haven,

TABLE 5–13. Prevalence/100 of Bipolar Disorder from Studies in Adolescents

Study	Country (Year)	Sample Size	Age Range (Years)	Diagnostic Method	Diagnosis	Time Period	Prevalence/100
NCS, unpublished	United States (1992)	468	15–17	CIDI	BP-I	Lifetime	1.4
MECA, unpublished	United States (1992)	1,285	9–17	DISC	Mania	6-month	1.2
					Hypomania	6-month	0.6
Lewinsohn et al., 1995	Western Oregon (1987)	1,709	14–18	KSADS/LIFE	BP	Lifetime	1.0
Wittchen et al., 1998	Bavaria, Germany (1988)	3,021	14–24	CIDI	BP-I	Annual	1.4
						Lifetime	0.4
					BP-II	Annual	0.4
						Lifetime	0.4
Aalto-Setälä et al., 2001	Helsinki, Finland (2000)	647	Follow-up of high school students, 20–24	SCAN	BP-I	1-month	0.2
					BP-II	1-month	0.5
					BP-NOS	1-month	0.2

Note: Only the MECA study included children.

BP = bipolar; BP-NOS = bipolar disorder–not otherwise specified; CIDI = Composite International Diagnostic Interview; DISC = Diagnostic Interview Schedule for Children; KSADS = Kiddie Schedule for Affective Disorders and Schizophrenia; LIFE = Longitudinal Interval Follow-up Evaluation; MECA = Methods for the Epidemiology of Child and Adolescent Mental Disorder; NCS = National Comorbidity Study; SCAN = Schedules for Clinical Assessment in Neuropsychiatry.

Connecticut; Westchester County, New York; and Puerto Rico). Lay interviewers administered a computer-assisted version of the NIMH Diagnostic Interview Schedule for Children (DISC) 2.3 and structured interviews to assess demographic variables, functional impairment, risk factors, service utilization, and barriers to service utilization (Lahey et al., 1996). Data were collected from both children and their parents. A clinician interviewer, again using DISC 2.3, reassessed 247 of these parent–child pairs 1 to 3 weeks later. The test-retest reliability of the interviews with the parents was generally good for most diagnoses but less satisfactory for the interviews with the children. The current (6-month) prevalence for mania was 1.2/100 and for hypomania was 0.6/100 (unpublished data). Annual rates were not available.

Gould and colleagues (1998) examined the relationships among suicidal ideation, suicide attempts, and mania in the MECA study. They found that 4.5 percent of youths having had suicidal ideation and 7.1 percent of those having made a suicide attempt had experienced manic symptoms, compared with 0.9 percent of those who had neither had suicidal ideation nor made an attempt. The comparison of these two groups was statistically significant. There were 16 children with mania—3 with suicidal ideation (18.7 percent), 3 who had made a suicide attempt (18.7 percent), and 10 who had neither had suicidal ideation nor

made an attempt (62.5 percent; $p < .005$ ideation versus none; $p < .001$ attempt versus none).

A community sample of 1,709 adolescents (aged 14 to 18 years) was randomly selected from nine senior high schools representative of urban and rural districts in western Oregon (Lewinsohn et al., 1995). The adolescents were interviewed initially between 1987 and 1989 using KSADS (with combined features of the epidemiologic and present state versions). Parents were not interviewed. At approximately 1 year, a follow-up interview (the Longitudinal Interval Follow-up Evaluation [LIFE]; Keller et al., 1987) and KSADS were administered to determine the presence of psychiatric disorders since the initial interview. The lifetime prevalence of bipolar disorder (primarily bipolar-II and cyclothymia) was approximately 1.0 percent. An additional 5.7 percent of the sample (termed "core positive subjects") reported experiencing a distinct period of abnormally elevated, expansive, and/or irritable mood, although they never met the criteria for bipolar disorder per se. Both bipolar and "core positive" patients exhibited significant functional impairment and high rates of comorbidity (anxiety and disruptive behavior), suicide attempts, and use of mental health services. The prevalence, age at onset, phenomenology, and course of bipolar disorder in adolescents were similar for both males and females.

To examine the course of adolescent depression, a follow-up was conducted to compare the rates of mood and other mental disorders between ages 19 and 24 for adolescents with a history of depression and those with adolescent adjustment disorder with depressed mood, those with nonaffective disorders, and those with no disorder. The study participants were followed-up again when they reached age 24. The follow-up sample (739 subjects) had low rates of dysthymia and bipolar disorder (less than 1 percent). In accord with other results, a small percentage (0.9 percent) of children and adolescents with major depression had experienced manic/hypomanic episodes.[8]

The same community sample in Oregon was used to compare the incidence and prevalence of bipolar disorder among adolescents and young adults, to explore the stability and consequences of adolescent bipolar disorder in young adulthood, to determine the rate of transition from depression to bipolar disorder, and to evaluate the significance of subsyndromal bipolar disorder (SUB) (Lewinsohn et al., 1995). The results show a lifetime prevalence of bipolar disorder of approximately 1.0 percent during adolescence and 2.0 percent during young adulthood. Lifetime prevalence of SUB was approximately 5.0 percent. Fewer than 1.0 percent of adolescents with depression had converted to bipolar disorder by age 24 (Lewinsohn et al., 2000). The bipolar disorder and SUB subgroups both had elevated rates of antisocial and other personality disorder symptoms. Both showed significant impairment in psychosocial functioning and had made greater use of mental health services. In general, adolescents with bipolar disorder showed significant continuity across developmental periods and had adverse outcomes during young adulthood. Adolescent SUB was also associated with adverse outcomes in adulthood, but not with increased incidence of bipolar disorder, a finding that questions the validity of the SUB diagnoses.

A study conducted in Bavaria, Germany, among a sample of 3,021 adolescents and young adults aged 14 to 24 using the CIDI and DSM-IV revealed a lifetime prevalence of 1.4/100 for bipolar-I and 0.4/100 for bipolar-II (Wittchen et al., 1998a). The annual rates were 1.3/100 and 0.4/100, respectively. The version of the CIDI used in this study also included questions about disabilities and impairment, operationalized as the assessment of economic, social, and leisure impairment during the worst episode and 1 month before the interview. Among those youths with any bipolar disorder, 94 percent considered themselves very impaired.

A 5-year follow-up of 647 high school students aged 20 to 24 in Helsinki, Finland, found 1-month prevalence rates of 0.2 percent for bipolar-I, 0.5 percent for bipolar-II, and 0.2 percent for bipolar-NOS, with a total rate of bipolar disorder of 0.9 percent (Aalto-Setälä et al., 2001). Given that these rates are monthly, they do not diverge greatly from the annual rates reported in Germany among a similar age group.

GLOBAL BURDEN OF DISEASE STUDIES

In recent decades the patterns of disease and mortality in developing countries have grown to resemble those of high-income countries, with a preponderance of burden resulting from chronic diseases. To quantify these changes the World Bank, in collaboration with WHO, undertook a systematic assessment of the global burden of disease (GBD) in 1990 (World Bank, 1993b; Murray et al., 1994; Murray and Lopez, 1996). The burden of disease was measured in disability-adjusted life years (DALYs), which are the sum of life years lost to premature mortality (YLL) and life years lost to disability (YLD). The 1990 GBD assessment confirmed a major epidemiological transition resulting from both decreasing birth rates and decreasing rates of death from communicable diseases. As the birth rate of a population drops, the number of adults increases relative to the number of children, and a greater proportion of health care resources is accordingly focused on adults. Then, as fatalities from acute diseases become increasingly preventable, and public health and medicine achieve growing success in controlling and stabilizing the effects of such chronic diseases as cancer, cardiovascular conditions, and AIDS, people live longer with the disabling effects of their illness. The disability from disease results in the inability to work or carry out daily activities of living.

A major assessment of the global burden of disease and risk factors, updated to 2001, has recently been published (Lopez et al., 2006). Self-inflicted injuries, overwhelmingly attributable to psychiatric illnesses—especially unipolar and bipolar disorders—are the sixth leading cause of death in adults 15–59 in low and middle-income countries and the second in high-income countries (Table 5–14). Unipolar depression ranks first in disability in both low and middle-income and high-income countries (Table 5–15).

Questions have been raised about the severity weights for mental disorders used in the GBD study and whether the weights for depression and substance abuse may have been overestimated (Andrews et al., 1998; Vos and Mathers, 2000). In a study from the Netherlands in which the burden of disease in 1994 in terms of DALYs was estimated by using data from Dutch vital statistics, registries, and surveys with Dutch disability weights, depression ranked eighth, accounting for 112,800 DALYs in that year. This figure represented 4.4 percent of the DALYs for all diseases, compared with a figure of 3.7 percent in established market economy populations from the GBD study (Melse et al., 2000).

TABLE 5–14. The 10 Leading Causes of Death in Adults Ages 15–59, by Broad Income Group, 2001

	LOW- AND MIDDLE-INCOME COUNTRIES				HIGH-INCOME COUNTRIES		
	Cause	Deaths (millions)	Percentage of total deaths		Cause	Deaths (millions)	Percentage of total deaths
1	HIV/AIDS	2.05	14.1	1	Ischemic heart disease	0.13	10.8
2	Ischemic heart disease	1.18	8.1	2	Self-inflicted injuries	0.09	7.2
3	Tuberculosis	1.03	7.1	3	Road traffic accidents	0.08	6.9
4	Road traffic accidents	0.73	5.0	4	Trachea, bronchus, and lung cancers	0.08	6.8
5	Cerebrovascular disease	0.71	4.9	5	Cerebrovascular disease	0.05	4.4
6	Self-inflicted injuries	0.58	4.0	6	Cirrhosis of the liver	0.05	4.4
7	Violence	0.45	3.1	7	Breast cancer	0.05	4.0
8	Lower respiratory infections	0.33	2.3	8	Colon and rectal cancers	0.04	3.1
9	Cirrhosis of the liver	0.32	2.2	9	Diabetes mellitus	0.03	2.1
10	Chronic obstructive pulmonary disease	0.32	2.2	10	Stomach cancer	0.02	2.0

Source: Mathers et al., 2006.

TABLE 5–15. **The 10 Leading Causes of Disability (Years Lived with Disability) by Broad Income Group, 2001**

LOW- AND MIDDLE-INCOME COUNTRIES			HIGH-INCOME COUNTRIES		
Cause	YLD (millions of years)	Percentage of total YLD	Cause	YLD (millions of years)	Percentage of total YLD
1 Unipolar depressive disorders	43.22	9.1	1 Unipolar depressive disorders	8.39	11.8
2 Cataracts	28.15	5.9	2 Alzheimer's and other dementias	6.33	8.9
3 Hearing loss, adult onset	24.61	5.2	3 Hearing loss, adult onset	5.39	7.6
4 Vision disorders, age-related	15.36	3.2	4 Alcohol use disorders	3.77	5.3
5 Osteoarthritis	13.65	2.9	5 Osteoarthritis	3.77	5.3
6 Perinatal conditions	13.52	2.8	6 Cerebrovascular disease	3.46	4.9
7 Cerebrovascular disease	11.10	2.3	7 Chronic obstructive pulmonary disease	2.86	4.0
8 Schizophrenia	10.15	2.1	8 Diabetes mellitus	2.25	3.2
9 Alcohol use disorders	9.81	2.1	9 Endocrine disorders	1.68	2.4
10 Protein-energy malnutrition	9.34	2.0	10 Vision disorders, age-related	1.53	2.1

Source: Mathers et al., 2006.

In a study from Victoria, Australia, rates of bipolar disorder were estimated from published studies by applying the Dutch disability weights (Vos and Mathers, 2000). The DALYs rates for depression were 7.7 for females and 5.3 for males, and those for bipolar disorder were 1.3 for females and 1.4 for males. These rates were lower than those for the established market economies in the WHO study—for depression, 10.7 for females and 6.0 for males, and for bipolar disorder, 2.1 for females and 2.2 for males. The burden of major depression was found to be higher for females than for males, but that of bipolar disorder did not differ by gender (Vos and Mathers, 2000), as determined from the gender ratios in the tables presented earlier.

Psychiatric disorders are expected to represent a greater global share of the disability burden than cardiovascular disease by 2020 (Murray and Lopez, 2000). Indeed, the results of the World Bank Development Study and the Murray and Lopez report caught the attention of the administration of WHO and helped spur the initiation of the World Mental Health Study, 2000, which is described next.

World Mental Health Study, 2000

The beginning of a new generation of cross-national studies of mental disorders was marked by a study in 2000 by the WHO International Consortium of Psychiatric Epidemiology (ICPE), which encompassed countries and geographic areas not included in previous cross-national studies.[9] The first prevalence rates, based on use of the CIDI to generate DSM–IV diagnoses, were from a sample of 29,644 persons participating in population surveys in North America (Canada and the United States [the NCS]), Latin America (Brazil and Mexico), and Europe (Germany, the Netherlands, and Turkey). Although the rates for bipolar disorder were not presented separately, the lifetime rates of any mood disorder (depression, dysthymia, and/or mania) are as follows: Turkey, 7.3 percent; Mexico, 9.2 percent; Canada, 10.2 percent; Brazil, 15.5 percent; Germany, 17.1 percent; the Netherlands, 18.9 percent; and the United States (the NCS), 19.4 percent. These, the first estimates from the consortium, show that mood disorders are highly prevalent throughout the world.

Additional surveys are to be conducted by the consortium in Mexico, Colombia, France, Italy, Belgium, the Ukraine, South Africa, Indonesia, China, and New Zealand and may include an adolescent sample. Data from the ICPE on individual mood disorders, including mania and disorder subtypes, are forthcoming (R.C. Kessler, Department of Health Care Policy, Harvard Medical School, personal communication, 2002). These data will encompass bipolar disorder and bipolar spectrum, as well as impairment, course, and current symptoms. Reappraisals of clinical data are also under way.

ASSOCIATED FEATURES

In this section, we summarize what is known about the correlates of bipolar disorder. These variables are often called "risk factors," but to avoid possible causal implications, we use instead the term "associated features." Some of this information has been presented earlier (e.g., in our review of cross-national studies or variation in rates by marital status or age), and some is discussed in detail in other chapters. Here we summarize that material, along with other information available from analytical epidemiologic studies. Analysis of data on associated features from community surveys is problematic except for such broad factors as age and gender because large samples are necessary for a disorder of relatively low prevalence. Therefore, few community-based epidemiologic studies of bipolar disorder are able to examine associated features beyond age, age at onset, and gender.

Temporal Variations

Gershon and colleagues (1987) observed birth cohort changes in mania among relatives of bipolar and schizoaffective patients. Using life table analysis, they found higher rates of bipolar disorder among those cohorts born after the 1940s, suggesting that the cumulative hazard for the disorder in a given age group is greater in those born after that decade. Gershon and colleagues (1987) concluded that cohorts with the highest rates of affective illness appear to have been born in the decades after World War II (these findings are the same for bipolar and major depressive disorders).

Somewhat similar findings were derived independently in the ECA (Lasch et al., 1990). Respondents were divided into eight birth cohorts, each spanning a 10-year interval. Actuarial life table analysis showed variations in the risk of mania by birth cohort, with the greatest risk seen among the post-1935 cohorts.

Various explanations have been proposed to account for these results (Klerman and Weissman, 1989). The temporal variations noted could be due to differential mortality and institutionalization, which could have removed older persons and earlier birth cohorts from the source populations, while changes in diagnostic criteria and the inclusion of persons with milder forms of bipolar disorder could have increased the rates in cohorts born after 1935. The onset of the "antidepressant era" in the early 1960s and the subsequent 10-fold increase in the use of this class of drugs, beginning with the appearance of "second-generation" antidepressants in the 1990s, may well have played a significant role. Dietary changes (including lower (compared with breast milk) concentrations of omega-3 fatty acids in infant formulas, discussed later, and younger age at first alcohol or drug use) and increased smoking in women must also be considered. It may be noted that there is some consensus that higher rates of bipolar disorder in the 1990 NCS compared with the 1980 ECA are due to methodological differences, as discussed earlier, rather than to temporal variations. Recall, memory, and a general reporting bias may also have contributed to the observed temporal variations in mania—specifically, a decline in the memory of lifetime events among the elderly or a conscious effort not to report them.

Gender

Mood disorders as a group are consistently more prevalent among women than men, but the difference is due to the higher prevalence of unipolar major depression in women. When only subjects with bipolar disorder are considered, nearly equal gender ratios have been found across most but not all national and cross-national studies, as reported earlier. Variations in one direction or another are likely due to the instability of small samples.

Social Class

In the first edition of this text, we reviewed more than 30 early studies of the association between social class and manic-depressive illness published between 1913 and 1989. We discussed in detail the considerable methodological problems involved in virtually every one of the studies but were impressed, nonetheless, by the overall association between bipolar illness and one or more measures reflecting upper social class.[10] The complexities are many, of course. We discuss in Chapter 12 the possible links among creativity, educational and occupational achievement, and certain behavioral, temperamental, cognitive, and behavioral characteristics associated with bipolar illness. Education and occupational achievement are, of course, associated with higher social class. It is also possible that characteristics associated with mild manic states, such as increased energy, risk-taking sexual drive, productivity, and social outgoingness, make some individuals more attractive and therefore, on occasion, more likely to marry into a higher social class.

More recent epidemiologic data show an equal distribution of the disorder among all social classes and educational levels. While bipolar illness in a small minority of patients may facilitate achievement and may aid the creative process (see Chapter 12), it is likely that most of the earlier association between bipolar disorder and higher social class had to do with diagnostic practices and inaccuracies in the concept. Upper- and middle-class people were more likely to be diagnosed as bipolar, whereas lower-class individuals, especially the urban poor, were (and still are) more likely to be diagnosed as schizophrenic (often mistakenly so) and consequently treated as such. Criteria for social class also varied widely across studies. Nonetheless, these investigations remain interesting for their span over many decades, their historical significance, and their great range across countries and cultures.

Most newer studies have failed to find a significantly lower than expected rate of bipolar disorder associated with indices of upper social class (educational status, occupation, economic status, or parental social class). In both the ECA and the NCS, lower educational level was not found to be associated with an increased risk of bipolar disorder. The NCS found an association between rates of bipolar illness and lower family income; it is unclear, however, whether the latter is a direct consequence of the illness or a trigger for its onset. Abood and colleagues (2002) examined 90 patients with bipolar-I disorder from a publicly financed service in Dublin to assess the association of the disorder with social advantage. Although not a representative sample, when compared with other psychiatric patients, excluding those with schizophrenia, the bipolar patients had similar demographic and socioeconomic characteristics (including more frequent residential moves).

On the other hand, a sample of 130 patients meeting DSM-III-R criteria for bipolar disorder and depression were compared on their and their relatives' occupational levels (Verdoux and Bourgeois, 1995). Occupational level did not differ significantly between unipolar and bipolar probands, although higher levels predominated among bipolar probands' brothers and children. A comparison of entire groups including probands and all their relatives revealed a social advantage for the relatives of bipolar patients. These results are consistent with the downward-drift hypothesis of bipolar disorder, which suggests that if there is any social advantage among bipolar patients, it may be reflected in the higher social class of their relatives. The devastation of the illness may erase these advantages and result in the association between the disorder and lower income seen in the NCS or the increased rates among the homeless discussed later. Consistent with this hypothesis is a recent study (Tsuchiya et al., 2004) finding that higher

parental educational level and greater parental wealth were associated with an elevated risk for bipolar disorder, but that the patients themselves were more likely to be unemployed and less well educated. The authors concluded that socioeconomic status may deteriorate as a result of the negative consequences of the disease (as described in Chapter 4). It may also be that milder forms of the illness on occasion lead to high achievement, but that the illness expressed in offspring of successful individuals is of a more severe nature (see Chapter 13, in particular the discussion of the phenomenon of anticipation).

Race/Ethnicity and Cultural Differences

A number of studies have examined racial similarities and differences in the prevalence and incidence of bipolar illness. Many factors apart from the previously discussed sources of variance cloud the accurate determination of these rates, including inadequate sampling from different socioeconomic groups, cultural differences and consequent problems regarding presentation, the misdiagnosis of schizophrenia noted earlier, and possible racial insensitivity among early researchers. These factors must be accounted for in such analyses.

Lewis and Hubbard (1931), Faris and Dunham (1939), Helzer (1975), and Weissman and Myers (1978) found equal rates of diagnosis of bipolar illness among African Americans and Caucasians. Likewise, the ECA revealed no significant difference in the prevalence or incidence of bipolar disorder among races (Robins and Regier, 1991). The NCS, on the other hand, indicated that African Americans had significantly lower rates of mania than Caucasians (Kessler et al., 1994). There is also some evidence that African Caribbean and African individuals are less likely to have experienced a depressive episode before the onset of first mania, and more likely to have more severe psychotic symptoms during their first mania, relative to Caucasian Europeans (Kennedy et al., 2004). In the study of the Cross-National Collaborative Group, the rates among the two Asian samples (Taiwan and Korea) and the Hispanic sample (Puerto Rico) were compared with those among the primarily Caucasian samples from Edmonton, Canada; West Germany; and Christchurch, New Zealand. The Asian samples clearly showed the lowest rates of bipolar disorder, but these rates were still within the same general range as those of the other sites. Moreover, the Asian sites (Taiwan, Korea, Hong Kong) generally showed the lowest rates for all psychiatric disorders.

In general, the newer epidemiologic data are consistent with the results of earlier studies in indicating no strong association between race/ethnicity and bipolar illness, with the possible exception of the unexplained lower rates of many psychiatric disorders in Asian countries. Too few Asians were included in the ECA and NCS to study the consistency of this finding among Asians living in the United States. Such data could aid in understanding whether low rates of bipolar disorder are intrinsic to Asian people or affected by environmental factors. Selective migration could also be at play in that families or persons with bipolar disorder may be more likely to emigrate. Future studies and the new worldwide epidemiologic study of the ICPE, described previously, may clarify this issue.

Marital Status

Epidemiologic studies investigating marital status among bipolar patients have revealed that the disorder is slightly more common among single and divorced persons. The ECA revealed that individuals who are separated or divorced are more likely to suffer from bipolar disorder as compared with married or never-married individuals (see Table 5–7). In a Hungarian national survey (Szadoczky et al., 1998), bipolar disorder was found to be more frequent among those who were separated and divorced. The rate among those never married was high as well. Early onset of the illness may contribute to the latter phenomenon, negatively influencing personality development and thus causing difficulties in establishing and maintaining interpersonal connections.

As Krauthammer and Klerman (1979) pointed out, marital status may change as a result of the disorder, rather than leading to its onset. On the other hand, it is plausible that being single or divorced constitutes a risk for bipolar illness in some populations; it is also plausible, indeed likely, that stressful marriages may precipitate affective episodes and, conversely, that supportive marriages may have a protective effect.

While persons with bipolar disorder are more likely than those in the general population to be single, divorced, or in a disrupted marriage, we know of no evidence to support a causal relationship between the disorder and marital status. The establishment of such a link is hampered by small sample sizes and a lack of clarity as to the direction of causality in studies addressing the question. Therefore, although it is likely that symptoms of untreated mania are disruptive to forming or sustaining intimate relationships, this hypothesis is not supported empirically. (See Chapter 10 for further discussion of the effect of bipolar disorder on interpersonal relationships.)

Urban/Rural Comparisons

No urban/rural differences in rates of bipolar disorder were found in the ECA or the NCS. In Taiwan, the lifetime prevalence was higher in metropolitan Taipei (1.6 percent) than in small towns (0.7 percent) and rural villages (1.0 percent) (Hwu et al., 1989). In Korea, the lifetime prevalence of mania was similar in metropolitan Seoul (0.4 percent) and in rural regions (0.4 percent) (Lee et al., 1990b). Urban/rural differences in prevalence rates of affective disorders, when they exist, may relate to the interplay among such factors as place of residence, migration patterns, socioeconomic status, diet, and environment, rather than just one variable.

The Homeless and the Institutionalized

Homelessness and mental illness among the homeless population have become a special interest of many mental health professionals. The homeless population itself is difficult to define, and ascertaining the prevalence of mental disorders within this community is even more problematic. In 1990, the lifetime and 5-year prevalence of all types of homelessness in the United States was estimated at 14.0 percent (26 million people) and 4.6 percent (8.5 million people), respectively. Lifetime "literal homelessness" (sleeping in shelters, abandoned buildings, bus and train stations, and the like) was 7.4 percent (13.5 million people). Among those who had ever been literally homeless, the 5-year (1985–1990) prevalence of self-reported homelessness was 3.1 percent (5.7 million people) (Link et al., 1994). More recent follow-up studies of the homeless, however, indicate that these figures overestimate the persistence of the problem and the number of homeless with psychiatric problems (Phelan and Link, 1999).

Among the mental disorders that exist within this population, schizophrenia, substance abuse, personality disorders, and affective disorders are the most prevalent (Arce and Vergare, 1984). Affective disorders make up 5 to 30 percent of mental disorders found among the homeless. The most comprehensive and standardized of the studies addressing this issue (Koegel et al., 1988) used the DIS to diagnose mental disorders among the mentally ill homeless in Los Angeles. Over the course of their lifetimes, these homeless individuals were 3.4 times more likely to have had any affective disorder, 17.7 times more likely to have had a manic episode, and 2.9 times more likely to have had a major depressive episode relative to people in the general population. Similarly, over a period of 6 months, the risk ratios for a mental disorder were many times greater among the homeless than in the general population (6.1, 37.5, and 5.0, respectively).

One must keep in mind when examining these data that these are prevalence rates within the mentally ill homeless population, and not within the general homeless population. Still, when these data are converted to rates within the general homeless population, the resulting proportions are higher than those among the general population. One other note regarding prevalence rates within this population is that substance abuse can easily coexist with or mask other underlying mental disorders, especially affective disorders. Therefore, these already high rates of bipolar disorder may be underestimates.

A more recent study of 1,022 homeless men living in shelters or on the street in Munich, Germany, using the SCID, also revealed high rates of mood disorders (lifetime prevalence of 32.8 percent for any mood disorder and of 5.2 percent for bipolar disorder). The highest rate was found for substance abuse (79.6 percent), particularly alcohol dependence (72.7 percent) (Fichter et al., 2001). A lifetime rate of bipolar disorder (3.6 percent), based on the CIDI, was found among 838 homeless men and women in a study conducted in Paris in 1996 (Kovess and Lazarus, 1999). Comparable studies in other European countries did not report bipolar disorder separately from other mood disorders (Vázquez et al., 1997; Muñoz et al., 1998; Babidge et al., 2002).

Some studies have oversampled the incarcerated (Buhrich et al., 2000) and the institutionalized (Robins and Regier, 1991). These groups were found to have higher rates of bipolar disorder than the general population. For example, Blazer (1985) found a lifetime prevalence of 5.4 percent for those living in prisons and 9.7 percent for those living in nursing homes. Yet the studies showed that the inclusion of these populations added only a small fraction (1.0 percent) to the estimated percentage of the general population having a mental disorder. Therefore, their inclusion or exclusion has little effect on community rates.

Pregnancy and Menopause

Childbearing represents a special risk for the onset of bipolar-I disorder in women. As shown by both epidemiologic and clinical studies, the first onset of bipolar disorder is almost always in the childbearing years (Blehar et al., 1998). As noted in Chapter 20, almost one-half of bipolar-I women who had been pregnant reported having experienced severe emotional disturbances in relationship to childbearing, with almost one-third citing episodes during pregnancy. Nair and colleagues (2000) hypothesized that subsets of women with a history of repeated reproductive-related mood disorders may be especially vulnerable to mood disturbances during perimenopause and menopause. In their study, two-thirds of perimenopausal bipolar-I women reported frequent mood disturbances, and almost 20 percent of postmenopausal bipolar-I women had experienced severe emotional disturbances during the menopausal transition.

Smoking

Bipolar disorder is associated with increased risk of smoking. A case-control study carried out in Alava, Spain, including patients with a DSM-III-R diagnosis of bipolar-I disorder found that smoking was more prevalent among bipolar patients than among the general population. Most patients had begun to smoke before the onset of bipolar disorder; thus vulnerability to bipolar illness (not the illness itself) may make subjects more likely to become smokers (Gonzalez-Pinto et al., 1998).

The NCS included questions on smoking. About 69 percent of respondents with bipolar-I were current smokers, and 82 percent had ever smoked. These rates were quite different from those among respondents without mental illness or with other psychiatric disorders (Lasser et al., 2000). For example, the 82 percent of bipolar respondents who had ever smoked is a significantly higher proportion than the 59 percent of subjects with major depression and the 72 percent of drug abusers who had ever done so. Analysis of the 2001–2002 National Epidemiologic Survey on Alcohol and Related Conditions found that nicotine dependence occurred in 40 percent of all cases (Grant et al., 2005). Moreover, studies that have addressed smoking in bipolar patients have noted their difficulty in quitting (Glassman, 1993).

Comorbid psychiatric and medical conditions are discussed in Chapter 7.

Omega-3 Fatty Acids

Essential fatty acids are crucial components of synaptic cell membranes (see Chapter 14). The essential long-chain polyunsaturated fatty acids, omega-3 and omega-6, cannot be formed in the human body, so dietary intake is their only source. Sources of omega-3 fatty acids include fish and seafood, particularly oily fish (cod, salmon, tuna, haddock, and scallops).

Hibbeln (1998) found that greater seafood consumption was related to lower lifetime prevalence rates of major depression across nine countries ($r = .84$, $p < .005$). Frequent fish consumption (at least twice a week) was revealed to be an independent factor for a reduced risk of depressive symptoms (odds ratio $= 0.63$) and suicidal thinking (odds ratio $= 0.57$) in a restricted geographic region within a single country. The use of omega-3 supplements in the treatment of depression and bipolar disorder is discussed in Chapters 19 and 20.

Relating data on fish consumption in a country to independently collected epidemiologic data on rates of a disorder requires many assumptions about the quality, time, and sample structure of both datasets and yields at best a rough estimate of correlations. However, the data are consistent with a growing body of literature. Tanskanen and colleagues (2001) reported lower rates of suicidal ideation among frequent consumers of lake fish in Finland and a decrease in suicide risk among daily fish consumers in

Japan followed over 17 years. Nonetheless, well-controlled studies in bipolar and unipolar patients are needed before definitive conclusions can be reached about the role of omega-3 fatty acids.

Family History

There is strong agreement that bipolar disorder is heritable. While family studies cannot determine heritability, one of the strongest predictors of first onset of bipolar illness is a family history of the disorder. Unfortunately, family history is excluded from epidemiologic studies, mainly because collecting accurate information on family history is time-consuming.

As detailed in Chapter 13, the morbid risk for bipolar disorder among first-degree relatives of bipolar probands is elevated substantially over the risk in the general population. Furthermore, adoption studies have shown that the monozygotic-to-dizygotic concordance ratio is higher for bipolar disorder than for unipolar depression, indicating greater genetic involvement in the former condition. A number of genetic linkage and association studies are under way to determine the genes involved.

CONCLUSIONS

In its calculations of rates of disability, WHO has ranked bipolar disorder among the top 10 disabling disorders in both developed and developing countries. It is not easy to summarize the results of epidemiologic studies of bipolar disorder from around the world, especially in light of a number of methodological problems. Nonetheless, it is possible to derive reasonable estimates of the prevalence and incidence of the disorder.

Findings of recent studies generally indicate an overall lifetime prevalence of bipolar-I disorder of about 1 percent. The range of rates is not great, even from diverse countries. In the United States, Europe, Scandinavia, the South Pacific, South America, and the United Kingdom, the lifetime prevalence of bipolar-I disorder ranges from 0.2 percent (Iceland) to 2.0 percent (the Netherlands and Hungary). Most rates are around 1 to 1.5 percent. The exceptions are Iceland (0.2 percent) and three Asian countries with lifetime rates of 0.015 to 0.3 percent. The reasons for the markedly low Asian rates, which are also low for a number of other mental disorders, are unclear. Studies of Asians living outside the continent are needed to determine whether these low rates are related to genetic differences, to living in Asian countries, or to ascertainment factors.

Studies that include a broad bipolar spectrum produce much higher lifetime prevalence rates of 3.0 to 8.3 percent. While there have been efforts to determine the rates of bipolar-II and milder forms of bipolar disorder

in community surveys, it is difficult to distinguish between normal moods and mild hypomania in nonpatient populations, making the validity of these findings questionable. Moreover, all of these rates for bipolar spectrum may be underestimates because they do not include patients with highly recurrent major depression, some of whom may fall within the bipolar spectrum (see Chapter 1).[11]

Several features associated with bipolar disorder have been studied. Most studies with large sample sizes have not shown strong differences in rates of bipolar disorder by gender. Persons who are separated or divorced have higher rates of the disorder than their married counterparts. Differences by social class and racial group have been less well studied. Smoking is more prevalent among those with bipolar disorder than among the general population. And pregnancy and menopause represent vulnerable periods for women in the development of manic episodes.

A family history of bipolar disorder in first-degree relatives remains the strongest predictor of risk of onset of bipolar disorder. However, it is also a risk factor not usually included in epidemiologic surveys.

NOTES

1. Cowley and Wyatt, 1993; World Bank, 1993a,b; Murray and Lopez, 1996.
2. In the ECA and the NCS, the diagnostic interviews (the DIS and the UM-CIDI, respectively) contained questions designed to determine the clinical significance of each symptom involved in the disorder (Narrow et al., 2002). Questions in the two surveys were similar, and information was obtained as to whether the symptom was severe enough to require telling a doctor or any professional about it, to take medicine for it, and/or to interfere with usual activities. Symptoms failing to meet any of these criteria were not identified as clinically significant and did not count toward making the diagnosis. The ECA used this approach for most disorders. However, neither the ECA nor the NCS applied these criteria at the symptom level for major depression or bipolar disorder. In both cases, questions about clinical significance were asked only after all symptoms had been obtained and diagnostic criteria met. Applying clinical significance criteria at the symptom level and not at the end of the diagnostic stage reduced the overall rates of mental disorders in both surveys. The impact was greater in the NCS, and the disparity in rates between the ECA and the NCS was reduced, with an estimated 18.5 percent annual rate of any disorder.

   Applying the clinical significance criteria in the ECA reduced the annual rate of unipolar depression by about 18 percent and that of bipolar disorder by 44 percent (see Table 5–1) (Narrow et al., 2002). The rate of unipolar major depression was reduced to 4.0 percent, compared with 4.9 percent without the clinical significance criteria. The clinical significance criteria had a greater effect on major depression prevalence rates in the NCS than on those in the ECA, drawing the two rates closer together. The annual prevalence estimate for unipolar major depression in the NCS fell from 8.9 to 5.4 percent. The annual prevalence of bipolar-I disorder did not change in the NCS and remained at 1.3 percent, but dropped to 0.5 percent in the ECA. Thus, the gap between the ECA and NCS widened. There is controversy about the manipulation of rates based on treatment need (Narrow et al., 2002). Wakefield and Spitzer (2002) noted that basing disorders on stringent impairment criteria, which led to reduced rates in the NCS, helped resolve discrepancies between the 1980 and 1990 surveys. However, they suggested that these revised prevalence rates are not necessarily a valid redefinition of the disorders, but may reflect an inadequate measure of treatment need. Use of the impairment or treatment criteria, they noted, means that disorders that are real but do not interfere significantly with life are ignored.

Another way of examining diagnostic validity, used in the NCS, is through a clinical reappraisal of potential mania cases. Kessler and colleagues (1997) concluded that validity was satisfactory on bipolar-I, as judged by the reappraisal, only for cases of mania with elevated mood or increased activity, decreased need for sleep, and elevated self-esteem or grandiosity. Requiring these symptoms reduced the prevalence of mania to 0.3 percent. However, the authors cautioned that, because of a significant number of CIDI false-negative findings in the clinical reappraisals, these clinically confirmed CIDI cases may underestimate by half the actual rate of mania in the community. If this statement holds true, the extrapolated estimate of 0.6 percent for bipolar-I disorder is closer to the ECA rate. The authors were unable to document an algorithm with acceptable concordance with clinical diagnosis for bipolar-II, and they concluded that bipolar-II prevalence was not valid in their sample.

Another analysis of factors that may have contributed to the differences between ECA and NCS rates was conducted by Regier and colleagues (1998). Their analysis produced rates of psychiatric disorder from each survey by controlling for demographic variables; standardizing the weights in both surveys to the age, sex, and racial distributions of the 1990 census; formulating diagnoses according to DSM-III; and restricting the age range to 18 to 54 years. Using this method, the lifetime rate of any DSM-III disorder for the first wave of interviews was 36 percent. Adding the cases from the second wave produced a rate of 47 percent, consistent with the rate of 48 percent from the single-wave NCS. Annual rates of mania produced in this way were almost identical to those in the ECA and the NCS. The annual rate of bipolar-I for the first wave of the ECA using these conventions was 0.9 percent; adding cases from the second wave produced a rate of 1.0 percent. The annual rate in the NCS was 1.1 percent with these conventions.

That such modifications can reduce or increase disparate rates concerns health policy planners and insurers, who base the direct costs of service delivery for a disorder on its prevalence rate. The WHO initiative to revise the CIDI by including impairment criteria for each disorder is addressing this issue (Regier and Burke, 2000). However, there is still no fully satisfactory method of calculating the actual rates.

3. Simpson et al., 1993; Benazzi, 1997; Koukopoulos and Koukopoulos, 1999; Dilsaver and Akiskal, 2005; Rybakowski et al, 2005; Sharma et al., 2005.

4. Dilling and Weyerer, 1984; Henderson et al., 2000; Murphy et al., 2000; World Health Organization International Consortium of Psychiatric Epidemiology, 2000.

5. Scully et al., 2000, 2002a,b; Baldwin et al., 2002.

6. Angst, 1978; Dunner et al., 1982; Akiskal et al., 2000; Cassano et al., 2000; Angst et al., 2002.

7. Research on minors often makes a distinction by pubertal status. Puberty has been shown to differentiate the onset and clinical course of mood disorders in longitudinal and epidemiologic studies (Angold et al., 1998, 1999; Weissman et al., 1999a,b). The rates and gender ratios of depression change dramatically at puberty, with a marked increase occurring in overall rates, especially among females. Some studies separate prepubertal children from adolescents, others focus on one or the other, and still others merge the two. Most studies use chronological age to designate pubertal status; a few use Tanner staging (see Angold et al., 1998, 1999). We recognize the importance of these age distinctions and make them where the necessary data are available. In the absence of such data or the need to make an age-specific point, however, we use the term *children* to describe minors.

8. Strober et al., 1993; Lewinsohn et al., 1995; Rao et al., 1995; Geller et al., 1998.

9. More information on the ICPE can be obtained from http://www.hcp.med.harvard.edu/icpe/.

10. For example, Hollingshead and Redlich, 1958; Parker et al., 1959; Rao, 1966; Hare, 1968; Rowitz and Levy, 1968; Bagley, 1973; Gershon and Liebowitz, 1975; Petterson, 1977; Coryell et al., 1989.

11. Indeed, Kraepelin's "manic-depressive illness" included both bipolar and highly recurrent unipolar subgroups.

6 Children and Adolescents

In rare cases the first beginnings can be traced back even to before the tenth year. . . . The greatest frequency of first attacks falls, however, in the *period of development* with its increased emotional excitability between the fifteenth and the twentieth year.

—*Emil Kraepelin (1921, p. 167)*

Bipolar disorder commonly manifests itself in adolescence or young adulthood, but classic descriptions and numerous case studies also demonstrate the existence of the disorder in children. In recent years, identification of these earliest forms of the disorder has been the subject of an explosion of interest among clinicians, scientists, the public, and the media.[1] This interest has been driven in part by the emerging hypothesis of bipolar disorder as a progressive neurobiological process that may worsen with succeeding episodes, so that early identification and treatment may have important implications for attenuating the course of illness. Increasingly, moreover, parents are seeking answers and help for their children who display bewildering or overwhelmingly severe symptoms and are at increased risk for serious behavioral and educational problems, as well as suicide (see Hellander and Burke, 1999; Lewinsohn et al., 2003). Aside from treatment considerations, childhood-onset bipolar disorder also raises important conceptual and etiological questions: Are there different subtypes with differing causes and courses? What are the defining distinctions between pediatric bipolar illness and other psychiatric disorders of childhood, such as attention-deficit hyperactivity disorder (ADHD)? Is the rate of childhood bipolar disorder increasing, and if so, why? Is the course of the disorder different for early versus adult onset? Although this book is about manic-depressive illness, which includes both bipolar and recurrent unipolar forms, the pediatric literature rarely distinguishes recurrent from nonrecurrent forms of unipolar depression; this chapter limits its focus to the bipolar subgroup.

We begin with a review of research on childhood- and adolescent-onset bipolar disorder. We then examine the epidemiology and implications of bipolar disorder in these populations. Finally, we present the findings of studies of high-risk subjects that have attempted to identify characteristics of children of bipolar parents, with particular emphasis on early markers of potential bipolar illness. Unfortunately, many unresolved issues remain. The interest in manifestations of bipolar disorder among children and young adolescents is far greater than the yield from research addressing the key questions involved.

Throughout the discussion, we attempt to identify problems with the methods used in existing studies, as well as research needed to address important issues. One of the most pervasive difficulties stems from the failure of many studies to distinguish between childhood- and adolescent-onset bipolar disorder; this occurs, for example, when vague terms such as "juvenile-onset bipolar disorder" and "pediatric bipolar disorder" are used or when child and adolescent samples are combined in the same study. This is a widespread problem in the study of adolescent bipolar disorder, where distinctions are seldom made between childhood and adolescent *onset*. Some studies of adolescents with bipolar disorder include patients whose symptoms actually first occurred before age 12 or before puberty. As detailed in chapter 4, age at onset is also defined differently in various studies—for example, as age at first diagnosable symptoms of mania or at first symptoms of any affective disorder, or as age at first actual diagnosis of mania or depression by a mental health professional. Studies have employed different diagnostic criteria as well, and many have included clinical populations with a mix of bipolar-I and other bipolar spectrum disorders, despite the fact that there is very little information specifically on bipolar-II disorder in children or adolescents (see Chapter 3). Finally, one of the greatest methodological gaps is the paucity of longitudinal studies of either childhood or adolescent bipolar disorder. Such studies are essential to clarify diagnostic controversies and to map the course of the disorder and the implications of its early onset.

CHILDHOOD-ONSET BIPOLAR DISORDER

Although occurrences of mania and depression in adolescence are well established, the frequency of early-childhood onset of bipolar disorder remains controversial. Kraepelin (1921) found that 0.4 percent of his patients had displayed manic features before age 10. Despite historical records of case studies documenting apparent bipolar illness in children, however, theorists believed for an extended period in the mid-twentieth century that bipolar disorder in children before puberty was not possible (reviewed in Faedda et al., 1995). For instance, Anthony and Scott (1960) examined the psychiatric literature from 1884 to 1954 and uncovered only 28 cases of alleged manic episodes in young children. After applying systematic diagnostic criteria to these clinical reports, they dismissed all of the cases as misdiagnosed and concluded that a classic clinical presentation of manic-depressive illness in childhood had yet to be demonstrated.

Recent years have seen a growing acceptance that prepubertal forms of mania can be identified. Opinions range from certainty that characteristic patterns of symptoms signal childhood bipolar disorder in substantial numbers, even if in a form that may not precisely follow that of classic forms of the disorder, to more cautious views that prepubertal mania exists, but that many such complex cases may be misinterpreted as bipolar disorder. Difficulty in applying the adult criteria for bipolar disorder in the *Diagnostic and Statistical Manual*, 4th edition (DSM-IV) to children is at the heart of the controversy. In the following sections, we present research on characteristics of bipolar disorder in children and discuss the controversies related to its diagnosis.

Symptoms and Clinical Presentation

Manic Features

The appearance and diagnosis of mania is considered a distinctive indicator of bipolar disorder in children. However, the diagnosis of mania in children is controversial and fraught with pitfalls, as reviewed below.

Even as young as preschool age, some children appear to present relatively classic manic symptoms, including DSM-IV–defined mania or hypomania with elated mood and/or grandiosity; flight of ideas or racing thoughts; poor judgment, such as excessive silliness, uninhibited people-seeking, hypersexuality, or daredevil acts; talking fast; and distractibility, with increased energy, activity, and agitation (e.g., Geller et al., 2000a, 2002c). In their study of 93 children

with prepubertal and early-adolescent onset of bipolar disorder (mean age at onset 7.3 years), Geller and colleagues (1998b, 2002c) found that five mania-specific symptoms were especially likely to discriminate bipolar children from children with ADHD or normal comparison groups: elation, grandiosity, flight of ideas/racing thoughts, decreased need for sleep, and hypersexuality. Table 6–1 presents examples of manic symptoms in children compared with normal characteristics of youngsters of similar age (Geller et al., 2002b).

Geller and colleagues (2002c) also found that 60 percent of their sample had symptoms of psychosis, including 50 percent who had grandiose delusions. In a later follow-up study, they found that psychosis predicted more weeks ill with mania or hypomania (Geller et al., 2004). In their review of psychotic symptoms in pediatric bipolar disorder, Pavuluri and colleagues (2004) found that the prevalence of psychotic features ranged from 16 to 88 percent; most common were mood-congruent delusions, especially of the grandiose type. Biederman and colleagues (2004c) found that nearly 1 in 4 of the 298 bipolar patients they studied were psychotic or had a history of psychosis. Likewise, in their study of 263 bipolar children and adolescents, Birmaher and colleagues (2005b) found that one-third (33.1 percent) of their subjects had a history of psychosis.

Geller and colleagues required elation and/or grandiosity for the diagnosis of mania in children, as did Leibenluft and colleagues (2003a). This is an important, if still preliminary, consensus of clinical researchers, although, as Carlson (2005) pointed out, uncertainty remains about what actually constitutes these two symptoms. Methods of assessment vary widely, as do cultural expectations and developmental factors, and all are likely to influence the ascertainment of both euphoria and grandiosity (Breslau, 1987; Shaffer, 2002; Harrington and Myatt, 2003). Some studies have defined mania by the presence of highly labile moods with intense irritability, rage, explosiveness, and destructiveness; extreme agitation; and behavioral dysregulation (e.g., Biederman et al., 2000a). Irritability, and indeed rage, are noted as prominent features in many bipolar children (e.g., Faraone et al., 1997b; Carlson and Kelly, 1998; Geller et al., 2002c). The children are often aggressive and frequently are described by their parents as "out of control." Not surprisingly, they are often seen in hospital settings, and overall their functioning is marked by severe impairment in social and academic as well as family roles (Geller et al., 2000a). Box 6–1 presents a mother's diary of the behaviors of her 9-year-old bipolar son, conveying a sense of the severe but characteristic features of the disorder. Suicidal thoughts and behaviors are not uncommon.

TABLE 6–1. Examples of Core Symptoms of Mania among Children

Normal Child	Child with Mania
	Elated Mood
Child was extremely happy on days family went to Disneyland, on Christmas morning, during grandparents' visits (joy appropriate to context, not impairing).	7-year-old boy repeatedly taken to principal for clowning and giggling in class; had to leave church for similar behaviors. 9-year-old girl continually danced around at home, stating, "I'm high, over the mountain high" after suspension from school.
	Grandiosity
After school hours, 7-year-old boy played at being a firefighter, directing other firefighters and rescuing victims. Child did not call fire station and tell firefighters what to do.	7-year-old boy stole go-cart because he wanted to have it; knew stealing was wrong, but did not believe it was wrong for *him* to steal. 8-year-old girl, failing in school, spent evenings practicing for when she would be the first female President. She was also planning how to train her husband to be the First Gentleman.
	Decreased Need for Sleep
Normal children sleep approximately 8 to 10 hours a night and are tired the next day if they sleep fewer hours than usual.	8-year-old boy chronically stayed up until 2 AM rearranging the furniture or playing games. He then awoke at 6 AM for school and was energetic throughout the day without evident fatigue.
	Poor Judgment: Hypersexuality
7-year-old child played doctor with a friend of the same age. 12-year-old boy looked at his father's pornographic magazines.	7-year-old girl touched the teacher's breasts and propositioned boys in class. 10-year-old boy used explicit sexual language in restaurants and public places. Girl faxed a note to the local police station asking police to____her.
	Racing Thoughts
Normal children do not report racing thoughts.	Children tend to give concrete answers to describe racing thoughts: A girl pointed to the middle of her forehead and stated, "I need a stoplight up there." Others: "It's like an energizer bunny in my head." "My thoughts broke the speed limit." "I don't know what to think first."

Source: Adapted from Geller et al., 2002a. Reprinted with permission from Mary Ann Liebert, Inc.

BOX 6–1.   Twelve Days in May: Diary of a Mother of a Nine-Year-Old Bipolar Child

5/11   Hypomanic, bizarre evening. "I hate me; kill me; Why am I like this?" Very rough with younger brother.

5/12   Good morning, dropped off well at school. Pretty good mood coming off bus, but more defiance in the afternoon. Uneventful evening. Went to bed well.

5/13   Up early, dressed well, good mood but problems on the bus. Kids teasing him. Teacher called and reported very bizarre behavior at school. She also reported a lot of ADHD symptoms—very fidgety, unable to remain seated in the afternoon, cruises around classroom, ran out of classroom, pestering other kids, unable to follow directions, not remaining on task or completing work.

5/14   Teacher reported a great day in school. Good mood after school.

5/15   Good A.M.—off to school well. Very defiant after school. Angered by new doctor. Got very angry in car—punching me, destructive to car, scribbling on dashboard, dumping over trash. Had to be restrained in office—punching, kicking, swearing—settled down at end of meeting and apologized.

5/16   Happy mood in A.M., but doing goofy, impulsive things—squirted water on dad's work shirt, squirted water on table and floor. Very aggressive after school—threatening me, hitting, increase in defiance. Aggressive toward other students.

5/17   Had a good time with grandparents. Crying a lot in the afternoon.

5/18   "Mixed," very irritable to hypomanic—increase in goal-directed activities, very easily frustrated and angered.

5/19   Good and uneventful day.

5/20   Very irritable in A.M.—threatened father—said: "I'm going to kill you someday." Manic after school—very goal-directed—taking all the tools out of the basement to use up in his room (hammer, sander, drill, staple gun). Very angry when I intervened—very loud, shouting, laughing, singing, dancing, "I don't feel good today. I want to kill myself. When I grow up, I am going to kill myself because being bipolar is bad." Hallucinating in afternoon—auditory and visual; goblin, clown, queen. "I hear the devil, I hear penises in your brain, Mom." Very hyperactive, and not rational. Gave him Risperdal and he went to sleep.

5/21   Hypomanic, happy in the afternoon.

5/22   Woke up laughing—found some needlepoint yarn and needles under the bed. "I'm giving myself a lab test"—trying to stick needles into his arm. Giddy, shouting "hubba, hubba, hubba, howdy, howdy" over and over again, very wound up. Settled down and watched some TV. Pleasant and more normal, but talkative in the afternoon. Easier to please. More irritable after dinner. Fascinated with knives, demonstrated how he would stab a wolf. Very quiet in my lap. He said: "I love you, Mom. You don't love me, you want me to die. I will if you want me to."

Source: Papolos and Papolos, 2002, pp. 22–23. © 2002 by Demitri Papolos and Janice Papolos. Used with permission of Broadway Books, a division of Random House, Inc.

Depressive Features

For many individuals, bipolar disorder first emerges in the form of depressive episodes in childhood (e.g., Geller et al., 1994; Lish et al., 1994). Although depression in children may be readily diagnosed using adult criteria, the majority of such cases probably go undetected and untreated. Even if they are detected, however, there is presently no certain way of knowing the extent to which early-onset depression presages childhood-onset bipolar disorder; the issue is an important question not only clinically but for research as well.

As noted previously, studies of bipolar illness have often combined childhood- and adolescent-onset populations, and longitudinal studies of the outcomes of depression in children have been rare. Given that unipolar depression in children is substantially more prevalent than mania and is characterized by marked clinical and etiological heterogeneity, it is difficult to identify predictors specific

to eventual bipolarity. Wozniak and colleagues (2004) compared 109 children with unipolar depression and 43 children with bipolar depression (all had been diagnosed with ADHD as well) and found that the bipolar children were more severely depressed and anhedonic, were more often suicidal, expressed greater hopelessness, and were more likely to need medication and hospitalization. They also had higher rates of comorbidity with conduct disorder, oppositional defiant disorder, agoraphobia, obsessive-compulsive disorder, and alcohol abuse (see Chapter 7 for a detailed discussion of comorbidity in bipolar disorder). A family history of bipolar disorder was more than twice as likely in the bipolar group as in the unipolar children (20 versus 8 percent).

Most follow-up studies of depressed children have yielded little information on predictors of bipolarity because of the limited size of samples that have converted to a bipolar course. Recently, Luby and Mrakotsky (2003) attempted to identify differences in symptoms among depressed preschoolers with and without a family history of bipolar disorder. Only one symptom (restlessness/"moves around a lot") distinguished the groups, but its association with the emergence of bipolarity remains to be seen. Geller and colleagues (1994) found that among a sample of 79 severely depressed children (ages 6 to 12), 32 percent switched to bipolar-I or bipolar-II during a 2- to 5-year follow-up. When the same subjects were recontacted in young adulthood (mean age 21), 49 percent were found to have switched to bipolar disorder, including 33 percent with bipolar-I (Geller et al., 2001b). The authors found that parental and grandparental mania was a significant predictor of bipolar switching.

Unfortunately, this information has sometimes been misstated. Although Geller and colleagues (2001b) did indeed find a 33 percent rate of switching to bipolar-I disorder among their severely depressed sample of children, their sample may be atypical and perhaps biased by high rates of referral for suspected bipolar disorder. The rate of switching is likely to be substantially lower in more typical outpatient samples. For instance, Weissman and colleagues (1999b) followed up on outpatient children with prepubertal depression an average of 11 years later, and found that only 6 percent had developed bipolar disorder, although this rate was much higher than that among comparison groups. Lewinsohn and colleagues (2000) found that fewer than 1 percent of adolescents with depression in a community sample switched to bipolar disorder. Differences in rates among these studies are likely due to differing diagnostic and exclusion criteria in the samples. Most clinical samples are small and can be greatly affected by variations in level of severity; family history of bipolar disorder; use of alcohol, stimulants, antidepressants, or other drugs; and other unspecified or unknown factors. Clearly, further research is needed on the predictors of switching among depressed children so as not to exaggerate, or even mislabel, bipolarity in children, yet provide accurate information to enable early treatment of those who truly have or are likely to develop the illness.

Diagnostic Controversies

Despite general agreement that bipolar disorder can emerge in childhood, several problems make it difficult to validate some of the assertions made about diagnosis of bipolar children. Three related issues are discussed here: comorbidity and indistinct diagnostic boundaries, the validity and meaning of a diagnosis of mania, and the lack of developmental guidelines.

Comorbidity and Indistinct Diagnostic Boundaries

As noted earlier, the great majority of cases of childhood-onset bipolar disorder also meet criteria for other disorders, including ADHD, conduct disorder, and oppositional defiant disorder.[2] Findings of the major studies of comorbidity in childhood-onset bipolar disorder are presented in Table 6–2. As can be seen in the table, many clinical investigations have documented a high rate of comorbid anxiety disorders as well.[3] (There is some indication that bipolar-II children and adolescents, like adults, are more likely to have comorbid anxiety disorders than those with bipolar-I disorder [Axelson et al., 2006].) Perhaps nothing has fueled the controversy as much as the potentially confusing overlap of symptoms between mania and disruptive behavioral disorders.

Many studies have shown that children with a bipolar diagnosis have a high probability of being diagnosed with ADHD. Geller and colleagues (2000a), for example, found this to be the case in 98 percent of their sample (see also Biederman et al., 2000a; Sachs et al., 2000; Spencer et al., 2001). Considerably lower rates have been found by other researchers, however (Masi et al., 2003; Faedda et al., 2004; Jaideep et al., 2006). Some investigators have argued that many children diagnosed with ADHD also have bipolar disorder. Biederman and colleagues (1996) identified psychiatrically referred children with ADHD, who were then assessed for the presence of mania at baseline and at 1 and 4 years later. Bipolar disorder was diagnosed in 11 percent of the ADHD children at baseline and in an additional 12 percent at the 4-year follow-up. Arguing that a substantial number of children diagnosed with ADHD may actually have unrecognized bipolar disorder, Biederman fueled a controversy that is still active (Wozniak et al., 1995; Faraone et al., 1997b; Biederman, 1998). Many investigators have also observed high rates of conduct disorder and oppositional defiant disorder (e.g., Biederman et al., 2000a; Geller et al., 2000b; Wozniak et al., 2001), as well as substance abuse and anxiety disorders (e.g., Birmaher et al., 2002), among bipolar children (see also reviews in Biederman et al., 2000a, and Papolos, 2003).

What is the meaning of the overlap between mania and ADHD (or other disruptive behavior disorders)? There are several different perspectives on this question. One general argument is that the comorbidity is simply an artifact of overlapping symptomatology. Three more specific arguments are that the ADHD–mania overlap is (1) true comorbidity (coexistence of separate disorders), potentially marking a genetically mediated subtype; (2) artifactual, reflecting severe psychopathology that is not specifically bipolar; and (3) artifactual, possibly reflecting a developmental manifestation of bipolar disorder in children.

The general argument that bipolar comorbidity may be a result of overlap of symptoms suggests that diagnostic inaccuracies are caused by indistinct symptom boundaries, clinician bias, or biased diagnostic expectations due to ascertainment source. Biederman and his colleagues at

TABLE 6–2. Comorbidities in Samples of Bipolar Children

Characteristic	Faraone et al., 1997a (child outpatient)	Carlson and Kelly, 1998 (child inpatient)	Tillman et al., 2003 (child outpatient)
Sample size	68	60	93
Source of sample	Outpatient psychopharmacology clinic	Children's inpatient unit	Research study, outpatient
Assessment used	KSADS	KSADS	WASH-U KSADS
Mean age (yrs)	7.9	8.7	10.9
% Male	78	91	61
Comorbidities			
% ADHD	93	66	87
% ODD/CD	91/38	75/54	79
% OCD	10		
Anxiety disorders	56	14	23 syndromal
% substance abuse disorders	—	None	Not stated
% psychosis	31	10	Not stated
% no comorbidity	Not stated	0	Not stated
% With >1 diagnosis	Probably high	Average: 3 diagnoses	98 (≥4 diagnoses: 20.4)

ADHD=attention-deficit hyperactivity disorder; KSADS=Kiddie Schedule for Affective Disorders and Schizophrenia; OCD=obsessive-compulsive disorder; ODD/CD=oppositional defiant disorder/conduct disorder; WASH-U KSADS=Washington University at St. Louis modification of KSADS.

Source: Updated from Geller et al., 1999. Reprinted with permission.

Massachusetts General Hospital studied large numbers of children with comorbid ADHD and bipolar disorder. They argued, through the use of various diagnostic algorithms, that the presence of the two separate diagnoses was valid and was not a result of overlapping symptoms such as talkativeness, hyperactivity–psychomotor agitation, or distractibility (e.g., Milberger et al., 1995; reviewed in Spencer et al., 2001). Moreover, Biederman and colleagues (1998) found that children with comorbid diagnoses of mania and ADHD ascertained from ADHD clinics and from a study of mania differed minimally in symptoms of either mania or ADHD.

Additionally, Biederman and colleagues (2004c) hypothesized that the comorbid combination of the two disorders may mark an etiological subtype. In family–genetic studies, Faraone and colleagues (1997b) found that first-degree relatives of children with bipolar disorder and ADHD had both disorders at rates greater than would be expected by chance alone. On the basis of these and other family patterns observed across several studies, they posited that the combination of ADHD and bipolar disorder is familially distinct and may be a marker of a subtype of very early–onset bipolarity.

Geller and colleagues (1998a, 2002b) also found high rates of comorbid ADHD and bipolar disorder. ADHD occurred among 97 percent of prepubertal bipolar children and 74 percent of bipolar adolescents. Even with ADHD, the bipolar children were distinctly different from ADHD-only children in symptoms of mania, as illustrated in Figure 6–1 (Geller et al., 1998b). As noted earlier, in a study comparing 93 participants with childhood- and early-adolescent–onset mania, 81 with ADHD and no mania, and 94 community controls, Geller and colleagues (2002b) found that, despite the high rate of ADHD–bipolar comorbidity, five symptoms distinguished most clearly between bipolar and ADHD samples: elation, grandiosity, flight of ideas/racing thoughts, decreased need for sleep, and hypersexuality. These findings appear to argue against the possibility that ADHD comorbidity is an artifact of overlapping symptoms—provided, as noted later, that children otherwise meet the full criteria for mania in DSM-IV.

Whereas Biederman and colleagues (1996) argued that the combination of ADHD and bipolar disorder in children marks a subtype of bipolar disorder, Geller and colleagues (1998a) suggested that ADHD in child bipolar samples may be a "phenocopy" ADHD, driven by developmentally prevalent high energy in children. That is, high energy combined with emerging bipolar symptoms promotes the hyperactivity, impulsivity, and attentional problems that are viewed as ADHD. Geller predicted that the

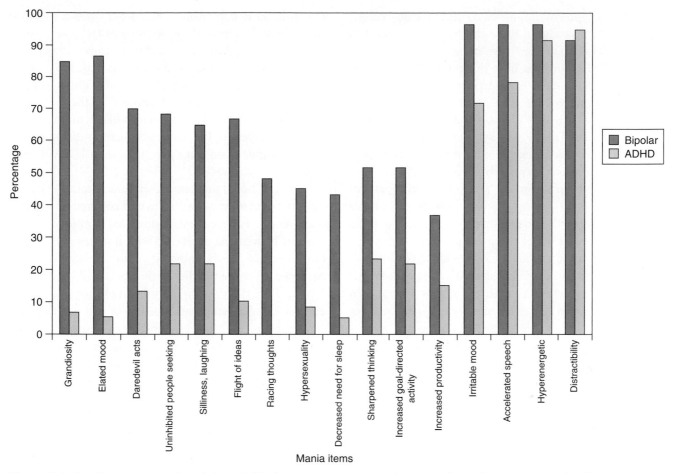

Figure 6–1. Baseline percentage of mania items in bipolar versus ADHD groups. (*Source:* Geller et al., 1998a. Reprinted with permission from Elsevier.)

ADHD will "decrease" to population levels by adulthood (e.g., Geller and Luby, 1997). Thus, ADHD may be a prodrome or developmentally expressed version of bipolarity in some children, rather than a separate disorder. Obviously, prospective longitudinal follow-up of samples of young bipolar patients would help resolve such diagnostic issues through clarification of clinical course and outcome (see reviews by Kim and Miklowitz, 2002; Kent and Craddock, 2003).

While it is doubtless likely that comorbid conditions can obscure the recognition of an underlying bipolar illness, the complex symptomatology involved may also have the opposite effect: clinicians are urged to consider bipolar disorder as an explanation for diffuse and difficult symptoms. A widely visible Web site for bipolar disorder in children, for example, listed the following as possible symptoms, among others more specific to typical mania: explosive, lengthy, and often destructive rages; separation anxiety; defiance of authority; hyperactivity, agitation, and distractibility; bed-wetting and night terrors; strong and frequent cravings; and daredevil behaviors.[4] Obviously,

although such symptoms may occur in children with bipolar disorder, each is also nonspecific. Precise diagnostic definitions that can help separate truly bipolar manifestations from overlapping conditions are needed to avoid misdiagnosis, as well as to facilitate recognition of bipolar illness.

Questions about the Validity of the Diagnosis of Mania in Children

Is severe behavioral dysregulation "mania," and does "mania" always mean bipolar disorder? Multiple, intense, and severe symptoms may be caused by brain injury, other forms of organic disorder (e.g., Carlson and Kelly, 1998), or severe disinhibition related to adverse medication responses (Carlson and Mick, 2003) (see also Chapter 3). Carlson (1998) noted that, in the child psychiatry literature, several nonspecific terms—such as "multidimensionally impaired" and "multiple complex developmental disorder"—are used to describe children with numerous, severe, disruptive behaviors that do not fit any typical diagnostic picture, as well as children suffering from some forms of head injury, pervasive developmental disorder, or other medical conditions. In the past, some of these children were labeled as "minimally brain damaged" or "hyperkinetic." Many of these historical syndromes have been described in terms that bear a marked resemblance to contemporary descriptions of childhood mania.

A related issue raised by Carlson and others is the possibility that mania or manic-like symptoms may occur as a dimension of disorder or serve as a marker of severe psychopathology without necessarily indicating the presence of a bipolar syndrome. Carlson and colleagues (1998) recruited a sample of boys aged 6 to 10 who had heterogeneous disruptive and/or depressive symptoms. The boys' mothers were asked about the presence of manic symptoms, and their responses led the researchers to distinguish three groups: those boys with at least two manic symptoms, and two matched comparison groups—those seen immediately next in the series of interviews but without manic symptoms, and those matched on the first group's comorbid disruptive symptoms (conduct disorder, ADHD, or oppositional defiant disorder) but without manic symptoms. The authors found that although the boys with symptoms of mania differed significantly from the nonmanic "next" control group, most of those differences disappeared in a comparison with the group with comorbid conditions. The presence of manic symptoms uniquely predicted significant emotionality and generally predicted more severe psychopathology (Carlson and Youngstrom, 2003). The investigators are continuing to study these children over time, attempting to determine whether some are truly bipolar, while in others the manic-like symptoms may serve mainly as markers for "behavioral and emotional multimorbidity." Similarly, Hazell and colleagues (2003) followed up boys aged 9 to 13 who met criteria for ADHD plus mania. When the boys were reevaluated after 6 years, there were no clear cases of bipolar disorder among those with prior manic symptoms; however, the boys with earlier manic symptoms had lower overall global functioning.

Geller and colleagues (2002) have reoperationalized several of the DSM criteria (most notably euphoria and grandiosity) to make them what the authors believe to be developmentally appropriate for children. Not everyone agrees with this reformulation, however (Harrington and Myatt, 2003). In a recent cross-national (United States and United Kingdom) study of five cases of children with mood symptoms in whom bipolar disorder might have been a diagnostic consideration, disagreement on diagnosis occurred in three of the five cases. The reason for this appears to be differing interpretations of specific symptoms. DSM's reliance on symptom counts (used in the United States) may result in a conceptualization that differs from the gestalt of bipolar disorder as described in the International Classification of Diseases (ICD)-10, used in the United Kingdom. Specifically, in a preadolescent patient with classic mania, agreement was close (96.4 percent of United States and 88.9 percent of United Kingdom physicians made a manic diagnosis). In the prepubertal child with both ADHD and manic-like symptoms, however, 86.2 percent of U.S. child psychiatrists diagnosed mania, in contrast to only 31.1 percent of their U.K. colleagues (Dubicka et al., 2005).

It may be noted that among adolescent samples in community populations, Lewinsohn and colleagues (1995) and Klein and colleagues (1996) observed manic-like symptoms or hypomania associated with impairment and various forms of psychopathology. Upon follow-up at age 24, those diagnosed earlier with bipolar disorder (mostly bipolar-II or cyclothymia) continued to show recurrent or chronic bipolar symptoms, but few of those with adolescent "subclinical" bipolar symptoms of mania/hypomania had developed full-blown bipolar disorder (Lewinsohn et al., 2000). Overall, studies of manic symptoms in children and adolescents may indicate true bipolar disorder in some cases, but in other cases these symptoms may be mainly markers for severe emotionality and disruptive behaviors.

Finally, a significant issue in the diagnosis of mania concerns the duration of affective cycles. Many children labeled "bipolar" may have numerous mood shifts within a day and have chronic symptoms and impairments not consistent with the adult concept of "episodes." As noted by Leibenluft and colleagues (2003a), in the absence of validated criteria for the duration of an episode in children, some investigators have defined episodes to be as brief as a few hours. Leibenluft and colleagues (2003b) suggested that within such brief periods, it is quite difficult to determine whether episodes are accompanied by the required DSM-IV criterion B changes in behavior. Thus, investigators' and parents' subjective impressions may be used to make diagnoses, contributing to the diagnostic confusion and heterogeneity in research samples. Tillman and Geller (2003) have proposed specific definitions of rapid, ultrarapid, and ultradian cycling, as well as distinctions between episodes and cycles. If used systematically in research, such definitions might help characterize the course of illness in bipolar children and contribute to diagnostic validity.

Lack of Data and Insufficient Knowledge of Developmental Issues

A further challenge to diagnosing bipolar disorder in children is the limited utility of applying to this population features of adult bipolar symptoms and course. Diagnostic confusion about how to interpret specific symptoms (e.g., hyperactivity, irritability) arises in part from developmental considerations for which little information is presently available. As Carlson (1998) noted, many of the other features of bipolar syndrome, such as grandiosity and elation, have not been systematically defined in developmentally appropriate and precise ways or evaluated in context. Simply hearing a child utter the words "I can fly," for instance, without considering the child's developmental stage and environmental context, could lead clinicians to misinterpret the statement as indicating grandiosity when it means nothing of the kind. Geller and colleagues (2002b) would argue that such states can be distinguished from normal childhood experiences; however, the issue must not hinge only on the experience and skill of a researcher or clinician, but rather on developmentally informed and validated criteria.

An intriguing suggestion that symptoms of bipolar disorder may have a developmental progression has been made by Post and colleagues (2002). These investigators studied three volunteer samples of parents: those with children who had been diagnosed with bipolar disorder or with psychiatric (nonbipolar) disorders, and those who were not ill. The parents were asked to identify their children's symptoms retrospectively during each year of life. Ages at which children displayed empirically derived clusters of symptoms were compared for the three groups. It appeared that among the bipolar children, an irritability–dyscontrol factor (e.g., impulsivity, tantrums, aggression, hyperactivity), emerging at age 1 to 3 years, was the first feature to distinguish among the groups. A depression factor began to differentiate the bipolar children from others by age 8 to 12. A mania factor (e.g., racing thoughts, grandiosity, mood elevations, bizarre behavior) did not begin to differentiate the bipolar children until ages 7 to 12, whereas a distinguishing psychosis–suicidality factor emerged at ages 9 to 12. Despite significant methodological limitations (including a lack of confirmatory diagnosis of the bipolar children, a mixed-disorder comparison group, and parental retrospective accounts), this study highlights the need for further investigation of the possible developmental progression of manifestations of bipolar symptoms.

Researchers have also urged further study of child-appropriate definitions of mania, as well as attention to traits and behaviors that may represent prodromal or subsyndromal forms of bipolar disorder (Shaffer, 2002; Coyle et al., 2003; Carlson, 2005). As we argue later, studies of children of bipolar parents may be an especially fruitful way to help identify some of the early indicators of mania and progression of symptoms in children known to be at risk for bipolar disorder.

Finally, it may be noted that boys tend to predominate in research samples of bipolar children (e.g., Faraone et al.,

1997b; Geller et al., 1998b). Indeed, this is true for most forms of childhood disorder, particularly disruptive disorders (ADHD, oppositional defiant disorder, conduct disorder), but also anxiety and depression prior to adolescence. Thus, gender differences may not be remarkable in young samples. In a study of 298 bipolar patients under the age of 18, Biederman and colleagues (2004a) found few significant differences in clinical features between males and females, although males were more likely to have ADHD as well as bipolar disorder; they were also less likely to have a chronic course. On the other hand, it is possible that this gender distribution in research samples signals under-recognition of mania in girls, inasmuch as they tend to be less aggressive and therefore may not attract as much attention as boys exhibiting destructive and risk-taking behaviors. Also, girls' initial mood disorder may more often be depression rather than mania. Therefore, developmental studies of bipolar disorder and manic symptoms need to address gender-relevant manifestations.

Current Suggestions for Assessment and Diagnosis of Bipolar Disorder in Children

In view of the varied opinions and relative paucity of data on assessment and diagnosis of bipolar disorder in children—and mindful of the high stakes involved in terms of accurate detection and early treatment—the National Institute of Mental Health (NIMH) convened the Bipolar Child Research Roundtable in 2000 (NIMH Research Roundtable on Prepubertal Bipolar Disorder, 2001) to share information and make recommendations. The roundtable members recommended that children who clearly meet current DSM-IV criteria for symptoms of bipolar-I or bipolar-II disorder—including core symptoms of grandiosity and/or elation (e.g., Geller et al., 2000a)—be distinguished from those with heterogeneous presentations who do not meet the full criteria but suffer from mood and behavior disturbances (prototypically, irritability or rage episodes) and severe impairment and *may* have bipolar disorder (e.g., Carlson et al., 1998; Biederman et al., 2000b). It was recommended that the latter be diagnosed as bipolar–not otherwise specified (NOS). The roundtable members noted that both of these groups are likely to have mixed states, chronic symptomatology, or long episodes with ultradian or continuous cycling. They speculated that many if not most suspected cases of bipolar disorder in children would be diagnosed bipolar-NOS, with a minority representing classic bipolar-I disorder. They also recommended that children be evaluated by clinicians who are well trained in mood disorders in youth, although there is a scarcity of such training (e.g., Coyle et al., 2003). The *Treatment Guidelines for Children and Adolescents with Bipolar Disorder,* published by the Child Psychiatric Workgroup on Bipolar Disorder, additionally stresses the importance of interviewing at least one parent, and ideally both; obtaining comprehensive school and medical histories; and encouraging family members to keep daily logs of the child's mood, energy, sleep, and unusual behaviors in the 2 weeks before the first visit to the clinician (Kowatch et al., 2005).

Leibenluft and colleagues (2003b) have suggested even further distinctions to improve the validation of diagnostic criteria for childhood bipolar disorder, proposing a phenotypic system of four categories ranging from narrow- to broadband subtypes. Their narrow phenotype includes the classic hallmark symptoms (e.g., elevated mood, grandiosity) and full-duration episodes. This phenotype is distinct from ADHD, despite overlapping symptoms, because ADHD is not episodic, and the associated symptoms occur only during hypomanic or manic episodes. At the broadest end of the spectrum, the system includes many children who are currently labeled as bipolar but do not meet criteria for the authors' narrower definitions. These children have severe mood and behavioral dysregulation, chronic hyperarousal, and negative reactivity to emotional stimuli, including severe rages, with no intervening periods of normal mood or adaptive functioning. Between these narrow and broad extremes lie two intermediate phenotypes: (hypo)mania-NOS, including hallmark symptoms but short episodes (although lasting at least 1 to 3 days), and irritable (hypo)mania, lacking elevated or expansive mood but with distinct episodes that meet DSM-IV duration criteria. Thus far, however, there are limited data to support these distinctions. Whether the proposal of Leibenluft and colleagues proves useful or not, it clearly addresses the crucial need for more homogeneous research samples that can help clarify and validate the construct of bipolar disorder in children.

Course of Disorder

Children diagnosed with bipolar disorder typically do not display course features commonly associated with classic bipolar disorder in adults, such as distinct mood episodes that endure for days or weeks (often clearly manic or depressive) separated by periods of being relatively well. Instead, bipolar children frequently display mixed mood states, extremely rapid cycling, and chronic psychopathology. The controversy over diagnostic criteria, including duration of episodes in children with purported bipolar disorder, is discussed further below.

Faraone and colleagues (1997b) found mixed states in 59 percent of children diagnosed with bipolar disorder, while Geller and colleagues (2002a) reported a rate of 55 percent. Geller's group (2002b) found that 87 percent of their sample had ultradian cycles (variation within a 24-hour period). Moreover, these children were chronically ill and

had been mood-disordered for an average of more than 3 years before entering the study. Craney and Geller (2003) concluded that typical youngsters with childhood-onset bipolar disorder in their sample were more severely ill than typical individuals with young adult–onset mania, and much more likely to display mixed mania, ultradian cycling, psychosis, and treatment resistance. Biederman and colleagues (2004a) found that the course of pediatric bipolar disorder was severe and chronic and was frequently characterized by severely impaired psychosocial functioning; they also observed chronic symptomatology in their bipolar–ADHD sample (Biederman et al., 1998). A prospective follow-up study of pediatric bipolar disorder in 22 boys with comorbid ADHD found that although 50 percent had remitted from the full syndrome of bipolar disorder at follow-up, 80 percent had failed to attain functional remission or euthymia over a course of 10 years (Biederman et al., 2004a). The course of the disorder, the investigators concluded, was "chronic, protracted, and dysfunctional" (p. 521). Many other investigators also have found that early onset of bipolar illness is associated with a poorer course (Carlson et al., 2002; Schneck et al., 2004; Birmaher et al., 2006). Some have argued that there may be periods of exacerbation of manic symptoms despite interepisode persistence of less severe mania, as is the case for many adult bipolar patients (Staton and Lysne, 1999).

Longitudinal research on the course of the disorder among carefully diagnosed bipolar children is sparse and greatly needed. Geller and colleagues (2000a) found 1-year mania recovery rates of 37 percent in their combined sample of youngsters with childhood- and early-adolescent–onset bipolar disorder, and substantial relapse rates within the year among those who recovered. At 2-year follow-up, the recovery rate was 65 percent, but 55 percent of those who had recovered relapsed (Geller et al., 2002a; Craney and Geller, 2003).

Thus the few outcome studies of childhood bipolar illness that exist indicate a highly pernicious course with substantial chronicity. Findling and colleagues (2001), for example, found that none of the 56 bipolar-I children they studied had interepisode recovery (defined as a 2-month period of remission of affective symptoms). Further longitudinal research is needed, however, to learn more about long-term course and outcome in children and their predictors, as well as to resolve some of the perplexing diagnostic issues in childhood bipolar disorder discussed above.

ADOLESCENT-ONSET BIPOLAR DISORDER

The onset and first diagnosis of bipolar disorder frequently occur in adolescence. For the most part, adolescent-onset bipolar disorder is clinically similar to adult bipolar disorder. Until recently, however, relatively little research had been conducted in adolescent populations.

Despite current awareness, adolescent bipolarity often was not recognized as such in the past. Diagnostic errors were common, reflecting biases of the time. These biases included the above-noted reluctance to accept the existence of youthful onset of bipolar disorder and a common tendency to assume that psychotic symptoms such as thought disorder, grandiosity, and bizarre delusional and hallucinatory phenomena are pathognomonic of schizophrenia (Carlson and Goodwin, 1973). Additionally, morbid preoccupations, frenzied behavior, moodiness or rapid mood swings, irritability, defiance, and a host of other disturbances were often regarded as exaggerations, if not typical manifestations, of adolescence. As discussed earlier, moreover, even when recognized as clearly pathological, disturbed behaviors in youths have been difficult to distinguish from alcohol and drug abuse disorders, conduct and other disruptive behavior disorders, and personality disorders. These diagnostic challenges remain today.

In recent years, however, several factors have contributed to the increased recognition and accurate diagnosis of adolescent bipolar disorder. These factors include greater awareness of the existence of severe mood pathology in adolescents, improved diagnostic criteria and interview methods for identifying depression and mania in younger populations, and increased availability of effective pharmacological and psychotherapeutic treatments for mood disorders. Increasingly, adult diagnostic criteria are being applied reliably and effectively to the diagnosis of bipolar disorder in adolescents. There is a general consensus that adolescent-onset bipolar disorder is a relatively common presentation and that, as noted, it essentially resembles the disorder in adults.

Symptoms and Clinical Presentation

Diagnosis

Adolescent onset of bipolar-I disorder may first present with major depression, mania, or a mixed state. The diagnosis is typically defined by DSM-IV criteria or by equivalent criteria used for adults (see Chapter 3; see also McClellan and Werry, 1997; Lewinsohn et al., 2003). Manic episodes, of course, provide the most unambiguous indicator of bipolar disorder. Symptoms such as elated mood, grandiosity, excessive activity, decreased need for sleep, hypersexuality, and racing thoughts are similar in both adolescents and adults, with differences only in developmental presentation. Geller and Luby (1997), for example, described grandiose beliefs in adolescents who, despite a lack of talent, believe they can become a rock star; whose excessive

activity takes the form of making curtains, illustrating a book, rearranging furniture, and making multiple phone calls all within a relatively brief period; or whose reduced need for sleep may take the form of sneaking out and partying all night. Engagement in high-risk pleasurable activities may involve a heightened interest in sex and risky sexual experiences, excessive spending through the use of parents' credit cards, taking dares, or driving more recklessly than their peers.

The assessment of bipolar illness in adolescents can be complicated. Tillman and colleagues (2004) found poor concordance between the symptom descriptions given by parents and offspring. Children and adolescents, for example, report the presence of racing thoughts and decreased need for sleep significantly more than do their parents, perhaps reflecting the reality that external and disruptive behaviors are more likely to be noted by parents. Other investigators have found high rates of bipolar spectrum in young people with recurrent depression (Smith et al., 2005), findings consistent with those of studies showing that adults with bipolar disorder tend to underreport hypomanic symptoms and impairment (Angst et al., 2003; Judd and Akiskal, 2003; Youngstrom et al., 2004). Supplemental assessment measures, such as the General Behavior Inventory and the Young Mania Rating Scale, add to diagnostic validity (Youngstrom et al., 2001, 2003; Findling et al., 2002). (See Chapter 11 for a more detailed discussion.)

Manic Features

Although the phenomenology of adolescent-onset mania has been studied incompletely, existing research clearly indicates a heterogeneity that may reflect different subgroups. Pooled data from several investigations of mania in adolescents have revealed pressured speech, euphoria, and hyperactivity to be the most common symptoms, similar to what has been found for adults (Faedda et al., 1995). Lewinsohn and colleagues (1995) noted a much higher frequency of elevated–expansive mood than irritability in their community sample (which, however, consisted primarily of those with bipolar spectrum rather than bipolar-I disorder). Faraone and colleagues (1997b), on the other hand, found relatively high rates of irritability and low rates of euphoria in their clinical sample of young manic patients. Both the Lewinsohn and Faraone subjects reported high rates of increased activity, grandiosity, and distractibility.

In an analysis of the symptoms of mania in 115 adolescents with manic or subsyndromal manic episodes, Lewinsohn and colleagues (1995) identified two factors: (1) behavioral disorganization, consisting of decreased need for sleep, flight of ideas, distractibility, and poor judgment; and (2) inflated self-esteem and increased activity. The former factor was correlated more highly than the latter with functional impairment (school, family, and social), and the authors speculated that individuals scoring high on this factor might be more likely to experience psychotic symptoms during severe manic episodes. Even in adolescents with only subthreshold bipolar disorder, Lewinsohn and colleagues (2003) noted substantial impairment, comorbidity, and increased risk of suicide attempts (18 percent, compared with 3 percent in never mentally ill controls).

Mania in adolescents often includes psychotic features (see Chapter 2). Several studies have found that between one third and one half of adolescent bipolar patients have prominent psychotic symptoms.[5] Kafantaris and colleagues (1998) found that half of the bipolar youths in their study who presented with psychotic mania had no prior psychiatric history and appeared to have experienced an acute onset after having functioned relatively well to that point. The authors suggested that this sudden-onset, psychotic subgroup may represent "classic" bipolar disorder. A recent study of 43 bipolar adolescents found that, in most, the prodromal onset was either slow with gradual deterioration (47 percent) or slow with quick worsening (39 percent). Rapid onset of illness was relatively uncommon (14 percent) (Correll et al., 2005). There is suggestive evidence that there are ethnic differences in psychotic features expressed during mania. A recent study compared clinical features in 17 bipolar African American adolescents and 61 bipolar Caucasian adolescents. Fully 90 percent of the African Americans had psychotic symptoms, as compared with only 30 percent of the Caucasian adolescents (p < .001) (Patel et al., 2006). These results are consistent with differences found between Caucasian and African American adult bipolar patients (Strakowski et al., 1996; Kirovetal, 1999).

Mixed mania and rapid-cycling mania are also common in those adolescents with bipolar disorder. Kutcher and colleagues (1998) studied a small, carefully ascertained clinical sample of 28 bipolar-I youths and found that the majority had mixed mania (74 percent), rapid cycling (76 percent), or both during their first (retrospectively assessed) episode. Fewer than 10 percent of the sample demonstrated a classic euphoric mania during their initial manic episode. Mixed episodes were reported by Faraone and colleagues (1997b) in 71 percent of a sample of 17 patients with adolescent onset of mania. McElroy and colleagues (1997) found that adolescents with bipolar disorder had a higher frequency of mixed episodes than was the case among comparison adult bipolar patients, but the investigators did not distinguish between childhood and adolescent onset in their adolescent sample. Findling and colleagues (2001) compared 56 children and 34 adolescents

with bipolar-I disorder and found that 56 percent of the adolescents had rapid cycling and 21 percent mixed states; proportions among children with bipolar-I disorder were similar. However, many of the adolescents with bipolar disorder in that study appeared to have had childhood onset. Finally, Strober and colleagues (1995) reported that the index episode in their inpatient sample (which was the first episode in 56 percent of the cases studied) was mixed in 19 percent and rapid cycling in 19 percent, with the other cases being "pure" depression or mania. An unresolved issue is whether rapid cycling or mixed states are particularly associated with bipolar adolescents with childhood onset, a typical developmental manifestation of bipolar illness in young people, or a subtype of bipolar-I disorder marking a course that may differ from more "classic" cycling episodes.

Depressive Features

For a substantial number if not the majority of individuals with adolescent-onset bipolar disorder, the illness starts with depression, thereby delaying recognition and diagnosis of the bipolar course. Kutcher and colleagues (1998) found that depressions were the first affective episodes in 75 percent of their sample of adolescents with bipolar-I disorder. Likewise, a community sample of adolescents with bipolar spectrum disorders revealed that 61 percent had experienced an initial depressive episode before mania or hypomania occurred (Lewinsohn et al., 1995). And among those who responded to a volunteer survey of members of the National Depressive and Manic-Depressive Association (now called the Depression and Bipolar Support Alliance), both early age at onset (childhood or adolescence) and female gender were associated with higher rates of initial depressive symptoms or both depressive and manic symptoms (Lish et al., 1994). The studies of Kutcher and colleagues (1998) and Lewinsohn and colleagues (1995) did not evaluate initial symptom presentation by gender status.

The switch rate of adolescent major depression to eventual mania or hypomania is quite variable across studies. Interpretation of this variation is complicated by the above-noted common practice of mixing children and adolescents in the same study samples. For instance, in a review of seven studies of more than 250 depressed children and adolescents followed for 2 to 4 years, Faedda and colleagues (1995) found a mean rate of switch from depression to eventual mania of about 25 percent. A review by Kovacs (1996) yielded a switch range of 8 to 37 percent; her own longitudinal study of 92 depressed children followed for 5 to 10 years yielded a rate of 21 percent. More recently, Birmaher and colleagues (2006) conducted a 2-year prospective study of 263 children and adolescents (mean age 13 years) with bipolar-I (n=152), bipolar-II (n=19), and BP-NOS (n=92). Of the bipolar-II subjects, 21 percent converted to bipolar-I; 20 percent of the bipolar-NOS subjects converted to bipolar I, and 10 percent converted to bipolar-II. Females were more likely to convert than males (odds ratio, 3.2; 95 percent confidence interval [CI] 1.33–7.50). The findings are of considerable interest but somewhat difficult to interpret because of the mixed age range of the sample. Such variations in rates of switching among studies may depend on the mean age and age ranges of the sample, the diagnostic criteria used, the ascertainment source (that is, whether the study involved community, outpatient, or inpatient populations), and the extent to which the initial depressive episode was treated with antidepressants (see Chapter 23). In contrast to the high switch rate in Kovacs' childhood sample, for instance, Weissman and colleagues (1999a) revisited 10 to 15 years later an outpatient sample that had been diagnosed with major depression during adolescence, and found that only 4.1 percent had developed bipolar-I disorder and 1.4 percent bipolar-II disorder. As discussed earlier, severe depression during childhood (rather than adolescence) may portend higher rates of eventual bipolarity (e.g., Geller et al., 1994).

Further studies are needed not just on adolescent depression switch rates, but also on characteristics that link adolescent and childhood depression to eventual bipolar disorder (e.g., State et al., 2002). Strober and Carlson (1982) studied 60 inpatient depressed adolescents and identified several features predictive of eventual bipolarity: rapid onset of the depressive episode, psychomotor retardation, psychotic features, family history of mood disorders (especially bipolar), and antidepressant-related onset of mania or hypomania. It should be noted, however, that a recent study of switching during a 2-year period among adults with first-onset psychotic depression showed no association of switching with medication use, earlier age at onset, or family history of bipolar disorder (DelBello et al., 2003). A 15-year follow-up study of 74 young adults hospitalized for major depression (average age 23) found that 27 percent of the study group had experienced at least one episode of hypomania and another 19 percent an episode of mania (Goldberg et al., 2001). Psychosis during the depressive episode was significantly correlated with a switch into manic states (see Chapter 19). Predicting bipolar switching in cases of adolescent depression is an important area for further study because of speculation that treatment with antidepressant medications in the absence of knowledge of underlying bipolarity precipitates switches from depression to mania or hypomania and predicts a more adverse course of bipolar disorder with rapid cycling (see Chapter 19).

Depressive symptoms in adolescents with bipolar disorder tend to be quite similar to those seen in adults, although psychotic features are more common in the younger age group (Carlson and Strober, 1979; Chambers et al., 1982; Friedman et al., 1983). Preoccupation with death and thoughts of suicide are common, and suicide attempts are frequent (see Box 6–2 for one 15-year-old bipolar girl's account of her experience during a suicidal depression). Lewinsohn and colleagues (2003), for example, found that 44 percent of the bipolar adolescents in their sample had attempted suicide; in comparison, 22 percent of the adolescents with major depression had attempted suicide, as had 18 percent of those with subsyndromal bipolar disorder syndrome (defined by the investigators as abnormally and persistently elevated, expansive, or irritable mood plus one other DSM-III-R manic symptom, but never having met criteria for full bipolar disorder).

Course of Disorder

Longitudinal studies of youths with bipolar-I disorder are rare; therefore, most data on the course of the illness come from retrospective accounts or short-term treatment outcome studies (e.g., Kafantaris et al., 1998; Kutcher et al., 1998). The latter studies certainly document the likelihood of further episodes and hospitalizations, but more information is needed to clarify the predictors of relatively better or worse outcomes and responsiveness to treatment in patients with adolescent onset.

Strober and colleagues (1995) conducted one of the few longitudinal studies, a 5-year naturalistic follow-up of 54 adolescents (mean age 16.0) who had been inpatients diagnosed with bipolar-I disorder (although age at first diagnosable episode was not reported). The rate of recovery from the index episode was high (96 percent), with only 2 of the patients failing to achieve recovery during the 5-year period. However, time to recovery was affected by the polarity of the index episode: median time to recovery was significantly longer for those who had pure depressive episodes (26 weeks) compared with those who had pure manic (9 weeks) or mixed (11 weeks) episodes. The majority (56 percent) of those who recovered remained free of major relapses during the follow-up period, and the probability of relapse did not vary by polarity of the index episode (although among those who had multiple relapses, most had mixed or cycling index episodes). Suicide attempts sufficient to require medical attention occurred in 20 percent of the adolescents during the 5-year follow-up (Strober et al., 1995). None of the clinical or demographic factors that were evaluated in the study significantly predicted relapse, and all participants were treated aggressively. Thus it is important to note that the information on course derived from this study cannot be generalized to untreated bipolar disorder in adolescents.

BOX 6–2.   **Drowning in My Personal Hell**

I'm being plunged into dark and murky waters
Someone or something is holding me there
I can't see—everything is black
I try to swim, to get away, back to the top, but the force
    is holding me too tight
Reluctantly I give up
I feel myself slipping down
Down, down, I am slipping down
My head aches with the pressure, but I keep sinking
With each inch, I grow colder
With each second, my lungs grow tighter
I pray to God to save me
There is no answer
I am deep now, buried under the layers of the sea
The water seems to be eating me
I wonder if I have entered Hell
All I want is to die
I want to relieve the pressure, the cold, the dark
I've already lost myself
My self is looking at me from above
She is miles from me
She is happy—she was me, but no more
It doesn't matter anymore
I'm not mad, not sad or scared
I am no one; I am nothing
I feel myself slipping down to the sea floor
And I watch shadows of the sun laugh at me as I die

—Katrina Skefos, 15-year-old girl with bipolar disorder. Reprinted with permission.

A 2-year prospective study of adolescent-onset psychotic disorders by McClellan and colleagues (1999) included a comparison of a small group of bipolar youths with patients who had schizophrenia. The results indicated that 50 percent of the bipolar youths had an episodic course, and 40 percent were chronically impaired (but fared significantly better than the schizophrenic youths). Rajeev and colleagues (2003) observed adolescent-onset patients with bipolar mania for 6 months; like Strober and colleagues (1995), but unlike McClellan and colleagues (1999), they found 96 percent recovery and very little chronicity. Recently, researchers at the University of Pittsburgh, Brown University, and the University of California-Los Angeles conducted a longitudinal study of 263 bipolar children and adolescents (13.0 ±3.1 years old); they interviewed their subjects on average every 35 weeks for 94.8 ±51.5 weeks using the Longitudinal Interval Follow-up Evaluation. Although two thirds of the subjects recovered

from the index episode, 50 percent had at least one syndromal recurrence (Birmaher et al., 2005b). Subjects were symptomatic for the majority (60 percent) of the follow-up period; almost one quarter (22 percent) of the time was spent in full syndromal episodes.

Additional research is needed on predictors of treatment responsiveness in bipolar adolescents (see Chapter 23). Moreover, given the potential for misdiagnosis of bipolar disorder in youths, further studies of the potentially adverse effects of antidepressant medications and stimulants used to treat ADHD are warranted (e.g., Soutullo et al., 2002).

Pre- and Postmorbid Adjustment and Functioning

Premorbid adjustment would appear to be an important clue to the possible presence of subclinical symptoms in childhood prior to the onset or diagnosis of bipolar disorder (see also Chapter 4). However, relatively few studies have reported information on prior adjustment. In the study by Kutcher and colleagues (1998), 90 percent of bipolar-I patients with adolescent onset had excellent or average peer relationships, and more than 60 percent had good to excellent academic achievement, before their diagnosis. Such findings suggest that many youths with adolescent-onset bipolar disorder have relatively good functioning before being diagnosed. In the study by McClellan and colleagues (1999), better premorbid functioning predicted higher levels of functioning over 2 years and was a more significant predictor than diagnosis in a sample of schizophrenic and bipolar adolescents.

Once initiated, however, the course of bipolar disorder in adolescents is associated with considerable impairment. Kutcher (2000) found that a bipolar-I adolescent-onset sample followed for a mean of 4.6 years after their initial manic episode had lower rates of high school graduation and lower full-scale IQ scores than those of unipolar and non-ill controls (see also Quackenbush et al., 1996). They also had significantly worse problems with peers and greater dissatisfaction with peer relationships than the comparison groups. Likewise, in a cross-sectional study that included adolescents with mania and distinguished between childhood and adolescent onset, Faraone and colleagues (1997a) found significantly worse functioning on most social, peer, recreational, and family variables, as well as school performance, among bipolar youths compared with normal controls. Few differences in functioning were observed between childhood- and adolescent-onset bipolar youths, except that manic adolescents generally had worse relationships with parents than did manic children. A recent comparison of 18 bipolar adolescents and 18 normal control subjects found that adolescents with bipolar

BOX 6–3.   One Adolescent's Experience with Bipolar Illness

The following is a first-person account of a hypomanic episode followed by severe depression in a 17-year-old girl. She went on to experience several further depressive and hypomanic episodes before becoming floridly manic in her 20s. This passage depicts the resilient recovery described by Carlson and Strober (1979), but it also underscores the disconcerting ability of some adolescents to continue the illusion of normal functioning even though seriously ill. It also illustrates many of the obscuring issues of adolescence and the effects of intense peer loyalties.

I was a senior in high school when I had my first attack of manic-depressive illness; once the siege began, I lost my mind rather rapidly. At first, everything seemed so easy. I raced about like a crazed weasel, bubbling with plans and enthusiasms, immersed in sports, and staying up all night, night after night, out with friends, reading everything that wasn't nailed down, filling manuscript books with poems and fragments of plays, and making expansive, completely unrealistic, plans for my future. The world was filled with pleasure and promise; I felt great. Not just great, I felt *really* great. I felt I could do anything, that no task was too difficult. My mind seemed clear, fabulously focused, and able to make intuitive mathematical leaps that had up to that point entirely eluded me. Indeed, they elude me still. At the time, however, not only did everything make perfect sense, but it all began to fit into a marvelous kind of cosmic relatedness. . . .

Unlike the very severe manic episodes that came a few years later and escalated wildly and psychotically out of control, this first sustained wave of mild mania was a light, lovely tincture of true mania; like hundreds of subsequent periods of high enthusiasms it was short-lived and quickly burned itself out; tiresome to my friends, perhaps; exhausting and exhilarating to me, definitely; but not disturbingly over the top. Then the bottom began to fall out of my life and mind. My thinking, far from being clearer than a crystal, was tortuous. I would read the same passage over and over again only to realize that I had no memory at all for what I just had read. Each book or poem I picked up was the same way. Incomprehensible. Nothing made sense. I could not begin to follow the material presented in my classes, and I would find myself staring out the window with no idea of what was going on around me. It was very frightening. . . .

Each day I awoke deeply tired, a feeling as foreign to my natural self as being bored or indifferent to life. Those were next. Then a gray, bleak preoccupation with death, dying, decaying, that everything was born but to die, best to die now and save the pain while waiting. I dragged exhausted mind and body around a local cemetery, ruminating about how long each of its inhabitants had lived before the final moment. I sat on the graves writing long, dreary, morbid poems, convinced that my brain and body were rotting, that everyone knew and no one would say. Laced into the exhaustion were periods of frenetic and horrible restlessness; no amount of running brought relief. For several weeks, I drank vodka in my orange juice before setting off for school in the mornings, and I thought obsessively about killing myself. It was a tribute to my ability to present an image so at variance with what I felt that few noticed I was in any way different. Certainly no one in my family did. Two friends were concerned, but I swore them to secrecy when they asked to talk with my parents. One teacher noticed, and the parent of a friend called me aside to ask if something was wrong. I lied readily: I'm fine, but thank you for asking.

I have no idea how I managed to pass as normal in school, except that other people are generally caught up in their own lives and seldom notice despair in others if those despairing make an effort to disguise the pain. I made not just an effort, but an enormous effort not to be noticed. I knew something was dreadfully wrong, but I had no idea what, and I had been brought up to believe that you kept your problems to yourself. Given that, it turned out to be unnervingly easy to keep my friends and family at psychological bay.

Source: Jamison, 1995, pp. 36–39. Reprinted with permission.

disorder displayed significantly more deficits in social skills performance; however, no significant differences emerged between the groups in social skills knowledge (Goldstein et al., 2006).

Thus whereas some individuals with adolescent-onset bipolar disorder—especially those with severe childhood psychopathology—may have a relatively poor course of illness and adjustment, many cases of more "classic" bipolar disorder emerge in adolescence. Such individuals may have relatively favorable outcomes in the long run and adequate if not excellent adjustment in the short run (Carlson and Strober, 1979). Box 6–3 presents a first-person account of a posthypomanic depressive episode in an adolescent who, although she subsequently developed full-blown psychotic manias, went on to have good academic and social functioning.

Comorbidity

Comorbidity complicates the diagnostic and clinical picture of adolescent-onset bipolar disorder, as it does for childhood-onset illness. Tables 6–3 and 6–4, respectively, display the results of the major studies of comorbidity among adolescent-onset and combined samples of adolescent- and child-onset bipolar subjects. Nowhere is the question of the meaning of comorbidity more complex than with adolescent-onset bipolar disorder, because the co-occurrence of psychiatric syndromes can be due to several factors. There are, for example, indistinct diagnostic boundaries and overlapping symptoms. Irritability, impulsivity, and excessive activity, for instance, are symptoms shared by bipolar and other syndromes. Moreover, there is a causal relationship between bipolar illness and other disorders, in that symptoms of mania or depression may lead to substance or alcohol abuse. (Likewise, substance abuse can precipitate mood disorders.) Too, there are shared genetic or other risk factors, such as parental assortative mating, and similar or related genes may be implicated in both ADHD and bipolar disorder. Considerable research, including carefully designed longitudinal studies, is needed to help clarify the meaning of comorbid conditions in those with childhood- and adolescent-onset bipolar disorder.

Comorbid conditions that commonly complicate differential diagnosis include drug or alcohol abuse, conduct disorder, and ADHD, all of which may involve manic-like symptoms of irritability, disruptiveness, hostility, impulsiveness, distractibility, antisocial behaviors, and the like. Psychotic symptoms may be mistaken for schizophrenia, and drug and alcohol abuse may obscure and complicate the diagnosis of mania, depression, or mixed states.

Comorbidity with personality disorders may also complicate the diagnosis of bipolar disorder in adolescents. Although relatively few studies of Axis II disorders in bipolar youths have been conducted, this important topic should be pursued because personality pathology not only makes differential diagnosis potentially difficult; it also affects the interpretation of studies of course and treatment outcome. A small study by Kutcher and colleagues (1990), for example, revealed a rate of 15 percent for borderline personality disorder among euthymic bipolar adolescents, and the presence of that disorder predicted worse responsiveness to lithium. Mood instability, impulsiveness, an inclination to suicide, irritability, and other characteristics of borderline personality disorder represent a conceptual challenge in determining the boundary between severe mood disorder and personality pathology. Such issues are pursued in greater detail in Chapter 10. It

TABLE 6–3. **Comorbidities in Samples of Bipolar Adolescents**

Characteristic	Faraone et al., 1997 (teen outpatient)	Kafantaris et al., 1998 (teen inpatient)
Sample size	17	28
Source of sample	Outpatient psychopharmacology clinic	Adolescent inpatient treatment
Assessment used	KSADS	KSADS
Mean age (yrs)	15.8	15.8
% male	65	44
Comorbidities		
% ADHD	59	21
% ODD/CD	71/35	
% OCD	38	
% anxiety disorders	59	33
% substance abuse disorders	35	Specifically excluded
% psychosis	35	48
% no comorbidity	Not stated	31
% With >1 diagnosis	Probably high	Not stated

ADHD = attention-deficit hyperactivity disorder; KSADS = Kiddie Schedule for Affective Disorders and Schizophrenia; OCD = obsessive-compulsive disorder; ODD/CD = oppositional defiant disorder/conduct disorder.
Source: Updated from Geller et al., 1999. Reprinted with permission.

TABLE 6–4. Comorbidities in Combined Samples of Bipolar Children and Adolescents

Characteristic	Kowatch et al., 2000 (child and teen outpatient)	Frazier et al., 2001 (child and teen outpatient)
Sample size	42	23
Source of sample	Outpatient treatment study	Outpatient olanzapine trial
Assessment used	KSADS	KSADS
Mean age (yrs)	11	10.2
% Male	62	57
Comorbidities		
% ADHD	71	78
% ODD/CD	38/7	100/35
% OCD	Not stated	35
% anxiety disorders	17	57
% substance abuse disorders	2	Not stated
% psychosis	Not stated	44
% no comorbidity	Not stated	Not stated

ADHD=attention-deficit hyperactivity disorder; KSADS=Kiddie Schedule for Affective Disorders and Schizophrenia; OCD=obsessive-compulsive disorder; ODD/CD=oppositional defiant disorder/conduct disorder.

is likely that mood instability and cognitive and behavioral dysfunction due to bipolar disorder in childhood and adolescence contribute to the development of personality pathology.

Studies vary in the rates of comorbid diagnosis reported among individuals with adolescent-onset bipolar disorder. Lewinsohn and colleagues (1995, 2003) found high rates of comorbid anxiety disorders (33 percent), substance abuse, and disruptive behavior disorders (22 percent each), as well as ADHD (11 percent), in their community sample of youths with bipolar spectrum disorders. Kutcher and colleagues (1998) found that 61 percent of their adolescent-onset sample had no psychiatric diagnoses other than mood disorders; among those who did, generalized anxiety disorder (21 percent), ADHD (11 percent), and conduct disorder (11 percent) were observed most frequently. Findling and colleagues (2001) also observed high levels of comorbidity (76 percent overall, including 62 percent with ADHD) among adolescents with bipolar-I disorder (many of whom, however, probably had had childhood onset). ADHD as a comorbid condition is of particular interest, as discussed earlier, because of the problem of differential diagnosis, markedly different treatment strategies, and the possibility that comorbid ADHD may identify a genetic subtype and predict a worse course and poorer response to lithium (e.g., Strober et al., 1998).

A recent European study of 98 consecutively referred bipolar children and adolescents found that 38 percent were comorbid for ADHD (Masi et al., 2006). The mean age at onset for bipolar disorder was 10.0 ±3.2 years and for ADHD was 3.7 ±1.1 years. The bipolar patients with comorbid ADHD were predominantly male (73 percent) and younger, had an earlier age at onset of their bipolar illness (8.1 ±2.8 years versus 11.1 ±2.9 years, p <.000), were more likely to exhibit a chronic rather than episodic course (67 versus 33 percent), were more likely to have irritable rather than elated mood (62 versus 36 percent), and were likely to have overall greater psychiatric impairment. As the authors of the study pointed out, these differences are important:

> An identification of ADHD may help to identify a specific subgroup of patients, with a more homogeneous course, outcome, and response to treatments. From a neurobiological standpoint, the identification of common biological pathways may help to more deeply define the links in the pathophysiology of both disorders, which are still under question. (p. 380) (see also Geller et al., 2006)

Neurodevelopmental Aspects of Adolescent Bipolar Disorder and the Issue of Puberty

Many studies use the term "prepubertal" or "pubertal" onset, but the vast majority have neither verified the pubertal status of research participants nor articulated a model of early-onset bipolar disorder in which "puberty" plays a role in pathophysiology. The issue is important, however, given the frequent onset of bipolar disorder in adolescence, apparently after pubertal changes.

A neurodevelopmental emphasis has emerged in the field of schizophrenia (e.g., Lenzenweger and Dworkin, 1998), helping to identify early markers of neurocognitive impairment that are predictive of eventual schizophrenia, as well as to generate etiological models pertinent to abnormal brain development. Benes (1999) and others have noted the significance of puberty for the development of neural circuits that are relevant to mental disorders. Walker (2002), for example, explored the role played by hormones in neuromaturation, speculating that vulnerability to mental disorders such as schizophrenia, severe depression, and bipolar illness is mediated in part by the effects of hormones on gene expression. Further research on the development of the brain and on the role of pubertal changes in neurodevelopmental processes might help clarify whether pubertal effects are indeed significant in triggering underlying vulnerabilities to bipolar disorder.

A small body of research has begun to emerge on the neurocognitive, neuroanatomic, and neurochemical correlates of bipolar disorder in adolescents (e.g., Davanzo et al., 2003; DelBello et al., 2004; see also Chapters 9, 14, and 15). Sigurdsson and colleagues (1999), for example, reviewed chart notes for a sample of bipolar adolescents and found significantly greater evidence of delays in linguistic, social, and motor development among bipolar youths compared with those with early-onset unipolar depression, and especially among those who developed psychotic symptoms. Although the neurodevelopmental differences were relatively general and nonspecific, these findings are compatible with the hypothesis that such impairments are indicators of neurocognitive vulnerability factors for bipolar disorder. A growing literature suggests that bipolar youths are more likely than controls to demonstrate impairment on a wide variety of neuropsychological measures, including executive functioning, sustained attention, and working memory (Dickstein et al., 2004; Meyer et al., 2004; Doyle et al., 2005). These deficits, in turn, contribute to substantial academic difficulties (Pavuluri et al., 2006). There is accumulating evidence that comorbid ADHD significantly contributes to the cognitive deficits (McClure et al., 2005; Rucklidge, 2006).

In related work, Friedman and colleagues (1999) conducted a magnetic resonance imaging (MRI) study of adolescent bipolar and schizophrenic patients compared with non-ill youths. They found few differences among the patient groups, but the schizophrenic and bipolar youths differed significantly from normal controls on various measures, including reduced intracranial volume and increased frontal sulcal prominence, among others. These results are consistent with neurodevelopmental abnormalities and

raise many intriguing questions for further study (see also Botteron et al., 1995, and the review by Todd and Botteron, 2002). It should be noted, however, that such studies need to verify age at onset and clarify whether state or trait markers of disorder are being identified. Recent studies by Blumberg and colleagues (2003a, 2003b) found that adolescents with bipolar illness show decreased volumes of medial temporal lobe structures (with greater effect sizes in the amygdala than in the hippocampus) and signal increases in the subcortical portions of the frontal striatal circuits. Additional discussion on the need to pursue potential markers of neurodevelopmental vulnerability for bipolar disorder is presented in our later review of the offspring of bipolar parents (see also Chapters 13, 14, and 15).

EPIDEMIOLOGY OF BIPOLAR DISORDER IN CHILDREN AND ADOLESCENTS

Three problems limit understanding of the prevalence of bipolar disorder in young populations: epidemiologic surveys encompassing children and adolescents have been rare (see Chapter 5); few have included bipolar disorder as an object of inquiry; and in most of the studies that are available, data have not been presented separately for children and adolescents or specified age at onset.

Chapter 5 (see especially Table 5–13) presents the results of community-based epidemiologic studies that have included children and adolescents, and those findings are not duplicated here. The sparse data available from representative community and psychiatric samples illustrate several patterns that are generally accepted and confirmed by clinical studies. First, childhood bipolar-I disorder is rare in community samples (although, of course, more prevalent in clinical samples). Second, bipolar disorder occurs among adolescents at about the same rate as in the general adult population. Third, subsyndromal forms of bipolar disorder can be identified in child and adolescent samples, and can reflect prodromal or stable dimensional traits of the bipolar spectrum that may be associated with impairment of functioning.

Some have asserted that the frequency of bipolar disorder in youngsters is increasing. There has been some evidence that rates of childhood- or adolescent-onset bipolar disorder have increased in more recent cohorts (e.g., Rice et al., 1987; Chengappa et al., 2003; Kessler et al., 2005) and that this increase is not due to increased ascertainment alone. It is difficult to determine the validity and generalizability of this conclusion, however, given the lack of epidemiologic surveys with comparable data over time, as well as the lack of consistent diagnostic criteria. Moreover, increasing rates of apparent mania in clinical samples of children and adolescents may reflect methodological matters, such as age-related changes in awareness and memory, temporal changes in morbidity and sample availability, and diagnostic practices (see Chapter 5).

At the same time, it has been argued that changes in health practices and environmental factors may induce earlier expression of bipolar disorder—or actual increased rates of bipolarity. Such factors may include widespread and increased use of stimulant and antidepressant medications (e.g., Zito et al., 2002) that could trigger bipolar rapid-cycling patterns in susceptible children or decrease the age at onset (DelBello et al., 2001); alcohol and drug use at younger ages, possibly inducing earlier onset of bipolar symptomatology; earlier onset of puberty; and exposure to maternal health risks during pregnancy (e.g., smoking, drug and alcohol intake, dietary reductions in omega-3 fatty acids, social stressors). Also, as noted in Chapter 13, genetic anticipation effects may promote earlier onset. These issues are clearly important, with critical implications for etiology and treatment, and require further study.

IMPLICATIONS OF CHILDHOOD AND ADOLESCENT ONSET OF BIPOLAR DISORDER

Other chapters in this volume address some of the implications of the onset of bipolar disorder in childhood and early adolescence, including effects of age at onset on course (Chapter 4), epidemiology and the possibility of cohort changes in age at onset (Chapter 5), genetic implications of early onset (Chapter 13), and treatment considerations (Chapter 23). A few important issues merit emphasis here, however, including the implications of childhood and adolescent onset for treatment and prevention.

Clinical Implications

Even apart from the goal of validating the diagnostic features of childhood bipolar disorder, it is important to study whether the outcomes and features of childhood-onset cases of the disorder differ from those of adolescent- and adult-onset cases. If, as discussed earlier, childhood onset reflects a particularly virulent form of the disorder, then relatively chronic symptomatology, mixed-state episodes, and rapid cycling might be expected to continue. It is possible, however, that such atypical features reflect developmental manifestations of nonspecific severe dysregulation, with maturity revealing a more recognizable episodic course with relatively better interepisode functioning. To answer this question, relevant longitudinal studies would need to separate out the effects on course and functioning that are due to comorbid childhood psychopathology—and indeed, to determine whether such

clinical conditions reflect true cases of multiple disorders or diffuse, severe bipolar symptomatology.

Preliminary studies suggest that early onset may indeed portend a worse course. Unfortunately, these studies do not always differentiate childhood from adolescent onset. Carlson and colleagues (2000) found that early-onset psychotic manic patients (onset before 21 years of age) had significantly poorer recovery between episodes, more manic episodes, and more time in the hospital during 2-year follow-up as compared with later-onset psychotic manic patients. Early-onset patients also were more likely than later-onset patients to have mixed episodes. The early-onset patients were significantly more likely to be male, high school dropouts, and never married. In a subsequent study of the same sample, Carlson and colleagues (2002) performed a separate analysis for the effects of "early onset" of bipolar disorder and comorbid childhood psychopathology. They determined that the two factors had somewhat independent effects in predicting outcome, with childhood disorders being more likely to predict poor functional outcome and early age at bipolar onset being related to continuing symptoms.

Similarly, Schurhoff and colleagues (2000) found that a group of bipolar patients with early onset (before age 18) was significantly more impaired, had more psychotic features, and had poorer response to lithium prophylaxis than a group with late onset (after age 40). Also, the early-onset group had more first-degree relatives with bipolar disorder. These findings are consistent with those of the above-noted retrospective self-report volunteer survey of members of the National Depressive and Manic-Depressive Association (Lish et al., 1994). Those who reported early (childhood/adolescent) onset (60 percent) were compared with adult-onset respondents on various indicators of functioning. Onset in childhood and adolescence was associated with significantly greater likelihood of social morbidity, as indicated by dropping out of school, financial difficulties, marital problems, being unmarried, alcohol and drug abuse, injury to self or others, and minor crime. Those with early onset also reported significantly more recurrent bipolar illness. Statistical analyses indicated that the effects on social morbidity were due to independent contributions by frequency of recurrences and early onset. Those with early-onset bipolar disorder reported that their initial symptoms were more likely to be depressive than manic and that their recurrences were predominantly depressive as well.

Neither the study of Schurhoff and colleagues (2000) nor the National Depressive and Manic-Depressive Association survey evaluated effects of childhood comorbid disruptive disorders. However, this is an important consideration in interpreting the effects of early age at onset, because those conditions may confound the results of such analysis, with outcomes perhaps being attributed inaccurately to bipolar disorder. A further consideration is that childhood or early-adolescent onset of bipolar disorder may cause later comorbid conditions (see the earlier discussion of comorbidity). For instance, Tohen and colleagues (1998) found that early age at onset, male gender, and the presence of mixed states predicted the development of substance abuse in bipolar patients (see Chapter 7).

Other methodological issues also need to be considered in studies of the effects of age at onset. As noted, few longitudinal studies exist; most data are therefore based on retrospective reports or short-term follow-up. Moreover, many studies have had small sample sizes. In addition, studies may differ as to whether they assess separately for psychotic features, effects of prior depressive histories and comorbid childhood disorders, and clinical presentation (such as mixed or cycling episodes)—all of which may affect prognosis. Despite these limitations, it appears that childhood and adolescent onset may portend greater functional impairment, and possibly a more difficult clinical course.

Implications for Treatment and Prevention

As noted elsewhere in this volume, two treatment issues are salient in considering the implications of childhood and early-adolescent onset of bipolar disorder (see Chapter 23). One is that misdiagnosis may worsen the course of bipolar illness. For instance, antidepressant-induced rapid cycling in adults may have a counterpart in children who have been erroneously diagnosed as having nonbipolar depression. It has been speculated that some cases of rapid or ultra-rapid cycling in children may stem from antidepressant treatment for depression—although the role of such treatments in this age group has not been thoroughly investigated. It has also been theorized that stimulants used to treat ADHD may worsen the course of bipolar disorder in children. Some have suggested that the widespread use of antidepressant and stimulant medications in U.S. children may have led to more cases of childhood onset of bipolar disorder in the United States than in European and other nations, where such medications are used less frequently in children (e.g., Reichart et al., 2000). These hypotheses require empirical validation, and in fact one review of the findings of preliminary studies casts doubt on notions of the negative impact of antidepressants and stimulants (e.g., Meyer et al., 2004). Further studies are vital to provide guidelines for maximally effective interventions for children with probable mood disorders.

The second treatment issue is the widely cited hypothesis that bipolar disorder is a progressive illness with neurobiological "kindling"—that is, episodes beget episodes (see,

for example, Post, 2006, and Chapter 4). If this were in fact the case, vigorous early intervention with mood-stabilizing drugs to prevent episodes would have critical and positive implications for long-term outcome. The successful use of such interventions would then depend on research aimed at identifying the earliest valid markers of bipolar disorder. At the very least, early recognition and diagnosis of established cases could have important consequences for treatment and eventual course. These are not easy tasks, however. Underrecognition of childhood disorders and underutilization of treatment are rampant problems in public health, not limited to mood disorders.

STUDIES OF CHILDREN AT HIGH RISK

Children at risk for bipolar disorder as a result of parental bipolar illness represent an ideal sample for the study of potential antecedents (see Chapter 13 for a full discussion of the genetics of bipolar disorder). The high-risk methodology in psychopathological research—that is, the study of children of psychiatrically ill parents—has been employed productively for more than 25 years to accomplish several interrelated goals. First, examination of early signs of a disorder in offspring helps clarify the course of the illness from its initial expression to its unfolding over the course of development. Identification of early signs of bipolar disorder in a prospectively followed high-risk sample is an especially useful approach to validation of the developmental manifestations of symptomatology and establishment of diagnostic certainty. Second, assessment of putative markers of a disorder can help flag those who will eventually develop it, and thereby identify possible targets for early intervention (a potentially important accomplishment for children with bipolar disorder, as discussed earlier). Third, study of such markers and other environmental and contextual factors that influence children's development can help clarify the psychological processes by which possible genetic predispositions are, or are not, manifested as disorders.

Despite their usefulness, however, offspring studies of bipolar disorder have limitations. For one thing, these high-risk children represent a unique sample not necessarily generalizable to the entire population of bipolar probands. By definition, youngsters in families with a bipolar parent experience both the genetic risk (perhaps a uniquely strong one) and the environmental impact of living with such a parent. The challenge to researchers is to disentangle these interrelated factors. Eventually, more precise knowledge of genetic factors will yield a greater understanding of the contributions of psychological and environmental factors to bipolar outcomes among those at risk. At the same time, while the majority of current offspring studies, as designed, do not clarify genetic contributions as such, they do shed light on early signs of bipolar disorder in children and young adolescents.

There are numerous methodological obstacles to be overcome in studies of high-risk children, including issues of diagnosis (how broad a spectrum of bipolarity to include, how comorbid conditions should be conceptualized and analyzed), evaluation of outcomes, and assessment of the many factors in families with bipolar illness that contribute to children's adjustment. Too, because the age range for the onset of bipolar disorder extends over decades, a cross-sectional evaluation of children is likely to be misleading (some children diagnosed with major depression or ADHD, for example, may later convert to bipolarity). Moreover, sample sizes in many high-risk studies have been small, and interviewers have not been blind to parental diagnosis. Finally, the majority of high-risk studies of children having a parent with bipolar disorder were not specifically designed to assess early signs of bipolarity and thus may not have realized their full potential. Research on children at risk for bipolar disorder is less well advanced than is the case for other major disorders, such as schizophrenia or unipolar depression. The latter fields have produced intriguing insights into the neurodevelopmental and neurocognitive markers of schizophrenia and of family and psychosocial risk factors in depression. Studies of families at high risk for bipolar disorder, by contrast, have been less common and less methodologically sophisticated. However, this situation is changing rapidly with improved diagnostic methods, theoretical developments to guide the search for potential markers and risk factors and mechanisms of action, and increased interest among researchers and affected families alike in learning more about options for early intervention.

Recent and Direct-Interview Studies of Children of Bipolar Parents

Early offspring studies were unsystematic or methodologically limited but still contributed important evidence regarding the risk to children of bipolar parents. Information from these early studies is presented in Box 6–4. In the following sections, we summarize the results of more methodologically sophisticated work. Before proceeding, however, we must make clear that the term "children" of bipolar parents refers generally to both preadolescent and adolescent offspring; as with the early-onset literature generally, the results of the great majority of studies have not been separated out by age.

Clinical Outcomes in Controlled Studies

Table 6–5 summarizes numerous high-risk studies that we selected because they had comparison groups and used adequate measures for assessing children's clinical status.

Specifically, both the child and a parent were interviewed, using well-established structured or semistructured interview methods to assign diagnoses. Many of the studies were attentive to matching bipolar and comparison families on demographic factors, and several also included diagnostic information on the nonproband parent. These studies represent the current state of the art of research on the offspring of bipolar parents.

The studies are relatively consistent in reporting higher rates of lifetime diagnosis among children of bipolar parents compared with those of non-ill controls. The diagnoses include the full range of childhood mood, anxiety, and behavioral disorders. Most of the studies found that children of bipolar parents were particularly likely to display mood disorders—chiefly depression, but also forms of bipolar disorder. A recent study (Klimas-Dougan et al., 2006) found slightly increased rates of major depressive disorder in children of mothers who had bipolar disorder (12 percent) or major depression (17 percent) as compared with children of mothers who were psychiatrically well (8 percent). Much more striking, however, the children of bipolar mothers showed far more neurocognitive deficits—in executive functioning, perceptual memory, and sustained attention—than the children of either the unipolar or psychiatrically well mothers. There were no differences in verbal memory between the high-risk and control children.

Only a few investigators looked for sampled subclinical manifestations of bipolar illness. Decina and colleagues (1983) observed the presence of subclinical symptoms—including expansiveness, excitability, need for constant attention and admiration, need for reassurance, and other traits potentially suggestive of hyperthymic or depressive personality—in half of nondiagnosed offspring. Depressive traits were observed in a substantial proportion of children of bipolar parents by Grigoroiu-Serbanescu and colleagues (1991). Reichard and colleagues (2005) administered the General Behavior Inventory (GBI) and the Kiddie Schedule for Affective Disorders and Schizophrenia (KSADS) to 129 adolescents and young adult offspring of bipolar parents at initial assessment and 14 months later. At 5-year follow-up, both the GBI and the Structured Clinical Interview for DSM (SCID) were administered. The scores on the Depression scale of the GBI for the offspring who later developed bipolar disorder were significantly higher than those for the offspring who did not. For the offspring with unipolar depression at the first assessment, the scores on the Depression scale were significantly higher for those who converted to bipolar disorder than for those who did not. Carlson and Weintraub (1993) found that young-adult offspring of bipolar parents scored significantly higher on a scale rating of subsyndromal bipolarity than

BOX **6–4.** **Early Studies of Children of Bipolar Parents**

The earliest studies of the impact on children of having a bipolar parent either were uncontrolled observations with no systematic comparison groups or consisted of psychiatric comparisons in studies of children of schizophrenic patients. Typically, the clinical studies had very small samples, and the assessment of the children was conducted by investigators who were not blinded to the parents' diagnosis. Early methods of assessing children typically relied on unsystematic observations or parent reports, which may be biased. In addition, the initial studies were generally guided by the assumption that risk was due exclusively to genetic factors, so that family (and spousal) characteristics were largely unreported. Despite these limitations, however, intriguing patterns began to emerge.

The earliest high-risk studies were conducted on schizophrenic patients and often included a comparison group of parents with affective disorders or psychotic mood disorders. As a result of the use of earlier diagnostic frameworks, such as DSM-I or DSM-II, the affective disorder groups contained a mix of unipolar and bipolar families, and some of those diagnosed as schizophrenic may have been bipolar. The St. Louis High-Risk Study (e.g., Worland et al., 1979) and the Stony Brook High-Risk Project (Weintraub and Neale, 1984) included hospitalized depressed comparison subjects, both unipolar and bipolar. The Stony Brook sample represents what is probably the largest comparative high-risk study, involving 113 children of unipolar parents, 73 of bipolar parents, 57 of schizophrenic parents, and 297 of normal parents.

Other studies were well designed in terms of careful diagnostic evaluations and comparisons with at least one other normal or psychopathological group but were limited in their assessment of the children (e.g., parent report only, nondiagnostic methods) or had small samples. These included studies by Conners and colleagues (1979) comparing children of 16 bipolar and 43 "other psychopathology" (primarily unipolar depressed) groups, and those by Greenhill and colleagues (1980) reporting on offspring of 7 bipolar and 2 unipolar parents. Other studies did not include a comparison group: Kuyler and colleagues (1980) studied 49 children of 27 parents, and Waters and colleagues (1983) sampled adult offspring of 17 bipolar parents. Investigations by McKnew and colleagues (1979) and Cytryn and colleagues (1982) were forerunners of later well-designed work by Gershon and colleagues (1985), which is listed in Table 6–2 as an example of a good case-control study with direct diagnostic evaluations of children. A study by LaRoche and colleagues (1987) that included 37 offspring of 21 bipolar families is unique because it reported 3 to 7 years of follow-up data on the children.

Virtually all of these studies found high rates of psychiatric disorders among children of bipolar parents—higher than in normal comparisons or than would be expected in the general population. Most of the studies specifically indicated higher levels of affective disorders in offspring. Among the adult offspring studied by Waters and colleagues (1983), 9 (17 percent) of 53 had been diagnosed as bipolar by young adulthood. The LaRoche and colleagues (1987) follow-up, including offspring up to age 25, found that 24 percent had been diagnosed, mainly in the affective disorder spectrum. Two studies compared offspring of bipolar and unipolar parents. Conners and colleagues (1979) found higher rates of symptoms and disorders among the children of unipolar depressed parents, whereas offspring of unipolar and bipolar parents in the Stony Brook sample did not differ from each other but were significantly more symptomatic than children of non-ill controls (Weintraub, 1987).

Two additional studies from the 1980s are informative. Zahn-Waxler and colleagues (1988) compared 7 children of bipolar parents with 12 control children. The unique features of this investigation were the inclusion of infants studied up to age 5 or 6 years and the intensive study of family relationships and children's psychosocial development. The offspring of the bipolar parents displayed a range of behavioral and adjustment difficulties that persisted at follow-up. This study was eventually expanded as the Radke-Yarrow and colleagues (1992) investigation, which is reported in the text, along with the data yielded on toddler development and parent–child relations.

An investigation by Akiskal and colleagues (1985) focused on affective symptoms in referred children who were known to be offspring or siblings of adult bipolar patients. Although not a traditional high-risk study, the work was aimed at identifying possible signs and symptoms of bipolarity in youngsters at risk. Using the investigators' Mood Clinic Data Questionnaire, which included diagnostic criteria as well as subclinical symptoms, the study revealed several features characteristic of the sample. Onset of systems before puberty was rare, and all bipolar diagnoses occurred after puberty. Acute depressive episodes and dysthymic-cyclothymic disorders were the most common symptom patterns. By the end of 3 years of follow-up, bipolar outcomes were prominent: 19 (28 percent) of 68 children were bipolar-I, and 12 (18 percent) were bipolar-II; 2 were rapid cyclers, and 6 were cyclothymic. There were no signs of bipolarity in 43 percent of the children; the authors argued, however, that 7 of these children were "pseudo-unipolar" and potentially at risk for bipolarity, as suggested by pharmacological hypomania.

TABLE 6–5. High-Risk Studies with Comparison Groups and Direct Assessment of Children: Clinical Findings

Study	HIGH RISK		COMPARISON		ASSESSMENT	
	Parents	Children	Parents	Children	Method	Findings
Decina et al., 1983	11 BP-I, 7 BP-II (7 fathers, 11 mothers)	14 M, 17 F (ages 7–14)	14 with no disorder	10 M, 8 F (ages 7–14)	Direct interview of child and parent; semistructured interview with some KSADS items.	Significantly higher rates of mood disorders in bipolar offspring than in offspring of non-ill parents; 50% of bipolar offspring had some psychiatric diagnosis. Presence of subclinical affective symptoms suggestive of depressive or hyperthymic personality.
Klein et al., 1985	24 BP (11 fathers, 13 mothers)	19 M, 18 F (ages 15–21)	14 with psychiatric disorders (outpatient) (10 fathers, 4 mothers)	13 M, 9 F (ages 15–21)	Direct interview of child; structured interview (KSADS) modified to include cyclothymia.	Significantly higher rates of mood disorders (38%) in offspring sample compared with psychiatric sample (5%). High rate of cyclothymia (9 of 16 youths). Higher risk of mood disorders if mother bipolar.
Gershon et al., 1985	19 BP-I (sex unspecified) and spouses; (12 had unspecified diagnoses)	12 M, 17 F (ages 6–17)	22 with no disorder (sex unspecified)	16 M, 21 F (ages 6–17)	Direct interview of child and parent; structured interview (KSADS-E); used "NIMH criteria," similar to RDC.	3 (10%) of 29 offspring of bipolar parents had mania/hypomania vs. none for controls. Overall, 66% of offspring of bipolar parents vs. 43% of controls had some diagnosis. No significant effect of two ill parents.

(continued)

TABLE 6–5. High-Risk Studies with Comparison Groups and Direct Assessment of Children: Clinical Findings (continued)

| | HIGH RISK | | COMPARISON | | ASSESSMENT | |
Study	Parents	Children	Parents	Children	Method	Findings
Nurnberger et al., 1988	(1) 23 BP or schizoaffective (sex unspecified; one parent ill); (2) 9 families with two ill parents (both BP or schizoaffective, or one ill and the other with "loaded" family history of disorder; sex unspecified)	(1) 15 M, 23 F (ages 15–25); (2) 9 M, 6 F (ages 15–25)	39 with no disorder (sex unspecified)	18 M, 21 F (ages 15–25)	Direct interview of child; structured interview (SADS-L adapted for children).	67–74% of offspring of one or two ill parents had disorders vs. 31% of normal controls. Over 1- or 2-year follow-up, increased rates of disorder were found in offspring of bipolar parents, including major affective illness and affective spectrum disorders.
Grigoroiu-Serbanescu et al., 1989	28 BP-I mothers, 19 BP-I fathers; spouses (34 no disorder, 13 other disorder)	34 M, 38 F (ages 10–17)	61 couples with no disorder	34 M, 38 F (ages 10–17)	Direct interview of child and parent; structured interview (KSADS-E); reported point prevalence.	7 (10%) of 72 offspring had affective disorder (1 bipolar); there were also significantly higher rates of anxiety disorders, ADHD, and personality disorders than in control offspring. Severity of illness in offspring was related to severity of illness in parent and psychopathology in spouse of bipolar parent.
Hammen et al., 1990	14 BP mothers[a] and spouses (7 fathers with no disorder, others with varied disorders)	8 M, 10 F (ages 8–16)	(1) 16 unipolar mothers and spouses (5 fathers no disorder, others with varied disorder); (2) 14 medically ill	(1) 10 M, 12 F; (2) 9 M, 9 F; (3) 19 M, 19 F (all groups ages 8–16)	Direct interview of child and parent; structured interview (KSADS-E).	Rates of current and past affective and disruptive behavior disorders were significantly higher in unipolar and bipolar groups. Cumulative probability of major depression was .67 in

Study	Sample	Measures	Results
	mothers and spouses (5 fathers no disorder, others varied disorders); (3) 24 non-ill mothers and spouses (15 fathers with no disorder, others varied disorders)		unipolar, .33 in bipolar, .45 in medical, and .12 in non-ill groups through 3-year follow-up. By age 19, the cumulative probability of any significant diagnosis in bipolar offspring was .75 (.85 in unipolar group). Bipolar offspring had later age at onset.
Radke-Yarrow et al., 1992	22 BP mothers[b] (5 BP-I, 17 BP-II) and spouses (14 unipolar fathers, 8 fathers with no disorder) — Sibling pairs: 22 ages 1½–3½[c], 22 ages 5–8[b] (gender not specified, stated as "approximately equal" in each group); (1) 41 unipolar mothers[d] and spouses (22 fathers with depression or anxiety disorder, 19 fathers with no disorder); (2) 37 mothers with no disorder and spouses (37 fathers with no disorder)[c] — (1) Sibling pairs: 41 ages 1½–3½[c], 41 ages 5–8[c]; (2) sibling pairs: 37 ages 1½–3½[c], 37 ages 5–8[c]	Age <4 yr: psychiatric evaluation based on observation of standardized play sessions, mothers' reports on CBCL; age >4 yr: CBCL, structured interview of child (Child Assessment Scale), DSM-III criteria	Outcomes varied by children's age and maternal group, mother or psychiatrist report. Generally, children of bipolar and unipolar mothers were more likely than control children to have disruptive and depressive disorders. Offspring of bipolar mothers had later onset than those of unipolar mothers. No differences between groups with one and two ill parents.
Carlson and Weintraub, 1993 (follow-up of Weintraub and Neale, 1984)	134 children of BP parents originally studied at ages 7–16; follow-up of 125 after age 18; 211 of 240 in original group of children of parents with unipolar depression, schizophrenia, substance abuse; 98 of 108 in original group of children of normal controls	Results reported on adult follow-up based on SCID interviews, DSM-III criteria.	4.8% of offspring of bipolar parents had definite bipolar disorder, 53% had some diagnosis overall. In childhood, 28% had behavior problems, 30% had attention problems (all significantly higher than normal controls but not "other" controls). Such problems predicted mood disorders in adulthood.

(continued)

211

TABLE 6–5. High-Risk Studies with Comparison Groups and Direct Assessment of Children: Clinical Findings *(continued)*

| Study | HIGH RISK | | COMPARISON | | ASSESSMENT | |
	Parents	Children	Parents	Children	Method	Findings
Todd et al., 1996	30 families selected because adult bipolar proband or proband's adult sibling was in bipolar pedigree study (NIMH Genetic Initiative Study); 12 parents affected: 8 BP-I, 1 BP-II, 3 unipolar depressed	Total sample across 30 families: 24 M, 26 F (ages 6–17); 23 offspring of affected families	18 sets of parents with no disorder	27 offspring of nonaffected families	Direct interview of child and parent, structured interview (Diagnostic Interview for Children and Adolescents-Revised) with revised mania sections.	9 offspring of 23 affected parents had affective disorder (including 5 bipolar), compared with 3 of 27 with unaffected parents.
Birmaher et al., 2005	132 BP: 56% BP-I, 36% BP-II, 8% BP-NOS or cyclothymia (79% mothers)	210: 49% F (average age=12.0 yr)	79: 29% MDD, 9% dysthymia (90% mothers)	138: 57% F (average age=11.5 yr)	Parental interview. Children assessed by KSADS-PL, K-MRS, KSADS-P. Family history obtained via FHRDC, DSM-IV diagnosis.	Offspring of BP parents showed 7.7-fold higher risk for any BP disorder, 4.0-fold risk for any mood disorder, and 2.2-fold risk for anxiety disorders.
Jones et al., 2006	19 BP-I, 1 BP-II (5 fathers, 15 mothers)	6 M, 19 F (ages 13–19)	19 with no disorder	6 M, 16 F (ages 13–19)	SADS-L, Self-report measures, actigraph, Social Rhythm Metric, diaries	Significantly higher rates of mood disorders in children of bipolar parents (CBP) (14/19) than in offspring of non-ill parents (CC) (2/19), p < .001. CBP had stronger ruminative coping styles and significantly greater self-esteem variation, but did not differ in positive affect. CBP exhibited shorter and less variable sleep latency.

| Klimas-Dougan et al., 2006 | 25 BP mothers | 43: 61% F (average age = 15.1 yr) | 26 psychiatrically well mothers | 50: 48% females (average age = 15.3 yr) | Administered a battery of neuropsychological tests, including Wisconsin Card Sorting Test, Trail Making Test, California Verbal Learning Task, Continuous Performance Task, and WISC-R/WAIS | Lifetime MDD diagnosis: children of bipolar mother, 12%; MDD mother, 17%; well mother, 8%. Children of BP mothers exhibited deficits in executive functioning, perceptual memory, and sustained attention, but not in verbal memory. These deficits were not found in children of MDD mothers or in healthy control mothers. |
| | 37 MDD mothers | 72: 64% F (average age = 16.0 yr) | | | | |

[a]3-year follow-up data reported here, with reduced sample numbers due to attrition (see Hammen et al., 1987, for initial results). Father data based on mothers' FHRDC reports; high rates of divorce in unipolar and bipolar families.

[b]n = 26 BP mothers reported later in study (Radke-Yarrow, 1998).

[c]3-year follow-up also.

[d]n = 42 unipolar mothers reported later in study (Radke-Yarrow, 1998).

ADHD = attention-deficit hyperactivity disorder; BP = bipolar; BP-NOS = bipolar-not otherwise specified; CBCL = Child Behavior Checklist (Achenbach, 1991); F = female; FHRDC = Family History Research Diagnostic Criteria; K-MRS = Kiddie Mania Rating Scale; KSADS = Kiddie Schedule for Affective Disorders and Schizophrenia for School-Age Children; KSADS-E = KSADS-Epidemiological Version; KSADS-P = KSADS-Present State; KSADS-PL = KSADS-Present and Lifetime version; M = male; MDD = major depressive disorder; NIMH = National Institute of Mental Health; RDC = Research Diagnostic Criteria; SADS = Schedule for Affective Disorders and Schizophrenia; SADS-L = SADS-Lifetime; SCID = Structured Clinical Interview for DSM. WAIS = Wechsler Adult Intelligence Scale; WISC-R = Wechsler Intelligence Scale for Children-Revised.

Source: Updated from Geller et al., 1998a.

did the offspring of both normal and "other" parents. A study by Klein and colleagues (1985) is noteworthy for the development and testing of a scale specifically for cyclothymic symptoms; it was found that more than half of the offspring of bipolar parents who had a diagnosis of affective disorder met criteria for cyclothymia.

Hirshfeld-Becker and colleagues (2006) compared 34 offspring of bipolar parents with 244 offspring of parents without bipolar disorder. Children (ages 2–6) had been classified in laboratory assessments as behaviorally inhibited, disinhibited, or neither. Offspring of bipolar parents had significantly higher rates of disinhibition than offspring of parents without bipolar disorder (53 versus 34 percent; odds ratio = 2.62, 95 percent CI = 1.22 − 5.62). The association between parental bipolar disorder was even stronger among the offspring of parents with bipolar-I illness (67 versus 34 percent; odds ratio = 5.01, 95 percent CI = 1.84 − 13.62). There was no difference in the rate of inhibition between the offspring of parents with and without bipolar disorder.

In one of the rare follow-up designs, Hammen and colleagues (1990) found that, despite relatively high rates of diagnosis over time, children of bipolar mothers were generally less chronically and severely impaired than those of unipolar mothers. The largest follow-up study, conducted by Carlson and Weintraub (1993) with 125 young-adult offspring of bipolar parents, found a rate of definite bipolar disorder of nearly 5 percent, as well as higher rates of diagnosis overall relative to normal comparison groups; generally, however, the bipolar offspring did not differ in symptoms and functioning from offspring of parents with other disorders (e.g., unipolar depression, schizophrenia, substance abuse).

A recent 5-year prospective study of adolescent offspring of parents with bipolar disorder found that the lifetime prevalence rate of bipolar disorder in the offspring increased from 3 to 10 percent at follow-up. The lifetime prevalence of overall mood disorders increased to 40 percent and of overall psychopathology to 59 percent (Hillegers et al., 2005). With the exception of one individual, all of the adolescent subjects subsequently diagnosed with bipolar illness first presented with a unipolar expression; this initial diagnosis occurred an average of 4.9 years (standard deviation = 3.4 years) before the first hypomanic or manic expression.

In their longitudinal study of young children of unipolar and bipolar mothers, Radke-Yarrow and colleagues (1992) initially found worse functioning in offspring of unipolar mothers, but in later analyses (Radke-Yarrow, 1998), the differences between unipolar and bipolar groups were negligible. This work is unique in that the sample was recruited to include mothers with sibling pairs—one of

toddler age (1½–3½) and the other of early school age (5–8); the families were studied at three points in time over a 10-year period. The young children of bipolar mothers, who suffered mainly from depression (bipolar-II), tended to have depressive and disruptive disorders; offspring in early adolescence had a diagnosis rate of 58 percent, especially for depressive and anxiety disorders, but they also had higher rates of disruptive disorders than children of well mothers. At younger ages, the offspring of unipolar mothers tended to have slightly more diagnoses than those of bipolar mothers, but both groups were substantially more likely to have disorders than the children of well mothers. By early adolescence, however, the children of bipolar mothers had similar rates of disruptive and anxiety disorders and higher rates of depression than children of unipolar depressed women. Of interest, it appeared that those offspring in all groups with early signs of disruptive disorders (20 percent) were more likely than those without such signs (2 percent)[1] to develop bipolar disorder by adulthood. The combination of a bipolar mother and an early history of chronic disruptive disorder was highly predictive of eventual bipolar disorder by adulthood— although the actual number of cases was small (Meyer et al., 2001).

A recent University of Pittsburgh study (Birmaher et al., 2005a) evaluated the lifetime prevalence of psychiatric disorders in 210 offspring of 132 parents with bipolar disorder. Rates of illness in these high-risk children were compared with those in 138 offspring of 79 community controls who were healthy or had nonbipolar psychiatric illnesses and who were matched by age, sex, and neighborhood. The offspring of parents with bipolar illness showed a 7.7-fold higher risk for bipolar disorder and a 4-fold increased risk for any mood disorder. The median age at onset for bipolar illness in the offspring was 9, but the rates of mood disorders rose steeply during adolescence. There were no differences in the rates of ADHD between the offspring of bipolar parents and those of controls.

The studies listed in Table 6–5 generally indicate few gender differences overall, although there may be gender-typical patterns of disorders, such as more disruptive behavior disorders in boys and more depressive disorders in girls. Moreover, although a few studies compared outcomes for children with one versus two ill parents, no definite conclusions could be drawn. There appears to be an increased likelihood that a bipolar adult will marry a person who also has a diagnosable disorder (nonrandom mating), thereby making it more likely that the couple's children will acquire a mix of genetic predispositions, in addition to being raised in a potentially disruptive family environment as a result of parental impairment or marital distress. There is a need for further evaluation of the impact of the marital relationship, as well as the gender and mental health of the spouse, as psychosocial contributors to outcomes among offspring (see Chapter 10).

The results of these case-control studies, along with those of other designs that did not include comparison groups but did report children's diagnoses, were summarized in a meta-analysis by Lapalme and colleagues (1997). They concluded that 52 percent of the offspring of bipolar parents met criteria for a diagnosis of at least one psychiatric disorder, compared with 29 percent of children of parents with no disorders—a highly statistically significant difference. (Note that these figures should be viewed as approximations because some of the samples overlapped, potentially causing cases to be counted more than once.) Aggregating across various samples makes it easier to see the specific concentration of mood disorders in the offspring. In total, 26.5 percent of the offspring of bipolar parents had an affective disorder (including major, minor, and intermittent depression and dysthymia, as well as mania, hypomania, cyclothymia, and hyperthymic states), compared with 8.3 percent of children of non-ill parents. Bipolar disorder occurred in 5.4 percent of the offspring of bipolar parents but in none of the children of non-ill parents. Obviously, this figure cannot be taken as a final estimate of risk for bipolarity because most of the children had not passed—or even entered—the age of risk. However, the figure does suggest that the majority of offspring of a bipolar parent fail to manifest diagnosable bipolar disorder at an early age.

Despite the overall consistency of the findings of these studies, there remain significant gaps in our knowledge of children's risk. Few of the studies included young children, while most included both older children and adolescents. The developmental manifestations of bipolar disorder, therefore, have not been fully tested in adequately large samples. The general lack of longitudinal studies means that the continuity or changes in symptom expression over time remain obscure. Although several studies attempted to evaluate subsyndromal symptoms of mood disorders or personality characteristics,[6] there is currently little consensus on the best and most valid instruments for this purpose. Additionally, future researchers will need to articulate theoretical models with specific variables—including both neurobiological and psychological factors—that might be measured as markers or mechanisms of risk. To date, little information exists about the predictive value of the bipolar parent's clinical history—including not only course subtypes, but also the role of the history of manic and depressive features of the illness, age at onset, and response to treatment. Moreover, virtually no studies have considered the potential impact on children of parental comorbidity, such as substance abuse or ADHD.

Most of the early studies and the case-control investigations discussed previously reported clinical diagnostic outcomes but did not include measures of children's personality, adaptive behaviors, and functioning in typical roles. Such variables are important to characterize potential markers of bipolar disorder—unique attributes that define both positive aspects of bipolar heritage and predictors of later adjustment, including coping capabilities that may affect mental health status. A brief review of relevant findings is presented in Box 6–5.

Recent Offspring Studies with Novel Designs

Several more recent studies have provided useful information about future directions for research on risk factors and mechanisms in bipolar families. Duffy and colleagues (1998) reported on a pilot study comparing adolescent children of bipolar parents who were characterized as responsive or nonresponsive to lithium monotherapy. Children of lithium-responsive parents had fewer psychiatric disorders and good premorbid adjustment, and their disorders tended to be mood related, compared with the children of lithium-nonresponsive parents, who had a broad range of psychopathology and more frequent comorbidity. Of interest, over follow-up of up to 5 years, all of the affectively ill children of lithium-responsive parents had remitting episodes and/or episodic courses, whereas the affectively ill children of lithium-nonresponsive parents had chronic mood disorders and continuing comorbidity (Duffy et al., 2002).

Todd and colleagues (1996) used a unique offspring design to examine psychiatric disorders in children with extended bipolar pedigrees (see Table 6–5). They evaluated children and adolescents from 14 extended families with at least two adult bipolar members. The sample included children in 12 families in which a parent was a bipolar proband or an affectively ill sibling of a bipolar proband, and 18 families in which neither parent had an affective disorder. As expected, offspring who had a parent with a mood disorder had a five-fold higher risk for developing an affective disorder than children of healthy parents. Degree of risk was associated with genetic relatedness to the affected members of the pedigree. Children of ill parents were also at apparent risk for anxiety disorders, but not for disruptive behavior disorders. The use of within-pedigree comparisons helps control for environmental factors that might contribute to disorder, and the results of such comparisons further support the hypothesis of genetic factors as a mechanism of risk.

Chang and colleagues (2000) documented initial results of a study of 60 offspring of 37 families (no comparison group). The mean age of the children was 11.1 years (standard deviation = 3.5 years), and the youngsters were evaluated by both parent and child interviews. Overall, 51 percent

In addition to the subclinical affective traits and related characteristics noted in the text, several early studies identified personality traits associated with children at high risk for bipolar disorder; these included aggressiveness (e.g., Worland et al., 1979; Kron et al., 1982), extraversion, introversion, and impulsiveness (Kron et al., 1982).

Data collected on participants in the Gershon and colleagues (1985) study and reported by Pellegrini and colleagues (1986) documented personal and social resources of the children of bipolar parents. There were no overall differences between offspring of bipolar versus control parents on such variables as IQ, social problem-solving ability, self-esteem, and perceived competence. LaRoche and colleagues (1987) also found no significant overall differences in self-esteem. However, Pellegrini and colleagues (1986), reported that those offspring of bipolar parents who did not have psychiatric disorders scored significantly in the more positive direction on the measures, relative to all the other groups, whereas those with psychiatric disorders had significantly less positive scores. Also, nondisordered offspring of bipolar parents reported significantly more supportive relationships and resources available to them than did the disordered youths. Although the direction of causality cannot be determined, superior competence and self-esteem may serve as resilience factors for children at risk and help protect them from the development of psychological disorders.

The findings of Pelligrini and colleagues (1986) are consistent with those of a Stanford study of 53 children and adolescent offspring of bipolar parents that found "super-normal" temperamental characteristics in the offspring who were diagnosis-free. That is, unaffected children and adolescents were more likely to approach new situations, things, and people; to have regular sleeping patterns; and to have lower energy and activity levels (Chang et al., 2003). The authors posited that these "exceptional" temperaments may protect against, or reflect an inherent brain chemistry that is resistant to, psychiatric disorders. Because there were no follow-up data on these offspring, however, it may be that the "exceptional" temperament only postpones onset, although that in its own right would be beneficial. It is possible that some of these well "super-normal" offspring may have inherited very mild subsyndromal variations of a hypomanic temperament; this may in turn provide a protective resilience and energy.

Nurnberger and colleagues (1988) included in their study measures of subsyndromal affective symptoms, as well as the personality trait of sensation seeking. On this measure, they found that children of bipolar parents displayed personality patterns suggestive of disinhibition, and they speculated that such offspring may be prone to respond to dysphoria with disinhibitory behaviors such as drug and alcohol abuse and high-risk behaviors.

Although based on only 7 boys of bipolar parents and 20 controls, a study by Zahn-Waxler and colleagues (1984a, 1984b) is unique in the intensity of its observations and in the young age (2–3yr) of the children involved. In laboratory observations of numerous real-life situations, the investigators found that the toddlers of bipolar parents displayed notable interpersonal difficulties and emotionality. For instance, they showed difficulties in peer interactions (e.g., sharing) and maladaptive aggression, as well as heightened distress and preoccupation in response to simulated conflict and suffering, among others. Although the children of bipolar parents did not display cognitive deficits, they did show more insecure attachment and deficits in taking another's perspective (Zahn-Waxler et al., 1984c). Radke-Yarrow's (1998) report on the expanded study also indicated significantly higher rates of insecure attachment among the children of bipolar mothers, compared with both the well and the unipolar groups. Nevertheless, these toddlers were seen as being relatively socially skilled. As they grew older, however, more disruptive and emotional disorders emerged that were associated with impaired functioning. For instance, peer relationships were rated as poor for 42 percent of the offspring of bipolar women, and 23 percent were doing poorly academically. The investigators found that, overall, 27 percent of the younger and 30 percent of the older siblings showed significant functioning problems in multiple areas (compared with very few of the children of well mothers). The findings of these studies suggest the value of intensive observation of high-risk children in stressful and challenging situations as a way of identifying potential deficits in emotional and behavioral regulation that may portend bipolar disorder.

Anderson and Hammen (1993) compared offspring in the University of California-Los Angeles (UCLA) high-risk study on social competence and academic functioning measures. They discovered that, although the offspring of unipolar mothers were the most impaired of all of the groups, the children of bipolar mothers were actually comparable to the children of non-ill mothers. The investigators predicted that, despite the symptomatology of the bipolar group and the likely increasing risk as they grew older, they were somewhat protected by positive social skills and successful academic achievement, compared with children in the unipolar group. Carlson and Weintraub (1993) evaluated young-adult functioning in their follow-up study of children of bipolar parents compared with a mixed group of offspring of parents with "other" psychopathology and with offspring of non-ill parents. They found that the Global Adjustment Scale scores of the young-adult offspring of bipolar parents were significantly lower than those of children from normal families but did not differ from the scores of offspring of parents with "other" psychopathology. Osher and colleagues (2000) compared the Rorschach responses of a small sample of offspring of manic-depressive parents and controls. They found indicators of thought disorder and unconventional perceptions, suggesting that these might be markers for manic-depressive illness.

The differing results across studies of offspring characteristics reflect a lack of standard batteries of measures (or theoretically driven explorations). The varying methods employed reveal an array of both positive and problematic attributes of children at risk for bipolar disorder. Future studies will be needed to determine whether there are consistent patterns of traits and characteristics that can inform predictions of eventual outcomes.

of the children had a definite diagnosis—chiefly ADHD, depressive disorders, and bipolar disorder (15 percent). Predictors of (childhood) bipolar disorder in the offspring were early onset of parental bipolar disorder and parental childhood ADHD. Children who had two parents with a mood disorder (bipolar or unipolar) tended to show somewhat different symptoms than those with only one ill parent, including increased severity of depressed mood and irritability and rejection sensitivity.

Egeland and colleagues (2003) reported on possible prodromal signs of bipolar disorder in 100 Amish children with a bipolar-I parent and matched controls. Annual evaluations of the children for 7 years, up to age 19 (mean age 14), were retrospectively reviewed and rated blindly by clinicians according to level of possible risk for future development of bipolar-I disorder. On the basis of their symptoms, 38 percent of the children of a bipolar parent were rated as being "at risk," compared with 17 percent of controls. The authors found many depression-related symptoms, as well as anxiety/fearfulness, hyperalertness, and anger dyscontrol, among others. In contrast to the findings of some other studies, however, they found little evidence of disruptive disorders, ADHD, or conduct problems in the Amish sample, and the symptoms observed had an episodic rather than a continuous and chronic course. Further follow-up of the offspring will be useful to determine whether the "risk" symptoms identified by these investigators do indeed portend bipolar-I disorder.

Relatively unremarkable rates of disorder among adolescent offspring were observed in a Dutch volunteer sample (largely from a manic-depressive association; see Wals et al., 2001). A 27 percent lifetime rate of mood disorders was found—not dissimilar to Dutch national norms—although there was no directly studied comparison group. The investigators speculated that the sample may have included relatively healthier bipolar parents than those ascertained primarily from treatment sources.

Mechanisms of Risk to Children of Bipolar Parents

Perhaps with the exception of the study of Todd and colleagues (1996), which linked children's psychopathology to the degree of genetic relatedness in a bipolar pedigree study, the high-risk offspring studies reviewed here cannot serve to confirm a genetic mode of transmission of risk for psychopathology. Rather, most of the studies were designed on the assumption of genetic transmission. Nonetheless, it is recognized that children in such families not only inherit whatever genes predispose to bipolar illness, but also "inherit" parents who are potentially impaired in the parental role at least periodically, and whose environments may be stressful because of instability in marital, occupational, and financial circumstances associated with the effects of

the illness. Moreover, a diathesis–stress perspective shared by most forms of psychopathology would lead to the expectation that even in the presence of genetic diatheses, information on additional variables, such as neurocognitive and biological factors, may be needed to determine whether—or when and how—an at-risk person develops a disorder. And because bipolar disorder manifests very different courses among affected individuals, it is important to link course and outcome features of the illness in parents to children's risk for disorder; also of interest are certain parental demographic features. Additional analyses are therefore needed to advance understanding of the varied outcomes of high-risk offspring of bipolar parents, and perhaps to shed light more generally on factors that affect the nature and timing of the course of the illness.

Family Life and Environment

Few bipolar high-risk studies have examined the association of children's psychiatric outcomes with characteristics of family life and environment. Marital conflict and disturbances of family climate and parent–child communication almost certainly have significant negative effects on children's adjustment. Obviously, the quality of relationships in families with bipolar parents is likely to play an important role in children's risk or resilience in the face of genetic predisposition (see Chapter 10 for further discussion of parenting characteristics in bipolar families).

A few bipolar high-risk studies have examined the role of such factors. LaRoche and colleagues (1987) found that among families with a bipolar mother, the father's report of marital dissatisfaction was the strongest predictor of the presence of a diagnosis in the offspring; in slightly different analyses, the mother's report of marital distress was also a significant predictor. The offspring who had disorders reported more negative quality of their relationship with both parents, compared with youngsters who did not have a diagnosis. Hammen (1991) also assessed marital functioning and other forms of stress in high-risk families. Both unipolar and bipolar mothers had high rates of divorce and current relationship stress compared with controls. In all groups, mothers' chronic stress and negative life events contributed to the prediction of worse outcomes in their children. Grigoroiu-Serbanescu and colleagues (1989) performed descriptive evaluations of "familial atmosphere" and determined that the greatest severity of psychopathology in offspring was associated with the highest levels of physical and verbal conflict within the family. Geller and colleagues (2002a) found that bipolar youths who lived in intact biological families were significantly more likely to recover than those in other living situations (Fig. 6–2).

A National Institute of Mental Health study found that bipolar women had higher levels of marital stress than

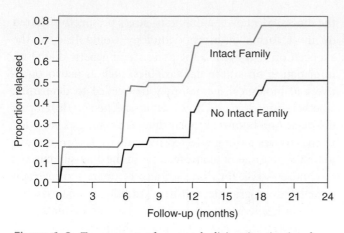

Figure 6–2. Two-year rate of recovery by living situation in subjects with a prepubertal and early adolescent bipolar disorder phenotype. Fifty-eight of the 89 subjects had recovered by 24 months. There was a significant difference between the 39 recovered subjects who lived with their intact biological families and the 19 who resided in other living situations (Cox model $\chi^2 = 7.40$, degrees of freedom [df] = 1, $p = .007$). The Kiddie Mania (K-M) estimate for recovery in intact families was 76.5% (95% confidence interval [CI] = 64.8–88.1), and for recovery in other living situations it was 50.0% (95% CI = 34.1–65.9). (*Source:* Geller et al., 2002. Reprinted with permission from the *American Journal of Psychiatry,* Copyright 2002, American Psychiatric Association.)

unipolar or well women; marital stress tended to be associated with other forms of family stress and maladaptive functioning as well, however, which made the effects difficult to disentangle (Radke-Yarrow, 1998). The combination of low maternal scores on global functioning and high indices of family stress (including marital conflict) was a strong predictor of depression in offspring, especially older children. In a more recent analysis, Meyer and colleagues (2004) reported that frequent maternal expressions of anger and irritability (perhaps themselves manifestations of mixed mania and therefore of genetic importance) during children's early years were associated with the development of mania in adulthood, even after controlling for maternal psychiatric features. Although based on a small sample, the results of this study hint that highly stressful family environments may contribute to the timing—or even the expression—of bipolar features in those at genetic risk (see also Miklowitz et al., 1988). In a 4-year prospective study of 86 prepubertal and early-adolescent bipolar patients, Geller and colleagues (2004) found that low maternal warmth predicted faster relapse after recovery from mania. In an earlier study, the same investigators had found that patients with prepubertal and early-onset adolescent bipolar disorder who were exposed to low levels of maternal warmth were four times more likely to relapse after recovery than those exposed to high levels of maternal warmth (Geller et al., 2002b). This effect

is clearly shown in Figure 6–3. It is not clear to what extent maternal warmth reflects an additional underlying vulnerability factor or if maternal warmth is decreased or adversely affected by the demands of caring for a child with bipolar illness.

One particularly dramatic example of family and environmental dysfunction concerns physical and sexual abuse. Analysis of data collected by the Stanley Foundation Bipolar Network showed that early traumatic abuse experiences were associated with a worse course of illness, including earlier onset, suicidality, and more rapid cycling (Leverich et al., 2002). Other investigators found elevated rates of childhood sexual abuse—significantly higher for males—among bipolar adults compared with those with unipolar depression (Hyun et al., 2000). There is also a highly significant association between those reporting childhood sexual abuse and auditory hallucinations (Hammersley et al., 2003). The findings of these studies suggest that among those with a predisposition to develop bipolar disorder, childhood trauma may play a role in the course of the illness; that parents who abuse children have a more severe or comorbid form that is genetically transmitted (as well as psychologically traumatic); or that children with early onset and impaired functioning may experience more severe abuse. It may be noted that self-reports

Figure 6–3. Two-year rate of relapse after recovery by high versus low levels of maternal–child warmth in subjects with a prepubertal and early-adolescent bipolar disorder phenotype. Thirty-two of the 58 recovered patients relapsed after recovery. There was a significant difference between the 21 relapsers with low maternal–child warmth and the 11 with high maternal warmth (Cox model $\chi^2 = 9.84$, degrees of freedom [df] = 1, $p = .002$). The Kiddie Mania (K-M) estimate for relapse by low maternal–child warmth was 100.0% (95% confidence interval [CI] = not applicable when K-M = 100.0%) and by high maternal–child warmth was 42.2% (95% CI = 23.2–61.2). (*Source:* Geller et al., 2002a. Reprinted with permission from the *American Journal of Psychiatry,* Copyright 2002, American Psychiatric Association.)

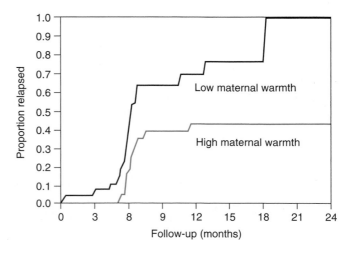

of trauma may overestimate its actual incidence, although this possibility has not been sufficiently investigated in bipolar illness.

A recent Dutch study of 132 offspring (mean age 16) of bipolar parents found that the relationship between stressful life events and the onset or recurrence of a DSM-IV mood disorder was almost entirely accounted for by the offspring's prior symptoms of depression and anxiety. The researchers concluded that the frequently hypothesized association between stressful life events and the precipitation of mood disorders may be a spurious one (Wals et al., 2005). The association between stressful life events and the onset or recurrence of a mood disorder was also independent of gender and familial loading. See Chapters 4 and 10 for a more complete discussion of life events and bipolar illness.

Neurocognitive and Biological Studies of High-Risk Youth

To date, few studies have included evaluation of potential neurocognitive and structural and functional brain markers of bipolar disorder. (See Chapters 9 and 15 for a detailed discussion of neurocognitive features of bipolar illness in general.) Because this approach has proven to be extremely fruitful in high-risk studies of schizophrenia, it is likely that such research on bipolar disorder will proliferate. Preliminary studies are beginning to emerge. For example, small samples of children at risk because of parental bipolar disorder or children/adolescents diagnosed with bipolar disorder have shown significant differences from normal controls on neurochemical abnormalities (Cecil et al., 2003), neuroanatomical features (DelBello et al., 2004), and neuropsychological performance (Dickstein et al., 2004). One study of neurocognitive effects in at-risk youth is especially interesting. Meyer and colleagues (2004) examined the outcomes after 23 years of offspring of bipolar, unipolar, and control women in the NIMH's longitudinal study of young children of women with affective disorders (Radke-Yarrow et al., 1992). They found that the majority of the offspring of bipolar mothers who later developed bipolar disorder had shown impairment on a neurocognitive test of executive functioning when they were adolescents.

In their analysis, Meyer and colleagues (2004) found that offspring in families with maternal bipolar disorder were substantially more likely to show impairment in neurocognitive functioning when tested in adolescence if they were also exposed to high levels of maternal anger and irritability during childhood. The investigators hypothesized that the maternal behavior was a potent stressor interacting with their offspring's genetic liability for bipolar disorder, potentially affecting brain development and increasing their risk for eventual development of the disorder. Direct causality has not been established, however, and it should be kept in mind that severely ill children have an impact on the degree of maternal irritability that is expressed. One study of 140 offspring of parents with bipolar disorder found lower birth weight in offspring to be significantly correlated with greater psychopathology (Wals et al., 2003); the authors suggested that this observed relationship might be due to a shared environmental or genetic factor that influences both. Other investigators have reported a more general association among birth weight, cognitive functioning, and psychopathology (Eaton et al., 2001).

Potential mechanisms underlying bipolar disorder were suggested by Leibenluft and colleagues (2003a), who specifically indicated possible applications to childhood-onset mania (and presumably, by extension, to children at risk because of parental bipolar disorder). Drawing on the work of various investigators, they suggested paradigms for physiological assessment, along with functional neuroimaging measures, of latency, magnitude, and recovery of emotional reactions to affective stimuli—as well as the relationships between attentional and emotional regulation processes in possibly bipolar children. Research aimed at clarifying underlying maladaptive processes in bipolar disorder that can be identified in at-risk samples of children holds promise for advancing understanding, and possibly detection, of bipolar disorder in the young.

Parents' Clinical and Demographic Features and Children's Outcomes

Findings thus far have been mixed on the extent to which there is increased risk to children if both parents are bipolar or if psychiatric disorder occurs in the first-degree relatives of a parent with bipolar disorder.[7] These mixed findings are likely attributable to design and sampling variations.

Few studies have examined features of parental bipolar course and their influence on children's disorders. An exception is Duffy and colleagues (1998), whose earlier-cited work suggests that parental responsiveness to lithium, which in turn is related to the presence of more "classic" bipolar illness, may be an important predictor. The most comprehensive analyses of clinical features as predictors of children's outcomes were reported by Grigoroiu-Serbanescu and colleagues (1989), who determined that severity of children's psychiatric disorders was significantly related to severity of the illness in the bipolar parent, number of manic and mixed (but not depressive) episodes, younger age at onset in the parent, and presence of psychopathology in the coparent. LaRoche and colleagues (1987) found that duration of parental illness was related to children's risk for disorder, but the nature of the episodes and the age at onset were not specified. Radke-Yarrow (1992) and Radke-Yarrow and colleagues (1998) reported a significant correlation between mothers' time in affective episodes and low levels of functioning (as assessed by the Global Assessment of Functioning) on the one hand and several measures of children's symptoms on the other, but did not distinguish between maternal manic and depressive symptoms.

Of interest, the study of Radke-Yarrow and colleagues (1992) included an evaluation of maternal Axis II disorders. It was found that two thirds of the bipolar mothers had at least one personality disorder, and personality disorder pathology measured dimensionally was significantly related to the extent of children's symptoms and disorders. Likewise, Hodgins and colleagues (2002) speculated that bipolar parents' high levels of trait neuroticism may expose their children to relatively stressful environments and models of poor coping, as well as to the genetic transmission of neuroticism that influences susceptibility to stress reactivity. Their proposal, similar to models of intergenerational transmission proposed by Hammen (1991), is that family discord and stress factors contribute to the risk of development of disorders in children.

It may be noted that there is a lack of information on the similarity of parent and child bipolar symptoms in cases of early-onset bipolar disorder. Follow-up studies are needed as well to evaluate possible similarities in course and treatment responsiveness.

Demographic factors have likewise not been fully explored, although they have been addressed in a modest number of studies. Grigoroiu-Serbanescu and colleagues (1989) found that gender of the bipolar parent did not make a difference in children's outcomes. On the other hand, Klein and colleagues (1985) found that bipolar mothers, compared with bipolar fathers, were more likely to have children with affective symptomatology. Several studies have included or controlled for socioeconomic status of bipolar parents. Grigoroiu-Serbanescu and colleagues (1989), for example, reported that lower socioeconomic status in their Romanian sample was associated with greater psychopathology in children.

Clearly, more research is needed to shed light on both clinical and demographic factors associated with bipolar parents that may moderate the effects of their disorder on outcomes among their offspring.

CONCLUSIONS

Increasing interest in mood disorders of children and adolescents has stimulated research and careful clinical observations aimed at identifying the clinical features, precursors, and course of bipolar disorder in these populations. However, numerous gaps in knowledge remain. For many years, unclear diagnostic criteria led to frequent misdiagnosis of bipolar disorder in children and adolescents. Today, pediatric bipolar disorders are increasingly being diagnosed and treated. Nonetheless, additional studies are needed to refine the predictive utility of age at onset of first symptoms, and to determine the correlates of illness course and level of functioning. Although "classic" bipolar features, including distinct affective episodes and good interepisode functioning, appear to be rare in children, some children display severe and chronic signs of emotional instability, behavioral dysregulation, and cognitive changes that are consistent with mania, and that appear to resemble bipolar mixed states and ultrarapid cycling. Whether such patterns mark developmentally consistent manifestations of bipolarity or reflect other traits or disorders not yet understood remains uncertain, however.

Diagnostic problems are compounded by the considerable overlap between presumed mania and ADHD, as well as other comorbid disorders, such as substance abuse, anxiety, and disruptive behavior disorders. Clearly, longitudinal studies are needed to determine the unique developmental manifestations of manic symptoms and whether possible manic syndrome or symptoms in children portend bipolar disorder in adolescence or later. Moreover, the significance of manic symptoms in children remains to be clarified, in particular whether they represent an especially severe and disabling form of the illness or a nonspecific indicator of psychopathology. Some have proposed that early-onset mania presenting with comorbid ADHD may represent an etiological subtype marked by familial concentrations of bipolar disorder and ADHD. Presently, it is recommended that a diagnosis of bipolar disorder be reserved for children who meet DSM-IV criteria for mania, and that bipolar-NOS be used for those with severe emotional and behavioral dysregulation when boundaries with disruptive behavior disorders are unclear.

Parental bipolar disorder in families of children with manic symptoms would appear to be a potentially validating criterion, but further research is needed to identify early markers (endophenotypes) of childhood bipolar disorder. The stakes are high for such severely ill children, because early valid diagnosis and empirically supported treatment could greatly improve their lives and future functioning. Studies of children of bipolar parents employing the high-risk methodology (that is, the study of children of psychiatrically ill parents) represent a design uniquely suited to refining the assessment and diagnosis of precursor forms of bipolar disorder. Moreover, such studies may prove crucial in identifying markers of risk processes that interact with genetic diatheses, although few studies to date have examined the neurobiological or developmental abnormalities that may signal onset of or vulnerability to bipolar disorder. The studies of high-risk children conducted thus far have clearly indicated that the offspring of bipolar parents have elevated rates of psychopathology, developing in childhood and adolescence. A significant proportion develop bipolar disorder—and the rate is likely to grow still higher as these offspring pass through the age of risk in late adolescence and adulthood. Longitudinal research on such samples is needed to help clarify the developmental progression of the disorder; its earliest symptoms; and predictors of its course, including adverse family and environmental experiences.

NOTES

1. See excellent reviews by Faedda et al., 1995; Geller and Luby, 1997; Coyle et al., 2003; Carlson, 2005.
2. See Biederman et al., 2000a, 2004c; Geller et al., 2000b; Masai et al., 2003.
3. Masi et al., 2001; Wozniak, 2002; Faedda et al., 2004; Harpold et al., 2005.
4. This statement appeared on the Web site of the Child and Adolescent Bipolar Foundation, http://www.bpkids.org (accessed August 31, 2006).
5. See Strober et al., 1995; Faraone et al., 1997a; McElroy et al., 1997; Kafantaris et al., 1998.
6. Decina et al., 1982; Gershon et al., 1985; Klein et al., 1985; Nurnberger et al., 1988; Grigoroiu-Serbanescu et al., 1989, 1991; Birmaher et al., 2005a,b.
7. See Gershon et al., 1985; LaRoche et al., 1987; Grigoroiu-Serbanescu et al., 1989; Radke-Yarrow et al., 1992; Todd et al., 1996.

7 Comorbidity

The patient who has for years before his illness shown morbid traits, who has been anxious, or quarrelsome, or suspicious, or odd, or solitary, or obsessional, or in some other way has shown that he is constantly at odds with himself, as well as with his surroundings—such a patient is not going to be cured of his maladjustment by having an affective flare-up. A sortie does not end a siege.

—*Sir Aubrey Lewis (1936, p. 997)*

Comorbidity in manic-depressive illness, in which the mood disorder is complicated by the presence of one or more additional disorders, is the rule rather than the exception, especially for the bipolar subgroup. Data from the Stanley Foundation Bipolar Network, a consortium of bipolar specialty clinics in academic health centers around the world, indicate that 65 percent of patients with bipolar disorder have a comorbid condition. Of these patients, almost a quarter have three or more diagnoses (Fig. 7–1) (McElroy et al., 2001).

Unfortunately, disorders that can accompany affective illness tend to be underrecognized and undertreated (Simon et al., 2004a). Poor recognition of comorbid conditions may be related to the way in which clinicians diagnose their patients. Psychiatric evaluation is often directed toward identifying a single diagnosis that will account for all or most of a patient's symptoms, rather than identifying multiple conditions. This expectation can lead to important disorders being overlooked, and the partially diagnosed and incompletely treated patient may be left with considerable symptomatology and disability, even after the primary disorder has been effectively treated. In the case of bipolar disorder, which can be destabilized by certain classes of medication, the clinician must also be wary of worsening one illness while treating another. For example, treating panic disorder with a selective serotonin reuptake inhibitor (SSRI) may trigger a switch to a manic or mixed episode. (The difficulties involved in the treatment of comorbid conditions are addressed in Chapter 24.) Proper attention to management of comorbidities can reduce their impact on a patient's functioning and general health. Unfortunately, even with the best treatment, the presence of one or more comorbid disorders tends to lead to a poorer outcome compared with uncomplicated manic-depressive illness.

Some investigators have evaluated the total burden of comorbidity by surveying multiple diagnostic categories, while others have focused in more detail on specific conditions. Studies taking a comprehensive approach to the presence of comorbidity have found that, especially for the bipolar subgroup, an uncomplicated recurrent mood disorder is unusual. The National Comorbidity Survey (NCS) of more than 58,000 individuals found that, among bipolar patients with "classic" features such as euphoria, grandiosity, and the ability to maintain energy without sleep, all met the *Diagnostic and Statistical Manual* (DSM)-III-R criteria for at least one other mental disorder. Fully 95 percent met the criteria for three or more disorders (Kessler et al., 1997). This, for reasons discussed below, is almost certainly a considerable overestimate. Another study, involving 3,258 randomly selected household residents of Edmonton, Alberta, found similarly high rates of comorbidity. Based on surveys performed by trained lay interviewers using the Diagnostic Interview Schedule (DIS), comorbidity with other disorders occurred in 92 percent of subjects who had experienced a manic episode. The generalizability of this particular study may be limited, however. The lifetime prevalence of mania identified by the lay interviewers was lower than in most other studies—only 0.6 percent. Consequently, the interviewers may have been identifying only a subset of patients with bipolar disorder who had more severe psychopathology. Also, as discussed later, there are significant discrepancies between the high rates of comorbidity identified by nonclinician versus clinician interviewers. For example, experienced clinicians in the Stanley Network identified social anxiety disorder in only 16 percent of their bipolar patients, compared with nearly 50 percent identified by nonclinicians in the NCS study.

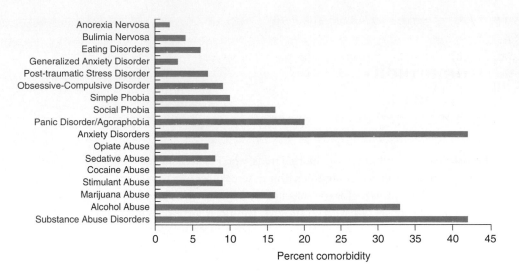

Figure 7–1. Axis I psychiatric comorbidities. Percent comorbidity in bipolar patients enrolled in the Stanley Bipolar Treatment Network. (*Source*: Adapted from McElroy et al., 2001. Reprinted with permission from the *American Journal of Psychiatry*, Copyright 2001. American Psychiatric Association.)

Guo and colleagues (2005) used a claims database to evaluate rates of bipolar comorbidity. They analyzed a large managed-care population of 123,292 patients who had been given an *International Classification of Diseases 9* (ICD-9) diagnostic code for bipolar disorder by their treating clinician. The prevalence of comorbid anxiety disorders was 36.7 percent, but the rate of comorbid substance disorders was only 12.0 percent. The low level of comorbid substance abuse/dependence in this population may have been due to the fact that individuals with commercial health insurance were more likely to be employed, whereas substance-related disorders often lead to the loss of a job or chronic unemployment (Leino-Arjas et al., 1999).

Data obtained from structured clinician interviews also reveal high levels of comorbidity in bipolar patients. Bauer and colleagues (2005) evaluated intake assessment data, obtained by clinicians using the Structured Clinical Interview for DSM (SCID), on subjects recruited as part of the Veterans Affairs (VA) Cooperative Study No. 430. In this sample of hospitalized bipolar veterans, 57 percent had at least one current comorbid disorder. More than one comorbid disorder was found in 30 percent of the patients, and 9 percent had three or more comorbidities. As in the preceding studies, the two most common comorbidities were anxiety and substance abuse disorders. At least one anxiety disorder was currently present in 38 percent of the sample; the lifetime rate was 43 percent. The similarity between current and lifetime rates suggests a high degree of chronicity. Post-traumatic stress disorder (PTSD) was present in 25 percent, panic disorder in 17 percent, and obsessive-compulsive disorder (OCD) in 8 percent. Current substance abuse disorders were present in 34 percent; alcohol (26 percent), marijuana (7 percent), and cocaine

(7 percent) were the most commonly abused substances. The lifetime rate for substance abuse disorders was considerably higher, 72 percent.

The VA investigators also evaluated correlates of anxiety and substance-related disorders and found them to be distinct. Compared with bipolar patients with no comorbidity, those with comorbid substance abuse/dependence had more marital problems and a higher probability of presenting with depression; they also had more medical conditions during the index hospitalization and were less able to work. Comorbid anxiety disorders were associated with earlier age at onset of bipolar disorder, rapid cycling, a greater likelihood of presenting with depression, a higher rate of suicide attempts, and a greater number of manic and depressive episodes in the year preceding hospitalization. Vieta and colleagues (2001), in their Barcelona Stanley Foundation Study of 129 bipolar-I outpatients in remission, found that comorbid bipolar patients had a higher number of mixed features, depressive episodes, and suicide attempts. The different patterns of correlates led Bauer and colleagues (2005) to speculate that distinct genetic subtypes of bipolar disorder were represented by patients who had comorbid anxiety disorders compared with those with comorbid substance abuse disorders. The association of discrete subtypes of bipolar disorder with specific comorbid presentations is discussed in further detail later.

Patients in the Bauer and colleagues (2005) VA study were all hospitalized and had either bipolar-I or bipolar-II disorder. However, it is not only the most severely ill patients who experience comorbid conditions. Patients with soft-spectrum bipolarity—those who, although they do not meet the full DSM criteria for bipolar disorder, nonetheless experience significant symptoms of depressed and elevated moods—also have high rates of comorbidity (Maremnani et al., 2006). For example, in the Zurich cohort study (Angst, 1998), a 15-year prospective study of 4,547 young adults, 78 percent of patients with brief hypomanic episodes had a lifetime prevalence of at least one anxiety disorder. Panic disorder was the most common anxiety disorder, affecting 12 percent of all patients; 32 percent experienced panic attacks without meeting the full criteria for panic disorder. Binge eating (13 percent) and alcohol abuse disorders (23 percent) were also common in this cohort. Patients with major depressive disorder have more anxiety and substance abuse disorders than the general population, but significantly fewer than patients with bipolar disorder (Chen and Dilsaver, 1995b).

Although comorbid conditions tend to be underdiagnosed, they can also be overdiagnosed. Manic-depressive illness, as we have emphasized, is highly variable in its presentation. Patients with completely different clinical presentations and courses are given the same DSM-IV diagnosis. Diagnostic criteria for mood disorders include symptoms of anxiety; conduct disturbance; cognitive impairment; and changes in eating, energy levels, sleeping, and sexual functioning. Comorbid diagnoses can be inflated by the confounding of symptoms with diagnoses. Nonclinician interviewers in particular, who estimate the presence of psychiatric disorders using a symptom checklist, are at greater risk for overestimating comorbidity than are experienced clinicians, who use pattern recognition to make diagnoses. Thus before one can properly interpret studies of comorbidity, the method used to establish diagnoses must be explicit.

In the remainder of this chapter, we review the findings of the literature on the major comorbid conditions in manic-depressive illness, with an emphasis on the bipolar subgroup. There is little published information on the more recurrent forms of unipolar depression per se. We address in turn alcohol and drug abuse/dependence disorders, anxiety disorders, other psychiatric illnesses, and medical illnesses.

ALCOHOL AND DRUG ABUSE/DEPENDENCE DISORDERS

Several general methodological issues arise in the study of alcohol and drug abuse/dependence in manic-depressive patients. We begin by considering these, and then turn to specific diagnostic issues. First, it is often difficult to obtain accurate histories of alcohol and drug abuse from patients; compounding the problem, clinicians tend to skirt this general line of inquiry. Second, patients vary tremendously in the development and expression of both manic-depressive illness and substance abuse/dependence disorders. Third, many studies do not adequately differentiate substance abuse from the more serious and persistent disorder of true alcohol or drug dependence.

Inconsistency and unreliability of diagnostic criteria are particular problems when investigators attempt to diagnose and study more than one disorder and then to determine which is primary and which secondary. Schuckit (1986) summarized several major sources of diagnostic confusion related to alcohol and mood disorders: (1) alcohol can cause depressive symptoms; (2) signs of temporary serious depression can follow prolonged drinking; (3) drinking can escalate during affective episodes in some patients, especially during mania; (4) depressive symptoms and alcohol problems occur in other psychiatric disorders; and (5) a subset of manic-depressive patients have independent alcohol abuse disorder. Differentiating symptoms caused by a primary psychiatric disorder from those secondary to substance abuse can be difficult. Affective, cognitive, and psychotic symptoms can result from alcohol and from a wide variety of classes of drugs, such as amphetamines, cocaine, and hallucinogens. Likewise, alcohol and other drugs can both mask and precipitate affective symptoms. Indeed, Kraepelin (1921) observed many years ago that manic attacks occasionally begin with delirium tremens. More recently, manic attacks induced by lysergic acid diethylamide (LSD) and phenylcyclidine (PCP) have been observed in biologically vulnerable individuals. These issues are discussed in more detail later in this chapter. Obtaining a detailed chronology of the onset of symptoms (i.e., whether difficulties with substance abuse predated affective symptoms or vice versa), ascertaining the severity of presenting symptoms, and taking a thorough family history can aid in making a correct differential diagnosis (Hesselbrock et al., 1985; Schuckit, 1986). Correct diagnosis, in turn, is essential to good medical and psychological care (see Chapter 24). In a 5-year prospective study of 27 bipolar-I patients in whom the onset of alcohol abuse disorder preceded the onset of bipolar disorder, and 33 patients in whom that order was reversed, Strakowski and colleagues (2005) found that those who abused alcohol first were more likely to recover and recovered more quickly. Those whose illness preceded their alcohol abuse spent more time affectively ill and experienced more symptoms of alcohol abuse.

Alcohol Abuse/Dependence

In a letter to a friend, the poet Edgar Allan Poe wrote about alcohol and mental illness from a deeply personal perspective:

> I became insane, with long periods of horrible sanity.
> During these fits of absolute unconsciousness I drank,
> God only knows how much or how long. As a matter of

course, my enemies referred the insanity to the drink, rather than the drink to the insanity.

Separating the insanity from the drink remains a difficult problem in the differential diagnosis and treatment of affective illness and substance abuse disorders. A relationship between alcohol and mood disorders has been observed for more than 2,000 years. Plato (cited in Ackerknecht, 1959) referred to alcoholism as a demonstrable cause of mania. Soranus (c. 100 AD, cited in Zilboorg, 1941) echoed the sentiment that excessive use of alcohol frequently caused mania and criticized those who prescribed it as a treatment. Aretaeus (c. 90 AD, cited in Whitwell, 1936) suggested that symptoms of mania may be produced by an excess of wine or opiates but concluded that the resulting states cannot properly be termed mania, just temporary deliria. Early in the twentieth century, Kraepelin (1921, p. 178) summarized his findings on alcohol dependence in manic-depressive illness as follows:

> Alcoholism occurs among male patients in about a quarter of the cases, but is to be regarded as the consequence of debaucheries committed in excitement, not as a cause.

Differing views about whether alcohol abuse disorder precedes or follows the onset of manic-depressive illness persist today, and there is a growing appreciation of the importance of recognizing this comorbidity (dual diagnosis).

Rates of Mood Disorders among Patients with Alcohol Abuse/Dependence

The lack of consistency in diagnostic criteria has led to widely disparate estimates of the rates of mood disorders in patients with alcohol abuse disorder. These estimates have ranged from 3 to 98 percent, depending on whether clinical scales or more formal diagnostic criteria were used (Keeler et al., 1979; Himmelhoch et al., 1983). Estimates of the prevalence of mood disorders in those with alcohol dependence range from 12 to 57 percent when mood disorders are defined by formal diagnostic criteria, but are as high as 98 percent when rating scales are used (Bernadt and Murray, 1986).

Rates of Alcohol Abuse/Dependence among Patients with Mood Disorders

The Epidemiological Catchment Area (ECA) data for alcohol abuse/dependence in patients with affective illness show a high lifetime prevalence rate (Table 7–1) of 17 percent in unipolar depressed patients (the proportion with recurrent depressions was not specified) and a strikingly higher rate, 46 percent, in bipolar-I patients (Regier et al., 1990). Three other studies (Freed, 1969; Morrison, 1974; Estroff et al., 1985) found that when bipolar patients in clinical settings were systematically queried, they reported rates of alcohol abuse/dependence of about 60 to 75 percent. Compared with patients with other psychiatric diagnoses, those with bipolar disorder were at particularly high risk of developing an alcohol problem during their lifetime. This can be seen in Figure 7–2, which shows the lifetime prevalence of alcohol abuse disorder in individuals with selected psychiatric diagnoses and in the general population.

Most studies have found alcohol abuse disorder comorbidity is more frequent in bipolar patients than in those with any other mood disorder. The ECA study of alcohol abuse/dependence and psychiatric comorbidity (Helzer and Pryzbeck, 1988) found that mania was strongly associated with alcohol abuse/dependence (odds ratio = 6.2) but

TABLE 7–1. **Lifetime Prevalence Rates for Alcohol and Drug Abuse/Dependence in Persons with Mood Disorders and in the General Population**

Type of Abuse/Dependence	Bipolar-I (%)	Bipolar-II (%)	Major Depression (%)	General Population (%)
Alcohol	46	39	17	13.5
Abuse only	15	18	5	
Dependence	31	21	12	
Drug	41	21	18	6.2
Abuse only	13	9	7	
Dependence	28	12	11	

Note: Data are from the Epidemiological Catchment Area (ECA) study and are based on DSM-III diagnosis.
ECA = Epidemiological Catchment Area.
Source: Regier et al., 1990.

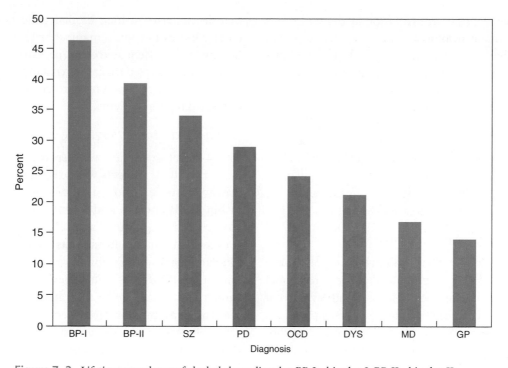

Figure 7–2. Lifetime prevalence of alcohol abuse disorder. BP-I = bipolar-I; BP-II = bipolar-II; DYS = dysthymia; GP = general population; MD = major depression; OCD = obsessive-compulsive disorder; PD = panic disorder; SZ = schizophrenia. (*Source:* Regier et al., 1990.)

that major depression was not (odds ratio = 1.7); more highly recurrent or cyclic depressions were not analyzed separately. Bipolar-I was associated with a higher lifetime rate of alcohol abuse/dependence than bipolar-II (46 versus 39 percent) or unipolar depression (17 percent) (Regier et al., 1990).

A study of 267 patients enrolled in the Stanley Foundation Bipolar Network found that, as in the general population, more men (49 percent) than women (29 percent) with bipolar disorder met the criteria for lifetime alcohol abuse. Likewise, a recent study of 211 bipolar patients found that men had significantly higher rates of comorbid alcohol abuse/dependence (Kawa et al., 2005). However, having bipolar disorder raised a woman's risk of having an alcohol-related disorder to a much greater degree than it did for a man. Compared with nonbipolar patients, the odds ratio of having an alcohol-related disorder among those with bipolar disorder was 7.35 for women and 2.77 for men (Frye et al., 2003). Men and women with bipolar disorder also have different risk factors for comorbid alcohol-related diagnoses. In men, the risk appears to be more associated with a genetic predisposition. Specifically, men with bipolar disorder and comorbid alcohol abuse/dependence have a more extensive family history of both disorders compared with men with noncomorbid bipolar disorder. Women with bipolar disorder and alcohol-related disorders, on the other hand, do not have as great a family loading. Comorbid alcohol

abuse/dependence in women is associated more with a greater familial burden of depressive episodes and anxiety disorders (Frye et al., 2003).

Elderly bipolar patients are also at increased risk for alcohol abuse. A community survey compared 84 elderly (ages ≥65 years) bipolar respondents with 8,121 elderly respondents without bipolar disorder; those with bipolar illness had a significantly higher lifetime and 12-month prevalence of alcohol disorders (p <.001) (Goldstein et al., 2006).

In summary, many studies, using a wide variety of diagnostic criteria and patient populations and conducted over a period of more than 50 years, have been quite consistent in finding significantly elevated rates of alcohol abuse/dependence in manic depressive illness, particularly the bipolar form. Conversely, they have found a significantly increased proportion of patients with manic-depressive illness within populations of alcohol abusers.

Drug Abuse/Dependence

The data on rates of comorbid bipolar illness and drug abuse/dependence are much less extensive and consistent than those on comorbid alcohol-related disorders, in no small part because of the illegal nature of drug-related disorders. The ECA data for drug abuse/dependence in patients with mood disorders show strikingly high lifetime prevalence rates of 18 percent in unipolar depressed patients and 41 percent in bipolar-I patients (Regier et al., 1990), nearly identical to the rates for alcohol-related disorders (see Table 7–1). In the general population, drug abuse/dependence is significantly less common than alcohol-related disorders (see also Table 7–2).

Determining the sequence of comorbid mood disorders and drug abuse/dependence presents the same methodological problems as those encountered in the case of alcohol-related diagnoses. The ECA data show that the affective disorder is 1.3 times more likely to occur before the drug abuse disorder (see the later discussion).

Cocaine

An interview study of patients voluntarily enrolled in a bipolar disorder case registry found that 3.4 percent met the diagnostic criteria for cocaine abuse, and 6.7 percent met the criteria for cocaine dependence (Chengappa et al., 2000). Consistent with other findings on drug abuse problems, more patients with bipolar-I than with bipolar-II abused cocaine.

Data of this sort cannot address the nature of the relationship between the mood and drug disorders. Clearly there are features of bipolar illness that can increase the likelihood of cocaine abuse, such as a desire to relieve the psychomotor retardation of bipolar depression and a desire to reinduce, prolong, or accelerate elevated mood and energy states. Weiss and Mirin (1986), for example, found that the majority of their bipolar patients reported using cocaine more often when manic than when depressed. This finding is consistent with that of Estroff and colleagues (1985), who observed that 58 percent of their manic bipolar patients abused cocaine, compared with 30 percent of their depressed bipolar patients.[1]

Opiates and Central Nervous System Depressants

In a study of 533 opiate and depressant abusers, 24 percent of the total subjects were diagnosed with major depressive disorder, and 5.4 percent were either bipolar-I or bipolar-II (Kosten and Rounsaville, 1986). Mirin and colleagues (1984) found a similar rate of unipolar depression among opiate addicts, but twice the rate of bipolar illness among abusers of these central nervous system (CNS) depressants. They also found that nearly three times more female than male opiate addicts were diagnosed as bipolar (10.8 versus 3.7 percent). These rates of bipolar illness are substantially higher than those found in the general population. Estroff and colleagues (1985) examined drug abuse in bipolar patients in their drug treatment clinic and reported that 25 percent of their manic patients abused heroin, compared with 20 percent of their depressed bipolar patients. The small sample size of this study limits its generalizability, however. Miller and colleagues (1989), studying a larger sample, found that only 5 percent of their manic patients abused opiates.

TABLE 7–2. **Rates of Drug Abuse/Dependence in the General Population**

Study	Total Population (%)	Male (%)	Female (%)	Prevalence
Regier et al., 1988 (ECA)				
Drug abuse/dependence	5.9			Lifetime
	2.0			6-month
Kessler et al., 1994 (NCS)				
Drug abuse	4.4	5.4	3.5	Lifetime
	0.8	1.3	0.3	12-month
Drug dependence	7.5	9.4	5.9	Lifetime
	2.8	3.8	1.9	12-month
Narrow et al., 2002 (ECA and NCS)	1.3	1.8	0.7	1-month
Drug abuse disorder using "clinical significance" criteria	1.7			12-month

ECA = Epidemiological Catchment Area; NCS = National Comorbidity Survey.

Overall, the rates of bipolar illness in opiate abusers, although not as dramatically high as in cocaine abusers, are greater than those found in the general population, but not as high as the rates of unipolar depression among those with opiate dependence.

Marijuana

Marijuana (cannabis) is the most widely abused illicit drug in the United States. According to the 2000 National Household Survey on Drug Abuse, 6.3 percent of Americans aged 12 or older were current abusers; approximately 59 percent of them abused only marijuana, and another 17 percent abused another illicit drug as well (Office of Applied Studies, 2001). Marijuana abuse is more prevalent among patients with bipolar disorder than in the general population. A study of 3,536 patients from 14 European countries, for example, found that 12 percent of patients being treated for mania were current abusers of marijuana (Reed et al., 2005). Other studies have found a wide range of rates of marijuana abuse in bipolar disorder—from 15 to 65 percent—but all rates have been high.[2] Marijuana, which has both sedative and psychedelic properties, can cause a variety of mood-related effects. Acute intoxication is associated with euphoria, anxiety, agitation, and grandiosity. Chronic abuse can lead to low-grade lethargy and depression, sometimes accompanied by anxiety, paranoia, and memory loss. A recent study of 52 bipolar alcohol-dependent patients found that 48 percent reported marijuana abuse; those that did had significantly more psychiatric comorbidity, in addition to more severe alcohol and other drug abuse (Salloum et al., 2005).

Hypotheses about the Relationship between Bipolar Illness and Alcohol and Drug Abuse

Relationship of Alcohol and Drug Abuse to Phase of Illness

Although it is perhaps more intuitive to link increased alcohol consumption with the depressed phase of bipolar illness, evidence suggests that the link is as or more common with hypomania, mania, and mixed or transitional states. Indeed, bipolar patients who increase their alcohol consumption generally do so during the manic phase (Zisook and Schuckit, 1987). Table 7–3 summarizes six studies of the relationship between alcohol intake and phase of illness. Alcohol, to a point, does appear to provide some relief for the irritability, restlessness, and agitation associated with mania. In this sense, although its use is damaging overall, it is not surprising that alcohol consumption increases during mania.

There is some evidence that bipolar patients (38 percent) are more likely than unipolar patients (15 percent) to increase their drinking when in a depressive episode (Bernadt and Murray, 1986). The tendency for bipolar patients to drink more heavily when depressed may reflect the increased agitation and perturbation associated with coexisting transitional or mixed states. In an early study, Winokur and colleagues (1969) found that the percentage of bipolar patients increasing their alcohol consumption was higher during mixed and manic states (43 and 42 percent, respectively) than during bipolar depression (27 percent). Himmelhoch and colleagues (1976a) noted that the major differ-

TABLE 7–3. Relationship between Alcohol Consumption and Phase of Bipolar Illness

Study	DEPRESSED PHASE (%)			MANIC PHASE (%)		
	Increase	Decrease	No Change	Increase	Decrease	No change
Minski, 1938	100	0	0	29	0	71
Mayfield and Coleman, 1968	26	43	31	83	0	17
Winokur et al., 1969	27	0	73	42	0	47
Reich et al., 1974[a]	3	0	97[a]	50	0	50[a]
Hensel et al., 1979[b]	21	22	57	14	7	79
Bernadt and Murray, 1986	38	25	36	20	23	57

[a]No information given as to decrease or no change.
[b]Depressed phase approximated, excluding unipolar patients.

entiating feature between patients in mixed and nonmixed states was their rate of alcohol and drug abuse; the former patients were twice as likely to abuse these substances.

As noted earlier, findings of clinical research suggest that bipolar patients abuse cocaine when depressed, but are even more likely to do so while hypomanic or manic. Patients increased their cocaine abuse during the latter states not only to alleviate associated dysphoria, but also to bring about, sustain, or heighten the high-energy, euphoric state. These mood-altering uses of cocaine have been discussed by several investigators. The use of cocaine in hypomanic states was described by Khantzian (1985, p. 1263) as a means "to augment a hyperactive, restless lifestyle." Gawin and Kleber (1986, pp. 110–111) discussed the use of cocaine by cyclothymic individuals:

> Cocaine use did not precipitate manic episodes, and it was initially well controlled. . . . Cocaine use early on reestablished hypomanic functioning during dysthymic cycles. However, cocaine use eventually was extended to continuously regulate mood state. When these subjects began to perceive that cocaine use was harmful, they successfully refrained from cocaine during dysthymic phases. Paradoxically, 80% described that when mood state improved toward hypomania, judgment of the seriousness of cocaine-related problems deteriorated, and cocaine use recurred.

The use of cocaine for control of both depressed and elated phases of bipolar illness was described by Weiss and Mirin (1984, pp. 49–50):

> We were impressed by the perceived utility of [cocaine] in the regulation of both dysphoric and elated mood. Typically, depressed patients reported symptom relief at moderate doses but also noted the need to gradually increase the dose or the frequency of drug administration. . . . Bipolar and cyclothymic patients hospitalized for chronic cocaine use reported that they used the drug most frequently to enhance endogenously elevated mood in the manic phases of their illness.

Self-Medication Hypothesis

The hypothesis that alcohol and drug abuse/dependence occurs in an effort to self-medicate mood disorders has been suggested in various ways for more than a thousand years. In 1884, Freud recognized that cocaine, with its mood-elevating properties, could be used as a potent antidepressant. Later, Milkman and Frosch (1973; quoted in Khantzian, 1985, p. 1260) wrote:

> [H]eroin addicts preferred the calming and dampening effects of opiates and seemed to use them to shore up tenuous defenses and reinforce a tendency toward withdrawal

and isolation, while amphetamine addicts used the stimulating action of amphetamines to support an inflated sense of self-worth and a defensive style involving active confrontation with their environment.

As we have seen, however, contrary to theories positing the use of stimulants to counter depressive states, most patients report using cocaine primarily when hypomanic or manic to enhance or induce euphoric moods associated with those states. Weiss and colleagues (1988), for example, found that the majority of their bipolar and cyclothymic patients abusing cocaine claimed that they were not self-medicating depression but lengthening and intensifying the euphoric effects of hypomania. These same authors had noted earlier (Weiss and Mirin, 1984, p. 50) that the manic phase of bipolar and cyclothymic cocaine abusers was characterized by euphoria, whereas "substance abusers who experienced dysphoria during mania or hypomania seemed to prefer to 'self-treat' their symptoms with opiates or other central nervous system depressants (including alcohol)."

This notion of using opiates to self-treat dysphoric feelings echoes similar results from Rounsaville and colleagues (1982) and Castaneda and colleagues (1989) and, in part, those of Khantzian (1974) and of Wurmser (1974, p. 358), who suggested that the abuse of opiates was a mechanism for combating the "psychologically disorganizing effects of overwhelming rage" (Weiss and Mirin, 1987). Evidence suggests, however, that alcohol and such drugs as heroin and PCP also may produce increased symptoms of dysphoria, irritability, and anxiety.

Why, then, do bipolar patients continue to abuse cocaine, even after they have alleviated the painful state from which they were trying to escape? Weiss and colleagues (1986) hypothesized that low to moderate doses of cocaine may make affectively ill patients feel better (as Post and colleagues, 1974b, found in depressed patients) by relieving anxious, agitated feelings, and that this effect promotes further drug use. Other factors then assume importance in maintaining drug-abusing behavior, and a chronic dependence often results (Castaneda et al., 1989). This may be true as well for opiate and alcohol abuse in manic and depressed patients who continue to drink or abuse drugs despite realizing the substances' adverse effects on mood (Weiss and Mirin, 1987).

Self-medication of affective illness by alcohol has been postulated, but it is less well supported by the evidence than such use of cocaine and opiates. Reich and colleagues (1974), like many other clinicians, observed that increased alcohol consumption appeared to be a type of self-medication, an attempt to slow down, relax, and take the edge off the dysphoria. They hypothesized that excessive alcohol use is a sign of more severe mania and represents an attempt to control manic symptoms, especially sleep disturbance and hyperactivity. Noting that patients with mixed states are twice as likely as other patients to abuse drugs and alcohol, Himmelhoch and colleagues (1976a) suggested that the switch phase could be dysphoric and uncomfortable, and substance abuse could be used to self-medicate this dysphoria. Weiss and Mirin (1987) posited that, in addition to self-medication, the increased use of drugs and alcohol during manic episodes could be attributed to impulsiveness, recklessness, and poor judgment. Liskow and colleagues (1982) suggested that "drinking may simply be another manifestation of mania—manics tend to do more of everything" (p. 145) and noted that "the self-medication hypothesis relating alcoholism to affective disorder appears to be simplistic if not entirely erroneous" (p. 146).

The self-medication hypothesis in substance abuse among affectively ill patients is likely to be debated for some time before being resolved. The ECA data discussed earlier show a greatly increased rate of major depression preceding substance abuse, rather than substance abuse preceding depression. Recently, a study of 45 patients with bipolar disorder and substance dependence found that nearly all patients said they had initiated substance abuse because of symptoms of bipolar disorder; of these, most (78 percent) cited depression, followed by racing thoughts (58 percent). Two thirds (67 percent) of the patients reported improvement in at least one symptom as a result of the substance abuse (Weiss et al., 2004).

In summary, not all studies have supported the validity of the self-medication hypothesis. It is probable that a subgroup of bipolar patients abuses alcohol and other drugs to intensify elevated mood and energy states, while another subgroup abuses the same substances to ameliorate or self-medicate their manic, depressive, or mixed symptoms. Some do both.

Precipitation of Illness

An underlying bipolar illness may be precipitated by alcohol or drug abuse. For example, the first manic episode in a biologically vulnerable individual may be triggered by hallucinogen or stimulant abuse. Interactions among predisposed individuals, their substance abuse patterns, and the onset of abnormal mood episodes have been observed by many clinicians and investigators.

The most demonstrable drug-induced psychoses in manic-depressive patients are those resulting from hallucinogenic drugs such as LSD and PCP. The psychotic symptoms associated with the abuse of these drugs have been well documented by several authors (e.g., El-Guebaly, 1975; Bowers, 1977; Erard et al., 1980). Amphetamine abuse was noted by Ellinwood and Petrie (1979) to be a precipitant of psychosis. Many of the presenting symptoms (e.g., delusions of persecution and grandeur and visual and auditory hallucinations) are present in manic psychoses. Evidence from animal studies shows that cocaine is a potent inducer of a process analogous to kindling in the CNS (sensitization) (Post et al., 1984). The role of kindling–sensitization processes in the pathophysiology of manic-depressive illness is discussed in Chapter 14.

There may be important differences between patients who develop substance abuse after the emergence of manic-depressive illness and those who develop substance abuse first. Since the literature on the sequential relationships between major depression and substance abuse typically does not differentiate more recurrent from less recurrent forms of depression, our focus once again is on the bipolar subgroup. In a retrospective study of 188 patients, those with bipolar disorder who later developed a substance abuse disorder had a younger age at onset of mood symptoms (13.5) compared with bipolar patients who never developed such a disorder (22.7) (Feinman and Dunner, 1996). As noted earlier, Strakowski and colleagues (2005), in a 5-year follow-up study of 144 bipolar-I patients, found that those whose alcohol abuse disorder preceded the onset of bipolar disorder were older and tended to recover more quickly than those whose bipolar illness proceeded their alcohol abuse disorder. This later age at onset in the alcohol-first group was found in the 2001–2002 National Epidemiologic Survey on Alcohol and Related Conditions as well (Goldstein and Levitt, 2006). This may mean that an early onset predisposes bipolar patients to future substance abuse, or there may be a subpopulation at risk for both an early onset of bipolar disorder and substance abuse. Of particular note in the Feinman and Dunner study, patients whose drug abuse came first had a later onset of mood symptoms than those with primary bipolar disorder, and later even than that of patients with uncomplicated bipolar disorder (i.e., no substance abuse at all). One might speculate that these patients had a less active form of bipolar disorder, perhaps one that required triggering by substance abuse before symptoms of abnormal mood could emerge.

Differences between primary and secondary substance abuse disorders were examined in a 5-year prospective follow-up study of 70 patients with alcohol abuse and bipolar disorder (Winokur et al., 1995). In this study, as in that conducted by Feinman and Dunner (1996), bipolar disorder that developed after exposure to alcohol abuse appeared to be less severe than that which developed spontaneously. Patients with primary alcohol abuse had fewer episodes of abnormal mood during the 5-year follow-up period.

The concept of activation of a latent bipolar vulnerability by the abuse of mood-altering substances illustrates the challenges involved in studying comorbid populations. As the two studies just discussed suggest, substance abuse may unmask a less severe form of bipolar disorder that might never have been expressed had the patient not been exposed to alcohol or drugs. Because these patients have an inherently less severe form of mood disorder, their inclusion in studies can lead to the occasional finding that comorbid patients have a more benign clinical course compared with non-drug-abusing patients with bipolar disorder. Alternatively, the indiscriminate blending of patients with secondary and primary bipolar disorder can lead to a washing out of potential differences between comorbid and noncomorbid groups. It appears to make a difference whether the substance abuse is a cause or a result of bipolar mood fluctuations. This methodological and diagnostic issue is one of many that complicate the study of the two illnesses.

From a clinical standpoint, if substance abuse is able to unmask a latent bipolar disorder, bipolar parents who pass along a genetic vulnerability to their children should be counseled on the importance of helping their children avoid substance abuse. Abuse of illicit drugs can cause significant morbidity and mortality in any child, but those who have a genetic predisposition toward development of a mood disorder are at particularly high risk of harm.

Modification of Course

Alcohol and drug abuse may modify the course and expression of manic-depressive illness. Substance abuse problems can lead to more severe psychopathology and less favorable outcomes in a number of ways, including higher rates of mixed states, rapid cycling, impulsivity, aggression, and destabilization of sleep patterns. They may also slow the time to recovery, increase the probability of treatment nonadherence, and decrease the effectiveness of prescribed medications. As reviewed in Chapter 8, the mortality associated with substance abuse and depressive disorders is cause for particular concern. More than 90 percent of suicides are associated with a psychiatric disorder (Institute of Medicine, 2002), but the association is stronger for some conditions than others. Two of the highest-risk conditions are bipolar disorder and substance abuse, and there appears to be an often dangerous interaction between the two. Harris and Barraclough (1997) examined the effect of comorbid substance abuse on suicide rates in 7,819 patients with bipolar disorder, unipolar depression, or schizophrenia. Substance abuse problems increased the lifetime risk of suicide in all of the patients, but the increase was greatest among those with bipolar disorder (recurrent unipolar patients were not identified separately).

Rapid-cycling bipolar disorder, defined by four or more mood episodes per year, tends to have a more treatment-resistant course, and a link between the risk of rapid cycling and substance abuse has long been considered likely. In the Systematic Treatment Enhancement Program for Bipolar Disorder (STEP-BD), a multicenter project designed to evaluate the longitudinal outcome of patients with bipolar disorder, the first 500 patients were evaluated for clinical characteristics associated with rapid cycling (Schneck et al., 2004). The investigators found a correlation between substance abuse and rapid cycling but concluded that the direction of causality was unknown; that is, it was not clear whether the substance abuse destabilized the bipolar disorder and led to rapid cycling, or the more severe psychopathology associated with rapid cycling predisposed to substance abuse. The authors did find that among rapid cyclers, those with bipolar-I were more likely than those with bipolar-II to abuse substances.

Mixed states, like rapid cycling, are characterized by greater psychopathology and associated with less favorable treatment outcomes than bipolar illness uncomplicated by these states (see Chapter 1). The observation that alcohol and drug abuse is significantly higher in patients with mixed mania has been reported by several authors (Winokur et al., 1969; Himmelhoch et al., 1976a; Himmelhoch and Garfinkel, 1986). Other investigators, however, have not found a higher frequency of substance abuse disorders in patients with mixed states (Cassidy et al., 2001; Brieger, 2005). Himmelhoch and colleagues (1976a, p. 1065) noted that "drug abuse (particularly alcohol and sedatives) alters the clinical presentation of manic-depressive swings, and the impact of oversedation or withdrawal or both on a 'pure' affective state is to make it dysphoric and mixed." More recently, Goldberg and colleagues (1999) studied the long-term effects of substance abuse on the course of bipolar-I disorder. They found that in a sample of hospitalized patients, substance abuse was more common among those who had mixed states. Remission during hospitalization was less likely among those with mixed mania, current substance abuse, or even a past history of substance abuse in the absence of current substance abuse. This finding raises the possibility that early or nonchronic substance abuse can have long-term negative effects on the course of bipolar disorder.

Although substantial data support the contention that alcohol abuse has a deleterious effect on mood disorders, less is known about the impact of moderate alcohol use. For healthy males, moderate alcohol use can have health benefits through a reduction in mortality from cardiovascular disease (Gaziano et al., 2000), but for patients with mood disorders, the negative effects on mood may outweigh the benefits. A study of 84 adult outpatients with bipolar-I or -II disorder who did not have active substance abuse disorders examined the relationship of moderate alcohol use to symptoms of mania and depression. On average, these patients consumed only 2.2 alcoholic beverages per week. Overall, beer consumption was not associated with mood symptoms; the consumption of distilled spirits, however, was associated with a lifetime number of manic episodes (Goldstein et al., 2005).

Comorbid substance abuse is reported to increase a bipolar patient's risk of experiencing a switch to mania when treated with an antidepressant (see Chapter 19). A recent controversial meta-analysis failed to find an increased risk of manic switch when the combination of a mood stabilizer[3] and an antidepressant was used to treat bipolar depression; however, all of the trials reviewed excluded patients with substance abuse disorder (Gijsman et al., 2004), and were therefore not representative of patients seen in clinical practice.

A smaller, retrospective investigation that did include substance abusers studied 53 DSM-IV bipolar patients. Fully 60 percent of those with comorbid substance abuse had a history of antidepressant-induced mania or hypomania, compared with 18 percent of patients with no substance abuse history. None of the patients without a substance abuse history switched into mania if they were taking a concomitant mood stabilizer during periods of antidepressant treatment. In the subgroup with comorbid substance abuse, however, 29 percent of the patients taking both an antidepressant and a mood stabilizer experienced antidepressant-induced mania or hypomania (Goldberg and Whiteside, 2002).

The effect of marijuana on mood changes was examined in a group of 50 patients with new-onset bipolar disorder. (Strakowski et al., 2000). Patients were followed for a period that ranged from 16 to 104 weeks. During this period, on average, patients met the full criteria for marijuana dependence or abuse 13 percent of the time. Patients who experienced a longer duration of marijuana abuse/dependence also had longer periods of mania. It is not clear whether the drug contributed to the maintenance of the manic state, or manic patients were more likely to abuse it as a result of symptoms associated with their elevated mood. A recent study carried out in the Netherlands, however, found that while use of marijuana at baseline increased the risk for manic symptoms during follow-up, manic symptoms at baseline did not predict the onset of marijuana use during follow-up (Henquet et al., 2006).

Evidence generally points to a destabilizing effect of marijuana. Its effect on mood was evaluated in participants in the 1980 ECA study, who were then questioned in a follow-up investigation conducted between 1994 and 1996 (Bovasso, 2001). Marijuana abuse was associated with subsequent depressive symptoms in individuals who had had no depression at the beginning of the study. Specifically, participants with no baseline depressive symptoms

who had a diagnosis of marijuana abuse were four times more likely than those with no marijuana abuse to have depressive symptoms at the follow-up assessment. Suicidal ideation and anhedonia were both associated with abuse of the drug. Shedding light on causality, depressive symptoms at baseline did not predict later development of marijuana abuse, supporting the theory that the abuse of the drug led to the depression, rather than the reverse. An Australian study of 81 patients with recent-onset psychosis (bipolar disorder, schizophrenia, delusional disorder, substance-induced psychosis) found that a higher frequency of marijuana use was predictive of psychotic relapse, after controlling for medication adherence, other substance abuse, and duration of untreated psychosis (Hides et al., 2006). An increase in psychotic symptoms was also predictive of relapse to marijuana use.

Treatment nonadherence may be a mediator of poorer outcome among manic-depressive patients with substance abuse. Personality factors, attitudes toward medication, and the experience of side effects have all been associated with nonadherence (see Chapter 21); it is only more recently that attention has been given to the role of comorbid substance abuse (Haywood et al., 1995; Swartz et al., 1998; Perlick et al., 2004). Patients with substance abuse are likely to have poor insight into both their substance abuse and their mood disorder, and the denial of the need for medication is a common reason for nonadherence in this population, especially in the bipolar subgroup (Keck et al., 1997). Calabrese and Delucchi (1990) found that poor medication adherence associated with comorbid alcohol, marijuana, or cocaine abuse led to poor outcomes in rapid-cycling patients being treated with lithium or valproate. The efficacy of these medications was not affected by comorbid substance abuse in medication-adherent patients.

The disorganized lifestyle that accompanies substance abuse, difficulties in personal relationships and employment, and the experience of more adverse effects due to the interaction between medications and alcohol and drugs (e.g., fatigue, headache, irritability, destabilized sleep, neurocognitive side effects) also contribute to the poorer clinical outcomes seen in bipolar patients with substance abuse problems. (See Chapter 4 for further details on the relationship between substance abuse and the clinical course of bipolar disorder.)

ANXIETY DISORDERS

While comorbidity implies the presence of two separate disorders, individual symptoms of anxiety—agitation, accelerated thought processes, restlessness, social anxiety, irritability, and dysphoric mood—are common features of depression, mixed states, and mania (Young et al., 1993; Gibb et al., 2005). In one study, 39 percent of a group of in-patients with bipolar disorder had symptoms of anxiety that were an integral part of their mood episodes (Cassidy et al., 1998). Thus it is not surprising that epidemiologic studies have found full-syndrome anxiety disorders to be common in bipolar populations. McElroy and colleagues (2001) observed a 42 percent rate of anxiety disorders in a group of 288 outpatients with bipolar-I or -II disorder, nearly the same rate noted earlier for anxiety *symptoms*. This rate was identical to the rate of substance abuse in the same clinical sample. The presence of at least one Axis I anxiety diagnosis was associated with a history of development of both cycle acceleration and more severe episodes over time. Table 7–4 summarizes the rates of comorbid anxiety disorders in this sample of bipolar patients.

In contrast to substance abuse, which is more common in bipolar-I than bipolar-II patients, comorbidity of anxiety disorders may be more common in patients with bipolar-II disorder (Judd et al., 2003a). In a recent Finnish study (Mantere et al., 2006), for example, rates of comorbid anxiety were similar in bipolar-II disorder and major depression (56.5 percent and 52.5 percent, respectively), but lower in bipolar-I patients (35.6 percent). This association may be related to the fact that bipolar-II patients have a more chronic course, more major and minor depressive episodes, and shorter well intervals between episodes.

Panic disorder and OCD are particularly common comorbidities in patients with bipolar disorder. In the ECA study, 21.0 percent of patients with either bipolar-I or bipolar-II disorder met criteria for lifetime panic disorder, and 21.0 percent met criteria for lifetime OCD, compared with 0.8 and 2.6 percent, respectively, in the general population (Robins and Regier, 1991). Table 7–5 provides an overview of studies of the comorbidity of bipolar and anxiety disorders.

Sociodemographic risk factors associated with bipolar–anxiety comorbidity were derived from the Netherlands Mental Health Survey and Incidence Study, a prospective epidemiological study of 7,076 adults aged 18 to 64 years. Comorbid mood and anxiety disorders, but not pure mood disorders (depression, bipolar disorder, and dysthymia), were associated with female gender, younger age, lower educational level, and unemployment (de Graaf et al., 2002).

There appears to be an interaction between mood and anxiety disorders in that each illness can be triggered or worsened by the other. Bipolar patients with high anxiety scores are more likely than those with low anxiety to have made suicide attempts, to abuse alcohol, and to respond less favorably to lithium treatment (Young et al., 1993). An analysis of a cross-sectional sample from the STEP-BD project found that the presence of a comorbid anxiety disorder was associated with younger age at onset of bipolar disorder, decreased likelihood of recovery, poorer role functioning, and lower quality of life (Otto et al., 2006). Comorbid anxiety and bipolar disorders were also associated with substance abuse and a greater risk of suicide attempts in the STEP-BD data.

TABLE 7–4. **Percent of 288 Bipolar Patients Who Also Met Criteria for Various Anxiety Disorders**

Disorder	Lifetime %	Current %
Anxiety disorders	42	30
Panic disorder/agoraphobia	20	9
Social phobia	16	13
Simple phobia	10	8
Obsessive-compulsive disorder	9	8
Post-traumatic stress disorder	7	4
Generalized anxiety disorder	3	3
Other anxiety disorders	3	2

Source: Sasson et al., 2003. Adapted from McElroy et al., 2001.

TABLE 7–5. **Overview of Studies of Comorbidity of Bipolar and Anxiety Disorders**

Study	Population	Sample Size	Comorbidity Findings
Savino et al., 1993	Patients with PD	108	Total comorbidity with BP was 13.5%; 2.1% had BP-I; 5% had BP-II; 6.4% had cyclothymia
Young et al., 1993	Patients with BP-I and -II	81	32% met criteria for PD and/or GAD
Bowen et al., 1994	Patients with PD	108	23.1% had comorbid BP
Kessler et al., 1994, 1997	NCS; noninstitutionalized civilian population, subgroup with BP-I	130	33.1% had comorbid PD; 47.2% had comorbid social phobia
Chen and Dilsaver, 1995b	ECA database, subgroup with BP	168	20.8% had comorbid PD; 21.0% had comorbid OCD
Keck et al., 1995	Patients with BP	71	10% had OCD; 17% had PTSD; 16% had "any" anxiety disorder (including PD, agoraphobia, social phobia, simple phobia)
Krüger et al., 1995	Patients with BP	37	35% had comorbid OCD
Lensi et al., 1996	Patients with OCD	263	1.5% had BP-I; 13.0% had hypomania (most after treatment with antidepressant)
Dilsaver et al., 1997	Patients with BP	129	Comorbidity with PD varied with episode: BP depression, 62.3%; pure mania, 2.3%
Perugi et al., 1997	Patients with OCD	315	15.7% had comorbid BP; 13.6% had BP-II; 2.0% had BP-I
Pini et al., 1997	Patients with BP depression	24	36.8% had PD; 21.1% had OCD; 31.6 % had GAD; none had social phobia
Szadoczky et al., 1998	Hungarian National Epidemiologic Survey, subgroup with BP	149	10.6% had comorbid PD; 3.2% had comorbid OCD; 7.8% had comorbid social phobia; 12.9% had specific phobia; 14.4% had GAD

(continued)

TABLE 7–5. Overview of Studies of Comorbidity of Bipolar and Anxiety Disorders *(continued)*

Study	Population	Sample Size	Comorbidity Findings
McElroy et al., 2001	Patients with BP	288	42% had a comorbid Axis I anxiety disorder; 20% had PD with agoraphobia; 16% had social phobia; 10% had simple phobia; 6% had GAD; 7% had PTSD; 9% had OCD

BP = Bipolar disorder; ECA = Epidemiologic Catchment Area; GAD = generalized anxiety disorder; NCS = National Comorbidity Survey; OCD = obsessive-compulsive disorder; PD = panic disorder; PTSD = post-traumatic stress disorder.
Source: Adapted from Freeman et al., 2002.

Not all studies of comorbid anxiety and bipolar disorders have found a less favorable outcome. In a French study that evaluated 318 consecutively hospitalized bipolar patients, co-morbidity with anxiety disorders was not correlated with severity of bipolar illness, as defined by number of previous hospitalizations, psychotic features, abuse of alcohol and drugs, and violent and nonviolent suicide attempts (Henry et al., 2003). This study also differed from other investigations in finding that comorbid patients, compared with bipolar patients without anxiety, responded less well to anticonvulsants but equally well to lithium; other studies have found anticonvulsants to be more effective than lithium in this population (see Chapter 24). The authors noted that only 21 percent of the patients in the study had a history of substance abuse. This relatively low rate of substance abuse may explain why the comorbid anxiety disorders had less of a negative impact on the clinical course of the bipolar disorder and its treatment than has been found in other studies.

Determining the prevalence of comorbid anxiety disorders and elucidating the nature of their interaction with bipolar disorder is scientifically important as well as clinically useful. Some investigators have suggested that genetic heterogeneity of bipolar illnesses may be responsible for the comorbidity with anxiety disorders (MacKinnon et al., 2003). That is, different forms or subphenotypes of bipolar disorder appear to aggregate in families and may be associated with different combinations of susceptibility genes and comorbid presentations (see Chapter 13). Ultimately, genetic research will provide a more fundamental understanding of comorbidity.

Panic Disorder

Panic disorder is one of the most common comorbid anxiety disorders seen in bipolar patients (McElroy et al., 2001). Data from the ECA study found that the lifetime prevalence of panic disorder among individuals with bipolar disorder was 21 percent, compared with 10 percent among those with unipolar depression and 0.8 percent of the general population (Chen and Dilsaver, 1995b). Conversely, patients with panic disorder have high rates of bipolar disorder, ranging from 6 to 23 percent (Savino et al., 1993; Bowen et al., 1994; Perugi et al., 1999).

Comorbid panic disorder can negatively affect the course of bipolar disorder. In a sample of 66 patients with bipolar-I disorder, comorbid panic symptoms were associated with more prior depressive episodes, higher levels of depressive symptoms, and greater suicidal ideation during the acute treatment phase. Patients who reported high life-time scores on the panic–agoraphobia spectrum took 27 weeks longer for their depressive episodes to remit than those who reported low scores (44 versus 17 weeks) (Frank et al., 2002).

Not only is the bipolar disorder more severe in comorbid patients, but so, too, is the anxiety disorder. The NCS found that the co-occurrence of bipolar disorder and panic attacks was associated with earlier onset of panic attacks (age 17.1 versus 22.0 years) and, not surprisingly, with significantly greater panic symptomatology (Goodwin and Hoven, 2002). Comorbid substance dependence, specific phobia, and generalized anxiety disorder were each independent correlates of the co-occurrence of bipolar disorder and panic attacks.

Evidence suggests that panic disorder may be genetically related to bipolar disorder. The National Institute of Mental Health's (NIMH) Bipolar Genetics Initiative, which focused on family members of probands with bipolar disorder, found that panic disorder occurred in 17 percent of relatives who had a recurrent major affective disorder, compared with only 3 percent of those who did not (MacKinnon et al., 2002). Conversely, 90 percent of first-degree relatives with panic disorder also had a major affective disorder (MacKinnon et al., 1997).

It has been observed that some forms of rapid cycling and panic disorder are phenomenologically linked by sudden shifts in affect. Consequently, a logistic regression analysis of rapid mood switching as a function of familial risk for panic disorder was performed on data gathered from subjects in the NIMH Bipolar Genetics Initiative (MacKinnon et al., 2003). The analysis found that familial panic disorder increased the odds of rapid mood switching, suggesting that this comorbid presentation may stem from a genetically distinct subtype of bipolar disorder. Similarly, family clusters or specific susceptibility genes have been identified for bipolar disorder with psychotic features (Potash et al., 2001) and for suicidality in the context of alcohol abuse/dependence and bipolar disorder (Potash et al., 2001). A study of bipolar patients that focused on siblings found that those who did not suffer from a mood disorder had a low rate of panic disorder (3 percent) compared with those who had bipolar disorder (32 percent) (Doughty et al., 2004).

The pathophysiology underlying the close relationship between the two disorders is not fully understood. Dysregulation of the serotonin system probably plays a role in the overlap of mood and anxiety disorders, and the fact that SSRIs are first-line agents in the treatment of panic disorder suggests a role for serotonin in the pathophysiology of that disorder. SSRIs and postsynaptic serotonin receptor antagonists are also commonly used to treat mood disorders, but the role of serotonin in bipolar disorder is complex. As detailed in Chapter 14, some studies have found abnormalities in levels of 5-hydroxyindolacetic acid (5-HIAA) in patients with bipolar disorder (Young et al., 1994); however, this finding is not consistent across all studies (Berrettini et al., 1985). Patients with both bipolar disorder and panic disorder have been found to have noradrenergic hyperactivity. Increased plasma levels of the main norepinephrine metabolite, 3-methoxy-4-hydroxyphenylglycol (MHPG), have been found in patients with mania and depression (Swann et al., 1983). Several lines of evidence suggest that catecholamines, especially norepinephrine, are also implicated in the etiology and symptomatology of panic disorder. Significantly higher baseline levels of norepinephrine excretion are seen in patients with panic disorder compared with healthy controls (Bandelow et al., 1997).

As reviewed in Chapter 24, SSRIs and serotonin/norepinephrine reuptake inhibitors (SNRIs) may be used to treat comorbid anxiety in bipolar disorder. However, they carry the risk of inducing manic and mixed episodes, as well as longer-term cycle acceleration.

The efficacy of benzodiazepines in panic disorder suggests that dysregulation of the gamma-aminobutyric acid (GABA) system may also contribute to the etiology of this illness. Evidence for GABA abnormalities in bipolar disorder, however, is uneven and conflicting. For example, effective mood stabilizers such as valproate have putative effects on the GABA system. Valproate increases functional levels of GABA in the brain, apparently by activating the biosynthetic enzyme glutamic acid decarboxylase and inhibiting the degradative enzyme GABA-transaminase. Other mood-stabilizing anticonvulsants also modulate the GABA system. However, the relevance of this neurotransmitter to unstable mood in bipolar disorder remains unknown. (See Chapter 14 for more information on the role of specific neurotransmitters in manic-depressive illness.)

Social Anxiety Disorder and Social Phobia

In the NCS, an epidemiologic study based on nonclinician assessments, nearly one-half of patients with bipolar disorder met criteria for a lifetime comorbid social anxiety disorder, compared with 13.3 percent of the general population (Kessler et al., 1994). However, data from the Stanley Foundation Bipolar Network, obtained by clinicians using structured diagnostic interviews with a clinical population, reveal social anxiety disorder in only 16 percent of bipolar patients (McElroy et al., 2001). As with panic disorder, there appears to be a mutual-risk interaction, such that patients with social anxiety disorder also have high rates of bipolar disorder. Symptoms of social anxiety tend to disappear during hypomanic episodes, when excessive social inhibition is replaced by disinhibition. There may be an underlying social behavior dysregulation connecting the two disorders (Perugi et al., 2001). A recent study of 57 patients with social anxiety disorder found that a subgroup improved while taking antidepressants, and indeed presented with clear hypomania. Without antidepressant therapy, the symptoms of social anxiety returned (Valengaet et al., 2005).

Although social anxiety disorder is a serious illness and is strongly associated with functional impairment, feelings of social isolation, and suicidal ideation (Olfson et al., 2000), it tends to go unrecognized and untreated (Weiller et al., 1996). Clinicians who treat patients with bipolar disorder should be particularly wary of failing to identify this potentially disabling disorder. However, just as with panic disorder, treatment decisions can be complex. For example, in a study of 32 patients with social anxiety disorder, 14 (78 percent) of 18 patients who responded to a monoamine oxidase inhibitor (MAOI) became hypomanic (Himmelhoch, 1998) (see Chapter 24).

Obsessive-Compulsive Disorder

Analysis of data from the ECA study showed a lifetime prevalence of OCD of 21.0 percent in patients with bipolar disorder; this was significantly higher than the rates of 12.2 percent in unipolar depression and 2.5 percent in the general population (Chen and Dilsaver, 1995a). As with anxiety disorders in general, bipolar-II is more common than bipolar-I among patients with OCD (Perugi et al., 1997, 2002). Among patients with bipolar-I disorder, those with episodes of mixed mania may be more likely to have comorbid OCD than those with pure euphoric mania (McElroy et al., 1995). The presence of comorbid OCD leads to greater bipolar morbidity and possibly to greater mortality due to suicide (Krüger et al., 2000). Compared with bipolar patients without OCD, those with OCD have more severe symptomatology, including more lifetime suicidal ideation, suicide attempts, and comorbid panic disorder.

The phenomenology of comorbid OCD is somewhat different from that of "pure" OCD. The onset of the illness is more gradual, and the course tends to be episodic rather than continuous. There are higher rates of sexual and religious obsessions and a lower rate of checking rituals (Perugi et al., 1997, 2002). The episodic nature of OCD in bipolar patients may be related to the course of the mood disorder. In one study (Strakowski et al., 1998), the symptoms of both OCD and bipolar disorder cycled together in 7 of 16 patients. There were no cases of OCD that persisted in the absence of an affective syndrome. These data showing such a tight correlation between the symptom emergence of the two illnesses suggest the possibility that the two represent variability in the expression of a single underlying CNS dysfunction.

Post-Traumatic Stress Disorder

Although PTSD is a less common comorbidity than some of the other anxiety disorders, it is substantially more common in bipolar patients than in the general population. A meta-analysis of eight studies representing a total of 1,214 bipolar patients found that the mean lifetime prevalence of PTSD in those patients was 16.0 percent, a rate roughly double that of the general population (Otto et al., 2004). Table 7–6 summarizes the seven studies.

Little is known about why there is a relatively high rate of comorbidity of the two disorders, but there are some characteristics of bipolar disorder that place a patient at risk for the development and exacerbation of PTSD and vice versa. Pretrauma psychiatric illness, including some symptoms of depression and hypomania, increase a patient's vulnerability to developing PTSD after trauma (Schnurr et al., 1993). Abnormal mood at the time of the trauma can reduce resilience. For example, unrealistic and exaggerated negative attitudes common in depression can aggravate a patient's response to stressful events.

The impulsivity and poor judgment associated with elevated mood states place patients at risk for the occurrence of traumatic events such as assault and motor vehicle accidents. In one study of the general population, 51 percent of women and 61 percent of men reported a history of exposure to trauma (Kessler et al., 1995), and while some studies have found no difference among bipolar patients (Neria et al., 2002), others have found rates as high as 98 percent (Mueser et al., 1998). The experience of psychosis, which may occur in the context of a manic or depressive episode, is often a highly traumatic event in itself. Psychosis fundamentally disrupts an individual's notion of self and expectations of the future. Psychosis as part of an abnormal mood episode occurs in the setting of a highly volatile

TABLE 7–6. Prevalence of Post-Traumatic Stress Disorder (PTSD) in Samples of Patients with Bipolar Disorder

Study	Sample Characteristics	Sample Size	Rate of PTSD (%)
Keck et al., 1995	BP patients admitted for mania or mixed mania	71	17
Kessler et al., 1997	National general population survey; respondents with BP-I characterized by euphoria, grandiosity, and excessive energy	29	39
Mueser et al., 1998	Inpatients and outpatients with BP	50	40
Strakowski et al., 1998	BP patients, manic or mixed; first admission for psychosis	77	21
McElroy et al., 2001	BP-I and BP-II outpatients recruited from the community	288	7
Neria et al., 2002	BP patients; first admission for psychosis	102	11
Simon et al., 2003	BP-I and BP-II, treatment-seeking outpatients	122	19

BP = bipolar disorder.
Source: Otto et al., 2004. Reprinted with permission from Blackwell Publishing.

emotional state that further diminishes a patient's capacity to adaptively tolerate this type of stress.

On the other hand, for some patients or situations, euphoria or an underlying hyperthymic temperament associated with bipolar disorder may increase resilience in the face of trauma. That is, some patients with bipolar disorder have temperamental features that protect them at least partially from the adverse psychological consequences of severe stress. Persistent optimism and self-confidence can enable an individual to avoid some of the emotional injury that occurs in the face of trauma and continue to function in an adaptive way in situations in which others would experience high levels of distress and functional impairment (Jamison, 2004). The tendency to shift focus rapidly, not always a positive attribute of a hyperthymic temperament, may be protective during periods of intense stress by allowing the individual to avoid ruminating and fixating on traumatic experiences. The hyperthymic individual is also future oriented, a trait that decreases the deleterious influence of past events.

Symptoms of PTSD can aggravate the course of bipolar disorder. Stress of any kind places bipolar patients at risk for the emergence of a mood episode. PTSD is commonly associated with chronic overarousal that occurs in addition to the acute overarousal experienced in response to environmental cues. One of the consequences of overarousal is sleep disturbance, which can have a direct impact on the course of bipolar disorder (see Chapter 16). Chronic symptoms of avoidance seen in patients with PTSD can lead to social isolation, which is associated with more depression and longer recovery times in bipolar patients (Johnson et al., 1999).

Like panic disorder and bipolar illness, PTSD has been associated with chronic noradrenergic hyperactivity (Kosten et al., 1987). One consequence of this abnormality is a decrease in the number and sensitivity of alpha-2-adrenergic receptors (Maes et al., 1999). The serotonin system is almost certainly involved as well. Large placebo-controlled trials have demonstrated the efficacy of SSRIs in the treatment of PTSD (see Chapter 24), supporting the view that pathology associated with the serotonin system plays an important role in the development and maintenance of the disorder.

The presence of comorbid PTSD increases the morbidity, mortality, and functional impairment associated with bipolar disorder. Data from the STEP-BD project reveal that patients with comorbid PTSD have a lower likelihood of being in remission from bipolar disorder, are more likely to abuse substances, have higher rates of suicide, and have lower role attainment and quality of life compared with bipolar patients without PTSD (Simon et al., 2004b).

OTHER PSYCHIATRIC ILLNESSES

Attention-Deficit Hyperactivity Disorder

The overlap of symptoms seen in bipolar disorder with those seen in attention-deficit hyperactivity disorder (ADHD) can make it difficult to separate the two illnesses. This is especially true in children, in whom mood disorders manifest somewhat differently than in adults, and who may have difficulty in accurately describing their internal affective states. Distractibility, physical hyperactivity, and pressured speech can be symptoms of either bipolar disorder or ADHD. See Chapter 6 for an extensive review of the comorbidity of ADHD and other disorders in children and adolescents. See also Chapter 9 for an in-depth discussion of the pervasive attentional deficits associated with bipolar illness, even when the illness is in remission.

The rate of comorbidity for ADHD is much lower in bipolar adults than in children. Most children aged 12 and younger with bipolar disorder meet the criteria for ADHD (Findling et al., 2001), whereas comorbid ADHD was found in just 9 percent of the first 1,000 adult patients enrolled in the STEP-BD project (aged 15 and older) (Kogan et al., 2004). Among adult patients with early-onset bipolar disorder (before age 13), the rate rose to 20 percent (Perlis et al., 2004). ADHD affects approximately 4 percent of adults in the general population (Kessler, 2004).

Data from a large claims database revealed that adults diagnosed with ADHD were significantly more likely to have a comorbid diagnosis of bipolar disorder or major depressive disorder than non-ADHD patients (Secnik et al., 2005). Adults diagnosed with ADHD had significantly higher outpatient, inpatient, and prescription drug costs than noncomorbid patients with a mood disorder. A study based on structured psychiatric interviews found that 88 percent of adults with comorbid ADHD and bipolar disorder had the bipolar-II subtype (Wilens et al., 2003). This is another example of a comorbidity that is chronic in nature, being associated with the more chronic form of bipolar disorder. Compared with patients with pure ADHD, those with both bipolar disorder and ADHD had more DSM-IV symptoms of ADHD (14.8 versus 11.4 percent), poorer global functioning, and more additional comorbid psychiatric disorders (3.7 versus 2.0 percent). Based on the outcome of their analysis, the authors concluded that the observed symptomatology in the comorbid group supported the construct of two separate disorders that were distinguishable clinically.

Eating Disorders

Only a few studies have assessed the co-occurrence of bipolar disorder and eating disorders in community samples. One study of 3,258 Canadian adults found no overlap between 22 individuals diagnosed with lifetime bipolar disorder and 4 individuals diagnosed with anorexia nervosa; other eating disorders were not assessed (Fogarty et al., 1994). More recent studies, which differed somewhat by including subthreshold hypomania and binge eating, did find associations. Among 891 randomly selected schoolgirls, approximately one-quarter of those with an eating disorder had subthreshold bipolar disorder, compared with 3.8 percent of those with no eating disorder (Lewinsohn et al., 2000). However, the rate of full-syndrome bipolar disorder was similar among the girls with and without an eating disorder. Binge eating has been found to be specifically associated with hypomania. A comparison of patients with a history of hypomania, patients with a history of depression, and a control group with no abnormal mood episodes found that the rate of binge eating was highest in the group with a history of hypomania (Angst, 1998).

Studies of clinical populations have also found connections between bipolar disorder and eating disorders. Data gathered from clinical populations may differ from community data, however, because subjects currently in treatment typically have higher levels of distress and comorbidity than do community samples.[4] Consistent with this pattern, bipolar-II disorder was found to be common among hospitalized patients with eating disorders. An evaluation of a group of 15 bulimics and 7 anorexics found that 19 of the 22 had a major mood disorder; 1 had bipolar-I disorder, and 13 had bipolar-II (Simpson et al., 1992). In a larger sample, patients with bipolar disorder were found to have a lifetime prevalence of bulimia of 4 percent (bipolar-I, 3 percent and bipolar-II, 6 percent) and a lifetime prevalence of anorexia nervosa of 2 percent (bipolar-I, 2 percent and bipolar-II, 4 percent) (McElroy et al., 2001). Analysis of the first 500 patients in the STEP-BD investigation found that the rate of bulimia in bipolar women was relatively high (12 percent), as was true for the rate in bipolar men (2 percent) (Baldassano et al., 2005). In the only study assessing binge eating and bipolar disorder (Krüger et al., 1996), the rate found in the bipolar patient sample (13 percent) was significantly higher than that reported for the general population (5 percent) (Spitzer et al., 1993). In a comprehensive review of comorbid bipolar and eating disorders, McElroy and colleagues (2005) found a particularly strong association between bulimia nervosa and bipolar-II disorder. Their summary of eating disorders in patients with bipolar disorder is given in Table 7–7.

Axis II Disorders

Affective instability is a common feature of certain personality disorders, especially those found in cluster B. Because of the frequency with which these disorders are seen in

bipolar patients and the effect they have on clinical course, Chapter 10 focuses specifically on this topic.

MEDICAL ILLNESSES

In addition to psychiatric disorders, bipolar patients experience certain general medical conditions at a higher rate than the general public. Some of this excess morbidity is associated with adverse effects of medications used to treat bipolar disorder and some with lifestyle. In other cases, the etiology of the comorbidity is not fully understood. Because many patients with serious mental illnesses have difficulty obtaining adequate medical care, the treating psychiatrist may be the only physician caring for these patients on a regular basis, and therefore should screen them for common medical problems.

Cardiovascular Disease

Cardiovascular disease accounts for the majority of the mortality seen with metabolic syndrome (discussed later). Obesity, glucose dysregulation, and dyslipidemia are all risk factors for cardiovascular disease, and consequently patients with bipolar disorder experience cardiovascular mortality at elevated rates compared with the general population (Weeke, 1979; Sharma and Markar, 1994). The mortality ratio of bipolar patients versus the general population for cardiovascular disease is 3.0. Additionally, when all the symptoms of the metabolic syndrome are controlled for, bipolar disorder continues to be an independent risk factor for cardiovascular mortality (Norton and Whalley, 1984). Before the modern era of psychopharmacology, death from manic exhaustion was not uncommon; many such deaths were attributable to cardiac events (Derby, 1933; Cade, 1979). In a long-term study that followed a group of 406 patients for more than 30 years, mortality due to circulatory disorders was second only to suicide as a cause of death among patients with bipolar disorder (Angst et al., 2002). A large study of 15,386 patients hospitalized in Sweden for bipolar disorder between 1973 and 1995 found that the most frequent cause of death was cardiovascular disease, followed by suicide and cancer. The observed number of cardiovascular deaths among male patients was 1.9 times the expected number. Among females, the mortality rate was 2.6 times the expected number (Osby, 2001).

Increased platelet aggregation and low-grade systemic inflammation seen in depressed patients may be mechanisms by which a mood disorder is a significant and independent risk factor for ischemic heart disease (Musselman et al., 1996). Patients with bipolar disorder also are more likely to smoke and to have a history of hypertension (Yates and Wallace, 1987; Johannessen et al., 2006).

TABLE 7–7. **Studies of Eating Disorders in Patients with Bipolar Disorder**

Study	Study Population	Assessment Instrument; Diagnostic Criteria	Eating Disorder Findings
Strakowski et al., 1992	41 inpatients with BP and first-episode mania (25 women)	SCID; DSM-III-R	7.3% had BN: 12.0% of women and no men had BN
Strakowski et al., 1993	60 inpatients with BP-I and first-episode mania	SCID; DSM-III-R	6.6% had BN
McElroy et al., 1995	71 inpatients with BP-I and acute mania (39 women)	SCID; DSM-III-R	8.5% had AN or BN
Krüger et al., 1996	61 euthymic outpatients with BP-I ($n=43$) or BP-II ($n=18$) (38 women)	Semistructured Clinical Interview; DSM-IV	13.1% had BED; 37.7% had recurrent binge eating episodes
Schuckit et al., 1996	14 women with BP and 1,176 with other psychiatric disorder[a]	SAGA; DSM-III-R	Of women with BD, none had AN and 7.1% had BN, compared with 0.3% and 0.6%, respectively, of controls ($p<.01$ for BN)
Cassano et al., 1998	47 inpatients with BP-I with psychotic features	SCID; DSM-III-R	6.4% had AN or BN
Edmonds et al., 1998	64 persons with BP-I ($n=44$) or BP-II ($n=11$) from a BP registry	DIGS; DSM-IV	7.3% had a DSM-IV ED
Pini et al., 1999	125 patients with BP-I with psychotic features (69 women)	SCID; DSM-III-R	4.0% had BN and 2.4% had AN
McElroy et al., 2001	288 outpatients with BP-I or BP-II (162 women)	SCID; DSM-IV	5.9% had AN or BN
Vieta et al., 2001	129 outpatients with BP-I (76 women)	SCID; DSM-IV	2.3% had BN
MacQueen et al., 2003	139 outpatients with BP-I or BP-II (94 women)	SCID; DSM-IV	15% had an ED

AN=anorexia nervosa; BED=binge eating disorder; BN=bulimia nervosa; BP=bipolar disorder; DIGS=Diagnostic Interview for Genetic Studies; ED=eating disorder; SAGA=Semi-Structured Assessment for the Genetics of Alcoholism; SCID=Structured Clinical Interview for DSM.

[a]Subjects were participants in the Collaborative Study of the Genetics of Alcoholism.

Source: Reprinted from McElroy et al., 2005 with permission from Elsevier.

Thyroid Dysfunction

Thyroid dysfunction associated with bipolar disorder is a significant problem. In addition to the medical morbidity associated with thyroid problems, mood states and affective stability are intimately connected to proper functioning of the hypothalamic–pituitary–thyroid axis (see Chapter 14). Patients with thyroid disease have higher rates of panic disorder, simple phobia, OCD, major depressive disorder, bipolar disorder, and cyclothymia than the general population (Placidi et al., 1998). Bipolar women have higher rates of comorbid thyroid disease than men; analysis of the first 500 STEP-BD participants, for example, found rates of 26.9 percent in females and 5.7 percent in males (Baldassano et al., 2005). Hypothyroidism is the most frequent manifestation of thyroid dysfunction. The most common psychiatric symptoms related to hypothyroidism are depression and cognitive dysfunction. Fatigue, weight gain, dry skin, hair loss, intolerance to cold, and irritability are also seen. Abnormally elevated levels of thyroid hormone can cause dysphoria, anxiety, restlessness, and emotional lability (Trzepacz et al., 1988).

Problems with the hypothalamic–pituitary–thyroid axis are more prevalent in patients with mood disorders than in the general population; however, many studies have included large numbers of patients taking lithium or carbamazepine, which may account for some of the high prevalence found. (The association between mood stabilizers and thyroid function is discussed in Chapter 20.) Nevertheless, the effects of lithium and carbamazepine do not fully explain the association between bipolar disorder and thyroid dysfunction. In a sample of bipolar patients who had never been treated with either lithium or carbamazepine, the rate of thyroid hypofunction was 9 percent (Valle et al., 1999). Hypofunction was determined on the basis of serum levels for total thyroxine (T_4), total triiodothyronine (T_3), and thyroid-stimulating hormone (TSH) levels. Bipolar-II patients showed significantly lower levels of thyroid functioning than those with bipolar-I disorder, as measured by higher TSH levels. Primary hypothyroidism was diagnosed in 3 percent of a general population sample (Flynn et al., 2004).

The relationship between thyroid hypofunctioning and rapid cycling is unclear. In the sample just described, no difference in thyroid parameters was observed between rapid-cycling and non-rapid-cycling bipolar patients. Other studies, however, have found hypothyroidism to be a risk factor for rapid cycling. For example, in a sample of 30 patients with rapid-cycling bipolar disorder, 60 percent also had hypothyroidism (Bauer et al., 1990). Subclinical hypothyroidism, in which thyroid hormone levels are low compared with controls but still fall within the broad normal range, has been found to be associated with rapid cycling (Kusalic, 1992), although more recently, doubt has been cast on this association (Post et al., 1997). Identifying subclinical hypothyroidism in bipolar patients may be almost as important as identifying overt dysfunction. In 1974, Wenzel and colleagues introduced a system for grading hypothyroidism. In this classification, grade 1 represents overt hypothyroidism, as defined by decreased serum T_4. Grades 2 and 3 define subclinical hypothyroidism. Grade 2 is characterized by increased TSH with normal T_4, and grade 3 by the presence of an isolated exaggeration of the TSH response to stimulation by thyroid-releasing hormone (TRH) (Wenzel et al., 1974).

Subclinical hypothyroidism can influence the outcome of mood disorders even in samples of patients with otherwise normal thyroid indices. Frye and colleagues (1999) assessed thyroid function prospectively in 52 outpatients with bipolar disorder. Even though their free thyroxine index (FTI) values were within the normal range, patients with lower mean FTI values had more affective episodes and more severe depressive symptoms. Cole and colleagues (2002) found less favorable treatment response in bipolar patients with low-normal FTI and high-normal TSH. Others have found subclinical hypothyroidism to be associated with an elevated lifetime prevalence of depression (Haggerty et al., 1993). The rate of subclinical hypothyroidism is particularly high (30 percent) in patients with refractory, treatment-resistant depression (Howland, 1993). The relationship between subclinical hypothyroidism and treatment response is discussed further in Chapter 19.

Hyperthyroidism has also been linked to depressive disorders in some studies (Kathol et al., 1986; Placidi et al., 1998), but not all (Fava et al., 1995; Engum et al., 2002; Thomsen and Kessing, 2005); it has also been linked to mania in a case series (Brownlie et al., 2000), but this finding was not confirmed in a controlled study (Cassidy et al., 2002). In a recent large historical cohort study of 133,570 patients with a clinical diagnosis of osteoarthritis, depressive disorder, or bipolar disorder (610 of whom had hyperthyroidism), patients with bipolar disorder had a hazard ratio for hyperthyroidism of 1.59 ($p < .052$) compared with the arthritis controls, and 1.86 ($p < .014$) compared with those with depression (Thomsen and Kessing, 2005).

Although the evidence for a link between mood disorders and decreased thyroid function is more consistent than that for a link to increased thyroid function, the hypothesis that some mood disorders may be linked to dysregulation of thyroid function is consistent with most of the data. Clearly, all patients with a mood disorder should be tested routinely for thyroid abnormalities, including abnormal levels of TSH and free T_4. Even in the context of normal T_4, elevated TSH should prompt a further workup and consideration of thyroid supplementation. The absence of abnormal TSH should not rule out hypothyroidism in a patient with clinical manifestations of the disease because many patients with both major depression and bipolar disorder fail to mount a TSH response to a TRH challenge (Gold et al., 1977). Evaluation of thyroid abnormalities is particularly appropriate in rapid-cycling and treatment-resistant patients.

Overweight and Obesity

Obesity is a leading cause of preventable death in the United States, and the prevalence of overweight and obesity is increasing. A survey of 4,115 adult men and women conducted in 1999 and 2000 as part of the National Health and Nutrition Examination Survey found that 64.5 percent of the U.S. population is overweight (body mass index [BMI] ≥25), and 30.5 percent is obese (BMI ≥30) (Flegal et al., 2002). A separate, smaller study of 50 bipolar patients, which used the same BMI standard, found an obesity rate that was only slightly higher (32 percent). The number of previous depressive episodes was correlated with the likelihood of being overweight or obese. Most of the weight gain occurred during acute rather than maintenance treatment, and the increase in BMI was related to the severity of the depressive episode, as measured by the patient's score on the Hamilton Rating Scale for Depression (Fagiolini et al., 2002). Although several studies have found significant obesity in bipolar patients (Elmslie et al., 2000, 2001; Fagiolini et al., 2002; McElroy et al., 2002), it is difficult to ascertain the degree to which the obesity is secondary to medications used to treat bipolar disorder or to the illness per se (see review by Toalson et al., 2004).

Longitudinal studies of children and adolescents have found a positive association of major depressive disorder with adult BMI. This association persisted even after controlling for age, gender, substance abuse, social class, pregnancy, and medication exposure (Pine et al., 2001). An important implication of the last of these factors (medication exposure) is that there is a baseline risk for elevated BMI that is independent of the weight gain associated with psychotropic medication. Yet despite the multiple etiologic factors that link mood disorders with obesity, of greatest concern to the clinician is the fact that mood-stabilizing medications frequently cause weight gain (see Chapter 20). Evidence for this conclusion comes from the Stanley Foundation Bipolar Network. Both current weight and the BMI of patients in this study were correlated with the number of weight gain–associated psychotropics to which patients had been exposed (McElroy et al., 2002). Atypical antipsychotic medications are associated specifically with central obesity, which occurs when the main deposits of body fat are localized around the abdomen. Accumulating evidence suggests that central deposition of body fat is a risk factor independent of overall obesity for mortality due to cardiovascular disease, hypertension, and type II diabetes (Donahue et al., 1987).

Other medications used to treat bipolar disorder, including lithium, valproate, and some antidepressants, have also been associated with weight gain. Thus far, there has been less concern regarding the development of metabolic syndrome with these drugs than with the atypical antipsychotics.

Beyond weight gain caused by medications, symptoms of bipolar disorder itself can lead to obesity. Depressed mood leads to lower levels of activity. Atypical features such as hyperphagia, hypersomnia, "leaden paralysis," and carbohydrate craving are seen more commonly in bipolar depression than in major depressive disorder and are more liable to lead to weight gain. It should be noted that manic syndromes are associated with loss of appetite, hypophagia, hyperactivity, and weight loss. In the majority of bipolar patients, however, depressive symptoms are far more frequent than manic symptoms (Judd et al., 2003b). Depression is often accompanied by hypercortisolemia, which is also associated with central obesity. Even in the context of normal body weight, hypercortisolemia has been associated with excess visceral fat deposition as measured by computed tomography (CT) scan (Weber-Hamann et al., 2002).

Overweight and obesity, in addition to being a result of bipolar disorder, can worsen the disorder by exacerbating depression. The Western emphasis on being thin as a desirable physical trait can lead to negative body-image problems among overweight individuals. Overweight and obese individuals may also be targets of discrimination. The socioeconomic effects of excess weight were studied in a group of 10,039 randomly selected young people, who were evaluated for weight and BMI and then followed-up 7 years later. Women who had been overweight had completed fewer years of school, were less likely to be married, and had lower household incomes than those who had not been overweight; these findings were independent of baseline socioeconomic status. Men who had been overweight also were less likely to be married. In contrast, people with other chronic health conditions did not differ in these ways from the nonoverweight subjects (Gortmaker et al., 1993).

Among individuals seeking weight loss treatments, rates of mood disorders have ranged from a low of 8 percent (Wise and Fernandez, 1979) to a high of 60 percent (Hudson et al., 1988). Although there can be an overrepresentation of psychopathology among treatment-seeking patients, studies using community samples have yielded similar results. A national survey of 40,086 adults examined the relationship between body weight and clinical depression, suicidal ideation, and suicide attempts. Among women, increased body weight was associated with major depression and suicidal ideation; in men, there was also an association with suicide attempts (Carpenter et al., 2000).

Diabetes

Because overweight and obesity are associated with diabetes, many of the risk factors that have been linked to weight gain apply also to the development of diabetes. The prevalence of reported diabetes mellitus was found to be approximately three times higher in a sample of 345 hospitalized bipolar patients (9.9 percent) than in the general population (3.4 percent) (Cassidy et al., 1999). Patients in this sample also had a more severe course of their mood disorder and significantly more lifetime psychiatric hospitalizations than the nondiabetic subjects. Age at first hospitalization and duration of psychiatric disorder were similar in the two groups. Patients with bipolar disorder and comorbid diabetes have also been reported to be more likely to experience rapid cycling and to have a chronic rather than an episodic course of illness (Ruzickova et al., 2003). A comparison of 26 diabetic and 196 nondiabetic subjects from a community-based project carried out in Canada found that the disability rates for bipolar disorder were significantly different (Ruzickova et al., 2003); 81 percent of comorbid patients were receiving disability compensation payments for bipolar disorder, compared with only 30 percent of bipolar patients without diabetes.

When patients with diabetes are being treated, lithium should be used with care. Patients with juvenile-onset insulin-dependent diabetes are susceptible to diabetic nephropathy, and the risk is increased by the presence of hypertension. On the other hand, there is evidence that when lithium is combined with an oral hypoglycemic medication or insulin, it has an assisting hypoglycemic effect in diabetic patients (Hu et al., 1997). Fasting blood glucose levels were found to be decreased in patients taking lithium combined with other therapy, but not in those being treated with a hypoglycemic agent alone. A possible explanation for this finding is that lithium increases the sensitivity of glucose transport to insulin in skeletal muscle and adipocytes (Tabata et al., 1994). The authors of this study noted that the effects of lithium on glucose transport and metabolism in skeletal muscle were strikingly similar to the effects of exercise.

Dysregulation of the hypothalamic–pituitary–adrenocortical axis occurs frequently in patients with mood disorders. Hypercortisolemia, associated with depressive states, can lead to insulin resistance. Conversely, diabetic vascular CNS lesions may contribute to mania. Weber-Hamann and colleagues (2002) found that postmenopausal women who had depression also had significantly higher levels of free cortisol than age-matched controls. Elevated levels of cortisol can lead to decreased insulin receptor sensitivity through currently unknown mechanisms (Perry et al., 2003).

A more hypothetical link between bipolar disorder and diabetes relates to intracellular signal transduction involving the enzyme glycogen synthase kinase-3-β (GSK-3β). Alterations in GSK-3β functioning play a role in insulin resistance. Insulin inhibits GSK-3β, which results in enhanced glucose transport into skeletal muscle. Insulin-mediated inhibition of GSK-3β leads as well to increased glucose utilization and the production of glycogen (Orena et al., 2000). GSK-3β is also one of the targets for lithium action. Lithium significantly inhibits brain GSK-3β at concentrations relevant for the treatment of bipolar disorder (Gould et al., 2004). In addition to its role in glucose regulation, active GSK-3β facilitates apoptosis in neurons, while inhibition of GSK-3β attenuates cellular apoptosis, resulting in a neuroprotective effect (Hetman et al., 2000). Disturbances in the GSK-3β signal transduction pathway associated with diabetes may affect the viability of neurons that play a role in mood stabilization. Diminished insulin-mediated inhibition of GSK-3β may have an effect opposite to that of lithium and may ultimately lead to an accentuation of psychiatric symptoms related to bipolar disorder. For a more detailed discussion of the neuroprotective role of lithium and its putative significance for lithium's mood-stabilizing effects, see Chapter 14.

Migraine Headaches

The lifetime prevalence of migraine is markedly higher among individuals with mood disorders (Swartz et al., 2000; Fasmer, 2001; Odegaard and Fasmer, 2005) than in the general population. Bipolar women especially are more likely to suffer from migraines (Blehar et al., 1998; Calabrese et al., 2002). The Canadian Community Health Survey (N = 36,984) found that individuals with bipolar disorder had a higher prevalence of migraine than the general population (24.8 versus 10.3 percent; $p < .05$); the sex-specific prevalence of comorbid migraine in bipolar disorder was 14.9 percent for males and 34.7 percent for females. Bipolar males with comorbid migraine reported an earlier age at onset of bipolar illness ($p < .05$) and a higher lifetime prevalence of comorbid anxiety disorders ($p < .05$) than bipolar males without migraine. Bipolar females with comorbid migraine had more additional comorbid medical disorders ($p < .05$) than bipolar females who did not have migraines (McIntyre et al., 2006). Most strikingly, bipolar-II patients are far more likely to suffer from migraines than bipolar-I patients (77 and 14 percent, respectively), leading Fasmer (2001, p. 894) to suggest that bipolar-I and bipolar-II are "biologically separate disorders [which points] to the possibility of using the association of bipolar II disorder with migraine to study both the pathophysiology and the genetics of this affective disorder."

The comorbidity of migraine in women with bipolar-I disorder may be mediated by shared hormonal mechanisms that influence the timing of recurrence or complicate treatment. Both clinical and community studies using standardized diagnostic criteria have provided evidence of this comorbidity, independently of which illness caused the patient to seek treatment (Angst and Merikangas, 1992). In another study (Merikangas and Angst, 1992), bipolar-II disorder in probands was associated with an increased risk of migraine in relatives.

CONCLUSIONS

The scientific principle of parsimony holds that one should not increase, beyond what is necessary, the number of entities required to explain an observed phenomenon. In many cases, attributing all of a patient's symptoms to a single diagnostic entity is an appealing strategy. Symptoms that might be caused by a comorbid illness—such as excessive worry (generalized anxiety disorder), social avoidance (social anxiety disorder), distractibility (ADHD), and low energy and fatigue (diabetes)—are consistent with a diagnosis of affective disorder. Nevertheless, a large body of evidence derived from rigorously conducted studies unambiguously supports the presence of extensive comorbidity in bipolar illness, although with what frequency and which diagnosis subtype is open to debate (while substance abuse is more common in bipolar-I than in bipolar-II patients, the opposite is true for anxiety and eating disorders). It is probably appropriate, therefore, to begin by assuming that symptoms such as those cited above are not part of the core bipolar or unipolar presentation, and then to evaluate the patient systematically for the presence or absence of suspected comorbid illnesses. At the very least, all bipolar patients should be screened routinely for both psychiatric and medical comorbidities.

This type of comprehensive evaluation is time-consuming. Complicating the clinician's task, one of the most common comorbidities—substance abuse—is likely to be actively concealed by a patient during psychiatric consultation. Self-report screening questionnaires are useful when well-validated instruments are available. If the patient fills out such a questionnaire before seeing the clinician, less time need be devoted to ruling out comorbid diagnoses. Additionally, as a clinician works with a patient over time, a deeper understanding of the patient's symptoms and level of functioning develops, increasing the likelihood of uncovering additional disorders or problems.

As with other psychiatric illnesses, patients with recurrent affective disorders often fail to experience a complete remission of symptoms and a return to premorbid levels of functioning. The widespread prevalence of comorbidities, often missed by the diagnosing clinician, offers an opportunity to improve outcomes substantially by identifying and treating such problems as substance abuse, thyroid dysfunction, and anxiety. Patients who fail to respond adequately to multiple trials of medication should not be considered treatment resistant until a comprehensive assessment for untreated comorbidities has been undertaken. (See Chapter 24 for a discussion of the treatment of comorbid conditions.)

NOTES

1. These percentages are substantially higher than noted in the bipolar case registry (Chengappa et al., 2000), because in the Estroff et al. (1985) study, cocaine abuse was observed during an active episode of either mania or depression.

2. Estroff et al., 1985; Winokur et al., 1998; Goldberg et al., 1999; Cassidy et al., 2001.

3. Nearly 70 percent of all of the patients included in the analysis were participants in a study in which the concomitant mood stabilizer was olanzapine, which was considered placebo for purposes of the analysis. A smaller, well-designed study of lithium with antidepressants versus placebo did find a higher switch rate in the antidepressant plus lithium group, but in the meta-analysis this study was overwhelmed by the huge olanzapine study. See Chapter 19 for additional discussion of this study.

4. As noted in the introduction to this chapter, however, there are biases that operate in the other direction, namely the tendency of nonclinician interviewers to overdiagnose when using symptom checklists.

Suicide

The patients . . . often try to starve themselves, to hang themselves, to cut their arteries; they
beg that they may be burned, buried alive, driven out into the woods and there allowed to
die . . . . One of my patients struck his neck so often on the edge of a chisel fixed on the ground
that all the soft parts were cut through to the vertebrae.

—*Emil Kraepelin (1921, p. 25)*

Patients with depressive and manic-depressive illness are far more likely to commit suicide than those with other psychiatric or medical illnesses. An analysis of nearly 250 studies, reported over a 30-year period, found that mood disorders carry the highest risk of suicide (Fig. 8–1; see also Juurlink et al., 2004). Yet despite this high risk, the lethality of manic-depressive illness is often underemphasized. We believe suicide is far too common in untreated, inadequately treated, or treatment-resistant manic-depressive illness. Suicide is often preventable if a correct diagnosis is made, if acute and chronic suicide risk factors are recognized and acted upon, and if appropriate treatment is provided (see Chapter 25).

We begin the chapter with a look at diagnostic and methodological issues related to the study of suicide in bipolar and unipolar depressed patients. Next, we present findings on suicide rates. We then address causes of suicide, including the contributions of genetic, family, biological, and psychosocial factors. Finally, we review psychiatric and medical comorbidities and other clinical correlates of suicidal states.

DIAGNOSTIC AND METHODOLOGICAL ISSUES

It has long been recognized that suicidal thinking and behavior are associated with both bipolar and unipolar major depressive disorders (see Chapter 2). More recently, the *Diagnostic and Statistical Manual*, 4th edition (DSM-IV) incorporated into its diagnostic criteria for major depression a specific criterion for suicidal potential: "Recurrent thoughts of death (not just fear of dying), recurrent suicidal ideation without a specific plan, or a suicide attempt or a specific plan for committing suicide" (p. 327).

Studies of suicide have used several outcome measures—ideation, suicide attempts, and completed suicide. Over the

years, researchers have recognized that these end points reflect a wide range of thoughts and behaviors. Today, the focus is on the use of more nuanced measures, such as the type (e.g., violent versus nonviolent) and the severity (e.g., Beck Scale of Suicidal Ideation, Schedule for Affective Disorders and Schizophrenia [SADS] suicide subscale) of the attempt. Suicidal ideation without particular information about plans or means is common in manic-depressive illness. Yet it is neither a sensitive nor a specific predictor of suicide, at least over the long term (see Chapter 25), and scales for rating suicidal ideation and intent therefore lead to high false-positive and false-negative rates (Jacobs et al., 2003). This chapter thus places greater emphasis on actual suicide attempts, especially those of high lethality (although, unfortunately, most studies of suicide attempts do not rate lethality), and completed suicide.

The approaches taken in research on suicide have generally ignored the presence of two distinct populations. The first comprises those individuals who commit suicide who have never been diagnosed with a psychiatric disorder. This group accounts for approximately 50 percent of all suicides, even though retrospective studies have found that a psychiatric diagnosis could be established in more than 90 percent of such cases (Henriksson et al., 1993; Cheng et al., 2000). This finding was the basis for *The Surgeon General's Call to Action to Prevent Suicide* (U.S. Public Health Service, 1999), which cited stigma, lack of public education about psychiatric disorders, and insufficient financial resources as barriers to diagnosis and treatment for those at risk of committing suicide. It also addressed the need to train physicians to recognize and treat conditions, such as depression or bipolar disorder, that can lead to increased suicide risk.

The other group of concern encompasses the remaining 50 percent of individuals who commit suicide despite

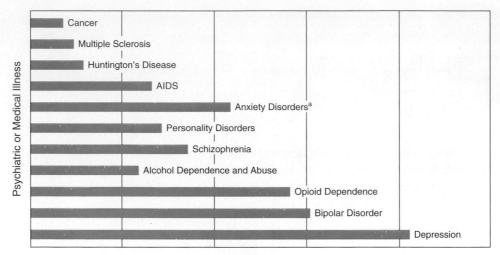

Figure 8–1. Suicide risk in psychiatric or medical illness: number of times the expected rate in the general population. [a]Obsessive-compulsive disorder and panic disorder. (*Source:* Adapted from Harris and Barraclough, 1997. Reprinted with permission from the *American Journal of Psychiatry*, copyright 2001, American Psychiatric Association.)

having been in recent contact with a clinician or diagnosed with or treated for a psychiatric disorder. Robins (1981) reported that 50 percent of his sample of suicides had seen a physician within 1 month of committing the act. Likewise, Barraclough (1970) found that 70 percent of those who had committed suicide had been in touch with a physician within 1 month, and nearly 50 percent within 1 week, of their death. And upon reviewing 40 published studies over the next decade, Luoma and colleagues (2002) concluded that 45 percent of those who had committed suicide had had contact with their primary care physician within 1 month of their death; 20 percent had been in contact with mental health services. Moreover, it has been reported that 6 to 10 percent of suicides occur in hospitals each year (Robins, 1981). Thus, despite ongoing treatment or health care contact, a significant number of patients are not being identified as being at acute risk for suicide. Others do not receive adequate treatment or fail to adhere to clinical recommendations (see Chapter 21). Many deaths could be prevented if physicians in both primary and specialty care settings became more alert to acute risk factors for suicide (see Chapter 25).

Other methodological problems limit interpretation of the findings of suicide studies. Diagnostic criteria often are unclear, and bipolar and unipolar distinctions only recently became standard in the literature. It is important to keep in mind that the definition of manic-depressive illness changed with the adoption of DSM-III in 1980 (see Chapter 3). The DSM-III nomenclature replaced the diagnosis manic-depressive disorder with that of bipolar disorder. Prior to this, a diagnosis of manic-depressive disorder had required a history or presence of recurrent depression *or* an episode of mania, thus encompassing the broader group of patients that is the focus of this volume (see Chapter 1). The narrower bipolar diagnosis required the presence or history of an episode of mania or hypomania; patients with recurrent depression were subsumed under the unipolar depression diagnosis, and recurrent unipolar was broadened to include anyone with more than one episode. This shift in diagnostic practice has made it more difficult to interpret secular trends. In this chapter, we employ the diagnostic terms relevant to particular studies, but otherwise (as throughout the volume) use "manic-depressive illness" to refer to the broader concept of recurrent major affective disorder; we use "bipolar disorder" to refer to the bipolar spectrum.

Particularly critical is the enormous range across studies in the length of follow-up periods; this broad range necessarily results in variable periods of risk for suicide. Moreover, when studies include only patients who have been hospitalized, suicide rates are likely to be higher, reflecting a greater severity of illness. Most early studies of suicide in manic-depressive illness were of hospitalized patients; many more recent studies are of outpatients or combinations of outpatients and inpatients. Because suicide risk is one of the most decisive criteria for admission to a psychiatric hospital, studies of hospitalized patients are necessarily skewed toward a greater likelihood of suicide.

SUICIDE RATES

In this section, we begin by reviewing suicide rates among the general population and among bipolar and unipolar depressed patients. We then present specific rates according to diagnosis (bipolar versus unipolar; bipolar-I versus bipolar-II), gender, and seasonality.

Rates in the General Population

In the United States in 2002, there were 31,655 deaths recorded as suicide.[1] This figure represents an overall suicide rate of 10.99 per 100,000 population (National Center for Injury Prevention and Control [NCIPC], 2005). Worldwide, an estimated 900,000 suicide deaths occur each year (World Health Organization [WHO], 2001); a figure of 1.5 million is projected for 2020 (Bertolote and Fleischmann, 2002). The estimated global suicide rate is 17.7 per 100,000 for males and 10.7 per 100,000 for females (Mathers et al., 2006). Many cultural factors, including religion and the adequacy of public health reporting systems, result in a wide range in the reporting and occurrence of suicide—from a low in Islamic countries to a high in Eastern Europe (the rates of suicide per 100,000 population are, for example, 33.1 in Hungary, 35.5 in the Russian Federation, and 41.9 in Lithuania [World Health Organization, 2001]).

Rates in Manic-Depressive Illness

Early studies documented a strikingly high lifetime rate of suicide, 15 percent, among patients with manic-depressive illness. The estimated rate today has dropped by about one half, except for patients early in the course of illness. The higher rates in most early studies (published before the mid-1980s) almost certainly reflect poorer clinical outcomes before the widespread use of lithium and other mood stabilizers, tricyclic antidepressants, and selective serotonin reuptake inhibitors (SSRIs). The figure of 15 percent lifetime risk also reflects suicide risk in clinical populations with severe, untreated manic-depressive illness.

Guze and Robins (1970) were the first to document systematically the extent of suicide risk in manic-depressive illness. They reviewed 14 follow-up studies, 2 population surveys, and 1 family study and found that at least 12 percent of all deaths among manic-depressive patients had been the result of suicide (in these early studies, patients with recurrent depressions were diagnosed as manic-depressive). In 9 of the studies, 12 to 19 percent of deaths had been due to suicide, and in the other 8 studies, the suicide rate ranged from 35 to 60 percent. The authors concluded that by the time all the patients in these studies had died, about 15 percent would have committed suicide, a rate at least 30 times that found in the general population.

Subsequent analyses buttressed these early findings. Our own review of 30 studies of completed suicide (1937–1988), presented in the first edition of this text, found a mean lifetime rate of 19 percent in patients with severe manic-depressive illness (range 9 to 60 percent). In 13 of the 30 studies, the figure was in the 10 to 30 percent range. In one fifth of the studies, at least half of the manic-depressive patients had died because of suicide. Similarly, a study of nearly 500 bipolar patients (mostly untreated or inadequately treated) over a 17-year period (1970–1987) found a suicide rate of 15 percent (Sharma and Markar, 1994).

The high suicide rate in manic-depressive illness is also documented by comparison with suicide rates in the general population. Harris and Barraclough (1997) calculated standardized mortality ratios (SMRs) in a meta-analysis of 14 studies reported from 1945 to 1992 (N=3,700 bipolar patients). They found that the SMR for suicide in bipolar disorder was about 15 times higher than expected (see Fig. 8–1). Increased risk was associated with recent hospital discharge, a suicide attempt within the previous 5 years, and current alcohol abuse. The authors found a somewhat higher SMR, 20.4, for suicide in patients with major depression.

More recent studies, however, have found significantly lower rates of suicide (in the range of 5 percent lifetime risk) among never-hospitalized patients with bipolar disorder of moderate severity (see Tondo et al., 2003, for a review). But these lower suicide rates do not apply early in the course of illness. A study from the United Kingdom found a lifetime suicide rate of 6 percent for patients with affective disorders (depression and bipolar disorder), but the rate increased to 23 to 26 percent early in the course of bipolar illness (Inskip et al., 1998) (see later discussion).

There are several possible explanations for this marked decrease over time in reported suicide rates in bipolar disorder. A major reason, alluded to earlier, is most likely the increased use of lithium and other medications in the treatment of manic-depressive illness since 1980 (see Chapter 25). Other reasons for the decline are probably methodological. The findings of newer studies, which often have focused on outpatient populations or mixed inpatient and outpatient populations, reflect suicide rates in less severely ill patients. In their review, Tondo and colleagues (2003) suggested that reported rates are lower because most of the patients among whom the rates were ascertained were never hospitalized. They also pointed out that more recent studies, by reflecting the milder range of illness severity, underestimate the risk in more severely ill patients. They noted as well that, compared with a general population of patients, there is a lower ratio of attempts to fatalities in patients with major mood disorders. In their view, this finding suggests a high lethality and intent in affectively ill patients. The SMR for bipolar patients, based on a review of 28 studies from 1945 to 2000, was 22.1. Rates of suicide averaged about 0.376 percent per year.

Bostwick and Pankratz (2000) directly calculated the rates of suicide in hospitalized affectively ill patients versus other groups. In their meta-analysis, they reanalyzed both the Guze and Robins (1970) study and our own analysis of 30 studies (cited earlier), in addition to more recent studies (up to 1998). Using a different metric (case-fatality prevalence) they found lifetime suicide rates of 8.6 percent for patients hospitalized for suicide risk, 4.0 percent for those not hospitalized, and 2.2 percent for mixed inpatient/outpatient populations; the rate was less than 0.5 percent for the non–affectively ill population. The authors did not separate the risk for bipolar and unipolar disorders.

Bipolar–Unipolar Differences

Most studies have tended to find somewhat higher suicide rates in unipolar depression than in bipolar disorder (e.g., Harris and Barraclough, 1997; Osby et al., 2001; Angst et al., 2002). Others, however, have found either no bipolar–unipolar difference[2] or higher rates among patients with bipolar disorder (e.g., Rihmer and Pestality, 1999; Bottlender et al., 2000). The reason for these disparate findings, in our view, lies largely in the heterogeneity of the unipolar population and the underdiagnosis of mixed states and other forms of bipolarity.

The broad definition of unipolar depression in today's nomenclature simply means that the diagnosis is not bipolar; that is, a unipolar diagnosis encompasses patients with all degrees of recurrence, ranging from single-episode depression to highly recurrent or cyclic depression (see Chapter 2). Yet the research literature rarely has distinguished among unipolar patients on the basis of differences in their patterns of recurrence, which may in turn reflect different suicide risks depending on comorbidities, course of illness, and other clinical factors noted throughout this chapter. We believe that patients with recurrent unipolar depression may be likely to have suicide rates as high as or higher than those with bipolar disorder, whereas patients with less recurrent forms of unipolar depression are likely to have lower rates. Because the majority of unipolar patients have at least some recurrence, their inclusion could be expected to skew the unipolar category to higher rates. This might explain why Harris and Barraclough's meta-analysis (see Fig. 8–1) and other studies have found somewhat higher rates in unipolar depression than in bipolar disorder. A compounding problem is that, as we have seen (see Chapter 19), a substantial percentage of patients with major depression eventually convert to bipolar

illness. Finnish researchers have found that these patients form a subgroup that is particularly prone to suicide (Sokero et al., 2005).

What also may contribute to the apparently higher suicide rates in unipolar illness is the tendency to misdiagnose bipolar-II disorder as unipolar depression. Rihmer and Kiss (2002) argued that patients with bipolar-II disorder are often misdiagnosed and then included as unipolar patients. The unipolar category would thereby be erroneously elevated because the suicide rate in bipolar-II is higher than that in unipolar depression (Rihmer and Kiss, 2002) (Table 8–1). A final problem is that some patients diagnosed as having "agitated depression" may in fact have mixed states associated with bipolar disorder. This, too, would falsely raise the suicide rate in unipolar depression, particularly because mixed states carry a relatively higher suicide risk (see later discussion). If suicide occurs early in the course of affective illness, it may well be that patients who otherwise might have gone on to have a recurrent or bipolar course will have been diagnosed as having had a single episode of depression, again spuriously elevating the rate in unipolar illness.

The search for bipolar–unipolar differences, while important, may obscure the more significant point that all studies show greatly elevated suicide rates in both unipolar and bipolar groups in comparison with other medical and psychiatric populations (Sharma and Markar, 1994; Harris and Barraclough, 1997; Juurlink et al., 2004). The most prudent approach is to assume a high suicide risk in both bipolar and unipolar patients.

Bipolar-I versus Bipolar-II Disorder

Identifying diagnostic subgroups with an increased incidence of suicide or suicide attempts is one of the first steps toward identifying individual bipolar patients who are at particularly high risk. Several investigations over the last three decades have found that patients with bipolar-II disorder have a higher risk of suicide attempts than those with bipolar-I. These studies were reviewed by Rihmer and Kiss (2002) (see Table 8–1).

In addition, Bulik and colleagues (1990) studied 67 patients with a history of recurrent depression and suicide attempts. In comparison with 163 patients with recurrent major depression and no suicide attempts, they found that attempters were distinguished by a history of bipolar-II depression. The findings of these studies suggest that bipolar-II depression confers a particularly high risk of suicide in patients presenting with major depression. A recent retrospective study of 90 bipolar-I and 10 bipolar-II patients, however, did not find a significant difference in rates of suicide attempts between the two groups (Valtonen et al., 2006).

TABLE 8–1. **History of Prior Suicide Attempts in Patients with Unipolar Major Depression and Bipolar-I and Bipolar-II Disorder**

Study	Patients with Unipolar Depression Rate (%)	Patients with Bipolar-I Disorder Rate (%)	Patients with Bipolar-II Disorder Rate (%)
Dunner et al., 1976	2/23 (9)	11/29 (38)	9/16 (56)
Endicott et al., 1985	26/204 (13)	30/122 (25)	15/56 (27)
Coryell et al., 1987	31/303 (10)	7/29 (24)	7/40 (18)
Cassano et al., 1992	60/558 (11)	9/35 (26)	17/94 (18)
Vieta et al., 1997	—	12/38 (32)	6/22 (27)
Tondo et al., 1999	24/126 (19)	34/353 (10)	7/25 (28)
TOTAL	143/1234 (12)	103/606 (17)	68/253 (24)

Note: Bipolar-I + bipolar-II versus unipolar: $X^2 = 21.32$, degrees of freedom $(df) = 1$, $p < .001$; bipolar-I versus unipolar: $X^2 = 9.41$, $df = 1$, $p < .01$; bipolar-II versus unipolar: $X^2 = 26.59$, $df = 1$, $p < 0.001$; bipolar-II versus bipolar-I: $X^2 = 5.85$, $df = 1$, $p < .02$.

Source: Rihmer and Kiss, 2002. Reprinted with permission from Blackwell Publishing.

In their review, MacQueen and Young (2001) noted a particularly high liability for comorbidity with personality disorders, substance abuse disorders, and anxiety disorders in bipolar-II patients with an elevated risk of suicide (see Chapter 7). Bipolar-II patients, who have higher rates of comorbid substance abuse and personality disorders than bipolar-I patients, may be at increased risk in large part because of the comorbidity. Rihmer and Kiss (2002) found that when lifetime prevalence in the general population is the comparator, bipolar-II patients have the highest prevalence of attempted and completed suicides. The evidence strongly suggests that bipolar-II patients have—relative to the general population and to those with bipolar-I or unipolar depression—the highest rate of suicide.

Differences by Gender

In the general population of the United States, approximately three times as many women as men attempt suicide; however, four times as many men actually kill themselves (NCIPC, 2005). The patterns of suicidal behavior among women and men with manic-depressive illness show both similarities to and differences from this pattern.

Like the general female population, bipolar women attempt suicide more often than bipolar men. In contrast to the general population, however, there is no clear predominance of males among bipolar patients who actually commit suicide; the completed suicide rate for males is generally equivalent to or lower than that for females.

Reviewing 28 studies conducted from 1945 to 2001, Tondo and colleagues (2003) found that among bipolar patients, the average SMR for suicide was 14.9 for males and 21.1 for females. And a recent Swedish study of mortality outcomes in 15,386 bipolar patients found very similar SMRs for suicide—15.0 for men and 22.4 for women (Osby et al., 2005). It may be that the risk of suicide associated with manic-depressive illness is so powerful that it overrides the male–female differences in the general population. With regard to suicide attempts, Tondo and colleagues (2003) found that the rate among females within the bipolar subgroup (15 to 48 percent) was about double that for men (4 to 27 percent). Evidence of differences by gender among suicide attempters may be distorted by reporting biases, however. When patients are asked about past suicidal behavior, women may be more likely than men to admit to or remember attempts; men, on the other hand, may be more prone to suicidal equivalents, such as extreme risk taking, involvement in car accidents, and substance abuse. These behaviors are less often explored in surveys.

In summary, women with manic-depressive illness attempt suicide more often than men. In contrast to the general population, the suicide rate in women with manic-depressive illness is higher than or equivalent to that in men.

Seasonality

Seasonality affects the timing of manic and depressive affective episodes (see Chapter 16). It also has a profound effect on suicide. There is a robust literature on suicide and seasonality, in part because it is easier to date a suicide than the onset of an affective episode accurately and precisely. Most of the literature reviewed here does not specify diagnosis, but at the end of the section we discuss studies that deal expressly with bipolar disorder and seasonal suicide patterns related to mood states.

We reviewed dozens of seasonality studies for the first edition of this text. Since that time, many more such studies have been published. Taken as a whole, this literature affirms a striking peak incidence of suicide in late spring–early summer. Many studies have also found a smaller peak in October, generally for women rather than men. Both peaks, however, have lessened in amplitude over time (Fig. 8–2). Findings of more recent studies add considerably more nuance to the overall pattern of a spring-to-summer peak in suicides.

Seasonality and Suicide Rates

Granberg and Westerberg (1999) analyzed suicide data from Sweden (1911–1993) and New Zealand (1975–1995) and found that suicides peaked in the spring months— May in Sweden and November in New Zealand. In other studies, carried out in the southern hemisphere (Takahashi, 1964; Parker and Walter, 1982), the seasonality of suicide was consistent with the pattern seen in the northern hemisphere (i.e., peaks in the spring), although for New

South Wales, Parker and Walter (1982) found two peak suicide periods (in May and November) among women rather than one. Chew and McCleary (1995), using time-series and cross-sectional data for 28 countries and employing bivariate plots and simple correlation techniques, found a sizable spring peak in suicide only in the temperate zones. More recently, Lee and colleagues (2006), utilizing the nationwide mortality database in Taiwan 1997–2003, found that suicides peaked in spring, regardless of gender or age. Ambient temperature was positively associated with suicide after adjustment for seasonality.

Fisher and colleagues (1997), studying 16,389 nationally registered suicide deaths between 1980 and 1989, found a peak in the spring in South Africa. Retamal and Humphreys (1998), reviewing 5,386 suicides in Chile for the period 1979–1994, found the highest rates in the "warm months" (i.e., the southern hemisphere's spring and summer), particularly December, and the lowest rates in the colder months, particularly June. Morken and colleagues (2002) studied all admissions in Norway for mania and depression during 1992–1996 ($N = 4,341$) and all 14,503 suicides in the years 1969–1996. They observed a significant peak in depression for women in November, with a secondary peak in April, and a peak for men in admissions for both depression and mania in April. Both genders showed a trough in admissions in July. Among men, the monthly occurrence of suicides correlated with the rate of admissions

Figure 8–2. Seasonal patterns of suicide. (*Source:* Jamison, 1999, *Night Falls Fast.* Reprinted with permission.)

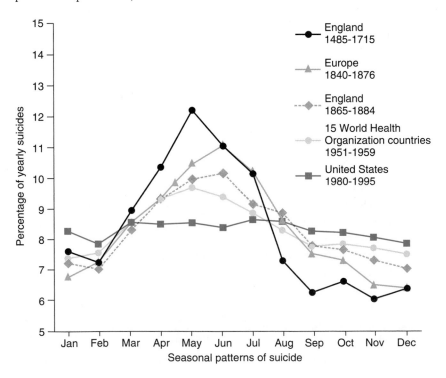

for depression and mania (a spring peak); no such correlation was found in women. It may be that women were admitted earlier in the course of their depressive episode and that the peak severity occurred later; men may have been more severely depressed at the time of their admission. This issue has not been studied systematically.

Maes and colleagues (1993a) found significant spring seasonality for violent suicides but not for nonviolent suicides in Belgium. They also noted seasonality in the severity of depressive symptomatology as measured by the Zung self-rating scale, with greater severity reported in the spring months. Preti and colleagues (1998, 2000), examining violent suicide attempts in Italy, found a peak in the spring months, but only for violent suicide attempts in males. No seasonal trend was observed in nonviolent suicides among males or females during 1984–1995.

Findings reported by Maes and colleagues (1994) and Linkowski and colleagues (1992) suggest that violent suicides and perhaps violent attempts may be more common in sunny weather or higher temperatures. It is known that violent suicides and attempts are much more common in males than in females, a fact that is consistent with the greater occurrence of seasonality patterns in males.

Rasanen and colleagues (2002) investigated the seasonal distribution of the specific suicide method for both genders ($N = 20{,}234$) in Finland for the years 1980–1995. In summer, significant peaks occurred in suicides by drowning, jumping, and gassing among males. In autumn, there were peaks in female suicides by poisoning and drowning. Traffic suicides showed substantial winter troughs for both genders. The results demonstrated that specific violent and nonviolent methods for suicide formed their traditional clusters on the basis of seasonality, except for suicides by gassing and shooting.

Gender differences in seasonal patterns of suicide in Italy were examined by Micciolo and colleagues (1989). They found cyclic fluctuations in the number of suicides in both sexes, but only one significant peak per year for men and two for women. The most significant peak for both men and women was in May; women had a second peak in October and November. Hakko and colleagues (1998) studied seasonal patterns of suicide in Finland using a database of 21,279 suicides and found a peak for males from April to July; the distribution for females was bimodal, with peaks in May and October. In the elderly, they found a significant excess of suicides in autumn. Violent suicides showed a single spring peak, whereas nonviolent suicides displayed a bimodal distribution. Marion and colleagues (1999) found that in British Columbia, suicides among the young were associated with a spring–summer peak, whereas those among the elderly appeared to be related to deviations from expected temperatures for the time of year. Salib (1997), studying suicide in an elderly population of 40,000 in Cheshire, England, over a 5-year period, found a positive relationship of suicide with hours of sunshine and humidity, rather than with extreme weather conditions. The findings of more recent studies have raised the question of whether the elderly may be affected more by rapid shifts in weather conditions than by seasonal effects. These findings raise the possibility that studies of seasonality should take into account age as well as violent versus nonviolent suicide methods, rather than simply merging groups of suicide cases.

There have also been suggestions that seasonal variation is greatest in rural as opposed to urban areas (e.g., Micciolo et al., 1991); one possible explanation for this difference is that urban living conditions, such as less direct exposure to natural light and more exposure to artificial light, may somehow reduce the seasonal effect. In their analysis of seasonal patterns of suicide in farmers and nonfarmers, Simkin and colleagues (2003) observed no significant seasonal patterns in violent suicides among nonfarmers.

The often-raised possibility of the effect of lunar cycles on suicide was addressed in a review of 20 studies by Martin and colleagues (1992), who found no evidence to support such a relationship. Likewise, Maldonado and Kraus (1991) found no effect of lunar phase in 4,190 suicides occurring between 1925 and 1983 among residents of Sacramento County, California. They did find that suicide occurred most frequently on Monday for both genders across age groups, and least frequently between the hours of 4:00 and 8:00 AM.

In short, it appears that seasonal variation in suicide applies most consistently to males, to the use of violent methods, and to those living in temperate zones. Seasonality may not be as much of a factor for females and males using nonviolent methods.

As noted earlier, a significant weakening of the association between seasonality and suicide over time has been observed in a number of studies. Rihmer and colleagues (1998), for example, found a link with seasonality in a (relatively small) sample of suicides from 1981–1986, but no such link in a sample from 1990–1996. Likewise, Hakko and colleagues (1998) found a decreasing frequency of seasonality in suicides in Finland after 1990. A reevaluation of seasonal variation in suicide in Australia and New Zealand led Yip and colleagues (1998) to conclude that seasonality was less of a determining factor than it had been. Tietjen and Kripke (1994) found no seasonal peaks in suicide in California's Los Angeles and Sacramento counties. Rock and colleagues (2003), on the other hand, found that seasonal amplitude had increased over time in Australia, contrasting this finding with those of contemporary European reports showing a decrease in seasonal amplitude over time. A recent study of suicides and seasonality in the Austrian prison system ($N = 412$), conducted over a 53-year period by Fruehwald and colleagues (2001), found no seasonal fluctuation in suicide rates. Parker and colleagues (2001) found no seasonal variation in 2,013 male and 1,382 female suicides in the equatorial region of Singapore.

Given the strength and breadth of the early findings of a strong seasonal component to suicide, an obvious question is why the seasonal effect has abated. In a review of the international literature on the seasonal incidence of suicide, Aschoff (1981) proposed that environmental factors play a role in the seasonal patterns observed. He found that during the nineteenth century, seasonal variation in suicide rates was greatest in the least industrialized nations and declined with greater industrialization. It is likely that certain aspects of industrialization (e.g., artificial light, central heating) may partially insulate patients from environmental risk factors for affective episodes. Seasonal variation in suicide rates, as we have seen, is greatest in the temperate latitudes as opposed to the north, with its extremes of light and temperature. Seasonal variation also is most correlated with hours of clear sunshine (not day length per se). Petridou and colleagues (2002), evaluating the traditional peak occurrence of suicide in June in the northern hemisphere and in December in the southern hemisphere, found an association between the seasonal amplitude of suicide and total sunshine. They suggested that suicide may be triggered by sunlight, perhaps through seasonally determined hormones such as melatonin (see later discussion). Papadopoulos and colleagues (2005) studied Greek suicide patterns and solar radiance data for a 10-year period and found that the solar radiance on the day preceding suicide was positively correlated with suicide risk, as was average solar radiance during the 4 days preceding that. They hypothesized that "sunshine acts as a natural antidepressant, which first improves motivation, then only later improves mood, thereby creating a potential short-term increased risk of suicide initially upon its application" (pp. 287–288).

Another likely explanation for the trend toward diminishing amplitude of the spring-to-summer peak in suicide rates is the greater use of mood-stabilizing medications. Rihmer and colleagues (1998) hypothesized that the link between seasonality and suicide has been weakened by the widespread use of lithium and antidepressants. Likewise, Oraveez and colleagues (2006) attributed the decrease in the seasonality of suicides in Slovenia to improvements in access to and effectiveness of psychiatric treatment following the 1991 war. Because major depression has such a strong seasonal component, the investigators argued that the decrease in the seasonality of suicide occurred as a result of improved treatment.

Neurobiological Factors in Seasonality

Clearly, profound biological changes occur in response to seasonal variations in light and temperature. Many neurobiological systems of relevance to mood disorders and suicide—including neurotransmitters, sleep and temperature regulators, melatonin, cholesterol, testosterone, estrogen, and thyroid hormone (summarized in Jamison, 1999; Institute of Medicine [IOM], 2002)—show pronounced seasonal fluctuation in their levels.[3]

A number of measures of serotonin function (see the later discussion of serotonin and suicide) have been reported to be correlated with the seasons.[4] This correlation may reflect a biological variable related to violent suicides, the effect of which may be diminished by older age, as well as urban living and perhaps even antidepressant treatment (see earlier discussion). Relating seasonal patterns in suicide to seasonal changes in various biological systems could thus yield greater insight into biological factors in susceptibility to suicide.

Timonen and colleagues (2004), studying 1,296 males and 289 females during the years 1988–2000, found the proportion of suicides in atopic (allergic) patients to be significantly higher than that in nonatopic patients. They further found that 72 percent of suicides in atopic patients occurred during the first 6 months of the year, and 28 percent during the second 6 months. By contrast, the distribution across the two periods was even in nonatopic patients. De Vriese and colleagues (2004) found a correlation between monthly variations in levels of the n-3 polyunsaturated fatty acids arachidonic acid and eicopentanoic acid and the mean weekly number of violent (but not nonviolent) suicides. A seasonal effect on factors likely to change levels of omega-3 essential fatty acids—such as fluctuating availability of foods and increased intake of fat-rich foods during the winter months—has been suggested by Hibbeln (1998, personal correspondence, 1999).

Seasonality in Bipolar Disorder

The seasonal pattern of suicide appears to run counter to that of bipolar depression, which is more likely to occur in the winter months in the temperate zones. (See Chapter 16 for extensive discussion of the seasonal patterns of mania and depression.) It may be that the increased activation associated with longer periods of light in the late spring months brings to a suicidal climax depressive episodes that begin in the winter months, particularly among those bipolar patients who are prone to developing dysphoric manic states. Cassidy and Carroll (2002a) analyzed the seasonal occurrence of 304 hospital admissions for mixed or manic bipolar states. They found that the frequency of all admissions for mania peaked in early spring, with a nadir in late fall. Admissions for mixed mania had a significantly different pattern, with a peak in late summer and a nadir in late November. Whitney and colleagues (1999) likewise found that mixed-state admissions in Canada peaked in the summer, but they did not find a seasonal pattern for mania and depression. D'Mello and colleagues (1995), studying the admissions of 377 bipolar patients in Michigan over a 6-year period, observed that women had a bimodal seasonal distribution, with peak admission rates in the spring and fall. They found that aggressive behavior peaked in the spring for both men and women. Several other investigators (Parker and Walter, 1982, in New South Wales; Mulder et al., 1990, in New Zealand; and Takei et al., 1992, in London) found a peak in admissions for mania in spring and summer.

These findings suggest a seasonal pattern in activation levels in bipolar disorder. Wehr (1992) observed that the risk for depression peaked at two opposite times of the year—spring/early summer and fall/early winter. These two periods are associated with opposite vegetative symptoms: sleep and appetite increases in winter depressions and decreases in spring/summer depressions. Maes and colleagues (1993b) observed that the severity of depression as measured by the Zung Self-Rating Depression (ZD) and Anxiety (ZA) scales showed a significant increase in the spring (April–May), with lows occurring in August–September; up to 31 percent of the variance in the weekly average of ZA scores could be explained by a circannual rhythm. In a subsequent study, Maes and colleagues (1995) noted a correlation between seasonal variations in serum L-tryptophan and suicide. Taken together, the studies reviewed here suggest an activation of manic-depressive illness (including mixed states, as well as unipolar recurrent depression) in the spring/summer months that roughly parallels the seasonal increase in suicides reported in the temperate zones, especially in males.

The second suicide peak in October may reflect an increase not only in unipolar depressive episodes, but also in suicidal depressions following the pronounced increase in manic episodes among bipolar patients during the summer months. That is, this second peak may represent suicidal postmanic depressions. It also may reflect the impact of mixed, transitional mood states. As patients recover from summer or autumn hypomania or mania, or as they switch from hypomania or mania into depression, mixed states are not uncommon. A recent study of depressed patients with mixed states found that the depressive episodes peaked in autumn (Sato et al., 2006). In vulnerable individuals, this may lead to periods of an acute, agitated suicidal state.

CAUSES OF SUICIDE

In this section, we review what is known about the biological, psychological, and social factors associated with suicide in bipolar illness. This growing body of research is focused on determining what role these factors play—as underlying causes, risk factors, or protective factors—and on ascertaining whether they can be modified through treatment. To date, while it is clear that suicide is caused by a potent combination of biological and psychosocial risk factors, research has not yet reached the point where any particular combination of factors can be identified as predictive of suicide.[5]

Genetic and Family Transmission

The tendency for suicides to run in families has been noted in writings dating back many hundreds, if not thousands, of years. Using modern methods, researchers have shown that suicidal behavior does indeed have heritable contributions. This has been demonstrated through three lines of inquiry: family studies, studies of suicide in monozygotic (MZ) versus dizygotic (DZ) twins, and studies of adoptees (for reviews see Roy et al., 1999; Baldessarini and Hennen, 2004). These types of studies allow us to draw inferences about heritability and genetic contributions to suicide. Yet while they help narrow the search for genes that may be implicated, they cannot, by design, be used to identify particular genes (candidate gene identification is discussed in the next section).

Family studies compare the risk of suicidal behavior (i.e., suicides or suicide attempts) in close relatives of index cases versus the risk in close relatives of nonsuicidal cases or normal controls. Tsuang (1977, 1983) was among the first of modern scientists to report clustering of suicide in families. Since the 1970s, dozens of such investigations have been undertaken. In a recent meta-analysis of 22 studies, Baldessarini and Hennen (2004) found a nearly three-fold higher risk of suicidal acts among relatives of index cases compared with controls (Fig. 8–3). The investigators used random-effects regression modeling with weighting for study size and interstudy variances.

In the original studies on which the meta-analysis was based, the index suicide cases were not limited to a particular psychiatric diagnosis; a few studies were limited to major depression, but only one to bipolar illness (with comorbid alcoholism) (Potash, 2000). This latter study found bipolar disorder, alcoholism, and attempted suicide to be clustered in some families. Among subjects with bipolar disorder, 38 percent of those with comorbid alcoholism had made a suicide attempt; 22 percent of those without alcoholism had attempted suicide ($p < .005$).

Family transmission of suicidal behavior is not necessarily tantamount to genetic transmission, for any linkage between suicide and families also could be through learned behaviors or shared environment (e.g., parenting, physical or sexual abuse). Identifying genetic transmission requires piecing together of additional evidence, such as studies of

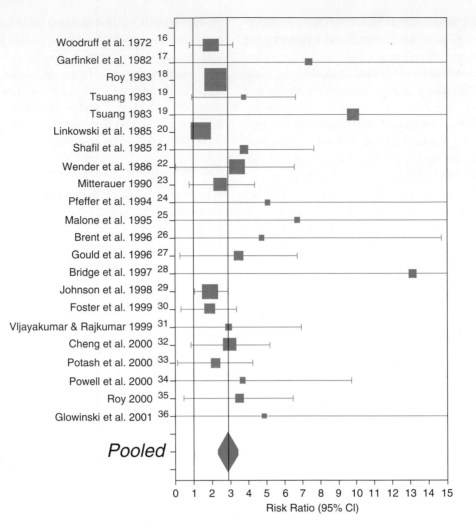

Figure 8–3. Meta-analysis of 22 studies of familial risk of suicide behavior based on random effects of modeling of relative risk (size of shaded squares reflects approximate weighting by sample size and variance measures) among families of suicidal probands versus controls and their 95% confidence intervals (CI; horizontal bars), with a pooled risk ratio and its CI (diamond). All 22 studies found increased familial risk associated with suicidal probands. The pooled risk ratio (vertical line with diamond) is 2.86 (CI, 2.32–3.53), which is highly significantly ($p < .0001$) greater than the null of 1.0 (vertical line). (*Source*: Baldessarini and Hennen, 2004.)

concordance rates in twins and adoptees, biological markers, and genetic polymorphisms, as well as linkage analysis.

Twin studies are designed to separate genetic from environmental contributions by comparing risks in MZ and DZ twins. Roy and colleagues (1999) compared concordance rates in 176 twin pairs with a suicide and found a greatly elevated rate among MZ (13.2 percent) versus DZ (0.7 percent) twins. His review examined only completed suicides, not attempts. In an analysis pooling seven twin studies, the rate of suicide or suicide attempts in MZ twin pairs (23 percent) was found to be much higher than that in DZ (0.1 percent) twin pairs (Table 8–2) (Baldessarini and Hennen, 2004). These rates yielded a relative risk of 175, but the investigators considered this figure to be unreliably high because the 0.1 percent rate in DZ pairs was cal-

culated from only 2 suicides among more than 1,000 pairs. The investigators concluded that case ascertainment was likely to have been incomplete because the rate among DZ twins should have been comparable to that found among siblings, which typically runs about 9 percent in most family studies. Substituting this expected rate of 9 percent for the actual rate of 0.1 percent among DZ twins, they found a more modest relative risk of 2.6 in MZ compared with DZ twins. The increased risk is similar in magnitude to that found in a large study of 3,416 female adolescent twins (relative risk [RR] = 1.9) (Glowinski et al., 2001).

Adoption studies compare the risk of suicidal behavior in biological versus adoptive relatives of index cases of suicide. This design gives adoption studies the advantage of controlling for shared environmental factors. Three adoption

TABLE 8–2. **Summary of Twin Studies of Suicidal Risk**

Study	REPORTED CO-TWIN SUICIDAL RATES		
	Identical (MZ)	Fraternal (DZ)	Risk Ratio
Kallman and Anastasio, 1947[a]	0/11	0/8	Not estimable
Haberlandt, 1967[b]	14/51	0/98	>27
Juel-Nielson and Videbach, 1970[a]	4/15	0/58	>15
Zair, 1981[a]	1/1	Not reported	Not estimable
Roy et al., 1991[a]	7/62	2/114	6.41 (95% CI, 1.38–30.0)
Statham et al., 1998[c]	365/1,538	0/1,199	>285
Roy et al., 1999[c]	10/26	0/9	>133
Total (7 studies)	401/1,704	2/1,486	174.8 (95% CI, 43.6–700.5)
Twin rates	23.5%	0.135%	175[d]
Family risk	Not applicable	8.98%[e]	2.62

Notes: The estimated risk (concordance) among DZ co-twins (0.135%) is 67 times lower than the average rate (8.98%) among the combined pool of first- and second-degree relatives in family studies summarized in Table 1 of Baldessarini and Hennen (2004), suggesting a more-plausible estimate of the MZ/DZ risk ratio of 2.62 (23.5%/8.98%; X^8 [1 df] = 276; p <.0001). Even with DZ and family rates pooled, the MZ/DZ risk ratio would be 23.5%/7.40%, or 3.18. For most studies, CIs are not provided because zero values appear in several numerators.

[a]Based on rate of suicides.
[b]Based on rate of suicides plus attempts.
[c]Based on rate of attempts only.
[d]Overall, Fisher's exact p <.0001 for the 7 studies.
[e]Based on raw data pooled from Table 1, column 3 (612/6811, or 8.98%), in Baldessarini and Hennen (2004).
CI = confidence interval; DZ = dizygotic; MZ = monozygotic.
Source: Baldessarini and Hennen, 2004. Reprinted from *Genetics of Suicide: An Overview* by Baldessarini and Hennen. Copyright 2004. Reproduced by permission of Taylor & Francis Group, LLC, http://www.taylorandfrancis.com.

studies have been undertaken, all of which used the same register of 5,483 adoptions in greater Copenhagen from 1924 to 1947 (Kety et al., 1968; Schulsinger et al., 1979; Wender et al.,1986). Pooling the data from these studies, Baldessarini and Hennen (2004) found that biological relatives of suicide cases are nearly five times more likely than adoptive relatives to commit suicide (risk ratio of 4.8) (Table 8–3).

What is being transmitted in the subjects of family, twin, and adoption studies? Is it the genes for a particular psychiatric disorder or some other factor (e.g., impulsivity, aggression) that may act independently of, or in an overlapping, additive, or catalytic manner with, a psychiatric disorder? For there to be overlap, some traits (and the genes underlying those traits) might be hypothesized to confer vulnerability to affective disorder as well as to suicidal behavior. Most of the research addressing the latter questions has not focused specifically on manic-depressive illness, however.

Several family studies have found that a higher risk of suicidal behavior holds true even after controlling for the effects of psychiatric disorders.[6] One of the largest and most recent studies was reported by Qin and colleagues (2002), who conducted a nested case-control study of 4,262 people who committed suicide between the ages of 9 and 45 during 1981–1997 and 80,238 population-based controls (matched for age, sex, and date of suicide). They found that a family history of suicide and psychiatric illness significantly and independently increased the suicide risk ratio by 2.58 and 1.31, respectively. This and the preceding studies are widely interpreted to suggest that there is an independent contributor to suicide risk beyond psychiatric illness.

In comprehensive reviews, Roy and colleagues (1999) and Mann (1998, 1999) and their colleagues proposed a stress–diathesis model of suicide in which an independent genetic/biologic factor predisposes to suicide risk only in

TABLE 8–3. **Summary of Adoption Studies of Suicide Risk**

Groups	REPORTED SUICIDE RATES IN RELATIVES		
	Biological	Adoptive	Risk Ratio (95% CI)
A. Kety et al., 1968[a]			
Suicides	5/156 (3.20%)	1/83 (1.20%)	2.67 (0.32–22.4)[b]
B. Schulsinger et al., 1979[c]			
Suicides	12/269 (4.46%)	0/148 (0.00%)	4.46[d]
C. Wender et al., 1986[e]			
Suicides + attempts	28/387 (7.24%)	8/180 (4.44%)	1.63 (0.76–3.50)
Suicides	15/387 (3.88%)	1/180 (0.56%)	6.93 (0.93–52.4)
Attempts	13/387 (3.36%)	7/180 (3.89%)	0.86 (0.32–2.13)
D. Pooled data from studies A and C	20/543 (3.68%)	2/263 (0.76%)	4.84 (1.14–20.6)

Notes: All three studies are based on a single Danish database. Study A data are for rates of suicides or attempts in biological or adoptive first-degree relatives of early-adopted probands who were diagnosed with schizophrenia-like disorders ($n = 33$), committed suicide ($n = 57$), or were diagnosed with an affective disorder (definite or probable DSM-III major depression or bipolar disorder; $n = 71$), compared with early-adopted controls matched for number, gender, socioeconomic class of adoptive parents, age at adoption, current age compared with proband age at suicide, and time living with biological mother. Study B data (involving suicidal adopted probands), although complementary to other analyses, are probably not independent and are therefore not included in D (pooled data from studies A and C).

[a]Schizophrenia-like probands.
[b]Fisher's exact $p = 0.0056$.
[c]Suicidal probands.
[d]CI is indeterminate because of zero numerator.
[e]Mood-disordered probands.
CI = Confidence interval.

Source: Baldessarini and Hennen, 2004. Reprinted from *Genetics of Suicide: An Overview* by Baldessarini and Hennen. Copyright 2004. Reproduced by permission of Taylor & Francis Group, LLC, http://www.taylorandfrancis.com.

association with psychiatric disorders or major life stressors. Psychiatric disorders and major life stressors, in other words, may trigger the genetic susceptibility to suicidal behavior.

Kety (1987) was among the first to hypothesize that a genetically influenced inability to control impulsive behavior might be a specific and independent susceptibility factor. Several family studies have lent support to the hypothesis that impulsive aggression, independently of psychiatric illness, increases suicide risk.[7] Impulsive aggression has been linked to low serotonin function (see reviews by Linnoila and Virkkunen, 1992; Oquendo and Mann, 2000), which is a biological marker of suicidal behavior (see later discussion).

Aggressiveness/impulsivity was one of a number of potential suicide risk factors studied by Oquendo and colleagues (2004). They tested the stress–diathesis model for suicidal behavior in a prospective investigation of 308 patients with major depressive or bipolar disorder. They found that the three strongest predictors of future suicidal acts were a history of suicide attempt(s), severe depression (according to subjective self-reports), and, for unknown reasons, cigarette smoking (although the National Comorbidity Survey—Replication [2001–2003] found no causal effect of smoking on suicidal behavior). Each of these factors posed an additive risk. The authors also determined that the tendency toward pessimism, as well as the presence of aggressive/impulsive traits, heightened future suicide risk in an additive manner. Swann and colleagues (2005) found that a history of severe suicidal behavior in 48 patients with bipolar disorder was associated with impulsivity, manifested as a tendency toward rapid, unplanned responses (as measured by impulsive errors on an immediate memory task and shorter response latencies).

Diathesis–stress models of suicide often assume that a predisposition to impulsive behavior provides the "diathesis" and the acute depressive or manic symptoms the "stress" that result in suicide.[8] However, there are virtually no longitudinal data on measures of impulsivity or aggression in bipolar disorder, and at the clinical level, rather than being invariant, impulsivity would be expected to be accentuated during manic and mixed states. Further, characterization of the essential deficit as being in the domain of impulsivity or aggressivity may be too narrow. An especially comprehensive neuropsychological study recently contrasted the profiles of medication-free depressed patients who had a history of a high-lethality suicide attempt, a low-lethality suicide attempt, or no suicide attempt with the profiles of healthy controls (Oquendo et al., 2003). The cognitive domains sampled included general intellectual functioning, motor functioning, attention, memory, and executive functioning. A discriminant analysis indicated that separate dimensions distinguished the total depressed sample from the healthy controls and the high-lethality attempters from the other patient groups. Impairment in attention and memory segregated the patients from controls, highlighting that a basic attentional disturbance may be a key factor in determining the cognitive sequelae of mood disorders, both unipolar and bipolar (see Chapter 9). Impaired executive function distinguished high-lethality attempters, with the executive function measures not restricted to indices of impulsivity. This work raised the possibility that a more broad-based deficit in executive function, perhaps related to self-monitoring functions, was disturbed in individuals with a history of a high-lethality suicide attempt.

In summary, there are strong genetic influences on suicidal behavior according to the findings of family, twin, and adoption studies. The findings of these studies also suggest that a family history of suicide and impulsivity/aggressiveness may increase the risk of suicide independently of transmission of psychiatric disorders. The possibility of independent risk factors should motivate clinicians, during their assessment of suicidal patients, to ask about family history of suicide, impulsivity, and aggression (see Chapter 25).

Neurobiological Factors

Serotonin Hypofunction

Many studies conducted over several decades have found an association between suicide and serotonin hypofunction. The first investigators to observe the association were Asberg and colleagues (1972), who found, in particularly violent suicide cases, low levels of 5-hydroxyindolacetic acid (5-HIAA)—the principal serotonin metabolite—in cerebrospinal fluid (CSF). A meta-analysis of 20 studies involving 1,002 psychiatric patients found that those with a history of attempted suicide, particularly violent attempts, had lower levels of 5-HIAA in CSF than did psychiatric controls (Lester, 1995). Lower serotonergic activity has

been localized to the prefrontal cortex in imaging studies of high-lethality suicide attempters (Oquendo et al., 2003). A recent prospective study of 27 bipolar depressed patients found that six subjects made suicide attempts during the 2-year follow-up period. These patients had higher aggression and hostility scores than the patients who did not make an attempt; CSF 5-HIAA, homovanillic acid (HVA), and MHPG levels were negatively correlated with the maximum lethality of the suicide attempts (Sher et al., 2006).

The robust finding of serotonin hypofunction, combined with the research discussed earlier pointing to genetic contributions to suicide, led to a search for candidate genes whose products control serotonin biosynthesis, degradation, or reuptake. Studies have sought to link higher prevalence of polymorphisms in serotonin-related genes to suicidal behavior.

Although serotonin hypofunction remains an important finding, studies of candidate genes have produced conflicting results and are beset by methodological problems (for reviews see Mann, 1998, 2002; Baldessarini and Hennen, 2004); moreover, few studies have focused specifically on bipolar patients. Consequently, a complete review of this subject is beyond the scope of this chapter. The recent studies highlighted here are illustrative of the complex range of findings regarding the enzyme tryptophan hydrolyase (TPH; the rate-limiting enzyme in serotonin synthesis), serotonin receptor subtypes, and the promoter region of the serotonin transporter. The serotonin transporter gene is responsible for reuptake of serotonin into the presynaptic neuron.

One explanation for finding low serotonin metabolites in individuals who have committed suicide is that less serotonin is being produced as a result of genetic defects affecting serotonin synthesis. Studying TPH, Turecki and colleagues (2001) found that one haplotype for the gene was significantly more prevalent among suicides involving violent methods than among living controls. Pooley and colleagues (2003) also found that a variation in the TPH gene was associated with deliberate self-harm. Other investigators, however, found no association between several TPH polymorphisms and suicidal behavior (Kunugi et al., 1999; Ono et al., 2000).

One of the earliest findings in autopsy studies was the higher number of serotonin 5-HT$_{1A}$ receptors, particularly in the prefrontal cortex, in suicide cases (Arango et al., 1995). Pandey and colleagues (2002) found an increase in another receptor subtype, the 5-HT$_{2A}$ receptor, in the prefrontal cortex and hippocampus of teenage suicide victims. In another study, one of the few with a distinct subgroup of bipolar patients, a polymorphism in the 5–HT$_{2A}$ receptor was found in this subgroup to be associated with a *lower* risk of suicidal behavior (Bonnier et al., 2002). On the other hand, Turecki and colleagues (2003), studying genes for seven serotonin receptor subtypes, found no differences in allelic or genotypic distributions. Schmauss (2003) found evidence of altered transcripts of the 5-HT2$_C$ gene in the brains of depressed suicide victims and hypothesized that the alteration reflects defects in regulation of ribonucleic acid (RNA) editing by synaptic serotonin.

The promoter region of the serotonin transporter gene has been found to be altered in several studies of suicidal behavior or violent suicides. Bondy and colleagues (2000) found increased frequency among suicide victims (with unknown diagnoses) of one or two short alleles of the serotonin transporter gene promoter (5-HTTLPR). The short allele, as compared with the long allele, has been linked to lower transcriptional efficacy (Lesch et al., 1996). In prior studies, the alleles were found to be associated with anxiety-related personality traits, affective disorders, or severe alcohol dependence. In a meta-analysis, Lin and Tsai (2004) also found a significant relationship between the short allele of 5-HTTLPR and suicidal behavior, especially violent suicide. But many studies have not found a relationship between the serotonin transporter polymorphism and completed suicide (Mann et al., 2000; Fitch et al., 2001) or suicide attempts (Geijer et al., 2000; Baca-Garcia et al., 2004) or in suicidal inpatients (Russ et al., 2000).

Two key studies sought to determine the predictive value of possessing the homozygous short (S/S) allele. Courtet and colleagues (2004) followed 133 patients hospitalized for a suicide attempt after first genotyping them for both A218C TPH and the functional S/L 5-HTTLPR polymorphism. Of the 76 patients they followed for 1 year, 20 reattempted suicide. The frequencies of the S or S/S allele were higher in those who had reattempted suicide, with elevated odds ratios (in comparison with the homozygous long [L/L] allele group) of 2.8 and 6.5, respectively. Impulsivity scores on the Baratt Impulsivity Scale (BIS) were significantly higher in patients carrying the S/S genotype than in those carrying the S/L genotype ($p = .026$). No differences were found in the TPH gene. The authors concluded that the SS genotype is a risk factor for future suicide attempts among those who have made a previous attempt.

A related study by Caspi and colleagues (2003) prospectively followed a cohort to test whether genetic vulnerability, as manifested by the short allele of 5-HTTLPR, would lead to depression or suicidality in individuals exposed to serious life stressors. Their hypothesis was supported by the finding that individuals with one or two copies of the short allele displayed, after exposure to stressful life events, more depressive symptoms, diagnosable depression, and suicidal ideation or attempts compared with individuals homozygous for the long allele. This study provides evidence of a gene–environment interaction, insofar as an individual's response to stressful life events is moderated by a particular aspect of his or her genetic makeup (in this case, the short allele of the promoter region of the serotonin transporter gene). It is noteworthy that the study found a relationship of genotype not only with depressive symptoms, but also with suicidal ideation or attempts.

While few studies of candidate genes have looked at possible gender differences, Baca-Garcia and colleagues (2003) published pilot data suggesting that females with the L/L allele are less likely to make suicide attempts than those with the S/S or S/L alleles. This protection may be lost, however, during life phases characterized by lower estradiol, such as menses or menopause.

The brain's serotonin system is highly complex. Although the findings of studies reviewed here point to genetic alterations in the serotonin system as having a relationship to suicidal behavior, the findings with respect to manic-depressive illness and suicide remain inconclusive.

Low Cholesterol

A number of studies have suggested a possible relationship between low cholesterol and impulsive aggression, including higher death rates from suicide. The link is hypothesized to occur through cholesterol's effect on serotonin activity (Mann, 1998). The findings of these studies, however, which include both large epidemiologic surveys and studies of suicidal individuals, have been mixed.[9] In some cases, an association was found only in violent suicide attempters (Alvarez et al., 2000). (See reviews by Boston et al., 1996; Hillbrand and Spitz, 1997.)

In those studies looking specifically at bipolar patients, the findings have again been mixed. Bocchetta and colleagues (2001) studied 783 consecutive patients admitted to a lithium clinic. They found that the proportion of men with a lifetime history of suicide attempts or a history of a suicide by a first-degree relative was significantly higher in the group with low cholesterol levels (in the lowest 25th percentile) than in those with higher levels. Cassidy and Carroll (2002a) found low fasting cholesterol in manic patients, particularly during mixed manic episodes, and hypothesized that this condition is secondary to immune activation. On the other hand, Tsai and colleagues (2002), studying 43 bipolar patients who died by suicide in Taiwan between 1985 and 1996, found no difference in cholesterol levels compared with controls, who were bipolar patients still living.

In summary, if there is a relationship between low cholesterol and suicide, it is likely to apply to violent suicide attempts and completed suicides. However, lowering cholesterol with statin medications does not appear to have increased suicide risk in the large samples studied (Manfredini et al., 2000; Muldoon et al., 2001), and it is unclear whether the association between low cholesterol and suicide risk will hold true in bipolar patients.

Hypothalamic–Pituitary–Adrenal Axis Hyperactivity

Hyperactivity of the hypothalamic–pituitary–adrenal (HPA) axis has long been hypothesized as a biochemical marker of suicide. The HPA axis is the preeminent modulator of the relationship between acute stress exposure and physiological activation. In studies dating back to the 1960s, researchers observed that, within days before suicide, patients with major affective disorders had elevated levels of urinary 17-hydroxycorticosteroid and serum cortisol.[10] Not all studies of suicide found these elevations, however (Levy and Hansen, 1969).

In a related finding, individuals who died from suicide had enlarged adrenal glands compared with controls who died from accidents (Dorovini-Zis and Zis, 1987; Szigethy et al., 1994). Findings of increased levels of corticotropin-releasing factor (CRF) in the CSF of suicide victims (Arato et al., 1989; Brunner and Bronisch, 1999), as well as evidence of downregulation of CRF receptors in the frontal cortex (Nemeroff et al., 1988), suggested increased CRF release prior to suicide. Hucks and colleagues (1997) found no decrease in CRF receptors, even when they compared those taking and not taking antidepressants before suicide. More recently, Hiroi and colleagues (2001) found a shift in the ratio of corticotropin-releasing hormone receptor 1 (CRH-R1) to corticotropin-releasing hormone receptor 2 (CRH-R2) in the pituitary gland of suicide victims.

Another measure of HPA hyperactivity studied in relation to suicide is the dexamethasone suppression test (DST), which shows a failure of exogenous dexamethasone to suppress levels of cortisol secreted by the adrenal glands. Most studies have found a relationship between DST nonsuppression and suicide completion, but the relationship to suicide attempts is not as strong.

Studying 65 patients with major depression, Brown and colleagues (1986) found no relationship between DST nonsuppression and suicide attempts. In contrast, Coryell (1990) observed that 76 depressed inpatients who were nonsuppressors at inpatient admission were more likely over a 5-year follow-up period to develop mania or hypomania and to make serious suicide attempts. Studying depressed inpatients, Norman and colleagues (1990) matched 13 patients who had committed suicide with depressed inpatients who had made suicide attempts before admission ($n = 25$) and those who had not made attempts ($n = 28$). More than half of the patients committing suicide were nonsuppressors, compared with lower proportions of

suicide attempters and nonattempters. Likewise, a meta-analysis found that DST nonsuppression was predictive of completed suicide (Lester, 1992).

Findings of a more recent study strengthened the relationship between nonsuppression and completed suicide. Coryell and Schlesser (2001) found that nearly half of 78 inpatients with affective disorders were DST nonsuppressors at admission. After being followed for 15 years, 26.8 percent of nonsuppressors eventually died by suicide, compared with only 2.9 percent of DST suppressors. Within this sample, a comparatively small number of bipolar patients had received a DST because most had been admitted in a manic state, which made cooperation in taking the DST more difficult. Data from studies of abused children and patients with post-traumatic stress disorder also suggest that these overwhelming stressors can persistently alter the responses of the HPA axis (Heim and Nemeroff, 1999, 2002).

Norepinephrine Function

Several studies have identified alterations in norepinephrine transmission in relation to suicide. Ordway (1997) and others (Arango et al., 1997; Gonzalez-Maeso et al., 2002) found reductions in norepinephrine levels in the locus caeruleus (LC) of suicide victims, as well as increased levels of tyrosine hydroxylase and supersensitivity of alpha-2 adrenoceptors. Ordway characterized the changes he found in suicide victims as being similar to those found in rats after LC activation. He hypothesized that suicide victims experience chronic activation of the LC, leading to depletion of norepinephrine and other compensatory changes. Recently, Ono and colleagues (2004) found evidence suggesting that a Val/Val polymorphism for the catecholamine-metabolizing enzyme, catechol-O-methyltransferase, may be protective against suicide.

Psychological Traits and Temperament

A passive sense of hopelessness is a chronic risk factor for suicide. This conclusion is supported by the findings of a 20-year prospective study (Beck et al., 1999; Brown et al., 2000); another large-scale prospective investigation, the National Institute of Mental Health's (NIMH) Collaborative Program on the Psychobiology of Depression-Clinical Studies, which studied 954 patients with affective disorders, including more than 300 with bipolar illness (Fawcett et al., 1990); and a meta-analysis of case-control, cohort, and cross-sectional investigations of attempted suicides (23 studies) or completed suicides (13 studies) in bipolar patients (Hawton et al., 2005). While hopelessness has generally been conceptualized as a symptom specific to depression, the NIMH study found baseline hopelessness to be trait-like (Young et al., 1996). The study also found that baseline hopelessness predicted a suicide attempt. In the 20-year prospective study, researchers found that severity of suicidal ideation at its worst point is predictive of suicide. The patients who scored in the high-severity category on this measure were far more likely to ultimately kill themselves than those in the lower-severity group (odds ratio [OR] = 13.8) (Beck et al., 1999). We are unaware of any studies concerning familial transmission of hopelessness. Hostility, which in an acute way is often associated with mixed states, is also associated with increased rates of attempted and completed suicide (so, too, relatedly, are impulsivity and aggression) (Michaelis et al., 2004; Rutter and Behrendt, 2004; Galfalvy et al., 2006).

Certain temperaments, such as novelty seeking and harm avoidance, have been hypothesized to show familial or genetic transmission. Such temperaments may also be related to suicide risk. According to Cloninger and colleagues (1993, 2000), novelty seeking is related to impulsiveness, while harm avoidance tends to be related to anxiety and anhedonia. Studying 758 sibling pairs from 177 nuclear families of alcoholics, Cloninger and colleagues (1998) demonstrated significant heritability for proneness to anxiety and harm avoidance. Likewise, the capacity for pleasure in an individual may be trait-like and connected to temperament (Clark, 1991). A strong harm avoidance trait could be related to both vulnerability to anhedonia and comorbid anxiety disorders. Engstrom and colleagues (2003) measured personality characteristics of bipolar patients with the Temperament and Character Inventory (TCI) and found that patients with early-onset bipolar illness scored significantly higher on harm avoidance than those with late onset. Suicide attempts also were significantly more common among patients with early onset. Bondy and colleagues (2000), as noted earlier, observed that the presence of one or two short alleles of the serotonin transporter gene was associated with anxiety-related personality traits as well as affective disorder. Caspi and colleagues (2003) found that individuals with one or two copies of the short allele exhibited more diagnosable depression and suicidality in response to stressful life events. Their study yielded evidence of a gene–environment interaction, in which the individual's response to major life stresses is mediated by his or her genetic makeup. As more evidence becomes available, vulnerability to suicide may be manifest in detectable familial–genetic traits associated with other biological markers that are triggered by psychiatric illness and major life stresses.

Social Factors

The impact of social factors, such as losing an important relationship or a job or facing legal or criminal proceed-ings, can be devastating to anyone; this is particularly true, however, for those with a major psychiatric illness such as bipolar disorder. Although rarely sufficient by themselves to cause suicide, social stressors can precipitate or determine the timing of the act. In this way, they act as risk factors that increase the likelihood of suicide. They may trigger suicide in individuals with certain biological vulnerabilities and psychological traits (e.g., Caspi et al., 2003, discussed earlier), but most studies have not teased apart their precise role in manic-depressive illness. Social stressors may also precipitate sleeplessness; this, in turn, has been shown in bipolar patients to increase the risk of an affective relapse.

Social factors not only can increase risk, but also may buffer individuals from suicide. For example, supportive families and friends and religious beliefs may, to a point, deter suicide by acting as protective factors (IOM, 2002). Religious beliefs and devotion—as opposed to practice and affiliation—have been shown to be protective for African-American women (Neeleman et al., 1998; Greening and Stoppelbein, 2002; Kaslow et al., 2004), the ethnic group with the lowest suicide rate in the United States (Kaslow, 2000). The potentially protective role of religious belief and practice has not been studied in relation to individuals with bipolar illness, however.

Social and cultural factors also shape an individual's willingness to seek help, styles of coping with adversity, and social support structures. On a societal level, social and cultural factors influence laws, regulations, and health policies that dictate the availability of resources for treatment and prevention (U.S. Department of Health and Human Services, 2000; IOM, 2002). Indeed, awareness of the potency of cultural and social factors prompted the U.S. Surgeon General, Dr. David Satcher, to mobilize clinicians, public health professionals, communities, families, and the media as part of a comprehensive strategy for suicide prevention (U.S. Public Health Service, 1999).

CLINICAL CORRELATES OF SUICIDE

In this section, we review research findings on correlations between suicide and various features of bipolar disorder: mixed states, depression, rapid cycling, and severe anxiety or agitation. We then examine suicide in bipolar disorder in relation to comorbid personality disorders, substance abuse, psychosis, and course of illness.

History of Suicide Attempts

There is an extensive literature documenting the strong correlation between a history of suicide attempts and subsequent completed suicide (see, for example, Nordstrom et al., 1995a,b; Tsai et al., 2002; Joiner et al., 2005). Harris and

Barraclough, in their extensive meta-analysis, found that a suicide attempt created a 37-fold risk for completed suicide; several large prospective studies also demonstrated a substantial increased risk for suicide in those who had previously attempted it (Jawcett et all., 1990; Marangell et al., 2006). In their meta-analysis of 13 studies of completed suicide and 23 studies of attempted suicide, Hawton and colleagues (2005) found that past suicide attempts were the factor most predictive of future suicidal behavior. In the Finnish Jorvi Bipolar Study, 191 bipolar patients were followed for 18 months, during which time 20 percent attempted suicide (Valtonen et al., 2006). Baseline previous suicide attempts were the most significant predictor (odds ratio [OR] = 3.8; 95 percent confidence interval [CI] = 1.7–8.8; p = 0.001) of a subsequent attempt.

During a 2-year follow-up period, 12 of 64 bipolar patients studied at Columbia University made at least one suicide attempt. All attempters had a history of past suicide attempts; none of the previously nonattempters made an attempt (Galfalvy et al., 2006).

Mixed States

Mixed states are a significant risk factor for suicide. Among the first to study the relationship between agitated, dysphoric states and suicide was Jameison (1936), who concluded that mixed states were the most dangerous clinical phase of illness for suicide risk.[11] In his investigation of 100 suicides (half with manic-depressive psychosis), he noted that the combination of depressive symptoms, mental alertness, and tense, apprehensive, and restless behavior was particularly lethal. Mixed states represent a potentially deadly combination of depressive affect and cognition, linked to dysphoric state, heightened energy level, and increased impulsiveness. Jameison's clinical account of mixed states and their association with suicide remains apt, as does his observation that those patients who were both tense and restless were at the greatest risk for suicide:

> Finally there are the patients with mixed manic-depressive states. The majority of these show the usual depression, numerous self-accusations, ideas of guilt and punishment and a varying degree of hypochondriasis. At the same time there is a mental alertness, associated with tense, apprehensive and restless behavior. The retardation of thought and action that paralyzes the acting out of the wish for death in the average depressed patient is entirely absent in these persons. They are, therefore, the most dangerous types of patients with mental disease, so far as suicide is concerned. The records of the fifteen patients in the group emphasize this strikingly. Three of these patients committed suicide twenty-four hours after leaving the hospital, two within forty-eight hours, another

within a week and still another within two weeks. The patient who was longest outside the hospital lived two months, and the average period for this group was fifteen days! (Jameison, 1936, p. 4)

Winokur and colleagues (1969) found that suicidal thoughts or attempts occurred in 13 percent of depressive episodes following mania and in a strikingly high proportion of mixed states (43 percent), although the latter finding applied only to women. Kotin and Goodwin (1972) also described the coexistence of suicidal behavior and mixed states, as did Kraepelin (1921) in his original clinical monograph.

In a series of studies, Dilsaver and colleagues (1994, 1997; Dilsaver and Chen, 2003) found that, compared with patients with pure mania, patients with depressive mania had significantly higher rates of suicidality. Suicidality was defined as a severity level of 3 to 7 on the suicide subscale of the SADS, which ranges from mild suicidality (frequent ideation, but without a specific method or plan) to suicide attempts. More recently, Dilsaver and colleagues (2005) studied suicidality in adolescents and determined that mixed states increased the probability of attempting suicide for girls only, in whom the increased risk was four-fold. In a study of 100 bipolar-I manic patients, Goldberg and colleagues (1998, 1999) found a significant relationship between dysphoric mania and suicidal ideation. They also noted that multiple suicide attempts were associated with nonremission of mixed mania. Sato and colleagues (2004), using the criteria for dysphoric mania developed by McElroy and colleagues (1992, 1995) and Strakowski and colleagues (1996), studied 576 patients hospitalized with acute mania. They found that mixed mania was strongly associated with suicidality.

Depression

It has long been known that depression is strongly correlated with suicide and suicide attempts (Jameison and Wall, 1933; Barraclough et al., 1974; Weeke, 1979). More recent findings strengthen the early clinical observations. Isometsa and colleagues (1994) studied a sample of 31 bipolar patients who committed suicide in Finland within a 12-month period, 74 percent of whom had been receiving psychiatric care at the time of their suicide. Among these patients, 79 percent were depressed at the time of death, 11 percent were in a mixed state, and 11 percent died during or immediately after remission of psychotic mania. Dilsaver and colleagues (1997) found bipolar depression to have been associated with suicidality somewhat more frequently than were mixed states, although both conditions were associated with greater suicidality than was pure mania. Grunebaum and colleagues (2004) compared suicide attempts among 347 patients with melancholic versus nonmelancholic major depression. They found that melancholic features during depression were correlated with more serious past attempts and the probability of suicide at follow-up.

The severity of depression is a factor as well (Arato et al., 1988; Henriksson et al., 1993; Isometsä et al., 1994). Swedish researchers psychiatrically assessed an entire rural population and then kept track of its mental health for the next 15 to 25 years (Hagnell et al., 1981). Virtually all of the men who committed suicide during the follow-up period had been diagnosed during their initial evaluations as having depressive illness. The suicide rate for men with no psychiatric diagnosis at all was 8.3 per 100,000, but for those with depression it escalated to 650. No one with mild depression committed suicide, but the rate rose to 220 per 100,000 for those who had been diagnosed with moderate depression and to 3,900 per 100,000 for those with severe depressive illnesses.

Weeke (1979) found that at the time of death, 58 percent of manic-depressive patients who committed suicide had been in a constant or worsening depressive state. Fully 30 percent of the patients, however, had been classified as "depressive state, recovering." Keith-Spiegel and Spiegel (1967) compared the clinician-rated mood states of 61 psychiatric patients immediately preceding their suicides with those of 51 matched control patients of comparable age and diagnoses who had not committed suicide or had no history of a suicide attempt. Those who killed themselves had histories of more frequent and more severe depressions, as well as more suicide attempts, threats, and suicidal ideation. Of particular significance, however, was that just before death, those who committed suicide had been assessed by their clinician as being calmer and in better spirits than members of the control group. An apparently unwarranted mood shift had been observed in those who killed themselves.

These findings add weight to the clinical observation, dating back hundreds of years, that improvement in depression is associated with an increased risk for suicide.[12] Several factors may account for this counterintuitive observation. The improvement may reflect a sense of calm once the decision has been made to die, a genuine calm before the storm brought about by biological changes, or a transition from one phase of the illness to another (e.g., from depression to hypomania, mania, or a mixed state). It also may reflect true clinical improvement, with a concomitant level of frustration when symptoms recur. In some instances, an improved clinical state enables a previously indecisive and lethargic patient to become more able to make an unambivalently lethal decision and to act on that decision. Finally, "improvement" may in fact be a patient's deliberate deception of physicians, hospital staff, and family so a suicide plan can be carried out. Problems

in assessing clinical improvement were described decades ago by Jameison (1936, p. 4):

> It is only when the depression is lifting, often some weeks before the morbid and self-accusatory ideas have disappeared, that the possibility of suicide is less remote. Unfortunately, at this time a tendency to project the inner distress on the environment leads to complaints and pleadings, so that relatives, noting the improvement, agree with the patient that the hospital restrictions are prolonging the illness. The patient is then removed at a time when he is potentially more suicidal than at any time before.

Rapid Cycling

Rapid cycling increases the risk of suicide and suicidal behavior. One of the first large studies to examine the relationship between suicide and rapid cycling was NIMH's Collaborative Study on the Psychobiology of Depression-Clinical Studies (Fawcett et al., 1987). Of the study's 954 patients, 569 had unipolar depression,[13] 185 had bipolar-I, 114 had bipolar-II, and the remaining 80 had schizoaffective disorder. The incidence of suicide over the 4-year study period was 3 percent. The rate did not differ by diagnosis. What did distinguish patients who died by suicide from those who did not was mood cycling during the index episode ($p < .002$). Mood cycling in this study meant that the patient had been admitted in one mood state, such as mania, and cycled into the other before recovery. While this is not synonymous with the classic definition of rapid cycling (i.e., four or more affective episodes in 1 year), there is overlap between the two groups. The authors of the study concluded that mood cycling, which is a feature of bipolar or schizoaffective disorder, is associated with suicide, particularly in men.

In a 5-year prospective study of 345 patients with bipolar-I or -II disorder, 89 patients were identified, using DSM-IV criteria, as having a pattern of rapid cycling for 1 year or more (Table 8–4; Coryell et al., 2003). The rapid-cycling patients were significantly more likely than the rest of the patients to have had onset of illness before age 17 and were twice as likely to attempt, but not to complete, suicide.[14] The differences between the groups were most pronounced for attempts rated as being of high lethality.

Brodersen and colleagues (2000) conducted a 16-year follow-up study of 133 patients with major affective disorders (defined as having two to three affective episodes in a 5-year period) treated with lithium. Most of the 11 suicides occurred among the "atypical" patients (those with schizoaffective disorder, bipolar-II disorder, mixed episodes, and/or rapid cycling). MacKinnon and colleagues (2005), in a study of 1,574 family members with bipolar disorder, also found that a history of rapid mood switching was

TABLE 8–4. **Relationship between Rapid Cycling, Suicide, and Suicide Attempts before Intake and during Follow-Up**

	Any Rapid Cycling ($n=89$)	No Rapid Cycling ($n=256$)
Before Intake, No. (%)		
Any attempt	51 (57.3)[a]	85 (33.2)
Any attempt of high intent	31 (34.8)[a]	38 (14.8)
Any attempt of high lethality	36 (40.4)[a]	35 (13.7)
After Intake, No. (%)		
Completed suicide	3 (3.4)	11 (4.3)
Any attempt	46 (51.7)[a]	70 (27.3)
Any attempt of high intent	27 (30.3)[a]	33 (12.9)
Any attempt of high lethality	30 (33.7)[a]	36 (14.1)

[a]Significant differences by chi square, $p < .001$.

associated with increased suicidality. Two other studies found trends for suicidal behavior and rapid cycling (Bauer et al., 1994; Maj et al., 1994). On the other hand, using retrospective chart reviews of 100 rapid-cycling and 120 non-rapid-cycling outpatients, Wu and Dunner (1993) found no association between suicide attempts and rapid cycling. Still, most studies have found that rapid cycling increases the risk of suicide and suicidal behaviors.

Anxiety and Agitation

Studies have shown high rates of comorbid anxiety disorder in bipolar patients, often reaching at least 40 percent (McElroy et al., 2001; Simon et al., 2004). The high incidence of comorbid anxiety disorders in both bipolar-I and bipolar-II patients calls for special attention to severe symptoms of anxiety in the assessment and management of suicide risk in bipolar patients (see Chapter 25).

Anxiety figured prominently in a major study of time-related risk factors for suicide. In their prospective study of 955 bipolar and unipolar patients, Fawcett and colleagues (1990) delineated a cluster of risk factors that were better predictors of suicide over the short term (acute risk factors) and others that were better over the long term (chronic risk factors). They found that anxiety symptoms were predictive both acutely (within 1 year of study entry) and chronically (after the first year of study entry). Among the 14 patients who committed suicide within 1 year of assessment, suicide was related to symptoms of severe psychic anxiety, panic attacks, anhedonia, and moderate alcohol abuse; the abuse of alcohol with another drug was a significant risk factor, especially in males (see later discussion). No difference was found between bipolar and unipolar depressed patients with regard to severe psychic anxiety, panic attacks, and suicide. Over the next 4 years, another 13 patients killed themselves. These later suicides were most commonly associated with severe hopelessness, somatic anxiety, suicidal ideation, and a history of one or more suicide attempts. These findings underscore the importance of assessing patients in terms of acute versus long-term suicide risk (see Chapter 25).

The identification of time-related factors helps address the difficult problem of predicting a relatively infrequent behavior in the midst of subtle and fluctuating mood states. This point is illustrated by the predictive role of past suicide attempts. While attempts carry a high chronic risk for suicide—with an SMR of 37, according to Harris and Barraclough (1997)—they do not confer a significant acute risk.

Numerous other studies underscore the role of comorbid anxiety/agitation in relation to suicide. Among a sample of 209 outpatients who had attempted suicide or been identified as being at high risk for continued suicidal behavior or eventual suicide, Rudd and colleagues (1993) noted a statistically significant incidence of comorbid panic disorder and post-traumatic stress disorder among suicidal bipolar patients. Likewise, MacKinnon and colleagues (2005) found that comorbid panic disorder increased the risk of suicidality in individuals with bipolar disorder. Among patients with major depression, Reich (1998) found that suicide attempts were correlated with higher levels of comorbid anxiety. Hall and colleagues (1999) found that severe anxiety was present in 90 percent and panic attacks in 80 percent of suicide attempters. Schnyder and colleagues (1999) reported similar findings showing the presence of severe anxiety in a study of 30 consecutive emergency room suicide attempters who were later admitted to a psychiatric inpatient unit (diagnoses not specified in the study). Likewise, Angst and colleagues (1998) found the presence of anxiety to be a suicide risk factor in a 5-year follow-up sample of 186 patients with unipolar and 220 patients with bipolar depression. And in an analysis of 76 inpatient suicides, Busch and colleagues (2003) found that 79 percent of patients had chart notes indicating severe anxiety/agitation within 1 week of their suicide.

One study attempted to ascertain what features of bipolar illness, including panic disorder, are related to suicidality. Dilsaver and colleagues (1997) divided their sample of 125 bipolar patients into three groups—those with bipolar depression, those with depressive mania, and those with pure mania. They examined the incidence of suicidality (rated using the SADS), psychosis, and intra-episode panic disorder (IEPD). IEPD was highly prevalent in the bipolar depression (79 percent) and depressive mania groups (56 percent) but rare (2.3 percent) in the pure mania group. Overall, the findings suggest a high degree of overlap among suicidality, IEPD, and bipolar depression or depressive mania, as opposed to pure mania.

Taken together, these studies argue for the assessment of severe anxiety or agitation and for aggressive anxiolytic treatment in the management of suicide risk in affective disorders (see Chapter 25).

Insomnia and excessive concern about sleep disturbances have been noted as correlates of increased potential for suicide,[15] as has pervasive hopelessness (see earlier discussion). The body of evidence has led to widespread acceptance that insomnia and hopelessness are risk factors for suicide. Global insomnia is considered an acute risk factor because it was found, in a prospective study, to be associated with suicide within the first year of study entry (Fawcett et al., 1990).

Comorbidity and Axis II Disorders

Suicide among individuals with comorbid psychiatric conditions is so prevalent that it is the norm rather than the exception. This point is best illustrated by a population-based study from Finland, which found that a small fraction—only 12 percent—of all 229 suicide victims had only one Axis I diagnosis with no comorbidity (Henriksson et al., 1993). Comorbid conditions and certain behavioral states dramatically increase the risk of suicide. Most of the studies reviewed here, however, did not study bipolar disorder separately. This may be an important limitation on the conclusions that can be drawn about the role of comorbid conditions in suicide among bipolar patients.

In a psychological autopsy study of 117 suicides, Foster and colleagues (1999) found that, in comparison with deceased community controls without a mental disorder, the risks were extraordinarily high for two groups of patients: those with comorbidity (an Axis I and Axis II disorder; OR = 346.0) and those with a single Axis I disorder (OR = 52.4). Kim and colleagues (2003), studying the records of 115 male suicides, found that the most common comorbidities in suicide completers were depressive disorders plus cluster B disorders[16] and substance dependence plus cluster B disorders (27.8 percent). In this study, those who committed suicide, compared with controls, were 22 times more likely to have three or more diagnoses (OR = 22.38, $p < .0000001$). Heikkinen and colleagues (1997) compared 56 suicides who had both Axis I disorders (most commonly major depression) and comorbid personality disorders with an equal number who had no comorbidity. The patients with personality disorders, cluster B type, had experienced multiple life events preceding their suicide compared with the noncomorbid patients who had died by suicide. It appears clear from these studies that comorbidity of Axis I and Axis II disorders strikingly increases the risk of suicide.

Substance Abuse

Comorbid substance abuse is another risk factor for suicide in both bipolar and unipolar patients, particularly in the young (Fawcett et al., 1987; Murphy, 1988). In their large, prospective study, Fawcett and colleagues (1987) found a significant increase in long-term risk with so-called "double abuse" (alcohol plus any other abused substance). They also found recent, moderate alcohol abuse to be a short-term (acute) risk factor (see Chapter 25).

Like Fawcett and colleagues, others have noted an association between alcohol abuse and suicide. Barraclough and colleagues (1974) found that as the number of suicide attempts increased, so did the chances that the attempter was alcohol dependent. In a study of 204 suicides, Rich and colleagues (1988) noted substance abuse and affective disorders to be the most frequent diagnoses for men and women. Morrison (1975) found that bipolar patients who were also alcohol dependent had a higher rate of suicide in their family histories than did nondependent bipolar patients. In a study of suicide among adolescents and young adults, Runeson (1989) observed a 47 percent rate of co-morbid substance abuse with any Axis I or II diagnoses. Depressive disorders were diagnosed in 64 percent of those who committed suicide (major depressive disorder = 41 percent).

Tondo and colleagues (1999) found an association between substance abuse disorders and suicide attempts in hospitalized patients, with substance abuse raising the suicide risk more than two-fold regardless of the disorder. In a study of 307 male veterans, Waller and colleagues (1999) noted that comorbidity of alcohol abuse and bipolar-I or unipolar depressive disorder was always associated with an increased risk of suicidality.

Pini and colleagues (1999) found that among 125 bipolar patients with psychotic features, the subgroup having substance abuse associated with other Axis I comorbidities had an earlier age at onset of their bipolar disorder, more frequent onset with a mixed state, and a higher risk of suicide. Oquendo and Mann (2001) observed that bipolar patients who attempted suicide had higher levels of aggression and comorbid substance abuse than nonattempters. Vieta and colleagues (2000) noted that among 40 patients with bipolar-II disorder, 21 percent had substance abuse comorbidity, and this group had significantly higher rates of suicidal ideation and attempts. Vieta and colleagues (2001) studied 129 bipolar outpatients in remission, finding comorbidity in 31 percent; these patients also had higher rates of mixed states, depressive episodes, and suicide attempts. Cornelius and colleagues (1995) found that suicidality was disproportionately higher among patients with comorbid depression and substance abuse than among those with either disorder alone.

The connection between suicide and substance abuse may be attributable to increased impulsivity or aggressiveness, impaired sleep, or destabilization of illness. As we have seen, low levels of the serotonin metabolite 5-HIAA are correlated with aggression and impulsivity, and it has been shown that patients making the most violent and impulsive suicide attempts have low 5-HIAA levels (see also Chapter 14). It is of interest that Rosenthal and colleagues (1980) found significantly lower levels of 5-HIAA among depressed patients with a family history of alcoholism than among those without such a family history. Low 5-HIAA levels also have been found in alcoholics after recovery (Ballenger et al., 1979; Linnoila and Virkkunen, 1992; Virkkunen and Linnoila, 1993). Therefore, not only do substance abusers have impaired judgment and decreased inhibition from the drugs themselves, but they may also bear a biological risk for suicide. Bipolar patients who are impulsive or more temperamentally prone to agitated states may be more inclined to use alcohol and other drugs than those who are not. Swann and colleagues (2004)

compared scores on a measure of impulsiveness (the BIS) in interepisode bipolar patients with and without substance abuse. Trait impulsivity was increased in interepisode bipolar disorder only in the case of current substance abuse.

Psychosis

The relationship between psychosis and suicide in mood disorders is unclear. An early, often-cited retrospective analysis of patients with unipolar depression hospitalized at the New York State Psychiatric Institute between 1955 and 1980 found an unusually high rate of delusions among those who committed suicide (Roose et al., 1983). Bipolar patients were not considered separately in this study, but the findings were suggestive of symptom patterns associated with a high risk of suicide. The authors noted that depressed inpatients who were delusional were five times more likely than those who were nondelusional to commit suicide, and that delusional males were particularly vulnerable. Two recent studies found that bipolar children and adolescents with a history of psychotic features were more likely to be suicidal than those who did not have such a history (Papolos et al., 2005; Caetano et al., 2006). The recent study from the Juvenile Bipolar Research Foundation (Papolos et al., 2005) also found that bipolar children and adolescents who threatened to commit suicide were far more likely to report having hallucinations than those who did not threaten suicide.

On the other hand, several studies suggest no such relationship. A study of 1,593 affectively ill patients revealed no increased risk of suicide among the 27.8 percent who had been psychotic at the time of their index hospitalization (Black et al., 1988). Likewise, Fawcett and colleagues (1987) found that psychotic patients diagnosed with affective illness did not have higher prospective rates of suicide over a 10-year follow-up. Dilsaver and colleagues (1997) found no association between the presence of psychosis and mild suicidality; a subsequent study found no association between psychotic features and suicidality in adolescents (Dilsaver et al., 2005). Similarly, Coryell and Tsuang (1982) and Frangos and colleagues (1983) found no increased risk of suicide in patients with delusional depression.

Course of Illness

There is consistent evidence of an increased risk of suicide and suicide attempts early in or just after the first episode of affective illness,[17] as well as in bipolar disorder more specifically. Among the first to study the time course of suicide attempts in bipolar patients were Johnson and Hunt (1979). They found in their very small sample that 30 percent of suicide attempts (90 percent of which warranted hospitalization) occurred at the onset of the illness or

TABLE 8–5. Suicide in Bipolar Patients with a Hospital Diagnosis of Bipolar Disorder (N = 15,386) in Sweden, 1973–1995

| Age | STANDARDIZED MORTALITY RATIO | |
	Males	Females
All ages	15.0	22.4
<30 yr[a]	81.6	71.7

[a]Age at first admission and in the first year of follow-up.
Source: Reprinted with permission from Osby et al., 2001. Copyright, American Medical Association. All rights reserved.

during the first episode of depression. Half of the serious suicide attempts occurred within 5 years of the onset of illness. In a related finding, Balazs and colleagues (2003), studying 100 suicide attempters in Hungary, observed that 60 percent were experiencing their first depressive episode. (Of this group, 35 percent had had mania or hypomania symptoms in the past.) In the largest study, Osby and colleagues (2001) documented suicide rates among all hospitalized patients in Sweden from 1973 to 1995, including more than 15,000 with bipolar disorder. The SMR was found to be especially high in patients whose age at first admission was less than 30 (81.6 for males and 71.7 for females) (Table 8–5).

Recent discharge from a hospital also carries a higher risk (Geddes and Juszczak, 1995, 1997; Appleby et al., 1999). A study was conducted of all suicides (N = 481) among discharged patients who had been receiving care in 128 Veterans Affairs hospitals in the United States from 1994 to 1998 (Desai et al., 2005). The patients had been diagnosed as having depression, bipolar disorder, schizophrenia, or post-traumatic stress disorder. The study found suicide deaths to be concentrated in the first 6 months after discharge, with almost 50 percent occurring within 3 months after discharge. Bipolar and unipolar rates were similarly high. A comprehensive investigation of all suicides committed in Denmark from January 1, 1981, to December 31, 1997 (N = 21,169) found that there were two sharp peaks of risk for suicide in relation to psychiatric hospitalization (Qin and Nordentoft, 2005). The highest peak, which was strikingly elevated in those patients with affective illness, was in the week immediately following discharge from the hospital. The second peak was in the week following admission to the hospital. Suicide was substantially more likely in patients who had shorter hospitalizations.

Several studies have examined suicide risk in relation to age at onset. Perlis and colleagues (2004) studied 983 subjects diagnosed with bipolar disorder on entry into the multicenter Systematic Treatment Enhancement Program for Bipolar Disorder (STEP-BD). For patients whose age at onset could be determined, the authors found that earlier onset of illness was associated with a greater likelihood of suicide attempts (Table 8–6). Based on multiple regression, the risk of making at least one suicide attempt was 2.85 times greater for those diagnosed with very early onset (before age 13) relative to those diagnosed after age 18. Early onset (ages 13 to 18) was also associated with higher rates of comorbid anxiety disorders and substance abuse, themselves risk factors for suicide (see earlier discussion). Grunebaum and colleagues (2006) found that suicide attempts in 96 patients with bipolar illness correlated with an earlier age at onset.

Engstrom and colleagues (2003) studied patients with bipolar-I and -II disorders and reported that in early-onset patients, treatment response was significantly lower (p = .005), and suicide attempts were more common

TABLE 8–6. Comorbid Conditions and Suicide Attempts in Bipolar Disorder by Age at Onset (percent)

	Onset Age <13 yr (n = 272)	Onset Age 13–18 yr (n = 370)	Onset Age >18 yr (n = 341)	Wald X^2 (2 df)	p Value
Suicide attempts[a]	49.8	37.0	24.6	32.58	<.0001[b,c,d]
Any anxiety disorder	69.2	53.9	38.3	48.87	<.0001[b,c,d]
Alcohol abuse/dependence	47.3	46.6	31.9	15.89	.0004[b,c]
Drug abuse and dependence	34.2	33.4	15.1	40.86	<.0001[b,c]

[a]These were past suicide attempts reported at study entry.
[b]p <.05 for pairwise comparison of prepubertal and adult-onset groups.
[c]p <.05 for pairwise comparison of adolescent and adult-onset groups.
[d]p <.05 for pairwise comparison of prepubertal and adolescent-onset groups.
Source: Adapted from Perlis et al., 2004, with permission from the Society of Biological Psychiatry.

(p=.001). Leverich and colleagues (2002, 2003) showed that a history of childhood sexual or physical abuse was associated with earlier age at onset; increased Axis I, II, and III comorbid disorders; more rapid cycling; and a higher rate and greater severity of suicide attempts (see Chapter 6). Similarly, Goldberg and Ernst (2004) found that a history of poor adjustment in childhood and adolescence was associated with both substance abuse and dependence and increased suicide attempts in adult patients with bipolar disorder.

The course of affective illness may have different effects on men and women. Johnson and Hunt (1979), in a very small but intriguing study, found that more men than women attempted suicide at the onset of manic-depressive illness (42 versus 17 percent), but that this gender difference later disappeared. Attempts by women were distributed more evenly across time. Although all attempts by women occurred within approximately 15 years after the onset of illness, those by men were distributed more extremely and bimodally: 60 percent of men who attempted suicide did so within 2 years after the onset of illness, and the other 40 percent 23 years or more after onset.

These findings underscore the importance of early recognition of bipolar disorder, accurate diagnosis, and aggressive treatment. They also highlight the need for ongoing reappraisal of suicidal risk (see Chapter 25).

CONCLUSIONS

Suicide is still far too common in manic-depressive illness. Patients diagnosed today face a lifetime suicide risk of at least 5 percent. While this figure is lower than in previous eras—a result in part of better treatments and in part of the inclusion of less severely ill patients in outcome studies—several groups of patients continue to bear a disproportionately high risk burden, including those who are hospitalized or recently discharged and those who are untreated, inadequately treated, or treatment resistant. Further, the suicide rate remains strikingly high early in the course of illness.

The precise causes of suicide remain elusive, although they most certainly entail an interaction between the underlying affective illness and additional biological and psychosocial risk factors. But research has not yet found any particular combination of risk factors to be sensitive or sufficient enough to predict a suicide. Salient risk factors include rapid cycling, mixed states, and severe depressive episodes. A significant advance has come with the identification of which of many risk factors operate in the short term (e.g., agitation, severe hopelessness, global insomnia) versus the long term (e.g., past suicide attempt, various comorbidities). Risk factors and their identification,

moreover, while far from perfect predictors of suicide, can serve as guideposts for clinicians confronting a complex clinical picture of an illness that encompasses the extremes of human emotions.

NOTES

1. National statistics tend to underestimate suicide deaths because of the difficulty of establishing suicidal intent in single-car accidents and other "accidental" deaths and because of cultural, financial, and religious disincentives to label a death as a suicide.
2. For example, Fawcett et al., 1987, 1990; Black et al., 1988; Angst et al., 1999.
3. Wetterberg et al., 1978; Carlsson et al., 1979; Oddie et al., 1979; Perez et al., 1980; Aschoff, 1981; Behall et al., 1984; Losonczy et al., 1984; Gordon et al., 1987; Lacoste and Wirz-Justice, 1989; Sarrias et al., 1989; Souêtre et al., 1989; Modai et al., 1992; Maes et al., 1995; Pine et al., 1995; Verkes et al., 1996; Zajicek et al., 2000.
4. Mann et al., 1992; D'Hondt et al., 1994; Maes et al., 1995; Pine et al., 1995.
5. Pokorny, 1983, 1991; Goldstein et al., 1991; IOM, 2002.
6. For example, Egeland and Sussex, 1985; Brent et al., 1996; Johnson et al., 1998; Statham et al., 1998; Johnson and Cameron, 2001; Fu et al., 2002.
7. Pfeffer et al., 1994; Brent et al., 1996, 2003; Johnson et al., 1998.
8. Mann et al., 1999; Keilp et al., 2001; Oquendo and Mann, 2001; Oquendo et al., 2004.
9. Fawcett et al., 1997; Partonen et al., 1999; Tanskanen et al., 2000; Ellison and Morrison, 2001; Golomb et al., 2002; Lester, 2002; Lalovic et al., 2004.
10. Bunney and Fawcett, 1965; Fawcett and Bunney, 1967; Bunney et al., 1969; Krieger, 1970.
11. Koukopoulos and Koukopoulos (1999) traced the history of the conceptualization of mixed states back to Kraepelin, who conceived them as a form of manic-depressive insanity; before that to the state of melancholia agitata described by Richarz (1858); and still further back to Hippocrates, who described the anxiety seen in agitated melancholia in *Diseases II*. This state, characterized by anxiety and agitation as primary symptoms, has gradually been separated from manic-depressive illness, appearing today as a subtype of major depression-agitated type.
12. Rush, 1812; Kraepelin, 1921; Clouston, 1915; Henderson and Gillespie, 1927; Jameison and Wall, 1933; Stengel, 1955; Copes et al., 1971; Copas and Fryer, 1980; Barner-Rasmussen, 1986; Schweizer et al., 1988.
13. Of the 569 with unipolar major depression, 210 were in first episodes, and 359 were in recurrent episodes.
14. There were too few completed suicides to permit meaningful comparisons.
15. Jameison and Wall, 1933; Slater and Roth, 1969; Barraclough et al., 1974; Motto, 1975; Fawcett et al., 1987, 1990.
16. Cluster B disorders are antisocial personality disorder, borderline personality disorder, histrionic personality disorder, and narcissistic personality disorder.
17. Guze and Robins, 1970; Tsuang and Woolson, 1977, Weeke, 1979; Inskip et al., 1998.

Part III

Psychological Studies

Neuropsychology

I seem to be in perpetual fog and darkness. I cannot get my mind to work; instead of associations "clicking into place" everything is an inextricable jumble; instead of seeming to grasp a whole, it seems to remain tied to the actual consciousness of the moment. . . . I could not feel more ignorant, undecided or inefficient. It is appallingly difficult to concentrate.

—*John Custance (1952, p. 62)*

In this chapter, we examine what can be learned from studies of the neuropsychology of manic-depressive illness. Two streams of neuropsychological investigation can be distinguished. One uses a battery of objective measures, focusing largely on the sensorimotor and cognitive functions, to characterize profiles of strength and weakness in the various phases of bipolar or recurrent unipolar illness. The other generates hypotheses about how affective states, normal and abnormal, are represented in the brain and what factors mediate their expression. We consider the contributions of this second stream of investigation after reviewing what has been learned from the first, the evaluation of sensorimotor and cognitive function in manic-depressive illness, with an emphasis on the bipolar form. In the final section, we assess the overall contribution of neuropsychology to the conceptualization of mood disorders.

CONTRIBUTIONS OF NEUROPSYCHOLOGICAL EVALUATION

The contributions of traditional neuropsychological testing to our understanding of manic-depressive illness pertain to four issues. Such investigation can (1) provide an empirical basis for and clarification of clinical phenomenological concepts; (2) determine which abnormalities are state dependent and which are state independent; (3) characterize the neuropsychological functions that appear to be most persistently impaired, providing a clue to pathophysiology; and (4) determine the burden of the illness and its treatments with respect to cognitive functioning in terms of both cross-sectional and longitudinal outcomes.

Objectifying Clinical Constructs

First, neuropsychological investigation can identify the constituent processes impaired in some of the classic symptoms of the disorder. For example, psychomotor disturbance is common in major depression and bipolar disorder, and depressed bipolar patients may be especially likely to manifest psychomotor retardation (Sobin and Sackeim, 1997). In turn, this motor disturbance is viewed by some as having special prognostic significance with respect to treatment outcome (Hickie et al., 1990a, 1996; Parker and Hadzi-Pavlovic, 1993). However, the term "psychomotor retardation" is itself an amalgam, and the slowness of movement seen in depressed patients may reflect slowing in any of a variety of cognitive or motor processes. Indeed, some success has been achieved in using objective measures to dissect the constituent processes of such retardation and to identify those disturbed in affective disorders (Sobin and Sackeim, 1997). Thus in principle, neuropsychological evaluation can determine just what is slowed in psychomotor retardation and quantify the extent of abnormality.

Similarly, disturbances in attention are rife in mood disorders, yet they can pertain to distinct cognitive processes such as vigilance or sustained attention, freedom from distraction, divided attention, and capacity to shift set.[1] Neuropsychological investigation can clarify the nature of what is typically referred to as impaired concentration.

Identifying State-Related and State-Independent Abnormalities

The above contribution involves clarifying and quantifying deficits described more generally by clinical characterization of key features of the disorder. However, neuropsychological evaluation also yields information on strengths and weaknesses that go beyond clinical phenomenology. For the past 40 years, there has been an unresolved debate about whether the bipolar subgroup of manic-depressive illness is overrepresented in individuals with higher levels of intelligence and/or creativity (Richards et al., 1983; Andreasen, 1987; Jamison, 1993) (see Chapter 12). This issue can be addressed by determining whether premorbid intelligence in individuals with bipolar disorder exceeds population norms, and whether such individuals exceed normative values on indicators of creativity, such as those assessed by measures of cognitive flexibility and idiosyncratic thought. In turn, findings in this area may be helpful in considering sociobiological questions, such as why the genes for bipolar disorder have been preserved.

More generally, through comparison of individuals in remission and in the depressed or manic state of bipolar disorder, neuropsychological investigation can provide new information on the sensorimotor and cognitive abnormalities that fluctuate with affective state or are invariant across the disorder. As noted above, the state of depression or mania can introduce serious confounds in neuropsychological evaluation. Therefore, a number of recent investigations have placed special emphasis on detailing the deficits characteristic of bipolar patients in remission,[2] of children at risk for the disorder (Decina et al., 1983; Dickstein et al., 2004; Meyer et al., 2004), and of other first-degree relatives (Sobczak et al., 2002; Ferrier et al., 2004; Zalla et al., 2004), including discordant monozygotic twins (Gourovitch et al., 1999). Indeed, the identification of abnormalities that persist across the phases of the illness or that precede its first expression as a mood disorder may provide markers of disease vulnerability and suggest neurobiological abnormalities responsible for disease expression.

Establishing Differential Deficits of Relevance to Pathoetiology

Perhaps the most common goal of neuropsychological evaluation is to identify the sensorimotor or cognitive processes that are most disturbed in patients with bipolar disorder, in contrast to either normative values or individuals with other neuropsychiatric disorders. The peaks and especially the nadirs of neuropsychological profiles are taken as evidence that certain neuropsychological processes are particularly disturbed, and therefore of particular relevance when considering pathoetiology.

The methods needed to establish such "differential deficits" were reviewed by Chapman and Chapman (1973) in the context of determining what aspect of information processing is most relevant in accounting for thought disorder in schizophrenia. Although there is intuitive appeal to a focus on abnormalities of greatest magnitude, what appears

to be most broken is not necessarily that which is in greatest need of repair. For example, intermittent dysfunction of the electrical system in a car may short out the radio, but the broken radio is not the fundamental problem. Other conceptual reservations concern the fact that cognitive processes are interdependent. Attention has a widespread impact on neuropsychological function. When one cannot attend adequately to information, encoding, learning, and memory are all impaired and, depending on other factors, perhaps more so than the attentional measures themselves. At a methodological level, the validity of comparisons across tests depends on the equivalence of the tests with regard to psychometric properties, particularly internal reliability (the extent to which one dimension is assessed) and difficulty level (overall performance level in the sample). These properties are partly intrinsic to a test and partly a function of the sample being assessed. Thus while it is common to view findings of differential deficit as indicating that one process is more impaired than another, such findings are commonly a psychometric artifact due to the fact that tests with greater power to discriminate among individuals detect larger differences. Thus, it can be argued that the prevalence of particular neuropsychological deficits, their persistence, and/or the extent to which particular deficits account for symptom severity may be as or more important than a gauge of the absolute level of deficit.

Documenting Neuropsychological Burden

Finally, neuropsychological evaluations have practical value in documenting the burden of the illness. Here as well, multiple approaches can be taken. Current theorizing suggests that states of depression and mania, especially when untreated, result in a destructive, atrophic process in the hippocampus due to excessive release of glucocorticoids (Brown et al., 1999; Lupien et al., 1999; MacQueen et al., 2003) (see Chapter 14). In turn, this progressive structural abnormality should be expressed in progressive deficits in declarative, episodic memory, the neuropsychological functions that are especially tied to hippocampal integrity. Indeed, it has been reported that, independently of age, hippocampal volume in euthymic unipolar women covaries with duration of lifetime exposure to the depressed state, as well as with verbal memory performance (Sheline et al., 1996, 1999).

Episode frequency is higher in bipolar than in most unipolar samples, and bipolar patients tend to express the most virulent forms of affective disturbance (e.g., psychotic depression). Thus it is possible that the neuropsychological consequences of manic-depressive illness are especially severe in bipolar relative to recurrent unipolar patients. In a recent study, performance on five tests of learning and memory was compared in young and elderly depressed unipolar and bipolar inpatients (Burt et al., 2000). Unipolar and bipolar patients within each age group had equivalent scores on the verbal and performance intelligence indices of the Wechsler Adult Intelligence Scale-Revised (WAIS-R) (Wechsler, 1981) and on the modified Mini-Mental State (mMMS) exam (Stern et al., 1987). All patients were tested during a major depressive episode, and symptom severity was found to be similar across the groups. The elderly bipolar patients were distinguished by a higher number of prior affective episodes and psychiatric hospitalizations compared with the other three groups. There was a tendency for the young bipolar group to outperform the young unipolar group on several memory measures. As illustrated by the findings obtained with the Complex Figure Test (Fig. 9–1), elderly bipolar patients decidedly showed the most marked deficits on four of the five tests.

While limited by a cross-sectional design, these findings suggest that deterioration in memory function may be a more prominent characteristic of bipolar than unipolar illness, broadly defined. It would be interesting to know whether there would be unipolar–bipolar differences in memory measures if the two groups were matched on total number of episodes. Given the neuroprotective effects posited for lithium (Manji et al., 2000a,b; Moore et al., 2000) and possibly other mood stabilizers (see Chapter 18), it becomes especially important to determine the impact of treatment on these putative longitudinal effects.

Neuropsychological burden not only results from disease expression and progression, but may also be an inadvertent outcome of treatment (as may neuroprotection). An especially frequent complaint of patients treated with lithium is that, in concert with a dampening of the peaks and valleys of mood fluctuation, creative processes are inhibited. Some individuals report that they are not as original or forward thinking when treated with lithium, or are less quick to see connections and less spontaneous (see Chapter 12). These claims have been tested in neuropsychological investigations, whose results have revealed adverse cognitive effects of lithium that are dose dependent and appear to reverse shortly after discontinuation of the drug (Shaw et al., 1986, 1987).

META-ANALYSIS OF FINDINGS ON NEUROPSYCHOLOGICAL DEFICITS IN MOOD DISORDERS

In the following sections, we present a critical evaluation of what has been learned from neuropsychological evaluations of samples of manic-depressive patients. Much of the literature on neuropsychological function in mood disorders, especially in the depressed phase, has failed to distinguish between bipolar and unipolar subgroups. Necessarily, some of the discussion of neuropsychological deficits in depression

Figure 9–1. Findings obtained with Complex Figure Test. Unmedicated unipolar (UP) and bipolar (BP) patients in an episode of major depression were divided into young and elderly groups. Across multiple measures of memory, the elderly BP patients were greatly impaired, while the young BP patients tended to have the best performance. Shown are scores for copying a complex figure and also for later reproduction of the figure from memory. The delayed reproduction scores show the special deficit in the bipolar elderly. (*Source*: Burt et al., 2000. Reprinted with permission from Lippincott Williams & Wilkins.)

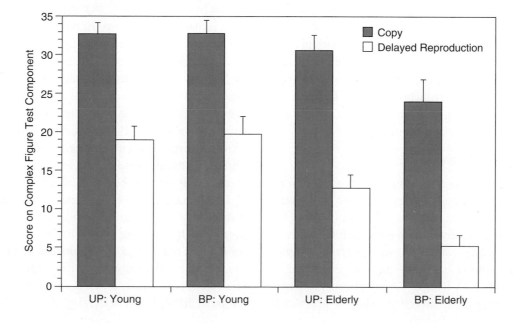

may not be specific to bipolar disorder, but to the extent that recurrent unipolar patients are included, these studies address the broader concept of manic-depressive illness. However, the major focus here is on those neuropsychological abnormalities that are consistent across manic, depressed, and euthymic phases of the bipolar form of the illness.

For the purposes of this chapter, we conducted a new meta-analysis of studies comparing neuropsychological functions in bipolar and healthy comparison samples. We identified 74 studies published since 1975 that entailed neuropsychological evaluations in a bipolar sample as compared with a healthy control or a psychiatric comparison sample (e.g., schizophrenia), and that met high methodological standards. For a study to be included, patients in the bipolar sample had to be described as predominantly in a depressed or manic state or in remission, and sufficient quantitative values had to be reported so that effect size could be computed. In addition, studies were labeled "mixed" if the bipolar sample included patients with a mix of manic, depressed, or euthymic states; did not specify the affective state; or provided no clear classification of state. Nonetheless, few of the studies classified as "mixed" actually focused on patients in a mixed state, and it is fair to assume that the bulk of patients in these studies were in a depressed state. The 74 studies thus identified yielded 1,216 statistical comparisons of a bipolar sample with another group on neuropsychological outcome measures. These comparisons pertained to multiple neuropsychological domains, sometimes with multiple tests sampling the same domain, and often with multiple outcome measures within a test.

The comparisons reported here concern only the performance of bipolar patients relative to normal control participants, and statistical comparisons were used in the meta-analysis only if they pertained to a major cognitive domain, such as attention. This filter reduced the number of studies examined to 52, and the number of neuropsychological comparisons to 614.[3] For each test, all outcome measures were examined so that the effect size assigned a test was the average of these measures. In our meta-analysis, effect sizes for different tests representing the same domain within any study (e.g., attention) were also averaged.[4]

Global Intellectual Functioning

Several key questions have been posed about general intellectual functioning in manic-depressive illness, a literature that focuses primarily on the bipolar subgroup. Most of the research in this area has centered on whether intelligence or global neuropsychological status is invariant across symptomatic states and remission, or the state of depression or mania is associated with deficits or enhancements. There has also been considerable interest in whether premorbid

levels of intelligence, or surrogate measures such as occupational achievement, differ from population norms.

Figure 9–2 presents a meta-analysis of recent studies contrasting the full-scale intelligence quotient (IQ) scores of bipolar patients and healthy volunteers obtained with the WAIS-R. Despite the relatively small number of studies, significant deficits were observed in the remitted, manic, and mixed samples relative to controls. (Only one study [Deptula et al., 1991] was classified as exclusively examining bipolar depressed patients.) Thus, preliminary evidence indicates that intelligence, as assessed by a well-validated measure, is reduced in bipolar illness in both the remitted and manic states. This conclusion is supported by a variety of early studies that found evidence for general intellectual impairment in symptomatic bipolar patients.

The above findings do not imply that variations in state have no impact on intelligence scores. Cross-sectional comparison with control samples can establish whether each state manifests abnormality, but can give only a rough indication of the magnitude of changes that may occur within the same individuals in different states. Indeed, there is evidence that some patients have higher intellectual functioning when hypomanic than when depressed (Donnelly et al., 1982). Furthermore, a variety of longitudinal studies have found the remitted state to be associated with higher IQ than the depressed state.[5] While such findings have been interpreted as indicating a state-dependent deterioration in IQ (Miller, 1975), much of this work was subject to the same confound: repeat IQ testing generally results in a modest increase in scores attributable to practice effects (Matarazzo et al., 1980). Most studies tested patients in a depressed or manic state, with later retesting during euthymia. Such an invariant order would bias results toward higher scores in the euthymic or remitted state relative to depression or mania.

The firmest conclusion that can be drawn from this literature is that samples of bipolar patients, whether remitted or not, show modest global cognitive impairment as reflected by diminished IQ scores. This conclusion is strengthened by findings obtained using broad-based clinical neuropsychological batteries, such as the Halstead-Reitan or Luria-Nebraska. Summary impairment scores on these batteries correlate highly with IQ scores. Several studies have found gross impairment, on a level comparable to that in schizophrenia, in manic samples, and moderate-to-severe impairment in unipolar and/or bipolar depressed samples.[6]

Interpretation of a global intellectual deficit in bipolar disorder is highly contingent on beliefs about the level of premorbid functioning. For example, an IQ deficit in the remitted state may reflect an impairment that preceded the expression of bipolar disorder, or may represent a form of deterioration resulting from the disorder or its treatments. On the other hand, it has been suggested that bipolar patients

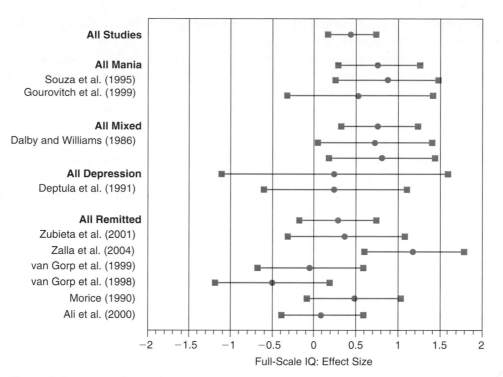

Figure 9–2. Meta-analysis of full-scale intelligence quotient (IQ) scores obtained with the Wechsler Adult Intelligence Scale-Revised (WAIS-R). Effect sizes (Hedges' G) are presented for individual study comparisons of a bipolar sample with healthy controls, as well as for samples of bipolar patients in remission, depression, mixed state, or mania and across all studies. Squares = confidence interval; circles = mean.

may be premorbidly advantaged; that is, their level of intelligence prior to disease expression tends to be above average. Were this the case, it would indicate that the deficits observed in comparisons with healthy volunteers underestimate the deterioration from premorbid values.

Unfortunately, while often discussed, this issue has received limited research attention. Mason (1956) contrasted the prerecruitment IQs of Army veterans hospitalized for schizophrenia and what was termed manic-depressive illness, which no doubt included some patients with recurrent unipolar depression. The schizophrenia sample had premorbid IQs below control values, whereas the IQs of mood disorder patients were significantly better than those of healthy subjects. Woodruff and colleagues (1968, 1971) found that bipolar patients and their brothers had higher levels of occupational and educational achievement than unipolar patients and their brothers, with the latter group not differing from healthy volunteers. Other work has similarly indicated that the families of individuals with bipolar disorder have an advantage relative to population norms for educational and occupational achievement (Petterson, 1977; Waters et al., 1981), as well as creativity (see Chapter 12). Indeed, limited research with children of bipolar probands before the first manifestation of frank mood disorder supports the possibility of an IQ elevation in the premorbid state (Decina et al., 1983).

This possibility of an elevation in premorbid intellectual abilities relative to population norms is reinforced by the literature on the relationship between social class and bipolar disorder. A number of studies, starting at the beginning of the twentieth century, have generally found that bipolar disorder is overrepresented in individuals with middle and high income levels and among business and other professionals. It is possible that these associations reflect an ascertainment bias. Individuals of a higher socioeconomic level may be especially likely to be diagnosed with a mood disorder instead of schizophrenia or schizoaffective disorder, with the reverse pertaining to those of lower socioeconomic levels. However, the fact that these associations are also observed among the family members of bipolar probands undercuts this hypothesis (Woodruff et al., 1971; Monelly et al., 1974; Eisemann, 1986; Coryell et al., 1989).

Thus there is reason to suspect that as a group, individuals with bipolar disorder are endowed with general intellectual abilities superior to the distribution in the general population and may be more likely to have backgrounds of middle and upper socioeconomic levels. Yet it also appears that bipolar disorder is characterized by poorer general intelligence across all phases of illness. If both of these views are correct, it would suggest that the disorder is associated with significant deterioration in general intellectual abilities or that there are compensatory cognitive advantages in a subgroup of individuals with bipolar illness (see Chapter 12). Studies contrasting patient samples with healthy volunteers likely underestimate the extent of deterioration because they do not account for the premorbid baseline.

Contexts in which a group differs in premorbid intellectual abilities present significant problems in interpreting comparisons with patients with other disorders or healthy volunteers. Neuropsychological tests differ in their sensitivity to the generalized effects of brain insult. For example, vocabulary and comprehension subtests of the WAIS-R are traditionally viewed as "hold" scales because of their relative immutability in providing an indication of premorbid ability in the face of brain damage. However, samples of patients with bipolar disorder have usually been matched to comparison groups on the basis of current demographic and neuropsychological features (e.g., age, sex, current IQ). This design may entail, therefore, that the two groups are mismatched with respect to premorbid levels. Thus patterns of apparently specific deficits seen in remitted or symptomatic states may be reflecting only the varying sensitivity of tests to a generalized destructive process.

Verbal and Performance IQ

The full-scale IQ score of the WAIS-R encompasses two composite scores: one for verbal IQ (VIQ) and one for performance (nonverbal) IQ (PIQ). It is well established that patients with mood disorders have a pattern of higher VIQ than PIQ. For example, a review by Kluger and Goldberg (1990) compared the VIQ–PIQ discrepancy in patients with bipolar disorder, right-hemisphere damage, left-hemisphere damage, and bilateral damage and healthy volunteers. Lower PIQ than VIQ was found in 19 of 22 studies of mood disorder patients (14 studies of bipolar and unipolar depressed patients, 4 of manic patients, and 4 of mixed groups), in 20 of 20 studies of patients with right-hemisphere lesions, and in 28 of 30 studies of patients with bilateral injuries. In contrast, PIQ exceeded VIQ in 15 of 20 studies of patients with left-hemisphere lesions. (See also our review of 25 studies in the first edition of this text.)

These effects were examined in the studies of bipolar samples included in our meta-analysis. Figure 9–3a presents the findings for VIQ and Figure 9–3b those for PIQ. Across studies and within studies grouped by state examined (mania, depression, mixed, remission), bipolar patients and normal controls evidenced no difference in VIQ. In contrast, across all studies ($z=3.36$, $p<.001$) and within studies grouped by state, bipolar samples showed a marked deficit in PIQ; the effect size (Hedges' G) across studies for PIQ was 0.71 (standard error [SE] $=0.21$), near the threshold for a strong effect. Specifically, the three studies of

bipolar patients in remission produced an effect size of 0.56 (SE $=0.25$).

The nature of the VIQ–PIQ discrepancy was closely examined in a study by Sackeim and colleagues (1992). They administered the full WAIS-R to 100 inpatients who were experiencing an episode of major depressive disorder and had been referred for electroconvulsive therapy (ECT), along with 50 matched healthy volunteers. In addition to age, gender, and race, the groups in this study were matched on indicators of premorbid function, specifically education and highest lifetime occupational level (sustained for 2 years). Based on an algorithm developed by Barona and colleagues (1984), estimates of premorbid full-scale IQ, VIQ, and PIQ were computed for all participants. A subset of patients was readministered the WAIS-R within 1 week ($n=26$) or 8 weeks after termination of ECT ($n=33$). Of the 100 patients, 25 were diagnosed with bipolar disorder, and 75 were unipolar. According to the Research Diagnostic Criteria (RDC) (Spitzer et al., 1978), 36 percent of the patient sample were psychotically depressed, 46 percent were of the retarded subtype, and all were of the endogenous subtype. Using a cap of 10, the bipolar patients averaged 5.3 (standard deviation [SD] $=3.2$) prior affective episodes and 3.1 (SD $=2.7$) prior hospitalizations. In contrast, the unipolar patients averaged 3.3 (SD $=3.4$) prior affective episodes and 1.8 (SD $=2.6$) prior psychiatric hospitalizations. Of the unipolar patients, 79 percent had recurrent illness.

Figure 9–4 presents the estimated premorbid IQ scores and IQ scores obtained with the WAIS-R for the total patient and healthy volunteer samples. The two groups did not differ in any of the three premorbid estimates. There was no consistent difference between estimated premorbid VIQ and PIQ in either group. In contrast, analyses of obtained IQ scores indicated that the patient group had significantly lower full-scale IQ. This result was attributable to low PIQ scores: the two groups did not differ in VIQ, but showed a marked difference in PIQ.[7] While the VIQ scores of the healthy comparison group averaged 4.7 points higher than their PIQ scores, the comparable figure in the patient sample was 12.7 points. The obtained VIQ among patients was less than 4 points lower than the premorbid estimate, while the obtained PIQ was more than 15 points lower than the premorbid estimate.

These effects pertained to patients with both unipolar and bipolar depression. Figure 9–5 plots the cumulative distribution of VIQ–PIQ discrepancy scores for the healthy control and bipolar and unipolar subgroups. Throughout the range of discrepancy scores, the two patient groups were generally shifted to the right of healthy controls by approximately 10 points. The only indication of a difference between unipolar and bipolar patients was a higher

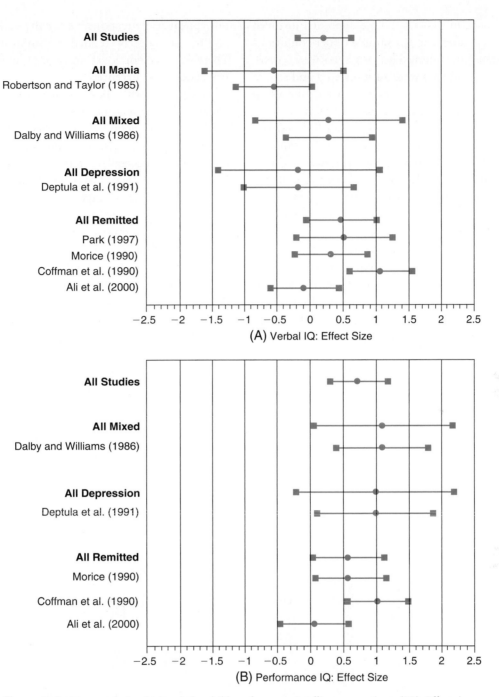

Figure 9–3. Meta-analysis of (a) verbal and (b) performance intelligence quotients (IQ). Effect sizes (Hedges' G) are presented for individual study comparisons of a bipolar sample with healthy controls, as well as for samples of bipolar patients in remission, depression, mixed state, or mania and across all studies. Squares = confidence interval; circles = mean.

frequency of marked discrepancies favoring VIQ in the bipolar group. However, the mean discrepancy in bipolar patients (14.52 ±14.22) was not different from that in unipolar patients (12.04 ±10.78).

Starting with Wechsler (1944), a common explanation for this discrepancy in mood disorder patients has concerned the effects of psychomotor retardation on task performance. Four of the PIQ subtests (picture arrangement, picture completion, object assembly, and block design) are timed tests, while this is true of only one VIQ subtest (arithmetic). Therefore, slowed processing or motor execution could conceivably lead to diminished performance. This issue was addressed in four ways. One approach involved testing the first 34 patients in the sample under conditions in which both timed and untimed performances were scored. In other words, the subtests were administered and scored in the usual manner, except that patients were allowed to complete each subtest after the standard time limit had expired. Scoring without time constraints had little impact on discrepancy scores, either before or after the course of ECT. The baseline discrepancy in the untimed condition averaged 11.35 (SD=11.06). Patients who met the RDC for retarded subtype (n=46) did not differ from the other patients (n=54) on this discrepancy score (retarded, 12.78±12.03; nonretarded, 12.56±11.54).

Another approach taken to this issue was to examine more broadly the relationships of symptom severity and other clinical features to the VIQ–PIQ discrepancy. A regression analysis was conducted on baseline discrepancy scores, with age, Hamilton Rating Scale for Depression (HAM-D) score (depression severity), duration of current depressive episode (chronicity), duration since onset of first affective episode, and number of previous affective episodes (recurrence) as predictors. Only baseline HAM-D scores showed a relationship. Greater symptom severity at baseline was associated with a smaller VIQ–PIQ discrepancy and lower VIQ scores. There were no other effects. Thus factors that varied with depression severity did not appear to be responsible for the VIQ–PIQ difference, and marked severity tended to diminish the discrepancy. There was no evidence of an association with chronicity or frequency of recurrence.

Compatible with these findings were those of analyses conducted after readministration of the WAIS-R 1 and 8 weeks after completion of ECT. The 1-week group ($n = 26$) showed a slight decrease in the discrepancy at retesting, with average scores decreasing from 12.12 ± 11.16 to 9.64 ± 13.22. Virtually no change was seen at the 8-week follow-up (n=33), with the average discrepancy decreasing from 13.48 ± 13.01 to 12.24 ± 12.86. Restricting the follow-up sample to patients in remission had no impact.

These findings suggest that the VIQ–PIQ discrepancy was manifested independently of affective state and characterized patients in remission. Indeed, it is possible that the discrepancy is expressed before the first episode of mood disturbance. This possibility is supported by the results of studies of children of bipolar probands aged 7 to 14 (Decina et al., 1983; Sackeim and Decina, 1983). None of the children had yet expressed bipolar disorder, and relatively few had other diagnosable mood disorders, although behavioral disturbance was common. Nonetheless, a marked VIQ–PIQ discrepancy was observed on the Wechsler Intelligence Scale for Children-Revised (WISC-R) in the high-risk sample relative to healthy comparison volunteers. Similar

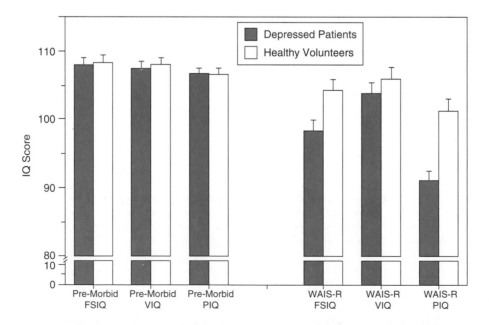

Figure 9–4. Premorbid intelligence quotient (IQ) estimates and IQ scores obtained with the Wechsler Adult Intelligence Scale-Revised (WAIS-R) in unmedicated patients with major depression and healthy controls. Premorbid estimates were identical in the patient (n=100) and control (n=50) groups. The patient group showed a marked discrepancy between verbal and performance IQ (VIQ > PIQ). FSIQ=full-scale IQ; PIQ=performance IQ; VIQ=verbal IQ. (*Source*: Sackeim et al., 1992. Reproduced with permission of Psychology Press.)

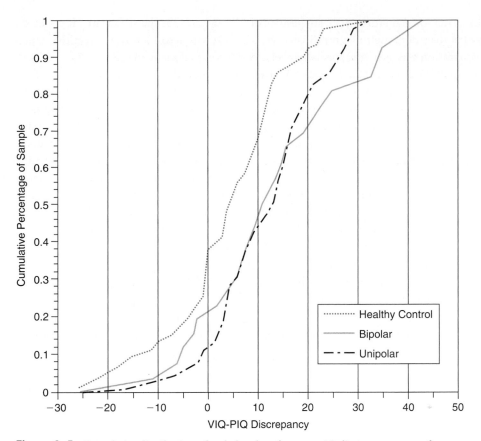

Figure 9–5. Cumulative distribution of verbal and performance IQ discrepancy scores for healthy controls and bipolar and unipolar depressed patients. Both patient groups are shifted to the right of healthy controls and have an average discrepancy favoring a verbal IQ approximately 10 points higher across the distribution in controls. (*Source*: Sackeim et al., 1992. Reproduced with permission of Psychology Press.)

results had been reported in an earlier, uncontrolled study of children at high risk (Kestenbaum, 1979).

Thus the notion that bipolar disorder is associated with a global intellectual impairment that is state independent should be revised. The reductions in full-scale IQ seen in mood disorders appear to be largely attributable to a decrement in PIQ, with preservation of VIQ. This differential deficit is relatively constant across states of euthymia, depression, and mania and may precede syndromal expression.

In interpreting this effect, it is important to consider whether the discrepancy arises from one or two subtests on the WAIS-R or WISC-R or reflects a more uniform difference in verbal and nonverbal task performance. In the study by Sackeim and colleagues (1992), a descriptive (canonical) discriminant analysis was conducted with diagnostic group (patient versus healthy volunteer) as the classification variable and scaled scores on the 11 subtests as the dependent measure. This analysis produced a single significant discriminant function, providing a description of the profile of subtests that distinguishes maximally

between the groups. Structure coefficients were determined for this linear function. These coefficients are more stable than the original weighting of subtests in the discriminant function (Huberty, 1984), and reflect the association between scores on a subtest and total scores on the composite discriminant function. The median structure coefficient for the five PIQ subtests was 0.53, with a range of 0.43 to 0.70. In contrast, the median structure coefficient for the six VIQ subtests was 0.13, with a range of 0.03 to 0.38. All five PIQ subtests made strong contributions to the differentiation between patients and controls. The comprehension (0.29) and digit span (0.38) VIQ subtests also contributed, but more weakly. Therefore, the results of this analysis suggest that the PIQ deficit in mood disorders is not specific to a particular PIQ subtest, but is expressed uniformly across all five PIQ subtests.

Thus the relative deficit in PIQ is uniform across the various subtests assessing this form of intelligence. The magnitude of this discrepancy appears to be independent of the phase of affective disorder, and may be a marker of a bipolar diathesis. Early work on children at risk indicated that children with behavioral disturbances suggestive of early signs of bipolar disorder, such as grandiosity, conduct disorder, or separation anxiety, are especially likely to manifest the discrepancy (Decina et al., 1983; Sackeim et al., 1983a). While many researchers attributed this phenomenon to a differential impact of psychomotor slowing on PIQ, this hypothesis can now be rejected given the discrepancy's persistence in remission, manifestation in at-risk samples, and persistence even when performance is not constrained by timing.

In this light, two hypotheses have been advanced. One posits that the PIQ deficit reflects a fundamental disturbance in visuospatial processing and implies a differential right hemisphere deficit (Flor-Henry, 1979). The second hypothesis is that the discrepancy has little localizing value and reflects the greater sensitivity of PIQ and other forms of "fluid" intelligence to generalized impairment, in contrast to the "crystallized" intelligence reflected in VIQ subscales (Kluger and Goldberg, 1990; Bearden et al., 2001).

Were the discrepancy to reflect a fundamental deficit in visuospatial processing, it could be compatible with a right-hemisphere insult, especially in parietal cortex. This classic formulation is compatible with evidence that manifestation of mania without a history of major depression (i.e., unipolar mania) is seen principally in the context of brain insult and most commonly with right-hemisphere damage, generally involving parietal tissue. Thus, bipolar illness would be viewed as especially likely to manifest a form of right-hemisphere dysfunction. However, the evidence in mood disorders clearly reveals that the discrepancy is also manifested in unipolar depression, at least in samples with severe and/or recurrent disorder. Thus if this discrepancy indeed reflects a lateralized insult, it must be viewed as characteristic of recurrent mood disorders—that is, manic-depressive illness in Kraepelin's terminology.

The second hypothesis is that the discrepancy per se has limited lateralizing value. It is seen with both bilateral and right-hemisphere brain damage. The effect size seen in mood disorder samples is comparable to that seen in patients with bilateral brain damage, itself a notable fact, and below that seen in patients with right-hemisphere lesions (Kluger and Goldberg, 1990). There is no reason to suspect, for example, that the pathophysiological process resulting in right-hemisphere dysfunction in mood disorders would produce the same level of differential deficit as that seen in patients with gross brain lesions.

A broader perspective on the neuropsychological profiles of mood disorder patients may help resolve this issue. The laterality hypothesis would stipulate that mood disorder samples show especially marked deficits in tests that rely heavily on visuospatial processing. The view that the discrepancy arises from generalized brain impairment would

suggest that the deficit in PIQ is of the same magnitude as deficits across a host of cognitive functions, including attention and memory.

Indeed, our examination of the profile of cognitive deficits in bipolar disorder raises a third, novel hypothesis. There is indeed evidence of widespread and generally uniform cognitive deficit across the phases of bipolar disorder, with little indication that visuospatial abilities are especially impaired. Rather, verbal skills appear to be consistently preserved. The implication is that the cognitive systems subserving language are spared with respect to an otherwise generalized disease process, are constitutionally endowed at higher capacity, or are complemented by compensatory cognitive advantages of an as-yet undetermined nature.

Psychomotor Functioning

The domain of psychomotor functioning reflects the integrity of processes determining the speed of information processing and the speed and organization of motor behavior. Individuals may appear to be "slowed" because of dysfunction in motor output and/or in the speed of thought. Alternatively, individuals may appear to be "dull" or "slow" because of poverty of mental content, in essence a lack of thought. This domain pertains to functions as diverse as manual dexterity, reaction time, and levels of spontaneous activity. As reviewed by Sobin and Sackeim (1997), a variety of experimental techniques have been developed to assess the component processes that may underlie psychomotor disturbance in mood disorders.

Disturbances of motility and speed of processing have long been considered central to the phenomenology of mood disorders. Psychomotor disturbance has generally been regarded as a cardinal feature of endogenous or melancholic depression, and some have contended that careful assessment of psychomotor disturbances has predictive value with respect to treatment outcome. The racing thoughts of the manic state suggest dysregulation in speed of processing that is opposite to that often seen in the depressed state. Thus psychomotor function, like mood and sleep, may be one of the few domains to show opposite symptom manifestations depending on phase of illness.

Some theorists have taken this overlap between the mood and motor output systems to suggest that mood disorders are essentially disorders of motility (Flor-Henry, 1983). While this is clearly an overstatement, it is noteworthy that mood disturbance occurs at especially high rates in patients with movement disorder. This observation is especially well documented for Parkinson's and Huntington's diseases. As indicated earlier, Huntington's disease is of special note as perhaps the only neurological illness to produce both depression and mania at some frequency. In contrast, imaging research has yet to relate psychomotor disturbance in mood disorders to basal ganglia dysfunction. Instead, the Hammersmith group found that psychomotor symptoms covary with the magnitude of regional cerebral blood flow deficits in prefrontal regions (Dolan et al., 1993). Indeed, they suggested that the prefrontal deficits commonly seen in both major depression and schizophrenia reflect a common psychomotor disturbance. Presumably, this disturbance pertains to executive functions that regulate the flow and speed of information processing.

Cognitive and Motor Speed

In a substantial literature over the last five decades, slowed reaction time has been documented in mood disorder patients during episodes of major depression relative to healthy participants (Marvel and Paradiso, 2004). The subgroups most likely to manifest this slowing were variously described in this work as manic-depressive, bipolar, psychotic, or presenting with endogenous depression compared with subgroups classified as neurotic, nonpsychotic, or reactive. Thus, there was a general impression that severity of illness was associated with psychomotor slowing. Frequently in this work, depressed samples had slower performance relative to healthy participants, nondepressed neurotic patients, and patients with acute schizophrenia. Nonetheless, the depressed samples were often less slowed than patients with chronic schizophrenia or brain damage. The investigators also found that clinical improvement was usually linked to improved speed of responding, suggesting that psychomotor slowing is largely a state-dependent phenomenon. In much of this work, time to complete tasks, such as the digit symbol subtest of the WAIS-R, was used to assess psychomotor slowing. Consequently, disturbances in cognitive processes and motor execution were confounded, and the source of the slowing was not identified.

While this issue is the subject of increasing attention (Sobin and Sackeim, 1997), it remains unresolved and may not have a simple answer. Cornell and colleagues (1984) varied cognitive load in a series of reaction-time measures when comparing patients who met diagnostic criteria for melancholia with nonmelancholic, nonendogenous depressed patients. They found that both groups manifested slow motor performance, and that this was a key abnormality independent of melancholia. In contrast, the melancholic subgroup was especially sensitive to the effects of cognitive load in further slowing motor response. This result was interpreted as reflecting an impairment in cognitive processing—a cognitive slowing—in melancholic patients.

Other dimensions to consider in studies of psychomotor speed concern the effects of distraction and the distinction between preferred rates of response and response speed when one is working at one's best. In a comprehensive study, Blackburn (1975) contrasted six groups of patients:

acutely symptomatic bipolar manic, bipolar depressed, and unipolar depressed and the same three groups at rest. Blackburn used separate tasks thought to measure principally mental and motor speed, although the motor task had more than nontrivial cognitive components. The mental task was administered with patients working both at their own speed (preferred speed) and as quickly as possible. The motor task was administered under conditions of no distraction, internal distraction (the patient counting), and external distraction (a news program played loudly during task performance). Acutely ill bipolar depressed patients were slower than all other groups on the motor task with no distraction. Surprisingly, both internal and external distraction resulted in improved performance among the bipolar depressed group but in deterioration among the unipolar patients, while results with the manic patients were equivocal. In contrast, on the mental speed test at the preferred rate of responding, the acutely ill manic patients were faster than the other two groups, but did not differ from the manic patients in remission. With instructions to respond as quickly as possible, the six groups had comparable scores.

The results of this study illustrate two points. First, most neuropsychological evaluations call for patients to perform at their best, which may obscure deficits in routine information processing. Second, this study provided evidence that bipolar depressed patients are especially likely to manifest marked psychomotor slowing. It has long been contended that psychomotor retardation is characteristic more of bipolar than of unipolar depression (Kotin and Goodwin, 1972; Dunner et al., 1976). We revisit this issue in reviewing the literature on spontaneous activity (see the later discussion).

Recent studies using reaction time measures have demonstrated that psychomotor disturbance is characteristic of elderly patients with bipolar disorder. Pier and colleagues (2004) manipulated task difficulty and contrasted speed of figure copying in 12 elderly depressed patients and matched healthy controls in an attempt to isolate cognitive from motor slowing. Pronounced psychomotor retardation was seen in the patient group, which reflected a cognitive and more pronounced motor slowing. However, patients were studied while medicated, and medication effects on psychomotor speed are commonly observed (Caligiuri et al., 2003).

Surprisingly, three recent studies of psychomotor speed in bipolar adolescents failed to find differences from controls or other clinical groups (DelBello et al., 2004; Dickstein et al., 2004; McCarthy et al., 2004). Furthermore, there is only equivocal evidence for psychomotor disturbance in the first-degree relatives of bipolar probands. Zalla and colleagues (2004) compared euthymic bipolar patients, patients with schizophrenia, the unaffected first-degree relatives of both patient groups, and healthy controls in performance on tests of verbal fluency—the Stroop Word Color Interference Test, the Wisconsin Card Sorting Test, and the Trail Making Test. Compared with healthy controls, patients with schizophrenia performed poorly on all measures. The only abnormality seen in the euthymic bipolar group and the two groups of unaffected relatives reflected increased slowness on the Stroop test. This deficit could have been attributable to an increased susceptibility to interference and/or psychomotor slowing in the context of increased cognitive demand. In contrast, Ferrier and colleagues (2004) found no evidence of psychomotor disturbance when contrasting the neuropsychological performance of 17 unaffected first-degree relatives of bipolar patients with that of matched controls. Instead, the relatives were significantly impaired in backward digit span, spatial span, and tasks of visuospatial declarative memory, while verbal declarative memory was intact.

It is premature to conclude that psychomotor disturbance is infrequent in children and adolescents manifesting bipolar disorder or in first-degree family members. These issues have been studied infrequently, and the extant research used relatively small samples, a key limitation in studies of familial transmission given heterogeneity in genetic diathesis. Furthermore, while there is substantial evidence that reaction time improves with clinical remission in mood disorders, as reviewed in the next section, there is also substantial evidence for persistent psychomotor disturbance in remitted bipolar patients on tasks that make significant motor demands in terms of both dexterity and speed (e.g., Purdue Pegboard). Little information exists on potential impairments in pediatric bipolar patients or first-degree relatives in the aspects of psychomotor dysfunction most persistent in adult patients with bipolar disorder.

There has been limited investigation of the neurobiological correlates of impairments in cognitive and motor speed in bipolar disorder. Caligiuri and colleagues (2003) conducted functional magnetic resonance imaging (fMRI) while patients in the manic or depressed phase of bipolar illness and healthy controls performed a manual reaction-time task. The study results implicated both basal ganglia disturbance and a dimension of laterality. Manic patients had higher blood oxygen level–dependent (BOLD) responses in the left globus pallidus and significantly lower activity in the right globus pallidus, while depressed patients showed the reverse pattern of asymmetry. Level of activity within the globus pallidus and caudate was associated with the severity of manic symptoms. Notably, patients not receiving antipsychotic or mood-stabilizing medications had higher BOLD responses throughout the motor

cortex, basal ganglia, and thalamus. These findings suggest that the depressed and manic states are related to excessive and lateralized activity within the basal ganglia, and that antipsychotics and mood stabilizers suppress cortical and subcortical hyperreactivity.

The results of subsequent research focused on the supplementary (SMA) and primary (M1) motor areas underscore the possibility of a disturbance in lateralized control over motor processes. Using fMRI and several reaction time tasks, Caligiuri and colleagues (2004) showed that healthy controls differentially activated the left and right SMA on right- and left-hand trials, respectively. In contrast, in the small samples of bipolar manic and depressed patients, the latter failed to suppress the ipsilateral right SMA in right-hand trials, while the former had bilateral SMA activation for both left- and right-hand trials. Both depressed and manic patients had greater activity in the left M1, and antipsychotic or mood-stabilizing medications were associated with increased reaction time, lower BOLD response in M1 and SMA, and a loss of normal hemispheric asymmetry. In addition to again raising the issue of a lateralized disturbance, the results of this work suggest that the psychomotor disturbance in bipolar disorder may be an outcome of excessive excitability in mediating brain regions. This formulation contrasts with the hypothesis, derived from resting positron emission tomography (PET) studies (Bench et al., 1992; Dolan et al., 1994), that psychomotor retardation reflects reduced activity in specific prefrontal cortical structures.

Recent work has also clarified the extent to which psychomotor disturbance in bipolar disorder reflects cognitive dysfunction that may interfere with the planning or initiation of movement and/or disturbance in the execution of movement. Caligiuri and Ellwanger (2000) administered a traditional psychomotor battery, as well as a measure of the integrity of motor programming, to 36 patients who met *Diagnostic and Statistical Manual* (DSM)-IV criteria for psychomotor retardation. The programming task assessed capacity to adjust velocity scaling of movement relative to movement distance. Compared with healthy controls, the patient group evidenced longer reaction time and impairment in velocity scaling. A significant subgroup had deficits that were akin to those observed with the bradykinesia associated with parkinsonian conditions. Thus the retardation was viewed as encompassing both the planning and the execution of movement. An earlier detailed review of this literature likewise suggested that psychomotor disturbance usually involves a mix of cognitive and motor deficits (Sobin and Sackeim, 1997).

Finally, limited attention has been given to the neurochemical imbalances that may result in disturbances in cognitive and motor speed. Swann and colleagues (1999) compared unipolar and bipolar depressed patients and manic and mixed-state patients with healthy controls in tests of psychomotor speed and accuracy of tracking. The depressed groups were impaired on all behavioral measures, whereas the manic and mixed patients did not differ from the controls. Cerebral spinal fluid (CSF) and urinary measures of catecholamines and their metabolites were obtained. For virtually all behavioral measures, increased catecholamine function was associated with poorer performance in bipolar but not unipolar patients. Further, psychomotor function was related to depression severity in bipolar but not unipolar depression. The results of this preliminary study raise the possibility that psychomotor retardation in bipolar disorder is accompanied by, if not an outcome of, catecholamine overdrive. This view may be congruent with imaging findings that suggest excessive excitability or failure of inhibition in the motor control systems of bipolar patients. Indeed, at a speculative level, it has long been thought that catatonia, which may be viewed as an extreme form of psychomotor retardation, reflects an internal state of excessive arousal, rapidly reversed by interventions with sedative or barbiturate properties (amobarbital, lorazepam, ECT).

Motor Skills

Traditional neuropsychological evaluations have placed little emphasis on assessment of reaction time per se. This situation is changing rapidly with the increasing use of computerized neuropsychological batteries, which allow more readily for trial-by-trial computation of reaction time. Instead, psychomotor function has typically been assessed with a range of performance measures that are sensitive to the dexterity or accuracy of motor execution, as well as speed. In the studies contributing to our meta-analysis, the psychomotor tasks employed included the Purdue Pegboard, Pursuit Rotor, mirror writing, and motor sequencing tasks, among others. Given this diversity of tasks, a deficit in psychomotor function may reflect some fundamental or general impairment in motor execution or output.

Figure 9–6 presents the findings on psychomotor function from our meta-analysis. It is evident that despite the diversity of tasks, there was a consistent effect across all studies, with bipolar samples showing impaired performance relative to healthy participants (overall effect size = 0.55, SE = 0.18, z = 3.12, p = .002). This effect is significant when the analysis is restricted to studies of patients in remission; the magnitude of the deficit in psychomotor function is near that for PIQ.

The source of the motor abnormalities seen in mood disorders is still unknown. In fact, relatively little work has been done to better characterize the phenomenology of this motor disturbance. Exquisite methodologies have been

Figure 9–6. Meta-analysis of psychomotor measures. Effect sizes (Hedges' G) are presented for individual study comparisons of a bipolar sample with healthy controls, as well as for samples of bipolar patients in remission, depression, mixed state, or mania and across all studies. Squares = confidence interval; circles = mean.

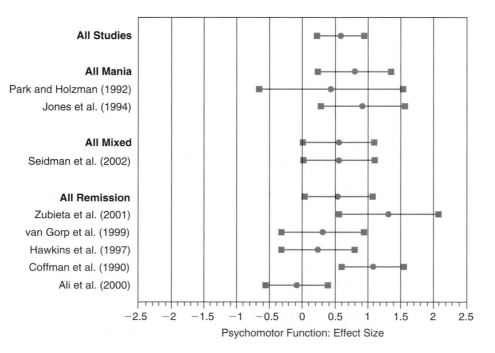

developed to assay components of motor control, but they have rarely been applied to mood disorder samples.

There are suggestions of a lateralized component to the motor disturbances seen in mood disorders. Indeed, there have been isolated reports of individuals whose handedness covaried with the phase of bipolar illness (depression, euthymia, mania). However, the relationship between handedness and bipolar illness is far from clear. Various researchers have reported that the frequency of left-handedness in mood disorders is increased (Fleminger et al., 1977), decreased (Merrin, 1984; Yan et al., 1985), or unchanged (Merrin, 1984; Yan et al., 1985). Sackeim and Decina (1983) took a different approach to this issue. They examined the possibility that handedness moderates genetic factors in the transmission of bipolar disorder. They found that the handedness of bipolar patients was associated with family history of affective disorder and not with family history of sinistrality. Among the bipolar-I subgroup, for example, 49 percent of strongly right-handed patients had a positive family history of affective disorder, compared with 89 percent of weakly right-handed and left-handed patients.

The possibility of a lateralized dimension to the motor disturbance of bipolar disorder is supported by the results of studies examining grip strength. Flor-Henry and Yeudall (1979) found that patients in either the manic or depressive phase of mood disturbance showed greater right-hand than left-hand grip strength, implicating right hemisphere dysfunction. They also found that speed of finger tapping was reduced primarily in the left hand. Merrin (1984) obtained similar results with respect to grip strength, and the asymmetry distinguished mood disorder patients from both patients with schizophrenia and normal controls. Merrin observed that patients with bipolar disorder and psychotic features were most likely to show the asymmetry. More recently, it was found that instability in maintaining stable force with the index finger placed on a strain gauge was greater for the left than the right hand in patients with bipolar disorder, whereas the opposite was true in patients with schizophrenia (Lohr and Caligiuri, 1995, 1997). These scattered results, along with the imaging findings in bipolar patients showing lateralized disturbances in activation patterns during motor tasks (Caligiuri et al., 2003, 2004), point to the need for systematic study of motor asymmetry.

Spontaneous Activity

Routine clinical evaluations of psychomotor disturbance and those conducted using formal rating instruments typically address a different level of behavior from that assessed with neuropsychological or information processing measures. For example, the CORE is a well-studied instrument that quantifies the extent of psychomotor disturbance. Box 9–1 lists the 18 behavioral manifestations assessed by

---

BOX 9–1.   Items in the CORE Measure of Psychomotor Disturbance

- Facial immobility (average across the interview)
- Postural slumping (average across the interview)
- Noninteractiveness (ability to respond to the social cues in the interview)
- Nonreactivity (rate any episode, not duration through the interview)
- Facial apprehension (rate any episode or fixed expression)
- Delay in responding verbally (average across the interview)
- Length of verbal responses
- Inattentiveness
- Facial agitation (movement; rate any episode—intensity rather than duration)
- Body immobility (amount, not speed; average across the interview)
- Motor agitation (rate any episode; intensity rather than persistence)
- Poverty of associations (ability to elaborate)
- Slowed movement (speed, not amount; average across the interview)
- Verbal stereotypy (rate any episode)
- Delay in motor activity (average across the interview)
- Impaired spontaneity of talk (ability to initiate conversation)
- Slowing of speech rate (average across the interview)
- Stereotyped movements (rate any episode)

---

the CORE. These aspects of psychomotor function are considerably more diverse than those assessed with the more atomistic approach of neuropsychological measurement. Further, these abnormalities are assessed in the normal course of interaction and not in relation to specific test demands. Of course, this sign- or symptom-based approach to assessment assumes a conceptualization of the boundaries and constituents of psychomotor disturbance. There would likely be strong consensus that some of the signs or symptoms in Box 9–1, such as facial immobility, delay in responding verbally, and slowed movement, reflect aspects of the construct. On the other hand, there could be considerable debate about the inclusion of other signs or symptoms, such as nonreactivity (lack of interest or pleasure), inattentiveness, and verbal stereotypy, in assessing the severity of psychomotor disturbance.

Parker and colleagues (1993, 1995a, 2000) contended that the assessment of signs and symptoms of psychomotor disturbance is of special importance in mood disorders. Specifically, they argued that such disturbance accounts for the lion's share of the variance in the diagnosis of melancholia. Melancholic and nonmelancholic depressed patients differ markedly in CORE scores, with the endogenity of symptoms accounting for a smaller portion of the variance.[8] Parker and colleagues claimed that the fundamental symptomalogical characteristic of the melancholic patient is psychomotor disturbance. They also found that the severity of psychomotor disturbance has predictive value with regard to treatment outcome with ECT and medications (Hickie et al., 1990b, 1996; Parker and Hadzi-Pavlovic, 1993), and that the psychomotor disturbance in melancholic unipolar patients shares features with the bradykinesia of Parkinson's disease in demonstrating difficulties with the initiation of movement in the absence of external cues (Austin et al., 2000; Rogers et al., 2000). The theoretical importance of some of these findings is challenged by the notion that the broad definition of psychomotor disturbance incorporates assessment of cardinal features of melancholia (such as lack of mood reactivity) that may not reflect psychomotor abnormalities. Thus the associations between the CORE and melancholic diagnosis may be partly tautological, and the linkage to treatment outcome could conceivably be associated with items influenced by melancholic manifestations that do not reflect psychomotor disturbance (e.g., inattentiveness).

A recent study contrasted the CORE ratings of bipolar and unipolar depressed patients. Parker and colleagues (2000) compared 904 unipolar and 83 bipolar patients using three methods for subtyping melancholia (DSM, clinical classification, and CORE). With all three methods, bipolar patients were considerably more likely to be diagnosed with melancholia and psychotic depression. Prevalence of psychomotor disturbance and pathological guilt were the signs or symptoms that distinguished the groups.

While it can be argued that studies of reaction time and other aspects of information processing may provide too narrow a view of psychomotor disturbance, it is also true that the use of rating scales such as the CORE is limited in that ratings may be contaminated by patient behavior reflective of domains other than psychomotor disturbance. Patient reports of lack of interest, loss of pleasure, or marked psychic anxiety may affect ratings of psychomotor disturbance. An alternative approach is to examine objective measures that reflect broader aspects of psychomotor function. Two such measures examine spontaneous activity and speech rate.

Various devices are available for continuous recording of the amount of motor activity. For example, activity monitors, worn like a wrist watch, can provide 24-hour data on fluctuation in movements of the wrist or arm. The potential utility of this approach is illustrated by findings in movement disorders. Although Huntington's disease is characterized by chorea, patients with this disorder have shown less daytime spontaneous movement than healthy controls. Further, this hypokinesia correlates cross-sectionally with impairment in voluntary movement, with disturbed posture and gait, and most robustly with reduced functional capacity (van Vugt et al., 2001). Over a 2-year follow-up period, van Vugt and colleagues (2001) also found that spontaneous activity remained unchanged in clinically stable patients, but worsened in those who deteriorated in functional capacity. Thus in this context, hypokinesia, as assessed by activity monitoring, showed a strong relationship with functional impairment.

A set of small-group comparisons reported by Kupfer and colleagues led to a number of explicit hypotheses about the patterns of gross motor activity in depression and mania.[9] These investigators suggested that (1) manic patients have higher activity levels than severely agitated depressed patients; (2) unipolar depressed patients have higher activity levels than bipolar depressed patients; (3) clinical remission in depression is accompanied by an increase in activity levels; and (4) manic patients manifest their highest activity levels in the late evening and early nighttime, whereas hypomanic patients peak during the daytime (see Chapter 2 for a discussion of the overlap between agitated depressive and mixed hypomanic states). These observations were based on small subgroups; lacked comparison with a normal control group; and were derived from work on a specialized inpatient unit at the National Institutes of Health (NIH), where hospital routine and regimentation may have affected activity levels. While there has been surprisingly limited further research in this area since the mid-1970s, the additional studies that have been done have substantially clarified the nature of the deficit in spontaneous activity during episodes of major depression.

In a study by Wolff and colleagues (1985), a group of 18 normal controls was housed on the same ward and shared in the same activities as a group of 30 euthymic patients (25 bipolar, 5 unipolar). In addition, 27 patients were studied through at least two phases of illness (depression, euthymia, or mania); the depressed state was consistently associated with lower 24-hour levels of activity than euthymia. This difference was significant for the within-subject comparison during daytime but not nighttime periods. Mania was associated with higher activity levels than depression, with the difference seen mainly in the late evening and nighttime hours (7:00 PM to 4:00 AM). Although mania tended to be associated with higher levels than euthymia, none of these comparisons were significant; however, the sample size for comparisons with euthymia was substantially smaller for mania ($n = 11$) than for depression ($n = 23$). Of special note is that, in comparison with controls, euthymic patients still manifested lower 24-hour activity levels, attributable mainly to the daytime period (2:00 PM to 12:00 AM).

Royant-Parola and colleagues (1986) followed a group of 12 patients with major depression, monitoring their activity throughout a hospital stay. In addition to the amount of activity, they assessed duration of immobility. Activity troughs and immobility peaks were bunched before noon and around 3:00 PM. With remission, activity levels increased, and immobility decreased. The authors suggested that immobility is a particularly sensitive measure, especially for patients with agitated depression, and that daytime manifestation may reflect release of an ultradian sleep–wake rhythm in major depression (see Chapter 16).

A reduction in daytime spontaneous activity does not appear to be an artifact of concomitant medications. Volkers and colleagues (2003) compared 67 unmedicated unipolar depressed patients with 64 matched healthy controls. Relative to the control sample, the patient group showed lower activity levels in daytime and higher activity levels and reduced immobility during sleep. It is not known whether this shift toward increased activity levels at night in depressed and manic samples contributes to or is an outcome of disrupted sleep, or both phenomena reflect the same underlying disturbance in rhythmicity.

As noted, these studies of spontaneous activity in mood disorders were conducted in inpatient samples, often with highly treatment-resistant patients. The generalizability of their findings to broader clinical populations was recently tested. Iverson (2004) conducted activity monitoring among 48 depressed patients being seen in primary care and 25 controls with general medical conditions. The depressed group was divided by a median split in scores on the Beck Depression Inventory (BDI) II (Beck et al., 1996). Patients with higher BDI scores had lower activity levels than the other depressed patients and the control group; this effect was most marked during 12:00 PM to 6:00 PM, in line with previous findings in the depressed state. However, the possibility of distinct subgroups was raised in a pilot study of geriatric patients with unipolar major depression. Teicher and colleagues (1988) compared eight geriatric depressed inpatients with eight elderly controls studied in similar settings and found that the depressed group had 29 percent higher mean total 24-hour activity levels, with no difference in circadian amplitude or frequency. Daily peak activity averaged slightly more than 2 hours later in the depressed sample, and the degree of this delay correlated with serum cortisol levels at 4:00 PM after earlier administration of dexamethasone. The heightened activity levels in this small geriatric sample contrast with the findings in unipolar and bipolar adult samples.

Overall, the findings in this area are consistent in indicating that episodes of major depression, whether bipolar or unipolar, are associated with reduced 24-hour activity, especially during daytime hours, and perhaps most markedly during the period 12:00 PM to 6:00 PM. There are suggestions in the study findings that bipolar depressed patients

manifest greater reductions in spontaneous activity than do unipolar patients, but work in this area with bipolar disorder has been limited in recent years. The evidence is robust and consistent that spontaneous activity levels improve with remission from the depressed state, although it is possible that this improvement fails to reach the levels of healthy controls. It is unknown whether the putative residual deficit is associated with the severity of residual depressive symptoms or is independent. The limited evidence indicates that mania is associated with increased activity levels relative to those of depressed patients, especially during the nighttime. However, it is not clear that the increase associated with mania exceeds the values obtained in healthy controls.

Clinical observation of psychomotor disturbance led to the original hypothesis that psychomotor retardation is more common and/or more severe in bipolar than unipolar patients (Kotin and Goodwin, 1972; Dunner et al., 1976). However, the need to ground such observations in objective measures is reflected in conflicting results obtained with the CORE. Mitchell and colleagues (1992) compared 27 age- and sex-matched pairs of unipolar and bipolar patients who met criteria for melancholia based on several diagnostic schemes. Bipolar patients were less likely to have slowed movement. In general, items reflecting psychomotor retardation were less common and agitation was more common in the bipolar cohort. In contrast, almost a decade later, Mitchell and colleagues (2001) compared the clinical features of 39 pairs of bipolar and unipolar patients using a similar methodology. The bipolar patients were more likely than the unipolar patients to manifest psychomotor-related melancholic features and symptoms of atypical depression. The authors suggested that psychomotor retardation, atypical features, and, less commonly, psychosis constitute the clinical signature of bipolar depression.

Speech Rate

Speech is a motor act. Clinically, it is common to observe severely depressed patients speaking in a halting, slow manner with frequent pauses, and often with a weak or raspy voice. It is also clear that manic patients often have racing speech along with racing ideas. Thus it is an empirical matter whether objective analysis of speech and voice characteristics will reveal abnormalities associated with mood disorders and/or provide information of prognostic significance.

The small literature in this area has presented consistent findings. The most common paradigm has been to examine automatic speech, as in counting from 1 to 10, where cognitive load is minimal,[10] although there have also been studies that involved taking samples of natural speech, as might occur during a diagnostic interview (Bouhuys and Mulder-Hajonides van der Meulen, 1984; Alpert et al.,

2001; Cannizzaro et al., 2004). The most common dependent measure has been speech pause time (SPT), the duration of the silent interval between phonations. Szabadi and colleagues (1976) and later Greden and colleagues (Greden and Carroll, 1980; Greden et al., 1981; Greden, 1982) first claimed that SPT was elongated in major depression without a change in phonation time, and that SPT shortened with clinical remission. These claims have received substantial support and have been extended to bipolar depressed patients. SPT has shown significant associations with depression severity, the Widlocher scale (Widlocher, 1983) for assessing psychomotor retardation, and reaction time.[11] Other aspects of speech, including total speaking time, various quantitative features of fundamental frequency and pitch, and speed of voice change, have shown less consistent associations with mood disorders. There is surprisingly little information on the impact of manic states on these measures, and comparisons of unipolar and bipolar depressed patients have shown limited power.

Attention

Impaired attention and insufficient motivation are the two most common reasons given for the pattern of widespread neuropsychological deficit in mood disorders (Miller, 1975; Bearden et al., 2001). To the extent that motivational impairments resolve with remission of depression or mania, persistent neuropsychological impairments are unlikely to be due to motivational factors. Attentional processes are in many respects the gateway to learning, memory, and other higher cognitive processes. While some forms of learning (e.g., procedural learning) undoubtedly occur outside of awareness and do not depend on the integrity of attentional processes, such is not the case for much of our knowledge of ourselves and the world.

Attention is a complex concept that encompasses multiple distinct processes. The concept of working memory denotes the capacity to hold in awareness for a limited time a limited number of visual or auditory representations. This type of attentional process, as in "keeping in mind" a telephone number, can be assessed with various "span" tasks, in which patients recall or recognize a serial list of digits, letters, or shapes just presented. In contrast, the capacity to detect a rarely occurring target is the form of attention commonly referred to as vigilance. The classic example here is the air traffic controller who monitors a screen for representations of two aircraft on a collision course. Although this event is infrequent, detecting its occurrence is of obvious importance. In psychiatric research, vigilance is commonly assessed with the Continuous Performance Test (CPT), originally developed by Beck and colleagues (1956) to detect lapses in attention among epilepsy patients. Another form of attention concerns freedom from distraction

or interference. The capacity to carry out more than one task simultaneously requires that one split attention between tasks (e.g., speaking on the phone while driving) or rapidly shift attention from one task to another. One method of assessing distractibility involves using dichotic listening; individuals must monitor for the occurrence of a target embedded in information delivered to one ear (as in vigilance tasks) but with other, sometimes conflicting, information presented to the other ear. In this context, freedom from distractibility involves the capacity to disattend to irrelevant but competing information channels. A similar phenomenon is tapped by the Stroop test. In one condition of this test, individuals identify the color of nonmeaningful stimuli, such as a series of X's. In another condition, they report the color of visual stimuli that are color names. These names may be in conflict with the appearance of the stimuli. For example, the word "green" may be presented for a stimulus in the color blue. The interference produced by such color–color word conflict is assessed by comparing reaction time in this condition with that for simple color naming. Disattending to the meaning of the word and focusing only on the color would optimize performance on the Stroop test.

It has long been thought that attentional processes are impaired in episodes of major depression in a state-dependent fashion (Cronholm and Ottosson, 1961; Sternberg and Jarvik, 1976) and that attentional deficits limit the extent to which learning may occur. Meta-analyses have consistently shown that attention and learning are among the most markedly impaired functions in episodes of major depression (Zakzanis et al., 1998).

Figure 9–7 presents the results of our meta-analysis of attentional measures in studies of bipolar disorder. The effect size (Hedges' G)[J] across all studies was 0.64 (SE = 0.063, $p < .001$) and was significant for studies of depression (effect size = 0.61, SE = 0.28, $p < .03$), mania (effect size = 0.75, SE = 0.15, $p < .001$), mixed states (effect size = 0.74, SE = 0.12, $p < .001$), and remission (effect size = 0.54, SE = 0.10, $p < .001$). While the effect size was smallest for studies of remitted patients and highest for studies of the manic state, formal testing failed to reveal a significant difference among the groups. Indeed, contrary to the notion that attentional disturbance is purely state dependent, deficits in this domain relative to healthy controls were seen in virtually all studies of patients in remission. This has been demonstrated in more recent studies of attentional deficits in euthymic patients as well.[12] A similar pattern of attentional deficits has been found in bipolar children and adolescents (see the review by Kyte et al., 2006; Kolur et al., 2006).

Our analysis of effects on attention involved 212 comparisons from 39 studies. Given that attentional processes are heterogeneous and are sampled by tasks differing radically

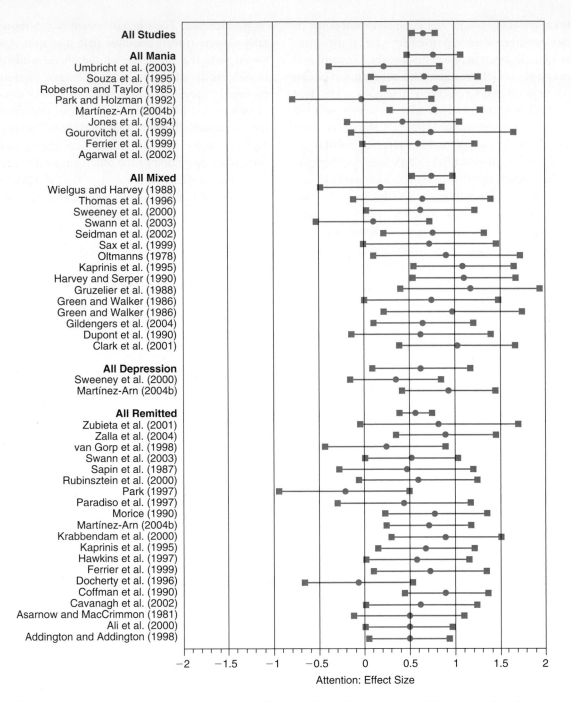

Figure 9–7. Meta-analysis of attention measures. Effect sizes (Hedges' G) are presented for individual study comparisons of a bipolar sample with healthy controls, as well as for samples of bipolar patients in remission, depression, mixed state, or mania and across all studies. Squares = confidence interval; circles = mean.

in their cognitive demands, averaging across distinct attentional measures could obscure more discrete patterns of deficit. Therefore, the analyses were predated for studies of patients in remission and for all studies as a function of the specific neuropsychological procedure used to evaluate attention. As seen in Figure 9–8, although the number of studies contributing to results for individual tests is often small, a consistent pattern is evident. Except for working-memory

tasks, all other tests showed a consistent deficit in both the remitted state and across remission and the phases of bipolar illness. Indeed, except for cancellation tasks, the effect sizes are uniform for the remaining tasks and essentially equivalent both for studies restricted to remission and for all studies. The failure to find a deficit in working memory may be related to the small number of studies that addressed this area and to the use of simple tasks, such as matching to sample (which may produce floor effects), to assess working memory. On the other hand, Harmer and colleagues (2002) noted that disturbance in sustained attention is a consistent finding in remitted bipolar patients, but that many vigilance tasks contain working components. By using tests of sustained attention that did and did not draw on working memory, they were able to demonstrate that the impairment in sustained attention did not derive from or depend on impairment in working memory.

Cancellation procedures require that targets embedded in an array of targets and foils be crossed out, with the rates of target identification (hits) relative to false identification (commission errors or false alarms) as the measure of performance accuracy. In brain-damaged individuals, right parietal injury is especially likely to disrupt cancellation performance, often producing a pattern of hemispatial neglect whereby failure to identify targets (false-negative errors) is overrepresented on the left side of arrays (Mesulam, 2000). While there was a robust effect size for deficits on cancellation tasks in patients in remission (effect size = 0.87, SE = 0.20, $p < .001$), the effect was even more robust when studies of patients in symptomatic states were included (effect size = 0.1.34, SE = 0.37, $p < .001$). This difference is due to the three studies of mania, which produced an especially high effect size (1.96, SE = 0.84). Again, the small number of studies providing cancellation test data calls for caution in placing emphasis on this specification. Rather, the conclusion most justified from the findings summarized in Figures 9–7 and 9–8 is that attentional disturbance is broadly manifested in bipolar disorder across multiple instantiations of this cognitive domain. Not only is the magnitude of deficit relatively uniform across tasks, but it is surprisingly uniform across the phases of bipolar illness, including remission. Furthermore, given the centrality of attentional processes to the integrity of many higher-order cognitive processes, the findings of attentional deficits in remission imply that broad or diffuse cognitive impairment should characterize many individuals with bipolar disorder in remission.

Learning and Memory

Disturbances in learning and memory may be divided into at least six categories of disturbance, each with its own pathoanatomical correlates (Kopelman, 2002; Stern and

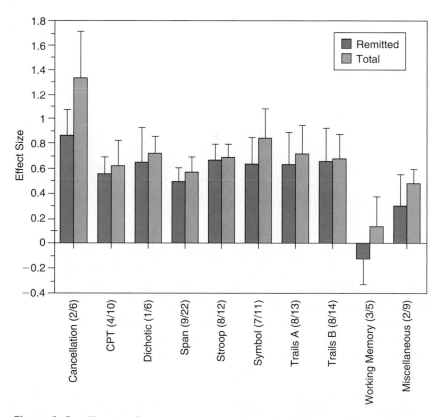

Figure 9–8. Effect sizes for various measures of attention. Effect sizes (Hedges' G) are shown for comparisons of bipolar patients in remission with healthy controls and for the total set of comparisons of bipolar patients across phases of illness with healthy controls. The numbers in parentheses indicate for each attentional measure the number of comparisons of remitted bipolar patients, followed by the total number of comparisons. CPT = Continuous Performance Test.

Sackeim, 2002; Squire et al., 2004): (1) Sensory memory deficits, involving modality-specific failures of preattentive information registration, at times associated with impairment of the reticular activating system or temporal or occipital neocortex; (2) Short-term or primary memory deficits, involving failures of acquisition and brief retention in a limited-capacity store, also associated with disturbance in prefrontal and temporal neocortex; (3) Abnormalities in acquisition and retention of long-term episodic memory, associated with prefrontal, medial temporal, and diencephalic impairment; (4) Disturbances of access to semantic memories, involving failures of storage or retrieval of language or knowledge that is not linked to temporal, sequential, or other contextual (episodic) information, and associated with disruption of posterior association cortex; (5) Deficits in the acquisition and retention of nondeclarative information, as reflected in procedural learning, priming, and classical conditioning (impairments in distinct neural systems are linked to the type of deficit, with striatal impairment tied to deficits in procedural learning and memory); and (6) Disturbances in the use of strategies mediating the acquisition and retention of information, with frontal cortex dysfunction linked to abnormalities in planning, encoding, and retrieval strategies.

When cast in this way, it is apparent that much of the landscape in learning and memory remains unexplored with respect to modulation by mood disorders. Although there has been some work suggesting subtle impairments of sensory and perceptual processes in major depression, including bipolar disorder, especially with respect to auditory processing (Yovell et al., 1995), investigation in this area has been extremely limited. The possibility of sensory memory deficits is largely untested, although not believed to be likely.

There is no evidence that mood disorder patients present with impairments of semantic memory, as tested, for example, by the information subtest of the WAIS-R. Memory for facts appears to be impervious to the effects of mood disorders.

In recent years, nondeclarative aspects of learning and memory, especially procedural learning, have been increasingly represented in neuropsychological batteries (Fig. 9–9). The preliminary evidence in bipolar disorder does not suggest impairment in procedural learning or memory, especially when remitted samples are examined (van Gorp et al., 1999; Altshuler et al., 2004). Preservation in this area may suggest that conscious awareness of mental contents is a property of the cognitive systems disrupted in mood disorders.

Of the six categories of memory disturbance, the focus of research in mood disorders has been on short-term memory, long-term episodic memory, and the strategies

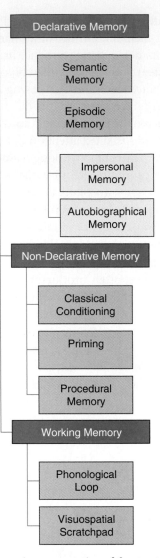

Figure 9–9. Schematic representation of the structure of memory. The main component systems are declarative, nondeclarative, and working memory. Each of these components comprises more elemental subcomponents. (Adapted from Stern and Sackeim, 2002).

used to acquire, retain, and recall declarative information. This focus has concerned almost exclusively the learning and retention of new information. Recall of information about the past, whether pertaining to autobiographical or public events, has rarely been assessed outside of studies of retrograde amnesia after brain insult. To establish a baseline for assessing the extent of amnesia following ECT, the Columbia University group compared unmedicated patients in episodes of major depression (bipolar and unipolar) with healthy controls on the "productivity" of memory for the past. Whether assessed in terms of autobiographical or public events and in terms of remembrance of the event itself versus details about the event, the depressed samples showed small but statistically significant deficits at baseline (McElhiney et al., 1995). The fact that these patients reported slightly fewer memories about themselves or the world could reflect little more than an impairment of the acquisition of information during the affective episode, since what was not learned cannot be remembered. Alternatively, it is also true that what has not taken place cannot be remembered. Relative to the experience of healthy controls, reduced activities during episodes of illness may lead to a relative paucity of events about which to have recent memories. In any case, these data suggest that mood disorder patients are unlikely to have a fundamental or clinically significant deficit in the recall of past events or the details of past events. Furthermore, McElhiney and colleagues (1995) found no indication of a bias in depressed samples toward differential recall of negatively charged events.

Short-Term Memory

The distinction between short-term and long-term memory is arbitrary, and is usually taken as representing the methodological distinction between memory for new information tested after a very short delay (usually less than 10 seconds) and after longer delays (tens of seconds to years) (Wickelgren, 1973). This distinction is consequential because holding information in short-term memory is thought to be mediated by prefrontal working-memory processes, while the consolidation and retention of this information are determined by the integrity of the medial temporal lobe and other structures. The distinction is reflected in the common experience of not being able to reproduce a phone number when attention is directed away. In the absence of continual rehearsal, some information is lost, and in the case of bilateral hippocampal damage, retention of new declarative information may be limited to the period of rehearsal. Retention of new information over delays greater than tens of seconds depends on the integrity of consolidation and retrieval processes that are thought to involve initially the hippocampus and other structures.

By far the most common method for assessing short-term memory has involved forward and backward auditory digit span procedures, although word, letter, block, and shape span tasks are also available (Lezak, 1995; Spreen and Strauss, 1998). The early literature is not consistent in addressing the elemental question of whether auditory digit span performance is abnormal in mood disorders.[13] However, as seen in Figure 9–8, more recent studies comparing patients with bipolar disorder and healthy controls have revealed a consistent deficit in the performance of span tasks, auditory or visual, and pertaining to digits, words, or shapes. Across 22 studies and all phases of bipolar disorder, the pooled effect size for this comparison was moderate: 0.58 (SE = 0.12, $p < .001$). In the 9 studies contrasting patients in remission, the effect size was 0.50 (SE = 0.11, $p < .001$).

It is conceivable that the impairment of span performance is specific to procedures not involving auditory presentation of digits. Baddeley (1986) proposed that the phonological loop challenged by digit span tasks is distinct from a visuospatial scratch pad, with both being key aspects of working or short-term memory (see Fig. 9–9). However, no differences are seen in a comparison of effect sizes in studies using digit span and those using other span procedures. Thus the conclusion is justified that bipolar patients, whether in remission or not, have a deficit in short-term memory, as reflected in span performance. This deficit is interpreted as reflecting impaired attention.

Verbal learning tasks present another context for assessing the integrity of short-term memory. However, recall or recognition after a single presentation of a list relies on both short- and long-term processes. This point is supported by the serial position effect, in which recall is best for the early (primacy effect) and late (recency effect) items in a list and poorest for the middle ones (Bayley et al., 2000). The recency effect reflects the integrity of short-term memory given the minimal interval between presentation of the last items on the list and recall. The primacy effect reflects the contribution of transfer to long-term memory and the consolidation process. Since many of the reports on learning in bipolar illness concern cumulative performance in recalling a list during repeated testing over several trials, such procedures, while involving minimal retention intervals since the last presentation of a list, nonetheless rely heavily on long-term memory.

Figure 9–10 illustrates the effect sizes obtained in comparisons of patients with bipolar disorder and healthy controls on learning tasks, both verbal and nonverbal. Across all studies, the effect size is 0.91 (SE = 0.11, $p < .001$). In comparisons restricted to remitted patients, the effect size is 0.81 (SE = 0.15, $p < .001$).

Without question, bipolar disorder is associated with a marked deficit in the acquisition of new information. This deficit is seen in all phases of the illness, and its magnitude does not appear to be lessened among patients in remission. However, cross-sectional comparison should be used only to establish the existence of deficits in specific phases of the disorder. Whether the deficits are truly comparable in mania, depression, or remission requires within-subject longitudinal investigation. For example, the reduced noise of measurement involved in neuropsychological assessment of remitted as opposed to acutely ill patients can inflate effect sizes indicating deficits in remission. Furthermore, it is common to evaluate clinical samples in a medication-free state when acutely ill at baseline, but to evaluate patients in remission who are medicated. Such a confound could also intensify the deficits observed in remitted patients.

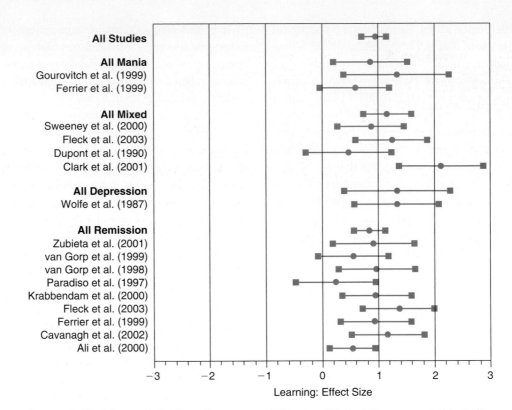

Figure 9–10. Meta-analysis of learning measures. Effect sizes (Hedges' G) are presented for individual study comparisons of a bipolar sample with healthy controls, as well as for samples of bipolar patients in remission, depression, mixed state, or mania and across all studies. Squares = confidence interval; circles = mean.

There has been very little investigation into bipolar-I vs. bipolar-II differences in attention, verbal learning and memory, and executive functioning. Recently, Torrent and colleagues (2006) compared 71 euthymic bipolar patients (38 bipolar-I, 33 bipolar-II) with 35 healthy controls on a battery of cognitive tasks. Both bipolar groups showed significant deficits in working memory, attention, and executive functions, with bipolar-II patients performing at a level between the bipolar-I patients and the healthy controls. Possibly confounding the results, bipolar-I patients were more likely to be taking lithium, carbamazepine, and/or antipsychotics; bipolar-II patients were more likely to be taking antidepressants. It is unclear which patients were taking more than one medication or what effects the medications may have had on performance.

Long-Term Memory

In recent years, it has been claimed that memory is the domain demonstrating the greatest impairment in mood disorders. Literature reviews and meta-analyses have indicated that relative to healthy controls, patients in an episode of major depression (bipolar or unipolar) manifest markedly inferior performance on tests involving the recall or recognition of information over a substantial delay or after

substantial training (Burt et al., 1995; Zakzanis et al., 1998). Further, it has been suggested that in recurrent unipolar disorder, lifetime duration of the depressive state is associated with both hippocampal atrophy and verbal memory deficits (Sheline et al., 1996, 1999). In line with this view, there is preliminary evidence that elderly bipolar patients show greater deterioration in memory processes than do elderly unipolar patients (Burt et al., 2000). Thus it would appear safe to conclude that long-term memory is especially impaired, that the impairment intensifies with disease progression, and that the impairment likely reflects dysfunction in medial temporal lobe structures.

The classic formulation of deficits in learning and memory in mood disorders presents a quite different view. Cronholm and Ottosson (1963) asserted that the depressed state is associated with a reduced capacity to acquire new information, but with no impact on the capacity to retain the information once it has been acquired. Thus in their work, patients were found to be notably deficient in learning verbal and nonverbal paired associates, but did not show proportionately greater loss of what was originally learned over a delay. In another influential study, Sternberg and Jarvik (1976) used similar tasks and also found that patients in an episode of major depression performed more poorly than controls on learning but not on retention, as measured by a "forgetting score," the mathematical difference in the number of items recalled before and after a delay. Following a pharmacological trial, the extent of clinical improvement covaried with improved learning (immediate memory).

One difficulty with this early work is that the integrity of long-term memory was assessed using a forgetting score that did not account for differences in the amount of material learned. Clearly the more one learns, the more material is available for forgetting. Steif and colleagues (1986a) raised conceptual and empirical issues in the assessment of these constructs. Despite more stringent controls, they also found that the primary deficit distinguishing unmedicated, depressed patients from controls was the learning or acquisition of new information, as opposed to the retention of what had been learned. Indeed, with retesting after a course of ECT, the authors were able to demonstrate a double dissociation. Whereas the state of depression involved impairment in learning and not retention, after ECT patients had a deficit in the retention of newly learned information, with no impact on learning. This type of effect is illustrated in Figure 9–11.

Figure 9–11. Dissociation in the effects of electroconvulsive therapy (ECT) on learning and retention of new information. Patients were randomly assigned to low- or high-dosage bilateral (BL) or right unilateral (RUL) ECT. Before and immediately after the course, they were administered a test of verbal list learning and retention using the selective reminding procedure (Buschke, 1973). Little change in immediate learning was seen when post-ECT values were compared with baseline values, with the exception of possible improvement in the low-dose RUL ECT group. In contrast, both low- and high-dose BL ECT resulted in clear-cut deficits in free recall of the list after a delay. The results illustrate the selective effect of ECT on the retention of newly learned information, which is thought to be due to a deficit in consolidation. (*Source*: Sackeim et al., 1993.)

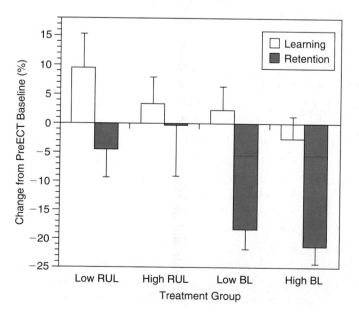

Why, then, are there conflicting views, with some recent work emphasizing long-term memory as a source of impairment and earlier work emphasizing impaired learning? It is quite likely that this apparent conflict stems from the fact that attentional deficits compromise the intake of information and disrupt learning. In turn, if little is learned, little can be remembered. For the most part, the work on impaired memory in depression has not taken into account the earlier stages of processing and their contributions. Thus in a concrete sense, being able to report only 3 of 15 items on a list after a 2-hour delay could reflect anterograde amnesia if 12 items were recalled during learning. On the other hand, if only 4 or 5 items were learned, impaired acquisition of the information would be the central deficit.

Figure 9–12 presents the effect sizes for comparisons of bipolar patients with healthy controls on a variety of memory measures. While the effect sizes for the subgroups and across all studies are substantial, they are virtually identical to the values obtained when assessing learning only (see Fig. 9–9). Again, it is hazardous to draw conclusions about within-subject effects using cross-sectional data. Nonetheless, the most parsimonious account of this literature is that impaired attention, which persists in remitted patients, is the major factor determining the adequacy of learning and memory.

Mediational Processes

Many processes determine whether a particular memory will be retrieved. Some of these processes relate to the infrastructure of memory, so that there is a contrast, for example, between deficits in the storage of information as assessed by recognition tasks and in the active retrieval of information as assessed by recall performance. Other processes, such as the organization imposed on newly presented information and the resultant depth of encoding, may determine whether information is learned and/or stored. Still other factors affect not so much whether new information will be retained, but how the choice is made whether to recall events from the past. For example, the issue is hotly debated as to whether being in the depressed or manic state biases retrieval toward memories that share the same affective valence. This form of mood-congruence effect addresses the question of whether depressed patients have preferential access to or are biased to retrieve negatively evaluated information.

Storage Versus Retrieval.   Assuming that information is acquired, failure to recall can be due to a breakdown either in consolidation or storage or in retrieval. Because recognition of information is far less demanding of retrieval processes but is dependent on the adequacy of storage, an

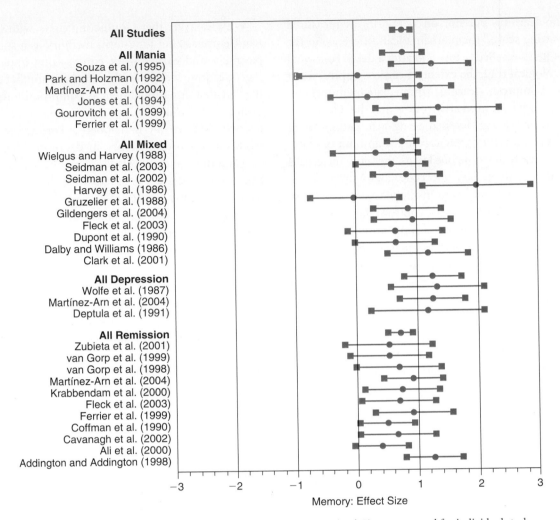

Figure 9–12. Meta-analysis of memory measures. Effect sizes (Hedges' G) are presented for individual study comparisons of a bipolar sample with healthy controls, as well as for samples of bipolar patients in remission, depression, mixed state, or mania and across all studies. Squares = confidence interval; circles = mean.

asymmetry whereby retrieval is impaired but recognition is intact could suggest a specific impairment in retrieval strategies—either the way information is organized for later retrieval or the way the search strategy is organized. However, recognition is intrinsically easier than retrieval, at least when the same information is tested, and claims of differential deficit are easily confounded with task differences in discriminating power and other psychometric properties.

A few authors have claimed that patients in an episode of major depression have a greater deficit in recall relative to recognition (Weingartner et al., 1977; Frith et al., 1983; Deptula et al., 1991). This work is problematic, however, because of the failure to compare recognition and recall paradigms directly or the lack of psychometric matching. These limitations were overcome by Calev and Erwin (1985), who used a matched-task paradigm. They found that depressed patients performed better on verbal recognition than on recall tasks, whereas healthy controls performed

similarly on both (demonstrating the adequacy of the matching). The recall disturbance was attributable to a reduced ability to organize the retrieval system. Thus, very limited data suggest the possibility of a particular deficit in retrieval processes in mood disorders. This deficit may be an example of a failure to engage in active, effortful processing.

Attention, Effort, and Levels of Processing. The deficits manifested by patients with mood disorders in tasks of learning and memory appear to be attributable largely to attentional dysfunction. Relevant here are well-established models from cognitive psychology that distinguish between automatic and effortful processing[14] and models of depth or levels of processing.[15] In the former models, attention is conceptualized as a limited-capacity resource. Automatic operations make minimal use of this resource and take place without intention or awareness. They do not interfere with ongoing cognitive operations and do not benefit from rehearsal. For example, remembering where one put one's keys is typically an instance of automatic or incidental learning. Typically, one does not consciously attempt to remember this information, and one is usually unaware of learning it. Skill or procedural learning and other nondeclarative forms of memory do not involve explicit, consciously mediated cognitive rehearsal. In contrast, effortful processes require the use of limited attentional capacities and interfere with other cognitive activities. The cognitive operations are initiated voluntarily and benefit from practice.

Similarly, a levels-of-processing approach emphasizes that the amount of attentional capacity allocated to the initial steps of information processing (e.g., encoding) influences the later retrievability of the information. The deeper the level of processing, the greater is the attentional allocation and the better the retrieval. For example, if one's task in listening to a set of words is to determine which words rhyme with a target (acoustic or shallow processing), later memory of the list will be poorer than if the task is to determine whether each word has the same meaning as a target (semantic or deep processing). The two models are convergent in that engaging in greater depth of processing is often an effortful, attention-demanding process.

The notion that individuals in episodes of major depression have a deficit in engaging spontaneously in effortful or deeper levels of processing has received substantial, although not unequivocal (Christensen et al., 1997), support. In a now-classic study, Weingartner and colleagues (1981) found that depressed patients did not differ from healthy controls in recalling words that had been acoustically (shallowly) processed, but were inferior in remembering semantically (deeply) processed words. The control group showed the typical advantage of better recall of the deeply processed words. In contrast, the patient group had equivalent scores on the two tasks, suggesting that despite the difference in task requirements, the patients' encoding on both tasks was shallow.

A second study reported by Weingartner and colleagues (1981) demonstrated that when deep encoding was provided externally on a verbal memory task, depressed patients performed similarly to healthy controls. Essentially, when given a list of random words, a depressed sample was shown to have markedly impaired recall. When presented a word list drawn from discrete semantic categories in which the word order was clustered, however, patients were not distinguishable in recall from healthy controls. Both the extent of categorization of words and the overt clustering within categories determined the magnitude of the difference in recall between patients and controls.

The implication of this work is that depressed patients, when exposed to new material, are less likely than healthy controls to apply preexisting knowledge and impose the organization that facilitates learning and memory. In this respect, the locus of abnormality is at the encoding stage and results in diminished learning. Fundamentally, the depth of encoding and the automatic versus effortful distinctions converge. Imposing organization is an effortful process, and in most circumstances, the automatic versus effortful distinction maps to shallow versus deep processing. This deficit pertains to the set of mediational processes termed by Moscovitch (1994) "working with memory." These processes involve the selection and execution of strategies used to enhance information processing and are thought to be heavily represented in prefrontal cortex. Further, effortful or deeper processing requires the allocation of attentional resources. Thus it is conceivable that the fundamental abnormality resides in an inflexibility or limited capacity of attentional mechanisms rather than difficulties with selecting or applying appropriate strategies for encoding or retrieval. Put another way, it would appear that the depressed state is characterized by a cognitive impairment likely to be most manifest on tasks that require complex processing, effortful processing, and/or independent structuring of information relative to preexisting knowledge.

This remains an active area of investigation, with repeated demonstrations that depressed patients are more likely than healthy controls to engage in shallow and/or noneffortful processing.[16] However, almost all of this work has focused on demonstrating the phenomenon and establishing its boundaries. There is little clarity regarding the neurobiological basis of this abnormality or its implications for therapeutics. Roy-Byrne and colleagues (1986) suggested that the deficit in effortful processing is dopaminergically mediated, but this hypothesis has yet to receive substantial investigation.

One thread in this literature ties the lack of effortful processing to an entirely different domain of behavioral limitation. Cohen and colleagues (1982) found that severity of depressive symptomatology correlated negatively with grip strength, as assessed with a hand dynamometer. Both symptom scores and grip strength correlated with performance on a verbal memory test, with less effort on the motor task being associated with poorer memory scores. The results of this work suggest that in major depression, there is a parallel between the diminished effort in physical activity and the diminished mental effort that results in inattention and lack of structuring of incoming information. Certainly, it would be noteworthy were this the case. While the effort expended in voluntary activity has a voluntary quality, as in how strongly one grips a dynamometer, this is not the conception regarding the mental effort leading to more extensive encoding. The failure to impose organization and process at deeper levels should be viewed as unconscious or automatic. Furthermore, the lack-of-effort analogy does not accord with what may be the most common reason for shallow processing in mood disorders. Under conditions of marked agitation or psychic pain, patients will often indicate that it is a struggle to get through the next 5 minutes, let alone attend to a task. With internal ruminations and marked distress, even reading a newspaper headline can be difficult. Thus it is probable that in some circumstances, the lack of effortful processing is due to the fact that the effort is being expended elsewhere.

It might be thought that this type of deficit in mediational processes should be fully state dependent. Otherwise, we would have to posit that patients with mood disorders engage in "shallow" processing even when in remission. Further, were this defect purely state dependent, it would have a rather limited role in accounting for the learning and memory deficits in patients with mood disorders. As described earlier, there is substantial evidence that attentional, learning, and memory deficits continue largely unabated during remission. Longitudinal investigation in this area has been limited, however. Hammar and colleagues (2003b) found that unipolar patients in a state of major depression were impaired in an effortful but not automatic visual search task. The deficit persisted for at least 6 months despite substantial clinical improvement. Further work of this type is needed.

Mood Congruence.   *Mood congruence* refers to the notion that the efficiency of mnemonic processing is biased by the congruence between the current affective state and the affective tone of the material being remembered. In general, it is believed that dysphoric or negative life events are recalled more easily when individuals are in a depressed state than when they are in a euthymic or manic state (Blaney, 1986).

This phenomenon has been examined mainly in studies using laboratory manipulations, such as rigged experiences of success and failure in completing laboratory tasks. These studies have yielded some evidence that depressed patients can be biased in recalling negative events or can exercise a mnemonic selectivity that emphasizes neutrality over positivity.[17] This type of mediational process, if of general consequence, would affect the content of remembrances, with the implication that this bias toward greater negativity in content may contribute to the monolithic experience of depression, and perhaps also to its maintenance. However, subtle demonstrations of bias in laboratory or real-world settings do not mean that this phenomenon is of general consequence. In intensive interviews regarding autobiographical events, severely depressed patients differ little from healthy controls in the richness of their reports of positive or negative events in their recent and remote past (McElhiney et al., 1995).

Summary

Deficits in learning and memory characterize unipolar depression and bipolar disorder through all its phases. The effect sizes for these deficits are the largest among neuropsychological domains. While it has been common in recent years to assert that episodes of major depression are associated with a memory deficit, there is little evidence that the deficits seen in learning and/or memory processes extend beyond attentional disturbance. This attentional disturbance may be structural in the sense of dysfunction in a limited-capacity store, or perhaps more likely, a disturbance in the allocation of attentional resources. The substantial literature on bipolar patients in remission indicates that the deficits in learning and memory persist during euthymia. There are compelling findings that mood disorder patients in episodes of major depression are more likely to engage in shallow processing and to fail to impose the organization on incoming information that assists in acquisition and retention. This "cognitive laziness" results from a failure of executive function—in this case, the utilization of strategies that facilitate learning and memory. Thus it becomes especially germane to inquire whether there is a more general impairment of executive functions.

Executive Functions

The concept of executive functions became a driving force in much thought about the core deficits in psychopathology, especially schizophrenia and bipolar disorder, starting in the 1980s. Fundamentally, disruption of these functions is deemed responsible for the lack of self-regulation on a variety of dimensions in patients with these disorders. Executive functions perform the brain's housekeeping, strategizing, and oversight roles, and come closest in principle to the neuropsychological concept of a neural homunculus in charge of neural resource allocation and other administrative functions or, perhaps, the concept of will.

The vagueness of definitions and descriptions of executive functions is to be expected given the vast and complex aspects of psychic functioning likely devoted to strategic, integrative, planning, inductive, and deductive activities. Indeed, at one level the type of executive functions involved in optimizing learning strategies by imposing conceptual organization (chunking) on incoming information automatically and without awareness must be quite distinct from the processes involved in making career choices, anticipating danger while driving, or inhibiting a prepotent response. Thus executive functions address our capacity to reason, to anticipate, to shift conceptual or perceptual sets, to solve problems, and so on.

Despite this richness of possibilities, a very limited range of executive functions has been studied in bipolar disorder. Figure 9–13 presents the results of our meta-analysis of comparisons involving executive functions other than reasoning. Tests of reasoning or concept formation were examined separately, partly because they are so strongly dependent on language and verbal abilities; these findings are presented in Figure 9–14. The instruments used most commonly to test the integrity of executive functions are the Wisconsin Card Sort Test (WCST) and the Category Test of the Halstead-Reitan battery. Both involve complex procedures in which individuals derive rules or abstractions from experience. The WCST also assesses the capacity to shift sets upon recognizing that the rules have changed. It is considered a test of executive functions in part because it requires strategic planning, organized searching, use of feedback to shift conceptual set, goal-oriented behavior, and the capacity to inhibit impulsive responding (Spreen and Strauss, 1998). Other instruments used to test executive functions include the Tower of London, which places heavy emphasis on planning (Shallice, 1982) and involves the rearrangement of balls in a vertical column to match a prespecified order using a minimum of moves, attentional set-shifting tasks, and decision-making tasks.

As seen in Figure 9–13, substantial deficits in executive functions were observed in all phases of bipolar disorder. Across the 25 studies contributing data, the overall effect size was 0.79 (SE = 0.13, $p < .001$). In the 14 studies that examined remitted bipolar patients, the effect size was 0.75 (SE = 0.18, $p < .001$), hardly suggestive of a state-dependent effect. Two recent studies also have found pervasive deficits in executive

Figure 9–13. Meta-analysis of executive function measures. Effect sizes (Hedges' G) are presented for individual study comparisons of a bipolar sample with healthy controls, as well as for samples of bipolar patients in remission, depression, mixed state, or mania and across all studies. Squares = confidence interval; circles = mean.

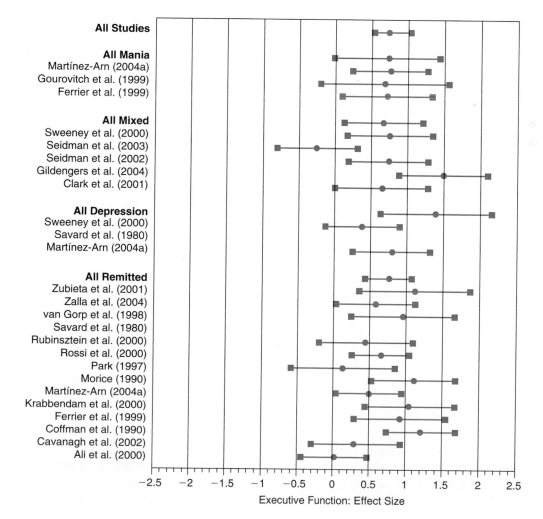

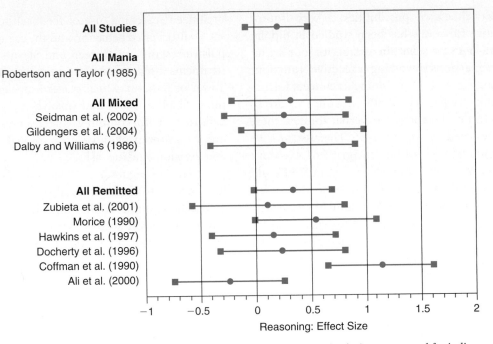

Figure 9–14. Meta-analysis of reasoning measures. Effect sizes (Hedges' G) are presented for individual study comparisons of a bipolar sample with healthy controls, as well as for samples of bipolar patients in remission, depression, mixed state, or mania and across all studies. Squares = confidence interval; circles = mean.

functioning in bipolar patients (Nehra et al., 2006; Robinson et al., 2006).

As in unipolar disorder, then, there is substantial evidence that periods of acute illness in bipolar disorder are associated with diminished executive functions, especially with respect to concept formation and set shifting. Recent studies have demonstrated this as well (Frangore et al., 2005; Goswami et al., 2006), including one that looked at executive functioning in patients with pediatric bipolar disorder (Pavuluri et al., 2006). Imaging studies have shown that, in healthy samples, the procedures examined in this domain result in activation of the dorsolateral prefrontal cortex (DLPFC). Abnormalities in DLPFC function in mood disorders have been reported from the earliest brain imaging studies of cerebral blood flow (CBF) or cerebral metabolic rate (CMR_{glu}), and more than 20 imaging studies have reported inverse relationships between depression severity and DLPFC, CBF, or CMR_{glu}.[18] It is noteworthy that these studies did not include significant sampling of ventral or orbital prefrontal cortex functions, notably inhibition of prepotent responses, as in "go–no go" tasks. In terms of what was studied, there is strong evidence for persistent impairment of executive functions despite remission. Indeed, it is noteworthy that the effect size for remitted patients is equivalent to that for patients in acute affective episodes.

However, inspection of Figure 9–14 suggests that the deficit in executive functions may not be uniform across various component processes. Values for one study (Robertson and Taylor, 1985) were omitted from the figure because they reflected an extreme outlier, in this case manic patients having clearly superior performance on a reasoning task compared with healthy participants. Inclusion of these values would further reduce the evidence for a deficit in reasoning. As it stands, the overall effect size is small, 0.21 ($SE = 0.14$, $p = .15$), and for studies of remitted patients is 0.33 ($SE = 0.18$, $p = .07$). A deficit in reasoning relative to controls was not significant within any of the four subgroups.

The tests that contributed to our meta-analysis on reasoning included the similarities and arithmetic subtests of the WAIS-R and tests of abstraction and concept attainment. Commonly, results of tests of reasoning correlate substantially with verbal abilities. The relative preservation of reasoning skills against a backdrop of marked deficits in other executive functions may reflect a pattern in which cognitive operations that are heavily dependent on language are among the least affected of the higher cognitive functions.

Verbal and Visuospatial Skills

The final cognitive domains subjected to this meta-analysis were verbal and visuospatial skills. Work in the verbal domain has been dominated by tasks assessing controlled oral word association (COWA). Such tests assess the spontaneous production of words beginning with a given letter, usually F, A, or S (FAS test), within a stipulated period of time. Alternatively, the tests may assess production of words as instances of a concept, such as animal naming. Verbal fluency, especially letter fluency, has often been taken as another type of executive function. Indeed, there is evidence that COWA is one of the last measures of prefrontal function to mature, with developmental improvement extending beyond age 12, whereas adult levels are achieved considerably earlier for many other measures (Lewis, 1983). There is some evidence from both imaging and lesion studies that temporal lobe regions may make more of a contribution to category than to letter fluency. However, this distinction and the stronger claim that letter fluency is subserved largely by prefrontal regions are supported only partially by lesion analysis and imaging

activation effects, with exceptional findings suggesting more widely distributed representations.[19]

The copy portion of the Complex Figure Test (Rey, 1941) is the task used most commonly to represent visuospatial functions. This task involves copying a detailed and complex figure, with accuracy of reproduction being scored for 18 portions of the figure. The copying portion of the procedure is followed by delayed reproduction purely from memory. To focus on visuospatial constructional ability, as opposed to visual memory, we included only copy procedures in this domain. Other tests commonly used to sample visuospatial functions are the WAIS-R block design subtest and tests of perceptual organization, such as line orientation, gestalt completion, and embedded figures.

Figures 9–15 and 9–16 present results of our meta-analysis for the verbal and visuospatial domains, respectively. The deficits seen in verbal skills are moderate at best

Figure 9–15. Meta-analysis of verbal skill measures. Effect sizes (Hedges' G) are presented for individual study comparisons of a bipolar sample with healthy controls, as well as for samples of bipolar patients in remission, depression, mixed state, or mania and across all studies. Squares = confidence interval; circles = mean.

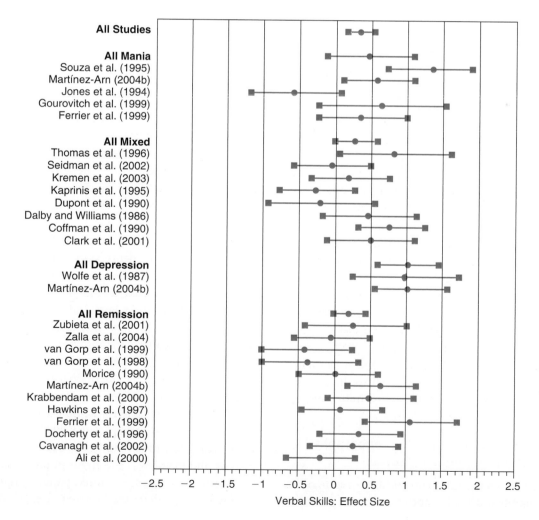

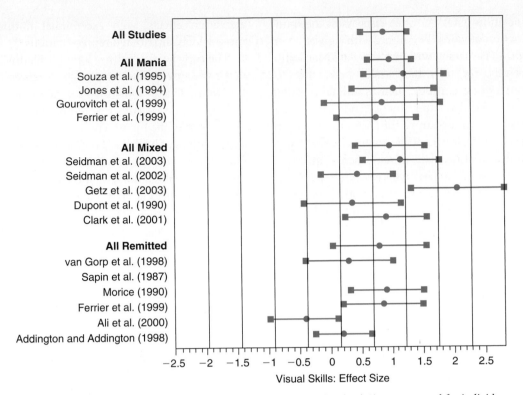

Figure 9–16. Meta-analysis of visual skill measures. Effect sizes (Hedges' G) are presented for individual study comparisons of a bipolar sample with healthy controls, as well as for samples of bipolar patients in remission, depression, mixed state, or mania and across all studies. Squares = confidence interval; circles = mean.

(see Fig. 9–15). The effect size (Hedges' G) for the comparison of bipolar and healthy control groups across all studies ($n = 26$) is 0.35 (SE = 0.09, $p < .001$). However, the effect is not significant across 12 studies of remitted bipolar samples (effect size = 0.22, SE = 0.12, $p = .064$) or 5 studies in mania (effect size = 0.495, SE = 0.31, $p = .11$). Relative to the pattern of widespread impairment across symptomatic and remitted states, verbal skills appear to have been preserved. In the few cases in which bipolar samples had inferior verbal fluency performance relative to healthy controls, the patient groups tended to make more incorrect responses (e.g., repeating the same word) and did not differ in number of responses (Wolfe et al., 1987; Coffman et al., 1990).

A different level of deficit is manifest in Figure 9–16, which summarizes our meta-analysis of visuospatial performance measures. One study (Sapin et al., 1987) was excluded because of an outlying value that only accentuated the deficit in remitted patients. Across all studies, the effect size is 0.65 (SE = 0.18, $p < .001$), and in remitted bipolar patients it is 0.57 (0.28, $p < .01$).

Comparisons across Domains: The Topography of Cognitive Deficit in Bipolar Disorder

Figure 9–17 combines the values on effect size reported for the various cognitive domains and presents the cognitive deficit profiles for the comparisons of depressed, mixed-state manic, and remitted samples with healthy controls, as well as for the comparisons across all phases of illness. The profile is relatively invariant across the phases of illness. Three central points can be made.

First, the same pattern of strengths and weaknesses is seen in remission and during episodes of affective disturbance. This invariance suggests that the core disturbance is state independent. Second, it is often claimed that the magnitude of deficit is generally greatest during mania, still marked during major depression, and least evident in remission. The deficit noted by investigators as residual during remission varied considerably among the studies included in our meta-analysis. Indeed, limited power, differences in the reliability of measurement, and other factors make it likely that different tasks would achieve statistical significance in separating remitted patients from controls. By combining these findings in a meta-analysis, it became evident that the remitted samples generally had the same level of deficit as the acutely ill groups in the areas most disturbed, and perhaps somewhat less marked deficits in the areas most disturbed in the acutely ill groups (e.g., learning and memory). The larger point is that the cognitive deficits observed in remitted patients were not a pale shadow of the deficits seen during affective disturbance, but were substantial, reliable, and of the same distribution as those seen during acutely ill states.

The third point is that against a background of generalized deficit, verbal processes as reflected in VIQ, verbal skills (i.e., verbal fluency), and reasoning are relatively preserved. This novel observation recasts the initial question about the meaning of the VIQ–PIQ discrepancy in bipolar disorder. The deficit in PIQ may not be of special note, and it may not signal, per se, a right-hemisphere abnormality. Rather, the effect sizes for PIQ and visuospatial skills are in the range of those for motor disturbance, attentional deficits, and other domains. What may be consequential is that verbal processes are preserved and, across the phases of illness, show less deterioration than virtually all other higher cognitive processes.

Why might this be, or better yet, what can this tell us about the neurobiology of bipolar illness? First, the fact that deficits in attention and concentration are reliably observed across the phases of bipolar illness means that cognitive impairment must be generalized. This point is underscored by the findings suggesting consistent impairment of executive functions. Attention and concentration may be seen as the fuel of higher cognitive processes, determining the capacity and efficiency limitations on processing. Executive functions determine resource allocation and thus also broadly shape the integrity of cognitive processing. Indeed, with respect to learning, memory, and visuospatial skills, there is little evidence that deficits reflect more than an attentional disturbance. Therefore, rather than positing multiple specific deficits in bipolar disorder, one could hypothesize that a persistent noradrenergic or dopaminergic disturbance gives rise to attentional impairment that in turn produces the widespread, more generalized pattern (Swanson et al., 1998; Cools and Robbins, 2004).

But why do we see the preservation of verbal processes? Surely attentional mechanisms also drive performance in this area. There are several possibilities. First, some of the areas of preservation concern aspects of cognition that are relatively protected against the effects of brain injury. The WAIS-R vocabulary and information subtests are often considered "hold" scores, indices more likely to reflect premorbid abilities than are tests more sensitive to the effects

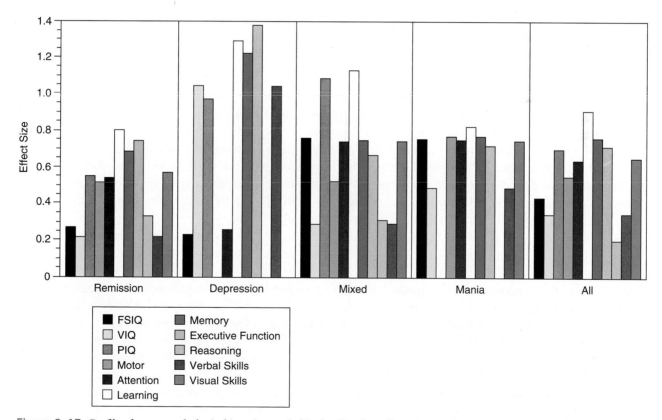

Figure 9–17. Profile of neuropsychological impairment in bipolar disorder. Effect sizes are shown for comparisons of a bipolar group (in remission or in a phase of depression, mixed state, or mania) with healthy controls for 11 cognitive domains. All bipolar subgroups, including remission, show deficits relative to controls. These impairments are most accentuated for the learning, memory, and executive function domains and are pronounced for all domains except those heavily involving verbal skills (verbal IQ, reasoning, and verbal skills). The preservation of verbal skills against a background of generalized impairment may be the salient dissociation. FSIQ = full-scale IQ; PIQ = performance IQ; VIQ = verbal IQ.

of brain damage (Lezak, 1995). These subtests assess semantic memory, or knowledge of facts, which has not been found to be impaired in bipolar disorder. Specifically, these subtests, by posing specific questions, may place few demands on attention or any form of new learning. This view posits, therefore, that the relative preservation of verbal skills is due to their escaping the deleterious and otherwise generalized impact of the core cognitive disturbance, presumably in the area of attention. However, the findings regarding verbal fluency and reasoning may belie this view since it is difficult to argue that attentional processes do not contribute to their performance.

A second alternative is to view this preservation of verbal processes as indicating a disassociation in the cognitive neural systems dysregulated in bipolar disorder. At the grossest level, this view would suggest preservation of left-hemisphere subsystems involved in verbal processing. How this could come about and the neurochemical and/or neurodevelopmental processes responsible for such a dissociation are a matter of speculation.

Finally, this asymmetry may be an endophenotype of bipolar disorder. We should not assume that the topography of cognitive function is a flat playing field in this patient population. As discussed at the outset, there is good reason to suspect that intellectual endowment is distributed differently in the families of bipolar probands than in the general population. Indeed, one of the earliest studies of children at risk found that the VIQ–PIQ discrepancy was robust before the onset of the first affective episode and was most common in children with prodromal symptoms (Decina et al., 1983; Sackeim and Decina, 1983). Thus the genetic transmission of bipolar disorder may confer a relative advantage for verbal processes. The insult that results in manifestation of the disorder may have a rather generalized effect, leading to impairments in multiple domains. This decrease in function is shared relatively equally, and verbal functions appear to be preserved only because their baseline was elevated. Research on the neuropsychological profiles of first-degree relatives of bipolar probands (Keri et al., 2001a) and of monozygotic twins discordant for bipolar disorder (Gourovitch et al., 1999) is in its infancy, but has indicated that impairments are evident in tests of learning and memory but not in verbal skills.

Other Neuropsychological Domains

A number of other cognitive functions have been studied in bipolar disorder, but with insufficient frequency to be included in our meta-analysis. These functions include auditory perception, somatosensory function, pain perception, impulsivity, processing of facial affective displays, and the extent of thought disorder. The paucity of research in these domains indicates a parochialism in the mapping of cognitive

functions in this disorder, with a strong focus on measures of attention, executive functions, and learning and memory. For example, rates of suicide are elevated in bipolar disorder, and diathesis–stress models of suicide often assume that a predisposition for impulsive behavior provides the "diathesis" and acute depressive or manic symptoms the "stress" that results in the act[20] (see Chapter 8). However, there are virtually no longitudinal data on measures of impulsivity or aggression in bipolar disorder, and at the clinical level, impulsivity would not be expected to be invariant, but to be accentuated during manic or mixed states. Further, characterization of the essential deficit as being in the domain of impulsivity or aggressivity may be too narrow.

An especially comprehensive neuropsychological study recently compared the profiles of medication-free depressed patients with a history of a high-lethality suicide attempt, a low-lethality suicide attempt, and no history of suicide attempt, and healthy controls. The cognitive domains sampled included general intellectual functioning, motor functioning, attention, memory, and executive functioning. A discriminant analysis indicated that different dimensions distinguished the total depressed sample from the healthy controls and distinguished the high-lethality attempters from the other patient groups. Impairment in attention and memory distinguished the patients from the controls, again highlighting that a basic attentional disturbance may be a key factor in determining the cognitive sequelae of mood disorders, both unipolar and bipolar. Impaired executive function distinguished high-lethality attempters, with the executive function measures not being restricted to indices of impulsivity. The results of this work raise the possibility that a more broad-based deficit in executive function, perhaps related to self-monitoring functions, is disturbed in individuals with a history of high-lethality suicide attempts.

Recent years have seen a movement away from the study of "cold" cognition to the study of "hot" cognition in bipolar disorder.[21] This distinction is thought to make neuropsychological investigation more ecologically valid and more likely to address core deficits in bipolar disorder. The movement to assess hot cognition is instantiated in studies in which the information being processed, such as facial emotional expression or the meaning of affectively laden words, has affective significance. Thus in both bipolar disorder and schizophrenia, there has been a significant increase in reports on facial emotion discrimination and other aspects of the processing of emotionally laden information. A particular emphasis in this work has been the extent to which such processing is biased by the affective state of patients (depressed versus manic) (Murphy et al., 1999).

Work in this area is insufficiently developed to yield conclusions. A cautionary note is in order, however, especially in light of the enthusiastic recommendations being made to incorporate affective processing tasks in studies of mood disorders. The processes involved in the regulation of mood appear to be wholly independent of the processes that subserve the "reception" of emotion (i.e., the processing of emotionally laden information). As noted earlier, brain injury can result in highly specific deficits in aspects of emotional processing and have no impact on the regulation of mood or emotional expression. Alternatively, there can be marked disturbance in mood without apparent impact on emotional processing. It is unclear to what extent determining that the intonation of a voice is sad differs fundamentally from determining that the speaker is male, that the voice is raspy, and so on. It is clear that the presentation of such stimuli rarely has an impact on affective state. Determining that a voice is sad does not require that one feel sad, and thus these procedures cannot be said to be indirect mood manipulations.

Often the outcome of such investigation is an indication of biased processing on the part of patient subgroups. Using an affective go–no go task, Murphy and colleagues (1999) alternated happy and sad words in blocks as either targets requiring response or distracters requiring inhibition of response. Compared with healthy controls, manic patients were slower to respond to sad but not to happy targets, whereas depressed patients were slower when responding to happy but not to sad targets. Manic patients also had an excess of response inhibition errors (responding to a distracter). Thus, the results of this study suggest a difference between depressed and manic patients in attentional bias as a function of affective valence. This effect was not seen in remitted patients in a subsequent study (Rubinsztein et al., 2000). Note that this effect can be distinguished from mood congruence effects. In the study by Murphy and colleagues (1999), patients were impeded in processing targets that did not correspond to their affective state. Mood congruence phenomena reflect privileged access to evaluations, memories, and so on that are congruent in emotional content with the current mood state.

Nonetheless, there is evidence that current affective state impacts the processing of ongoing affectively charged information. More broadly, mood congruence effects also pertain to the differential retrieval of memories, the attributions made for ongoing positive and negative events, and other aspects of complex cognitive function. For example, the depressed state is frequently characterized by a marked cognitive bias, referred to as depressive realism. When healthy controls, or for that matter patients with schizophrenia, are confronted with success, the tendency is to assume that they caused this outcome, they should be

praised, and the outcome was very good. In contrast, when confronted with failure, healthy controls will often state that the outcome was uncontrollable, they should not be blamed, and it was not so bad anyway. While patients with major depression might be expected to show a reverse bias, to overaccentuate the negative, their attributions tend to be much more even-handed than those of controls, and thus by most accounts, more realistic (Sackeim and Wegner, 1986). Therefore, it is fair to say that the states of depression and euphoria are characterized by a gross alteration in cognitive schema, reflecting diminished or absent self-serving biases in the depressed state (Taylor and Brown, 1988, 1994; Colvin and Block, 1994). If the objective of recent work on hot cognition in mood disorders is to address state-related biases in information processing, it is far from clear that studies of facial emotional identification provide the optimal models.

FACTORS AFFECTING COGNITIVE FUNCTION

Treatment

In many of the studies included in our meta-analysis, bipolar patients were tested in an unmedicated state when depressed or manic, but were medicated when studied in the remitted state. This convention arises from the fact that a period of medication withdrawal in acutely ill patients is considered acceptable before starting a new treatment. Indeed, in some cases such withdrawal is of clinical value. On the other hand, the risks of relapse are so high that withdrawal of treatment in recently remitted patients is unacceptable. Consequently, this pattern introduces a potentially serious confound in much of the neuropsychological and neurobiological investigation of state-independent phenomena in bipolar disorder. Specifically, could the widespread neuropsychological impairment seen in remitted patients be a result of an adverse and generalized cognitive effect of continuation and maintenance treatment? Could lithium, the anticonvulsant medications, or the antidepressants be responsible for this cognitive profile? To the extent that patients in some studies are abruptly withdrawn from psychotropics, what impact does drug withdrawal have on cognitive function?

For example, Martinez-Arán and colleagues (2004a) conducted a comprehensive study of cognitive impairment in euthymic bipolar patients, contrasting 40 such patients with 30 healthy controls and accounting for the effects of subsyndromal symptomatology. After controlling for age, premorbid IQ, and subsyndromal symptomatology, the patient sample still manifested deficits on several measures of memory and executive functions. The extent of verbal memory impairment was related to a longer duration of illness, a higher number of manic episodes, and prior psychotic symptoms. However, 38 of the 40 patients were receiving psychotropic medications at the time of testing: 33 of the 40 were being treated with lithium carbonate, 12 with carbamazepine, and 7 with valproate; 11 patients were receiving more than one mood stabilizer; 23 were also being treated with antipsychotic medications (15 of which were on atypical antipsychotics), 17 were being given benzodiazepines, and 8 were receiving antidepressants. The complexity of these medication regimens is characteristic of the long-term treatment of bipolar disorder and illustrates the difficulty of ruling out adverse medication effects or interactions in naturalistic studies.

The most rigorous way of addressing this question is to conduct a randomized, placebo-controlled trial. Given the possibilities of state-related changes in cognition, fluctuating clinical symptomatology, effects of ancillary medications (e.g., benzodiazepines), practice and order effects, and other factors, adverse cognitive effects of primary mood-stabilizing or adjunctive sedative medications could easily be falsely accentuated or underestimated. Especially in clinical populations, however, the feasibility and ethics of such a study are questionable.

The best alternative in such a circumstance is longitudinal investigation using an ABA design, with patients being tested while on (A) and off (B) medication. Perhaps the most critical study in this area used such a design. Shaw and colleagues (1987) studied 28 outpatients with mood disorders maintained on lithium prophylaxis. Of these 28, 22 completed the protocol, 6 being dropped because of clinical deterioration; a criterion for participation was maintaining euthymia throughout. On average, patients had been maintained on lithium for 9.4 years (SD = 5.8 years), with an average level of 0.80 mEq/L (SD = 0.23 MEq/L). Patients were tested at the same time each week at each of five weekly sessions. The first session took place while patients continued to receive lithium, the second and third while they received substituted placebo, and the fourth and fifth after they had returned to lithium. Motor speed was assessed using the finger-tapping procedure, and the Buschke Selective Reminding Test was used to evaluate effects on learning and memory.

Over the 5 weeks of this study, depression and mania symptom scores were flat and in the euthymic range. Lithium levels went from a mean of 0.83 mEq/L at the first session to 0.05, 0.04, 0.71, and 0.74 at sessions 2 through 5, respectively. Figure 9–18 presents the results for the finger-tapping task and Figure 9–19 those for the memory test. Motor speed was quantified as the mean number of taps per five 10 s trials with both the dominant and nondominant hand. There was a significant difference in tapping performance across the 5 weeks, with motor speed improving after

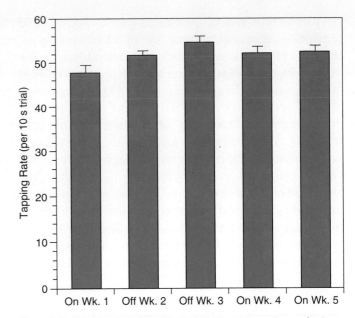

Figure 9–18. Tapping rate with lithium discontinuation and reinstatement. Twenty-two patients were retested for tapping speed weekly for 5 weeks. Lithium was discontinued after the first week and reinstated by the fourth week. Tapping speed improved in weeks 2 and 3 off lithium and slowed with lithium reinstatement. (*Source*: Shaw et al., 1987.)

discontinuation of lithium and deteriorating with its reintroduction. The magnitude of this effect, while consistent, was small. For example, the deterioration between weeks 3 and 5 ($p < .02$) averaged a 4.2 percent reduction in tapping rate.

The study by Shaw and colleagues (1987) constituted the first report of reversible lithium-induced motor speed impairment. Several previous studies of patients and healthy participants had suggested that lithium had a negative effect on performance of the WAIS-R digit symbol test and possibly on perceptual-motor tasks (Demers and Heninger, 1971; Judd, 1979; Squire et al., 1980). The digit symbol subtest is usually regarded as an attentional measure. Given its timed nature, however, motoric slowing would have a negative impact. Thus the findings of the Shaw et al. (1987) study raise the possibility that lithium resulted in a subtle slowing of basic motor movement, which could affect any timed procedure.

The findings obtained with the Buschke Selective Reminding Test are illustrated in Figure 9–19. This test produces a variety of indices of the adequacy of short- and long-term memory, and a representative index of each is plotted in the figure. Short-term recall is heavily influenced by attention and reflects the recall of items just recently presented, as in the reminding procedure. Long-term recall concerns the number of words recalled at some interval since original presentation or reminding. No impact of

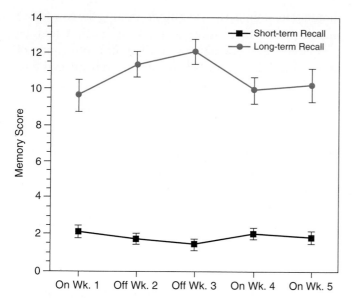

Figure 9–19. Short- and long-term recall on a verbal learning and memory test with lithium discontinuation and reinstatement. Lithium was discontinued after the first week and reinstated by the fourth week. Short-term or immediate memory was unaffected by lithium status. Long-term recall was reduced when patients were given lithium. (*Source*: Shaw et al., 1987. Reprinted with permission.)

remission, in whom learning and memory appear to be equally disrupted (see Fig. 9–17). Other research has yielded findings that support this framework. Two studies of healthy participants found that retrieval of information after a long delay (7 to 14 days) was impaired by lithium (Karniol et al., 1978; Kropf and Muller-Oerlinghausen, 1979). And in a study of 18 bipolar patients, Christodoulou and colleagues (1981) found no effect of a 16-day placebo period on short-term memory measures.

In this light, the findings of naturalistic studies of cognitive impairment in bipolar disorder may take on different meaning. Lund and colleagues (1982) found that chronic bipolar patients stabilized on lithium performed in the low-average range on tests of attention and memory, below expectations given their educational achievement. This pattern in remitted patients could reflect both a trait-level deficit in attentional and executive functions and a specific deleterious effect of lithium on long-term retrieval. Kessing (1998) found that both the number of affective episodes and treatment with lithium were associated with inferior performance on two of five tests of diffuse cognitive function. In this case, exposure to lithium and the effects of chronicity could not be separated. Finally, Engelsmann and colleagues (1988) conducted a longitudinal cognitive investigation of bipolar patients treated with lithium. They found little evidence of a cumulative deleterious effect, as there was significant decline over a 6-year follow-up period in only 1 of 10 memory subtests. However, evidence from discontinuation and reinstatement studies indicates that adverse effects of lithium on cognition are expressed immediately, and reverse at least partially with discontinuation. The findings of Engelsmann and colleagues (1988) are critical in suggesting that any short-term negative impact is not cumulative.[22]

Cognitive impairment is a common complaint of patients treated for bipolar disorder, and undoubtedly contributes considerably to nonadherence to treatment regimens (see Chapter 21). It has been common for clinicians to dismiss such complaints of clouded thinking, slowed processing, or memory impairment as reflecting the ravages of the illness, somatization and negativism on the part of the patient, and the like. Teasing out which if any cognitive effects reflect disease processes and which indicate adverse pharmacological effects is next to impossible for any individual patient. Given the neurotoxicity of lithium at high doses, it should not be unexpected if some individuals show cognitive sensitivity and experience a range of cognitive impairments while receiving the drug. In some cases, these effects can be addressed through dosage reduction. However, especially for patients in whom lithium is clearly more effective than alternative maintenance agents, there may be no choice but to accept these side effects as part of the price of maintaining

lithium withdrawal or reintroduction on the short-term memory measures was observed. Instead, substantial improvement in long-term memory measures occurred when lithium was removed, and deterioration when it was reintroduced. At face value, these data suggest that lithium had little impact on the attentive processes involved in the immediate recall of new information, but produced a significant compromise (about 20 percent) in the amount of information that could be recalled with a delay since presentation. In other words, these data suggest that lithium produced a mild anterograde amnesia.

In fact, although negative findings have been reported regarding lithium's effects on memory (Squire et al., 1980), a substantial literature is consistent with these effects. Reus and colleagues (1979) compared 17 bipolar manic patients receiving lithium with 7 other patients who had discontinued lithium for at least 3 weeks (5 because of pregnancy). Using procedures similar to those of Shaw and colleagues (1987), they found that the lithium group had a deficit in long-term recall. Specifically, this deficit pertained to the capacity to recall consistently material for which earlier learning had been established. This finding supports the possibility that lithium has negligible effects on attention and the intake or encoding of new information, but interferes with the retrieval of what has been learned. Were this the case, it would represent a neurocognitive profile distinct from that which appears to characterize bipolar patients in remission. In this respect, the absence of evidence that lithium per se has a cumulative deleterious influence and the clear evidence of reversal of deficits once the drug is discontinued should be reassuring. So, too, should the accumulating body of evidence indicating that lithium exerts a neuroprotective effect (see Chapter 14).

As noted earlier, an especially common complaint of patients receiving long-term treatment with lithium is blunting of creativity. Similar to the notion that lithium can blunt the peaks of extreme dysphoric and euphoric states, some patients report that lithium interferes with the highest levels of creativity. Given the apparent overrepresentation of bipolar illness among individuals in the creative arts, the frequency of this complaint is not surprising (see Chapter 12).

Evaluating the validity of this claim is difficult, however. Enhanced creativity is frequently reported in hypomanic states, with a concomitant increase in productivity. Rather than a reduction in creativity being attributable to lithium, effective treatment of bipolar disorder and the maintenance of sustained remission may have this untoward consequence. Were this the case, however, complaints about reduced creative abilities should be reported for any agents that produce or sustain remission. Yet experience indicates that such complaints are especially common among those being treated with lithium as opposed to other mood stabilizers. Indeed, a preliminary and, as far as we know, as yet unreplicated case study, has been reported in which complaints of diminished creativity were reduced by switching from lithium to sodium divalproex (Stoll et al., 1996).

The obvious difficulty here involves operationalizing the construct of creativity. No single neuropsychological test fully captures this construct. Shaw and colleagues (1986) conducted a critical study in this area, which is one of the only controlled studies to date of lithium's effects on the creative process. When given a word association task, such as providing associations for the word "camera," individuals will differ in the number and in the novelty or idiosyncrasy of the associations they report. Norms in fact exist for the frequency of particular associations. "Photograph" would be a highly common association for the stimulus "camera," whereas "chamber," "private," "stealth," or "subrosa" would be understandable but idiosyncratic responses. Using the same methodology over a 5-week testing period involving discontinuation and reinstatement of lithium, Shaw and colleagues (1986) found that upon discontinuation, remitted patients were more generative and also showed an increase in idiosyncrasy of association. Both effects reversed when lithium was reinstituted (see Chapter 12 for further discussion of this and related studies). In a subsequent study, this effect of discontinuation was reaffirmed (Kocsis et al., 1993). Therefore, the extremely limited data available suggest that lithium may result in a diminution of unusual associations, making the case for an impact on creativity more plausible. The effect may be complicated in those patients in whom discontinuation of lithium precipitates a rapid relapse to hypomania and thus an increase in associational fluency secondary to mood state.

This focus on the cognitive sequelae of lithium should not be taken as implying that the major alternatives to lithium, anticonvulsant mood stabilizers, do not present similar issues. Rather, it is only in the case of lithium that there is a substantial empirical literature on potential adverse cognitive effects. Indeed, examination of the neuropsychological effects of the anticonvulsants is standard in evaluating their use in seizure disorders.

Clinical Features

A good deal of medical research involves searching for clinical–pathological correlations in an effort to identify individuals at heightened risk or to further our understanding of disease processes. Once it has been accepted that manic-depressive illness, especially its bipolar form, is associated with a profile of cognitive deficits, a host of questions arise regarding the factors that influence the expression of such neuropsychological disturbances. For example, do all individuals manifest the cognitive deficits characteristic of bipolar illness, or do subgroups manifest these effects more intensely? Alternatively, does the manifestation of cognitive deficits change with development? In particular, does chronicity of illness affect the expression of such deficits? Is the adult pattern of cognitive deficit seen in pediatric bipolar disorder or in children at risk for the disorder? If so, does this obviate the potential confound of medication effects? And to what extent does the severity of cognitive deficits covary with structural abnormalities of the brain, especially the burden of hyperintensities as revealed by fMRI?

Psychotic Features

A number of studies have found a link between the presence of psychotic features and a more chronic and severe course of bipolar illness with respect to both symptomatic and functional outcomes.[23] Especially since cognitive impairment is linked to poorer functional outcomes in bipolar disorder (Zarate et al., 2000), one might surmise that psychotic features are predictive of poorer neuropsychological outcome. This conjecture has received some empirical support. Albus and colleagues (1996) failed to find differences in cognitive performance between first-episode nonpsychotic patients with mood disorders and healthy controls. In contrast, mood disorder patients with psychotic features performed as poorly as patients with first-episode schizophrenia. Thus in this study, the presence of psychosis was found to be a greater determinant of neuropsychological profile than the diagnosis of mood disorder or schizophrenia. In light of the neuropsychological deterioration often seen early after the onset of psychosis in first-episode schizophrenia and the hypothesis that psychotic states are intrinsically toxic (Wyatt, 1991, 1995), it is especially important to examine the validity of this association and to determine whether early intervention can improve cognitive and other long-term outcomes in patients with bipolar disorder with psychotic features. The duration of untreated psychosis in patients with first-episode schizophrenia is associated with both the quality of symptomatic outcomes and the extent of cognitive deterioration (Norman and Malla, 2001; Amminger et al., 2002).

Chronicity and Other Developmental Effects

An active effect of psychiatric illness on brain structure and function need not be restricted to psychotic subtypes. Altshuler (1993) and others have contended that episodes of depression and mania may have similar consequences. Indeed, a particularly popular view is that the release of excessive glucocorticoids during such episodes leads to hippocampal atrophy and consequent disruption of declarative memory processes (Brown et al., 1999) (see Chapter 15). This possibility accords with data indicating that the lifetime duration of depression is associated with hippocampal volume and verbal memory performance in euthymic women with recurrent major depression (Sheline et al., 1996, 1999). A role for interventions is supported by recent evidence that the linkage between lifetime duration of days depressed and structural and functional outcomes holds only for periods without active antidepressant treatment (Sheline, E., personal communication, May 2004).

Bipolar patients can vary in the chronicity of their disorder, differing in the number of episodes, type of episodes, number of hospitalizations, duration of episodes, and severity of symptoms. The directions of these effects are not necessarily uniform. An unremitting, continuous episode of illness may indicate greater chronicity than a history of recurrent but responsive episodes. Adequate metrics by which to evaluate the course of bipolar illness are unavailable. Nonetheless, patients with more severe symptomatic presentations and with courses of illness lacking long periods of remission (e.g., chronic and/or recurrent) tend to have poorer neuropsychological outcomes.[24] Cognitive outcomes in bipolar patients have been linked to a rapid-cycling course (McKay et al., 1995), number of prior hospitalizations (Tham et al., 1997), and lifetime duration in episodes of mania or depression (van Gorp et al., 1998). Denicoff and colleagues (1999) found that number of episodes, longer duration of illness, and more frequent hospitalizations were each associated with performance on tests of attention, abstraction, and memory. Kessing (1998), using regression techniques, found a linkage to cognitive dysfunction for number of episodes and not for duration of illness (see Chapter 4).

While the consensus on this issue is impressive, each of the supportive studies used a cross-sectional design. Two observations illustrate the problem: (1) a more virulent course is associated with neuropsychological deterioration, and (2) patients in remission manifest a profile of cognitive dysfunction, noteworthy mainly for the relative sparing of verbal functions, but otherwise widespread. It is conceivable that the abnormalities seen in remitted patients reflect the deterioration associated with chronicity and are not present from the onset of illness. If so, longitudinal evaluation should detect this change over time. Unfortunately, longitudinal investigation of cognitive function in bipolar disorder has rarely been conducted. An exception in this regard is a study conducted by Dhingra and Rabins (1991). They followed for 5 to 7 years 25 bipolar patients who initially presented in a manic state with no signs of cognitive impairment. At long-term follow-up, approximately one third of the sample had clinically significant cognitive impairment.

Another approach can be taken to determine whether the cognitive deficits seen in euthymia precede the classic expression of illness, accompany the onset of the first affective episode, or are a result of the expression of the disorder. Evaluating family members of bipolar probands, children at risk for bipolar disorder, or pediatric manifestations of bipolar disorder can provide clues to the unfolding of cognitive deficits in this illness. For example, Dickstein and colleagues (2004) compared 21 bipolar children with 21 age- and gender-matched controls on the Cambridge Neuropsychological Test Automated Battery. The bipolar children had a profile of deficits similar to that seen in adults, with deficits in attention, set shifting, and visuospatial memory. Post hoc analyses indicated that these deficits could not be attributed to manic symptoms or the presence of attention-deficit disorder. The average age of the bipolar sample was 12.7 years (range 6 to 17 years), and it is conceivable that the medications used to treat the condition or other ancillary factors distorted cognitive performance. Clarification of the neuropsychological profiles of children at risk (as well as family members) could help clarify these issues while minimizing the confounding effects of illness expression and treatment.

Results of a study by Burt and colleagues (2000) suggest that neuropsychological course may be quite different in bipolar and unipolar patients. The authors compared young and elderly unipolar and bipolar patients in an episode of major depression on the performance of a variety of memory measures. No differences in performance were found between the young bipolar and unipolar groups, while the elderly bipolar patients had markedly inferior performance compared with all other groups. The authors speculated that the history of more frequent affective episodes and the earlier age at onset in the bipolar group resulted in a more pronounced deteriorative process.

The evidence, reviewed earlier, that lithium has negative but quickly reversible cognitive effects does not contradict the possibility that the drug also exerts neuroprotective effects (Manji et al., 2000a,b) (see Chapter 14). To date, there is no evidence that long-term exposure to lithium, as opposed to any other agent, has a specific or general impact on the cognitive deficits characteristic of bipolar disorder. Research to address these issues is essential.

Structural Brain Abnormalities

The fact that some neurocognitive effects reverse with the discontinuation or reinitiation of lithium demonstrates a causal pathway. However, medication effects are unlikely to account for the bulk of the deficits seen during symptomatic or remitted states. There appears to be a core pattern of cognitive deficit that is manifested across the phases of illness. Some evidence indicates that duration of lifetime exposure to major depression covaries with hippocampal volume and a measure of verbal memory. More generally, the evidence for persistent cognitive deficit raises the issue of neuroanatomical correlates (see Chapter 15). There are particular reasons for investigating the relations of MRI hyperintensities (HI) to cognitive manifestations in bipolar disorder.

In comparison with healthy controls and other neuropsychiatric groups, elderly patients with major depressive disorder have consistently shown high rates of abnormality in MRI evaluations. These abnormalities appear as areas of increased signal intensity in both balanced, T_2-weighted and fluid-attenuated inversion recovery (FLAIR) images. T_1-weighted sequences maximize the contrast between gray and white matter and provide fine anatomic detail. In contrast, T_2-weighted and FLAIR sequences are particularly sensitive in identifying fluid-filled areas, which appear as areas of high signal intensity.

The abnormalities can be classified into three types. Periventricular hyperintensities (PVH) are a halo or rim adjacent to ventricles that in severe forms invades surrounding deep white matter. Alternatively, single, patchy, or confluent foci may be observed in deep white matter hyperintensities (DWMH), with or without PVH. HI may also be found in deep gray structures, particularly the basal ganglia, thalamus, and pons. These abnormalities have been referred to as leukoencephalopathy, leukoariosis, subcortical arteriosclerotic encephalopathy, encephalomalacia, and unidentified bright objects (UBOs). Because the HI in major depression are not restricted to white matter and their etiology has not been established, we use the term encephalomalacia.

Figure 9–20 illustrates a moderate-to-severe case of encephalomalacia. FLAIR images are presented for a patient with late-onset, first-episode major depression. The image on the left illustrates PVH, with thick bands of high signal intensity (white) adjacent to the lateral ventricles. Note that on the left side of this image, the HI are extending into the deep white matter. The image on the right is of a higher MRI slice from the same patient and shows multiple confluent HI through the DWMH. In patients presenting with these MRI findings, clinicians typically receive radiological reports that emphasize ischemic small-vessel disease.

In one of the largest prospective MRI series in major depression, all 51 elderly patients (aged >60) referred for ECT presented with HI, more than half rated moderate to severe, and 51 percent had lesions of subcortical gray nuclei (Coffey et al., 1990). These rates of abnormality greatly exceeded those found in a healthy control sample, with basal ganglia abnormalities being most discriminative (Fig. 9–21). The depressed samples studied to date have often included patients with comorbid medical illnesses, without adequate controls for risk factors for cerebrovascular disease (CVD), medications being taken, or drug abuse. Nonetheless, in the work of Coffey and colleagues (1990), when depressed patients with preexisting neurological conditions were excluded, the rate of encephalomalacia greatly exceeded that found in normal controls. In a replication study, patients with major depression showed marked increases in the frequency of PVH, DWMH, and basal ganglia and thalamic HI relative to controls matched for CVD risk factors (Coffey et al., 1993). The age-adjusted odds ratio for PVH was 5.32. In other, often large population studies of elderly healthy controls, when the halos or caps commonly seen at the top and bottom of the lateral ventricles were excluded, approximately 10 to 30 percent presented with MRI white matter abnormalities, with typically mild severity and low rates of subcortical gray matter abnormalities (Breteler et al., 1994).

The rate or severity of encephalomalacia in geriatric depression may equal or exceed that in Alzheimer's disease (Erkinjuntti et al., 1994) and may be comparable to that in multi-infarct dementia (Zubenko et al., 1990; see Sackeim et al., 2000a, for a review). Meta-analyses have supported the excess of HI in geriatric unipolar depression (Videbech, 1997). These abnormalities tend to be overrepresented in frontal lobe white matter and in the basal ganglia, perhaps with a left-sided predominance (Greenwald et al., 1998). For instance, Greenwald and colleagues (1998) found that left frontal DWHI and left putamen HI discriminated between an elderly unipolar sample and a matched healthy comparison group.

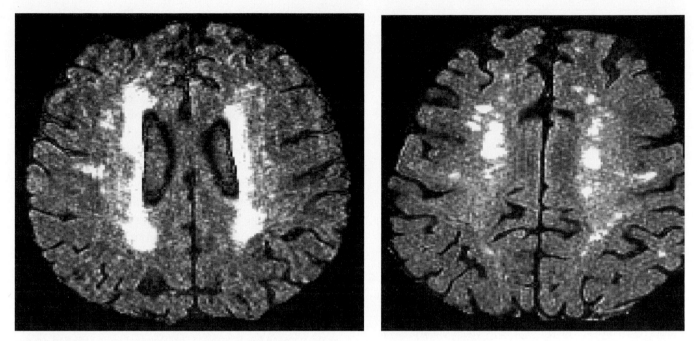

Figure 9–20. Fluid-attenuated inversion recovery (FLAIR) images of a patient with late-onset major depression. White or bright areas show magnetic resonance imaging (MRI) hyperintensities. The image on the left demonstrates periventricular hyperintensities, with a broad band of increased signal adjacent to the lateral ventricles and invading the deep white matter. The image on the right, from the same patient at a higher level, shows multiple, confluent foci of hyperintensities in the deep white matter (centrum semiovale).

Several correlates of HI burden have been suggested in studies of elderly unipolar patients. The excess of HI appears to be most marked in patients with late- as opposed to early-onset mood disorder.[25] In turn, this association may be due to a greater rate of cerebrovascular risk factors in the late-onset population. Indeed, as in normal and neurological samples, the strongest predictors of encephalomalacia in unipolar depression are age and cerebrovascular risk factors. There are also suggestions that, in addition to late onset, absence of a family history of mood disorder is predictive of HI burden (Krishnan et al., 2004). This finding regarding transmission of mood disorder would suggest determination of whether family history of CVD is overrepresented in unipolar or bipolar patients with significant encephalomalacia, an issue yet to be resolved.

In unipolar patients, the presence of encephalomalacia has predictive power with respect to treatment outcome and subsequent course. In naturalistic studies, greater HI burden has been associated with poorer acute response to antidepressant medications and ECT.[26] The limited information on longitudinal follow-up suggests that encephalomalacia in unipolar disorder may be a marker for cognitive decline and the development of dementia (Hickie et al., 1997; Baldwin et al., 2000).

In normal, nonsymptomatic subjects, some degree of encephalomalacia may be observed, and its prevalence and extent are linked to aging. It is unclear whether the limited encephalomalacia in normal samples is associated with cognitive impairment, and there may be threshold effects for HI volume (Boone et al., 1992). Nonetheless, in normal and neurological samples, there is a body of replicated findings associating encephalomalacia specifically with deficits in attention, motor speed, and executive function (e.g., Breteler et al., 1994; see Sackeim et al., 2000a, for a review). As noted earlier, these are hallmark deficits in unipolar and bipolar depression. In nonpsychiatric patient samples, the most common neurological abnormalities associated with encephalomalacia are gait disturbances, tendency to fall, extensor plantar reflex, and primitive reflexes.[27]

There has been limited investigation of the neuropsychological correlates of encephalomalacia in unipolar major depression. Ebmeier and colleagues (1997) found that the severity of DWMH was inversely related to global cognitive function (Mini-Mental State scores) in elderly depressed patients. In an especially comprehensive study, Lesser and colleagues (1996) compared 60 late-onset (>50 years of age) unipolar depressed patients, 35 early-onset (<35 years of age) depressed patients, and 165 normal controls. All subjects were at least 50 years of age. The late-onset group had greater DWMH than either of the other groups. Cognitive deficits were most marked in the late-onset group and pertained to nonverbal intelligence, nonverbal memory, constructional ability, executive function,

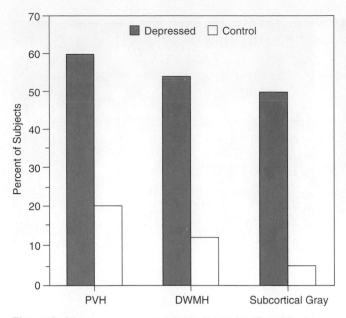

Figure 9–21. Representation of the findings of Coffey and colleagues (1990). The percentages of patients with major depression and control subjects are contrasted in rates of periventricular hyperintensities (PVH), deep white matter hyperintensities (DWMH), and hyperintensities in subcortical gray matter structures.

and speed of processing. Patients with greater severity of DWMH had significantly poorer executive function.

Jenkins and colleagues (1998) found that elderly depressed patients with HI showed poorer performance on a number of learning and memory indices, with the pattern of deficits resembling that observed in subcortical degenerative disorders (i.e., Huntington's and Parkinson's diseases). Simpson and colleagues (1997b) conducted neuropsychological assessment after treatment of an elderly unipolar depressed sample. Signal abnormalities in the pons were associated with reduced psychomotor speed, basal ganglia HI were linked to impaired category productivity (executive function), and PVH were associated with recall deficits. It should be noted that since the severity of encephalomalacia in this study was also associated with clinical outcome, the findings regarding neuropsychological correlates may have been confounded with clinical state. Yet the findings of these and other studies indicate that in general, encephalomalacia in elderly unipolar patients is associated with impairments of psychomotor function, attention, executive function, and learning and memory. There is also evidence that specific cognitive domains may be affected by the anatomic location of HI (deep white matter, periventricular, or subcortical gray matter structures).

The characterization of encephalomalacia in bipolar disorder is less certain, in part because it has received less research attention. Nonetheless, encephalomalacia clearly has different meanings in bipolar and unipolar disorder.

In considerably younger samples than those studied in unipolar disorder, several groups have reported that MRI HI are more common among young bipolar patients than controls.[28] Aylward and colleagues (1994) found that older (> age 38) and not younger bipolar patients had an excess of HI. Brown and colleagues (1992) failed to detect an excess in young bipolar patients, although they did observe that severe HI were overrepresented in elderly patients with major depression. In a sample of 600 psychiatric patients who underwent MRI, Breeze and colleagues (2003) failed to observe a difference in rates of DWMH in bipolar patients compared with other psychiatric groups. However, in the same sample, this group reported that bipolar patients had a clear excess of *severe* DWMH compared with other groups (Lyoo et al., 2002). In relatively small samples, Silverstone and colleagues (2003) compared bipolar depressed, unipolar depressed, and healthy participants and found that the bipolar patients had twice the rate of severe DWMH relative to unipolar patients or healthy controls. Ahn and colleagues (2004) recently confirmed an excess of DWMH in bipolar adults relative to healthy controls, with the discrimination being strongest for more severe structural abnormality.

The findings of two recent studies are particularly revealing. Pillai and colleagues (2002) compared rates of white matter HI in adolescents with bipolar disorder and schizophrenia and matched healthy controls. These HI were more common in the bipolar group (67 percent) relative to the schizophrenic (37 percent) and comparison (32 percent) groups. HI occur in individuals with early-onset bipolar disorder and have been reported at first psychiatric contact. Ahearn and colleagues (1998) conducted MRI examinations of the affected and unaffected first-degree relatives of bipolar probands. Of the 21 family members examined, 15 had HI, including 6 of 10 family members with no history of mood disorder and all of those with bipolar disorder. Lesions of both white matter and subcortical gray nuclei were seen. The authors raised the possibility that these HI serve as a biomarker of bipolar disorder.

The literature on encephalomalacia in bipolar disorder is somewhat less consistent than that in unipolar disorder in demonstrating this structural abnormality. On the other hand, some authors claim that encephalomalacia is especially marked in bipolar disorder. The reasons for this discrepancy are not well understood. Nonetheless, reports demonstrating differences from healthy participants and other psychiatric groups are sufficient for us to conclude that bipolar disorder is characterized by an excess of these structural abnormalities. In their meta-analysis, Bearden and colleagues (2001) found a pooled odds ratio of 7.2 for the likelihood of HI in bipolar patients relative to healthy participants.

The striking thing is that the correlates of these abnormalities appear to differ in bipolar and unipolar disorder. There is a dramatic difference in age at manifestation. In all populations studied to date, HI burden increases with advancing age. This may also be true in bipolar disorder. What is exceptional, however, that adolescents with bipolar disorder show the abnormality (Botteron et al., 1995; Lyoo et al., 2002; Pillai et al., 2002). In unipolar patients and neurological samples, the presence and severity of HI are linked to CVD. Indeed, the predominant view is that encephalomalacia is an outcome of ischemic changes in white matter watershed areas that are fed by tiny arterioles and have limited collateral vascular supply. Rigidification of these small vessels or blockage through arteriosclerosis will result in ischemic damage. Not surprisingly, then, age and cerebrovascular risk factors would be key determinants. Further, given this hypothesized vascular etiology, it is not surprising that encephalomalacia is especially prevalent in late-onset depression in patients without a family history of mood disorder. It is CVD that is the primary agent, and not a genetic liability to depression. Indeed, the invasion of fibers in the white matter by HI must be a random process. If the right fibers are damaged, major depression may result as disconnection syndrome (Geschwind, 1965). Further, it makes sense that encephalomalacia, by reflecting ischemic brain changes, is associated with specific forms of cognitive impairment and predicts future course.

The young age at which many bipolar patients show this abnormality makes it unlikely that these HI are the outcome of an ischemic disease process. Indeed, the notion that the severity of the MRI abnormalities covaries with cerebrovascular risk factors has not been established in bipolar samples. Excluding patients or controlling for CVD risk factors still results in an excess of HI in bipolar samples relative to controls (Altshuler et al., 1995; Hickie et al., 1995). Thus while a vascular, age-related etiology for encephalomalacia is most likely in unipolar disorder, a different etiology may be at play in bipolar disorder. In turn, it cannot be assumed that HI burden is associated with neuropsychological impairment in bipolar disorder.

Limited investigation has been done in this area. In a small sample, Dupont and colleagues (1990) found that bipolar patients with HI were more impaired than bipolar patients without HI or healthy controls on tests of attention, letter fluency, visuospatial skills, and memory. In contrast, Krabbendam and colleagues (2000) compared matched groups of remitted patients with bipolar disorder, patients with schizophrenia, and healthy controls. The groups did not differ in the presence or severity of HI. More surprisingly, no differences in cognitive performance were found between patients with and without white matter lesions. Clearly, this area needs further attention, and the pathoetiology of encephalomalacia in bipolar disorder remains a mystery.

NEUROPSYCHOLOGY AND THE CONCEPTUALIZATION OF MOOD DISORDERS

However revealing about the disorder, a detailing of the areas of cognitive strength and weakness in manic-depressive illness is a highly incomplete account of the neuropsychological contribution to theories of the nature of the illness. The application of psychometrics to affective processes lags considerably behind advances in cognitive assessment. However, the study of brain–behavior relationships with respect to the regulation of emotion draws on a vast clinical and experimental literature involving psychiatric, neurological, and healthy samples to derive conclusions about how emotional states are represented in the brain and what may go wrong such that some individuals are subject to recurrent bouts of depression or mania. The remainder of this chapter is devoted to a brief review of some of the key questions addressed in this literature.

Are Mood Disorders Deficit States or Release Phenomena?

Theorists such as Donald Klein have viewed major depression as a deficit state, the affective equivalent of an aphasia (Klein et al., 1980). The depressed patient is characterized by an inability to feel pleasure, lack of interest, sleep and appetite disturbance, lack of energy, immobility, and so on. By this view, then, basic appetitive, motoric, and hedonic functions are disturbed, much as sensation, movement, or speech is lost in neurological disorders resulting from destructive brain lesions.

An alternative view is that these affective states are manifested as highly integrated behaviors with mood, motor, cognitive, and conative components. Normal states of sadness and euphoria or, by extension, depression and mania are "positive symptoms" in the sense of Hughlings Jackson (1985), reflecting "hyperfunction" more than "hypofunction," and are expressed through excitatory or disinhibitory mechanisms (Head, 1921). By this view, depression and mania are more akin to automatic speech than to speech arrest (Sackeim, 1986).

What type of evidence might support such a view? First, complex affective states can reliably be provoked by stimulating specific regions of the brain. Indeed, they can be turned on and off by changing the electrical stimulation. During the course of deep-brain stimulation for movement disorders, it has become clear that stimulation at a particular contact on an electrode in the subthalamic nucleus (or elsewhere) can provoke an overwhelming feeling of depression, accompanied by crying, beliefs of worthless-ness or hopelessness, and other classic phenomena associ-ated with the depressed state.[29] Turning the stimulation off turns off the emotional display. The importance of such demonstrations lies not so much in the hints about local-ization, but more in the fact that the immediacy of the de-pressive mood and of the changes in emotional expression and worldview indicate the triggering of an integrated "de-pressive system" that alters the content of both mood and thought. Thus the brain, at least in this context, behaves in a way envisaged neither by James (1890) nor by Schachter (Schachter and Singer, 1962). We do not come to have a feel-ing because we are expressing the emotion (e.g., we know we are afraid because we are running), as suggested by James. Nor do we come to have a feeling because of an ap-praisal we have made about our surroundings that explains why we are aroused, as suggested by Schachter. In the case of deep-brain stimulation, mood, expression, and thought present simultaneously as integrated psychic phenomena triggered by a manipulation of brain tissue. None has pri-macy, as would be demanded by these earlier theories.

Depressive-catastrophic reactions during the Wada procedure are another example of provoked and transient mood disorder. This procedure involves injecting a barbi-turate into the internal carotid artery to temporarily "bar-biturate" the ipsilateral hemisphere (Snyder and Harris, 1997; Wada, 1997). Contralateral flaccid hemiplegia or hemi-paresis and homonymous hemianopsia soon result. The procedure is used to establish laterality of language and verbal memory in individuals scheduled for neurosurgery (Branch et al., 1964; Cohen-Gadol et al., 2004; Takayama et al., 2004). At a point when sensorimotor function and cog-nition return toward baseline, some patients report de-pressed mood and catastrophic beliefs (e.g., their lives are ruined, the world is coming to an end). Since the 1950s, some investigators have claimed that left-side injections are more likely to produce this outcome, whereas right-side injections are more likely to result in a euphoric reac-tion.[30] While this idea is subject to controversy (Kolb and Milner, 1981; Kurthen et al., 1991), results of a recent study using masked ratings of facial expression during the Wada procedure support the notion that depressive reactions are more common with left-side injection.

Normal functioning is characterized by its own mood swings. Profound sadness, as during mourning or other losses, is a normal variant and shares virtually all the symp-toms of the clinical disorder. What distinguishes major de-pressive episodes from the normal experience of intense dysphoric states is not so much the phenomenology of these presentations as the fact that major depression does not re-solve as quickly. Viewing these phenomena in normal indi-viduals as a deficit state strains credibility. Furthermore,

states of euphoria and mania also involve integrated man-ifestations in mood, motor function, cognition, and cona-tion, with many of these functions appearing to be in overdrive.

Another argument regarding the status of depression and mania as release phenomena concerns the fact that the disorders most clearly reflecting deficits in emotional pro-cesses are distinct from depression and mania. Individuals may have agnosias for emotional communications. In other words, they may be incapable of identifying affective intonation or emotional facial expressions. For example, prosopoaffective agnosia refers to the inability to discern fa-cial emotional expression without an accompanying deficit in processing of facial identity (Vuilleumier et al., 1998). Other neurological disorders can result in an incapacity to display emotions, either voluntarily or spontaneously (Borod et al., 1988; Ghacibeh and Heilman, 2003). And alexithymia is a disorder involving the capacity to feel or process affectively laden information (Becerra et al., 2002; Kano et al., 2003; Larsen et al., 2003); some refer to this condition as emotional blunting or emotion blindness. If affective disorders have a form of negative symptoms re-flecting a fundamental defect or incapacity, these condi-tions would be exemplars.

Are We Wired to Be Depressed, and What Are the Therapeutic Implications?

The difference in conceptualization discussed above is not academic. The release model essentially claims that we are wired to be depressed and euphoric. Depressive or manic states do not arise because of a disruption of vari-ous discrete functions, such as sleep and appetite, but represent the expression of excitatory or disinhibitory re-lease of distributed networks that subserve the integrated features of mood disorder (Tanaka and Sumitsuji, 1991). Concretely, this conception posits that there are depres-sion and euphoria circuits in the brain, just as there are circuits for fear.

By positing that excessive excitation or disinhibition leads to release of the affective states, this perspective also has im-plications for our understanding of therapeutics. ECT is the most effective short-term treatment for both the depressed and manic phases of bipolar disorder. As reviewed in Chap-ter 19, bipolar depressed patients remit at the same rate as unipolar patients but require fewer treatments (Daly et al., 2001). Regardless of the form of ECT that was used in a se-ries of randomized, controlled trials at Columbia University, bipolar patients on average required about 1.5 fewer treat-ments than unipolar depressed patients, with optimal forms of ECT resulting in immediate remission rates of 60 to 80 percent (Fig. 9–22). The immediate remission rate in mania is also on the order of 80 percent, and improvement is often

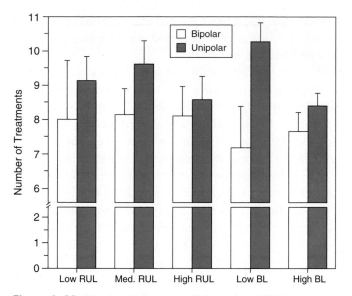

Figure 9–22. Number of electroconvulsive therapy (ECT) treatments for bipolar and unipolar depressed patients. Based on data pooled across four studies at the New York State Psychiatric Institute/Columbia University, 78 bipolar patients required on average about 1.5 fewer treatments than 185 unipolar depressed patients. Patients were randomly assigned to forms of ECT that differed in electrical dosage (low, medium, and high) and electrode placement (right unilateral [RUL] versus bilateral [BL]). An analysis of variation (ANOVA) was conducted on the number of treatments administered, with diagnosis (bipolar versus unipolar), treatment condition (five levels), and the interaction of those two factors as between-subject terms, and age and pre-ECT Hamilton Rating Scale for Depression (HAM-D) score as covariates. The main effects of diagnosis ($p = .0008$) and pre-ECT HAM-D score ($p = .0002$) were significant. (*Source*: Adapted from Sackeim et al., 1987, 1993, 2000b, and Sackeim, 2004.)

brisker than in major depression (Mukherjee et al., 1994). Why is ECT unique among therapeutics in both the breadth of its therapeutic action and its success rate? Why is a treatment that results in a hyperexcited state of the brain effective in treatment conditions that we posit reflect the release of function?

ECT is a profound anticonvulsant.[31] The induction of the seizure initiates a set of endogenous inhibitory processes that terminate the seizure (Madsen et al., 2000); the leading theories on what mediates this anticonvulsant effect involve increased transmission of gamma-aminobutyric acid (GABA), endogenous opioids (Sanacora et al., 2003), or other peptides (Tortella and Long, 1985). ECT raises the seizure threshold for itself and all agents that trigger seizures through GABAergic antagonism (Green et al., 1982). It also results in progressive shortening of seizure duration and weakening of seizure expression (Sackeim, 1999). Increasing the threshold for seizures and blocking or weakening seizure expression are the two conditions to be satisfied in determining whether a drug has anticonvulsant

properties. In a variety of animal models, including kindling, electroconvulsive shock (ECS) exerts more powerful anticonvulsant properties than drugs such as carbamazepine or valproate. In this light, it is not surprising that ECT has been of value in the treatment of resistant seizure disorders, including status epilepticus (Sackeim et al., 1983b; Lisanby et al., 2001).

The therapeutic properties of ECT have been linked to its anticonvulsant effects. Forms of ECT that result in the most marked increases in seizure threshold tend to be the most effective (Sackeim, 1999). The strength of the inhibitory process immediately after the seizure can be indexed by the presence or absence of postictal suppression of the electroencephalogram (EEG). Postictal suppression (bioelectric silence) is predictive of a favorable outcome (Nobler et al., 1993; Suppes et al., 1996; Perera et al., 2004). Most critically, since Kety's work initiated the field of brain imaging (Kety et al., 1948), it has been clear that ECT results in marked reductions in CBF (and CMR_{glu}).[32] Recent work has revealed powerful relationships between the extent of this suppression in prefrontal regions and clinical outcome in both major depression and mania (Nobler et al., 1994, 2000b, 2001). Consonant with this perspective, ECT results in a marked increase in slow-wave (delta) activity. The efficacy of the procedure has been linked to a topography dominated by increased slow-wave activity in prefrontal regions (Sackeim et al., 1996a). Thus depressed and manic patients may have "bad brakes," resulting in a failure to diminish activation in the released mood circuitry. ECT, at least temporarily, enhances inhibitory tone, reducing expression of the released mood circuitry.

The large imaging literature on antidepressant effects is mainly in keeping with this view (Mayberg et al., 1999; Drevets et al., 2002; Seminowicz et al., 2004). Although there are disagreements about the sites of inhibition that are most critical, the antidepressant effects of ECT, sleep deprivation, and antidepressant medications have commonly been tied to reductions of regional cerebral blood flow (rCBF) or CMR_{glu} in specific brain regions. Frontal pole, medial orbital prefrontal cortex, anterior cingulate, and amygdala have been identified as primary in reflecting the covariation between reduced CBF or CMR_{glu} and clinical outcome.[33]

Of course, this view readily accommodates the fact that several anticonvulsant agents have mood-stabilizing properties. Thus to the extent that depressed or manic patients can be said to have "bad brakes," treatments with prophylactic properties may exert tonic inhibition.

Does the Brain Regulate Depression and Mania Differently?

Bipolar disorder is one of the few illnesses in which polar-opposite symptoms (euphoria and depression) are experienced as part of the same illness. It is tempting to view these abnormal states as the ends of a seesaw, such that when one side is up, the other is down. This analogy presumes that some force is tilting a balance toward or away from depression or mania, thus regulating both. However, the nature of regulatory control probably differs for euphoric and dysphoric states. Take the example of uncontrollable laughing and crying. In the context of destructive, silent (nonepileptic) lesions, pathological crying is more frequent than pathological laughing (Mills, 1912; Davison and Kelman, 1939; Tateno et al., 2004). Uncontrollable outbursts of laughter as a prodrome or during seizures are referred to as gelastic epilepsy (Daly and Mulder, 1957; Gascon and Lombroso, 1971). As peri-ictal manifestations, these highly organized behavioral displays occur in the context of excessive cerebral excitability, during states of hypersynchronous neuronal firing (Arroyo et al., 1993). Dacrystic epilepsy refers to the occurrence of crying as a prodromal or ictal event. When we collected the world literature on gelastic and dacrystic epilepsy, we found a pattern with pathological laughing and crying: there were 91 cases of laughing as a peri-ictal event, but only 6 cases of crying outbursts and 6 cases that presented laughing and crying outbursts to an equal extent (Sackeim et al., 1982b).

It is unlikely that the paucity of dacrystic epilepsy and excess of gelastic epilepsy case studies reflects only a reporting bias. As noted, in the context of silent, nonirritative lesions, reports of pathological crying are common. Taken at face value, this difference in rates of occurrence suggests that uncontrollable crying is released more readily through disinhibitory mechanisms as opposed to an excitatory process, while laughter is readily released through "irritative" or excitatory as well as disinhibitory mechanisms.

Even granting such a possibility, it is not evident that the pattern of neural control over these emotional displays is of consequence for the regulation of mood. At issue is whether these examples of dysregulation of spontaneous emotional expression should serve as a model for the pathophysiology of abnormal mood states. Three key arguments support the validity of this model.

First, as noted earlier, in a substantial minority of patients with pathological laughing and/or crying, mood is altered during the outbursts in a manner that is consonant with the expressive outburst. Thus these individuals report marked sadness during pathological crying and euphoria during pathological laughter. This same pattern holds for gelastic and dacrystic epilepsy. This would suggest that in some cases, the physiological state that results in release of the expressive outbursts also releases these organized mood states (Black, 1982). Precise data are lacking on the prevalence of mood alterations during ictal events. It is noteworthy that fear and euphoria are commonly reported.

For example, Dostoyevsky stated that he would give up 10 years of his life for the brief period of ecstasy he experienced as a peri-ictal event.

Second, the therapeutics of pathological laughing and crying supports the concept that mood and emotional expression are part of an integrated emotion circuit. In controlled trials, antidepressant medications, including tricyclic antidepressants and selective serotonin reuptake inhibitors (SSRIs), have been found to be effective.[34]

Third, the lateralization of brain damage (or seizure foci) in these cases of uncontrollable emotional display matches that seen for depressive and euphoric mood changes that occur after destructive, silent lesions. As with the Wada procedure, and also not without controversy, a significant body of research has linked acute depressive reactions following brain insult to damage in left-sided regions, especially in frontal cortex, and euphoric mood changes to right-sided damage.[35] Figure 9–23 presents ratings of the predominant side of lesion in cases of pathological laughing and crying; the raters were blinded to the nature of the affective display (Sackeim et al., 1982a). As in the literature on mood change, crying outbursts are associated with an excess of left-sided lesions, and laughing outbursts with an excess of right-sided lesions.

Sackeim and colleagues (1982b) hypothesized that the opposite pattern would obtain when these outbursts occurred in the context of epilepsy as prodromal or ictal events. Focal seizure activity has unique localizing value. For example, lateralized somatosensory alterations have 100 percent correspondence to contralateral seizure activity in somatosensory cortex. Hughlings Jackson (1985) described the "homunculus," the ordered representation of the body in motor and somatosensory cortex based on the march of motor symptoms during Jacksonian seizures, a description later validated by Penfield with direct electrical stimulation of motor cortex (Penfield and Jasper, 1954). Sackeim and colleagues had further hypothesized that depressive and euphoric mood states following lateralized silent (nonepileptic) lesions reflect disinhibition in contralateral brain regions that subserve depressed or euphoric states—that is, breaking a brake over contralateral regions. Thus, for example, they posited that euphoria results from right-sided brain damage due to release of the left-sided regions that subserve this affective state. This hypothesis derived partly from data indicating that right hemispherectomy (removal of the anterior two thirds of the cerebral hemisphere) often results in a syndrome of increased jocularity, poor judgment, lack of responsibility, and so on (Sackeim et al., 1982b). These affective changes cannot be mediated by the broad expanse of cortex that has been removed, but only by remaining subcortical regions in the ipsilateral hemisphere or by release of the

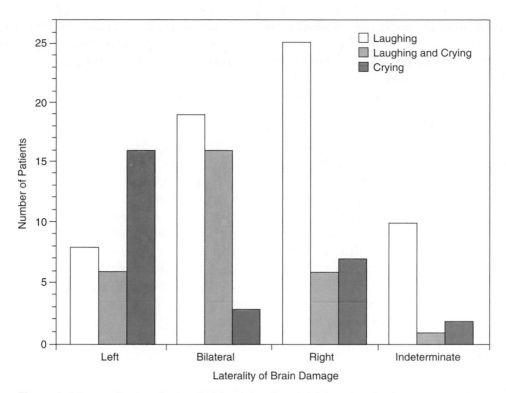

Figure 9–23. Distribution of primarily left-sided, right-sided, bilateral, and indeterminate nonirritative lesions in patients with pathological laughing only, laughing and crying, and crying only. Left-sided and right-sided lesions are associated with pathological crying and laughing, respectively, whereas bilateral lesions are associated with presentation of both uncontrollable laughing and crying. (*Source*: Sackeim et al., 1982b.)

regions in the contralateral hemisphere. Likewise, the affective changes seen after barbituration of the left or right hemisphere suggest that contralateral disinhibition may be at play.

Figure 9–24 presents findings regarding the lateralization of epileptic foci in cases of gelastic epilepsy. There was an overwhelming excess of left-sided foci, as predicted—the opposite of what was seen with pathological laughing in the context of silent lesions. Thus, the model offered by Sackeim and colleagues (1982b) stipulated that depressed and euphoric states are under reciprocal inhibitory control. Depressive phenomena are released mainly by disinhibitory mechanisms, while euphoric mood changes and laughter are released by disinhibition or direct excitation. The model did not require that the inhibitory control mechanisms be reciprocal. Including this element implied a partial seesaw effect. Reciprocal regulation would mean that depression and euphoria cannot be experienced simultaneously, an issue that is key to the conceptualization of mixed states.

Our conceptions of how emotional processes are represented in the brain are rudimentary. Undoubtedly the model of Sackeim and colleagues is overly broad and, at best, an echo of the true state of affairs. Nonetheless, the

evidence that led to this model was consistent and illustrated the power of using experimental invasive techniques (e.g., deep brain stimulation, Wada test, hemispherectomy), along with experiments in nature (lateralization of epileptic foci and silent lesions), to constrain theorizing

Figure 9–24. Distribution of left-sided, right-sided, and indeterminate epileptic foci in patients with gelastic (laughing) epilepsy. Foci were more than twice as likely to be left-sided than right-sided. (*Source*: Sackeim et al., 1982b.)

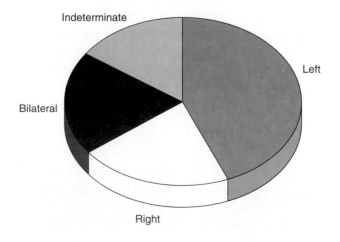

about fundamental mechanisms in the regulation of emotion.

There are other speculative grounds for postulating a fundamental difference in the neural control of euphoric and dysphoric states or, as some have suggested, emotional states involved in approach or avoidance (Davidson, 1995). A long list of pharmacological agents, including laughing gas, stimulants, opioids, cocaine, and others, can reliably induce euphoric mood in the majority of people. Many of these effects are immediate, occurring within seconds or minutes after exposure. In contrast, despite intensive research efforts and standard surveillance techniques during drug screening, not a single pharmacological agent has been identified that can reliably induce depression in the majority of naïve individuals. In only a minority of individuals with a family history of mood disorder, reserpine will elicit a depressive reaction (Kraemer and McKinney, 1979). Similarly, tryptophan depletion has no impact on mood in healthy individuals, except for a small change in a minority of individuals with a positive family history (Ellenbogen et al., 1996; Shansis et al., 2000). This discrepancy in the likelihood that pharmaceutical agents can provoke depression or mania is curious, and its significance is reinforced by the psychometrics of psychological mood manipulation.

Symbolic representations can drive mood change. Being told that one is deficient, unloved, corrupt, or ineffective affects mood. Clearly, we are built such that our ideas about the world and ourselves can alter our mood. Indeed, a small industry has developed that uses psychological manipulations to produce mood changes in specific directions (e.g., from sadness to euphoria) (Velten, 1968; Bouhuys et al., 1995; Richell and Anderson, 2004). This literature suggests that the range or intensity of affect produced by psychological manipulations is often greater for inductions of sadness than those of happiness. In other words, it appears to be much easier to induce clear-cut sadness as opposed to euphoria through words or music (symbolic representations).

If these observations are valid—and much work needs to be done on the psychometrics of mood change—they may advance our understanding of how pharmacological agents and psychological manipulations constitute intrinsically different types of triggers or pathways for mood alteration, perhaps because of intrinsic differences in modulating disinhibitory versus excitatory processes.

Functional Brain Asymmetry and the Localization of Mood Systems

In the first edition of this text, laterality and kindling were identified as key concepts in theories about the neural origins of manic-depressive illness. At the time, it was common to hypothesize that schizophrenia was an outcome of left-hemisphere dysfunction, while manic-depressive illness derived from right-hemisphere deficits (Flor-Henry, 1976). Another view was that a cumulative history of stress, affective episodes themselves, and biological predisposition fueled a kindling process that resulted in manifestation of mood disturbance and progressively more frequent and intense episodes of illness (Post, 1990, 2002).

Neither hypothesis has remained the focus of mainstream research. In both cases, this shift in attention reflects in part advances in basic neuroscience that have produced research tools and concepts with the potential to provide great explanatory power with respect to fundamental abnormalities in clinical populations, as well as opportunities for designing new interventions. Understanding of intracellular cascades and the factors that promote cellular resilience or the expression of neurogenesis has led to new conceptualizations of pathoetiology and potential avenues for treatment (see Chapter 14).

In a number of respects, the lateralization view was a dead end. On the one hand, linking disorders to dysfunction at the level of a hemisphere, even if true, was hardly precise in terms of localization. The total right hemisphere could not be abnormal in mood disorders. Furthermore, this hypothesis was imprecise as to whether this right-hemisphere dysfunction is the core problem resulting in periodic manifestations of depression and mania or in an expression of these affective states.

Perhaps the greatest limitation of the laterality hypothesis was its lack of practical application for diagnosis or treatment or for the development of a direct method for testing validity. Until recently, psychiatry had no means other than ECT of targeting biological treatment to specific brain areas. Systemic administration of medications allows no control over the neural systems being modulated. In contrast, left and right unilateral ECT produce profound asymmetries in the physiology and function of the brain. Unilateral ECT produces marked decreases in CBF and CMR_{glu} and marked increases in EEG slow-wave activity in the hemisphere ipsilateral to the side of stimulation (Kriss et al., 1978; Nobler et al., 1994; Sackeim et al., 1996b). It also produces marked disjunctions in neuropsychological measures. For example, assessment of orientation and language functions in the postictal period immediately following left and right unilateral ECT is as reliable as the Wada test in identifying laterality of language (Pratt et al., 1971; Pratt and Warrington, 1972). Thus the view that euphoric and depressed states reflect release of function in the left and right hemispheres, respectively, would imply that left unilateral ECT is more effective than right unilateral ECT in the treatment of mania, with the reverse holding true for depression. Although some findings in the ECT literature support both predictions (Small et al.,

1993), the larger point is that left and right unilateral ECT both show considerable efficacy in the treatment of mania and depression, and that any difference in therapeutic effects is relatively minor compared with the shared variance. Given the asymmetrical physiological and cognitive effects of unilateral ECT, the efficacy data largely contradict a prominent role for functional brain asymmetry in treatment mechanisms and, by extension, in the pathophysiology of depression and mania.

A key observation that promoted interest in lateralization effects was the association between localization of stroke and other forms of brain damage and manifestation of mood disturbance. Clinically, as mentioned earlier, it has long been noted that "unipolar mania" (i.e., manifestation of mania without prior or subsequent episodes of major depression) occurs almost exclusively in the context of coarse brain injury (Jorge et al., 1993; Fujikawa et al., 1995; Robinson, 1997). Further, it is generally agreed that such lesions are predominantly right-sided (Cummings and Mendez, 1984; Starkstein et al., 1988a).

In contrast, the relationships between location of brain lesion and manifestation of depression have become less certain with additional research. Interest in the laterality of emotion was sparked by findings relating side of brain injury to affective state (Gainotti, 1972) and to uncontrollable emotional expressions (Sackeim et al., 1982a), by the demonstration of asymmetry in the emotional expressions of the human face (Sackeim et al., 1978), and by the linkage of disturbances in the processing of affectively laden information to right-sided brain damage (Heilman et al., 1975). However, the relevance of a laterality dimension to mood disorders was contingent on reliable associations between side of brain damage and manifestations of mood disturbance.

Gainotti (1969, 1972) was the first to examine systematically the distinct differences in emotional reactions of patients with left- and right-hemisphere stroke. Right-sided damage was associated with anosognosia (denial of illness) or anosdisaphorie (lack of concern about illness, i.e., a carefree attitude) and a "euphoric-indifference reaction." Robinson's research, however, catalyzed interest in this area. In a seminal paper, Robinson and colleagues (1984) linked the severity of depressive symptoms shortly after stroke to damage to left-sided prefrontal regions. The closer the lesions were to the left frontal pole, the more severe was the depressive syndrome. Right parietal lesions were also linked to depression, but at lower incidence and with lesser intensity of depressive manifestations. This work had important methodological limitations, such as the exclusion of patients with significant aphasia, which possibly distorted the sample of patients with left-sided injury, and problems in the blinding of assessment given the motor,

sensory, and cognitive deficits that reveal the side of lateralized brain damage. Most of the subsequent studies failed to replicate Robinson's core findings, and some meta-analyses of this literature contested the existence of an association between lesion location and depressive manifestations (Carson et al., 2000; Narushima et al., 2003; Yu et al., 2004).

Missing from this perspective were the results of long-term follow-up of individuals with penetrating head wounds after World War II. Mood disturbance was common in such patients. In particularly careful work, Lishman (1968) noted that right posterior head wounds were far more likely to be associated with depressive and manic manifestations than were injuries to any of the remaining three quadrants. It hardly appeared likely that different forms of nonirritative brain insult—stroke versus head wound—could fundamentally alter the linkage between side of brain insult and depressive symptoms.

One possibility accounting for the discrepancies in this literature concerns the issue of time since stroke. Robinson's early work involved patients who were examined very soon after stroke, recruited at emergency room presentation. Later studies often examined patients months to years after their cerebrovascular accident. There has been little longitudinal work addressing whether localization of damage is related to the persistence (chronicity) and/or late emergence of depressive symptoms. Nelson and colleagues (1994) evaluated affective symptoms in patients with lateralized stroke at 2-week, 2-month, and 6-month time points. Initially, the group with left-hemisphere stroke experienced a slower rate of recovery from depressive symptoms. At the 6-month time point, however, the emotional functioning of the right-hemisphere group worsened. The evidence regarding temporal interval as a moderator of the relationship between lesion location and affective disturbance is not consistent, and considerably more work is necessary (Carson et al., 2000). Nonetheless, the positive findings in this area introduce a dynamic element to the relationships between brain injury and altered affective states.

One interpretation of this literature would be to argue that in the acute poststroke period, depressive symptoms are most severe when the lesion is closest to the left frontal pole. The most recent meta-analysis (Narushima et al., 2003) supports this association. However, manifestation of this syndrome is time-limited, and depressive symptoms spontaneously remit within a few months. In contrast, right parietal lesions result in milder depressive symptoms in the acute period. Yet this disturbance is more likely to be chronic, and these lesions may also result in late-emerging affective disturbance. Following the disinhibition model for nonirritative lesions, both left anterior and right posterior stroke may disinhibit right prefrontal areas critical to the manifestation of depressed mood. Prefrontal-parietal connectivity is well established, and reciprocal inhibitory pathways have been demonstrated (Goldman-Rakic, 1987; Woods et al., 1993). Thus this view, albeit post hoc in accounting for discrepancies, leads to the assertion that the functional consequences of brain lesions are time dependent, and this temporal effect may differ based on laterality. That such temporal effects can occur is amply demonstrated in the neurosurgical literature on the treatment of highly resistant mood disorders. Therapeutic benefit from psychosurgery usually is manifest only months after the intervention.

Dissociating Therapeutics and Pathophysiology

Although the linkage of right-sided damage to mania remains uncontested, there is uncertainty about the role of lateralized brain damage in the manifestation of depressed states. Indeed, one possibility yet to be raised is that the strength of association for lateralized effects is stronger for euphoric or manic than for dysphoric or depressed states. As seen in Figure 9–22, the association between pathological laughing and right-sided silent lesions is stronger than that between pathological crying and left-sided lesions. As seen in Figure 9–24, there is also a robust association between laterality of epileptic focus and uncontrollable laughter as a peri-ictal phenomenon.

Until recently, data-driven formulations of this type had little possibility of being tested experimentally. The common denominator in this sort of theorizing is that disinhibition of right prefrontal structures is the common final pathway for depressive manifestation. If that were the case, selective suppression of such activity would be expected to have antidepressant properties, and left prefrontal suppression to have antimanic effects.

The development of noninvasive methods for focal neuromodulation resulted in new life for this area of research. For example, repetitive transcranial magnetic stimulation (rTMS) offers a means of suppressing or enhancing activity in regions under the coil or at a distance through patterns of connectivity. Because the scalp and skull are transparent to the magnetic field, it is possible through use of appropriate coil geometry to restrict stimulation to target brain areas. There is considerable evidence that slow-frequency rTMS (one or fewer pulses per second) produces an inhibitory effect, whereas fast-frequency rTMS (five or more pulses per second) has a poststimulation excitatory effect (Wassermann et al., 1993; Terao and Ugawa, 2002; Wu et al., 2002).

There is now a substantial literature on sham-controlled studies testing the efficacy of rTMS in major depression, and the meta-analyses of this literature have all reached the same conclusions (Holtzheimer et al., 2001; McNamara et al., 2001; Burt et al., 2002). The active rTMS conditions compared with sham have been fast-frequency left DLPFC stimulation and slow-frequency right DLPFC stimulation. Both interventions yield moderate to large effect sizes for antidepressant properties; in other words, both are consistently superior to sham. However, these findings are of greater theoretical than practical importance. In absolute magnitude, the therapeutic effects in the active conditions, although superior to those in sham, have commonly been modest, and the durability of the benefit derived has rarely been tested. For rTMS to have a role in routine practice, these issues must be addressed (Sackeim, 2000b).

From a theoretical perspective, however, it is extraordinary that a highly lateralized intervention can display these antidepressant properties, and moreover, that antidepressant effects can be achieved with opposite physiological alterations (inhibition versus excitation) that are dependent on the laterality of the brain region stimulated. Taken at face value, for example, these effects could indicate that the key to exerting antidepressant properties is the state of the "seesaw": any intervention that tips the seesaw toward greater left prefrontal or reduced right prefrontal expression in the DLPFC will have antidepressant properties. This formulation could mean that mood states are not attributable to the physiological status of a specific brain region, but are an emergent property reflecting the balance of activity among regions in a distributed network. Another possibility is that different individuals benefit from slow right or fast left rTMS, and that left-sided hypofunction and right-sided hyperfunction are alternative routes to major depression (Kimbrell et al., 1999; Speer et al., 2000).

Focal brain stimulation offers an experimental means of testing key concepts about the neuroanatomy and neurophysiology of mood disorders and their treatment. Two caveats are in order about the state of knowledge in this area. First, while it is established that slow right and fast left rTMS have antidepressant properties, however modest, it is assumed that fast right and slow left rTMS are ineffective, something that has never been adequately tested. For example, were slow left DLPFC to exert equal antidepressant properties, a fundamental role for laterality in generating therapeutic effects would be seriously questioned. The key experiment, in which depressed patients are randomly assigned in a 2×2 design to slow- or fast-frequency stimulation and left or right DLPFC, has not been conducted, and is essential to further understanding of the effects of this intervention on mood.

The second caveat is more general. It is often assumed that knowledge of the mode of action of a therapeutic agent (e.g., serotonin reuptake blockade) dictates conceptualization about the underlying pathophysiology (or vice versa). However, there are many examples in medicine in which the optimal treatment for a condition acts through a mechanism distinct from the pathoetiology of the illness. It is doubtful that anyone ever became depressed because of lack of a seizure, and yet ECT is the most effective antidepressant. Put more forcefully, many of our pharmacological interventions produce chronic alterations in brain neurochemistry and other aspects of physiology that are simply not seen otherwise in nature and do not restore the brain to a normative state. Thus the circuitry involved in achieving an antidepressant effect may be distinct from that responsible for manifestation of the mood disorder. The therapeutic properties of interventions such as rTMS may reveal a great deal about the pathways that modulate or ameliorate the experience of major depression. However, these pathways may be distinct from those that generate the abnormal mood state.

Ultimately, progress in genetics and molecular biology is likely to produce breakthroughs in our understanding of the pathoetiology of bipolar disorder and recurrent unipolar depression and in our ability to provide more effective therapeutic interventions. Nonetheless, these disorders need to be understood at a system level. Discrete aspects of emotional life have neural representation. System theories draw on evidence from neurological, psychiatric, and normal populations to constrain hypotheses about the neuroanatomy and physiology that subserve abnormal mood states and that mediate therapeutic outcomes. We are just entering an era in which these hypotheses can be tested through the controlled use of anatomically targeted alterations of physiology and neurochemistry. It can be anticipated that the formulations presented here will be refined or undone, and that the next edition of this text will offer superior descriptions of the neural networks dysregulated in manic-depressive illness.

CONCLUSIONS

Normal Findings in Bipolar Patients

Bipolar patients have normal VIQ, a finding that challenges the idea that bipolar disorder is associated with pervasive intellectual impairment. One possible explanation is that the cognitive systems underlying language are spared from the otherwise generalized bipolar disease process; or they may be constitutionally endowed at higher capacity. Likewise, preliminary evidence indicates that procedural learning and memory are not significantly affected by bipolar illness, while limited data suggest that the ability to recall past events, or details of past events, is not significantly impaired in bipolar patients.

Alone among the executive functions, reasoning remains relatively preserved in bipolar illness. Because the results of tests of reasoning correlate substantially with the results of tests of verbal ability, this finding may reflect a pattern in which cognitive operations heavily dependent on language are among the higher cognitive functions least affected by bipolar disorder.

Neuropsychological Deficits in Bipolar Patients

Intelligence is somewhat reduced in bipolar illness in both the remitted and manic states as reflected in diminished IQ scores. Reasoning remains intact. The marked deficit in PIQ among bipolar patients is commonly ascribed to the effects of mood-dependent psychomotor retardation on task performance, but the presence of the deficit during remission and in individuals at risk for bipolar disorder, as well as its persistence when performance is untimed, argues otherwise. It now appears that the discrepancy is independent of the affective state and may even be present before the first episode of mood disturbance. The above proposed explanation for normal VIQ scores in bipolar patients can also help account for the deficit in PIQ: although the cognitive systems underlying language are spared by the disease or are constitutionally endowed at higher capacity, those underlying other components of intelligence, including performance, are not.

Attention comprises several distinct processes, and its overall integrity is central to the normal functioning of higher cognitive processes such as learning and memory. Disturbances of attention ("impaired concentration") are typical of bipolar disorder, and attention is among the most dramatically impaired functions in patients during episodes of major depression, and indeed across all phases of the illness, including remission. With respect to learning, memory, and visuospatial skills, there is little evidence that deficits reflect more than an attentional disturbance. Short-term memory deficits are typical of bipolar patients, even in remission. It is possible that these deficits result from impaired attention. Bipolar patients also have decided and uniform difficulty in acquiring new information during all phases of the illness, including remission.

Executive functions come closest to the idea of a neural homunculus in charge of administering neural resources. Only a very limited range of executive functions in bipolar disorder has been studied, however. The studies that have been conducted have found substantial deficits in all phases of bipolar disorder. Severe illness has been associated in particular with difficulty in concept formation and set shifting.

NOTES

1. Corwin et al., 1990; Rubinsztein et al., 2000; Sweeney et al., 2000; Murphy and Sahakian, 2001; Quraishi and Frangou, 2002; Martinez-Arán et al., 2004b; Marvel and Paradiso, 2004.

2. Martinez-Arán et al., 2000, 2002a,b, 2004a,b; Rubinsztein et al., 2000; Zubieta et al., 2001; El-Badri et al., 2001; Yen et al., 2002; Altshuler et al., 2004; Dixon et al., 2004.

3. The 52 studies that contributed to the meta-analysis were Oltmanns, 1978; Savard et al., 1980; Asarnow and MacCrimmon, 1981; Robertson and Taylor, 1985; Dalby and Williams, 1986; Green and Walker, 1986; Harvey and Brault, 1986; Sapin et al., 1987; Wolfe et al., 1987; Gruzelier et al., 1988; Wielgus and Harvey, 1988; Coffman et al., 1990; David and Cutting, 1990; Dupont et al., 1990; Harvey and Serper, 1990; Morice, 1990; Deptula et al., 1991; Park and Holzman, 1992; Jones et al., 1994; Kaprinis et al., 1995; Souza et al., 1995; Docherty et al., 1996; Thomas et al., 1996; Hawkins et al., 1997; Lohr and Caligiuri, 1997; Paradiso et al., 1997; Park, 1997; Addington and Addington, 1998; van Gorp et al., 1998, 1999; Ferrier et al., 1999; Gourovitch et al., 1999; Sax et al., 1999; Ali et al., 2000; Krabbendam et al., 2000; Rossi et al., 2000; Rubinsztein et al., 2000; Sweeney et al., 2000; Clark et al., 2001; Zubieta et al., 2001; Agarwal et al., 2002; Cavanagh et al., 2002; Seidman et al., 2002, 2003; Fleck et al., 2003; Getz et al., 2003; Kremen et al., 2003; Swann et al., 2003; Umbricht et al., 2003; Gildengers et al., 2004; Martínez-Arán et al., 2004b; Zalla et al., 2004.

4. The effect size measure used throughout was Hedges' G, and the z-value associated with the point estimate (effect size across studies) and the variance of this estimate were computed to determine significance. All computations were conducted with a beta version of Comprehensive Meta-Analysis II. Dr. Michael Borenstein made upgrades to the program that enabled this meta-analysis.

5. Davidson, 1939; Fisher, 1949; Callagan, 1952; Miller et al., 1981; Donnelly et al., 1982.

6. Flor-Henry and Gruzelier, 1983; Rush et al., 1983; Silverstein and Meltzer, 1983; Taylor and Abrams, 1983.

7. This specification was supported by a significant interaction between group (patient vs. normal control) and IQ component (VIQ vs. PIQ) in a repeated measure analysis of covariance (ANCOVA).

8. Ashton et al., 1995; Parker et al., 1995a,b; 2000; Mitchell et al., 1996.

9. Kupfer and Foster, 1973; Kupfer et al., 1974, 1975; Weiss et al., 1974a,b; Foster and Kupfer, 1975; McPartland et al., 1975; Goode et al., 1979.

10. Szabadi et al., 1976; Greden and Carroll, 1980; Greden et al., 1981; Godfrey and Knight, 1984; Hardy et al., 1984; Hoffmann et al., 1985; Nilsonne, 1987, 1988; Alpert et al., 2001.

11. Bouhuys and Mulder-Hajonides van der Meulen, 1984; Hardy et al., 1984; Hoffmann et al., 1985; Alpert et al., 2001; Cannizzaro et al., 2004.

12. Clark et al., 2002, 2005; Liu et al., 2002; Strakowski et al., 2005.

13. Whitehead, 1973a,b; Strömgren, 1977; Breslow et al., 1980; Gass and Russell, 1986.

14. Hasher and Zacks, 1979; Roy-Byrne et al., 1986; Thomas et al., 1999; Hammar, 2003.

15. Craik and Tulving, 1975; Craik and Jennings, 1992; Mandzia et al., 2004; Newell and Andrews, 2004.

16. Roy-Byrne et al., 1986; el Massioui and Lesevre, 1988; Hartlage et al., 1993; Christensen et al., 1997; Thomas et al., 1999; Den Hartog et al., 2003; Hammar, 2003; Hammar et al., 2003a,b; Politis et al., 2004.

17. Nelson and Craighead, 1977; Breslow et al., 1981; Gotlib, 1981; Clark and Teasdale, 1982; Coyne and Gotlib, 1983; Gotlib and Olson, 1983; Yang and Rehm, 1993; Murray et al., 1999; Winter et al., 2000.

18. Sackeim and Prohovnik, 1993; Soares and Mann, 1997; Haldane and Frangou, 2004; Rogers et al., 2004.

19. Joanette and Goulet, 1986; Bayles et al., 1993; Schlosser et al., 1998; Spreen and Strauss, 1998; Spence et al., 2000.

20. Mann et al., 1999; Keilp et al., 2001; Oquendo and Mann, 2001; Oquendo et al., 2004.

21. Phillips et al., 2003a,b; Schaefer et al., 2003; Tavares et al., 2003; Chamberlain and Sahakian, 2004.

22. One study (Joffe et al., 1988) found no difference among bipolar patients treated with lithium, carbamazepine, or no medication on tests of attention, visuomotor function, and memory. However, this study also failed to find differences between the bipolar groups and healthy controls on the cognitive measures, raising doubt about the sensitivity or reliability of the neuropsychological assessment. Other studies yielding negative findings on the cognitive effects of lithium include Telford and Worrall, 1978; Kjellman et al., 1980; and Ghadirian et al., 1983.

23. Tohen et al., 1990a,b, 2000; Albus et al., 1996; Atre-Vaidya et al., 1998.

24. McKay et al., 1995; Tham et al., 1997; Kessing, 1998; van Gorp et al., 1998; Denicoff et al., 1999.

25. Lesser et al., 1993; Salloway et al., 1996; Dahabra et al., 1998; Kumar et al., 1998.

26. Hickie et al., 1995, 1997; Simpson et al., 1997a, 1998; Baldwin et al., 2000.

27. Steingart et al., 1987; Junqué et al., 1990; Cadelo et al., 1991; Baloh et al., 1995.

28. Dupont et al., 1987, 1990, 1995; Swayze et al., 1990.

29. Bejjani et al., 1999; Berney et al., 2002; Stefurak et al., 2003; Okun et al., 2004.

30. Terzian and Cecotto, 1959; Alema and Donini, 1960; Terzian, 1964; Rosadini and Rossi, 1967; Rossi and Rosadini, 1967.

31. Sackeim et al., 1983a, 1987b; Sackeim, 1999, 2004.

32. Engel et al., 1982; Rosenberg et al., 1988; Volkow et al., 1988; Silfverskiöld and Risberg, 1989; Nobler et al., 1994, 2001; Henry et al., 2001.

33. Wu et al., 1992, 1999; Mayberg et al., 1999; Teneback et al., 1999; Nobler et al., 2000a; Drevets et al., 2002.

34. Andersen et al., 1993; Benedek and Peterson, 1995; Jeret, 1997; McCullagh and Feinstein, 2000; Kaschka et al., 2001; Smith et al., 2003; House et al., 2004.

35. Hommes, 1965; Gainotti, 1970, 1972; Robinson and Szetela, 1981; Robinson et al., 1984; Narushima et al., 2003.

10   Personality, Personality Disorders, and Interpersonal Functioning

Those only, who lived for some time with [Lord Byron], could believe that a man's temper, Proteus like, was capable of assuming so many shapes. It may literally be said, that at different hours of the day he metamorphosed himself into four or more individuals, each possessed of the most opposite qualities; for, in every change, his natural impetuosity made him fly into the furthermost extremes. In the course of the day he might become the most morose, and the most gay; the most melancholy, and the most frolicsome . . . the most gentle being in existence, and the most irascible.

—*Julius Millingen (Byron's physician), 1831*

The intense emotions and troubling thoughts and behaviors of manic and depressive states often confound the person who has bipolar disorder and family members alike: What is due to the illness? What is due to personality? Where does one end and the other begin? Will treatment alter not only the disorder, but also personality? Do pathological mood states reflect the real self, or is there a coherent self despite the mood swings that characterize the disorder? Scientists and clinicians ask related questions: Are there unique and characteristic personality styles associated with bipolar disorder, and are they present when the person is not affectively ill? Are there predisposing or precursor "traits"? Do personality characteristics affect the course of the disorder? (Related questions concerning the mild forms of bipolar disorder that may be continuous with personality patterns are discussed separately in Chapter 2.)

Questions about "personality" are both personally meaningful and clinically and theoretically important because they may help shed light on the enormous variability among individuals with bipolar disorder and aid in achieving a fuller understanding of the disorder's development. Issues of personality have been addressed in various ways by psychologists and psychiatrists, and in the first section of this chapter we review both the complexities of the questions examined and the research results.

We next address the issue of personality disorders, the enduring and dysfunctional patterns of behaviors and traits defined by Axis II of the *Diagnostic and Statistical Manual* (DSM), that may accompany Axis I diagnoses of any kind. Personality disorders may profoundly color the experience of the coexisting psychological disorder, as well as affect both the clinical and social adjustment of the individual and the success of treatment. They have been the focus of many recent studies in the field of bipolar research, and the results of these studies may help inform patients and clinicians about how individuals with a diagnosis of bipolar illness can be so different from one another in presentation and prognosis.

Finally, we discuss the interpersonal functioning of individuals with bipolar disorder in major role areas, such as intimate relationships, social behavior, and family relations. There is increasing interest not only in the clinical manifestations of bipolar disorder, but also in the ways in which individuals with the disorder live their lives and cope with their condition. What are the unique interpersonal patterns and challenges for the bipolar patient, and what does the social milieu itself contribute to the understanding of the course of the disorder? Of particular importance is growing awareness of the discrepancies that sometimes exist between social functioning and clinical status.

Prior to DSM-III the term "manic-depressive illness" could either mean what we now call bipolar disorder or include all recurrent affective disorders. When the context of the older literature makes clear that it is referring to bipolar disorder, we use that term. Because the literature relevant to this chapter rarely distinguishes recurrent from nonrecurrent forms of unipolar depression, we focus on the bipolar subgroup of manic-depressive illness.

PERSONALITY AND BIPOLAR DISORDER

In this section, we begin by reviewing a number of conceptual and methodological issues associated with studies of the relationship between personality and bipolar disorder. We then examine, in turn, the findings of studies addressing personality during mania and depression, comparisons of two major dimensions of personality—neuroticism and extraversion–introversion—among remitted bipolar patients and normal groups, comparisons of the personality traits of bipolar and unipolar patients, effects of medication on personality, and predictive associations between personality characteristics and the development and outcome of bipolar disorder.

Conceptual Issues and Key Definitions

The terms *personality, character,* and *temperament* are sometimes used interchangeably. They differ in important ways, however.

Personality generally refers to the unique aspects of an individual, especially those most distinctive or likely to be noticed by others in social interactions. Personality theorist Gordon Allport (1961, p. 35) suggested that personality is simply "what a person 'really is' "—his or her most typical and deeply characteristic features. Yet there are as many psychological definitions of personality as theorists writing about the subject. Two prominent theorists summarized these many definitions succinctly as focusing on one or more of the following facets: "the individual's social stimulus value; the integrative or organizational function of personality; an individual's general adjustment; the unique or individual aspects of behavior; and the essence of man" (Hall and Lindzey, 1970, p. 8). In the absence of any universally accepted definition, most personality theorists define the construct by the assessment instruments they use to measure it. Clearly, some theories of personality lend themselves more readily to empirical research than others.[1]

Personality has traditionally been viewed as having several qualities: it is stable across time and situations; it encompasses an organized set of traits forming a coherent personality style; and it is the underlying psychological "cause" of a person's specific behaviors and beliefs. These assumptions have been challenged because we have learned that behaviors and beliefs are overtly and subtly determined by experiences, by current environmental demands, by cognitive capacities and styles, by genetic and constitutional factors, and certainly by affect and emotion. Nevertheless, researchers are increasingly attempting to account for the complexities involved by defining a few traits that can be used to describe most people and by taking into account the biological, temperamental features of personality and the environmental determinants that greatly shape its expression.

Character has been defined as "personality evaluated"—that aspect of an individual which bears a moral stamp and reflects the person's integrative and organizing functions. The concept of character is employed less frequently in the United States than in Europe, although it is often used interchangeably with that of personality. In part, the concept of personality disorder addresses the issue of a person's character traits.

Temperament has always been viewed as having a more constitutional, genetic, and biological basis than either personality or character. Hippocrates and Galen, for example, based their theories of temperament on the four humors of the body. According to Allport (1961, pp. 33–34), "Temperament refers to the characteristic phenomena of an individual's emotional nature, including his susceptibility to emotional stimulation, his customary strength and speed of response, the quality of his prevailing mood, and all peculiarities of fluctuation and intensity in mood, these phenomena being regarded as dependent upon constitutional make-up, and therefore largely hereditary in nature."

The affective temperaments that reflect the milder manifestations of the bipolar spectrum are discussed extensively in Chapter 2. Although there is overlap between the topics of personality and the bipolar spectrum, we attempt in this chapter to limit the discussion to several specific issues detailed in the following sections.

Relationship of Personality to Affective Disorders

Several researchers (Akiskal et al., 1983; Clark et al., 1994) have noted the complex relationship and interactions between personality and affective illness, especially depression. From their work and that of many others, four major models have been formulated:

- Personality is a *predisposition* to affective illness. This model assumes that personality patterns precede and therefore predispose an individual to develop affective illness. This view, fundamental to psychoanalytical thought and writing, also is reflected to varying degrees in the writings of cognitive and behavioral psychologists who have formulated various theories about predisposing characteristics for depression, such as negative views of the self and depressive attributional style. There is a relatively small literature on personality antecedents of bipolar disorder.
- Personality is an *expression* of affective illness. Personality patterns are viewed as manifestations of mild to moderate forms of the underlying affective illness. The individual's temperament is assumed to be intricately bound up with the genetic predisposition to mania and depression. This view, integral to the work of Kraepelin and Kretschmer, is shared in part by most of the modern researchers who posit a continuum of affective states (see Chapters 1 and 2).
- Personality is a *modifier* of affective illness. Many investigators (Chodoff, 1972; Klerman, 1973; von Zerssen, 1977) have emphasized the role of personality in determining the clinical presentation of affective symptom patterns (especially in obsessive, dependent, or hysterical person-

ality types), the response to psychotherapy and medication, the tendency to become dependent on alcohol or other drugs, and adherence to prescribed treatment regimens. They have also identified personality as an important determinant of the nature and extent of interpersonal relationships. These relationships, in turn, can affect both precipitating events and the likelihood of emotional support during and after affective episodes. The ability to handle the enormous stress and complications of affective illness is assumed to be strongly influenced by premorbid personality and character structure.

· Personality is *altered* by affective illness. In this model, personality is assumed to be altered by the experience of affective illness. Various consequences of the illness—including changes in self-esteem and social interaction patterns; difficulties in sustaining meaningful relationships and employment; and frequent fluctuations in mood, energy, perception, and thinking—are all thought to both cause and reflect short- or long-term personality changes that may be reversible or irreversible. The obvious importance and impact on personality of such illness variables as frequency, duration, severity, and nature of episodes have not been well studied.

These models of the association between affective illness and personality are not mutually exclusive, and they may be difficult to disentangle in practice. Moreover, research has not tested all of the models with respect to bipolar disorder, leaving many questions unanswered. Recent research has generally addressed several largely descriptive issues. One such issue concerns the stability of personality traits and whether they vary by manic or depressed state. A related issue is whether there are unique personality characteristics of bipolar patients that differ from those of unipolar depressed or well individuals. Still another set of issues has to do with the predictive association between personality features and clinical course. Before turning to a review of studies that address these matters, however, a further caution concerning methodological issues is in order.

Methodological Issues

In addition to the conceptual issues raised above, many specific methodological problems are intrinsic to the study of personality and bipolar disorder. The most central of these is the problem of *trait and state*, or disentangling manifestations of illness from the more stable and lasting structures of personality. Specific problems include the substantial difficulties of separating the current clinical state from measured personality traits, of assessing the effects of medications on personality (independently of their effects on the underlying affective illness), of sorting through the personality effects of previous manic and depressive episodes, and of delineating the effects of subclinical episodes on personality. Fundamental issues of measurement and philosophy emerge when two pivotal questions are posed. First, what aspects of personality are being studied when one is assessing the successfully treated person with bipolar illness—true premorbid ones or affectively changed and attenuated ones? Second, to what extent is personality a function of medication level or of the cumulative effects of disease?

Another set of problems concerns issues of *diagnostic and illness heterogeneity*. Heterogeneity is well recognized in the unipolar depressive disorders (in symptom patterns, etiology, severity, episodic patterning, and frequency). Although bipolar illness is more homogeneous, it, too, can be confusingly varied. Few investigations of personality distinguish between bipolar-I and bipolar-II, and fewer still consider other issues related to the full spectrum of bipolarity, such as the stage or severity of manic and depressive illness at the time of testing, the ratio of manic to depressive episodes, the age at illness onset, the frequency and nature of mixed states, the duration and patterning of episodes, and the characteristic nature of the manic episodes (euphoric and expansive, for example, rather than paranoid and dysphoric). All of these variables are likely to have both long- and short-term effects on the expression of personality. Other variables generally not controlled for in personality studies of affective illness include seasonal factors of importance to studies done during both remission and illness (see Chapter 4); the competence and sophistication of clinical care, including such common problems as prescribing incorrect medications or dosages; and selection factors intrinsic to the nature of remission studies—that is, a selection bias favoring healthier, more normal bipolar patients.

Measurement and design also are problematic. Until recently, comparison groups were inadequate. Early studies compared manic-depressive (predominantly bipolar) with schizophrenic patients; more recent studies have used unipolar depressed patients as controls. Studies using subjects from the general population as controls, although a clear improvement, too often have not controlled for family history of affective illness or for important demographic variables, such as age, IQ, socioeconomic status, and gender. Standard problems of measurement, such as the reliability and validity of the psychometric tests used, are well reviewed elsewhere. We note here, however, that much of the earlier research employed assessment methods based on questionable assumptions and validity (e.g., Rorschach), or on instruments that may no longer be widely used now that newer and more empirically and conceptually based approaches are available. In the sections to follow, older work is noted briefly, with greater emphasis on more contemporary methods.

Several study designs have been used to investigate personality and bipolar illness, including studies of patients across different mood states. In addition, comparisons have been made between affectively ill bipolar and unipolar patients, remitted bipolar and unipolar patients, and remitted bipolar patients and members of the general population. These design strategies are generally appropriate to address simple, descriptive questions, but more complex designs, including longitudinal studies, are greatly needed to pursue questions relating personality characteristics to the clinical and course features of bipolar disorder and social adjustment. Heterogeneity of comparison groups (for example, the tendency not to distinguish melancholic from nonmelancholic unipolar depression) is a significant problem (Parker et al., 2004).

Psychoanalytic Perspectives

Prior to the psychoanalytic era, most early clinical investigators assumed that personality structure in bipolar disorder reflected the underlying disease process.[2] Psychoanalytic theorists considered two major issues in their writings on manic-depressive illness: the etiology of mania and depression and the underlying personality structure of patients with bipolar illness. Most psychoanalysts focused primarily on the origins and nature of depression rather than mania. Their findings on this subject are well known and are not presented here. Instead, we briefly outline psychoanalytic concepts of mania and the manic-depressive personality. Although neither time nor research has supported the psychoanalytic perspective on bipolar illness, it is historically important, especially in the United States, because it deeply influenced generations of psychiatrists, psychologists, and social workers.

From a psychoanalytic perspective, mania can best be understood as a defense against underlying depressive affect. This fundamental concept has been stated in different ways by many authors.[3] Although interesting, the psychoanalytic perspective suffers from the usual difficulties involved in analyzing open-ended, clinical observations: such observations are retrospective, interpretive, and highly speculative. Comparison groups are lacking, and there are few, if any, ways of subjecting the theory to test. Finally, as (Kotin and Goodwin, 1972, p. 684) concluded from their data-based studies of mania:

> Our data suggest that if mania is a defense against depression, it is often an inadequate defense, since depressive symptoms remain prominent during the manic phase.

The manic-depressive personality has been viewed by psychoanalysts as narcissistic (Freud, 1917; Fenichel, 1945), masochistic (Gerö, 1936; Jacobson, 1953; Garma 1968), extraverted,[4] and highly conventional.[5] Rado (1928) discussed at length the belief that manic-depressive individuals have an "obsessive need for the approval of others."[6] Alexander (1948) described the manic-depressive individual as warm, outgoing, and practical—a person who prefers the concrete to the abstract. Not surprisingly, he noted a tendency for the emotions to rule reason. English (1949) characterized the manic-depressive patient as perfectionist, egocentric, logical, wise, talented, afraid to hate (except when manic), and rigid. Other writers (Dooley, 1921; Wilson, 1951; Cohen et al., 1954) highlighted somewhat different constellations of traits and the problems they pose for the therapist and others.[7] Obviously inadequate as an etiological model, what psychoanalysts have historically viewed as "personality" often appears from our modern perspective to be the expression of symptoms of bipolar illness.

Personality during Mania and Depression

Studies contrasting personality functioning during manic or hypomanic and depressive states often—not surprisingly—reveal dramatic differences. Rather than a core, stable personality as assumed by psychoanalytically oriented theorists, observations made during episodes reflect the powerful influence of fluctuating mood and energy levels, as well as behavioral changes, brought about by the illness.

Comparisons between Manic/Depressive Episodes and Periods of Remission

Bipolar patients tested during remission show clear changes relative to personality profiles obtained during depressive episodes. Early studies focused in particular on neuroticism as measured by Eysenck's (1959) Maudsley Personality Inventory (MPI) (e.g., Perris, 1971; Liebowitz et al., 1979; Hirschfeld et al., 1983). The majority of studies showed significant decreases in neuroticism during remission, as well as increases in extraversion. A review of the stability of neuroticism scores during clinical states of depression and remission (mainly among unipolar depressed patients) suggested that neuroticism captures two elements: (1) a depressive-state influence and (2) an underlying vulnerability dimension that predicts the development and severity of depression (Clark et al., 1994). Neuroticism has also been conceptualized as a general factor termed *negative affectivity*, defined as a temperamental sensitivity to stimuli associated with a range of negative emotional states, negative perceptions and expectations, and low self-esteem (Clark et al., 1994).

In a combined sample of bipolar and unipolar patients, Hirschfeld and colleagues (1983) found that impulsivity scores were unchanged from depression to remission, and that no state-dependent changes occurred in measures of rigidity, obsessionality, restraint, reflectiveness, demandingness, and dominance. They also found, however, that patients who had recovered from a depression scored lower than when depressed on measures of emotional lability, neuroticism, passivity, hypersensitivity, and interpersonal dependency and higher on measures of emotional strength, resiliency, and extraversion. For a subgroup of patients who had not recovered from depression at the time of follow-up, scores on the personality tests did not change, lending credence to the authors' interpretation that "the changes recorded for the recovered patients reflect the influence of the depressed state" (Hirschfeld et al., 1983, p. 698).

A few studies have examined personality profiles across all three major affective states: mania, depression, and euthymia. Researchers (Lumry et al., 1982) administered the Minnesota Multiphasic Personality Inventory (MMPI) to a small sample of bipolar-I patients. The MMPI profiles obtained from 12 patients when manic or hypomanic and from 10 of these patients when depressed were classic manic and depressive profiles. The mean profile for the 12 euthymic patients was entirely within normal limits. The mean MMPI profiles obtained during hypomania or mania and depression are shown graphically in Figure 10–1. The authors concluded that the normal profile pattern obtained during euthymia in most of their lithium-stabilized patients indicated "complete restitution of normality."

Perceptions of Self across Affective States

Widely discrepant views of the self emerge during mania, depression, and normal functioning. Indeed, these differences in self-perception have been incorporated into the DSM-IV diagnostic criteria for mania and depression ("inflated self-esteem or grandiosity" and "feelings of

worthlessness or excessive or inappropriate guilt," respectively). In an attempt to study alternating views of the self in depression and mania, Platman and colleagues (1969) administered the Emotions Profile Index weekly to 11 bipolar patients. This psychological measure was designed to assess eight primary emotions: fear, anger, acceptance, rejection, surprise, exploration, joy, and deprivation. Twelve staff members were asked to provide their conceptions of mania and depression. This collective profile was then compared with the profiles produced by patients while manic or depressed.

The staff's and patients' conceptions of depression were strikingly similar on all eight dimensions. For both groups, depression was characterized by decreases in sociability, in interest in new experiences, and in feelings of acceptance, as well as by increases in feelings of deprivation, in aggression, and in rejection of others. Mania, on the other hand, was perceived in very different ways by staff and patients, with seven of eight mean scores showing highly significant differences (at the $p < .01$ level). Patients while manic saw themselves as sociable, trusting, moderately impulsive, and cautious and not at all stubborn or aggressive. Staff members, however, saw them as only moderately sociable, somewhat distrustful, extremely impulsive and aggressive, quite rejecting of others, and completely incautious and unafraid. Response patterns from patients were far more variable than those from staff members, suggesting a more stereotypical (or accurate) view from the latter group.

Patients were asked, when normal, to recall their previous manic and depressive episodes. Their recalled depressive profiles were similar to those produced while actually depressed, and both resembled the staff-generated depressive profile. By contrast, profiles of recalled manic episodes did not resemble those actually obtained during mania. The patients' recall of mania was far more highly correlated with staff perceptions of mania ($r = .95$) than with their own ratings produced while manic ($r = .35$). The authors concluded:

> These facts imply that the self-critical judgmental process is severely impaired in the manic state but not in the depressed state. This is consistent with the well-known fact that manic patients do not usually admit to any illness, or that they deny the maladaptive nature of their behavior. This is also why it is difficult to detect the presence of manic states by means of self-description type inventories; these usually show that the manic patient is normal.

One interesting theoretical question posed by these findings is whether the manic patient is deliberately misrepresenting his feelings and behavior, or whether he is simply unable to discriminate the specific feelings and behaviors which are judged by an outside observer as pathognomonic of mania (Platman et al., 1969, p. 213).

Figure 10–1. Mean Minnesota Multiphasic Personality Inventory (MMPI) profiles of bipolar probands during a hypomanic/manic phase (blue circles; $n = 12$) and during a depressive phase (black circles; $n = 10$); 5 cases overlap. (*Source:* Adapted from Lumry et al., 1982.)

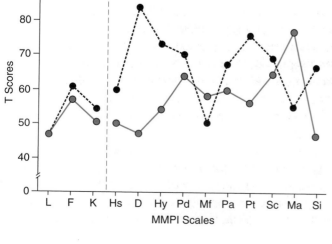

Jamison and colleagues (unpublished data) examined self-perceptions across affective states in 69 euthymic bipolar patients using the Semantic Differential, a combination of associational and scaling procedures. Patients were tested with 22 pairs of opposite adjectives (e.g., good–bad, strong–weak, complex–simple), shown as the polar ends of a seven-point continuum. Patients indicated their perceptions of themselves when manic, hypomanic, depressed, and normal by marking the most descriptive point between each polar pair. Analyses of variance by gender, with repeated measures of mood phase, were performed on the adjective pairs. The phase of illness affected virtually all pairs, indicating that changes in self-perception across the affective states of bipolar illness were consistent and widespread (Fig. 10–2). Statistical comparisons, conducted to identify significant differences between each pair of different mood phases, revealed a number of consistent patterns, particularly for the adjective pairs reflecting a positive–negative, or valuative, dimension.

For all these pairs, self-perceptions in the depressed phase were significantly more negative than those in the other phases. More interesting, for all except two pairs (serious–humorous and cautious–rash), the ratings for the hypomanic phase did not differ significantly from those for the euthymic phase. Compared with men, women rated themselves overall as less active and as more "cold" and "boring" during the depressed phase, and more "exciting" and "warm" during the manic phase. Women also perceived themselves as more changeable overall relative to men.

Of interest, men's and women's perceptions of their masculinity–femininity in various phases of illness also changed (not shown). Women felt less feminine and men less masculine in the depressed than in the euthymic phase; the opposite was true for the hypomanic and manic phases. In other words, depression had a neuterizing effect and hypomania or mania a polarizing or enhancing effect on sexual identity.

Figure 10–2. Perceptions of self in 69 bipolar patients as a function of affective state. Squares=normal state; diamonds=depressed state; circles=hypomanic state. (*Source*: Jamison et al., unpublished data.)

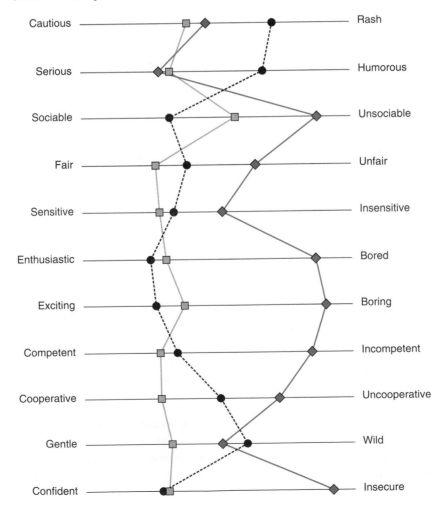

Throughout their bipolar cycles, patients underwent not only mood swings, but also substantial changes in their perception of self, self-esteem, energy expenditure, and interpersonal conduct. The study revealed that, as expected, bipolar patients had high self-esteem in the hypomanic or manic phase and low self-esteem in the depressive phase. Of more interest, self-esteem in the euthymic state did not differ substantially from that in the hypomanic phase. That is, bipolar patients generally held themselves in high regard; their apparently low self-esteem during the depressive phase was encapsulated, without perceived long-term adverse effects. Interpersonal conduct was perceived by patients to be less socially desirable in the hypomanic phase than during euthymia. Such findings are especially revealing in light of the common conception that bipolar patients are outgoing and socially engaging during their highs; this suggests that patients may have some insight into the one-sidedness of their social engagement in the manic and hypomanic phases.

Comparisons of Remitted Bipolar Patients and Normal Groups

Two major dimensions of personality—neuroticism and extraversion—have been compared between remitted bipolar patients and normal groups.

Neuroticism

Measures of neuroticism, typically using the MPI (or its later version, the Eysenck Personality Inventory [EPI]), identify significant differences between each pair of different mood phases (e.g., Clark et al., 1994). The neuroticism scale of the MPI/EPI is more likely to reflect changes in clinical state than is the extraversion scale. Several investigators have shown that neuroticism scores decrease following recovery in patients with endogenous depression (Crookes and Hutt, 1963; Coppen and Metcalfe, 1965; Ingham, 1966). In normal populations, neuroticism and extraversion are independent factors, but in psychiatric patients, the correlation between the two is usually quite high.

Eysenck and colleagues (Eysenck and Eysenck, 1963a,b) have defined neuroticism as "a largely inherited lability of the autonomic nervous system" and as a general measure of emotionality. Its principal components include mood swings, a sense of inferiority, poor emotional adjustment, lack of social responsibility, suspiciousness, lack of persistence, social shyness and hypochondriasis, and lack of relaxed composure. Moodiness, which has the single highest loading on the neuroticism factor in the EPI, is illustrated by positive answers to the following sample items: "Do you sometimes feel happy, sometimes depressed, without any apparent reason?" "Are you inclined to be moody?" and "Do you have frequent ups and downs

in mood, either with or without apparent cause?" Because of this measure of affective lability, the construct has frequently been investigated as a potential indicator of bipolar disorder.

Only one of several early studies[8] comparing neuroticism scores on the MPI/EPI found significant differences between remitted bipolar patients and normal populations (Hirschfeld and colleagues [1986] found lower neuroticism among never-ill relatives of bipolar patients than among the patient group). This apparently anomalous finding was replicated in a more recent study conducted within the same program (the Collaborative Program on the Psychobiology of Depression). Solomon and colleagues (1996) compared 30 individuals diagnosed with bipolar-I disorder who were first-degree relatives or spouses of the patients in the Hirschfeld study and 974 never-ill relatives. They found that the bipolar patients, who were currently in remission, scored significantly higher on neuroticism than did the controls. Thus although most of the early studies indicated no stable traits of elevated neuroticism for remitted bipolar patients, results of more recent investigations suggest that some samples of such patients may in fact show elevated levels of the trait.

Extraversion–Introversion

As with neuroticism, the primary psychological measure of the extraversion–introversion dimension used in research on affective illness is the MPI/EPI. Extraversion was originally characterized in the MPI/EPI by impulsivity (typical item: "Are you inclined to be quick and sure in your actions?") and sociability (typical item: "Would you be very unhappy if you were prevented from making numerous social contacts?"). In normal populations, impulsivity and sociability correlate at 0.5, producing a second-order factor of extraversion. More recently, impulsivity has been recognized as a separate factor, and it is not included in contemporary assessments of extraversion. Thus there may be some discrepancy between results of older and newer studies (Watson et al., 1994). Introversion can be further subdivided into social introversion (characteristic of those who prefer not to have much social contact with others) and neurotic introversion (characteristic of those who are afraid to have contact with others and are basically unsure of themselves and their interpersonal competence) (Eysenck, 1956). Just as neuroticism has been conceptualized as negative affectivity (as discussed earlier), extraversion has been conceptualized as positive affectivity—a stable, heritable, temperamental trait (Clark et al., 1994).

Based on the typical conceptualization of extraversion, many researchers have expected to find greater levels of this trait among bipolar patients. The authors of the MPI/

EPI (Eysenck, 1959; Eysenck and Eysenck, 1963a,b) described a typical extravert as one who:

> [is] sociable, likes parties, has many friends, needs to have people to talk to . . . craves excitement, takes chances . . . is generally an impulsive individual . . . [is] easy going, optimistic . . . prefers to keep moving and doing things . . . and [loses] his temper quickly.

A typical introvert, on the other hand:

> [is a] quiet, retiring sort of person, introspective, fond of books rather than people . . . reserved and distant except to intimate friends . . . tends to plan ahead . . . distrusts the impulse of the moment . . . does not like excitement . . . likes a well-ordered mode of life . . . keeps his feelings under close control . . . does not lose his temper easily . . . [and is] reliable, somewhat pessimistic.

As noted earlier, the extraversion–introversion scale of the MPI/EPI, unlike the neuroticism scale, is relatively impervious to the effects of mood or clinical state. Most studies comparing extraversion in remitted bipolar patients and normal individuals have found no significant differences between the two groups. One study of 45 bipolar patients, using the Cattell 16 Personality Factor Inventory, reported that remitted bipolar patients were more extraverted than the general population (Popescu et al., 1985). Two studies, however, found remitted female bipolar patients to be less extraverted (more introverted) than published norms or never-ill relatives (Hirschfeld, 1985; Hirschfeld et al., 1986). There was no significant difference for men (Hirschfeld et al., 1986).

Cyclothymia and Hyperthymia

Several investigators have found that an underlying cyclothymic temperament is particularly associated with bipolar-II disorder (Hartouche et al., 1998; Benazzi and Akiskal, 2005), as well as being elevated in healthy relatives of bipolar probands (Mendlowicz et al., 2005). Other investigators have confirmed Kraepelin's observation of a high rate of hyperthymic temperament in both bipolar-I and bipolar-II patients (Cassano et al., 1992; Perugi et al., 1998), although the interpretation of this observation is confounded by the fact that elevated rates of hyperthymic temperament have been demonstrated in control subjects as well (Evans et al., 2005; Matsumoto et al., 2005; Mendlowicz et al., 2005). Other researchers have found that individuals with bipolar disorder score significantly higher than controls on measures of novelty seeking (a tendency to seek out new situations, to be curious and impulsive, a trait discussed further in the next section) (Cronin and Zuckerman, 1992; Young et al., 1995; Nowakowska et al., 2005). A similar elevation in novelty-seeking behavior has been

shown to occur in pediatric bipolar patients and in the offspring of bipolar patients (Chang et al., 2003).

In summary, there are few significant differences between remitted bipolar patients and normal individuals on the two most frequently assessed personality dimensions, neuroticism and extraversion–introversion. Other studies that have included different measures of personality traits have also failed to find significant differences (e.g., Lepkifker et al., 1988). However, Solomon and colleagues (1996) found that the bipolar-I group scored significantly lower than never-ill controls on measures of emotional stability, ego resiliency, and ego control. They cautioned that their comparison group had been screened for absence of psychopathology, whereas prior disorders may not have been ruled out for control groups in other studies. They also noted that nearly 50 percent of their bipolar group had a history of substance abuse. The results of early studies require caution as well because their samples were small, and probably differed as to the extent of their predominance of mania and depression, as well as their social role functioning. Thus some samples of bipolar patients may indeed differ from normal controls during remission, perhaps depending on the composition and clinical features of the sample. In particular, it is likely that elevated neuroticism and introversion characterize those with prominent depressive episodes. (See Savitz and Ramesar, 2006, for an excellent review of personality research in bipolar disorder.)

Significant differences are found between bipolar patients and controls on measures of temperament. Several studies have found that cyclothymia and novelty seeking are more elevated in bipolar samples.

Comparisons of Bipolar and Unipolar Patients

Of historical interest in the pursuit and eventual recognition of the unipolar–bipolar distinction was a series of studies conducted in the 1970s comparing depressed unipolar and bipolar patients. Donnelly and colleagues (e.g., Donnelly and Murphy, 1973, 1974; Donnelly et al., 1976) found several differences between the groups: when acutely depressed, bipolar patients exhibited a greater social desirability response set with more "normal" profiles and less neuroticism, less impulse control, and less anxiety relative to unipolar patients. Many other studies found that unipolar patients scored higher in the direction of neuroticism and low self-esteem, or emotional instability.[9] Two studies using alternative measures of neuroticism concluded that bipolar patients were more neurotic than unipolar patients (Abou-Saleh and Coppen, 1984; Popescu et al., 1985). However, many studies that specifically pursued comparisons of unipolar and bipolar patients in remission on neuroticism using the MPI/EPI failed to show differences between the groups.[10]

In several studies of extraversion using the MPI/EPI[11] and two using the extraversion factor from the Cattell 16 Personality Factor Questionnaire (Murray and Blackburn, 1974; Popescu et al., 1985), remitted bipolar patients scored higher on extraversion than did remitted unipolar patients. More recent and more tightly designed studies also found that remitted bipolar patients scored significantly higher on extraversion than remitted unipolar patients (e.g., Sauer et al., 1997; Janowsky et al., 1999). Preliminary findings suggest that not only bipolar–unipolar differences but also differences between bipolar subtypes may be associated with specific temperamental and personality profiles. Akiskal and colleagues (2006) administered a large battery of self-report personality scales to 78 bipolar-I, 64 bipolar-II, and 251 unipolar patients, all remitted. Most of the bipolar-I patients described themselves as essentially normal in emotional stability and extraversion, and they scored low on measures of neuroticism. In contrast, both the bipolar-II and unipolar patients scored high on neuroticism, although in the bipolar-II subgroup, the neuroticism scores were elevated as a result of mood lability, while in the unipolar group, the elevation was due to subdepressive traits. Two studies (Bech et al., 1980; Hirschfeld et al., 1986) found no significant differences in extraversion between the two groups. Hirschfeld and colleagues (1986) found no significant bipolar-unipolar differences in women, but they did find that bipolar men scored higher on extraversion measures than did unipolar men. Three studies of dominance, a closely related personality factor, found that bipolar patients were more dominant than unipolar patients (Strandman, 1978; Abou-Saleh and Coppen, 1984; Popescu et al., 1985).

A more recent comparison of depressed unipolar and bipolar patients failed to find greater "normality" in the bipolar group (Wetzler et al., 1995). In general, across testing with the MMPI and the Millon Clinical Multiaxial Inventory-II (MCMI) (Millon, 1987), few consistent differences were observed. Bipolar patients scored higher on indicators of narcissism, antisocial behaviors, and compulsive personality style, but Wetzler and colleagues (1995) noted that such elevated scores could be due to residual aspects of mania, such as grandiosity.

Cloninger (1987) developed a personality assessment system (the Tridimensional Personality Questionnaire [TPQ]) purporting to link heritable temperaments with underlying brain monoaminergic pathways. Three dimensions—harm avoidance (HA; pessimistic and shy versus carefree and outgoing), reward dependence (RD; sentimental and tender-hearted versus insensitive and practical), and novelty seeking (NS; curious and impulsive versus stoical and orderly) are presumed to relate to, and perhaps predict, forms of psychopathology.

A consistent finding in the literature, for example, is an association between elevated HA and unipolar depression (Strakowski et al., 1992), even during remission. Strakowski and colleagues (1993) found that bipolar patients, by contrast, scored significantly lower on HA than did unipolar depressed patients, and did not differ from controls. Young and colleagues (1995) suggested, however, that the patients in the Strakowski sample were not recovered from mania at the time of testing, and they therefore undertook a study of carefully defined "remitted" bipolar patients compared with recovered unipolar patients and controls. They found no significant differences between unipolar and bipolar patients on HA, and both patient groups had significantly higher HA than did the controls. Bipolar patients scored significantly higher on the NS scale than did unipolar and control subjects. The results suggest that HA may be a nonspecific indicator of mood disorders (perhaps like neuroticism), whereas NS may be more specific to bipolar disorder. The cross-sectional design of the Young et al. study makes it impossible to determine whether the traits result from manic episodes, are subsyndromal symptoms, or represent premorbid personality characteristics. There is suggestive evidence that bipolar patients with an earlier age at onset are more harm avoidant (Engström et al., 2003). A recent study of type A behavior in 23 bipolar-II and 42 unipolar patients found that the bipolar patients had significantly higher scores, largely attributable to greater impatience, time urgency, and irritability (Oedegaard et al., 2006).

Another study employing the TPQ compared 50 bipolar patients considered to be euthymic with U.S. norms. Like Young and colleagues (1995), Osher and colleagues (1996) found that the patients had significantly elevated scores on HA, as well as on RD, including the "persistence" subscale of RD. Unlike Young's group, however, Osher and colleagues found no differences on NS.

Overall, few general conclusions can be drawn. Although bipolar patients in remission may differ from unipolar patients on extraversion, there is little indication that they are "healthier" than unipolar patients, and there is mixed evidence on normalcy during remission compared with well controls. Inconsistencies in study findings derive in part from heterogeneity among populations (due to use of differing diagnostic or inclusion criteria), variations in type and degree of illness (including manic/depressive states and response to treatment, as well as degree of recurrence within unipolar patients), inconsistent criteria for "remission," and inclusion or exclusion of patients with "double depressions" (concurrent major depressive episode and dysthymia). The search for descriptive differences therefore appears unproductive, at least at this point in time, and more interesting questions of prediction and the implications of various traits are increasingly the focus of research, as discussed in the next section.

Predictive Associations between Personality Features and Clinical Outcome

Premorbid Traits and Vulnerability

Although the topic of premorbid traits and vulnerability is a well-developed area of research in unipolar depression, it is rarely addressed in bipolar samples, perhaps because of the general assumption of a genetically based biological predisposition to bipolar disorder. Nevertheless, as suggested in Chapter 2, there may be early traits that portend the development of bipolar illness, or characteristics that might be viewed as risk factors given the appropriate biological vulnerability. An obvious research strategy would be assessment of premorbid characteristics, ideally in longitudinal studies involving subjects who are at high risk by virtue of having one or both parents with bipolar disorder. As indicated in Chapter 6, however, such work is in its infancy.

Although several studies have attempted to evaluate personality characteristics or subsyndromal symptoms of mood disorders,[12] there is little consensus on the best methods and instruments to use for the purpose. Several early studies identified personality traits associated with high-risk children: aggressiveness (e.g., Worland et al., 1979; Kron et al., 1982); extraversion, introversion, and impulsiveness (Kron et al., 1982); and sensation seeking (e.g., Nurnberger et al., 1988). Long-term follow-up studies are needed to determine whether such traits predict eventual bipolar disorder in high-risk populations. One such study of premorbid functioning was conducted by Clayton and colleagues (1994), who reviewed military records of performance on the Freiburg Personality Inventory of men who were later diagnosed with bipolar disorder. No differences in premorbid personality were observed as compared with controls who did not develop bipolar disorder.

Temperament and Vulnerability

As noted earlier, neuroticism may be conceptualized as a broad temperamental construct of negative affectivity, which has been linked empirically to general emotional distress (anxiety and depression) reflecting both current mood state and vulnerability to developing depression (Clark et al., 1994). Extraversion, conceptualized as positive affectivity, may be predictive of depression (with low positive affectivity being associated with depression and introversion). Persons with high positive affectivity/extraversion "feel joyful, enthusiastic, energetic, friendly, bold, assertive, proud, and confident," whereas those with low positive affectivity/introversion "tend to feel dull, flat, disinterested, and unenthusiastic" (Clark et al., 1994, p. 107). While low positive affectivity/

introversion has been linked to depression, other theorists have recently proposed that high positive affectivity/extraversion may be linked to a biologically based approach system that activates behavior in response to signals for reward—also called the behavioral activation system (Gray, 1982). According to Depue and Iacono (1988), the behavioral activation system is similar to what they term the behavior facilitation system, which they believe underlies bipolar disorder. The latter system is believed to include locomotor behavior, incentive motivation, interest and alertness, and level of pleasure or excitement seeking. Poor regulation and the tonic level of the system have been speculated to predict mood disorders and their specific manifestations. Depue and colleagues (1994) also proposed a link between temperament and neurotransmitter functioning, and found preliminary evidence of an association between dopaminergic functioning and positive emotionality. The association among positive affectivity, bipolar temperament, and emotional resilience was addressed at length by Jamison (2004).

Johnson and colleagues developed a polarity-specific model of mood states and hypothesized that behaviors and traits consistent with the behavioral activation system may differentially predict manic symptoms (see, e.g., Johnson et al., in press). They specifically tested the hypothesis that extraversion and achievement striving would predict manic symptoms over time in bipolar-I patients, whereas neuroticism would predict increases in depressive symptoms (Lozano and Johnson, 2001). Using a version of the NEO Five-Factor Inventory (Costa and McCrae, 1992) that includes all of these constructs, Lozano and Johnson (2001) followed 39 bipolar patients over a 6-month period. Controlling for initial manic symptoms, they found that achievement striving predicted increased manic symptoms (although extraversion did not); likewise, controlling for initial depressive symptoms, they found that level of neuroticism predicted increases in depression. Thus their findings provided some support for their polarity-specific model.

Partially consistent data were obtained by Strakowski and colleagues (1993) in investigating their hypothesis regarding recovery from first-episode mania among 27 bipolar patients. They found that, although personality measures in the form of TPQ scores did not predict time to clinical recovery, *functional* recovery (which was uncorrelated with symptom status) was predicted by level of novelty seeking on the TPQ. Novelty seeking was significantly higher among those who failed to attain premorbid levels of adjustment, a finding consistent with the view that this dimension reflects impulsiveness and pleasure seeking. The authors noted, however, that they could not rule out the possibility that high scores on novelty seeking reflected subsyndromal symptoms. (Although bipolar patients score higher than unipolar patients on novelty seeking, Parker and colleagues

[2004] made the critical point that the heterogeneity among unipolar depressed patients is a confusing and confounding source of inconsistency in studies.)

An additional predictive study, by Carpenter and colleagues (1999), examined the association between neuroticism and affective symptoms, self-confidence, and marital satisfaction among a sample of married bipolar patients. Using the NEO Five-Factor Inventory of personality (Costa and McCrae, 1985), administered when the patients were not in an episode, they found that greater neuroticism predicted more severe illness during the 2 years before entry into the study and during the first year of treatment, worse Global Assessment Scale (GAS) scores during treatment, and lower self-confidence. Neuroticism also predicted Axis II (personality disorder) dimensional scores. Of interest, extraversion—but not neuroticism—predicted marital distress. The authors noted that in general, the personality scores were not especially deviant as a group, although there was considerable variability; they also observed that extremely high neuroticism scores could be indistinguishable from personality disorder.

Effects of Medication on Personality

Evidence for a strong effect of medication on personality functioning relates almost entirely to lithium and comes from several sources: studies of lithium's effects on normal subjects; prima facie evidence derived from both clinical and systematic observation of the drug's profound effects on behavior, mood, and personality in affectively ill patients; and comparisons of personality studies completed in the prelithium era with those completed after lithium treatment became widespread. Results of the latter studies indicate that personality differences between bipolar patients and other groups pale considerably, and often entirely, when lithium is used effectively.

We raise here several important philosophical and treatment issues. Does lithium make the personality of a bipolar individual revert to pre-illness levels, or does it decrease variability in mood and personality functioning beyond those levels? Does lithium create an abnormally stable personality and mood system? To what extent is personality in lithium-treated patients a function of blood level? Does a patient who is inadequately treated with or only partially responsive to lithium show premorbid personality or subsyndromal disease? How does lithium's influence on personality affect medication adherence?

Several authors have examined the effects of lithium on personality function in normal subjects. Schou (1968) was the first to describe systematically the cognitive, behavioral, and personality effects of the drug in normal people. At relatively low blood levels, lithium had minimal effects on personality functioning in medical student volunteers.

In three researchers taking lithium at higher levels, however, effects were more pronounced. They noted occasional hypersensitivity but also decreased responsivity to their environment, increased indifference and malaise, greater passivity, and cognitive changes (discussed further in Chapters 12 and 21). Judd and colleagues (1977a), studying lithium's effects on normal male volunteers, found that in addition to reporting a mood-lowering effect, their subjects cited less inclination and desire to "deal with the demands of the environment." Normal men studied by Kropf and Müller-Oerlinghausen (1979) showed, while on lithium, decreased social involvement, activity, and concentration, as well as increased boredom and lethargy. When White and colleagues (1979) administered the Profile of Mood States (POMS) to 10 normal volunteers treated with lithium, the subjects reported a reduced sense of well-being and fewer social interactions; they also complained of fatigue, anxiety, lack of initiative, and decreased efficiency. In an indirect measure of lithium's ability to attenuate emotional responsiveness, Belmaker and colleagues (1979) found that, while taking lithium, neither normal subjects nor patients experienced the predicted increased heart rate generally caused by participation in cognitive tasks. Both of these studies, although intriguing, were relatively short-term trials (1–3 weeks and 2 weeks, respectively), and there is some indication that longer periods of time on lithium result in at least partial accommodation to some of these effects.

The most clear-cut influences of lithium on bipolar personality were evident in personality studies done on euthymic, lithium-stabilized patients. Additionally, a few studies have examined personality and mood stabilization over time in lithium-treated, affectively ill patients. Bonetti and colleagues (1977) administered the EPI and the Marke-Nyman Temperament Scale to 33 recurrent (minimally three episodes) unipolar and 28 bipolar patients at the end of the index episode and at least 3 months later. They found that personality changes were more pronounced in the bipolar patients, especially on measures of sociability, initiative, and impulsiveness. Neuroticism scores decreased most dramatically within the unipolar group (test–retest differences, $p < .001$). The authors speculated that lithium both reduced symptoms and altered habitual patterns of personality, such as high activity levels and impulsiveness in bipolar patients and anxious–neurotic traits in unipolar patients.

In an interesting and important study of the relationship between lithium blood level and personality change, Kropf and Müller-Oerlinghausen (1985) conducted a double-blind study of lithium dose reduction (20 percent) in 14 long-term lithium-treated patients (5 unipolar, 9 bipolar), all of whom were euthymic when tested. Eleven patients (3 unipolar, 8 bipolar) maintained at their regular lithium levels served as controls. The patients receiving higher levels of lithium tended to be less active, less obsessive, and less elated. Specifically, those taking lower levels of lithium scored higher on Von Zerssen's measures of initiative and assertiveness ($p < .05$) and of social resonance (social acceptance and assertiveness), transparency (social openness and sensitivity), and social potency (sociability and "ability for devotion"). However, a significant proportion (29 percent) of the patients in the experimental group became affectively ill at a reduced lithium level.

Mood stability in lithium-treated patients, although not a direct measure of personality, clearly is related to personality functioning. Folstein and colleagues (1982) administered the Visual Analogue Mood Scale (VAMS) for 30 days to 65 euthymic bipolar patients on chronic lithium therapy and to 36 nonpatient control subjects. The mean mood ratings for the two groups were similar; the patients, however, reported significantly less mood variability. The authors attributed this unusual degree of mood stability to the effects of lithium treatment and suggested that euthymic patients might view this change as an undesirable aspect of lithium therapy. DePaulo and colleagues (1983) administered the VAMS to 17 euthymic bipolar patients and 21 nonpatient controls. Like Folstein and colleagues (1982), they found that the mean mood ratings were similar in the two groups and that the patients' moods were less variable than those of the controls. Three bipolar patients were studied separately, during and after lithium treatment. Two became manic, and the third, who remained euthymic while off lithium, showed markedly increased variability in daily mood ratings. The authors were uncertain whether these results reflected baseline differences in reporting between affectively ill patients and normal controls, lithium's therapeutic effects, or a medication effect.

PERSONALITY DISORDERS

Axis II (personality) disorders occur relatively frequently in clinical populations (with a range of about 5 to 40 percent, varying by personality disorder type) (Widiger and Rogers, 1989). Although epidemiologic studies of personality pathology in community samples have been infrequent and limited in scope, Weissman's (1993) review of such studies suggests that the population prevalence is 10 to 23 percent. Researchers have raised the question of the rates of personality disorders in bipolar samples and explored the correlates of Axis II pathology.

Early studies of the comorbidity of personality disorder with bipolar illness were hampered by methodological shortcomings, such as shifting diagnostic criteria for assessing Axis II disorders, assessment methods of uncertain validity, unclear or mixed samples of bipolar patients (e.g.,

comingling bipolar-I and -II), and small patient samples. A particularly serious problem was the failure to evaluate bipolar patients during euthymic states, so that reported "personality disorders" may have reflected largely mood state–related symptoms rather than stable underlying personality pathology.

Table 10–1 presents recent studies that attempted to verify bipolar-I diagnoses in patients while making an effort to control for mood state at the time of the assessment of Axis II disorders. For the most part, these studies used validated structured interview methods for assessing personality disorders. The samples included outpatients as well as inpatients, and those of varying ages and social/cultural circumstances. However, these studies employed relatively small samples, and some failed to control for other comorbid conditions, such as substance abuse. It is important to note that age at onset of bipolar disorder has not been explored (see Chapter 6), and early age at onset may be a significant predictor of Axis II symptomatology. Moreover, many of the studies were based on samples in tertiary care treatment, and may therefore reflect relatively more severe or complex cases of bipolar disorder.

Despite the significant variability in sample characteristics among these studies, however, they yield evidence of rates of comorbid personality disorders that, although relatively consistent with those of other diagnostic groups in clinical populations, exceed the rates in the general population. Several studies involved a unique sample not generalizable to the overall population of persons with bipolar-I disorder; for example Kutcher and colleagues (1990) included only adolescents, Carpenter and Hittner (1995) only married patients, and Kay and colleagues (1999) only male veterans. Overall, the rates of personality disorders across all the samples ranged from 22 to 62 percent, as listed in Table 10–1.

According to the studies reported in Table 10–1, somewhat higher rates of personality disorders were found among bipolar patients who had experienced more previous episodes and those who had a history of alcohol abuse, and when self-report questionnaires or informant reports (rather than clinician interviews) were used as the basis for symptom assessment. At least two studies found an association between greater levels of depressive symptoms and personality disorders (Brieger et al., 2003; George et al., 2003). One additional study—not included in the table because it appears to have combined bipolar-I, bipolar-II, and cyclothymic patients in unknown proportions—found that participants with dysthymia or bipolar disorder were more likely to have personality disorders (70 percent) than patients in treatment for other disorders, such as anxiety disorder (Flick et al., 1993). A recent study of young adults with affective illness found significantly higher median levels of

TABLE 10–1. **Personality Disorders in Bipolar-I Patients**

Study	Sample	Method	Clinical State	Comparison Group	Overall Rate[a] (%)	Most Common Diagnoses
Kutcher et al., 1990	20 adolescents/outpatients[b]	Personality Disorders Examination (PDE) (interview)	Euthymic		35	Borderline, narcissistic
Pica et al., 1990	26 inpatients (16 bipolar-I, 10 bipolar schizoaffective)	Structured Interview for DSM-III Personality Disorders (SIDP-III)	Current symptoms not controlled	33 patients with schizophrenia	62	Histrionic, antisocial, borderline
O'Connell et al., 1991	50 outpatients	Personality Diagnosis Questionnaire-Revised (PDQ-R)	Current symptoms not controlled but "stable"		58	Borderline, histrionic
Carpenter et al., 1995	23 outpatients (married or cohabiting)	PDE	Few or no current symptoms		22	Dependent, borderline, obsessive-compulsive
Peselow et al., 1995	66 patients	Structured Interview for DSM-III-R Personality Disorders (SIDP-III-R)	Interviewed when manic or hypomanic, then again when euthymic		53 manic or hypomanic, 45 euthymic	Borderline, schizoid, histrionic
Dunayevich et al., 1996	33 first-episode, 26 multiple-episode inpatients	Structured Clinical Interview for DSM (SCID-II)			48	Avoidant, Cluster B (mixed)[c]
Barbato and Hafner, 1998	42 outpatients	International Personality Disorders Examination (IPDE) (interview)	"In remission"		45	Histrionic, borderline, avoidant, compulsive
Ucok et al., 1998	90 outpatients	SCID-II	Euthymic	58 normal controls	48 bipolar patients, 16 controls	Histrionic, compulsive, paranoid
Kay et al., 1999	61 Veterans Affairs (VA) outpatients	SCID-II PDQ-R	Euthymic	Compared patients with and without history of alcohol abuse disorder	38[d]	Cluster A, Cluster C[c]
Brieger et al., 2003	60 inpatients	SCID-II NEO Five Factor Personality Inventory	"Mostly in remission"	117 unipolar depressed inpatients	38 bipolar, 51 unipolar	Compulsive, narcissistic, borderline
George et al., 2003	52 outpatients	PDE	"In remission"		29	Histrionic, compulsive

[a]Estimates of personality disorders in general clinical populations range from 5 to 40 percent (Widiger and Rogers, 1989), and in community samples from 10 to 23 percent (Weissman, 1993).

[b]There were no differences in rates of Axis II disorders between bipolar-I and schizoaffective patients, so the authors combined the groups in their analysis.

[c]Cluster A: paranoid, schizoid, schizotypal; Cluster B: antisocial, borderline, histrionic, narcissistic; Cluster C: avoidant, dependent, obsessive-compulsive.

[d]Highest in patients with history of alcohol abuse.

borderline characteristics in the bipolar patients than in those with major depression (Smith et al., 2005). Three of the borderline characteristics differentiated bipolar from unipolar depression: "I've never threatened suicide or injured myself on purpose"; "I have tantrums or angry outbursts"; and "Giving in to some of my urges gets me into trouble." A study of 40 bipolar-II patients (Vieta et al., 1999) found that 33 percent met diagnostic criteria for a personality disorder. Overall, therefore, the typical bipolar patient sample appears to have relatively high rates of Axis II comorbidity.

Table 10–1 also indicates the most frequent individual personality disorder diagnoses. A number of studies found multiple disorders in bipolar patients, as is generally typical of diagnoses on Axis II. Viewed individually, however, the Cluster B disorders—especially borderline and histrionic—were most common among the bipolar samples. Rossi and colleagues (2001) also reported high rates of borderline as well as compulsive personality disorders; however, their bipolar sample included only those with recent depressive episodes, excluding those with recent mania.

Despite the general consistency in frequency and types of personality disorders observed across studies, the meaning of the results remains elusive. Conceptually, it is widely recognized that rates of comorbidity may be inflated because of the overlap of symptoms across disorders. Despite various efforts to assess for personality pathology during euthymic states, it is nonetheless possible that the personality disorders reported may reflect the symptoms of hypomania or depression. For instance, histrionic or borderline pathology may be difficult to distinguish from attention seeking, intense or exaggerated emotional expression, intense irritability, impulsive or provocative behaviors, and affective instability and rapidly changing mood. (See MacKinnon et al., 2006, for an excellent review of the centrality of affective instability to both bipolar illness and borderline personality disorder.) Peselow and colleagues (1995), comparing personality pathology assessed in the same patients during hypomania and euthymia, found a reduction in such pathology when the patients had recovered from the hypomanic state. Thus personality pathology may be inflated as a result of overlapping symptoms in Axis I and II categories containing manic, mixed, and depressive symptoms and behaviors.

A related conceptual question, noted previously, is the issue of whether personality pathology may be a consequence of bipolar disorder. Thus, for example, the unstable self-image or identity disturbance or the recurrent suicidal or parasuicidal behaviors of the borderline personality may be a reaction to the cumulative unpredictable and massively destructive mood swings of bipolar illness. It is possible that the onset of bipolar disorder in childhood or early adolescence may exacerbate identity difficulties and impair the ability to form solid and sustaining relationships, thereby contributing to diffuse Axis II symptomatology. Thus the maladaptive behaviors reflected in personality disorders may in some cases be dysfunctional coping methods or adaptations to the illness.

A third conceptual consideration concerns sampling: patients included in the studies reported in Table 10–1 may reflect those who are most disturbed, and who are seen in research-oriented settings that may draw more difficult patients not readily managed in community or private care. As noted, clinical samples in general (compared with epidemiologic samples), and especially those in tertiary care settings, may not be representative in terms of comorbidity because they are likely to be sicker.

Finally, as discussed in Chapter 3, some would argue against conceptualizing Axis II disorders as conditions comorbid with bipolar disorder. Instead, it is argued, they may represent forms of disorder in the bipolar spectrum (e.g., Akiskal et al., 1985, 2000; Deltito et al., 2001). Gunderson and colleagues (2006) recently reported the results of a 4-year prospective investigation of 196 patients with bipolar disorder and 433 patients with personality disorders. They found that bipolar-I and bipolar-II disorders were significantly more common in patients with borderline personality disorder (19.4 percent) than in patients with other types of personality disorder (7.9 percent). The presence of co-occurring bipolar disorder had no significant effect on the course of the borderline personality disorder, as measured by remission rates, functional adjustment, or treatment utilization rates (hospitalization and medication usage). The investigators concluded that there was only a modest association between bipolar disorder and borderline personality disorder, "thereby making a strong spectrum relationship with bipolar disorder extremely unlikely" (p. 1177). We do not know enough at the present time to draw firm conclusions on this question.

Despite uncertainty about the conceptualization of personality disorder comorbidity, one meaning of comorbid Axis II pathology is not ambiguous: bipolar (or any psychiatric) patients who have personality pathology typically have worse outcomes. Kay and colleagues (2002) found significantly lower rates of employment, more complex medication regimens, and greater likelihood of substance and alcohol abuse among bipolar-I male veterans who had diagnosed personality disorders (but no differences between the groups in age at onset or duration of disorder). Over time, Carpenter and colleagues (1995) found that patients with personality disorder had significantly more symptoms and worse social adjustment scores than those without such disorder. Others have also found this to be the case (Bieling et al., 2003). Kutcher and colleagues (1990) found that adolescent bipolar patients without personality disorder had a better response to lithium treatment.

Although Ucok and colleagues (1998) did not find differences in lithium responsiveness among their bipolar patients with and without personality disorder, they did find that patients with Axis II comorbidity had made more severe suicide attempts. Barbato and Hafner (1998) found that bipolar-I patients with personality disorder had significantly more lifetime days hospitalized and more severe symptomatology than those without personality disorder, and were more likely to report that their medications were "unhelpful." Others (Dunayevich et al., 1996) have reported that patients with multiple episodes were more likely than first-episode patients to have personality disorder. Moreover, in a 12-month follow-up of these patients, those diagnosed with personality disorder were less likely to show syndrome or symptom recovery and had achieved significantly less functional recovery (Dunayevich et al., 2000). The authors speculated that poor medication adherence may mediate the link between personality disorder and poor outcome (see Chapter 21). Poor adherence, in turn, may reflect poorer response to treatment. Finally, Vieta and colleagues (1999) reported that those in their bipolar-II sample with personality disorder had earlier age at onset of bipolar disorder and more severe suicidal ideation. In general, these findings are consistent with those of research on other psychiatric populations, indicating that, whether true "comorbidity" is involved or mainly more severe general symptomatology, patients with Axis II disorders typically have worse illness course and are more difficult to treat effectively.

INTERPERSONAL FUNCTIONING

No one has the slightest idea of what I've been through with Cal [Robert Lowell]. In 4½ years, counting this present breakup, he has had four collapses! Three manic, and one depression. These things take time to come and long after he is out of the hospital there is a period which can only be called "nursing." The long, difficult pull back—which does not show always to others. I knew the possibility of this when I married him, and I have always felt that the joy of his "normal" periods, the lovely time we had, all I've learned from him, the immeasurable things I've derived from our marriage made up for the bad periods. I consider it all a gain of the most precious kind. But he has torn down this time everything we've built up . . . how difficult these break-ups are for both of us. (Elizabeth Hardwick[13])

Moods are by nature compelling, contagious, and profoundly interpersonal. Mania and depression alter the perceptions and behaviors not only of those who have them,

but also of those who are related or closely associated. Bipolar illness—marked as it is by extraordinary and confusing fluctuations in mood, personality, thinking, and behavior—inevitably has powerful and often painful effects on relationships. Violence, poor judgment, and indiscreet financial and sexual behavior are almost always destructive and embarrassing to spouses, children, family members, and friends. Trust is not easily restored in the wake of mania, nor are goodwill and love always regenerated after months of severe, depleting, and unremitting depression.

Mood-related changes in interpersonal functioning are not the whole story, however; increasing evidence points to persisting social, marital, and family difficulties even when individuals are not in the throes of an episode. Such impairments in interpersonal relationships may affect subsequent clinical functioning in a complex, reciprocal pattern. In this section, we review issues and studies concerned with bipolar patients and their relationships with other people. It should be emphasized that the studies reviewed focused exclusively on the impaired functioning associated with symptoms and episodes. As is typical of most psychopathology studies, little research has been conducted on aspects of marital and family functioning that may be associated with positive moods and behaviors, such as optimism, energy, and infectious enthusiasm (Jamison, 2004).

Social Functioning

Impairment during Mania and Depression

The complex, subtle, and potentially infuriating aspects of manic interpersonal behavior were observed by most early clinical investigators (see Chapter 1). Hypomanic behavior, especially, was noted for its powerful and confusing influence on others. The positive, engaging, and occasionally charismatic qualities of many individuals with bipolar illness are discussed at length in Chapters 2 and 12. Here we describe some of the more detrimental interpersonal features of bipolar illness.

Kraepelin (1921, p. 61) wrote of the skill of hypomanic patients in manipulating fellow patients:

It is just the peculiar mixture of sense and maniacal activity, frequently also an extensive experience of institutions, which makes them extremely ingenious in finding out means to satisfy their numerous desires, to deceive their surroundings, to procure for themselves all kinds of advantages, to secure the property of others for themselves. They usually soon domineer completely over their fellow-patients, use them for profit, report about them to the physician in technical terms, act as guardian to them, and hold them in check.

Psychoanalytic writers, with rare exceptions, regarded the interpersonal lives of bipolar patients as unstable and chaotic, narcissistically based, bereft of empathic regard for the rights of others, too dependent or independent, singularly rigid, and full of rage. These conclusions are not surprising given that they were based substantially on experiences with patients in the prepharmacotherapy era. Understandably, such perceptions led most psychoanalysts to be wary of and reluctant to treat these patients. Since the psychoanalytic relationship with bipolar patients was seen as superficial and distant, countertransference was the subject of considerable discussion and writing about such patients (see Chapter 22). Most psychoanalytic writers were interested primarily in the origins of the illness and the personality structure of bipolar patients, but we present here a brief review of their observations and interpretations of interpersonal behavior.

Abraham (1911, 1924), one of the earliest writers to formulate psychodynamic principles in bipolar illness, described what he perceived to be the patients' abnormal character development and inability to maintain good relationships. These features, he speculated, were coupled with an ongoing sense of impending loss of objects, which produced a "rageful" stance toward these objects and their inability to "gratify narcissistic demands." Freud (1917), for the most part, concurred: "Manic-depressives show simultaneously the tendency to too-strong fixations to their love-object and to a quick withdrawal of object cathexis. Object choice is on a narcissistic basis."

The attitude of bipolar individuals toward others was described by Blalock (1936, p. 342) as "a selfish one serving in its several aspects the narcissistic needs of the patient." Equally critical in his views, Fenichel (1945) regarded bipolar patients as "love addicts," narcissistic, and incapable of love. To English (1949, p. 131), the bipolar patient was egocentric, incapable of relating warmly to others, rigid, afraid to hate except when manic, and powerfully influenced by the intensity of feelings:

> The manic-depressive is afraid of extremes of emotion, of great love, or of hostility, and yet these are the very things he may show in his illness. One patient . . . said, "To live is like opening all my pores on a cold day and subjecting myself to a catastrophe." The manic-depressive therefore has a defect in catching the feelings of others. He ignores what others feel and want as long as he can. Thus in trying to avoid being hurt he avoids the strengthening influence of friendship.

Fromm-Reichmann (1949), in a similar vein, described a "lack of subtlety," a "lack of any close interpersonal relatedness," and a tendency to exaggerate the intensity of interactions with other people. While describing manic-depressive patients as manifesting a "particular kind of narcissistic dependency on their love objects," Jacobson (1953, p. 66) provided a perspective at variance with that of the earlier psychoanalytic writers:

> We are also surprised to see that as long as they are not sick, they may be delightful companions or marital partners, a feature that Bleuler mentioned especially. In their sexual life they may show a full . . . response, and emotionally, in contradistinction to schizoid persons, a touching warmth and unusual, affectionate clinging to people they like . . . [they] are potentially able to function extraordinarily well.

Cohen and colleagues (1954, p. 119), however, commented on what they viewed as the illusion of normal relationships in manic-depressive patients:

> The appearance of closeness is provided by the hypomanic's liveliness, talkativeness, wittiness, and social aggressiveness. Actually, there is little or no communicative exchange between the hypomanic and any one of his socalled friends. . . . The concept of reciprocity is missing; the needs of the other for similar experiences are not recognized.

Finally, Gibson and colleagues (1959, p. 1,102) stressed the dependent nature of the manic-depressive patient—the difficulties in dealing with feelings of envy and competition and the "common use of denial as a defense, there being a notable lack of subtlety, and of awareness of their own or the feelings of others in their interpersonal relations."

Janowsky and colleagues (1970, 1974), in an attempt to measure more objectively the interpersonal behavior of patients during the manic phase of their illness, assessed the interactional style of acutely manic patients with tape recordings of psychotherapy sessions (both group and individual), physician and social worker notes, observations of milieu therapy, and nurses' behavioral descriptions and ratings of patients. The manic person's interpersonal maneuvers are, according to these authors, "simultaneously cementing and distancing." Although their study presumes too much conscious control and manipulation on the part of the patient, it is one of the few clinical reports to describe in detail the interpersonal behavior of hospitalized manic patients. We quote, as an example, from their work on the manic patient's perceptiveness with regard to vulnerability and conflict (Janowsky et al., 1970, p. 254):

> Intimately related to the manic's ability to appeal to the self-esteem systems of others is his extraordinary perceptiveness. In interpersonal encounters, the manic possesses a highly refined talent for sensing an individual's vulnerability or a group's area of conflict, and exploiting this in

a manipulative fashion. This sensitivity may be utilized in dealing directly with a given individual or in focusing on areas of conflict between others. In either case, the manic patient is able to make covert conflicts overt, causing the person or group with whom he is dealing to feel discomfort. . . . What he says cannot be dismissed as untrue or unreal, for the areas attacked truly do exist and, indeed, are areas of vulnerability.

The playful, high-energy, and extraverted behaviors associated with mania are often irritating. So, too, are the interpersonal qualities usually present during depression. Interviews with roommates of college students identified by clinical assessments as falling in the bipolar spectrum (cyclothymia as well as bipolar-I or -II) found that bipolar students were perceived as excessively excitable, showed poor judgment, were argumentative when hypomanic, and were irritable and socially withdrawn when depressed (Depue et al., 1981). It is not surprising, given the number of negative social behaviors exhibited by the bipolar students, that 58 percent of the roommates reported that they avoided the subject, finding him or her "noxious."

Fluctuations in levels of sociability almost define bipolar illness. Energetic seeking out of other people and uninhibited social behavior are common features of mania. Winokur and colleagues (1969, p. 63) described this in their monograph:

> A most characteristic sight when the patient is brought to the hospital is a frightened and exhausted family, which has frequently been awake for 1 or more nights being lectured to by a bright-eyed and excited patient.

In their study of 30 bipolar patients, Murphy and colleagues (1974) found two distinctive behavioral characteristics of mania: noticeably increased psychomotor activity and, of relevance here, a need for increased interpersonal contact ("people seeking"). Akiskal and colleagues (1977) reported that half of their cyclothymic patients alternated periods of uninhibited people seeking with periods of introverted self-absorption.

During depressive episodes, maladaptive patterns of relating to others are common, including social withdrawal, loss of enjoyment and pleasure, irritability, increased criticism of and negativism toward others, and sensitivity to criticism or rejection by others (see Chapter 2; Benazzi, 2000). Depressed people are often highly dependent on others for reassurance and support, yet appear paradoxically to reject the support or view it as untrustworthy and insufficient. Friends and family may be frustrated by the exaggerated dependence of the depressed patient, especially when they seem unable to relieve his or her despondency. Moreover, the depressed person may be particularly sensitive to perceived rejection or criticism, and minor or even nonexistent slights are exaggerated or interpreted inaccurately. All of these common symptoms of depression can thwart the best intentions and efforts of friends and family members.

Interpersonal tension may be further intensified by the depressed individual's marked guilt and feelings of worthlessness and self-blame for real or perceived negative social encounters. Indeed, when depressed, individuals may correctly perceive that they are a burden to others, a reality that may serve to heighten their depression (e.g., Coyne et al., 1987). Moreover, depression tends to elicit negative reactions even from strangers or acquaintances; many studies (reviewed in Gurtman, 1986) have demonstrated that others tend to reject depressed persons and express preferences for avoiding interactions with them.

Impairment despite Remission and Treatment

Compared with the clinical states and symptomatology of individuals with bipolar disorder, relatively little attention has been devoted to understanding social and interpersonal aspects of the disorder. Increasingly, however, research supports prior clinical observations of the extent to which social impairment persists even during stable, euthymic periods. For instance, Cooke and colleagues (1996) identified a sample of bipolar patients who were euthymic as well as free of recent substance abuse, personality disorder, or medical illness. The patients were administered the self-report functioning scales of the Medical Outcomes Study, and their results were compared with those previously obtained for a large number of individuals in treatment for a variety of chronic medical illnesses. Cooke and colleagues found that the bipolar patients scored lower on social functioning than did the medically ill patients. Similarly, Romans and McPherson (1992) interviewed remitted bipolar-I patients about their social functioning, and found that they scored significantly lower on availability and perceived adequacy of close relationships and had significantly fewer general social contacts and interactions than did a random community sample. A recent multicenter European study of 144 remitted bipolar patients found that, compared with normal subjects, patients were less well adjusted in general and, more specifically, in their leisure activities, relationships with extended family, marital relationships, and work activities (Blairy et al., 2004).

A study comparing outpatients in treatment for schizophrenia or bipolar disorder found that the two patient groups showed relatively similar levels of cognitive and social impairment on a battery of measures (Dickerson et al., 2001). Although the schizophrenic patients generally performed worse on most measures, the bipolar group was nearly as impaired. However, the clinical state of the bipolar patients at the time of testing was not specifically noted. Coryell and colleagues (1993) reported on 5-year follow-ups of patients from the National Institute of Mental Health (NIMH) Psychobiology of Depression sample, including 148 bipolar patients. Both unipolar and bipolar probands showed deficits in their relationships with friends, children, and relatives, and they also displayed less involvement in and enjoyment of social and recreational activities compared with non-ill controls. Although Coryell and colleagues did not report on the clinical status of the bipolar probands during the follow-up period, they noted that the majority were being treated for their disorder. Thus despite treatment and variations in the course of the disorder, the bipolar patients fared relatively poorly compared with matched controls. It may be noted that several studies comparing unipolar and bipolar probands on social functioning have yielded inconsistent results, probably because of variability in clinical histories, mood states during assessment, premorbid functioning and temperament, age and demographic factors, and methods of measuring interpersonal functioning.[14]

Overall, therefore, it appears that bipolar disorder is associated with a variety of general indicators of social impairment. Even when the individual is not in an affective episode, these interpersonal difficulties appear to persist. The direction of causality remains unclear, however. Are the maladjustments in social functioning due to bipolar disorder, or might they be related to clinical variables such as comorbid substance abuse or early age at onset? In the following sections, we review research addressing the predictors of social functioning and the predictive relationship between social functioning and subsequent clinical status.

Clinical Predictors of Social Functioning

The relatively sparse literature aimed at understanding the conditions under which bipolar disorder is associated with good or poor interpersonal functioning is also limited by relatively small samples, varying definitions and methods of assessing functioning, and a narrow range of potentially key variables. Nevertheless, these studies provide intriguing glimpses of issues warranting further study.

O'Connell and colleagues (1991) evaluated predictors of general functioning in 248 bipolar patients using the GAS. Several variables correlated with outcome and were evaluated in a multiple-regression equation. Number of prior admissions was the strongest predictor, followed by family attitudes and social class. Family attitudes of hostility and criticism imply poor interpersonal relationships in the family, suggesting in turn poor general functioning associated with interpersonal difficulties. Bauwens and colleagues (1991) explored correlates of social adjustment in 27 remitted bipolar patients. They found that a composite overall measure of social adjustment was significantly related to

episode frequency, and poorer social/leisure activity was associated with more episodes and hospitalizations. Scores on depression symptomatology were also associated with lower levels of social/leisure activity.

Several studies have found that depression is more linked to difficulties in functioning than is mania. In a study aimed at exploring the mutual influence of social and clinical functioning, Gitlin and colleagues (1995) evaluated the impact of both past episode history and subclinical symptoms on indicators of social functioning in a sample of 82 bipolar patients followed for at least 2 years. Social (close relationships) and family functioning were significantly related to number of past and recent depressive episodes but not to manic or hypomanic episodes. In all the analyses, subclinical symptoms were more strongly predictive of poorer social functioning than was number of clinical episodes. The researchers also determined that depressive episodes were significantly more (negatively) predictive of the quality of relationships with family members than were manic episodes, with a similar trend toward a greater association of depression with social (close) relationships. In contrast, occupational functioning was negatively associated with both depressive and manic episodes.

A recent review and investigation of functional outcomes in bipolar patients revealed depression to be one of the few fairly consistent predictors of social, family, and marital (as well as occupational) functioning (Bauer et al., 2001). This study is noteworthy for its careful assessment of symptoms and functioning over 48 weeks in a sample of 43 male Veterans Affairs outpatients. The amount of time depressed and average depression symptom scores—but not mania scores—were significantly correlated with social and work functioning. Other researchers (Cooke et al., 1996) also found that bipolar patients' low scores on social functioning were associated with subclinical depressive symptoms (subclinical mania/hypomania was not assessed), and social functioning was lower in bipolar-II than in bipolar-I patients. Different investigators (Romans and McPherson, 1992), in contrast, found that a subgroup of patients with a predominantly manic course reported less adequate close relationships and less available social contacts than did those with depressive episodes, although the effect was not statistically significant. Perhaps consistent with the previously cited studies, Romans and McPherson found that patients with a longer history of illness reported fewer close and general social contacts.

A study of 40 bipolar-I patients' social functioning (Lam and Wong, 1997) included ratings of relationships with intimate partners and friends and "social presentation." The investigators evaluated recognition of prodromes of mania and depression and scored the patients' reports of how they coped with prodromal symptoms of depression and mania. Generally, those with good awareness of prodromal symptoms and good coping methods had better overall social functioning. A multiple-regression analysis to predict overall social functioning indicated that lower current subclinical depression scores and good reported coping with prodromes of mania and depression significantly predicted good functioning, whereas number of past hospitalizations and current subsyndromal manic symptoms did not.

Social Predictors of Clinical Outcomes

The question of the origins of and contributors to social adjustment in those with bipolar disorder takes on particular urgency in view of studies now beginning to demonstrate a functional link between social and clinical outcomes. As evidence accumulates of enormous variability in the clinical course of bipolar disorder, even in those who are adequately or aggressively treated pharmacologically,[15] studies have increasingly been exploring predictors of diverse clinical outcomes by including social variables.

Among recent longitudinal outcome studies, several indicate the importance of interpersonal functioning. Table 10–2 summarizes several studies of social predictors of clinical outcomes in patients with bipolar disorder. In all of these studies, patients were in treatment, and many of the studies controlled for medication adherence. The studies differ considerably in the social functioning variables assessed, but they are consistent in finding that indicators of interpersonal adjustment play an important role in clinical outcomes, independently of clinical history factors. Note that several of the studies found social impairment to be especially predictive of depressive symptoms. Coryell and colleagues (1998) hypothesized that a "prevailingly depressive subtype" of bipolar patients may mark a particularly poor prognosis group with considerable social dysfunction.

Several of the studies listed in Table 10–2 identified family discord or negative family attitudes toward the patient with bipolar disorder as a predictor of worse clinical outcomes (Miklowitz et al., 1988; see also O'Connell et al., 1991). Research on the effect of family attitudes (particularly those of the caretaker or spouse) on the course of bipolar disorder, including "expressed emotion" and related constructs, is reviewed below in the section on marital functioning.

A particular focus of several of the studies in Table 10–2 is the role of the quality and availability of social support in predicting clinical outcomes among individuals with bipolar disorder. Generally, social support refers to individuals' perceptions of the extent to which others are available to provide emotional and material assistance and to their satisfaction with the perceived supportiveness offered by others. O'Connell and colleagues (1985) found that a global measure of social support was the strongest correlate of clinical

outcome, social adjustment, and overall GAS score. Other researchers (Stefos et al., 1996) found that social support and social functioning variables predicted outcome, but clinical factors did not. They observed that 69 percent of patients with good social support, compared with 25 percent of those with low support, remained episode-free during a 4-year period of assessment. Similar results have been reported more recently.[16] Of interest, several investigators[17] have found the effects of social support to be polarity-specific, with lower social support at baseline predicting more increase in depressive symptoms over time, but no significant association with changes in manic symptoms was found. The relationship between social support and clinical outcome is complicated by the likelihood that support is more likely to be given to those who are less overtly or chronically ill. It may well be that patients who experience primarily euphoric manias or hypomanias garner more support than those who have predominantly mixed states. This issue has not been adequately addressed in the research conducted to date. Clearly, premorbid functioning and temperament are relevant, albeit poorly studied, factors in predicting how individuals will cope with their illnesses and maintain or develop personal relationships.

Conceptualization and Methodology

Although the studies discussed above generally indicate a link between clinical and interpersonal functioning, there is clearly a need for more exploration of the origins of poor or good social functioning. One promising pattern concerns the role of depression, with most studies indicating an association between depressive symptoms and social functioning. While several studies suggest that depressive symptoms may be especially impairing, however, the specific contributors and features of social functioning are not known. For instance, do symptoms prevent individuals from engaging in social relationships and activities, or do symptoms affect the quality (and eventually the availability) of such pursuits? Do symptoms emerge subclinically during developmentally important periods of life to an extent sufficient to impair normal acquisition of social skills and attributes, or are the social impairments consequences of repeated episodes that devastate the individual's coping capacities?

There is a need to explore the origins of social impairments, as the question of whether they predate or follow bipolar episodes is unresolved. The topic of "premorbid social adjustment," although well established in schizophrenia research and a potent predictor of disorder and functioning, is relatively less well studied in bipolar samples. An exception is the work of Cannon and colleagues (1997), who clearly demonstrated that the social functioning of bipolar patients when they were children and adolescents

TABLE 10–2. Social Predictors of Clinical Outcomes

Study	Sample	Significant Predictors of Poorer Outcome
O'Connell et al., 1985	60 bipolar-I outpatients	Episode intensity–duration score over a 1-yr period was correlated with less social support and worse social adjustment scores. Social factors were correlated more strongly with outcome than were demographic or clinical variables.
Miklowitz et al., 1988	23 bipolar inpatients	Relapse during a 9-mo follow-up was associated with family negative expressed emotion and negative interactions (affective style). Social variables predicted outcome independently of demographic and clinical factors.
Gitlin et al., 1995	52 bipolar-I outpatients	Relapse over a mean follow-up period of 4 yr was associated with both clinical features (prior episodes) and worse social adjustment. Strongest associations were between depressive symptoms and prior depressive episodes and poor family and social functioning.
Stefos et al., 1996	14 bipolar-I and 7 bipolar-II patients	A higher rate of major recurrences over a 4-yr follow-up period was associated with less social support, impaired social and leisure activities, and poor quality of relationships with the extended family, but clinical predictors were not significant.
Coryell et al., 1998	113 bipolar (with mania) inpatients and outpatients	Depression at 15-year follow-up was predicted by poor social (functional) adjustment before the study and persisting depression in the first 2 yr of follow-up. Earlier manic symptoms were generally unrelated to functional or clinical outcomes at 15-yr follow-up.
Kulhara et al., 1999	118 bipolar-I outpatients	A higher rate of recurrence over the follow-up period was associated with more depressive episodes before lithium treatment, more life events, and less social support.
Johnson et al., 2000	59 bipolar-I patients	Longer time to recovery over a 2-yr follow-up period was associated with lower social support. Depressive symptoms over time were predicted by life events and lower social support, but manic symptoms were not predicted by lower social support or stressors.
Johnson et al., 2003	94 bipolar patients	Those who relapsed over a 12-mo follow-up period had significantly lower perceived social support. Those with lower perceived support were also more likely to have partial rather than complete remission before relapse.
Cohen et al., 2004	52 bipolar-I outpatients	Episode recurrence over a 1-yr follow-up period, after controlling for clinical variables, was predicted by low social support and life events. Depressive episodes were more strongly predictive than manic episodes.

(continued)

TABLE 10–2. **Social Predictors of Clinical Outcomes** (continued)

Study	Sample	Significant Predictors of Poorer Outcome
Kim and Miklowitz, 2004	125 bipolar outpatients (116 bipolar-I, 9 bipolar-II)	Patients from families with high expressed emotion (EE) relatives did not experience higher rates of relapse over 2-yr follow-up, but they did experience higher levels of depression.
Yan et al., 2004	47 bipolar-I outpatients	High EE in collaterals (romantic partners, parents, friends) predicted depressive but not manic recurrence. After controlling for prior symptom severity, patients with high EE were five times more likely to have a depressive recurrence than those with low EE.

(as reported retrospectively by their mothers) was significantly worse than that of normal comparison subjects of similar age. Appropriate social behavior, quality of peer relations, and pursuit of interests appeared to be impaired in the prebipolar lives of patients. It is unclear, however, whether these individuals were actually symptomatic at young ages. Moreover, variability in reported adjustment suggests differing subgroups, including some with exceptionally good functioning. Such patterns warrant further study—as does clarification of the role of childhood disorders (see Chapter 7) in later social adjustment.

In view of the apparent impact of depressive symptoms on social adjustment, it may be noted that research on unipolar depression is focused increasingly on interpersonal functioning. Social variables are seen as playing a role in vulnerability to onset of the disorder and in the prediction of relapse, recurrence, and chronicity, and also as resulting from the impact of depression on the relationships of the depressed person with others. A large body of research has begun to document the role of social factors in depression, presumably operating both as cause and consequence of the disorder (e.g., reviews in Hammen and Brennan, 2002; see also Joiner and Coyne, 1999). This research may provide guidelines for further studies of bipolar samples.

There is a related need for further study of the specific effects of depression and mania on interpersonal relationships. Are there conditions under which manic and hypomanic symptoms portend decrements in social connections, as appears to be the case with depression? Or can they under some circumstances facilitate social contacts and friendships? Can the optimism and positive affectivity often associated with bipolar patients who have an underlying hyperthymic temperament lead to more opportunity for relationships that may prove to be sustaining and meaningful?

Marriage

I am tired of papering over the cracks and pretending to friends and relatives that life is wonderful. It is the nearest and dearest who come in for the bulk of the barrage. . . . It is the Jekyll and Hyde syndrome. I never know which is going to walk in through the door, and the unpredictability is most unnerving. It is like living on a knife-edge. You can never relax or take anything for granted and any thought of lapsing into "placid serenity" is completely out of the question. (Anonymous[18])

To understand some of the important clinical as well as research issues that arise in addressing the topic of bipolar disorder and marital relationships, a brief discussion of research on unipolar depression and marital functioning is useful. This is followed by a review of descriptive studies of bipolar disorder and marital functioning and a consideration of the complex and reciprocal relationship between marital and clinical functioning. The section ends with a review of the literature on sexual behavior in bipolar illness, assortive mating among bipolar patients, and effects on marriage of treatment of bipolar spouses.

Unipolar Depression and Marital Functioning

There has been considerable research on depression and marital functioning in recent years, corresponding to a growing focus on the interpersonal causes and consequences of depression, as well as the development of effective psychotherapies aimed at treating interpersonal and marital dysfunction in depressed individuals. Two themes and sets of findings in particular are potentially relevant to bipolar disorder.

First, the phenomenology of depression may contribute to problematic marriages. Weissman and Paykel (1974) were among the first to characterize the marriages of depressed women as fraught with friction, inadequate communication, dependency, overt hostility, resentment and guilt, poor sexual relationships, and a lack of affection. For both men and women, depressive symptoms such as irritability, loss of energy and enjoyment, heightened sensitivity to criticism, and defeatist and pessimistic attitudes all may erode the initial concern and patience of the spouse. The depressed person's exaggerated negative interpretations of self, the world, and the future may seem irrational and inexplicable, while an unwillingness to engage in typical or enjoyable pursuits and unresponsiveness to encouragement may be frustrating to the spouse and may even appear to reflect willfulness or resistance. Spouses and partners often are especially troubled by the restrictions on social and leisure activities and by the depressed person's withdrawal, worry, and suicidal thoughts (e.g., Coyne et al., 1987; Fadden et al., 1987).

As Coyne (1976) noted, there may be a deteriorating marital process in which initial concern and caring by the spouse is eventually replaced by resentment and impatience— reactions likely perceived by the depressed person as rejection and lack of sympathy, provoking further depression. As might be expected, observed communications between depressed individuals and their partners are characterized by relatively more negativity and fewer positive interactions than those of nondepressed couples (Johnson and Jacob, 1997). Such patterns have been found to be particularly pronounced among depressed women compared with depressed men (Gotlib and Whiffen, 1989; Johnson and Jacob, 1997). Over time, depression in a spouse may be perceived as a significant burden, and may even cause distress and symptoms in the nondepressed spouse (Coyne et al., 1987). Not surprisingly, depressed individuals are less likely than nondepressed controls to be married, and if they are married, they are more likely to divorce or to report the marriage as being of poor quality (Fadden et al., 1987; Coryell et al., 1993; Whisman, 2001).

A second set of findings in the unipolar field that is salient for bipolar disorder indicates that depressive episodes often result from environmental precipitants, among which marital conflict and difficulties may be especially common and potent. For example, Weissman (1987) noted a 25-fold increase in the relative risk for major depressive episodes among those in unhappy marriages, based on Epidemiological Catchment Area data for 3,000 respondents (see also Brown and Harris, 1986; Coryell et al., 1992; Anderson et al., 1999). Thus the consequences of depression for relationships may include the creation of a context that is stressful and unfulfilling, contributing to increased risk for further symptomatology.

The self-perpetuating cycle of depression and marital distress may be further complicated by some individuals' vulnerabilities in the form of maladaptive dependency or the need for frequent reassurance, dysfunctional skills in resolving interpersonal problems and conflicts, and maladaptive mate selection (Hammen, 1997, 1999). Moreover, there is evidence that the impaired interpersonal relationships of depressed persons may not be confined to periods of depression. For instance, several studies have shown that even in remission, formerly depressed patients and community members continue to show social impairment, including marital dissatisfaction and conflict (Weissman and Paykel, 1974; Billings and Moos, 1985; Hammen and Brennan, 2002).

The link between depression and marital distress may be reciprocal: some individuals may be particularly vulnerable to developing depressive reactions because of dysfunctional needs and skills with regard to intimate relationships. As suggested earlier, increased recognition of the link between depression and marital distress has led to the development of several therapeutic approaches based on addressing marital difficulties as a way to treat depressive disorders. Interpersonal psychotherapy (Klerman et al., 1984; Weissman et al., 2000) and behavioral marital therapy (Beach and Jones, 2002), for example, have proven successful both in reducing depression and in improving marital functioning.

Bipolar Disorder and Marital Functioning

The marriages of untreated, inadequately treated, or treatment-nonresponsive bipolar patients tend to be turbulent, fluctuating, and uncertain. An overall clinical description was given by Janowsky and colleagues (1970, p. 259):

> Diametrically opposed styles of marital relating, occurring during depressed or manic phases respectively, seem intolerable to the spouse. The depressive phase is usually viewed by the spouse as an illness over which the patient has little control. Here, spouses offer significant physical care and emotional support. The patient, during the depressive phase, often expresses much guilt and self-blame and sometimes speaks of the spouse in laudatory and absolving terms. . . .
>
> In contrast, the attitude of the spouse undergoes a marked change when the patient is manic. The manic phase is perceived as a willful, spiteful act. Lip service only is given to seeing the mania as an illness. There is always an underlying feeling that the manic can control his actions, and does not do so out of maliciousness, selfishness, and lack of consideration. This impression is fostered by the fact that the manic often has periods of seeming reasonableness. . . .
>
> Related to the issue of the spouse feeling betrayed and experiencing diminished self-esteem is the problem of marital infidelity. Often, manic patients speak of divorce, make sexual advances to other people, become engaged in affairs. . . .

In all these situations, the spouses felt trapped in what they perceived as an impossible situation. They felt caught in a whirlwind of activity, personally threatened, powerless to enforce limits. . . . Their moods and feelings were intimately related to the disease state of the sick partner.

Not all would agree with this characterization of spousal perceptions. Nevertheless, the turmoil associated with marriage to someone who undergoes unpredictable severe mood shifts clearly is highly stressful and challenges the coping capabilities of the partner. As we shall see, the attitudes expressed within the intimate relationship may also create conditions that may influence the course of bipolar illness.

At present, research on and conceptualization of marital functioning is less well developed for patients with bipolar disorder than for those with unipolar depression. Some of the earliest bipolar studies simply compared the marital functioning of unipolar and bipolar patients, yielding mixed findings as to which group had the "worse" outcomes (Janowsky et al., 1970; Brodie and Leff, 1971; Ruestow et al., 1978). The more crucial questions, however, concern marital functioning in treated patients, the impact of clinical features of bipolar disorder on intimate relationships, and effects of the quality of relationships on outcomes among bipolar patients.

Studies of treated patients provide ample but perhaps unsurprising evidence that marital functioning is often impaired among those with bipolar disorder. For instance, in one of the largest follow-up studies (5 years) of bipolar patients, Coryell and colleagues (1993) found that 148 such patients were only half as likely to be married by the end of the follow-up period as matched well controls (32 percent never married, compared with 15 percent of controls). Those who had married were twice as likely to be divorced as controls (45 percent divorced, compared with 18 percent of controls). Similarly, the Stanley Foundation Bipolar Network reported rates of divorced/separated or single status exceeding U.S. national norms (Suppes et al., 2001). It should be noted, however, that there is no evidence of higher divorce rates among those with bipolar disorder than among those with unipolar depression.

Corresponding to the high rates of divorce and reduced frequency of marriage among bipolar patients, couples in which one spouse is bipolar commonly report dissatisfaction. Several studies have obtained such information from the patient. For instance, Radke-Yarrow (1998) interviewed bipolar women in a study of offspring and family interactions. She found that women with bipolar disorder (a mix of bipolar-I and -II) reported higher rates of marital disorder at all follow-up assessments (62 to 76 percent) compared with non-ill women (7 to 13 percent) or women with

unipolar depression (53 to 59 percent). She speculated that psychiatric illness in many of the fathers of bipolar women may have contributed in part to the high rates of marital discord. Bauwens and colleagues (1991) collected Social Adjustment Scale information on 27 remitted bipolar, 24 remitted unipolar, and 25 control individuals. They found that bipolar patients scored midway between the unipolar (worst) and control (best) subjects in overall marital adjustment. Frequency of hospitalizations per year tended to be correlated with poorer marital adjustment, but there was no indication of the specific features of the course of illness that might have a particular association with marital difficulties.

A limited number of studies have examined the perceptions of spouses of bipolar patients. Hoover and Fitzgerald (1981) compared reported marital interactions of 42 bipolar and depressive inpatients and their spouses with those of 30 normal couples from the community. Using the 67-item Conflict in Marriage Scale (designed to measure resolution of conflicts, ways of dealing with anger, and content of disputes), they found that couples with an affectively ill spouse scored significantly higher on expressed conflict than did the community controls. Within the affectively ill group, couples with a bipolar-I member expressed more conflict than those with a unipolar or bipolar-II member, but the effects were not statistically significant. Of interest, there was low agreement between spouses in couples that included a member with mood disorder, with the ill member typically reporting much higher levels of conflict. Hoover and Fitzgerald (1981, p. 67) proposed several possible explanations for this discrepancy:

> It may be that conflict with an ill partner is more difficult to acknowledge and express. . . . Another possibility is that the spouses of manic-depressive patients derive some personality reinforcement, a tested sense of ability or moral fulfillment, from caring for a recurrently sick partner. Or perhaps some spouses need to be a trifle oblivious and not too sensitive to remain with a manic-depressive patient through the years. . . . Finally, there remains the possibility that, in a complementary sense, mercurial persons seek out cheerful, denying persons to marry whereas stolid maintainers of the peace search for more spontaneous, mood-varying types.

Levkovitz and colleagues (2000) collected reports from 34 spouses of bipolar and unipolar patients during remission and from 34 non-ill control spouses. Unfortunately, results were not reported separately for the two diagnoses. Overall, however, patients' spouses perceived significantly more negative characteristics in their marriage, lower marital satisfaction, and more negative and fewer positive traits in their partner. There was some suggestion that these more negative views were associated with unemployment status and prior history of suicide attempts on the part of the ill spouse, but generally there were no associations with clinical features of the disorder.

Few studies have attempted to shed light on the particular concerns of the spouse married to a bipolar patient. In a small-scale study, researchers administered the Family Attitudes Questionnaire to 19 bipolar patients and their well spouses to determine their attitudes and beliefs about the etiology, familial risk, and long-term burden of bipolar illness, as well as their attitudes toward marriage and childbearing (Targum et al., 1981). The reported long-term burdens of the illness included financial difficulties, home and child neglect, marital problems, loss of status and prestige, tension, and fears of recurrence of acute illness. The researchers concluded that the bipolar patients compared with their spouses tended to minimize problems associated with their illness and were more likely to deny the role of genetic factors in the disorder.

When the investigators asked the couples whether they would have married their spouses if they had known more about bipolar illness, 5 percent of the bipolar patients but fully 53 percent of their spouses said they would not have, a statistically significant difference. Similarly, when asked whether they would have had children, 5 percent of the bipolar patients and 47 percent of their spouses said they would not have. Both patients and spouses perceived violent behavior as the most troubling characteristic of mania. Patients also were especially worried by their poor judgment during mania. Spouses were particularly concerned about impulsive spending, overtalkativeness, and decreased need for sleep. Both groups saw suicide threats and attempts as the most troubling aspect of depression, and patients were also bothered by the hopelessness and poor concentration accompanying that state; spouses, on the other hand, were most disturbed by the patient's lowered self-esteem and withdrawal from others. Overall, the most troublesome long-term social problems resulting from bipolar illness were financial difficulties, unemployment, marital problems, recurrences of illness leading to rehospitalization, and social withdrawal due to depression. The researchers concluded:

> Well spouses who have coped with affective illness for many years perceived bipolar illness as a profound burden that had seriously disrupted their lives. . . . The regrets of the well spouse are a most striking feature of this study. . . . Whereas affective episodes may not be directly associated with major persistent psychological deficits, the damaging effects of these episodes may still yield psychological and economic consequences, particularly for the spouse. The spouse is the person who bears the brunt of manic episodes. . . . In depression, the spouse is the most frequent target of demands and hostility, and often feels inordinate responsibility for the mood state of the patient. (Targum et al., 1981, p. 568)

Targum and colleagues (1981) were the first to examine and compare systematically the attitudes of bipolar patients and their spouses and to highlight spousal distress. Yet other studies (e.g., Frank et al., 1981, in a study of 16 couples) have not found such negative effects. It should be noted that the study by Targum and colleagues did not employ a comparison group; moreover, most of the couples had been married for many years, increasing the chances that the bipolar spouse had not been treated with lithium or another mood stabilizer. In a study conducted in India, Chakrabarti and Gill (2002) found that caregivers (mainly spouses) of bipolar patients reported experiencing less of a burden than that reported by caregivers of people with schizophrenia; the burden they did experience involved mainly physical and mental health problems.

Perlick and colleagues (1999) studied perceived burden in a large sample of caregivers of 266 bipolar-I and -II and schizoaffective (manic) patients. Patients' depression was perceived as being associated with a greater burden relative to mania; caregiver distress was especially pronounced when the patient displayed symptoms of "misery, irritability, and withdrawal." The authors also found that the association between severity-of-illness factors and perceived burden was mediated by caregivers' beliefs and attitudes. Specifically, perceived burden was higher among those who believed the patient with bipolar disorder could control his or her symptoms whereas the caregiver could not, and among those with an accurate awareness of the nature and prognosis of the disorder.

Others have likewise speculated that a critical factor in attitudes toward partners with bipolar disorder is the extent to which the patient is perceived as willfully causing or controlling the symptoms. A study conducted by Hooley and colleagues (1987), which included both schizophrenic and bipolar patients and their spouses or family members, revealed that spouses or family of patients with florid, positive symptoms (auditory or visual hallucinations; grandiosity; agitation; speech disorganization; delusions; elated mood; silliness; or inappropriate affect, appearance, or behavior) reported significantly higher levels of marital satisfaction than spouses of patients with negative symptoms (social isolation, depression, lack of emotion, or routine or leisure-time impairment). The authors attributed this difference to the fact that the more bizarre and flagrant positive symptoms, unlike the negative ones, were perceived by the spouse as being caused by an illness and thus beyond the patient's volition. It is likely that milder symptoms of hypomania and depressive symptoms are especially likely to be attributed erroneously to the patient's personality and behaviors. As discussed later, the attitudes of spouses and family members may play a significant role in clinical outcomes and therefore may be an important factor in treatment effectiveness.

A study of caregiver burden among spouses of bipolar patients was conducted in New Zealand (Dore and Romans, 2001). The caregivers were, for the most part, partners or parents of 41 bipolar patients. Virtually all reported that the patient was difficult and irritable or more distant during an affective episode, and that this caused the caregiver considerable distress. Nearly half reported experience with or concern about violence when the patient was in the midst of an episode. Marital difficulties were common and sometimes persistent. Fully 62 percent of the partners said they would probably not have entered into the relationship had they had more knowledge and understanding of the illness beforehand. Nevertheless, most caregivers felt that the relationship was good when the patient was in remission, and few were experiencing significant distress symptoms themselves at the time of the assessment.

Marital Functioning, Family Attitudes, and Predictors of Outcome

Clinical experience suggests that mood stabilizers have a positive effect on marriages involving bipolar individuals because the drugs partially or totally eliminate both highly volatile and disruptive manic episodes and frightening and depleting depressive episodes. These benefits appear to be corroborated by the few existing studies of marital interaction among adequately treated bipolar patients (McKnight et al., 1989). As the results of one early study suggest, however, improvements may be perceived differently by the spouse and the patient. Demers and Davis (1971) found that most of the well spouses participating in their study perceived improvements associated with lithium treatment, including enhanced marital satisfaction, as well as observed decreases in nervousness, violent or threatening behavior, withdrawn or demanding behavior, and sadness. Yet only a minority of the patients themselves perceived such positive changes—perhaps because they were still experiencing subsyndromal episodes or, in some instances, because of their perceived loss of the positive experiences associated with hypomania.

Although the improved clinical status of a bipolar spouse may greatly relieve the patient's partner and family, there is, as noted earlier, a reciprocal impact: increasing evidence indicates that the quality of marital and family functioning may contribute to the patient's clinical outcome during treatment. Results of several studies suggest that good marital functioning or just being married may contribute to the effectiveness of treatment in reducing episodes. For instance, Yazici and colleagues (1999) found that being married was associated with good response to lithium; 27 percent of good-response patients and 48 percent of poor-response patients were unmarried. Similar results have been reported by others (O'Connell et al., 1991). It is important to note, however, that these findings cannot clarify the direction of causality of effects, inasmuch as good response to lithium may be more likely among more well-functioning individuals, as well as those whose manic episodes are relatively more euphoric in nature (see Chapter 18). Likewise, medication adherence and stable sleep may be more likely in the context of a good marriage.

Several studies have found that the "expressed emotion" or "affective style" of partners (the overall negativity or positivity of attitudes toward the patient) may predict relapse and outcome in treated patients over time (Mundt et al., 2000). Miklowitz and colleagues (1988), for example, first demonstrated that bipolar patients whose spouses or parents expressed negative attitudes about them during hospitalization for mania were significantly more likely to have a relapse in the ensuing 9 months than were those patients whose spouses or parents expressed more benign or positive attitudes. O'Connell and colleagues (1991) also found that attitudes of family members, including those of spouses, were significantly related to outcome in a lithium treatment outpatient clinic. More negative attitudes were expressed by partners of patients with poor outcomes (40 percent) than by partners of patients with good outcomes (12 percent). Perlick and colleagues (2001) found that greater perceived caretaker burden, which, as noted, reflects in part attitudes toward the patient and the illness, predicted depressive relapse at follow-up, even after controlling for baseline symptoms. Furthermore, over a 15-month period of mood stabilization, those patients who had fewer symptoms but whose caretakers reported a high perceived burden were more likely to experience a recurrence of their illness. The investigators suggested that stressful family environments contribute to caretaker burden and possibly to depression, as well as to patient relapse.

A family-focused psychoeducational treatment program was devised by Miklowitz and Goldstein (1997) to improve the attitudes of spouses and family members toward the bipolar patient by increasing their knowledge and understanding of the disorder and improving their skills in communicating and solving family-related problems. An evaluation of the treatment suggested that it was effective in improving positive nonverbal communication, and that such improvements accounted in part for the progress seen in patients' symptoms over a 1-year period (Simoneau et al., 1999; Miklowitz et al., 2003) (see Chapter 22). The effectiveness of psychosocial treatments that include spouses is increasingly being demonstrated (e.g., Clarkin et al., 1998), including their potential role in helping to extend the duration and quality of the beneficial effects of medication on the outcome of bipolar disorder (see Chapter 22).

Sexual Behavior

> Again judging from my own experience, the sexual symptoms of the manic state seem to be the most powerful and important of all. . . . The normal inhibitions disappear, and sexual activity, instead of being placed, as in our Western Christian civilization, in opposition to religion, becomes associated with it. This release of the underlying sexual tension . . . seems to me to be the primary and governing factor of all the ecstasies and many other experiences of the manic state. (John Custance, 1952)

Changes in sexual desire, thought, and behavior during depression and mania were observed centuries ago. Aretaeus of Cappadocia (150 AD), for example, observed that "a period of lewdness and shamelessness exists with the highest type of [manic] delirium" (Jelliffe, 1931, p. 20). In the nineteenth and twentieth centuries, Tuke (1892), Kraepelin (1921), Bleuler (1924), Campbell (1953), and Mayer-Gross and colleagues (1955) also described heightened sexuality during mania and decreased sexuality during depression (see Chapter 2).

Fluctuations in sexual drive are sufficiently important in bipolar illness to warrant inclusion as diagnostic criteria in DSM-III and/or DSM-IV ("sexual indiscretions" for manic episodes and "decrease in sexual interest or drive" for depressive episodes). Items pertaining to sexual behavior are on most self- and observer-rating instruments for both mania and depression (see Chapter 12). Beigel and colleagues (1971), for example, required nurses to judge 26 items most characteristic of manic behavior, thought, and affect. Of those items, the 2 pertaining to sex ("talks about sex" and "is sexually preoccupied") had high concordance with independent ratings on both a psychiatrists' global mania scale and a nurses' manic-symptom checklist.

The actual data on changes in sexual behavior and thinking during different phases of bipolar illness are relatively limited. Quantified observational data are presented in Chapter 2 and can be summarized here. Hypersexuality was observed or reported in 57 percent of manic patients (averaged across seven studies, with a range of values from 25 to 80 percent), and actual nudity or sexual exposure was reported in 29 percent (averaged across three studies, with a range of values from 23 to 33 percent). Akiskal and colleagues (1977) reported that 40 percent of their cyclothymic patients had "episodic or unexplained promiscuity or extramarital affairs." Allison and Wilson (1960) studied the sexual behavior of 24 manic patients using data based on physician observations and on historical information from patients and their relatives. They found no relationship between

sexual display during mania and age, religion, duration of illness, previous episodes, or social class. Women were far more sexually provocative and seductive than men (58 and 0 percent, respectively) on a 5-point rating scale. However, women and men were equally likely to have both increased "libidinal drives" and increased frequency of sexual relations. In 78 percent of the patients, the frequency of sexual intercourse increased substantially during manic episodes.

A recent study of sexual satisfaction in 37 partners of bipolar patients found that partners were less satisfied when the patient was affectively ill (Lam et al., 2005). The investigators attributed this finding to illness-related changes in sexual interest, affection, and responsiveness.

Winokur and colleagues (1969) found that 65 percent of manic episodes were characterized by increased sexuality. In 32 percent of cases, the sexuality was of a socially approved type, that is, within marriage or a long-lasting relationship. In 10 percent of patients, the increased sexuality was in thought or discussion only, and in 11 percent it was manifested in socially disapproved behavior. In this latter group, patients were homosexually or heterosexually promiscuous or both; in all cases, the hypersexuality was clearly associated with being ill. Like those patients studied by Allison and Wilson (1960), the women (18 percent) in the study of Winokur and colleagues were more likely to have increased sexual contacts (noncoital) than the men (3 percent), but women and men were equally likely to have an increased frequency of intercourse (30 and 35 percent, respectively).

Spalt (1975) studied lifetime sexual behavior in 42 patients with unipolar depression, 19 with bipolar illness, 56 with secondary affective illness, and 38 with nonaffective illness. Extramarital sexual experiences were more frequent among bipolar patients (29 percent had more than 10 experiences) than among unipolar patients (12 percent). Bipolar patients (21 percent) also were more likely than unipolar patients (10 percent) to have had more than 10 sexual partners during their lifetime. These figures almost certainly reflect many other behavioral differences between the two groups, including hypersexuality and differences in sexual drive during normal periods, as well as differences in levels of gregariousness, sociability, and interpersonal turmoil.

Jamison and colleagues (1980) studied changes attributed to affective illness in 35 bipolar and 26 unipolar patients. Twice as many women (41 percent) as men (20 percent) reported that sexual intensity was "very much increased" during hypomania; 40 percent of the men and 18 percent of the women stated that sexual intensity during hypomania was "somewhat increased." Women rated increased sexual intensity as the most important or enjoyable change they experienced during hypomania.[19] Bipolar patients were significantly more likely than unipolar patients ($p < .01$) to feel that increased sexual intensity was a lasting characteristic attributable to their mood disorder.

As noted, bipolar illness also can be associated with decreased sexual drive. For example, Winokur and colleagues (1969) reported that 63 percent of patients with bipolar mixed states reported decreased sexual interest. Indeed, approximately three-fourths of bipolar depressed patients have been found to experience a loss of sexual interest: 73 percent reported by Winokur and colleagues (1969) and 77 percent by Casper and colleagues (1985).

Sexual responsiveness can also be dampened in patients taking lithium.[20] Sheard (1971, 1975) and Lion (1975) attributed this phenomenon to a common effect on aggressive and sexual behaviors, both often occurring together in bipolar patients. Lorimy and colleagues (1977) reported that half of their patients taking prophylactic lithium experienced troublesome side effects affecting their sexual activities, including decreases in sexual intensity, frequency of sexual drive, and frequency of sexual intercourse. However, patients reported that once intercourse began, there was no decrement in enjoyment or orgasmic ability.

What accounts for these lithium-induced changes is unclear. Among the possible explanations are lithium-induced hypothyroidism, decreased frequency or intensity of hypomanic episodes, or the direct effect of lithium on the central mechanisms underlying sexual drive and behavior. Yet another possible reason for these changes is vacillation in interpersonal relationships brought about by lithium, with secondary manifestation in the sexual domain.

Assortative Mating among Bipolar Patients

An additional challenge to marital adjustment among individuals with bipolar disorder is the increased likelihood of nonrandom mate selection. Specifically, research, although limited, suggests that bipolar individuals have an increased likelihood of marrying a partner with affective illness (see Chapter 13). For instance, in a sample of 56 married inpatients with mood disorders, Merikangas and Spiker (1982) found a higher degree of assortative mating among bipolar than unipolar patients. They noted high diagnostic concordance between patients and spouses for both affective disorders and alcoholism. The effects could not be attributed to spouses' symptomatic reactions to marriage to an ill spouse because the spouses appeared to have a predisposition to the disorders based on elevated rates of psychiatric and mood disorders in their own relatives. Colombo and colleagues (1990) studied assortative mating in a large sample of more than 1,000 patients with mood or anxiety disorders. They observed that while patients with bipolar illness were less likely to marry overall than were those with unipolar disorder, there was a specific

assortative mating pattern such that bipolar men were more likely than controls to have wives with mood disorders.

Most of the few studies examining assortative mating have had methodological limitations, such as small sample sizes, lack of direct comparison groups, and differing diagnostic criteria. A meta-analysis approach is especially helpful for evaluating pooled effects across several small studies. One such analysis (Mathews and Reus, 2001), based on the six best-designed studies, confirmed the commonly reported finding of assortative mating for bipolar individuals, with higher rates than for those with unipolar depression. Specific analyses based on husbands and wives were inconclusive because of limited data, but suggested that data supporting the marriage of bipolar men to women with mood disorders are much more robust than is the case for the marriage of bipolar women to men with mood disorders. The authors also noted the paucity of evidence of mood disorders in mates before the marriage; thus depressive reactions to stress in marriage to a bipolar partner cannot be ruled out.

Although these studies raise a number of questions to be pursued in further research, they support the often-observed pattern of the marriage of bipolar individuals to those who also have mood disorders. Such dual-disorder pairings may promote shared understanding, but may also give rise to marital discord and instability by contributing to stressful home environments and potentially to limited skills for resolving interpersonal disputes. While not confined to bipolar disorder, such pairings may present a treatment challenge requiring family or couple interventions. Obviously if confirmed, assortative mating also has considerable genetic significance.

Effects on Marriage of Treatment of Bipolar Spouses

Clinical experience suggests that lithium, the only mood stabilizer that has been studied systematically for its effect on marital stability, has a highly stabilizing effect on the marriages of patients with bipolar illness because it partially or totally eliminates both highly volatile and disruptive manic episodes and frightening and depleting depressive ones. These benefits appear to be corroborated by the few marital studies of adequately treated bipolar patients,[21] although they were not observed in the study by Targum and colleagues (1981).

Demers and Davis (1971) administered the Marital Partner Attribute Test to 14 married bipolar patients and their spouses. Lithium produced a highly significant decrease in spouses' negative ratings of the patients but no significant changes in patients' ratings of their spouses. In fact, 13 (93 percent) of 14 bipolar patients were rated by their spouses as improved and as having significantly fewer undesirable attributes ($p < .01$) after lithium treatment. Spouses particularly noted decreases in nervousness; bizarre, threatening, and violent behavior; withdrawn or demanding behavior; guilt; sadness; and undue exaggeration of abilities. But they also reported missing the enthusiasm and heightened sexuality associated with hypomanic phases:

> Hypomanic joviality, enthusiasm, and spontaneity are often regarded as social pluses; and manic-depressives and their spouses complain about the loss of these valued attributes. When pressed to discuss the sexual compatibility of the marriage, frequently they will say it is worse since lithium treatment started, as the lithium-treated spouse has less libidinal strivings. (Demers and Davis, 1971, p. 352)

Although 77 percent of the spouses rated the marriage as considerably improved, only 43 percent of the bipolar patients expressed this opinion. Patients may be more sensitive to the loss of positive experiences associated with bipolar illness, whereas their spouses may be more aware of lithium's beneficial effects. Such a possibility would be consistent with the discrepancies in perceptions reported by Targum and colleagues (1981). These results again underscore the importance of sophisticated clinical management and subtle titration of lithium to the lowest possible level consistent with efficacy.

O'Connell and Mayo (1981) studied the effects of lithium treatment on 12 bipolar patients and their families. They found that lithium increased the direct care of children by both patients and spouses, significantly alleviated marital friction, and resulted in increased cooperative planning, communication, and trust.

Holinger and Wolpert (1979) found that the majority (59 percent) of their 56 manic-depressive patients showed improvement in their relationships with spouses, families, or friends as a result of taking lithium; slightly more than one-third (39 percent) showed no change. The primary changes observed by the authors were decreases in impulsivity, fragility, and erratic behavior; confidence in relationships increased. The bipolar patients were far more likely than the lithium-treated unipolar patients to demonstrate a change in interpersonal behavior (59 and 11 percent, respectively). In a study by Lepkifker and colleagues (1988), psychiatrists' ratings of marital and other interpersonal relationships were significantly higher for the 50 bipolar and 50 unipolar patients (all of whom were euthymic and lithium-treated) than for 50 psychiatric controls with personality disorders. There were no significant bipolar–unipolar differences.

Finally, Ruestow and colleagues (1978), in a study cited earlier, suggested that bipolar manic-depressive patients, especially men, could have good marriages if stabilized by lithium. While emphasizing the importance of adjunctive use of marital therapy, they also suggested "that patients be treated with medication . . . prior to the initiation of marital therapy and that the need for intensive marital therapy be reassessed after the patient's illness has been stabilized."

Bipolar Disorder and Family Functioning

In addition to the genetic risk imparted by bipolar parents to their children, there is a potential risk due to the children's exposure to parents' moods and maladaptive child rearing. This is an understudied research topic in bipolar samples; however, there is an important and well-developed literature linking the effects of parental depression and the commonly associated environmental conditions with diagnosable disorders in children and disturbances in their functioning.[22] The vast majority of these studies involved mothers with diagnosed unipolar depression or nondiagnosed women who displayed elevated symptoms of depressed mood; the samples included children of all ages, from infancy to young adulthood. Across the wide array of samples with varying demographic characteristics in these studies, the results have been quite consistent. Infants display a variety of indicators of distress and discomfort while interacting with depressed mothers. School-age children with clinically depressed mothers show high rates of major depression, as well as anxiety and disruptive behavior disorders, with studies indicating that 50 percent or more of such children may have diagnosable disorders during childhood and adolescence (Hammen, 1991; Beardslee et al., 1998). The offspring of depressed parents have also been found to be impaired in academic and social functioning, and indicators of maladjustment and psychopathology appear to suggest further dysfunction over follow-up periods of several years (Anderson and Hammen, 1993; Weissman et al., 1997; NICHD Early Child Care Research Network, 1999).

While children's maladjustment may in part reflect genetically transmitted disorder, it has been widely speculated that depressed parents, particularly depressed mothers, are impaired in their parental roles in ways that have substantial negative impacts on their children, ways likely to be linked to the chronicity and severity of and perhaps the timing of the child's exposure to the parent's depression. Depressed women may be apathetic and withdrawn, display less physical affection, or be irritable and critical with their children. Not only do the symptoms of depression interfere with the kinds of warm, consistent, responsive, and available nurturing believed to be optimal for children's development, but the depressed parent may also be unable to assist the child in coping with stressful life events that befall the child or family and may fail to model effective strategies for coping with interpersonal and stressful challenges. In addition, the lives of depressed women are commonly characterized by a variety of factors that may have a negative impact on the developing child, including marital conflict or divorce, as well as work and financial difficulties that create stressful conditions in the family.

As noted, far less research has been conducted on the parenting characteristics of women with bipolar disorder than on those of women with depression. Moreover, parenting behaviors are likely to differ as a function of mood state. While depressive symptoms may be associated with maladaptive parenting, it is less clear that bipolar parents who are euthymic or even hypomanic display dysfunctional behaviors. Additionally, significant changes in parenting style, perhaps resulting from mood shifts, may themselves have important effects on children. It is also important to distinguish the potentially detrimental effect on children of such cofactors of bipolar disorder as exposure to violence, psychosis, and substance abuse from outcomes associated with typical functioning while not in the midst of episodes. Thus parenting characteristics should be explored as a function of current, typical, and potentially changing clinical status, with attention to the considerable differences in outcomes that may be associated with each.

As noted in Chapter 7, relatively few studies addressing high risk for bipolar disorder have examined psychosocial mechanisms of children's risk in bipolar families. Radke-Yarrow (1998), reporting the results of an approximately 10-year follow-up of children of unipolar and bipolar mothers, summarized the results of several observational sessions involving mothers and their children. She and her colleagues attempted to characterize two mechanisms by which a mother's disorder affected her children—maternal symptomatology, and socialization and caregiving functions. Both unipolar and bipolar women were frequently observed to be irritable and angry with their youngsters (42 percent), and some of the bipolar women displayed an overall uninvolved or unavailable style (19 percent). Bipolar women also evidenced boundary issues, "unstable enthusiasms," and impulsive behavior in their interactions (61 to 69 percent). Overall, the maternal styles observed were fairly stable over the years of the study and were predictive of maladaptive outcomes in the children. It should be noted that because most of the bipolar women in the study had bipolar-II disorder, their symptoms were chiefly depressive, and the specific role of mania was not examined.

A study of the family environments of bipolar parents of 56 children aged 6 to 18 was conducted by Chang and colleagues (2001). They collected parents' reports on the Family Environment Scale, and found significantly lower scores on the cohesion and organization subscales and higher scores on the conflict subscale compared with normative data. The scores were unrelated to whether the children had diagnoses of Axis I disorders, however, so child psychopathology was not directly associated with family functioning.

One of the rare studies of mother–infant behavior involving women with bipolar disorder compared ratings of mother–child interactions during hospitalization among unipolar, bipolar, and schizophrenic women (Hipwell and Kumar, 1996). All groups displayed erratic or dysfunctional interactions at first, but improved over time. While the scores of the bipolar women were initially similar to those of the schizophrenic women, they showed greater improvement over the course of hospitalization: by the time of discharge, 77 percent of bipolar and 86 percent of unipolar mothers fell within the normal range, compared with only 33 percent of schizophrenic women. It appeared that the impairments associated with bipolar disorder were symptom related and became normalized with clinical improvement.

The University of California-Los Angeles (UCLA) High Risk Study observed mother–child interactions among bipolar, unipolar, and medically ill and well women during discussions involving typical family disagreements. The researchers found that the bipolar women largely resembled the normal comparison women in their interaction styles, whereas the unipolar depressed women were significantly more negative, critical, and withdrawn from the discussion task with their children (Gordon et al., 1989). Analysis of the findings of this study revealed that overall, depressive mood was a strong predictor of maternal behavior, as well as of children's symptoms (Hammen, 1991). Regardless of diagnosis, women with more severe depressive symptoms had more disturbances in their interactions with their children, and their children were less well adjusted in various roles. Bipolar women had significantly fewer depressive episodes over the course of the study (3 years) than did unipolar women, and thus the phenomenology of the family experiences was quite different for the two groups. Anderson and Hammen (1993) reported that the offspring of bipolar mothers had better social adjustment and academic achievement relative to those of unipolar depressed mothers; indeed, their adjustment resembled that of children of normal community women. Similar results were reported by Klein and colleagues (1986), who found normal social adjustment in the adolescent offspring of parents with bipolar disorder. However, if the offspring themselves had cyclothymic behavior and mood disturbances, they tended to have impaired social adjustment. Thus the sparse evidence available suggests relatively good adjustment in children of bipolar parents (unless the children themselves are symptomatic) and provides little indication of significant parenting impairment, except among those with chronic depression.

One hypothesis that should be pursued in future research is that the reactions of children and other family members to depression, mania, and mixed states are almost certainly quite different. As discussed earlier, a manic episode may be viewed as being more clearly beyond the individual's control than a depressive episode and therefore may be more likely to elicit alternative caretaking for children. The predominant mood state of the parent's mania—euphoric versus angry and highly volatile—is certainly relevant but has not been studied in this context. Also, of course, the parent's psychological and social functioning between episodes is likely to be a strong predictor of children's adjustment, inasmuch as stable and euthymic periods may help repair disruptions caused by periods of symptomatology. Not only the specific effects of depression and mania, but also the level of chronicity or recovery between major episodes, are of considerable predictive significance in understanding the overall effects of parenting behavior.

Clearly, further studies are needed to evaluate the parental functioning of adults with bipolar disorder. Of particular importance is the quality of parenting when the patient is not in the midst of a major episode. As in research on the effects of unipolar depression on children's risk, it is also important to measure and evaluate the environment in which families live, including parents' marital status, economic conditions, and the spouse's mental health and adjustment, as well as general resources for coping with the illness.

CONCLUSIONS

Personality

Contemporary research generally dispels the idea that the personalities of bipolar patients are fundamentally different from those of people without mood disorders. Descriptive studies comparing bipolar patients with other groups have yielded few consistent results and clearly suggest enormous variability, depending in part on the instruments used and individuals' current mood status. The major drawback of such studies is their limited utility. Nevertheless, the close and likely bidirectional association between personality and mood disorders suggests that many behaviors and attitudes we regard as personality may in fact be somewhat unstable and highly colored by affective experiences. The field now appears ready to proceed to more conceptually and practically challenging questions and prospective methods concerning the predictive utility of personality constructs: Do they tell us something important about the course of disorder, treatment responsiveness, and functional outcome

beyond that attributable to symptoms or psychosocial context? Are there premorbid signs of eventual bipolar disorder that might help in both understanding the risk for illness and altering its course? What are the underlying neurobiological processes of normal mood and temperament that may help us understand mood disorders?

Personality Disorders

Research on personality disorders—the enduring, pervasive, and dysfunctional styles measured on Axis II of the DSM—has increased in sophistication in the bipolar field. As with most Axis I disorders, studies of bipolar patients evaluated during remission indicate relatively high rates of personality disorders, and such disorders generally predict a relatively worse course of illness and functional adjustment. However, the overlap among bipolar symptoms, mood states, and personality pathology may obscure the question of whether a bipolar patient truly has an Axis II disorder.

Interpersonal Functioning

Interpersonal functioning is commonly a casualty of bipolar disorder, although there is tremendous variability in individuals' abilities to sustain close friendships and family relationships. It is unclear whether the effects of bipolar disorder on interpersonal functioning are the result of episodes or of underlying impairment of social skills. There is, however, ample evidence that poor social functioning may negatively affect clinical outcomes. Thus interventions targeting social and family relationships may potentiate the effects of psychopharmacology and, of course, benefit the loved ones greatly affected by their relative's disorder.

NOTES

1. These differences were well summarized by Hall and Lindzey (1970): the relative importance of the uniqueness of the individual (the idiographic-nomothetic controversy), whether man should be viewed as possessing purposive or teleological qualities, the importance of group membership, the relative importance of conscious and unconscious determinants of behavior, the number of motivational concepts, the importance of the principles of reward and association, the relative emphasis on stable structures or the process of change in personality, the functional independence of personality structure at any particular point in time, the relative importance of genetic factors in determining behavior, and the relative importance of early developmental experiences.

2. Thus Kraepelin (1921) delineated four fundamental types of temperament: *depressive, manic, irritable,* and *cyclothymic.* Kretschmer (1936) stressed the overlap among these personality types in the prepsychotic, *cycloid personality* of manic-depressive patients: "they form layers or patterns in individual cases, arranged in the most varied combinations." Campbell

(1953), too, described a cycloid personality, which could occur in one of three forms—*hypomanic, depressive*, and *cyclothymic*—"with innumerable gradations and mixtures between the three." He, like Kraepelin, regarded all of these personality types as "part of the same disease process, and that any one of these may change into any other." Leonhard (1957), who separated major affective illness into unipolar and bipolar types, also regarded many personality patterns in manic-depressive patients as subclinical, or "diluted," forms of the primary illness itself. Mayer-Gross and colleagues (1955) derived personality topologies similar to those of Kraepelin (1921), Kretschmer (1936), and Campbell (1953): *cyclothymic* (social, good-hearted, kind, and easy-going), *hyperthymic* (elated, humorous, lively, and hot-tempered), and *hypothymic* (quiet, calm, serious, and gentle). Rowe and Daggett (1954) and Von Zerssen (1977) summarized premorbid personality traits of manic and depressed patients, which are quite consistent with the earlier clinical topologies.

3. Dooley (1921, p. 167) wrote:

> The behavior found in the manic attack, in which the patient throws himself with almost equal vim into every possible avenue of expression, is in itself a defense reaction. By thus taking the offensive he keeps himself safe from the approach of the painful thought or feeling which is usually a realization of some failure or degradation, or fundamental inferiority of his own. When he is depressed his defense is no longer possible and he is weighed down by the pain of the acknowledged defect.

More specifically, Schwartz (1961, p. 244) described the dynamic purpose for hyperactive behavior and grandiose thought:

> The hypermotility in mania may have a twofold purpose. First, it may serve as a method for distracting attention from the perception of deprivation; second, it is a diffuse and multidirectional effort to obtain pleasure, in which some realistic basis for the denial of deprivation may be grasped. . . . Grandiosity as a defense by denial against emptiness, however . . . may even represent, additionally, an intellectual attempt at a further regression, in the service of the ego, to the stage of omnipotence.

Grotstein (1986) described the manic mechanism of denial in terms of power and self-regulation:

> The psychical state which is set up to regulate this primal state of powerlessness is that of a fraudulent state of power, including that of a severe superego and/or compulsive and/or hypomanic defenses which seek to create an artificial "floor" over a "floorless" psyche.

4. Dooley, 1921; Wilson, 1951; Arieti, 1959; Stone, 1978.
5. Cohen et al., 1954; Arieti, 1959; Gibson et al., 1959; Smith, 1960.
6. This concept was explained in a different way by Arieti (1959, p. 431):

> The receptiveness to others and willingness to introject the others determines, at this early age, some aspects of the personality of the patient. He tends to become

an "extrovert"; at the same time he tends to become a conformist, willing to accept what he is given by his surroundings (not only in material things but also in terms of habits and values).

7. According to Dooley (1921, p. 39, 166):

> The personality of the manic depressive individual also presents an obstacle. Those who manifest frequent manic attacks are likely to be headstrong, self-sufficient, know-it all types of persons who will not take suggestions or yield to direction. They are "doers" and managers, and will get the upper hand of the analyst and everyone else around them if given the opportunity . . . . The manic-depressive character is extroverted, he tries always to relate himself to his environment, he minimizes the subjective element and makes use of every object in the range of his senses.

Wilson (1951, p. 362) further discussed the therapist's problems in treating the manic-depressive patient:

> From the psychiatrist's point of view he is uninteresting because he is hard to get at. He is friendly and superficially cooperative, but soon personality investigation ceases because the patient refuses to be self analytical. When the patient is depressed or manic, his illness seems to explain his unapproachableness, and when he is well he will have nothing to do with you except in a very superficial way. This impenetrable shell is characteristic of persons with this illness and sets them apart from those having other forms of depression.

Cohen and colleagues (1954, p. 120) described the manic-depressive personality as dependent, even during states of normal functioning:

> We see, then, in the adult cyclothymic, a person who is apparently well adjusted between attacks, although he may show minor mood swings or be chronically overactive or chronically mildly depressed. He is conventionally well-behaved and frequently successful, and he is hardworking and conscientious; indeed, at times his overconscientiousness and scrupulousness lead to his being called obsessional. He is typically involved in one or more relationships of extreme dependence, in which, however, he does not show the obsessional's typical need to control the other person for the sake of power, but instead seeks to control the other person in the sense of swallowing him up. His inner feeling, when he allows himself to notice it, is one of emptiness and need. He is extremely stereotyped in his attitudes and opinions, tending to take over the opinions of the person in his environment whom he regards as an important authority. Again this contrasts with the outward conformity but subtle rebellion of the obsessional. It should be emphasized that the dependency feelings are largely out of awareness in states of well-being and also in the manic phase; in fact, these people frequently take pride in being independent.

8. Frey, 1977; Hirschfeld and Klerman, 1979; Liebowitz et al., 1979; Bech et al., 1980; Hirschfeld, 1985, 1986.

9. Perris, 1966; Murray and Blackburn, 1974; Hirschfeld and Klerman, 1979; Liebowitz et al., 1979; Winters and Neale, 1985.

10. Perris, 1971; Frey, 1977; Bech et al., 1980; Matussek and Feil, 1983; Hirschfeld, 1985; Hirschfeld et al., 1986.

11. Frey, 1977; Hirschfeld and Klerman, 1979; Liebowitz et al., 1979; Abou-Saleh and Coppen, 1984.

12. Kron et al., 1982; Gershon et al. 1985; Klein and Depue, 1985; Nurnberger et al., 1988; Grigoroiu-Serbanescu et al., 1989, 1991.

13. Cited in Hamilton, 1982, p. 214.

14. See, e.g., Bauwens et al., 1991; Coryell et al., 1993; Mundt et al., 2000; Dorz et al., 2002.

15. Harrow et al., 1990; Tohen et al., 1990; Keller et al., 1993; Gitlin et al., 1995.

16. Kulhara et al., 1999; Johnson et al., 2000, 2003; Cohen et al., 2004.

17. Johnson et al., 2000; Cohen et al., 2004; Kim and Miklowitz, 2004; Yan et al., 2004.

18. Published in *The Times* (London), January 24, 1986.

19. Stoddard and colleagues (1977) studied eight affective episodes in a 39-year-old rapid-cycling woman. They collected systematic behavioral data twice a day and observed that she became sexually provocative during mania. Conversely, a significant predictor of her switch into depression was a decrease in sexual preoccupation ($p < .05$).

20. In addition to the references in this paragraph, see Demers and Davis (1971).

21. Demers and Davis, 1971; Ruestow et al., 1978; Frank et al., 1981; O'Connell and Mayo, 1981.

22. Downey and Coyne, 1990; Gelfand and Teti, 1990; Hammen, 1991; Goodman and Gotlib, 1999; NICHD Early Child Care Research Network, 1999.

Assessment

Our customary grouping into manic and melancholic attacks does not fit the facts, but requires substantial enlargement, if it is to reproduce nature.

—*Emil Kraepelin (1921, p. 191)*

Standardized measures of mania and depression provide the common language by which clinicians and researchers can communicate. By minimizing differences in the way clinicians record their observations, such instruments contribute to the widespread sharing of information and provide yardsticks for a variety of observers in very different settings. The measures discussed in this chapter vary in their goals and uses. Some help in determining the severity of episodes or symptom states, providing information about treatment response, and ascertaining the incidence of different types of affective states. Quantitative rating scales for mania and depression can be especially important in longitudinal studies (e.g., to describe the natural course of the illness and individual manic and depressive episodes) for identifying the progression and resolution of symptom patterns; studying euthymic states in bipolar patients; and correlating manic and depressive states with other aspects of behavior, cognition, personality, and neurobiology. The assessment literature focuses on bipolar disorder or major depression; there are no measures of depression that focus on the highly recurrent forms that, along with bipolar disorder, make up what we mean by manic-depressive illness. Accordingly the focus of this chapter is on the bipolar subgroup.

There are several additional uses of assessment instruments in the field of bipolar disorder. With the abundance of longitudinal studies of bipolar course, as well as treatment outcome studies, procedures for systematic mapping of the course of the disorder have been developed. Less focused on symptoms as such than measures of severity of mood states, such procedures have the primary aim of capturing changes in and patterns of mood episodes over time. Another relatively new development is the search for measures of risk for bipolar disorder. The potential utility of procedures that could be used to assess subsyndromal or preclinical states lies in their ability to predict who will develop bipolar disorder over time. Because those with the disorder may be untreated and underdiagnosed, it would be useful to have screening measures to identify such individuals in general psychological, psychiatric, or medical settings. Also discussed in this chapter are measures of functional outcomes in work and social relationships; we note the paucity of such approaches relative to those with a clinical focus. Gaining a fuller understanding of bipolar disorder—as well as helping patients improve in key areas that affect the quality of their lives—requires attention to the development and application of such measures.

Several general types of measures have been developed to classify and quantify changes in affective states. The major categories, delineated by von Zerssen and Cording (1978), are (1) self-ratings, made by patients; (2) observer ratings, usually made by clinicians; (3) analyses of behavior (including linguistic analyses of speech or written productions); and (4) objective measurements, either of spontaneous activities (physical activity) or of reactions within a standardized situation (objective psychometric tests). This chapter necessarily is limited to an overview of self-rating and observer rating scales constructed to measure manic, depressive, mixed, and cyclothymic states. Measurement issues specific to particular topics are covered in the relevant chapters of this volume. For example, diagnostic evaluation is covered in Chapter 3, assessment of course and outcome in Chapter 4, assessment of neuropsychological functioning in Chapter 9, and measures of personality in Chapter 10. This chapter includes those generic rating scales that have been used or replicated most widely, as well as several instruments with potential utility for specific goals, such as screening for bipolar disorder.

We begin by describing conceptual and methodological issues involved in the assessment of manic and depressive states. We then review in turn instruments used for assessment of the two states, and analyze and compare the scales used for both purposes. The following sections describe instruments used for combined assessment of manic and depressive states, assessment of bipolar risk and screening for bipolar disorder, charting of the course of bipolar disorder, assessment of psychosocial adjustment, and assessment of bipolar symptoms in children and adolescents.

CONCEPTUAL AND METHODOLOGICAL ISSUES

Conceptual Challenges

There are a number of difficulties associated with the measurement of manic and depressive conditions. Moods may be highly unstable, fluctuating rapidly over days or even hours. Bipolar conditions by definition include patterns over time, requiring longitudinal data gathering, which is fraught with its own pitfalls. Moods may be mixed, including both manic and depressive elements, and may include or reflect other emotional states and comorbid conditions, such as anxiety, substance abuse, and Axis II disorders (see Chapters 7 and 10). Bipolar conditions themselves are highly heterogeneous, including a wide range of syndromal and subsyndromal states, which vary in course and episode features. Continuing changes and refinements in diagnostic criteria and elucidation of potential subtypes suggest that no "gold standard" criteria currently exist against which to validate new instruments. Generally, there is reliance on convergent validation—agreement between the results of two instruments or of newer and older instruments. Additionally, most measures attempt to include a multitude of clinical symptoms of the syndromes of mania or depression. However, refinements of models of etiology and targeted treatment-related functional outcomes will likely require greater attention to specific clusters of symptoms—such as anhedonia, excessive activity, or distractibility—that are poorly conceptualized and lack adequate measures. Most of the instruments described in this chapter are used largely for clinical assessment and may not be sufficient for other research purposes. Finally, a further challenge, even for well-established measures, is the need for empirically derived endpoints that would be widely accepted and consistently employed as markers of meaningful clinical change in treatment outcome studies (Baldessarini, 2003).

Methodological Issues

Added to these conceptually challenging issues are numerous psychometric hurdles that must be overcome by any good measure, including establishment of various forms of reliability and validity. As discussed later, clinical activity and research in the field of bipolar disorder have brought to light a number of gaps in existing tools for measuring manic and depressive states, indicating that much progress has yet to be made.

One methodological challenge is clarification of the goals of assessment. What do we mean, for example, by the measurement of "depression," a term that variously denotes a mood state, a constellation of symptoms, and a diagnostic entity? Instruments designed to assess a constellation of symptoms of depression, such as the Beck Depression Inventory (BDI), are sometimes used erroneously as diagnostic tools, identifying "depression" if respondents score beyond a certain cutoff point. Yet a diagnostic instrument, such as the Structured Clinical Interview for DSM (SCID), used to identify major depressive episodes, may do a limited job of measuring the mood state "depression." Numerous instruments, as we shall see, purport to assess syndromic features of depression or mania. Nonetheless, they may differ considerably in their item content, with varying emphases on cognitive, behavioral, mood, and somatic features (e.g., Snaith, 1993). The goals and limitations of each instrument must be clearly conceptualized so its uses will be appropriate to the purposes at hand, and conclusions based on a particular assessment strategy must be specific to that instrument.

Selection of appropriate instruments for specific purposes also requires determination of the validity of an assessment approach for a particular goal. Instruments appropriate for selecting patients for a treatment study or investigating an etiological mechanism may not be valid for measuring changes in mood state or evaluating outcomes over time. Thus different assessment procedures may be required to diagnose, measure severity, observe course features, and assess elements of a particular symptom.

In addition to such issues regarding the goals and meaning of various instruments, methodological challenges are inherent in the very assessment of manic and depressive mood states. Mood states color subjective reports of experiences and behavior, as well as memory of the past and expectations of the future; when depressed, for example, an individual may report having "always" been depressed and may exaggerate symptoms of past depressive episodes. Transient mood states may not only vary with clinical conditions, but also be affected by seasonal, diurnal, menstrual, and other cyclic variations. As noted, moreover, mixed states are more common than previously believed, and they confound the utility of bipolar scales—those constructed on the assumption that mania and depression are, in all respects, opposite states. Mood states also are often highly nonspecific across diverse clinical populations. It has been demonstrated that depressed patients, although distinguishable from normal populations on most scales, may not be readily distinguished by mood symptoms from other clinical populations, such as general medical patients, schizophrenic patients, or other psychiatric patients (Mendels et al., 1972; Murphy et al., 1982). Similarly, certain manic symptoms, such as impulsivity, irritability, and distractibility, may occur in various diagnostic groups.

In the discussion that follows, these and related methodological problems are examined in greater detail. As a first step, we outline the advantages and disadvantages of the two major methods for measuring manic and depressive states: self-rating and observer rating.

Self-Rating of Affective States

There are obvious advantages to using self-ratings by affectively ill patients. Foremost, as Murphy and colleagues (1982) pointed out, patients are in a unique position to provide information about their feelings and moods—key symptoms in any assessment of mood disorders. The value of self-ratings was confirmed by Raskin and colleagues (1970), who found that a mood scale completed by patients was one of the best measures of significant treatment effects. The patient is also, for the most part, free of the theoretical biases that affect the development and use of observer ratings, and "has access to the totality of his experience, rather than only a subset of behavior that the observer views" (Murphy et al., 1982). For example, in an early study, Zealley and Aitken (1969) analyzed independent mood recordings made by patients and nursing staff; an example of the results of their analysis is shown in Figure 11–1, which illustrates the lag between a patient's self-ratings and a nurse's ratings of the patient. The results of this study indicate that patients' mood symptoms changed from depressed to normal to hypomanic more rapidly than the staff detected, and suggest that the staff may have been unaware of patients' mood states day to day. In addition to improved accuracy, there are several practical advantages to using patient self-report measures: they require relatively little professional time and expense, can be completed rapidly, and can be used for repeated measurement (Hamilton, 1976; Murphy et al., 1982).

Self-ratings have obvious disadvantages, however. Patients must be literate, cooperative, not too depressed or too manic, and able to concentrate (Hamilton, 1976; Snaith, 1981; Murphy et al., 1982). Other difficulties derive from patients' idiosyncratic interpretations of the language of rating scales, their highly variable degrees of insight, and the scales' inability to differentiate clearly between symptoms (e.g., mood and energy changes) when they occur simultaneously (Pinard and Tetreault, 1974; Snaith, 1981). Finally, there is some evidence that severely depressed patients tend to underestimate the severity of their psychopathology (see, e.g., Paykel et al., 1973). For instance, Prusoff and colleagues (1972b) assessed 200 depressed patients using semistructured clinical interviews and self-reports. They found that self-report ratings, although useful in measuring the presence or

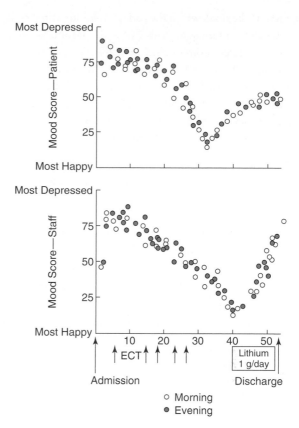

Figure 11–1. Visual analogue scale scores obtained from nursing staff and from a patient with manic-depressive illness. ECT = electroconvulsive therapy; open circles = morning observations; filled circles = evening observations. (*Source*: Adapted from Zealley and Aitken, 1969.)

absence of symptoms, were not a reliable index of symptom severity. Self-reports and clinically obtained measures were far more highly correlated at follow-up than during an acute episode. In a related study, Prusoff and colleagues (1972a) examined the nature of the discrepancy in scores derived from self- and clinician ratings. They found that patients whose ratings of symptoms were higher than those of clinicians tended to be younger, less severely depressed, and more histrionic. Conversely, those who minimized their symptoms tended to be older, more severely depressed, and obsessive. These results may reflect in part variations among patients with differing clinical and demographic characteristics, ranging from acute emotional turmoil with exaggerated subjective suffering to withdrawn, perhaps passive detachment and more physical manifestations.

Observer Rating of Affective States

In summarizing the advantages of observer ratings, Hamilton (1976, p. 158) cited the observer's ability to:

evaluate the intensity of any one symptom by comparing it against the background of experience which he has . . .

penetrate the mask which the patient holds up, whether deliberately or unintentionally . . . [and] rate and assess certain manifestations of illness which the patient would find impossible or extremely difficult to do. [These include] loss of insight . . . mild retardation . . . [and] hypochondriasis and delusions. An observer can rate all grades of severity of an illness . . . whereas a patient can be too ill to complete a questionnaire.

At the same time, however, observer ratings have significant potential drawbacks, as discussed at length by both Lorr (1974) and Bech (1981). Lorr noted that variability in the degree of the patient's disturbance from one interview to another affects both self- and observer ratings. Furthermore, observers may differ in efficiency and their manner in relating to the patient, and rating scales may be worded ambiguously or require too much inference. Bech (1981) stressed sources of variance in observer ratings, including differences that occur because information is not gathered from the same sources, differences in multiple observers' perceptions of the same phenomena, and variations in the terminology used to report results of observations of the same phenomena. Variations in the mood of the observer also affect ratings for some items (Bunney and Hamburg, 1963); this is the case especially for anger and anxiety ratings, which may be distorted if the observer confuses his own feelings with those of the patient.

ASSESSMENT OF MANIC STATES

Self-Rating Scales

Self-rating scales have rarely been used to measure manic states. Poor judgment, uncooperativeness, cognitive impairment, distractibility, and denial combine to make meaningful measurement problematic. Platman and colleagues (1969), for instance, found a very low correlation (0.35) between self-ratings of patients during manic episodes and ratings by staff. After recovery, however, the patients' recall of mania was highly correlated (0.95) with staff perceptions. An early instrument designed to assess the less severe, hypomanic range of symptoms was the M-D Scale, developed by Plutchik and colleagues (1970). It had 16 items scored in a yes/no format (e.g., "Lately I feel like breaking things"; "I've been telephoning a lot of friends recently"). This instrument demonstrated discrimination of hypomania from normality, but little reliability or validity information is available.

Recently, renewed attempts have been made to develop and employ self-rating scales for mania because of their obvious advantages. Shugar and colleagues (1992; see also Braunig et al., 1996) reported on the development and

initial validation of a Self-Report Mania Inventory (SRMI). This instrument currently consists of 47 items rated true or false. Its developers based the scale on behavioral items indicative of severity and DSM-III-R criteria, on the assumption that these would be reported more accurately than would inferences about symptoms. Examples include the following: "I started things I didn't finish"; "I partied more"; "I was getting into arguments"; and "I thought I could change the world."

Braunig and colleagues (1996) found that manic patients were able to report reliably on such behaviors over various intervals on the SRMI. Self-report scores correlated highly with results of the Young Mania Rating Scale (YMRS) assessed by observers, and also reflected clinical improvement in hospitalized manic patients. In one study of 20 rapid-cycling bipolar patients, the SRMI results correlated with YMRS ratings, but the SRMI was found to be more sensitive than the latter scale to milder mood fluctuations in the euthymia to hypomania range (Cooke et al., 1996). A study of manic inpatients by Altman and colleagues (2001) found that the SRMI showed good sensitivity in detecting severe cases (86 percent) and was also sensitive to post-test treatment effects; however, its results did not correlate significantly with interviewer-based ratings at initial evaluation. The authors suggested as one possible explanation for this discrepancy that at least eight of the items on the SRMI refer to behaviors that would be prohibited in an inpatient setting (e.g., drinking alcoholic beverages), and thus the instrument might underestimate the severity of manic symptoms in such settings.

Altman and colleagues (1997) reported on the development and preliminary psychometric characteristics of the Altman Self-Rating Mania Scale (ASRM). Five content items based on DSM-IV criteria (cheerful, self-confident, sleep less, talk more, and activity) remained after specificity analyses, and each is presented with five response options. In a later study, Altman and colleagues (2001) compared the ASRM with the SRMI and a visual analogue scale (VAS) (the Internal State Scale [ISS], discussed later, used to record patients' subjective impressions of their mood states) in a sample of manic patients. The ASRM was found to have the highest sensitivity (93 percent) for detecting acute manic symptoms, showed good agreement with an interviewer-rated severity scale, and was also sensitive to treatment-related changes. The authors noted that further studies of patients with mixed states are needed.

Visual analogue scales are discussed later in the section on combined assessment of depression and mania. We note here, however, an application of the VAS methodology to self-reported manic symptoms in a French study using the Ahearn and Carroll (1996) Multiple Visual Analog

Scales of Bipolarity (MVAS-BP) (Akiskal et al., 2001). This instrument, based on a model of mania proposed by Carroll and Klein (Carroll, 1991), comprises 26 VAS items on global mood state; anger; and subscales of "consummatory reward," "incentive reward," "psychomotor pressure," and "central pain." A study of 104 hospitalized manic patients found that patient self-reports were especially likely to correlate with clinician reports on emotional factors of depression and elation. In a related analysis of the same sample, Hantouche and colleagues (2001) found that the MVAS-BP was particularly useful in detecting dysphoric mania, with such patients scoring significantly lower than euphoric manic patients on the psychometrically derived subtypes of symptoms.

The examples cited here provide evidence of the utility of self-reported manic symptoms. Further work is needed, however, to develop the psychometric features of the scales, as well as to identify their limitations.

Observer Rating Scales

Considerably more effort in assessment of manic states has focused on observer ratings, including methods based on patient interviews and behavioral observations. The following sections describe several of the more commonly used instruments and their historical predecessors. Readers are referred to a review by Livianos-Aldana and Rojo-Moreno (2001) for psychometric details and reproduction of various instruments. We begin by discussing observation-based scales (typically used by medical and nursing staff in inpatient settings) and then turn to clinician-administered interview-based scales (which may also include observations of the individual during the interview).

Early Efforts to Develop Rating Scales for Observations of Mania

One of the first systematic observer rating scales for the measurement of mania—the Manic State Rating Scale (MSRS)—was developed at the National Institute of Mental Health (NIMH) (Beigel et al., 1971; Murphy et al., 1974). The scale is made up of 26 items, rated from 0 to 5 on both frequency and intensity dimensions. It was designed to be used by trained research nursing staff in inpatient settings (Table 11–1). The nine superscripted items in Table 11–1 were found to be core features of mania—elements present in all patients and most characteristic of manic severity. The reliability and validity of the MSRS are generally good (Livianos-Aldana and Rojo-Moreno, 2001), and the evidence suggests that the scale can easily be taught to new nursing staff. On the other hand, the MSRS has been criticized as being too extensive to be practical. It is also thought to contain inadequately defined items and scale steps; to require too much time to complete; and to exclude certain

core features of mania, such as sleep changes (Petterson et al., 1973; Tyrer and Shopsin, 1982).

The Modified Manic Rating Scale (MMRS) (Blackburn et al., 1977; Loudon et al., 1977) was based largely on the MSRS. It comprises 28 items and uses a six-point rating scale for information derived from interviews and from nursing staff and case notes. The authors found good validity when using a global rating scale as an independent measure, and the scale was highly reliable when employed in a structured interview by several independent raters.

Attempting to develop a shorter but still reliable observation-based rating scale for mania, Petterson and colleagues (1973) devised a seven-item scale that uses a five-point severity system. The behaviors assessed are motor activity, pressured speech, flight of ideas, noisiness, aggressiveness, orientation, and elevated mood. As with the other scales that measure only mania, the Petterson Scale is flawed both theoretically and empirically in not assessing mixed (simultaneous manic and depressed) states. Although the scale rates fewer symptoms of mania than does the MSRS, its measures of severity are far more precisely defined, and because of its relative brevity, it can be readministered easily to obtain serial ratings. Interrater reliability is good, and validity measures generally indicate good correspondence with other measures of mania and treatment outcome. However, several salient aspects of mania, such as sleep and work disturbances, are not assessed.

Young Mania Rating Scale

Presently, the YMRS is the most commonly used interviewer-based measure of severity of manic symptoms. Young and colleagues (1978) sought to develop a mania rating scale broader than the Petterson Scale but shorter and with more explicit ratings of severity than the MSRS. To this end, they devised an 11-item checklist, modeled on the Hamilton Rating Scale for Depression (HAM-D) (discussed later in the section on observer rating scales for depressive symptoms). They based their choice of items on published descriptions of the core symptoms of mania—those cutting across the entire spectrum of illness severity, although dysphoria is not included. Items assessed during the 15- to 30-minute interview are elevated mood, increased motor activity (energy), sexual interest, sleep changes, irritability, speech (rate and amount), language–thought disorder, language content, disruptive–aggressive behavior, appearance, and insight. Ratings are based on subjective reports by patients and on behavioral observations made by the clinician during the interview. Seven of the items are rated on an explicitly defined severity scale of 0 to 4. Four items (irritability, speech rate and amount, language content, and disruptive–aggressive behavior) are scored on a broader scale of 0 to 8. The authors reported that, based on their published results for relatively

TABLE 11–1. **Manic State Rating Scale**

Part A—Frequency (How much of time?)	The Patient	Part B—Intensity (How intense is it?)
0 to 5		0 to 5
—	1. Looks depressed	—
—	2. Is talking[a]	—
—	3. Moves from one place to another[a]	—
—	4. Makes threats	—
—	5. Has poor judgment[a]	—
—	6. Dresses inappropriately	—
—	7. Looks happy and cheerful	—
—	8. Seeks out others	—
—	9. Is distractible[a]	—
—	10. Has grandiose ideas	—
—	11. Is irritable[a]	—
—	12. Is combative or destructive	—
—	13. Is delusional	—
—	14. Verbalizes depressive feelings	—
—	15. Is active[a]	—
—	16. Is argumentative	—
—	17. Talks about sex	—
—	18. Is angry[a]	—
—	19. Is careless about dress and grooming	—
—	20. Has diminished impulse control[a]	—
—	21. Verbalizes feelings of well-being	—
—	22. Is suspicious	—
—	23. Makes unrealistic plans	—
—	24. Demands contact with others[a]	—
—	25. Is sexually preoccupied	—
—	26. Jumps from one subject to another	—

[a]Core feature of mania.
Source: Adapted from Beigel et al., 1971. Reprinted with permission from the *American Journal of Psychiatry.* Copyright 1971, American Psychiatric Association.

small samples, the scale is a reliable, valid, and sensitive measure of mania. More recent data showed that interrater reliability averaged .68 across items (Altman et al., 1994). The YMRS is increasingly being employed in bipolar clinical trials and treatment outcome studies because of its ease of use (e.g., Tohen et al., 2000; Leverich et al., 2001). The following is a sample from the YMRS developed to assess elevated mood:

Elevated Mood

0 = absent

1 = mildly or possibly increased on questioning

2 = definite subjective elevation; optimistic, self confident; cheerful; appropriate to content

3 = elevated, inappropriate to content; humorous

4 = euphoric; inappropriate laughter; singing

Bech-Rafaelsen Mania Scale

The main purpose of the Bech-Rafaelsen Mania Scale (MAS) (Bech et al., 1979; Bech, 2002) is to assess the severity of current manic symptoms. There are 11 items rated on a five-point scale, with highly specific ratings of severity; for example, a score of 1 on the sleep item represents a reduction of sleep by 25 percent, and a score of 2 represents a reduction by 50 percent. To control for diurnal variation in mood and behavior, the investigators specified that the 15- to 30-minute interview should always take place at a fixed hour. The scale items are motor activity, verbal activity, flight of thoughts, voice/noise level, hostility/destructiveness, mood (feelings of well-being), self-esteem, contact with others, sleep changes, sexual interest, and work activities. Data demonstrating the scale's adequate interrater reliability and a high degree of item homogeneity were presented in an article by Bech and colleagues (1986). An example of the motor activity item follows:

0: Normal motor activity, adequate facial expression.
1: Slightly increased motor activity, lively facial expression.
2: Somewhat excessive motor activity, lively gestures.
3: Outright excessive motor activity, on the move most of the time. Rises one or several times during interview.
4: Constantly active, restless, energetic. Even if urged, patient cannot sit still.

The MAS is commonly used in treatment outcome trials. For instance, it is being used in ongoing trials of adjunctive interpersonal and social rhythm therapy for bipolar patients (Frank et al., 1999). Results of recent research also indicate the scale's validity and internal consistency (e.g., as reviewed by Bech [2002]), as well as its sensitivity to changes in bipolar patients participating in a drug trial (e.g., Licht and Jensen, 1997). It might be noted that Bech (2002; see also Rossi et al., 2001) has recommended using the MAS in conjunction with the Bech-Rafaelsen Melancholia Rating Scale (reviewed later) to capture the frequent co-occurrence of depressive and manic symptoms.

Clinician-Administered Rating Scale for Mania

The Clinician-Administered Rating Scale for Mania (CARS-M) (Altman et al., 1994) was derived from the Schedule for Affective Disorders and Schizophrenia (SADS) and DSM-III-R to characterize the severity of manic symptoms. The 15 items are each rated on a six-point severity scale ("insight" is rated on a five-point scale). Preliminary validity data were based on comparisons with the YMRS; the correlation with the latter was .94. Test–retest and internal consistency reliabilities were found to be adequate. Factor analyses revealed two subscales, mania and psychoticism, which are scored separately.

Additional Interviewer-Based Scales for Mania

Several additional scales for rating mania have been developed, but appear to be used relatively infrequently and may be limited in their testing of psychometric properties. The Manic Diagnostic and Severity Scale (MADS) was developed by Secunda and colleagues (1985) as part of the NIMH Collaborative Program on the Psychobiology of Depression-Clinical Studies. The authors aggregated previously developed items from physician- and nurse-rated instruments to create the MADS. Two subscales taken from physician-rated scales—the Schedule for Affective Disorders and Schizophrenia–Change (SADS-C) Scale 17 and the Global Severity Scale (Katz and Itil, 1974)—correspond, respectively, to the elated–grandiose

and paranoid–destructive indices proposed by Beigel and Murphy (1971). Two factors derived from the nurse-rated Affective Disorder Rating Scale (ADRS) (Murphy et al., 1982) also address items designed to measure these two major subtypes of manic symptoms. The MADS subscales measure elevated mood, sleep and energy changes, grandiosity, guardedness, anger, disturbances in insight and judgment, negativism, restlessness, impulsivity, and distractibility. Detailed reliability and validity data have not yet been published (see Livianos-Aldana and Rojo-Moreno [2001] for further discussion).

Several general rating scales measure features of mania even though they were not developed specifically for that purpose. These scales include the Inpatient Multidimensional Psychiatric Scale, the Brief Psychiatric Rating Scale, and the Clinical Global Inventory. The Differential Diagnostic Scale, Bellevue Differential Inventory, and SADS, devised for differentiating mania from schizophrenia and not directly relevant to the measurement of mania per se, are not reviewed here.

ASSESSMENT OF DEPRESSIVE STATES

Self-Rating Scales for Depressive Symptoms

Several self-report instruments are available for assessment of depressive symptoms, syndromes, and mood states. A few of those most widely used in clinical and research applications are discussed here. Further information on these and numerous other measures was provided by Ronan and colleagues (2000). Many additional instruments have been developed for use with specific populations, such as children and adolescents and the elderly, and for assessment of specialized content areas related to depression, such as hopelessness, suicidality, and self-esteem. These instruments are beyond the scope of the current discussion.

Beck Depression Inventory

The Beck Depression Inventory (BDI) is the most widely used self-rating scale for depression for both research and clinical purposes. Developed by Beck and colleagues (1961) and revised as the BDI-II for consistency with DSM-IV (1996), the scale consists of 21 items, each containing four response options with content ranging in severity from not depressed to severely depressed. Individuals select the one response per item that best corresponds to their current clinical state "over the past 2 weeks," and the options are scored on a scale of 0 to 3, yielding a total across all items. For the BDI-II, a score below 13 suggests minimal depression, a score of 14 to 19 mild depression, and so on. Like all self-report scales in which a cutoff is used to indicate significant symptoms, the scale is not a diagnostic instrument, and scores may be elevated temporarily as a result of environmental, medical, or other difficulties. The items assessed include mood, guilt, irritability, social withdrawal, indecisiveness, fatigability, sleep and appetite changes, and loss of libido. The original BDI tended to emphasize the mood and cognitive features of depression, with less assessment of the more somatic symptoms, whereas the BDI-II includes modifications that permit individuals to indicate whether they have experienced an increase or decrease in sleep and appetite. The following sample item illustrates the range of severity assessed:

14. Worthlessness
    0 I do not feel that I am worthless.
    1 I don't consider myself as worthwhile and useful as I used to.
    2 I feel more worthless as compared to other people.
    3 I feel utterly worthless.

The original BDI had excellent psychometric properties, including internal consistency and test-retest reliability. It was shown to be a valid indicator of severity of depressed mood, having good correspondence with other measures and diagnostic criteria for depression (e.g., Beck et al., 1988). The BDI-II likewise has been well tested. It shows good correspondence with the HAM-D (Hamilton, 1960) and with other measures of depression-related constructs (Beck et al., 1996).

Zung Self-Rating Depression Scale

The Zung Self-Rating Depression Scale (Zung SDS), a 20-item scale with a four-point severity range, measures somatic, psychological, and mood aspects of depression. It is a modified version of the earlier Zung Depression Scale (Zung et al., 1965; Zung, 1974). For an item such as "I have trouble sleeping through the night," the patient is expected to indicate which of the following responses is most appropriate: "none or a little of the time," "some of the time," "good part of the time," or "most or all of the time." Note that the graded response to this question applies only to frequency, not to the extent of sleep loss. Further, the scale does not rate hypersomnia, a frequent symptom among patients with bipolar depression.

The Zung SDS does not show consistently high correlation with the HAM-D (Murphy et al., 1982). It has been criticized on the grounds that depressed patients have difficulty judging the degree and frequency of their symptoms, and endogenous symptoms are underrepresented (Rush et al., 1986). Hamilton (1988) also reported as a major shortcoming of the Zung SDS its relative insensitivity to clinical improvement after treatment (Rickels et al., 1968; Feighner et al., 1984). However, its brevity may enhance its value as a quick screen for severity of depressive symptoms.

Carroll Depression Rating Scale-Revised

The original Carroll Rating Scale was developed to parallel closely in item content the observer-scored HAM-D (Carroll et al., 1981; Feinberg et al., 1981; Smouse et al., 1981). The Carroll Depression Rating Scale-Revised (CDS-R) (Carroll, 1998) is a 61-item self-report questionnaire with items concerning 17 areas of depressive symptoms over the past few days, each rated yes or no. The revised version attempts to make the scale more compatible with DSM-IV. Examples include the following:

2. I have dropped many of my interests and activities.
7. I feel worthless and ashamed of myself.

Both the original and revised scales were based on Carroll's observation that neither existing self-report nor clinician-based scales were adequate for diagnosis of depressive symptoms (Carroll et al., 1981).

Most empirical evaluation of the Carroll scales has been based on the original version, but the author has indicated that the evaluation results are also applicable to the CDS-R. The scales appear to have excellent convergent validity with both self-report and clinician-based measures (e.g., correlation with the BDI, $r=.86$; correlation with the observer-rated HAM-D, $r=.71$ [Carroll, 1998]). Because it is similar in structure and content to the HAM-D and is less time-consuming and less expensive to administer, it may be a good alternative (see Smouse et al., 1981; Tandon et al., 1986). Correlations with other depression scales suggest that it is as sensitive to bipolar as to unipolar depression. Carroll and colleagues (1981) suggested that a cutoff of 10 can serve as a screen for the presence of significant depression.

Hamilton Depression Inventory

A different self-report instrument based on the observer-rated HAM-D was developed by Reynolds and Kobak (1995). The Hamilton Depression Inventory consists of 38 questions covering the original items of the HAM-D; there is also a melancholia subscale for evaluating the severity of DSM-IV melancholia symptoms. The instrument attempts to measure both the frequency and severity of symptomatology over the preceding 2 weeks. Its psychometric properties are promising, including a correlation of .94 with scores on the clinician-administered HAM-D in a sample of 403 adults (Reynolds and Kobak, 1995). It has not been extensively used in research or clinical settings, however, and its value therefore awaits confirmation.

A briefer version (19 items) of the same scale, the Reynolds Depression Screening Inventory (RDSI) (Reynolds and Kobak, 1998), is intended to take only 5 to 10 minutes to complete. Using a clinical cutoff score of 16, it has the potential to identify major depression among nonreferred community adults with a high degree of sensitivity and specificity. Therefore, it may serve as a useful screening instrument. Its research uses have been limited to date, however.

Inventory of Depressive Symptomatology

Another recent addition to self-report measures of depression is the self-report version of the Inventory of Depressive Symptomatology (IDS-SR), devised by Rush and colleagues (1986, 1996b). It was based on the authors' clinician-rated scale (IDS-C, discussed later), which was developed to improve on the HAM-D and was recently revised to include symptoms compatible with DSM-IV. The IDS-SR includes 30 items assessed over the preceding week, rated 0 to 3, measuring three factors: a cognitive/mood factor; an anxiety/arousal factor; and a sleep, appetite, and leaden paralysis factor (confirmed by Corruble et al., 1999). Both the self-report and clinician-administered versions take approximately 30 to 45 minutes to complete. Excellent psychometric properties have been reported, including good convergent validation with other measures of self- and clinician-reported symptoms (Rush et al., 1996b; see also Trivedi et al., 2004). Research has demonstrated that the measures are sensitive to treatment-related changes. Recently, Rush and colleagues (2003) developed a shortened form of the two versions of the IDS, called the Quick IDS (QIDS, with self-report and clinician versions), consisting of 16 items from the original 30-item scale—those needed to assess DSM-IV criteria for major depression. Trivedi and colleagues (2004) reported on the use of these shorter versions with a large sample of outpatients with major depression or bipolar disorder. They concluded that the brief instruments corresponded closely to the longer IDS measures, had solid psychometric properties, and were sensitive to treatment-related change.

Additional Self-Report Scales

Several additional self-report scales for depressive symptoms merit mention. The Center for Epidemiologic Studies-Depression (CES-D) scale (Radloff, 1977) is used extensively in community surveys and as a screening measure for depression. It was designed to be administered quickly and easily in research and epidemiologic settings, but has limited clinical utility. Normative information on its use in various samples was reported by Weissman and colleagues (1977). Furukawa and colleagues (1997) reviewed studies of the CES-D and the limitations of its psychometric properties, and presented data on potential cutoff scores to be used in various settings to predict the probability of depressive disorder given a specific individual score.

The Inventory to Diagnose Depression (Zimmerman et al., 1986) was developed to serve as a self-report diagnostic instrument for assessing the attainment of syndromic features of major depressive disorder based on DSM-III features; the authors presented initial evidence of its validity. Recently, noting changes in the DSM-IV criteria, Zimmerman and colleagues (2004a) developed a new 38-item self-report measure called the Diagnostic Inventory for Depression (DID), which includes symptoms, severity, duration, and impairment due to depressive symptoms. The authors reported on initial psychometric evaluation of the measure based on 626 psychiatric outpatients. The DID showed significant agreement with the SCID on diagnoses of depression, as well as convergent and discriminant validity. The instrument also showed sensitivity to change in symptom severity in follow-up assessments.

Bech and colleagues (2001) similarly developed a self-report scale for diagnosing major depressive episodes. A preliminary study based on 43 psychiatric patients and controls indicated a sensitivity of 1.0 and a specificity of .82 in comparison with DSM-IV/*International Classification of Diseases 10* (ICD-10) diagnoses. Further work is warranted to determine the validity of the procedure for screening and other clinical purposes.

Depressed Mood Self-Rating Scales

There are a number of scales for measuring depressed mood state, not including associated symptoms and syndromic features of depression. Such scales have been widely used in research on moods and emotions, may capture short-term changes in mood, and in some cases may be useful for limited clinical purposes.

- Visual analogue scales, mentioned earlier, are used to measure both manic and depressive states, and therefore are discussed in the section on combined measurement instruments (Hayes and Patterson, 1921; Zealley and Aitken, 1969).
- The Depression Adjective Check Lists (DACL) have both state and trait versions and have been studied extensively, including among clinical populations (Lubin, 1994).
- The Medical Care Outcomes Study (MOS) Screener (Burnam et al., 1988) was developed as an eight-item scale to screen for symptoms of depression in the MOS, in order to identify those with likely depressive disorders. It is not suitable as a measure of severity, and its use for diagnosis requires application of a complex formula for weighting items. Nevertheless, it appears to have acceptable validity and has been used extensively in epidemiologic and health policy research.

Observer Rating Scales for Depressive Symptoms

It is often argued that, while self-report instruments are uniquely suited to capturing the subjective experiences of depression, certain aspects of the depressive syndrome may be characterized more accurately by observers. As suggested earlier, self-reports may be biased not only by the cognitive capabilities or awareness, as well as mood-related perceptions, of depressed individuals, but also by their motives to present themselves in certain lights. Thus, for instance, evaluation of treatment outcomes may require objective ratings by trained clinicians. The drawback of such methods—and the reason for the relative paucity of such instruments compared with self-report questionnaires—is the requirement for training and the establishment of adequate expertise and reliability.

Hamilton Rating Scale for Depression

The HAM-D remains the most widely used observer-rated scale for depression. It was developed by Hamilton (1960) to measure severity and changes over time in the clinical state of depressed patients, and has been amended several times over the years. Although not developed as a diagnostic tool, it has been used with success in making retrospective diagnoses from chart reviews (Thase et al., 1983). It has been widely used as well to evaluate treatment response, correlate depression severity with biological parameters, and evaluate depression subtypes.

The HAM-D is focused much more on somatic and behavioral symptoms than on mood and cognitive symptoms. In its most commonly administered form, it consists of 17 items (9 on a five-point scale [0 to 4] and 8 on a three-point scale [0 to 2]) that measure mood, guilt, suicidal ideation, sleep disorders, changes in work and interests, psychomotor agitation and retardation, anxiety, somatic symptoms, hypochondriasis, loss of insight, and loss of weight. In later versions, additional items were added, so that it is essential to indicate which version is being reported. Note that, in contrast with most depression assessment instruments, the content includes several items pertaining to anxiety states. These features may be somewhat less relevant to bipolar than to unipolar depression.

Interobserver reliability is good, although various factor analyses have extracted inconsistent numbers and types of factors (see Hedlund and Vieweg, 1979). The HAM-D's high reliability, ease of administration (taking approximately 30 minutes), and emphasis on somatic symptoms have been cited as reasons for its enormous popularity (Murphy et al., 1982). On the other hand, critics believe that somatic symptoms are disproportionately represented in the HAM-D, that the differential weighting of symptoms is arbitrary, and that anchor points are ambiguous. Furthermore, certain symptoms, such as hypersomnia, increases in weight and appetite, and changes in quality of mood, are not assessed (Bech, 1981; Rush et al.,

1986). This last point may be an especially important limitation in the assessment of bipolar depression. As noted earlier, Rush and colleagues (1996a) developed a clinician-administered version of what they believe is an improved HAM-D addressing several of the shortcomings noted. The IDS-C is currently being used in the multisite NIMH–Stanley Foundation Bipolar Network study (Leverich et al., 2001), and its scores correlate highly with those on the HAM-D. A study of depressed inpatients reported by Corruble and colleagues (1999) confirmed the IDS-C's strong psychometric properties and suggested that it is more sensitive to treatment-related changes than the Montgomery-Asberg Depression Rating Scale (MADRS) (discussed later). The brief, 16-item clinician version of the QIDS was also found to have excellent psychometric properties in a large-scale study of unipolar depressed and bipolar outpatients (Trivedi et al., 2004). Finally, there is a Revised HAM-D (Warren, 1994). It remains to be seen whether alternatives to the HAM-D will flourish in clinical research over time.

Bech-Rafaelsen Melancholia Rating Scale

The Bech-Rafaelsen Melancholia Rating Scale, developed to combine the HAM-D and the Cronholm-Ottosson Depression Scale, comprises 11 items rated at five degrees of severity (Bech et al., 1979; Bech and Rafaelsen, 1980; Rafaelsen et al., 1980). Items are decreased motor activity, decreased verbal activity, intellectual and emotional retardation, psychic anxiety, suicidal impulses, lowered mood, self-depreciation, sleep disturbances, tiredness and pains, decreased motivation, and decreased productivity in work and interests. The interview is designed to be completed within 15 to 30 minutes, and to control for possible diurnal variation, is to be administered at approximately the same time of day each time. Guidelines for ratings are highly specific; for example, the guidelines for intellectual retardation are as follows:

0 Normal intellectual activity.
1 The patient has to make an effort to concentrate on his work.
2 Even with a major effort it is difficult for the patient to concentrate or make decisions. Less initiative than usual. The patient easily experiences "brain fatigue."
3 Marked difficulties with concentration, initiative and decision-making. For example, can hardly read a newspaper or watch television. Score 3 as long as the retardation has not clearly influenced the interview.
4 When the patient during the interview has shown marked difficulties in following normal conversation.

The interobserver reliability of the Bech-Rafaelsen Melancholia Rating Scale has been found to be as high as that of the HAM-D (Rafaelsen et al., 1980), and the item–total score correlations are adequate (Bech and Rafaelsen, 1980).

Montgomery-Asberg Depression Rating Scale

Yet another observer rating scale for depression is the MADRS of Montgomery and Asberg (1979), developed to measure changes in depression after antidepressant treatment. Easily administered by clinicians, the scale's 10 items measure the major components of clinical depression: apparent sadness, reported sadness, inner tension, reduced sleep, reduced appetite, concentration difficulties, lassitude, inability to feel, pessimistic thoughts, and suicidal thoughts. Items are rated on a seven-point scale (0 to 6), with illustrative anchor points given for ratings of 0, 2, 4, and 6. For example, ratings for the item measuring pessimistic thoughts are as follows:

> *Representing thoughts of guilt, inferiority, self-reproach, sinfulness, remorse and ruin*
>
> 0 No pessimistic thoughts.
>
> 1
>
> 2 Fluctuating ideas of a failure, self-reproach or self-depreciation.
>
> 3
>
> 4 Persistent self-accusations, or definite but still rational ideas of guilt or sin. Increasingly pessimistic about the future.
>
> 5
>
> 6 Delusions of ruin, remorse or unredeemable sin. Self-accusations which are absurd and unshakable.

The MADRS exhibits construct validity and concurrent validity relative to the HAM-D (Davidson et al., 1986; Khan et al., 2004). Further, it is easily and relatively quickly administered, has well-defined items, and provides for equal weighting of symptoms (Rush et al., 1986). The MADRS has been shown to demonstrate considerable clinical relevance as well (Williamson et al., 2006). On the other hand, its unidirectional rating of sleep change (i.e., decreased sleep) may be a disadvantage in rating bipolar patients. It may be noted that a self-report version of the MADRS (the MADRS-S) has been developed and shown to correlate highly with the BDI (Svanborg and Asberg, 2001).

Additional major observer rating scales for depression include the Cronholm-Ottosson Depression Scale (Cronholm and Ottosson, 1960); the Inpatient Multidimensional Psychiatric Scale (Lorr, 1974); the Physicians' Global Assessment Scale (GAS) (Carney et al., 1965; Endicott et al., 1976); and the Newcastle Rating Scales (Roth et al., 1983), which have been of special interest in biological studies because of their sensitivity to endogenous or melancholic items. As one might expect from the symptomatic differences

reviewed in Chapters 1 and 2, bipolar and unipolar depressed patients show different patterns of response to some of the same standard rating instruments (Paykel and Prusoff, 1973). In this light, it is unfortunate that there have been no systematic studies of the differential sensitivity of rating scales to bipolar depression. To our knowledge, the only scale designed specifically with bipolar patients in mind is the ADRS (Murphy et al., 1982), described later.

Instruments for assessment of depression are being refined and developed with increasing frequency and psychometric sophistication. The tension between having well-developed and empirically sound measures on the one hand and the capacity for widespread use and communicability on the other will doubtless grow. Most of today's instruments continue to be validated by comparison with older instruments (e.g., the HAM-D) without sufficient consideration of sources of invalidity of the latter. A further significant problem is the heterogeneity of the scales' contents, with some being far more focused on somatic or cognitive symptoms than others (see the later discussion). This variation leads to discrepancies in the results of treatment and clinical studies. Moreover, given the heterogeneity among clinical presentations of depressive syndromes, there have been calls for the development of more "narrowband" instruments that can be used to assess individual or clusters of symptoms, such as energy and fatigability, sleep difficulties, and hopelessness. Such more narrowly focused assessments could potentially facilitate advances in treatment or in understanding of depressive subtypes.

Perhaps the greatest limitation of most well-established self-report and observer rating scales for depression is their failure to capture potentially unique aspects of bipolar depression. This shortcoming, discussed at length in Chapter 2, is of obvious concern to most researchers in the field (see Berk et al., 2004, for a review of the subject). Further research on the clinical features of bipolar depression is needed to help identify factors that should be developed or refined in assessment instruments.

ANALYSIS AND COMPARISON OF SCALES FOR MANIA AND DEPRESSION

There are many ways of comparing rating scales; here we focus primarily on differences in item content. Content profiles of the items included in observer rating scales for mania and in self-report and observer rating scales for depression are presented in Figures 11–2 through 11–5. The classification of items is, of necessity, occasionally arbitrary. For example, symptoms of mood and cognition (hopelessness and pessimism) often overlap, as do symptoms of behavior and activity level. Working within these and

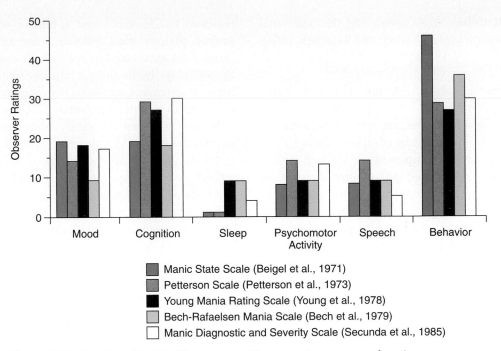

Figure 11–2. Relative weighting of item content: Observer rating measures of mania.

other constraints, it is possible to develop item-content profiles—that is, the items in each scale that are designed to assess a particular feature of mania or depression.

Content of Mania Scales

Figure 11–2 illustrates relative weightings for mood, cognition, sleep, psychomotor activity, speech, and behavior in observer rating scales for mania. The CARS-M (Altman et al., 1994) is not included; its 10 mania items are based on DSM-III-R and SADS criteria, with a separate psychoticism–insight subscale. Figure 11–3 portrays content profiles for more specific types of manic behavior—aggression and hostility, hypersexuality, impaired judgment, seeking out others, impulsivity, and appearance. Mood items represent approximately 15 percent of the total number of observer-rated mania items. The greatest emphasis is placed on euphoric and expansive mood, although all but two scales (the Petterson Scale and the Bech-Rafaelsen MAS) also include items measuring dysphoric, angry, irritable, or negativistic mood.

Despite the frequency of depression during mania (see Chapter 2), this mixed mood state is assessed in only one scale—the MSRS. The proportion of cognitive items is high on all scales, especially the MADS and the Petterson Scale. Sleep disorder symptoms, although integral to the diagnosis and pathophysiology of mania, are the least represented of all symptoms on the various scales; indeed, two scales do not inquire about sleep changes at all. Psychomotor activity and speech symptoms are measured by all of the mania scales. Behavior changes, like cognitive symptoms, are

widely represented, especially on the MSRS. The breakdown of behavior symptoms shown in Figure 11–3 reveals that the symptoms represented most widely and consistently are aggression and hostility, followed by hypersexuality and seeking out others. Impaired judgment, impulsivity, and appearance are assessed less consistently.

The decision to use a particular rating scale for mania is based not only on the item content, but also on the nature of the patient population and the training of the raters administering the scale. The YMRS and the MAS, for example, are more appropriate for less severely ill patients and require a less experienced rating staff, whereas the MSRS is more comprehensive, but also requires sophisticated nurse raters. If patients are only hypomanic rather than manic, additional useful subjective information may be obtained by using self-rating forms.

Content of Depression Scales

Relative weightings for item content in self-rating scales for depression are shown in Figure 11–4 and for item content in observer rating scales in Figure 11–5. Mood and cognitive symptoms are the best represented of symptom groups in both types of scales. The BDI is particularly weighted toward cognitive items, and the MADRS toward both mood and cognition. Somatic and sleep symptoms are represented most strongly on the HAM-D and on its self-rating parallel, the CDS-R. There are no other major differences in relative weightings of item content. Behavior items are not substantially represented on either self-rating

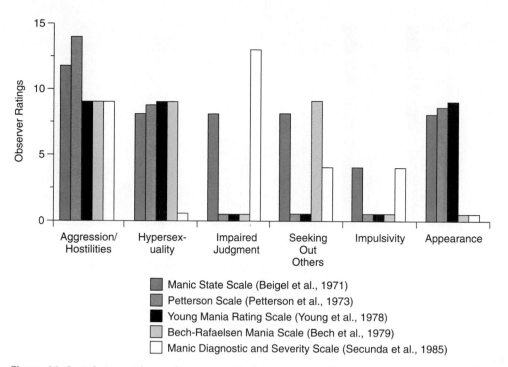

Figure 11–3. Relative weighting of item content for behavior items: Observer rating measures of mania.

Figure 11–4. Relative weighting of item content: Self-rating measures of depression.

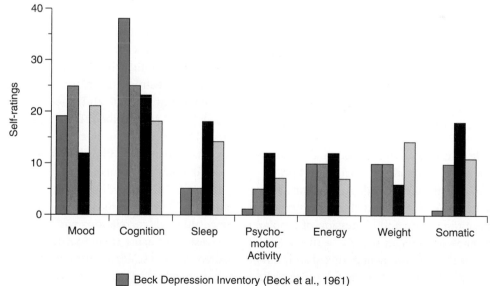

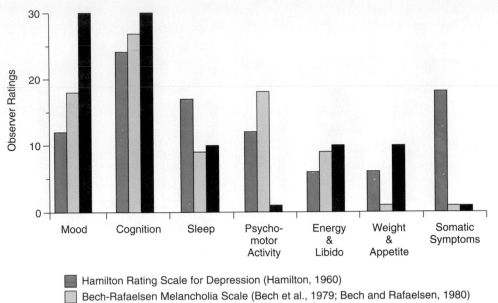

Figure 11–5. Relative weighting of item content: Observer-rating measures of depression.

or observer rating scales with the exception of work activities and interests, which together make up 7 percent of the total self-rating and 6 percent of the total observer rating items (all of the latter are on the HAM-D). As in the assessment of mania, the choice of instruments for assessment of depression depends on the patient population being evaluated, the level of interviewer training required, and the nature of the clinical or research issue being addressed. It is often useful to combine a self-rating with an observer rating measure.

COMBINED ASSESSMENT OF MANIC AND DEPRESSIVE STATES

A single rating scale that measures depression and mania along one continuum creates both theoretical and practical difficulties because it implies that depression and mania are opposite states—an assumption clearly contrary to what is known about the nature and expression of bipolar disorder (see Chapter 2). Monopolar scales (e.g., Bech, 1981) also generally preclude the measurement of mixed and transition states, rapid-cycling states, and diurnal or other cyclic variations in mood, behavior, and activity. A combination of individual measures of depression and mania or other combined measures, such as those discussed later, can be used to mitigate these problems.

Visual Analogue Scales

In their most commonly administered form, visual analogue scales (Hayes and Patterson, 1921; Zealley and

Aitken, 1969) are composed of a 100-mm line anchored at either end with opposite descriptors (e.g., "Worst I have ever felt" and "Best I have ever felt"). The patient is asked to place a mark or line across the point on the scale that best characterizes his or her mental state. Ratings are made frequently, typically once or twice a day, a characteristic that makes visual analogue scales especially appropriate for longitudinal studies of mood and treatment effects. Further advantages include the rapidity of assessment, economic feasibility, involvement of patients in their research and treatment protocols, a relative lack of cultural and educational bias, and good reliability and validity (Zealley and Aitken, 1969; Folstein and Luria, 1973; Luria, 1975). The simplicity of the test makes it ideal for depressed patients who are very ill or indecisive.

Moderately high correlations exist between visual analogue scales and the Zung SDS, the HAM-D, and global ratings by psychiatrists (Folstein and Luria, 1973; Luria, 1975), although correlations with clinical judgment tend to decrease after acute treatment (Zealley and Aitken, 1969). Moreover, such scales are not sensitive at lower levels of depression and other types of psychopathology. The most important limitation of the simple versions of these scales is that they are global measures not designed to assess specific psychopathological states or symptoms. As noted previously, however, Ahearn and Carroll's bipolar scales use the VAS format for self-report across a variety of symptoms (e.g., Akiskal et al., 2001).

A more recent application of the VAS format, involving development and rescaling of the Internal State Scale (ISS), was reported by Bauer and colleagues (2000). The 15-item self-report covers items from subscales called "activation," "well-being," a "depression index," and "perceived conflict," measuring patients' subjective impressions of mood states. In a Veterans Affairs medical center study of bipolar patients, scores on the subscales were able to identify and distinguish among groups that were euthymic, manic/hypomanic, mixed, and depressed. Glick and colleagues (2003) recently developed a Likert-based scoring system that they believe is easier to use than the VAS method and results in characteristics similar to those of the original ISS. With respect to its use for self-rating of mania, however, Altman and colleagues (2001) found that the ISS well-being scale was not sensitive to treatment effects in manic inpatients, although the activation scale did show significant changes from pre- to post-treatment. Most important, the ISS had relatively poor sensitivity, detecting only 45 percent of patients with moderate or severe symptomatology at baseline.

Affective Disorder Rating Scale

The ADRS (Murphy et al., 1982) comprises 34 specific items assessing mania and depression, using a 6-point scale for the frequency and intensity of the behavior and global ratings (on a 15-point scale) of mania, depression, psychosis, anxiety, and anger. For the global ratings, specific guidelines for assigning scores are provided. For example, in the mild range (within normal limits), scores of 2 or 3 on the mania scale reflect "especially talkative, active, enthusiastic, gregarious or boisterous behavior," while at the extreme end of the scale, scores of 13 to 15 reflect "nearly continuous manic activity and other symptoms, with uncontrolled, impulsive behavior requiring close supervision and often seclusion for the majority of the day." Although preliminary psychometric data suggest good convergent validation with other scales of depressive and manic symptoms, little information exists about the properties and use of this instrument.

Comprehensive Psychopathological Rating Scale

The Comprehensive Psychopathological Rating Scale (CPRS) was developed in 1971 by the Swedish Medical Research Council to measure treatment effects (Asberg et al., 1978). Four scale steps, each described in detail, are allocated for each item. The scale, designed for use by all trained mental health workers, can be used to assess both reported and observed behaviors. Items include elevated and sad mood states, indecision, lassitude, fatigability, concentration difficulties, reduced or increased sexual interest, ideas of grandeur, and ecstatic experiences. Reliability studies among depressed patients in the United Kingdom (Montgomery et al., 1978a) and among cross-cultural populations of Swedish and British depressed patients (Montgomery et al., 1978b) indicated that the CPRS is "highly reliable and highly sensitive [and] easily communicable" (Perris, 1979).

ASSESSMENT OF BIPOLAR RISK AND SCREENING INSTRUMENTS

Risk for Bipolar Disorder

There is considerable interest in detecting risk for bipolar disorder. The aim is to enable early intervention to alter the course of the illness and prevent the severe psychosocial consequences of the disruption of normal social development typically associated with the disorder. Several such instruments have been developed for use in research studies.

General Behavior Inventory

The General Behavior Inventory (GBI), a self-report inventory for nonpatients, was developed to identify individuals at high risk for developing bipolar disorder, particularly adolescents and young adults (Depue et al., 1981). Five dimensions of bipolarity are defined as characterizing the disorder: its core behaviors and symptoms; their intensity, frequency, and duration; and rapid shifts in mood and behavior. Sample questions (taken from a longitudinal mood-rating study), with their extreme polar descriptors, are presented in Table 11–2. Each item is rated on a four-point frequency scale.

The GBI, uniquely designed to measure subsyndromal variants of bipolar disorder (see Chapter 1), was validated in an initial series of studies through interview-derived diagnoses, interviews with college roommates, family histories of affective illness, clinical characteristics, and longitudinal mood-rating investigations (Depue et al., 1981). The GBI was originally viewed as a measure of subsyndromal cyclothymia or prodromal signs of bipolarity. Klein and colleagues (1986) predicted that it would identify youths at risk for bipolar disorder in a sample of offspring of bipolar-I parents; they found that half of the offspring had significant cyclothymic features identified by the GBI. The authors noted that offspring with cyclothymic features had significantly poorer social adjustment relative to noncyclothymic offspring and children of control parents. A follow-up study of 45 college students identified by the GBI as being at risk for bipolar disorder was conducted 19 months later (Klein and Depue, 1984); the investigators found that high scorers continued to exhibit significant impairment of functioning. Two patients had been hospitalized for major depressive episodes, and overall, the group reported higher suicidal ideation and treatment seeking.

Table 11–2. **Sample Items from the General Behavior Inventory**

Question Content	Extreme Polar Descriptions
Stimulus-seeking/excitement (receptivity toward and stimulation by the world)	• Passionately absorbed in the world's excitement; my sensations and feelings incredibly intensified; I seek out novel stimulations. • Life is too much trouble; sick of everything.
Flight of ideas/thought retardation (thought processes)	• Brilliant penetrating ideas emerging spontaneously and with great rapidity. • My mind is cold, dead; nothing moves.
Decisiveness/doubt	• Supremely confident in my judgment and strength of mind; I can instantly see problems which confuse others and solve them. • Utterly immobile, frozen by doubts; nothing is certain or solid for me.

Source: Depue et al., 1981. Reprinted with permission from the *American Journal of Psychiatry.* Copyright 1981, American Psychiatric Association.

Noting that the GBI appeared to identify those at risk for unipolar as well as bipolar depressive conditions, Depue and colleagues (1989) subsequently revised the GBI specifically to identify subgroups of unipolar (46 items) and bipolar (hypomanic/biphasic, 26 items) affective conditions. They reported that in a university sample, high scorers for the two conditions were identified and diagnosed by blind interviewers. The GBI's unipolar and bipolar scales showed adequate sensitivity (.78 and .76, respectively) and high specificity (.99 for both) for research use in nonclinical samples.

Hypomanic Personality Scale

Eckblad and Chapman (1986) developed the Hypomanic Personality Scale (HPS), a self-report scale for use in identifying those with gregarious and overactive behavior styles characteristic of episodes of hypomanic euphoria and hypothesized to indicate potential risk for developing bipolar disorder. The scale consists of 48 true–false items, such as "Sometimes ideas and insights come to me so fast that I cannot express them all" and "I would rather be an ordinary success in life than a spectacular failure" (scored in hypomania direction if false-rated). Internal consistency and test–retest reliabilities were shown to be high among a student population. The scale was validated among a university population against standardized diagnostic assessments; high scorers were significantly more likely to have experienced hypomanic episodes and depressive symptoms, drug and alcohol use, and psychotic-like symptoms. A longitudinal study of 36 high scorers on the HPS and 31 controls followed the groups for 13 years (Kwapil et al.,

2000). As predicted, significantly more high scorers than controls developed bipolar disorder (25 percent versus none) and experienced major depressive episodes (28 versus 19 percent); this was the case in particular for those who also scored high on the impulsive–nonconformity scale (Chapman et al., 1984). High scorers also had more severe psychotic-like symptoms, borderline personality disorder symptoms, and substance abuse disorders relative to the controls. A more recent study of 224 German university students found that the HPS was more effective in ascertaining individuals with a history of hypomanic or manic episodes than those with a history of depressive episodes (Meyer and Hautzinger, 2003).

An abbreviated version of the HPS was included in the Oregon Adolescent Depression Project (Klein et al., 1996), where it was found to be predictive of a wide range of psychosocial impairments; mood, disruptive, and substance abuse disorders; and suicide attempts. Among youths with a history of depressive disorders, the HPS appeared to predict for high scorers significantly more severe symptoms of depression and worse functional outcomes. Hofmann and Meyer (2006) studied three groups of young adults with high (n=17), medium (n=19), and low (n=18) scores on the Hypomanic Personality Scale. Those at elevated risk for bipolar disorder reported greater mood instability, as well as higher levels of both positive and negative affect. Although the sample has not yet been followed long enough to validate use of the HPS as a predictor of bipolar disorder, the scale appears to be valid for predicting mood and behavioral dysfunction that is potentially indicative of the disorder.

More recently, researchers have developed measures to assess bipolar spectrum disorder on the assumption that categorical measures are intrinsically limiting. These assessment systems—the Bipolar Affective Disorder Dimension Scale (Craddock et al., 2004) and the Bipolar Spectrum Diagnostic Scale (Ghaemi et al., 2005)—are promising but need further validation and replication. Also promising but preliminary are measures developed to assess dysfunctional beliefs that may predispose to bipolar disorder (Mansell and Jones, 2006) and positive self-dispositional appraisals linked to both hypomanic personality and bipolar disorder (Jones et al., 2006). Measures of temperament, beyond the scope of this chapter, have been studied by many groups[1] (see Chapter 10).

Screening for Bipolar Disorder

Noting that many cases of bipolar spectrum disorder may go undetected and undiagnosed, Hirschfeld and colleagues (2000, 2002) developed the Mood Disorder Questionnaire (MDQ), a brief self-report screening instrument for use in primary care, community agency, and psychiatric settings (Table 11–3). Based on DSM-IV criteria, it contains 13 yes–no items, as well as 2 additional questions designed to verify whether symptoms occurred during the same time period and caused significant problems. The questionnaire originated with a sample of 198 patients from five outpatient mood disorders clinics, who were then interviewed by telephone using the SCID for bipolar-I, bipolar-II, and bipolar–not otherwise specified (NOS) disorders. Using a threshold of seven or more yes responses, along with an indication that the symptoms occurred during the same time period and caused moderate or severe problems, the sensitivity was .73 and the specificity .90. This suggests a basis for the instrument's use in psychiatric settings, but how useful it will prove to be in general medical or community settings (where screening instruments should have the most utility) remains to be seen. When the same investigators conducted a population-based replication study, for example, the sensitivity of the MDQ (identification of true positive cases) was found to be .28, much lower than that found in the original study (Hirschfeld et al., 2003b). A recent study of 1,157 patients at a general medicine clinic found that although the specificity of the MDQ was lower than found in mood disorders clinics, the measure was helpful in identifying bipolar patients who would not otherwise have been recognized (Das et al., 2005). On the other hand, in a review of studies of screening instruments, Phelps and Ghaemi (2006) concluded that where there is likely to be a low prevalence of bipolar disorder, such as in community or primary care settings, screening measures such as the MDQ can rule out bipolarity but do not effectively rule it in.

As discussed, Hirschfeld's group reported on a population-based replication study in which the sensitivity of the MDQ was found to be much lower than that found in the original study (Hirschfeld et al., 2003b). Replication and further validation studies are well-warranted in view of the overlap of bipolar symptoms with those of other mood, substance, and behavioral disorders.

Despite ongoing concerns about its utility outside of mood disorders clinics, the MDQ has been widely disseminated, appearing in psychiatric publications and on Web sites, in the hope that it can facilitate the identification and treatment of bipolar disorder. It was tested in a French population of bipolar patients, with the investigators finding much greater sensitivity in bipolar-I than in bipolar-II patients (90 and 52 percent, respectively) (Rouget et al., 2005). It also served as the basis for an epidemiologic survey of bipolar spectrum disorder (see Chapter 5) (Hirschfeld et al., 2003a). But given the evidence to date that the MDQ appears to be insufficiently accurate to be used as a case-finding measure in community studies or as a screening scale in clinical practice, further research and refinement of the instrument are needed (Zimmerman et al., 2004b). Given that many bipolar patients lack insight into the hypomanic and manic phases of their illness, one helpful refinement might be a version of the instrument that could be filled out by family members. We recommend that the MDQ, while promising, be viewed with some skepticism until further validation and replication studies have been completed.

A somewhat similar scale, the Manic Depressiveness Scale, was documented by Thalbourne and colleagues (1994). The 19-item questionnaire, assessing manic and depressive experiences, was administered to normal college students and to a sample of bipolar patients. Despite significant mean differences between the groups and relatively good internal consistency and reliability, however, the scale showed overlapping distributions between the two populations, apparently precluding its use to identify bipolar disorder among nonpatient samples. A later revision (9 manic experience items and 9 depressive experience items) was found to correlate with severity of illness and number of hospitalizations for bipolar patients, but not for unipolar depressed patients (Thalbourne and Bassett, 1998).

Recently, Solomon and colleagues (2006) reported the development of a brief instrument to screen for bipolar disorder in patients acutely ill with major depression. The Screening Assessment of Depression-Polarity (SAD-P) consists of 3 items demonstrating the greatest disparity between bipolar-I and unipolar depression: presence of delusions during the current episode of major depression, number of prior episodes of major depression, and family

Table 11–3. **Sample Items from the Mood Disorder Questionnaire**

Question	Response	
1. Has there ever been a period of time when you were not your usual self and . . .		
• you felt so good or so hyper that other people thought you were not your normal self or you were so hyper that you got into trouble?	○ yes	O no
• you were so irritable that you shouted at people or started fights or arguments?	○ yes	○ no
• you felt much more self-confident than usual?	○ yes	○ no
• you got much less sleep than usual and found you didn't really miss it?	○ yes	○ no
• you were much more talkative or spoke much faster than usual?	○ yes	○ no
• thoughts raced through your mind or you couldn't slow your mind down?	○ yes	○ no
• you were so easily distracted by things around you that you had trouble concentrating or staying on track?	○ yes	○ no
• you had much more energy than usual?	○ yes	○ no
• you were much more active or did many more things than usual?	○ yes	○ no
• you were much more social or outgoing than usual; for example, you telephoned friends in the middle of the night?	○ yes	○ no
• you were much more interested in sex than usual?	○ yes	○ no
• you did things that were unusual for you or that other people might have thought were excessive, foolish, or risky?	○ yes	○ no
• spending money got you or your family into trouble?	○ yes	○ no
2. If you checked YES to more than one of the above, have several of these ever happened during the same period of time?	○ yes	○ no
3. How much of a problem did any of these cause you—like being unable to work; having family, money, or legal troubles; getting into arguments or fights?		
• No problem		
• Minor problem		
• Moderate problem		
• Serious problem		

Source: Adapted from Hirschfeld et al., 2000. Reprinted with permission from the *American Journal of Psychiatry*, Copyright 2005, American Psychiatric Association.

history of major depression or mania. The investigators found that the screening instrument was easy to use and, in a cross-validation sample, correctly identified a substantial proportion of subjects with bipolar or unipolar illness (bipolar major depression was identified in the bipolar-I index sample with a sensitivity of 0.82 and in the cross-validation sample with a sensitivity of 0.72).

Screening for Bipolar Spectrum Disorders in Youths

As noted previously, the GBI (Depue et al., 1981) was initially developed for use with college-age young adults. Recently, it has been used in younger samples. A study of clinically diagnosed children and adolescents, for instance, found that both youth- and parent-reported symptoms on the bipolar scale of the GBI were sensitive to the detection of actual bipolar disorder (Youngstrom et al., 2001; Findling et al., 2002). Results of various studies suggest that a cutoff score of 13 and higher for adults, and of 17 and higher for children and adolescents may be useful in screening for bipolar spectrum disorder or risk. Reichart and colleagues (2005) in the Netherlands used the GBI to assess psychopathology among 129 adolescent and young adult children of a bipolar parent over a 5-year follow-up period. They found that the depression scale of the GBI discriminated well between the development of new bipolar disorder and no disorder or unipolar disorder.

Also as noted previously, a version of the HPS (Eckblad and Chapman, 1986) was used in the Oregon Adolescent Depression Project (Klein et al., 1996), where it identified youths with clinical features and functional impairment who may have been in the bipolar spectrum. Further research is needed, however, to validate diagnostic status over time.

CHARTING THE COURSE OF BIPOLAR DISORDER

Because bipolar disorder is recurrent by definition, it is essential to have methods for capturing the phenomenology of the course of the illness to supplement methods used to characterize individual episodes. Indeed, Kraepelin (1921) used life charts with many of his patients and, from the study of these charts, made critical observations about the course of manic-depressive illness. Figure 11–6 is a case history used by Kraepelin to illustrate periodic mania with isolated episodes of depression. Such procedures yield charts of the past or recent history of changes in the illness, permitting examination of both clinical and research issues based on details of

those patterns. There are several methods for systematically assessing—either retrospectively or prospectively—the details of the topology and course of bipolar disorder.

Longitudinal Interval Follow-Up Evaluation

The contribution of the Longitudinal Interval Follow-up Evaluation (LIFE) to characterization of the course of bipolar disorder is noted only briefly here because this method is a procedure widely used for all DSM-related disorders. Developed by Keller and colleagues (1987), it is a semistructured interview procedure whose purpose is to provide a continual (e.g., weekly) charting of symptomatology, psychosocial functioning, and treatment based on regular follow-up evaluations. Severity of psychopathology is rated on a six-point Psychiatric Status Rating (PSR) scale tied to Research Diagnostic Criteria symptoms; several areas of psychosocial functioning (e.g., employment, relationships with family members) are also rated on five- or seven-point scales. The PSR scale and psychosocial ratings have been shown to have high interrater reliability (e.g., Keller et al., 1987). The LIFE charts provide an excellent basis for characterizing landmark clinical events, such as time to recovery or duration of episodes. The LIFE methods are widely used, especially in research on unipolar depression, as in the NIMH Collaborative Program on the Psychobiology of Depression-Clinical Studies (e.g., Judd et al., 2000; Solomon et al., 2000); they are also used to study anxiety disorders (e.g., Warshaw et al., 1994).

Life Chart Method

The Life Chart Method (LCM) was designed as a brief, easily administered, and flexible approach for mapping the course

Figure 11–6. Relapsing mania with isolated periods of depression. Light blue = depression; dark blue = manic excitement. (*Source*: Kraepelin, 1921, p. 143) Reprinted with permission.

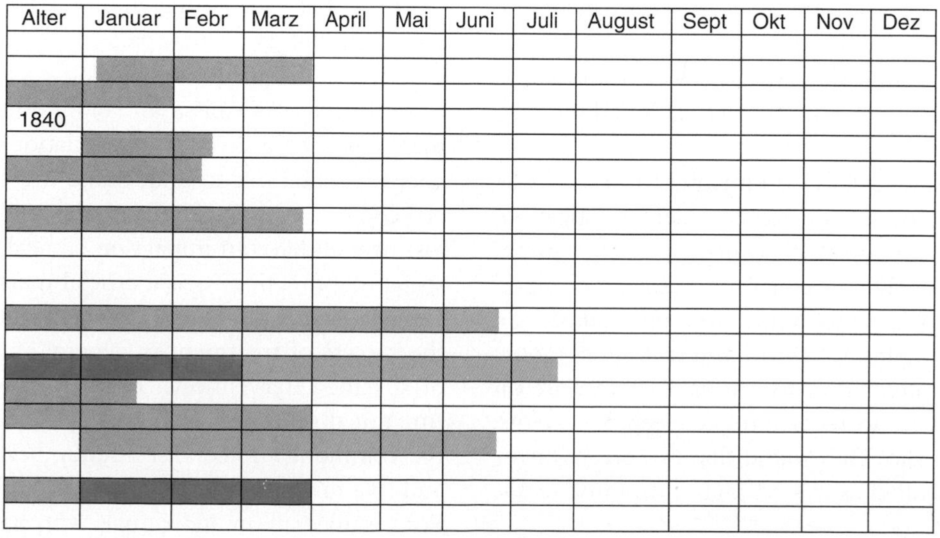

Alter	Januar	Febr	Marz	April	Mai	Juni	Juli	August	Sept	Okt	Nov	Dez
1840												

of bipolar disorder. In the original development of the approach, Post and colleagues (e.g., Squillace et al., 1984; Roy-Byrne et al., 1985) identified several goals for such a methodology: to systematize retrospective clinical history data; to capture meaningful episodes that might be missed because of incomplete memory; and, of course, to provide detailed phenomenological and descriptive information about the clinical course of mood disorders. The methodology bases the definition of an episode on functional impairment rather than symptomatic criteria, on the assumption that the former information is recalled more readily than whether a particular symptom occurred during a given time frame. Moreover, definitions based on functional impairment may capture a more detailed picture of variations in mood than can definitions based on strict adherence to DSM criteria. Accordingly, manic and depressive episodes are each measured on a three-point scale: mild, with only subjective distress and no or minimal functional impairment; moderate, with clear impairment in functioning in usual roles; and severe, involving incapacitation or resulting in hospitalization. Manic episodes are defined by any level of severity, and depressive episodes by moderate or severe ratings. The investigators noted that subjective reports were supplemented by the observations of others, especially for mild mania, a state often overlooked or denied by patients themselves.

The LCM has the advantage that it can be applied flexibly, so that different studies or contexts may involve different duration criteria (e.g., Kramlinger and Post, 1996; Denicoff et al., 1997), may be prospective or retrospective (or both), and may include staff ratings as well as patient reports. Denicoff and colleagues (1997) presented reliability and validity data on a prospective version of the LCM, developed during 2 years of a clinical trial on bipolar-I and -II outpatients. Daily ratings of mood severity based on functional impairment were provided by patients, supplemented by information from other sources (including spouses). Interrater reliabilities were very high. Validity was supported by significant associations with both self- and clinician-rated mood measures that included the BDI, YMRS, HAM-D, and GAS.

It may be noted that daily administration of the LCM using a palmtop handheld device is under investigation. Initial feasibility data indicate that this approach is useful and might greatly facilitate frequent monitoring of mood states and psychosocial functioning (Scharer et al., 2002). In a related development, Whybrow and colleagues (2003) devised the ChronoRecord, software patients can use on their home computers to record mood, sleep, life events, and medication intake. They found that 83 percent of the 96 patients they studied expressed high acceptance of the computer format.

Average Mood Symptom Score

The Average Mood Symptom Score (AMSS) is a somewhat similar method of prospective charting of mood patterns, adapted from the LCM (Gitlin et al., 1995). Hammen and colleagues (1989) first reported use of the procedure as a method for characterizing the timing and features of changes in symptoms of unipolar depression and bipolar disorder in relation to stressful life events. The goal is to systematize the severity and duration of mood states over time during ongoing follow-up. To this end, clinicians' chart notes of clinical status and dates of changes are translated into a time line, with dates on the horizontal axis and a vertical axis indicating nine levels of severity of mania or depression (where the zero midpoint is euthymia). Based on DSM criteria, manic states are rated as M1 (only one or two symptoms) through M4 (severe, hospitalized mania) above the zero point, or D1 (only one or two symptoms) through D4 (severe major depressive episode involving hospitalization or suicide attempt) below the zero point; mixed states can also be indicated. Figure 11–7 presents an example.

In addition to time lines that can be used to identify dates of onset or significant changes in severity or polarity of symptoms, the method yields a quantitative score of symptomatology per unit of time. A total mood score for a defined period may be calculated as level of symptoms multiplied by duration in days; the AMSS is the total mood score divided by days in the period of interest. A series of studies has employed such methods in samples of both unipolar and bipolar patients to characterize course of illness in relation to psychosocial factors, such as role functioning and episodic stressful life events (Ellicott et al., 1990; Hammen et al., 1992, 2000).

ASSESSMENT OF PSYCHOSOCIAL ADJUSTMENT

There has been increasing emphasis on the need for characterization of psychiatric patients' functional outcomes as a critical supplement to the relatively exclusive focus on clinical status. As Weissman (1997) noted, since the 1960s there has been a growing appreciation that for all disorders, it is necessary to understand individuals in their social contexts because family, social, and occupational adjustment all have an impact on clinical course. Moreover, social role functioning is a crucial marker by which individuals, their families, and the community at large judge the success of treatment in general and the effectiveness of specific interventions. Further impetus for studying functional outcomes in bipolar populations comes from the commonly noted discrepancy between clinical state and role functioning among people with mood disorders. For instance, many individuals who have recovered from

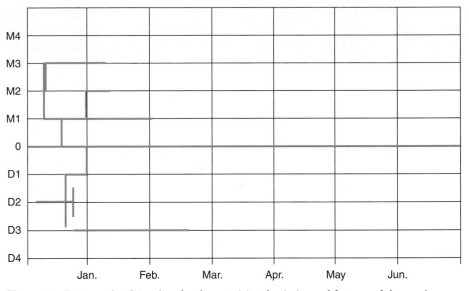

Figure 11–7. Example of time line for characterizing the timing and features of changes in symptoms of unipolar depression and bipolar disorder (see text for explanation).

episodes or have not experienced recurrences nonetheless display functional impairment,[2] especially in family and work adjustment. Maladjustment in important roles, moreover, may contribute—presumably as a stressor—to further clinical episodes and debility. Consequently, interest in the measurement of functioning in major roles and the use of such data to evaluate treatment outcomes has grown. In this section, we briefly review some of the methods used for these purposes and the resultant findings, noting that such issues are by no means specific to bipolar illness.

Unfortunately, actual progress in mapping social adjustment among those with mood disorders has been relatively limited, owing to the complexity of the constructs involved and the resulting problems in collecting reliable and valid information in relevant areas. The widely used GAS or its variant, the Global Assessment of Functioning (GAF) scale, employed as Axis V of DSM-IV, has been criticized for confounding clinical symptoms and psychosocial functioning (Williams, 2000). The single-item GAS and GAF scales provide no specificity in ratings for different areas of functioning. Similarly, the Clinical Global Impressions Scale for Bipolar Illness (CGI-BP) (Spearing et al., 1997), while providing clinician judgments specifically of illness severity and changes in mania, depression, and overall bipolar illness, does not yield information about functioning and changes in particular roles. Similar concerns may arise with regard to many "quality-of-life" scales, which provide general information about the adverse effects of clinical and medical states but less information about particular areas of discomfort (e.g., Vojta et al., 2001).

Weissman and colleagues (1981) reviewed a number of scales that specifically address social functioning and found their quality and utility to be relatively poor. Thus although many such scales exist, few have provided the utility and psychometric qualities necessary for their survival (see Williams, 2000).

Currently, three patient-report scales are used relatively widely in research on quality-of-life issues for those with mood disorders. The Social Adjustment Scale-Self Report (SAS-SR) (Weissman and Bothwell, 1976; Weissman et al., 1978) assesses instrumental and emotional role functioning in six areas: work, social and leisure, marital–sexual, relationships with extended family, parenting, and family unit. It includes a total of 54 items and yields both subscale and overall adjustment scores. An example is the following:

How have you been getting along with the children during the last 2 weeks?
1. I had no arguments and got along very well.
2. I usually got along well but had minor arguments.
3. I had more than one argument.
4. I had many arguments.
5. I was constantly in arguments.

The SAS-SR has been shown to have excellent reliability and validity (reviewed by Williams, 2000). The initially developed clinician-rated version of the SAS employs a semi-structured interview format and is especially suitable for use when there is concern that patients' mood status may distort their responses and perceptions.

The Social Adaptation Self-Evaluation Scale (SASS) (Bosc et al., 1997) was developed for use in clinical trials. It contains 21 self-report items covering current functioning in various psychosocial domains. As noted by Weissman (1997), its content emphasizes subjective aspects of functioning, including motivation and self-perception, drive, and mastery, but focuses less on role performance. Instrumental functioning, such as work behavior and family and parental role functioning, is not specifically included. However, to the extent that the scale taps interest and enjoyment in functional roles, it adds an important dimension beyond clinical status.

The Short-Form Health Survey (SF-36) (Ware and Sherbourne, 1992) of the MOS includes several items specific to role functioning, such as loss of work functioning due to medical or depressive conditions. Data from the MOS have provided an important comparison between people with depressive conditions and those experiencing a variety of major medical syndromes (e.g., Wells et al., 1989; Hays, 1995). However, what is measured is largely global functioning, and the self-report format makes it difficult to disentangle actual psychosocial behavior and adjustment from depressive mood state.

Clinician-rated social adjustment scales include the Weissman Social Adjustment Scale (the precursor to the SAS-SR) and the social functioning scales of the LIFE method discussed previously (e.g., Keller et al., 1987). Both scales have solid psychometric properties but generally lack sufficient behavioral detail to fully characterize functioning in specific domains, such as work, parenting, and marital life.

ASSESSMENT OF BIPOLAR SYMPTOMS IN CHILDREN AND ADOLESCENTS

Measurement of Mania

As noted in Chapter 6, there is considerable controversy regarding the diagnosis of mania and manic symptoms in children (see also Chapter 3). The NIMH Bipolar Child Roundtable (2001) recommended the use of well-established interview diagnostic procedures for this purpose. One such instrument is the Kiddie Schedule for Affective Disorders and Schizophrenia (KSADS), specifically the Washington University version (WASH-U-KSADS), which contains items developed to assess childhood mania and other syndromes, including onset and offset of individual items and syndromes for current and lifetime disorders. Geller and colleagues (2001) reported excellent interrater reliability, including high kappa values between expert observers and off-site blind evaluators on ratings of mania and rapid cycling. At this time, the majority of NIMH-funded studies of bipolar disorder in children use the WASH-U-KSADS sections on mania and rapid cycling.

There is obviously a long way to go in developing an array of measures of mania symptoms in children that will parallel those available for adults. Considerable work is still

needed to assess individual manic symptoms in children validly and reliably; to establish developmentally appropriate indicators; and to distinguish them from those of other disorders, such as attention-deficit hyperactivity disorder (ADHD). For instance, it is necessary to address symptoms that occur in bipolar children but not in those with ADHD, including hypersexuality and grandiosity, while also distinguishing overlapping symptoms, such as distractibility and hyperactivity. Parents of 268 subjects (93 with a prepubertal or early-adolescent form of bipolar disorder, 81 with ADHD, and 94 healthy controls) completed the 10-item Conners' Abbreviated Parent Questionnaire before the WASH-U-KSADS was administered (Tillman and Geller, 2005). The results are shown in Table 11–4. Items 7, 8, 9, and 10 significantly distinguished between those children and adolescents with bipolar illness and those with ADHD. The authors concluded that the Conners' Abbreviated Parent Questionnaire (sensitivity = 0.73, specificity = 0.86) is a promising tool as a screen for early- and adolescent-onset bipolar disorder. The NIMH Research Roundtable on Prepubertal Bipolar Disorder (2001) recommended that researchers develop operational criteria for frequency and severity of various behaviors and symptoms potentially relevant to juvenile mania and the co-occurring disruptive behavior disorders and impairing symptoms.

To date, little information exists on the use of adult rating scales for manic symptoms with children. Gracious and colleagues (2002) reported on a parent-completed version of the YMRS, noting that it discriminated well among diagnostic groups aged 5 to 17, including those with ADHD. They found good psychometric properties for an eight-item version (eliminating three items, such as sexual interest, that did not contribute to the total scores) (see also Youngstrom et al., 2002, 2003). The agreement between the reports of children and adolescents and those of parents is problematic, however. Children, for example, are more likely than parents to report racing thoughts and decreased need for sleep (Tillman et al., 2004), and adolescents with bipolar disorder tend to underreport manic symptoms (Youngstrom et al., 2004).

Measurement of Depression

The assessment of depressive symptoms and syndromes in children and adolescents has been well described elsewhere (e.g., Nezu et al., 2000). In general, self-report questionnaires about symptoms and diagnostic interviews can be administered reliably and yield valid conclusions about symptom severity and the presence of depressive disorders. For example, a Children's Depression Inventory (CDI) was developed by Kovacs (1981); it has a three-response options format with content appropriate for those aged 7 to 17. The BDI, discussed earlier, is suitable for most patients aged 13 and older.

TABLE 11–4. Scores on Items of the Conners' Abbreviated Parent Questionnaire for Subjects with a Prepubertal and Early Adolescent Bipolar Disorder (BP) Phenotype, Subjects with Attention-Deficit Hyperactivity Disorder (ADHD), and Healthy Comparison Subjects

Questionnaire Item	SUBJECTS WITH A BP PHENOTYPE ($n=92$)		SUBJECTS WITH ADHD ($n=80$)		HEALTHY COMPARISON SUBJECTS ($n=92$)	
	Mean	Std. Dev.	Mean	Std. Dev.	Mean	Std. Dev.
1. Restless or overactive	2.9[a]	0.9	3.0[a]	0.8	1.2	0.5
2. Excitable, impulsive	3.2[a]	0.8	3.1[a]	0.8	1.3	0.5
3. Disturbs other children	2.7[a]	1.0	2.5[a]	0.8	1.1	0.3
4. Fails to finish things he or she starts—short attention span	2.9[a]	1.0	2.9[a]	0.9	1.2	0.4
5. Constantly fidgeting	2.7[a]	1.0	3.1[a]	0.8	1.2	0.4
6. Inattentive, easily distracted	3.2[a]	0.9	3.3[a]	0.7	1.2	0.4
7. Demands must be met immediately—easily frustrated	3.3[a,b]	0.9	2.9[a]	1.0	1.2	0.4
8. Cries often and easily	2.5[a,c]	1.0	1.9[a]	0.9	1.2	0.5
9. Mood changes quickly and drastically	3.2[a,c]	0.9	2.3[a]	1.0	1.2	0.4
10. Temper outbursts, explosive and unpredictable behavior	3.1[a,c]	1.0	2.3[a]	1.0	1.2	0.4

Note: See Tillman and Geller (2005) for a scoring algorithm and age-specific cutoffs for use of the Conners' Abbreviated Parent Questionnaire as a screening tool. Std. Dev. = standard deviation.

[a]Significant difference compared with the healthy comparison group ($p<.0001$).
[b]Significant difference compared with the ADHD group ($p<.003$).
[c]Significant difference compared with the ADHD group ($p<.0001$).

Source: Tillman and Geller, 2005. Reprinted with permission from the *American Journal of Psychiatry*, Copyright 2005, American Psychiatric Association.

Two major issues are associated with assessment of depression in children. First, most diagnostic interview procedures assume that children's reports of their symptoms should be supplemented by information collected from caretakers. Most diagnostic methods for assessing depression, such as the clinician-administered KSADS (Ambrosini, 2000) or the Diagnostic Interview Schedule for Children (DISC), which is administered by trained laypersons (Shaffer et al., 2000), prescribe separate interviews for children and parents. KSADS commonly uses a "best clinical estimate" method, combining information from the child and the parent weighted by the type of information given, according to the clinician's judgment. For example, internal symptoms, such as depressed feelings and negative thoughts, cannot readily be detected by parents, and there-

fore the child's report on these symptoms might be given greater weight in a diagnosis of depression. The DISC is a highly structured interview, with a computer-based scoring algorithm often being used to combine information about diagnostic criteria.

A second, related issue concerns the relatively low agreement among informants (the child or adolescent, parents, and teachers). This problem occurs for all childhood disorders, not just depressive illnesses. It has been speculated, however, that reports of depression may be associated with systematic biases in the reports of certain informants. Specifically, some research has indicated that relatively depressed women may distort or exaggerate their children's behavior as more negative than it actually is. However, a review of 22 studies by Richters (1992) revealed that such claims were based largely on inadequate designs, including simple associations between mothers' and children's symptoms that could be accurate given the common finding of disorders in offspring of depressed women. Subsequent studies using sophisticated methods, such as covariance structure analysis with latent variables formed from different informants, have supported the hypothesis that depressed mothers may report more negative behaviors. As these studies have shown, the fact that maternal depression truly is associated with more child disorder makes the conclusion of "bias" unclear (Fergusson et al., 1993; Boyle and Pickles, 1997). Other researchers who have evaluated parent–child concordance over time (Renouf and Kovacs, 1994; Boyle and Pickles, 1997) have suggested that maternal bias, if any, may be more pronounced for younger than for older children.

CONCLUSIONS

The status of assessment methods in bipolar disorder varies by topic:

- Diagnostic procedures, not specifically discussed in this chapter, are administered relatively reliably but are only as valid as our evolving conceptualization of bipolar disorder.
- Evaluation of states of depression has been a significant achievement in recent years, making use of a number of well-supported self-report and clinician-rated procedures that measure the presence and severity of various depressive symptoms. Instruments vary, however, in their coverage of particular symptoms.
- Measurement of states of mania is less well developed. The experience of manic symptoms interferes with obtaining valid self-reports by questionnaire, but even clinician-based measures are relatively sparse. Several self-report and clinician-rated instruments for measuring mania are currently available, but psychometric studies of their merits lag behind those used for depressive symptoms.
- There is a significant potential gap in measurement of particular symptoms or clusters. This gap is particularly pronounced in the assessment of mixed states. It might be anticipated that further developments in both conceptualization and instrumentation for specific symp-

toms would improve evaluation of the treatment of bipolar conditions (e.g., sleep disturbances, mixed states, cognitive–intellectual functioning).
- Several methods are for characterizing the course of bipolar disorder, based on symptom levels, episode status, and functional impairment. These methods of longitudinal or retrospective charting have proved valuable for understanding features of the course of the disorder, and potentially they can play an important role in treatment decision making.
- Preliminary steps have been taken to evaluate hypomanic personality, or risk for future bipolar disorder. Similarly, there have been some positive steps toward the development of screening instruments to help identify in nonclinical populations those who are at risk or have already experienced bipolar states.
- Initial steps have also been taken to describe functioning in important roles—areas of living that may be relatively independent of symptom levels. Further work is needed to provide scales that capture both objective features of how individuals live their lives and the contexts in which they struggle with their illness, as well as methods for capturing the motivations and perceptions of people with bipolar disorder.
- Research on the assessment of mania and manic symptoms in children is at a relatively preliminary stage. Diagnostic assessments require careful attention to clinical and course features, such as rapid cycling and mixed states, that differ between children and adults with bipolar disorder. There is a great need for developmentally appropriate indicators of symptoms, as well as for indicators that can distinguish among groups with overlapping disorders, such as ADHD.

NOTES

1. Many of these studies were reported in a special issue of the *Journal of Affective Disorders* in 2005: Akiskal et al., 2005a,b,c; Akiyama et al., 2005; Erfurth et al., 2005a,b; Matsumoto et al., 2005; Mendlowicz et al., 2005.
2. Paykel and Weissman, 1973; Harrow et al., 1990; Mintz et al., 1992; Gitlin et al., 1995.

12   Creativity

[Edgar Allan Poe's alcoholism] was one of the methods by which he fought the intolerable morbidity of his manic-depressive state of mind . . . Had this been his only weapon to relieve the depressions that overtook him, he would, like thousands of others similarly affected, have lived his life unknown and gone unsung by posterity. But he had a second weapon—his pen.

—W. R. Bett (1952, pp. 74–75)

HISTORICAL BACKGROUND

The notion of a relationship between creativity and extremes in mood states is an ancient one, described in pre-Grecian myths and later by Plato and Socrates. Divine madness and inspiration were thought to be obtainable only during particular states of mind, such as loss of consciousness, affliction with illness, or fits of "possession." In his speech on divine madness in *Phaedrus*, Socrates said:

> Madness, provided it comes as the gift of heaven, is the channel by which we receive the greatest blessings . . . [T]he men of old who gave things their names saw no disgrace or reproach in madness; otherwise they would not have connected it with the name of the noblest of all arts, the art of discerning the future, and called it the manic art. (Plato, 1974, pp. 46–47)

He went on to discuss artistic "madness" in particular (p. 48): "If a man comes to the door of poetry untouched by the madness of the Muses, believing that technique alone will make him a good poet," he proclaimed, "he and his sane compositions never reach perfection, but are utterly eclipsed by the performances of the inspired madman."

Madness, as understood by Plato and Socrates, encompassed a wide range of states of thought and emotion, not just psychosis, but the emphasis was on a profoundly altered state of thinking, awareness, and feeling. Aristotle, writing in the 4th century BC, focused more specifically on the relationship among melancholia, madness, and inspiration. "Why is it," he asked, "that all men who are outstanding in philosophy, poetry or the arts are melancholic?" This was true of Ajax and Bellerophontes, he said: "The former went completely insane. . . . And many other heroes suffered in the same way as these. In later times also there have been

Empedocles, Plato, Socrates and many other well-known men. The same is true for most of those who have handled poetry" (1936, pp. 155–157).

The Renaissance saw a resurgence of interest in the relationship among genius, melancholy, and madness, but an important distinction was made between sane melancholics of high achievement and individuals whose insanity prevented them from using their gifts. The eighteenth century witnessed a sharp change in attitude, with rational thought seen as essential to genius, a view then sharply reversed by the nineteenth-century Romantics, who once again emphasized extremes in mood and experience as critical to artistic inspiration and expression. In 1812—the same year that Byron, the personification of Romantic, melancholic intensity, published *Childe Harold's Pilgrimage*—physician Benjamin Rush, author of the first major psychiatric treatise in the United States, recorded his clinical observations about the relationship between acute manic and creative states (Rush, 1812, pp. 153–154):

> From a part of the brain preternaturally elevated, but not diseased, the mind sometimes discovers not only unusual strength and acuteness, but certain talents it never exhibited before. . . . Talents for eloquence, poetry, music and painting, and uncommon ingenuity in several of the mechanical arts, are often involved in this state of madness. . . . The disease which thus evolves these new and wonderful talents and operations of the mind may be compared to an earthquake, which, by convulsing the upper strata of our globe, throws upon its surface precious and splendid fossils, the existence of which was unknown to the proprietors of the soil in which they were buried.

An ironic exception to the nineteenth-century writers who emphasized deep, mysterious, and irrational forces giving rise to genius was the essayist Charles Lamb, himself institutionalized for what would now be called bipolar illness, and companion to a sister intermittently insane with the same illness. In *The Sanity of True Genius*, Lamb argued for a balance of faculties, much as the eighteenth-century writers had done (Lamb, 1987, pp. 212–213):

> Far from the position holding true, that great wit (or genius, in our modern way of speaking), has a necessary alliance with insanity, the greatest wits, on the contrary, will ever be found in the sanest writers. It is impossible for the mind to conceive a mad Shakespeare. The greatness of wit, by which the poetic talent is here chiefly to be understood, manifests itself in the admirable balance of all faculties. Madness is the disproportionate straining or excess of any one of them. . . . The ground of the mistake is, that men, finding in the raptures of the higher poetry a condition of exaltation, to which they have no parallel in their own experience, besides the spurious resemblance of it in dreams and fevers, impute a state of dreaminess and fever to the poet. But the true poet dreams being awake. He is not possessed by his subject, but has dominion over it.

The late nineteenth and early twentieth centuries saw a moderation of earlier Romantic views, due in part to the inevitable swing from any extreme and in part to the more circumspect reasoning of academic psychologists and psychiatrists. William James and Emil Kraepelin, for example, emphasized positive features associated with certain kinds of madness, or "psychopathy," and speculated on how these features might combine with other talents in some instances to produce an extraordinarily creative or accomplished person. They also stressed, however, the debilitating extremes of mental illness—psychosis or morbid depressions, for example—in addition to the milder, potentially productive hypomanias and more reflective, philosophical melancholias. These scholars underscored the need for sustained attention, discipline, and balance in the truly accomplished individual. This more moderate view has characterized most modern thinking about the relationship between psychopathology and genius.

Kraepelin, a contemporary of William James, was acutely aware of the dire consequences of untreated manic-depressive illness. But like many who had observed and studied it, he wrote of its occasional positive aspects as well (Kraepelin, [1921] 1976, p. 17):

> The volitional excitement which accompanies the disease may under certain circumstances set free powers which otherwise are constrained by all kinds of inhibition. Artistic activity namely may, by the untroubled surrender to momentary fancies or moods, and especially poetical activity by the facilitation of linguistic expression, experience a certain furtherance.

Swiss psychiatrist Eugen Bleuler concurred, and further drew the parallel between manic and artistic thought (Bleuler, 1924, pp. 466, 468):

> The *thinking* of the manic is flighty. He jumps by by-paths from one subject to another, and cannot adhere to anything. With this the ideas run along very easily and involuntarily, even so freely that it may be felt as unpleasant by the patient. . . .
>
> Because of the more rapid flow of ideas, and especially because of the falling off of inhibitions, artistic activities are facilitated even though something worthwhile is produced only in very mild cases and when the patient is otherwise talented in this direction. The heightened sensibilities naturally have the effect of furthering this.

William James, like his brother Henry and other members of their family, was subject to profound, debilitating depressions. Nonetheless, he wrote about the potentially valuable combination of an ardent, excitable temperament with talent (James, 1902):

> The psychopathic temperament [by which James meant "border-line insanity, insane temperament, loss of mental balance"], whatever be the intellect with which it finds itself paired, often brings with it ardor and excitability of character. . . . His conceptions tend to pass immediately into belief and action . . . [W]hen a superior intellect and a psychopathic temperament coalesce—as in the endless permutations and combinations of human faculty, they are bound to coalesce often enough—in the same individual, we have the best possible condition for the kind of effective genius that gets into the biographical dictionaries. Such men do not remain mere critics and understanders with their intellect. Their ideas possess them, they inflict them, for better or worse, upon their companions or their age.

Myerson and Boyle, writing from Boston's McLean Hospital in the 1940s, reiterated the basic position of William James; as Kraepelin and Rush had done, they focused on manic-depressive illness. In discussing affective psychosis in socially prominent families, they concluded (Myerson and Boyle, 1941):

> It does not necessarily follow that the individuals who appear in these records were great because they had mental disease, although that proposition might be maintained with considerable cogency and relevance. It may be that the situation is more aptly expressed as follows. The manic drive in its controlled form and phase is of value *only* if joined to ability. A feebleminded person of hypomanic temperament would simply be one who carried on

more activity at a feebleminded level, and this is true also of mediocrity, so the bulk of manic-depressive temperaments are of no special value to the world, and certainly not of distinguished value. If however, the hypomanic temperament is joined to high ability, an independent characteristic, then the combination may well be more effective than the union of high ability with normal temperament and drive might be. The indefatigability, the pitch of enthusiasm, the geniality and warmth which one so often sees in the hypomanic state may well be a fortunate combination and socially and historically valuable.

EVIDENCE FOR A LINK BETWEEN MANIC-DEPRESSIVE ILLNESS AND CREATIVITY

Any relationship between manic-depressive illness and creativity would appear to be unlikely, especially in light of recent and overwhelming evidence that pervasive cognitive deficits mark many if not most individuals afflicted by the bipolar form of the disorder (see Chapter 9), although it should be noted that standard measures of intellectual functioning, such as IQ tests, show only a modest association with creativity (see, e.g., Ochse, 1990; Piirto, 1994; Simonton, 1994). (Anecdotally, it is of interest that scientists Richard Feynman and James Watson scored 120 on their respective IQ tests.) It is counterintuitive that such a destructive illness could be associated with imagination or great works of art. Yet the perceived association is a persistent cultural belief and one that is backed by data from many studies. All of these studies are limited by their methods, but as we shall see, their findings—converging as they do from across varied methodologies and different populations—are certainly suggestive. It may be, of course, that there is no relationship. Or there may be a link, but not a causal one. If there is a link, it may be that creativity or the creative lifestyle leads to instability (for example, through highly irregular sleep patterns, financial and other stresses, alcohol and drug abuse, or a social milieu with an excessive tolerance for erratic behavior), rather than the instability's facilitating creativity. Indeed, there may be a selection factor for those who choose a life within the arts.

We argue here that there is a causal link whereby the cognitive styles, temperaments, and intense, cyclic moods associated with bipolar spectrum disorders cause some who are already creative and productive to be even more so. The argument is not that manic-depressive illness and its related temperaments are essential to creative work; clearly they are not. Nor do we argue that most people who have bipolar or recurrent depressive illness are creative; they are not. The argument is, rather, that a *disproportionate* number of eminent writers and artists have suffered from bipolar spectrum disorders and that, under some circumstances, creativity can be facilitated by such disorders. Indeed, great creative accomplishment is by definition a rare merging of temperament, intellect, imagination, happenstance, energy, and discipline.

While we focus here on mood, cognitive, and temperamental aspects of great achievement, the role of hard work and discipline cannot be overemphasized. Lord Byron is a good example of this point. There can be little question that his poetry was strongly affected by his extreme moods and indisputable mental anguish, but his personal discipline was extraordinary. Byron's extensive reworking of a single stanza from *Don Juan*, for example, is illustrated in Figure 12–1 and Box 12–1. "His reason was punctuated, even disturbed, by passion," wrote another poet, "but whatever he was in person he was not, as an artist, passion's slave. In the poetry Byron masks his passion and makes it into endurable art" (Bold, 1983, p. 13). Byron himself wrote: "Yet, see, he mastereth himself, and makes / His torture tributary to his will."[1]

Methodological Issues

There are several ways to examine the relationship between manic-depressive illness and creativity, but until recently, apocryphal speculation far outweighed systematic study. Criticism of work purporting to find a link has been justified. Biographical studies—while intrinsically fascinating, irreplaceable, and deeply instructive sources of information about moods, their extremes, and their roles in the lives of artists—are fraught with difficulties (Jamison, 1993).[2] This criticism has been discussed at length elsewhere (see, e.g., Jamison, 1993; Post, 1994; Ludwig, 1995).

Writers and artists, for example, however brutally honest they may be in some of their self-assessments, are of necessity subjective and biased as well. The reliability of letters, journals, and memoirs can be limited because they are written from a single perspective or because the writer was fully mindful of future biographers and posterity. Biographers, too, write with biases and under the influence of prevailing or idiosyncratic viewpoints. Historical context and existing social customs also determine which behaviors are culled or emphasized for comment. Certain lifestyles provide cover for deviant and bizarre behavior, and the arts, especially, have long given latitude to extremes in behavior and mood. The assumption is prevalent that within artistic circles, madness, melancholy, and suicide are somehow normal, making it difficult at times to distinguish truth from expectation.

Biographical or posthumous research poses other problems as well. Any historical perspective dictates that a listing of highly accomplished, affectively ill individuals will be illustrative, but by no means definitive. Always in the analysis of individual lives, problems arise. It is fairly easy

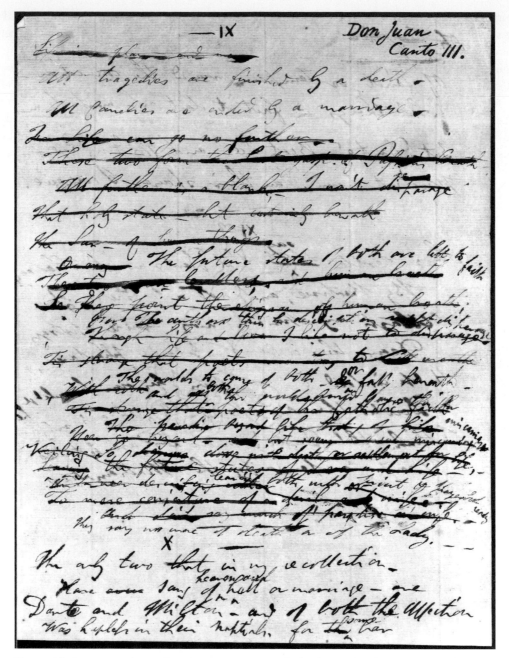

Figure 12–1. Autograph page from stanza 9, canto III, of Byron's *Don Juan* (reduced by one-third). (*Source*: Reproduced by permission of the Pierpont Morgan Library, New York. MA56-57.)

to identify any number of major nineteenth-century British or American poets who were manic-depressive, for example, but it is more difficult to determine what proportion of the total pool of "great poets" they represent. (In many instances, of course, the individuals under study are sufficiently important to be interesting in their own right, independently of any general grouping.) Also, more detailed information exists for some individuals than for others (for example, those more in the public eye, those living in relatively recent times, those institutionalized, or those writing more extensively about themselves).

The tendency for highly accomplished individuals to be, almost by definition, inordinately productive and energetic creates a problem of another sort—a bias toward underdiagnosis of the manic side of bipolar illness. Biographical studies indicate that writers, artists, and composers often describe their periods of melancholy or depression in great detail, but that other aspects of mood swings, such as hypomania and even at times overt psychosis, are subsumed under "eccentricity," "creative inspiration," or "artistic temperament." Thus many individuals with clear histories of profound or debilitating depressions are

BOX 12–1. Reworking by Byron of Stanza 9, Canto III, from *Don Juan*

1. ~~Life is a play and men~~
   All tragedies are finished by a death,
2. All Comedies are ended by a marriage,
3. ~~For Life can go no further~~
   ~~These two form the last gasp of Passion's breath~~
4. ~~All further is a blank—I won't disparage~~
5. ~~That holy state—but certainly beneath~~
6. ~~The Sun—of human beings~~
3. ~~These two are lovellers, and human breath~~
   ~~So~~ ~~These point the epigram of human breath,~~
   ~~Or any~~ The future states of both are left to faith,
4. ~~Though Life and love I like not to disparage~~
   ~~The~~ For authors ~~think~~ description might disparage
                         fear
5. ~~'Tis strange that poets never try to wreathe~~ [sic?]
   ~~With eith~~ ~~'Tis strange that poets of the Catholic faith~~
6. ~~Neer go beyond~~ ~~and~~ ~~but seem to dread miscarriage~~
7. ~~So dramas close with death or settlement for life~~
   ~~Veiling~~ ~~Leaving the future states of Love and Life~~
   ~~The paradise beyond like that of life~~
8. ~~And neer describing either~~
   ~~To mere conjecture of a devil—and—or wife~~
5. The worlds to come of both ~~—&~~ or fall beneath,
6. And ~~all—both the worlds would blame them for miscarriage~~
   And then both worlds would punish their miscarriage—
7. ~~So leaving both with priest & prayerbook ready~~
   So leaving ~~Clerg both a~~ each their Priest and prayerbook ready,
8. They say no more of death or of the Lady.

Source: Steffan, 1971, p. 345. Reprinted from Byron's *Don Juan: Volume 1, The Making of a Masterpiece*, 2nd Edition, edited by Truman Guy Steffan, Copyright 1957, 1971, renewed 1985. Courtesy of the University of Texas Press.

labeled "melancholic" rather than manic-depressive, despite their episodic (and often seasonal) histories of extremely high energy, irritability, enthusiasm, and increased productivity (periods often accompanied by costly lapses in financial, social, and sexual judgment). Paradoxically, the more chronically hypomanic the individual, the more noticeable and relatively pathological the depression will be. Diagnostic biases in the opposite direction also occur. Some researchers tend to overdiagnose bipolar illness because they observe patterns of behavior common to both hypomania and normal accomplishment (for example, enthusiasm, high energy, and the ability to function with little sleep) and then label as manic-depressive anyone displaying these "symptoms."

Despite the difficulty of conducting diagnostic studies based on biographical material, valid and useful research can be carried out by using in a systematic way what is known about bipolar illness: its symptomatic presentation (for example, pronounced changes in mood, energy, sleep, thinking, and behavior); associated behavior patterns (such as alcohol and drug abuse, pathological gambling, violence, pronounced and repeated financial reversals, and chaotic interpersonal relationships); its association with suicide[3]; its natural course[4]; and a family history, especially in first-degree relatives (parents, siblings, or children), of depression, mania, psychosis, or suicide. Psychiatric and medical conditions that can have similar symptoms (for example, thyroid and other metabolic disturbances, drug-induced states, or complex partial seizures and related epileptic conditions) need to be considered, and ruled out, as well. Making a retrospective diagnosis is, in many ways, like putting together the pieces of a three-dimensional puzzle or solving a mystery by a complicated but careful marshaling of evidence. Biographical diagnoses must ultimately, of course, be more tentative than diagnoses made on living individuals, being circumstantial by nature, but they can be made, reliably and responsibly and with an appreciation for the complexities of anyone's life, especially that of an artist.

Studies of living artists, writers, and composers have had serious methodological flaws as well, including small sample sizes, inconsistent definitions of creativity and psychiatric illness, and nonrandom or nonspecified selection of subjects. These issues are discussed in greater detail later in the chapter.

Biographical Studies

Many case-history studies of psychopathology in eminent writers and artists were conducted during the late nineteenth and early twentieth centuries. Lombroso (1891) found an overrepresentation of manic-depressive illness in his study of geniuses and attributed it to his belief that those who suffered from the illness "feel and notice more things and with greater vivacity and tenacity than other men, their recollections are richer, and their mental combinations more fruitful" (p. 27). Babcock (1895), writing a few years later, observed that the geniuses he had studied were more likely to be emotionally unstable and given to extremes in moods. Jacobson (1912), White (1930), and Lange-Eichbaum (1932) found high general rates of insanity in their biographical studies of genius. The latter concluded that within the group defined as geniuses, artists and poets tended more to insanity than scientists and statesmen. Reid (1912) and Onuf (1918) found that manic-depressive illness was strongly overrepresented in their eminent subjects.

In a more quantitative analysis, Juda (1949) studied 113 German artists, writers, architects, and composers; she was one of the first to undertake an extensive, in-depth investigation of not only artists and writers but also their relatives.

TABLE 12–1. Biographical Studies of Depression, Mania, and Suicide in Eminent Writers, Composers, and Artists

Study	Subjects	Findings
Juda, 1949	113 German artists and writers	Two-thirds were "psychically normal"; more suicides and "insane and neurotic" individuals in artistic group than general population. Highest rates of psychiatric abnormalities in poets (50%), musicians (38%), painters (18%), and architects (17%). First-degree relatives of artists and writers were more likely to be cyclothymic, commit suicide, or have manic-depressive illness. Psychosis was much more common in grandchildren of artists and writers.
Martindale, 1972	21 eminent English poets (born 1670–1809); 21 eminent French poets (born 1770–1909)	55% of English poets and 40% of French poets had significant psychopathology ("nervous breakdown," suicide, and/or alcoholism). One in 7 had been placed in asylum or had suffered from severe "recurring and unmistakable symptoms," such as hallucinations or delusions.
Trethowan, 1977	60 eminent composers	Mood disorders "easily the commonest and most important of psychiatric illnesses" in composers; approximately 50% had a "melancholic temperament."
Jamison, 1993	36 eminent/most anthologized British and Irish poets (born 1705–1805)	17% had been committed to insane asylum; 22% had a history of psychosis; 39% had a strong family history of psychosis, suicide, and/or melancholia; 6% committed suicide.
Schildkraut et al., 1994	15 abstract expressionist artists (New York School)	More than 50% had a depressive illness; 40% received treatment; 20% hospitalized; 13% committed suicide; 2 paternal suicides.
Post, 1994	100 eminent American and British writers	5% had history of bipolar psychosis; 2% unipolar psychosis; 16% severely disabled by depression; 8% committed suicide. Total of 82% with "affective abnormalities."

(continued)

TABLE 12–1. **Biographical Studies of Depression, Mania, and Suicide in Eminent Writers, Composers, and Artists** *(continued)*

Study	Subjects	Findings
Ludwig, 1995	1,004 eminent individuals across all fields of accomplishment	Compared with other professions (business, science, public life), artistic group had 2–3 times the rate of psychosis, suicide attempts, mood disorders, and substance abuse. Those in the artistic group were 6–7 times more likely to have been involuntarily hospitalized.
Post, 1996	45 scientists, 52 composers, 48 artists, 50 writers	Severe depressive illness: scientists (18%); composers (15%); artists (8%); writers (36%).
Czeizel, 2001	21 eminent Hungarian poets (born 1554–1925)	Bipolar-I (14%); bipolar-II (53%); major depression (9%); committed suicide (9%).
Wills, 2003	40 eminent American modern jazz musicians	Psychotic illness (7.5%); major affective illness (28.5%); inpatient treatment for depression (10%); committed suicide (2.5%).

She found a high rate of what she called manic-depressive psychosis (4.3 percent) in her comparison sample of scientists (a broadly defined group), but no manic-depressive illness in the artists. (Not uncommon for the times, there was diagnostic confusion between schizophrenia and manic-depressive illness.) The artists, instead, showed a disproportionate rate of "undetermined psychoses" (2.7 percent) and schizophrenia (2.7 percent). First-degree relatives of the artists and writers, however, were disproportionately likely to be cyclothymic, to commit suicide, or to have manic-depressive illness. Juda's findings, together with those from more recent systematic biographical studies, are presented in Table 12–1. The methods and populations used across these studies varied enormously, as did the selection criteria and means used for diagnostic ascertainment.

The inconsistencies and methodological flaws in these studies were substantial, but the individuals studied were of indisputable artistic ability, and most had made lasting contributions to their fields. What is of interest is the consistency of the findings—the strikingly increased rates of psychosis, institutionalization, and suicide in eminent artists and writers. The markedly elevated rates for depressive illnesses are particularly noteworthy given that the overwhelming majority of the subjects were men, who have a considerably lower rate of depression than women.

To study the occurrence of mood disorders and suicide in a consecutive sample of all of the most eminent British and Irish poets born within a 100-year period (the most frequently represented poets in 15 anthologies of eighteenth- and nineteenth-century verse), Jamison (1993) examined autobiographical sources, contemporary accounts, and medical records (where available) for poets born between 1705 and 1805. She examined the available letters, journals, and medical records for symptoms of depression, mania, and mixed states; seasonal or other patterns in moods, behavior, and productivity; the nature of the course of the illness (for example, age at onset, duration, and patterns of recurrence); and evidence of other psychiatric or medical illnesses (for example, substance abuse or syphilis) that might confound the diagnostic picture. She placed a strong emphasis on both the severity and the recurrence of symptoms. In all cases it was the *patterning* of mood, cognitive, energy, sleep, and behavior symptoms that formed the focus of the study. The results are summarized in Table 12–2. Jamison's findings—a disproportionately high rate of psychosis, manic-depressive illness, institutionalization, and suicide—are consistent with those of other biographical studies, such as Martindale's (1972) of eminent English and French poets; Trethowan's (1977) of composers; Schildkraut and colleagues' (1994) of visual artists; Ludwig's (1992) of artists, writers, composers, and eminent nonartists (see Table 12–3); Post's (1994, 1996) of American and British writers and of scientists, composers, artists, and writers, respectively;

TABLE 12–2. **Mood Disorders and Suicide in Eminent British and Irish Poets Born 1705–1805**

Poets	Comments
Samuel Johnson 1709–1784	Severe recurrent melancholia. Perceived himself as intermittently mad and had a terror of insanity. First serious breakdown at 20, lasting more than 2 years. Experienced tics, obsessions, and phobias as well. Felt he had inherited his "vile melancholy" from his father.
Thomas Gray 1716–1771	"Habitual melancholy" and attacks of depression that grew more frequent over time. Father "subject to intermittent fits of insanity"; extravagant, alcoholic, and violent.
Williams Collins 1721–1759	Psychotic melancholia and possible mania. First complete breakdown at 29. Confined to lunatic asylum; "accustomed to rave much and make great moanings." Dissipation, intemperance, and excess while undergraduate at Cambridge. Little known about family history.
Christopher Smart 1722–1771	Ecstatic, grandiose, and religious mania. First confined to asylum in his early thirties, but financial extravagance, instability, and dissipation apparent while an undergraduate at Cambridge. Spent several years in "madhouse" on "incurable ward."
Joseph Warton 1722–1800	No indication of a significant mood disorder.
Oliver Goldsmith 1730–1774	Violent temper, fitfully melancholic, financially extravagant, compulsive gambler. Increasingly irritable, melancholic, and subject to "violent alternations of mood" as he grew older. Little known about family history except that Goldsmiths were perceived as "strange" and "eccentric."
William Cowper 1731–1800	Recurrent psychotic melancholia and repeated suicide attempts. Delusions and hallucinations. First signs of mental instability while in his twenties; confined to asylum in his early thirties. Family history of melancholia.
James Macpherson 1736–1796	No indication of a significant mood disorder.
Robert Fergusson 1750–1774	Cyclothymic temperament progressed to psychotic melancholia and then maniacal excitement (possibly exacerbated by head trauma). Died "furiously insane," at age 24, in the Edinburgh Bedlam.
Thomas Chatterton 1752–1770	Committed suicide at age 17. Extremely moody even as a child. Subject to severe melancholia as well as periods of frenzied energies, occasionally incoherent enthusiasms, and extreme grandiosity. "Wild" fluctuations in mood. Sister confined to asylum, and niece suffered from unspecified psychiatric condition.
John Bampfylde 1754–1796	Confinement in private "madhouse" for 20 years. "Fell into dissipation" after Cambridge studies. Little known about nature of his psychiatric problems. "A disposition to insanity in the family," including a sister who became insane.

(continued)

TABLE 12–2. **Mood Disorders and Suicide in Eminent British and Irish Poets Born 1705–1805** (continued)

Poets	Comments
George Crabbe 1754–1832	By age 24 described an "annual woe and dread"; suffered throughout his life from fits of depression. Daily opium use (initially prescribed for tic douloureux) for more than 40 years. Father, described as "a man of imperious temper and violent passions," became increasingly and more irrationally violent as he became older.
William Blake 1757–1827	Hallucinations and delusions from an early age. Periods of exaltation and grandiosity, as well as periods he described as "a deep pit of melancholy—melancholy without any real reason." Excessive irritability and attacks of rage, suspiciousness, and paranoia. Little information about family history although one brother, who spoke of visions of Moses and Abraham, was described as a "bit mad."
Robert Burns 1759–1796	Severe, recurrent, often seasonal melancholia (described by Burns as "the miseries of a diseased nervous system" and a "deep incurable taint which poisons my existence"). Mercurial, agitated, and volatile temperament. Both parents described as "subject to strong passions," fiery, and irascible.
Joanna Baillie 1762–1851	No indication of a significant mood disorder.
William Lisle Bowles 1762–1850	No indication of a significant mood disorder.
Samuel Rogers 1763–1855	No indication of a significant mood disorder.
William Wordsworth 1770–1850	Self-described as "of a moody and violent temper." Subject to hypochondriacal aches and pains. Described by some biographers as suffering from severe depressions "to the verge of a mental breakdown," but their nature and severity are unclear. Sister's "insanity" likely to have been due to dementia rather than to a psychiatric illness.
Sir Walter Scott 1771–1832	At various times described himself as suffering from a "disposition to causeless alarm—much lassitude—and decay of vigor and intellect," a *morbus eruditorum*, and a "black dog" of melancholy.
Samuel Taylor Coleridge 1772–1834	Extended and recurrent melancholia. Mercurial, restless, extravagant, grandiose, and agitated. Fitful enthusiasms and despairs. Opiate addiction. Visionary states. Family history of affective illness and suicide.
Robert Southey 1774–1843	Described as unduly excitable, with a history of "nervous fever" and an unbalanced state of "nerves"; however, unclear indication of recurrent mood disorder of any significant severity.
Walter Savage Landor 1775–1864	Violent, restless, and unstable temperament. Litigious and impulsive. "Very much disposed" to melancholy. Expelled from both Rugby and Oxford. Thought by others to have had "at least a touch of insanity." "Ungovernable temper" and financially extravagant.

(continued)

Poets	Comments
Thomas Campbell 1777–1844	Recurrent and severe melancholia, "aggravated fits of despondency." First attack when 18. Violently irritable, financially extravagant, and "alternately excited and depressed within short-periods of time." Insanity in his and his wife's families. Son placed in asylum, suffering from melancholia, "capricious fits of temper," paranoia, and "leap-frog play of thoughts."
Leigh Hunt 1784–1859	Autobiography describes a "nervous condition," a "melancholy state," which lasted, the first time, for several months. "I experienced it twice afterwards, each time more painfully than before, and for a much longer period . . . for upwards of four years, without intermission, and above six years in all."
Thomas Love Peacock 1785–1866	No indication of a significant mood disorder.
George Gordon, Lord Byron 1788–1824	Recurrent, often agitated, melancholia. Volatile temperament with occasional "paroxysms of rage." Mercurial and extravagant; worsening depressions over time. Strong family history of mental instability and suicide.
Percy Bysshe Shelley 1792–1822	Recurrent, agitated, and occasionally suicidal melancholia. "Hysterical attacks" followed by periods of listlessness; often seasonal. Ecstatic episodes and "violent paroxysms of rage." Self-described as "tormented by visions," the psychiatric nature of which remains unclear. Probable transient delusions. Intermittent laudanum use for "nerves."
John Clare 1793–1864	Spent 25 years in insane asylum. Long periods of inertia and melancholia interspersed with episodes of frenzied, violent, and extravagant activity. Hallucinations, as well as delusions of persecution and grandeur. Cause of madness listed as "hereditary" by asylum physician.
John Keats 1795–1821	"Violent and ungovernable as a child"; described by brother as nervous, "morbid," and suffering from "many a bitter fit of hypochondriasm" [melancholy]; periods of depression often followed by periods of intense activity and "exhilaration." Described himself as having a "horrid Morbidity of Temperament." Rapidly shifting moods predated symptoms and diagnosis of tuberculosis.
George Darley 1795–1846	Recurrent, occasionally suicidal melancholia. Increasing periods of depression and social withdrawal. Described extreme mood swings, ranging from "causeless and unreasonable" periods of "frolic, extravagance, and insane" actions to "crazed" periods of despair.
Hartley Coleridge 1796–1849	Recurrent melancholia; severe mood swings alternating between "depression and extravagant hilarity." Lifelong struggles with alcoholism, "heavings of agony," and "paroxysms of rage." Expelled from Oxford for dissipation. Eccentric and visionary. Under conservatorship toward end of life. Insanity on both sides of his family.

(continued)

TABLE 12–2. **Mood Disorders and Suicide in Eminent British and Irish Poets Born 1705–1805** *(continued)*

Poets	Comments
Thomas Hood 1799–1845	Periods of morbidity, melancholia, and lethargy, but diagnosis complicated by severe, recurrent physical illness.
Thomas Lovell Beddoes 1803–1849	Committed suicide at 45 after at least one earlier attempt. Volatile, extravagant, eccentric, and subject to severe recurrent melancholia. Father, also a physician, was highly eccentric and of an "extremely ardent" temperament.
Robert Stephen Hawker 1803–1875	"Fits" of depression throughout his life. Deep depression and "brain fever" after wife's death; possible psychosis. Volatile, extravagant, and eccentric. Intermittent opium habit. Physician had "never encountered in all his practice so excitable a tissue as that which held [his] Brain." "My Grandfather and Father," Hawker wrote, "were both of the same excitable temperament."
James Clarence Mangan 1803–1849	Recurrent and prolonged psychotic depressions. Hallucinations, agitation, "great overcurtaining gloom." Extreme eccentricity: "with one voice they all proclaimed me mad." Probable opiate abuse. Father described as extravagant, financially dissolute, and of "quick and irascible temper."

Note: Poets selected for inclusion were the most frequently represented in 15 anthologies of eighteenth- and nineteenth-century British and Irish verse.
Source: Adapted from Jamison, 1993.

Czeizel's (2001) of Hungarian poets;[5] and Wills' (2003) of the lives of American jazz musicians. These studies are necessarily subjective in many respects—although suicide, psychosis, and institutionalization are relatively objective phenomena—but they are notable for the eminence of the subjects involved and for the consistency of their findings. Suicide rates were markedly elevated in all of the studies (see Fig. 12–2).

Studies of Living Writers and Artists

There have been fewer studies of psychopathology in living writers and artists. Andreasen and colleagues undertook the first such inquiries into the relationship between creativity and mental disorders (Andreasen and Canter, 1974; Andreasen and Powers, 1975; Andreasen, 1987). These studies, using structured interviews, the Research Diagnostic Criteria (RDC), and matched control groups,

TABLE 12–3. **Rates of Suicide, Depression, Mania, and Psychosis in a Sample of Writers, Artists, and Composers**

		LIFETIME RATES (%)			
	Sample Size	Depression	Mania	Psychosis	Suicide
Poets	53	77	13	17	20
Fiction writers	180	59	9	7	4
Nonfiction writers	64	47	11	8	1
Artists	70	50	9	4	6
Composers	48	46	6	10	0

Source: Adapted from Ludwig, 1992.

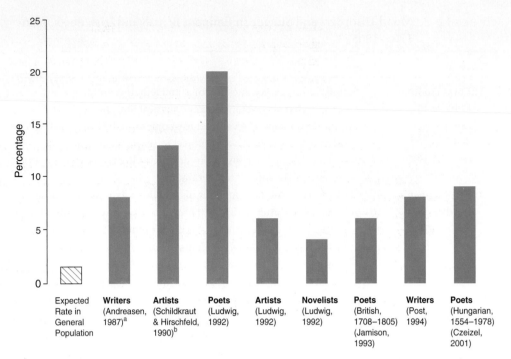

Figure 12–2. Suicide rates in writers and artists. [a]Suicide rate at the time of study completion. [b]Two other artists died in single car accidents.

represented significant methodological advances over prior, anecdotally based research. The size of the sample of writers was relatively small (N=30), however, and the subjects were of varying levels of creative accomplishment (all were participants in the University of Iowa Writers' workshop, but some were nationally acclaimed writers, while others were graduate students or teaching fellows not nationally or internationally recognized). Andreasen noted that because she studied only writers, her results could not be generalized to other groups of creative individuals, such as philosophers, scientists, or musicians. Although this is true, and writers may be disproportionately likely to have affective disorders, the homogeneity of the sample is valuable in its own right.

The results of the Iowa research are summarized in Table 12–4. Clearly, the writers had an exceptionally high rate of affective illness and alcoholism. Fully 80 percent of the study sample met standardized (RDC) diagnostic criteria for a major affective disorder. In contrast, 30 percent of the control sample (individuals outside the arts who were matched for age, education, and gender) met the same criteria (*p* < .001). Although this is a much lower figure relative to the study sample, it still represents a rate greater than that expected for the general population. It is unclear whether this discrepancy reflects an overrepresentation of affective illness in the control sample, or the diagnostic criteria were overly inclusive for both the

creative and control groups. Almost one-half (43 percent) of the creative sample met the diagnostic criteria for bipolar-I or bipolar-II disorder.

In a study of eminent British writers and artists, Jamison (1989) examined rates of treatment for affective illness within these groups and looked at seasonal patterns of moods and productivity, the nature of intense creative episodes and the similarities between such episodes and hypomania, and the perceived role of very intense moods in the writers' or artists' work. Subjects were chosen for the study on the basis of having won at least one of several specified top prizes or awards in their fields. Thus, all painters and sculptors were either Royal Academicians or Associates of the Royal Academy, and the work of 9 of the 18 poets in the study sample had already been anthologized in *The Oxford Book of Twentieth Century English Verse*. Six of the eight playwrights had won the New York Drama Critics Award and/or the Evening Standard Drama Award (the London Critics' award); several had won both or had won one of these awards more than once.

The artists and writers were asked whether they had ever received treatment for a mood disorder and, if so, what that treatment had consisted of. The results, shown in Figure 12–3, indicate that a large proportion of the total sample (38 percent) had been treated for an affective illness. Three-fourths of those treated had been given antidepressants or lithium or

TABLE 12–4. **Lifetime Prevalence of Mental Illness in Writers and Control Subjects**

Diagnosis (Research Diagnostic Criteria)	Writers (n = 30) (%)	Controls (n = 30) (%)	p
Any affective disorder	80	30	.001
Any bipolar disorder	43	10	.01
Bipolar-I	13	0	NS
Bipolar-II	30	10	NS
Major depression	37	17	NS
Schizophrenia	0	0	NS
Alcoholism	30	7	.05
Drug abuse	7	7	NS
Suicide	7	0	NS

NS = not significant.
Source: Adapted from Andreasen, 1987. Reprinted with permission from the *American Journal of Psychiatry*, American Psychiatric Association.

had been hospitalized. Poets were most likely to have received medication for depression (33 percent) and were the only ones to have received medical intervention (hospitalization, electroconvulsive therapy, and/or lithium) for mania (17 percent). Thus, one-half of the poets had been treated with drugs or hospitalized for mood disorders. This rate is strikingly high when compared with rates in the general population (see Chapter 5). It is even higher when one considers the fact that the proportion of those in the general population so seriously ill as to actually seek and receive treatment is much lower, perhaps one-third to one-half the rates reported in prevalence studies using diagnostic criteria alone (Andreasen and Canter, 1974; Robins et al., 1984). A further probable underestimate of the total rate of affective illness in the study sample derives from the sample's being comprised largely of men, who, as noted, are less likely than women to suffer from depression, as well as less likely to seek treatment. The playwrights had the highest total rate of treatment for mood disorders (63 percent), but a very high percentage (38 percent) had been treated with psychotherapy alone; it is unclear whether this was due to a difference in illness severity or in treatment preference. Visual artists and biographers had relatively lower rates of treatment (13 and 20 percent, respectively); all treatment was with antidepressants.

Although, with the exception of the poets, the subjects reported being treated for depression, not mania or hypomania, the design of the study did not allow systematic inquiry into hypomanic or manic episodes. About one-third of the writers and artists reported histories of severe mood swings, however, and one-fourth reported histories of extended elated mood states. The novelists and poets most frequently reported elated mood states, whereas the playwrights and artists were the most likely to report severe mood swings. Biographers reported no history of severe mood swings or elated states, an interesting finding since of the five groups, they were the least likely to be associated with creativity and thus provide a natural comparison group (i.e., one highly proficient in writing but perhaps less outstandingly creative by the nature of their work).

One of the major purposes of the British study was to look at the similarities and dissimilarities between periods of intense creative activity and hypomania. Hypothesized similarities were based on the episodic nature of both; the overlapping nature of the behavioral, mood, and cognitive changes associated with both; and a possible link between the duration and frequencies of the two types of experiences. The vast majority of the subjects (89 percent) reported having had experienced intense creative episodes (100 percent of the poets, novelists, and artists; 88 percent

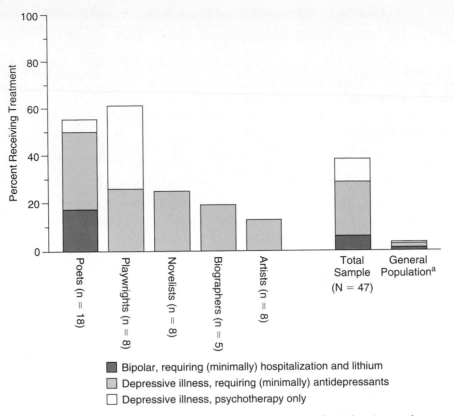

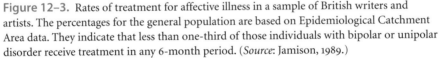

Figure 12–3. Rates of treatment for affective illness in a sample of British writers and artists. The percentages for the general population are based on Epidemiological Catchment Area data. They indicate that less than one-third of those individuals with bipolar or unipolar disorder receive treatment in any 6-month period. (*Source*: Jamison, 1989.)

of the playwrights; and, consistent with results reported earlier, only 20 percent of the biographers). The modal duration of these episodes was 2 weeks (35 percent); 55 percent of the episodes lasted 1 to 4 weeks, 20 percent 1 to 24 hours, and 25 percent longer than 1 month. The episodes were characterized by increases in enthusiasm, energy, self-confidence, speed of mental associations, fluency of thoughts, elevated mood, and a sense of well-being. Mood and cognitive changes showed the greatest degree of overlap with the episodes characterized as "intense creativity." Approximately half of the subjects described a decreased need for sleep and increased sensory awareness, but several of the more behavioral changes typically associated with hypomania (hypersexuality, increased talkativeness, and spending of money) were reported by only a minority of subjects.

When asked open-ended questions about changes before these intense creative episodes, 89 percent reported less need for sleep. (Coincident with the timing of the switch process in bipolar illness, 28 percent spontaneously reported waking abruptly at 3:00 or 4:00 AM and being unable to return to sleep.) Fifty percent of the subjects reported a sharp increase in mood just

before the beginning of an intensely creative period; for example, "I have a fever to write, and throw myself energetically into new projects"; "excited, anticipatory, energetic"; "more optimistic"; "elated"; "uplifted"; "euphoric"; and "ecstatic." Dysphoria preceded creativity in 28 percent of the subjects; that is, subjects reported feeling "more anxious"; "near suicide"; "increased irritability and tension"; "fearfulness, general mood of distress and slight paranoia"; and "irritable, antisocial." Finally, 22 percent reported mixed mood changes and psychomotor restlessness; for example, "mixture of elation together with some gloominess, feeling of isolation, sexual pressure, fast emotional responses"; "restlessness"; "low ebb bordering on despair often precedes good phase when work will flow almost as though one is a medium, rather than an originator"; "restless, dissatisfied." When asked specifically about the importance of very intense feelings and moods in their work, almost 90 percent stated that such feelings and moods were either integral and necessary (60 percent) or very important (30 percent). More poets than any other group regarded these intense moods as integral and necessary to what they did and how they did it.

Yet another link between creativity and affective illness may be the seasonal patterns underlying both moods and artistic productivity (as discussed more extensively by Jamison, 1993). Subjects rated their moods and productivity over a period of 36 months. Figures 12–4 and 12–5 show mood and productivity curves for the study sample (broken down by those writers and artists with a history of treatment for an affective illness and those with no such history). Very different seasonal patterns emerged. Those with a history of treatment demonstrated inversely related curves for summer productivity and moods, whereas those in the group with no history of treatment showed mood and productivity curves more directly covarying. In the treatment group, the peaks for productivity preceded and followed the mood peak by 3 to 4 months.

There are several possible explanations for these differences. First, increased productivity associated with elevated mood is almost certainly less likely to lead to treatment-seeking behavior than low productivity associated with elevated or any other mood. Second, the elevated mood of the treatment group may reflect more true hypomania (i.e., greater distractibility, increased stimulus and people seeking), which may well lead to less productivity in the acute phase. Indeed, Andreasen (1980, p. 381) found this in several of the writers in her study: "Some of their periods of hypomania were clearly counterproductive. The increased energy that they experienced could not be focused and controlled so that it could be expressed creatively, and so that energy was dissipated in social or personal outlets."

The British study of writers and artists revealed many overlapping mood, cognitive, and behavioral (especially sleep) changes between hypomania and intense creative

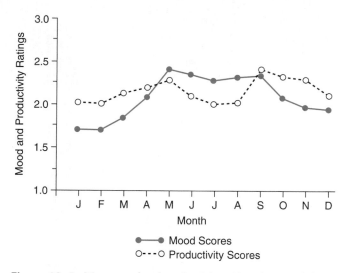

Figure 12–5. Mean mood and productivity ratings (36 months) in British writers and artists with no history of treatment for affective illness (N = 32). (*Source*: Jamison, 1989.)

states. Cognitive and mood changes showed far more overlap than behavioral ones, indicating that the milder forms of hypomania may represent the more productive phase. The affective continuum that ranges from normal states through hypomania and then mania is very important, but poorly understood (Jamison, 2004). It remains unclear whether the overlap in cognitive and mood changes represents etiologically related syndromes or phenomenologically similar but causally unrelated patterns of expression. It also remains unclear to what extent writers and artists are simply more sensitive than the general population to their own mood states and are therefore more able, and perhaps also more willing, to articulate and report them.

In the no-treatment group, the periods of intensified mood and increased productivity may represent a milder form of hypomania, with cognitive and mood changes only. These milder forms of hypomania or intensified normal functioning may result in simultaneous peaks for mood and productivity. In the treatment group, the execution of work may have preceded and lagged behind the mood component.

In another study of psychiatric disorders in living writers, Ludwig (1994), using the *Diagnostic and Statistical Manual* (DSM)-III-R and the Lifetime Creativity Scales developed by Richards and colleagues (1988, discussed below), compared 59 female writers with 59 female nonwriters matched for age, educational level, and father's occupational status. The writers were far more likely to meet the diagnostic criteria for depression and mania, and five times more likely to have made a suicide attempt (see Fig. 12–6). They were also more likely to have had a history of panic attacks, drug abuse, or an eating disorder.

Figure 12–4. Mean mood and productivity ratings (36 months) in British writers and artists with a history of treatment for affective illness (N = 15). (*Source*: Jamison, 1989.)

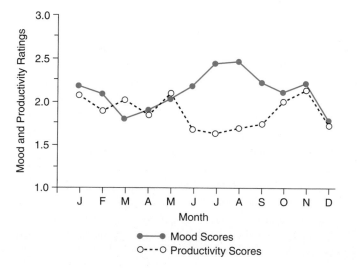

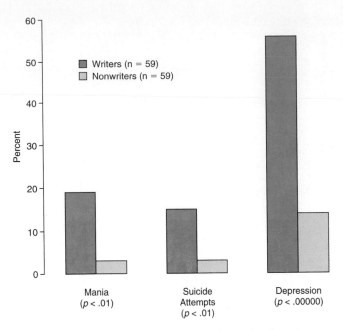

Figure 12–6. Lifetime rates of mood disorders in female writers and nonwriters. (*Source*: Adapted from Ludwig, 1994. Reprinted with permission from the *American Journal of Psychiatry*, American Psychiatric Association.)

Family Studies

A familial association between psychopathology and creativity has been found in several studies. Early biographical work by Lombrosa (1891), Galton (1892), and Lange-Eichbaum (1932) suggested that both psychopathology and creative accomplishment ran in the families of eminent writers, artists, and composers. Juda (1949), as we have noted, found that first-degree relatives of artists and writers were more likely to have had manic-depressive illness, committed suicide, been cyclothymic, or been psychotic. This finding is supported by the results of Jamison's (1993) study of first-degree relatives of eminent British and Irish poets, as well as by the extensive family history (often multigenerational) of suicide, manic-depressive illness, and psychosis in the pedigrees of, among others, George Gordon, Lord Byron; Alfred Lord Tennyson; Robert Schumann; William and Henry James; Herman Melville; Samuel Taylor Coleridge; Virginia Woolf; Ernest Hemingway; Mary Shelley and Mary Wollstonecraft; James Boswell; Samuel Johnson; Vincent van Gogh; Théodore Géricault; Gustav Mahler; Robert Lowell; John Berryman; Anne Sexton; August Strindberg; Tennessee Williams; and Eugene O'Neill.

More systematic investigations have provided a valuable supplement to these case studies. Karlsson (1970), at the Institute of Genetics in Iceland, showed that first-degree relatives of psychotic patients, as well as the patients themselves, were far more likely than the general popula-

tion to be eminent across many fields of artistic and intellectual endeavor. He also showed that there was a significantly increased risk of mental illness in distinguished Icelandic scholars and their relatives. Although Karlsson posited a familial relationship between schizophrenia and creativity, later investigators have concluded that his data actually show a very strong relationship between mood disorders, especially bipolar illness, and creativity (Richards, 1981; Andreasen and Glick, 1988; George et al., 1988).

Other researchers have looked at familial patterns of creativity and mood disorders in living artists and writers. Andreasen (1987) investigated the family histories of the University of Iowa Writers' Workshop writers and controls discussed earlier (see Table 12–5). Consistent with the elevated rate of affective illness in the writers, there was a significantly higher rate of affective illness in the primary relatives of the writers than in the primary relatives of the controls ($p < .001$). The overall prevalence for any type of psychiatric disorder was also much higher in the relatives of the writers (42 percent) than in the relatives of the controls (8 percent). Additionally, more first-degree relatives of writers than of controls showed histories of creative accomplishment (20 versus 8 percent).

Using a very different research design to study the relationship between creativity and psychopathology, Richards and colleagues (1988) at Harvard investigated creativity broadly defined in a sample of patients and their relatives. They hypothesized that a genetic vulnerability to manic-depressive illness may be accompanied by a predisposition to creativity, which may be more prominent among close relatives of patients with bipolar spectrum disorders than among the patients themselves. Such a compensatory advantage, they speculated, would be roughly analogous to the resistance to malaria found among unaffected carriers of the gene for sickle-cell anemia. To test their hypothesis, the researchers selected 17 bipolar and 16 cyclothymic patients, along with 11 of their normal first-degree relatives, using criteria that would ensure inclusion of a spectrum of disorders. These patients and their relatives were compared with 15 normal control subjects and with 18 controls who had a psychiatric diagnosis but no personal or family history of major affective disorder, schizophrenia, or suicide. Unlike other studies in the field, which limited the definition of creativity to significant, socially recognized accomplishment in the arts or sciences, these investigators attempted to measure the disposition toward originality manifested in a wide range of everyday endeavors. They administered the Lifetime Creativity Scales, a previously validated instrument that assesses the quality and quantity of "everyday" creative involvement in both work and leisure activities.

TABLE 12–5. Mental Illness in First-Degree Relatives of 30 Writers and 30 Control Subjects

Family History Diagnosis (Research Diagnostic Criteria)	ALL RELATIVES			PARENTS			SIBLINGS		
	Of Writers (n=116) (%)	Of Controls (n=121) (%)	p	Of Writers (n=60) (%)	Of Controls (n=60) (%)	P	Of Writers (n=56) (%)	Of Controls (n=121) (%)	p
Any affective disorder	18	2	.001	7	2	.001	20	3	.001
Bipolar disorder	3	0	.056	2	0	NS	5	0	NS
Major depression	15	2	.01	5	2	.05	14	3	.05
Alcoholism	7	6	NS	8	7	NS	5	5	NS
Suicide	3	0	NS	3	0	NS	2	0	NS
Any illness	42	8	.0001	42	8	.00003	43	8	.001

NS=not significant.

Source: Adapted from Andreasen, 1987. Reprinted with permission from the *American Journal of Psychiatry*, American Psychiatric Association.

Richards and colleagues found significantly higher combined creativity scores among the bipolar and cyclothymic patients and their normal first-degree relatives than among the control subjects (see Fig. 12–7). The normal index relatives showed suggestively higher creativity relative to the bipolar patients, and the cyclothymic patients were close to the normal relatives. Modifying their original hypothesis, the authors concluded (p. 287):

Overall peak creativity may be enhanced, on the average, in subjects showing milder and, perhaps, subclinical expressions of potential bipolar liability (i.e., the cyclothymes and normal first-degree relatives) compared either with individuals who carry no bipolar liability (control subjects) or individuals with more severe manifestations of bipolar liability (manic-depressives). . . . There may be a positive compensatory advantage . . . to genes associated with greater liability for bipolar disorder. The possibility that normal relatives of manic-depressives and cyclothymes have heightened creativity may have been overlooked because of a medical-model orientation that focused on dysfunction rather than positive characteristics of individuals. Such a compensatory advantage among the relatives of a disorder affecting at least 1% of the population could affect a relatively large group of people.

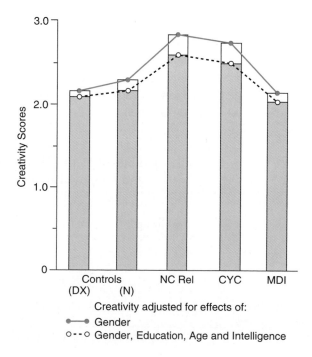

Figure 12–7. Mean creativity in selected diagnostic groups. Mean overall peak creativity scores for controls with a diagnosis (DX), normal controls (N), normal first-degree biological relatives of cyclothymes and manic-depressives (NC Rel), cyclothymes (CYC), and manic-depressives (MDI). (*Source*: Richards et al., 1988.)

More recently, Simeonova and colleagues (2005) examined the potential familial connection between bipolar illness and creativity in a different way. They compared creativity in bipolar parents (n=40), their offspring with bipolar disorder (n=20), and bipolar offspring with attention-deficit hyperactivity disorder (ADHD) (n=20) with healthy control adults (n=18) and their healthy control children (n=18). The investigators found that parents with bipolar disorder and their bipolar offspring scored higher than healthy controls on measures of creativity. They suggested several interpretations for their findings, which are consistent with those of studies discussed earlier: bipolar disorder could "cause" creativity; bipolar disorder and creativity could be transmitted independently from parents to children; family environment may affect the putative familial cotransmission of creativity and bipolar disorder; or the genes for bipolar disorder and creativity may be "linked and co-segregate through generations, accounting for their co-occurrence in people with BD [bipolar disorder]" (p. 624). The study was unable to ascertain which of these hypotheses was the most viable, and its measure of creativity (the Barron-Welsh Art Scale) is not commonly used for that purpose, but the findings suggest that children with familial bipolar illness are more creative than healthy control children. The researchers also found that creativity in bipolar children was negatively correlated with duration of illness, which they attributed to the deleterious effects of prolonged illness and/or protracted exposure to medications.

In earlier, related research, Coryell and colleagues (1989) found that, although affectively ill groups (major depression, n=442; bipolar-I, n=64; bipolar-II, n=88) did not differ from one another in occupational or educational achievement, the first-degree relatives of the probands with bipolar disorder had significantly higher mean levels of achievement compared with the first-degree relatives of the probands with major depression. Earlier, Woodruff and colleagues (1971) had shown that bipolar probands and their brothers had higher status ratings than probands with major depression and their brothers.

The results of these studies suggest that creativity and mental illness, especially bipolar disorder, may tend to aggregate in certain families and not in others, but they do not show decisively that genetic factors are operating; that is, they demonstrate that there is a familial association, but not necessarily that the characteristics under discussion are heritable. It could be, for example, that the family and its environment, rather than the genetic inheritance itself, are exerting the primary influence. McNeil (1971), using an adopted-offspring research design, attempted to clarify this nature-versus-nurture problem. All of his subjects were adults who had been adopted shortly after birth and were part of a larger Danish psychiatric genetics study. They were classified as being "high creative" (most of the individuals in this group had achieved national prominence in the arts), "above average," or "low creative." Their rates of mental illness were then compared with those found in their biological and adoptive parents. The results are summarized in Table 12–6. The rates of mental illness were highest in the "high creative" group and their biological parents. The rates of psychopathology in the adoptive parents did not vary significantly from one level of adoptee creativity to another. Although the size of the sample was necessarily small, and the type of psychopathology was not rigorously ascertained, the study is both an interesting and an important one; its significance lies in the reasons given by McNeil in his summary remarks (p. 405):

Mental illness rates in the adoptees were positively and significantly related to their creative ability level, substantiating the hypothesized relationship between creative ability and mental illness. The mental illness rates of the biological parents were positively and significantly related to the creative ability of the adoptees. Mental illness rates among the adoptive parents and the adoptive and biological siblings were independent of the adoptees' creative ability level. The data were interpreted as evidence for the influence of prebirth factors on the relationship between creative ability and mental illness. No evidence of family-related postbirth influence was found.

TABLE 12–6. **Rates of Mental Illness in Adoptees and their Biological and Adoptive Parents**

Adoptee Group	Adoptees (%)	Biological Parents (%)	Adoptee Parents (%)
High creative	30	27.7	5.3
Above average	10	8.3	5.0
Low creative	0	12.1	5.1

Source: Adapted from McNeil, 1971. Reproduced with permission from Blackwell Publishing Ltd.

Hypothesized Relationships between Manic-Depressive Illness and Creativity

In hypothesizing possible relationships between manic-depressive illness and creative accomplishment, several general areas need to be explored: characteristics of the illness, such as acute and long-term cognitive, temperamental, and mood changes; experiences due to having the illness; and the relative importance of different aspects of the illness to various types of accomplishment.

Characteristics of the Illness

Profound changes in mood, cognition, personality, sleep, energy, and behavior can occur during all phases of manic-depressive illness. Even during normal states, many individuals experience subtle and not-so-subtle fluctuations in the intensity of their perceptions and feelings. All of these changes have potentially important effects on creativity and productivity, but perhaps most relevant to our discussion here are those changes that occur during the milder manic states. The DSM-IV-R criteria for hypomania are given in Chapter 3; even the most casual review suggests prima facie reasons for a possible connection between hypomania and accomplishment. There is some truth in the easy, glib question that often arises in clinical teaching situations: Who would not want an illness that numbers among its symptoms elevated and expansive mood, inflated self-esteem, more energy than usual, decreased need for sleep, and enhanced sexuality? (Notably, DSM-III criteria for hypomania also included "sharpened and unusually creative thinking" and "increased productivity" as diagnostic criteria.)

Many creative individuals describe their mood states during moments of greatest inspiration and productivity as elated, expansive, and, on occasion, ecstatic. Although it is unclear whether these mood changes precede or follow creative thought, there is some evidence that expansiveness of thought and grandiosity of both mood and thought—common features of mild mania—can result in an increased fluency and frequency of ideas that is highly conducive to creative achievement. The similarities between intense creative episodes and hypomania were discussed earlier; these are periods when many successful artists and writers report powerful mood and sleep changes, often just preceding times of intense creative activity. This period of elated and expansive mood is described by many individuals as a time of faster and more fluid thinking, new ideas, and novel connections between thoughts. The fluency of thought common to hypomania and creative activity was reported by Kraepelin (1921, p. 15) in his citation of the experimental work of Isserlin:

> Isserlin has specially investigated the duration of ideas in manic patients. He found that their associations show

heightened distractibility in the tendency to "diffusiveness," to spinning out the circle of ideas stimulated and jumping off to others, a phenomenon which in high degree is peculiar to mania.

The increase in speed of thoughts—ranging from a very mild quickening, to flight of ideas, to psychotic incoherence—may exert its influence on creative production in several ways. Speed per se, or the quantity of thoughts and associations, may be enhanced. Also significant, however, may be the effect of this increased quantity on the qualitative aspects of thought; that is, the sheer volume of thought may produce unique ideas and associations.

Guilford's (1957) systematic psychological studies of the nature of creativity led to the conclusion that creative thinking encompasses several components (many of which relate directly to cognitive changes that take place during mild manias as well). *Fluency of thinking* is defined operationally by Guilford through several related concepts, each with tests to measure it: (1) word fluency, or the ability to produce words each containing a specified letter or combination of letters; (2) associational fluency, or the production of as many synonyms as possible for a given word in a limited amount of time; (3) expressional fluency, or the production and rapid juxtaposition of phrases or sentences; and (4) ideational fluency, or the ability to produce ideas to fulfill certain requirements in a limited amount of time. In addition to fluency of thinking, Guilford developed two other concepts important to creativity: *spontaneous flexibility*, or the ability and disposition to produce a great variety of ideas, with freedom to switch from category to category, and *adaptive flexibility*, or the ability to devise unusual types of solutions (relative to the frequency of response occurrences in the general population). Guilford (1959) also concluded, as did Hudson (1966) in his later work, that creative individuals are far more characterized by "divergent" thinking ("a type of thinking in which considerable searching about is done and a number of answers will do") than by "convergent" thinking ("thinking toward one right answer").

More recently, several researchers have shown that manic patients, unlike normal individuals or patients with schizophrenia, tend to exhibit pronounced *combinatory thinking*. Characterized by the merging of "percepts, ideas, or images in an incongruous fashion," the ideas formed in this way become "loosely strung together and extravagantly combined and elaborated" (Shenton et al., 1987; Solovay et al., 1987). Manic subjects show highly combinatory thought patterns—often characterized by humor, flippancy, and playfulness—in sharp contrast to the response patterns exhibited by normal subjects and by patients with schizophrenia (see Chapter 2, particularly Table 2–4).

Andreasen and Powers (1975) compared manic patients, schizophrenic patients, and writers from the University of Iowa Writers' Workshop on measures of conceptual overinclusiveness (the tendency to combine test objects into categories in a way that tends to "blur, broaden, or shift conceptual boundaries"). They hypothesized that creative writers might show thinking styles similar to those seen in schizophrenic individuals, but this notion was found to be groundless; instead, they observed that the writers showed conceptual styles quite like those of the manic patients: "Both writers and manics tend to sort in large groups, change dimensions while in the process of sorting, arbitrarily change starting points, or use vague distantly related concepts as categorizing principles" (p. 72). The subjects differed primarily in the degree of control they were able to exert over their patterns of thought, with the writers able to carry out "controlled flights of fancy during the process of sorting, while the manics tend to sort many objects for bizarre or personalized reasons" (p. 72).

Schuldberg (1990) found that several hypomanic traits contributed to performance on tests measuring creativity; of particular relevance here, he found that creative cognition was far more similar to hypomanic flight of ideas than to the loose associations that are characteristic of schizophrenia. Relatedly, people having strong emotional responses in general, who also tend to score higher on measures of being at risk for developing bipolar illness, often have more elaborate and generalizing cognitive operations (Larsen et al., 1987). Early studies had found that rhymes, punning, and sound associations increase during mania, and that many patients spontaneously start writing poetry while manic (Kraepelin, 1921; Murphy, 1923). Welch and colleagues (1946), in an early study of associational fluency in 101 inpatients at the Payne Whitney Psychiatric Clinic, found that patient groups that would today be called bipolar scored higher when elated than other clinical groups; all patient groups scored higher when elated than when less elated (see Table 12–7).

Nearly 150 years ago, Richarz noted that "in mania thoughts tend to form strings of ideas . . . that link together by their content, alliteration, or assonance. In racing thoughts, the ideas come and go rapidly as if they were hunting each other or continuously overlapping without any link between them" (1858; quoted in Koukopoulos and Koukopoulos, 1999, pp. 557–558). The predominant difference between the two states described is mood; that is, the elated mood of mania probably is more likely to result in a linking of ideas than is the dysphoria associated with racing thoughts.

Likewise, in studies of word-associational patterns, researchers have found that the number of original responses

TABLE 12–7. **Average Score on the Association Test for Elated and Nonelated Patients When Classified According to Clinical Groups**

Clinical Group	Mean Score When Elated	Mean Score When Not Elated
Anxiety neurosis	—	3.5
Depression	—	2.3
Manic excitement	8.8	—
Manic-depressive	9.9	4.2
Manic-depressive, psychopathic	7.6	3.1
Paranoid reaction	—	5.4
Psychopathic personality	4.3	2.8
Schizophrenia	6.9	3.8
All groups	7.9	3.2

Source: Adapted from Welch et al., 1946.

to a word-association task (in which an individual is asked to give as many associations as possible for a particular word) increases three-fold during mania; the number of statistically common, or predictable, responses falls by approximately one-third (Henry et al., 1971; Pons et al., 1985). Henry and colleagues (1971) found that the change in word-association patterns was directly proportional to the severity of manic symptoms. Other researchers have found that acutely manic patients score much higher on a word-association task than patients acutely ill with schizophrenia or control subjects (Levine et al., 1996) (see Fig. 12–8). Hypomania also has been found to increase intellectual functioning on the Wechsler Adult Intelligence Scale (Donnelly et al., 1982). Many mood-induction studies have shown that a strongly positive, or "up," mood facilitates creative problem solving[6]; relatedly, the majority of the British writers and artists in Jamison's (1989) study reported pronounced elevations in mood just prior to their periods of intensive creative activity. Richards and Kinney (1990) at Harvard found that the overwhelming majority of bipolar patients they studied reported being in a mildly or very elevated mood when experiencing their greatest periods of creativity. Several features closely linked to elevated mood states in their subjects clearly overlapped with those found in the British writers and artists; these included

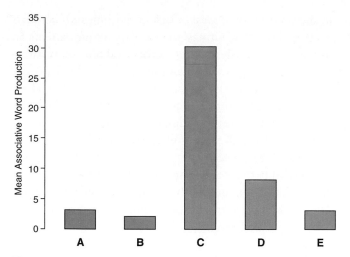

Figure 12–8. Mean associative word production—differential findings in acute manic versus acute schizophrenic patients. Given for each group are mean (± standard error [SE]) of associative words produced to 12 stimulus words. Mean associative word production by bipolar patients with acute mania (C) was higher in a statistically significant manner than in patients with acute schizophrenia (D) ($t=2.43$, $p<.05$). Both patients with mania and patients with acute schizophrenia showed significantly higher associative word production than control subjects (A) ($t=4.5$, $p<.001$; $t=4.5$, $p<0.001$, respectively). Patients with unipolar depression (B) or residual schizophrenia (E) showed mean associative word production similar to the control values. (*Source*: Levine et al., 1996. Reproduced with permission from Karger Publishing.)

increased speed of association, ease of thinking, new ideas, and expansiveness. Although the tendency has been to assume that creative periods lead to "high" or elevated moods and noncreative periods to depressed ones, the results of these studies suggest that the reverse may be true. It may be that elevations in mood such as those caused by hypomania result in more creative thought; likewise, depressed mood and thinking usually lead to periods relatively bereft of creative work.

In all these facets of creative thought, the elements of fluency and flexibility of cognitive processing are emphasized. Clearly, the mere quickening and opening up of thought in an otherwise unimaginative person will not result in creative achievement. If the cognitive processes of an otherwise creative individual are hastened and loosened by hypomania, however, a qualitatively different result may well emerge. Hyperacusis, so often experienced during manic states, may contribute to creativity as well. Characteristics of a noncognitive nature—such as boldness, grandiosity of spirit and vision, disinhibition, impatience, abandonment of normal judgment and restraint, and recklessness—also link bipolar illness and creative accomplishment. The temperamental characteristics observed to be common in highly creative individuals—persistence, wit, self-confidence, a

pleasure in taking risk, high energy, independence, exuberance, rebelliousness, and playfulness[7] are also characteristic of many who have hypomanic and cyclothymic temperaments. Stanford researchers, for example, found that bipolar patients and highly creative individuals have more personality traits in common than do healthy normal controls and creative individuals (Nowakowska et al., 2005; see also Jamison, 2004).

It may be that the combination of experience, potentiating personality characteristics (see Chapter 10), and cognitive changes that occur during hypomania and may facilitate original thought gives rise to a subgroup of individuals with bipolar illness that is unusually creative. Two critical components of creativity—an independent, risk-taking, restless, and enthusiastic personality, and a fluent, disinhibited cognitive style—are found at an increased frequency in the bipolar population, thus producing some of the conditions that may lead to a disproportionate rate of creativity in a group otherwise characterized by damaging moods and behavior. Recent research lends credence to the importance of disinhibition, or an openness to incoming stimuli from the surrounding environment, to creativity. Carson and colleagues (2003), for example, found that highly creative Harvard students were seven times more likely to have low inhibition scores than less creative Harvard students. The investigators hypothesized that low inhibition, when coupled with extreme flexibility of thought, may lead to mental illness in some individuals and to creative accomplishment in others. Presumably it could also lead to the coexistence of creativity and mental illness in yet others. Likewise, the ability to function well on a few hours of sleep and to work at a high energy level are integral to most hypomanic states; they are also integral to putting ideas into action. In her studies of outstanding artists and scientists, for example, Anne Roe (1946, 1951, 1952) found one trait that stood out: the willingness and ability to work hard and to work long hours.

Throughout this book, we stress the recurrent, cyclic nature of manic-depressive illness—its natural course, pathophysiology, subjective experience, and seasonal and diurnal patterns. Integrally linked to this conception and of particular consequence here is the significance of contrasting, recurrent mood states. Cyclic patterns are common to both mood disorders and the nature of creative work. The ebbing and flowing character of inspiration, described so often, bears a striking resemblance to changes from the vitality to nonvitality of different seasons, death and rebirth, and the antithetical qualities of the bipolar mood states.

Clinical characteristics such as changes in mood, thinking, energy, and behavior are usually opposite in mania and depression. This is true for linguistic and artistic patterns as well. Manic patients, for example, tend not only to speak more and more rapidly, but also to use more colorful and powerful speech, including more action verbs and adjectives (see Chapter 2). Artistic expression also changes across mood states (see Table 12–8 and Plates 15–18). Manic patients tend to use vivid and highly contrasting colors; depressed patients, on the other hand, use primarily black and cold, darker colors (when the depression begins to clear, the palette tends to lighten accordingly). The content of paintings produced during mania tends to be more sexual, filled with motion and bright portrayals of natural phenomena such as fires, waterfalls, and landscapes; in contrast, paintings done during the depressed phase tend to show a paucity of ideas, a lack of motion, and themes of death and decay. Paintings produced by manic patients are usually done rapidly and impulsively and often have an agitated or swirling quality; paintings produced by depressed patients are relatively barren, are painted slowly, and exhibit less imagination. The contrasting nature of the elated and depressive states provides, for those with artistic or literary ability, a rich variety of experiences and sensations from which to create.

The ability to reconcile opposite states, whether they are of mood, thought, or vitality, is critical to any creative act.[8] Thomas Moore (1832), himself a poet, described this ability in his friend Byron:

TABLE 12–8. **Artistic Expression during Mania and Depression**

Feature	Mania	Depression
Color	Vivid, hot, sharply contrasting (Zimmerman and Garfinckle, 1942); wild (Reitman, 1950); highly colored, without the time to use a variety of colors (Dax, 1953); vivid (Plokker, 1965); bright, warm, optimistic (Enâchescu, 1971); color did not differentiate manic patients as a diagnostic group (Wadeson and Carpenter, 1976).	Somber (Reitman, 1950); somber, usually black with upper portion darkest (Dax, 1953); dark colors, upper portion of picture generally darker than lower, lightening of palette as depression begins to clear (Plokker, 1965); dark, dirty, cold, somber (Enâchescu, 1971); bipolar more colorful than unipolar (Wadeson and Carpenter, 1976).
Content	Sexual, setting sun, orifices (Zimmerman and Garfinckle, 1942); often obscene (Dax, 1953); flowers, landscapes, sunrises, fires, waterfalls, animals, people, dance scenes (Enâchescu, 1971).	Poverty of ideas (Reitman, 1950); immobile figures with sunken heads, signs of death, starless nights rather than days, trees broken off, no flowers (Dax, 1953); representations of delusions (sin, poverty, hypochondriasis), torture, suicide (Plokker, 1965); mourning scenes, physical or moral disaster, abandonment, physical decompensation (Enâchescu, 1971).
Affect	Positive, assured (Zimmerman and Garfinckle, 1942); excitement (Reitman, 1950); careless (Dax, 1953); euphoric (Enâchescu, 1971).	Useless, depressive, cold, gloomy (Enâchescu, 1971).
Form and activity	Extreme agitation, productive, fluid composition, swirl-like forms (Zimmerman and Garfinckle, 1942); restless, disordered, incoherent lines (Reitman, 1950); rapidly produced, lacking in restraint (Dax, 1953); deterioration in composition (Plokker, 1965); rapid and expansive, far more productive than in depressed phase; lines are rash, thick, and crossed (Enâchescu, 1971).	Bareness and lack of detail (Dax, 1953); rarely engaged in artistic activity (Plokker, 1965); less creative activity (Enâchescu, 1971).

It must be perceived by all endowed with quick powers of association how constantly, when any particular thought or sentiment presents itself to their minds, its very opposite, at the same moment, springs up there also; if anything sublime occurs, its neighbour, the ridiculous, is by its side; across a bright view of the present or the future, a dark one throws its shadow; and, even in questions respecting morals and conduct, all the reasonings and consequences that may suggest themselves on the side of one of two opposite courses will, in such minds, be instantly confronted by an array just as cogent on the other. A mind of this structure—and such more or less, are all those in which the reasoning is made subservient to the imaginative faculty—though enabled, by such rapid powers of association, to multiply its resources without end, has need of the constant exercise of a controlling judgment to keep its perceptions pure and undisturbed between the contrasts it thus simultaneously calls up.

The manic-depressive, or cyclothymic, temperament carries with it the capacity to react strongly and quickly; it is, in a biological sense, an alert and excitable system. It responds to the world with a wide range of emotional, perceptual, intellectual, behavioral, and energy changes, and it creates around itself both the possibilities and chaos afforded by altered experiences and fluctuating tempos. The constant transitions can be painful and confusing. Such chaos in those able ultimately to transcend it or shape it to their will can, however, result in an artistically useful comfort with transitions, an ease with ambiguities and with life on the edge, and an intuitive awareness of the coexisting and oppositional forces at work in the world.

Of interest, two recent studies found increased cyclothymia in creative individuals (Akiskal et al., 2005; Nowakowska et al., 2005). The relationship between the cyclic and contrasting nature of manic-depressive illness and creative work is discussed in much further detail by Jamison (1993).

Experiences Derived from Having the Illness

I do strongly feel that among the greatest pieces of luck for high achievement is ordeal. Certain great artists can make out without it, Titian and others, but mostly you need ordeal. My idea is this: The artist is extremely lucky who is presented with the worst possible ordeal which will not actually kill him. At that point, he's in business. Beethoven's deafness, Goya's deafness, Milton's blindness, that kind of thing. And I think that what happens in my poetic work in the future work will probably largely depend not on my sitting calmly on my ass as I think, "Hmm, hmm, a long poem again? Hmm," but on being

knocked in the face, and thrown flat, and given cancer, and all kinds of other things short of senile dementia. At that point, I'm out, but short of that, I don't know. I hope to be nearly crucified.—John Berryman (1976, p. 322)

Berryman, a contemporary of Robert Lowell and Theodore Roethke, was, like them, a winner of the Pulitzer Prize for poetry and someone who suffered from bipolar illness. At the end of a full but highly painful and tumultuous life, he committed suicide (as had his father and aunt before him). He was far from alone in believing that suffering could be conducive to creative work. Learning through intense and deep emotional experiences and using that learning to add meaning and depth to creative work is probably the aspect of the relationship between mood disorders and accomplishment most widely accepted and written about. The influence of pain's dominion fills novels, biographies and autobiographies, sermons, and canvases; there is no shortage of portrayals.

Profound depression or the suffering of psychosis can, and often does, fundamentally change expectations and beliefs about the nature and length of life, God, and other people. Many writers have described the impact of their long periods of depression, how they have dealt with them, and how they have used them in their work. Anne Sexton, a contemporary of Lowell, Roethke, and Berryman, was also a Pulitzer Prize winner in poetry and someone who almost certainly had bipolar illness. After many hospitalizations for both mania and depression, she, like Berryman, committed suicide. She described the importance of using pain in her work:

> I, myself, alternate between hiding behind my own hands, protecting myself any way possible, and this other, this seeing ouching other. I guess I mean that creative people must not avoid the pain that they get dealt. . . . Hurt must be examined like a plague. (Sexton and Ames, 1977, p. 105)

Robert Lowell, who wrote of depression, "I don't think it a visitation of the angels but a weakening in the blood," also wrote:

> Depression's no gift from the Muse. At worst, I do nothing. But often I've written, and wrote one whole book—*For the Union Dead*—about witheredness. . . . Most of the best poems, the most personal, are gathered crumbs from the lost cake. I had better moods, but the book is lemony, soured and dry, the drought I had touched with my own hands. That, too, may be poetry—on sufferance. (quoted in Giroux, 1987, p. 287)

Both Lowell and Sexton wrote of their heightened psychological sensitivity and vulnerability in graphic and quite similar physical metaphors: "seeing too much and feeling it/with one skin-layer missing" (Lowell) and "even illusion breaks its filament wings/on the raw skin of all I wouldn't know" (Sexton).

Hypomania and mania often generate ideas and associations, propel contact with life and other people, induce frenzied energies and enthusiasms, and cast an ecstatic, rather cosmic hue over life. Melancholy, on the other hand, tends to force a slower pace; cools the ardor; and puts into perspective the thoughts, observations, and feelings generated during more enthusiastic moments. Mild depression can act as ballast; it can also serve a critical editorial role for work produced in more fevered states. Depression prunes and sculpts; it also ruminates and ponders and, ultimately, subdues and focuses thought. It allows structuring, at a detailed level, of the more expansive patterns generated during hypomania.

Relative Importance of Different Aspects of the Illness to Various Types of Accomplishment

Changes brought about by bipolar illness—during hypomania, mania, depression, and normal states—produce different advantages and disadvantages in various fields of creative work and other types of accomplishment. Although there are no systematic data, a review of available studies strongly suggests that the actual prevalence of bipolar illness is distributed unequally across professions; for example, poets appear to have an unusually high rate, scientists a lower one. To a poet, the cognitive, energy, mood, and experiential advantages of the elated and depressive states may outweigh the disruptions, chaos, turmoil, and inconsistent productivity that would be insurmountable to most scientists. Pragmatic issues of education and job requirements also probably affect the rates of bipolar illness in various occupations. Composers and poets, while increasingly likely to obtain graduate levels of education or professional training, do not absolutely require it. On the other hand, medical and graduate schools—particularly those with highly structured programs, such as those for medicine and law—tend to select students who, by and large, have demonstrated an ability to conform to strict requirements for consistently high levels of performance over long periods of time. This may well exclude many individuals at risk or those with an actual history of bipolar illness, since they are more likely to show greater variability in their performance across seasons and years.

The risk period for a first manic or depressive episode overlaps considerably with the period of advanced education, eliminating some bipolar individuals from being selected. Further selection bias exists in the decisions made about those individuals who have actually had an affective episode, especially a manic one, while in training. The professional consequences of a psychotic break are generally different for those in medicine, clinical psychology, nursing, or law school than they are for those writing poetry or composing music.

Even within the field of literary accomplishment, differences in the characteristics of bipolar illness are likely to produce relative gains and losses for various types of writers. Poets may benefit much more than novelists from mood and cognitive changes, for example, because the language and rhythms of poetry are more akin to primitive thought processes and psychosis and because the nature of sustained work is probably different in poetry and fiction.

Certain aspects of bipolar illness probably are important and helpful in other fields of accomplishment as well. It is likely that mood changes (elevated and expansive mood, inflated self-esteem, increased enthusiasm, increased emotional intensity, and infectious mood) are equally, if differently, important to those who create and to those in business or positions of leadership. This is probably true as well for increased energy levels and a decreased need for sleep. On a very general level, however, cognitive changes (sharpened and unusually creative thinking, flight of ideas, and hyperacusis) are likely more useful to those in the arts and sciences than to those in positions of political and military leadership. Conversely, interpersonal changes brought about by hypomania (enhanced liveliness, uninhibited people seeking, interpersonal charm, the ability to find vulnerable spots in others and to make use of them, increased perceptiveness at the subconscious or unconscious level, and increased social ease) are probably more likely to benefit those in leadership positions than those in the arts and sciences.

IMPORTANCE OF STUDYING POSITIVE ASPECTS OF MANIC-DEPRESSIVE ILLNESS

Although it certainly is possible to exaggerate or romanticize the positive aspects of mood disorders, it is important not to minimize their beneficial features or deal with them in only a perfunctory way. Understanding the assets that may accompany manic-depressive illness—the characteristics linking it to the arts, leadership, and society at large—is important to a thorough understanding of the illness. Three principal areas of consideration are relevant to the study of the positive features of manic-depressive: theoretical, clinical, and social–ethical.

Theoretical Considerations

Positive aspects of manic-depressive illness, including associations with accomplishment, are, of course, interesting in their own right. At first glance, the notion of advantage gained from an otherwise catastrophic illness may appear counterintuitive, yet both history and clinical experience affirm the reality of this paradox. The association may be an infrequent one, but it is important. Most clinical research understandably has focused on the depressive spectrum and given relatively little emphasis to the manic continuum. There has been next to no study of the spectrum of elated states most relevant to the discussion here. Of the many still unexamined aspects of bipolar illness that could profitably be studied, its positive features are particularly germane. There has been little research into subtle oscillations in perception, mood, behavior, and cognition across the elated states. Quantitative and qualitative differences between the milder hypomanias and manias also require more study. Likewise, we need to learn to differentiate characteristics of high-functioning normal individuals—those with decreased need for sleep coupled with high energy, productivity, and mood—from the characteristics of individuals with hyperthymia, cyclothymia, or bipolar illness.

The existence of elated states also provides an opportunity for cognitive psychologists to study a long-standing theoretical question: Does cognition precede or follow mood change? The considerable body of literature on this question is based on studies of depression and, because of psychological assumptions about etiology, tends to assume that cognitive changes precede—indeed cause or facilitate—depressive affect. Similarly, many creative individuals and students of creativity assume that inspiration, creative ideas, and fluency of thinking precede euphoric affect. That is, many believe that the creative act generates euphoria, not that heightened mood facilitates the increased flow of thoughts and ideas. Notwithstanding these assumptions, evidence indicates that in a sizable proportion of highly creative writers and artists, elevated mood changes precede cognitive and behavioral changes, and that intense creative episodes are, in many instances, indistinguishable from hypomania (Richards and Kinney, 1990; Schuldberg, 1990; Jamison, 1993, 2004).

Yet another important theoretical issue, one with enormous practical ramifications, centers on the highly seductive, if not actually addictive, qualities of the elated or euphoric states. Such altered states of consciousness and mood can be highly potent reinforcers during euthymic or depressed periods, creating in some patients a strong desire to induce or recreate such conditions. This phenomenon is roughly analogous to drug self-administration, in which a highly pleasurable and often immediate state can be obtained. Thus for some patients, the positive aspects of the illness may be similar to stimulant addiction.

Clinical experience suggests that patients may attempt to induce mania by discontinuing lithium not just at times when they are depressed but also when they face problematic decisions and life events. Because the negative consequences are delayed, it is not always clear to the patient that the costs outweigh the benefits. The clinical implications of this phenomenon are discussed in the next section and in Chapters 21 and 22. Here it is important to mention that the addictive or addictive-like qualities of the elated states raise fascinating issues about the means used to self-induce these states (sleep deprivation, medication nonadherence, or psychological means), the relevance of this phenomenon to kindling models, and, of course, the use of cocaine and other stimulants to self-medicate or to induce euphoric and high-energy states. The high rate of affective illness in cocaine abuse (see Chapter 7) may reflect not only self-medication per se, but also an attempt to recapture a known, previously experienced and highly pleasurable mood state, a reality that makes bipolar individuals perhaps uniquely vulnerable to cocaine addiction on both psychological and biological grounds.

Clinical Considerations

The existence of potentiating positive features in bipolar illness, perceived to be or actually associated with increased creativity and productivity, affects the willingness of some afflicted with the illness to seek and comply with treatment. Many highly accomplished individuals in the arts, the sciences, and business are reluctant to seek treatment for their mood disorders because they are reluctant to give up the edge they feel they obtain from it. Others view their serious mood problems as part of the human condition, the price one pays for being "too sensitive," having an artistic temperament, or leading an artistic lifestyle. Indeed, many such individuals see emotional turmoil as essential to their identity as performing or creative artists. Additionally, many writers and artists are concerned that psychiatric treatment will erode or compromise their ability to create. An appreciation of the potentially productive or "up" side of mood disorders may lead to greater credibility on the part of the treating clinician, as well as a stronger therapeutic bond. Strict adherence to an often arbitrary distinction between psychopathology on the one hand and a chaotic, tumultuous, and artistic lifestyle on the other can lead to unnecessary suffering and treatment resistance.

Writers and artists frequently express concern about the effects of psychiatric treatment on their ability to create and produce; these concerns are especially pronounced when it comes to taking medication. Some of this mistrust no doubt reflects unfounded preconceptions, fears of altering long-established work patterns and rituals, or simple resistance to treatment. In some instances, however, these concerns are grounded in reality. A review of the literature on mood-stabilizing medications reveals disturbingly little research on the effects of the drugs on productivity and creativity.

Even the early lithium researchers were well aware of problems created by lithium's effects on certain useful or enjoyable qualities of the illness (e.g., decreasing or eliminating the highs of hypomania, decreasing sexuality and energy levels), as well as by the drug's untoward side effects (possible cognitive slowing and memory impairment) (see Chapters 9 and 21). Schou (1968, p. 78) described the subjective effects of lithium in three "normal" subjects (medical researchers). This description has relevance to highly creative individuals who are dependent on the mind and the senses for their work:

> The subjective experience was primarily one of indifference and slight general malaise. This led to a certain passivity. . . . The subjective feeling of having been altered by the treatment was disproportionately strong in relation to objective behavioral changes. The subjects could engage in discussions and social activities but found it difficult to comprehend and integrate more than a few elements of a situation. Intellectual initiative was diminished and there was a feeling of lowered ability to concentrate and memorize; but thought processes were unaffected, and the subjects could think logically and produce ideas.

It should be noted that Schou's study involved a relatively short-term trial of lithium, and there is some indication that patients partially accommodate to lithium's cognitive effects. Many patients, of course, experience no significant cognitive side effects, and for those who do, the risks of no treatment must always be weighed against those side effects.

What is actually known about the specific effects of lithium and other medications on productivity and creativity? Polatin and Fieve (1971, p. 864) described their clinical experience of using lithium in creative individuals:

> In the creative individual who does his best work in the course of a hypomanic period, the complaint regarding the continued use of lithium carbonate is that it acts as a "brake." These patients report that lithium carbonate inhibits creativity so that the individual is unable to express himself, drive is diminished, and there is no incentive. These patients also indicate that when they are depressed, the symptoms are so demoralizing and so uncomfortable that they welcome the "mild high" when the depression disappears and prefer to settle for a cyclothymic life of highs and lows rather than an apathetic middle-of-road mood state achieved through the use of lithium carbonate.
>
> Their argument is that if lithium carbonate prevents the high and may possibly prevent the "low," they prefer not to take lithium carbonate, since never to have a high as a result of the drug seems equivalent to being deprived

of an "addictive-like" pleasurable and productive state. Some of these patients are terrified of having a low again, but insist on taking their chances without lithium carbonate therapy, knowing that sooner or later they will be compensated by the high, even if they do go into a low state.

No controlled studies of lithium's effects on productivity have been conducted, but Marshall and colleagues (1970) and Schou (1979) studied a total of 30 artists, writers, and businessmen taking lithium. Their findings are summarized in Table 12–9. More than three-quarters (77 percent) of the patients reported no change or an increase in their productivity while on lithium. Approximately one-quarter reported a decrease. In 17 percent, lithium was seen as leading to problems sufficient to warrant refusal to take it. It is not known how accurately these figures reflect artists and writers at the upper end of creative accomplishment. Most of these subjects, although earning their living by their creative work, were not at that level. Schou (1979) pointed out that lithium may affect inspiration, the ability to execute, or both, and saw the following as contributing factors in a creative individual's response to lithium: the severity of illness, the type of illness, the artist's habits of using manic periods of inspiration, and individual sensitivity to the pharmacological action of the drug.

Three other studies of particular relevance for artistic creativity yielded conflicting results. Judd and colleagues (1977) found no effects of short-term lithium treatment on creativity in normal subjects. A study using bipolar patients as their own controls, however, found substantial detrimental effects of the drug on associational productivity and originality of responses (Shaw et al., 1986; see Fig. 12–9). These differing results may be due in part to the fact that lithium's effect on cognition is probably quite different in bipolar patients and normal controls (Pons et al., 1985). Lithium exerts effects not only on cognition, but also on drive and personality (see Chapter 10); although cognitive side effects are undeniably important to creative work, so, too, are these noncognitive effects. Kocsis and colleagues (1993) found that lithium discontinuation resulted in improvement on memory and creativity measures (although not idiosyncratic word associations), as well as motor performance. In an open, nonrandom case series of seven bipolar patients who reported cognitive dulling during lithium therapy, Stoll and colleagues (1996) concluded that the partial or full substitution of divalproex sodium for lithium as the primary mood stabilizer "reduced the cognitive, motivational, or creative deficits attributed to lithium" (p. 359). To our knowledge,

TABLE 12–9. Productivity While Taking Lithium

	Marshall et al. (1970)	Schou (1979)	Combined Number	%
Subjects	6 artists and businessmen	24 artists and writers	30	
Productivity on lithium				
Increased	5	12	17	57
No change	0	6	6	20
Decreased	1	6	7	23
Refused to continue lithium treatment	1	4	5	17

however, there has been no replication of this preliminary finding. Individual differences in clinical state, serum lithium levels, sensitivity to cognitive side effects, and the severity, frequency, and type of affective illness clearly affect the degree to which an individual will experience impairment in intellectual functioning, creativity, and productivity. Artists, writers, and many others who rely on their initiative, intellect, emotional intensity, and energy for their life's work underscore the need for a reexamination of this problem.

Artists and writers represent a group at high risk for affective illness and should be assessed and counseled accordingly. Ideal treatment requires a sensitive understanding

Figure 12–9. Associational patterns and lithium level. (*Source:* Adapted from Shaw et al., 1986. Reprinted with permission from the *American Journal of Psychiatry*, American Psychiatric Association.)

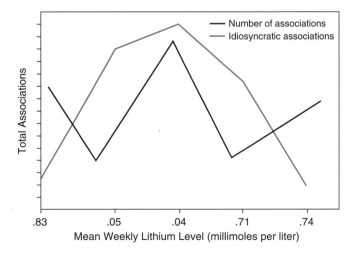

of the possible benefits of mood disorders to creativity and also the severe liabilities of untreated depression and mania, including the risk of suicide, hospitalization, and substance abuse. Moreover, the clinician must be aware of available medications and side effects that could potentially be damaging to the creative process. Physicians should minimize medication levels whenever possible.

Social and Ethical Considerations

As noted in Chapter 13, genetic research has progressed to the point that ethical issues are now arising about prenatal screening and selective abortion, as well as the identification and treatment of individuals at high risk for developing bipolar illness. It becomes particularly important under these circumstances to have at least some broad notion of the possible benefits, as well as catastrophic outcomes, of bipolar illness not only for potential parents and the unborn child, but also for society at large. The implications of losing societal variance in such basic characteristics as drive, cognitive style, energy, risk taking, and temperament have not yet been examined in any systematic way, although evolutionary perspectives on depression and bipolar illness have been discussed at some length.[9] Ironically, these issues were considered, to some extent, in the 1930s; in one study, carried out in Germany, the advisability of sterilizing manic-depressive individuals was examined. Luxenburger (1933) found manic-depressive illness to be greatly overrepresented in the higher occupational classes and recommended against sterilizing these patients, "especially if the patient does not have siblings who could transmit the positive aspects of the genetic heritage." Myerson and Boyle (1941, p. 20), in their study of manic-depressive psychosis in socially prominent American families, concurred:

> Perhaps the words of Bumke need to be taken into account before we embark too whole-heartedly on any sterilization program: "If we could extinguish the sufferers from manic-depressive psychosis from the world, we would at the same time deprive ourselves of an immeasurable amount of the accomplished and good, of color and warmth, of spirit and freshness. Finally only dried up bureaucrats and schizophrenics would be left. Here I must say that I would rather accept into the bargain the diseased manic-depressive than to give up the healthy individuals of the same heredity cycle."

Treatable common illnesses such as bipolar illness—ones that may confer societal and individual advantage and that vary greatly in the nature of their expression and their severity—are particularly problematic. Francis Collins (1990), director of the U.S. National Human Genome Research Institute and a scientist who was instrumental in identifying the genes for cystic fibrosis and neurofibromatosis, was asked in an interview about prenatal testing for diseases that vary in severity or that first occur only later in life:

> This is where it gets muddy, and everyone is going to draw the line differently. Consider the situation with manic-depressive illness, a reasonably common disorder. It is clearly genetically influenced, though not in a simple way. Now, manic-depressive illness can be a terrible cross to bear. The swings into depression are awful, and the highs can be very destructive. Yet a substantial number of highly creative people have suffered from this disease. Suppose we find the gene responsible for manic depression. If every couple has a prenatal test to determine if a fetus is at risk for manic depression, and if every time the answer is yes that fetus is done away with, then we will have done something troubling, something with large consequences. Is this what we want to do?

CONCLUSIONS

There is strong scientific and biographical evidence linking mood disorders to artistic creativity. Biographies of eminent poets, composers, and artists attest to the prevalence of extremes of mood in creative individuals. Systematic studies are increasingly documenting the link as well. It should be emphasized, however, that most creative writers, artists, and musicians have no significant psychopathology. Conversely, most individuals with manic-depressive illness are not unusually creative.

We have considered the issue of the reliability—indeed, the advisability—of making a posthumous diagnosis of manic-depressive illness. This concern is important and valid. Labeling as manic-depressive anyone who is unusually creative, accomplished, energetic, intense, moody, or eccentric both diminishes the notion of individuality within the arts and trivializes a very serious, often lethal illness. We have been careful to base our conclusions and suggestions on what is known clinically and scientifically about depression and bipolar disorder.

That the illness and its related temperaments are associated with creativity appears clear; the clinical, ethical, and social implications of this association are less so. We have tried to convey that bipolar disorder and depression are destructive, painful, sometimes fatal, and yet intriguing and important illnesses. In the great majority of instances, the effective treatments now available will not hinder creative ability. Indeed, treatment almost always results in longer periods of sustained productivity. One of our concerns, however, remains the study, public discussion, and development of treatments that will minimize the side effects of currently available medications.

The neurochemical and anatomical processes responsible for the cognitive changes occurring during manic and highly creative states are poorly understood. It remains for molecular biology, neuropsychology, and quickly evolving neuroimaging techniques to provide us with a more sophisticated understanding of the underlying changes in thought and behavior that are enhanced, left unaffected, or impaired by shifting patterns of mood (see, e.g., Hoffman et al., 2001; Folley et al., 2003; Ghacibeh et al., 2006).

Perhaps some suffering must always accompany great artistic achievement. Certainly, depth and intensity of human feeling must be a part of creation in the arts. But modern medicine now allows relief of the extremes of despair, turmoil, and psychosis. It allows choices not previously available. Most of the writers, artists, and composers discussed in this chapter had no such choices.

NOTES

1. George Gordon, Lord Byron. "Manfred," act II, scene 4, lines 160–161. *Lord Byron: The Complete Poetical Works*, vol. 4, p. 86. Edited by Jerome J. McGann. Oxford: Clarendon Press, 1986.
2. Much of the discussion of manic-depressive illness and creativity in this chapter is based on Jamison's elaboration, in *Touched with Fire*, of the arguments originally presented in the first edition of *Manic-Depressive Illness*.
3. Fully 70 to 90 percent of all suicides are associated with bipolar or depressive illness; therefore, if an individual has died by suicide, it is usually the case that a mood disorder was at least contributory.
4. An episodic, cyclic course of symptoms with normal functioning in between; usual onset of symptoms in the late

teens or early twenties, with temperamental signs often exhibited much earlier; seasonal aspects to the mood and energy changes; and if untreated, a worsening of the illness over time. (See Chapter 4.)

5. This study was brought to the attention of the authors by Dr. Zoltán Rihmer.

6. Isen and Daubman, 1984; Isen et al., 1985, 1987; Greene and Noice, 1988; Fodor, 1999; Isen, 1999; Fodor and Laird, 2004.

7. Roe, 1946, 1951, 1952; MacKinnon, 1962; Getzels and Jackson, 1963; Hudson, 1966; Barron, 1968; Welsh, 1977, Gardner, 1993; Winner, 1996; Jamison, 2004.

8. Among the many writers who have emphasized the importance of the reconciliation of opposite states in the creative process are Aristotle, "On the Art of Poetry," *Classical Literary Criticism*, translated by T. S. Dorsch, London: Penguin, 1965; Percy Bysshe Shelley, "A Defence of Poetry," *Shelley's Critical Prose*, edited by B.R. McElderry (1821; reprint, Lincoln: University of Nebraska Press, 1967); Maurice Bowra, *The Romantic Imagination*, Cambridge: Harvard University Press, 1950; J.P. Guilford, Traits of creativity, in H.H. Anderson (Ed.), *Creativity and its Cultivation*, New York: Harper, 1959; F. Barron, *Creative Person and Creative Process*, New York: Holt, Rinehart & Winston, 1969; A. Koestler, *The Act of Creation*, New York: Dell, 1971; A. Storr, *The Dynamics of Creation*, London: Penguin, 1972; A. Rothenberg, *The Emerging Goddess*, Chicago: University of Chicago Press, 1979; J. Carey, *John Donne: Life, Mind and Art*, London: Faber and Faber, 1981; K. Miller, *Doubles: Studies in Literary History*, Oxford: Oxford University Press, 1985.

9. Price, 1967, 1972; Gardner, 1982; Jamison, 1993; Wilson, 1993; Price et al., 1994; Brody, 2001; Watson and Andrews, 2002; Gilbert, 2004, 2006; Keller and Nesse, 2005; Keller and Miller, 2006.

RESOURCES FOR INFORMATION ABOUT BIPOLAR DISORDER AND RELATED TOPICS

Organizations

American Academy of Child and Adolescent Psychiatry
3615 Wisconsin Avenue, N.W.
Washington, D.C. 20016-3007
Phone: 202-966-7300
Fax: 202-966-2891
http://www.aacap.org/

American Foundation for Suicide Prevention
(AFSP)
120 Wall Street, 22nd Floor
New York, NY 10005
Phone: 888-333-2377
Fax: 212-363-6237
www.afsp.org

Anxiety Disorders Association of America
8730 Georgia Avenue, Suite 600
Silver Spring, MD 20910-3604
Phone: 240-485-1001
Fax: 240-485-1035
www.adaa.org

American Psychiatric Association
1000 Wilson Blvd., Suite 1825
Arlington, VA 22209-3901
Phone: 888-357-7924
www.psych.org
www.healthyminds.org

American Psychological Association
750 First Street, N.E.
Washington, DC 20002-4242
Phone: 800-374-2721
www.apa.org
www.apahelpcenter.org

Bipolar Disorders Information Center
http://www.mhsource.com/bipolar/

Bipolar Kids
http://www.geocities.com/enchantedforest/1068/

Bipolar News
http://www.bipolarnews.org/

Bipolar Significant Others
http://www.bpso.org/

Centers for Disease Control and Prevention
National Center for Injury Control
and Prevention
Mailstop K65
4770 Buford Highway NE
Atlanta, GA 30341-3724
Phone: 800-232-4636
Fax: 770-488-1667
www.cdc.gov/ncipc

Center for Mental Health Services
P.O. Box 42557
Washington, DC 20015
Phone: 800-789-2647
Fax: 240-747-5470
http://www.mentalhealth.samhsa.gov/

Child and Adolescent Bipolar Foundation (CABF)
1000 Skokie Blvd., Suite 570
Wilmette, IL 60091
Phone: 847-256-8525
Fax: 847-920-9498
www.cabf.org

Depression and Bipolar Support Alliance (DBSA)
730 N. Franklin Street, Suite 501
Chicago, IL 60610-7224
Phone: 800-826-3632
Fax: 312-642-7243
http://www.dbsalliance.org

Depression and Related Affective Disorders
Association (DRADA)
8201 Greensboro Drive, Suite 300
McLean, VA 22102
Phone: 888-288-1104
http://www.drada.org/

Expert Consensus Guideline Series
http://www.psychguides.com/

International Foundation for Research
and Education on Depression (iFred)
7040 Bembe Beach Road, Suite 100
Annapolis, MD 21403
Phone: 800-789-2647
Fax: 443-782-0739
http://www.ifred.org/

Juvenile Bipolar Research Foundation (JBRF)
550 Ridgewood Road
Maplewood, NJ 07040
Phone: 866-333-5273
Fax: 973-275-0420
http://www.bpchildresearch.org/

Medscape Psychiatry & Mental Health
http://www.medscape.com/psychiatry

Mood Garden
www.moodgarden.org

National Alliance for Research on Schizophrenia
and Depression (NARSAD)
60 Cutter Mill Road, Suite 404
Great Neck, NY 11021
Phone: 800-829-8289
Fax: 516-487-6930
http://www.narsad.org/

National Alliance on Mental Illness (NAMI)
Colonial Place Three
2107 Wilson Blvd., Suite 300
Arlington, VA 22201-3042
Phone: 703-524-7600
Fax: 703-524-9094
www.nami.org

National Institute of Mental Health (NIMH)
Public Information and Communications Branch
6001 Executive Boulevard, Room 8184, MSC 9663
Bethesda, MD 20892-9663
Phone: 866-615-6464
Fax: 301-443-4279
www.nimh.nih.gov

National Institute on Alcohol Abuse
and Alcoholism (NIAAA)
5635 Fishers Lane, MSC 9304
Bethesda, MD 20892-9304
www.niaaa.nih.gov

National Institute on Drug Abuse
National Institutes of Health
6001 Executive Boulevard, Room 5213
Bethesda, MD 20892-9561
Phone: 301-443-1124
www.nida.nih.gov

National Mental Health Association (NMHA)
2000 N. Beauregard Street, 6th Floor
Alexandria, VA 22311
Phone: 703-684-7722
Fax: 703-684-5968
http://www.nmha.org/

Parents Med Guide
www.parentsmedguide.org.

Pendulum Resources
http://pendulum.org/

Screening for Mental Health, Inc.
One Washington Street, Suite 304
Wellesley Hills, MA 02481

Phone: 781-239-0071
Fax: 781-431-7447
www.nmisp.org

Stanley Medical Research Institute
8401 Connecticut Avenue, Suite 200
Chevy Chase, MD 20815
Phone: 301-571-0760
Fax: 301-571-0769
http://www.stanleyresearch.org/

Substance Abuse and Mental Health Services
Administration
1 Choke Cherry Road
Rockville, MD 20857
Phone: 800-273-8255
www.samhsa.gov

Suicide Awareness Voices of Education
9001 E. Bloomington Freeway, Suite 150
Bloomington, MN 55420
Phone: 952-946-7998
www.save.org

Suicide Prevention Action Network USA (SPAN USA)
1025 Vermont Avenue, N.W., Suite 1066
Washington, DC 20005
Phone: 202-449-3600
Fax: 202-449-3601
www.spanusa.org

Surgeon General of the United States
www.surgeongeneral.gov

Systemic Enhancement Program for Bipolar
Disorder (STEP-BD)
http://www.stepbd.org/

Recommended Reading for Patients and Families

Barondes, S.H. (1998). *Mood Genes: Hunting for Origins of Mania and Depression*. New York: Oxford University Press.

Basco, M.R., and Rush, A.J. (1996).*Cognitive-Behavioral Therapy for Bipolar Disorder*. New York: Guilford Press.

Bauer, M., and McBride, L. (1996). *Structured Group Psychotherapy for Bipolar Disorder: The Life Goals Program*. New York: Springer Publishing Company.

Beers, C. (1981). *A Mind that Found Itself*. Pittsburgh: University of Pittsburgh Press (first published, 1908).

Casey, N. (2001). *Unholy Ghost: Writers on Depression*. New York: Harper Collins.

Coate, M. (1964). *Beyond All Reason*. London: Constable.

Copeland, M.E. (1994). *Living without Depression and Manic-Depression: A Workbook for Maintaining Mood Stability*. Oakland, CA: New Harbinger Publications.

Cronkite, K. (1994). *On the Edge of Darkness: Conversations about Conquering Depression*. New York: Doubleday.

Custance, J. (1952). *Wisdom, Madness, and Folly: The Philosophy of a Lunatic*. New York: Farrar, Straus & Cudahy.

Danquah, M.N.-A. (1998). *Willow Weep for Me: A Black Woman's Journey through Depression*. New York: W. W. Norton.

Dees, M., Canfield, C., and Rowe, V. (1999). *Texas Medication Algorithm Project (TMAP) Consumer-to-Consumer Discussion Materials Peer Facilitator Guide*. Austin, TX: Texas Department of Mental Health and Mental Retardation (TDMHMR).

DePaulo, R., and Horvitz, L.A. (2002). *Understanding Depression: What We Know and What You Can Do About It*. New York: John Wiley & Sons.

Duke, P., and Hochman, G. (1992). *A Brilliant Madness: Living with Manic-Depressive Illness*. New York: Bantam Books.

Evans, D.L., and Andrews, L. W. (2005). *If Your Adolescent Has Depression or Bipolar Disorder: An Essential Resource for Parents*. New York: Oxford University Press.

Fieve, R.R. (1997). *Moodswing*, 2nd Edition. New York: Bantam Books.

Fitzgerald, F.S. (first published in 1936; reissued in 1965). *The Crack-Up. In: The Crack-Up with Other Pieces and Stories*. Middlesex, London: Penguin.

Goodwin, G. and Sachs, G. (2004). *Fast Facts: Bipolar Disorder*. Oxford: Health Press, UK.

Hamilton, I. (1982). *Robert Lowell: A Biography*. New York: Random House.

Head, J. (2004). *Standing in the Shadows: Black Men and Depression*. New York: Broadway.

Hinshaw, S.P. (2002). *The Years of Silence Are Past: My Father's Life with Bipolar Disorder*. Cambridge, MA: Cambridge University Press.

Irwin, C., with Evans, D.L., and Andrews, L.W. (2007). *Monochrome Days: A Firsthand Account of One Teenager's Experience with Depression*. New York: Oxford University Press.

Jamieson, P.E., with Rynn, M.A. (2006). *Mind Race: A Firsthand Account of One Teenager's Experience with Bipolar Disorder*. New York: Oxford University Press.

Jamison, K.R. (1993). *Touched with Fire: Manic-Depressive Illness and the Artistic Temperament*. New York: Free Press.

Jamison, K.R. (1995). *An Unquiet Mind: A Memoir of Moods and Madness*. New York: Alfred A. Knopf.

Jamison, K.R. (1999). *Night Falls Fast: Understanding Suicide*. New York: Alfred A. Knopf.

Logan, J. (1976). *Josh: My Up and Down, In and Out Life*. New York: Delacorte Press.

Manning, M. (1994). *Undercurrents: A Therapist's Reckoning with Her Own Depression*. New York: Harper Collins.

McDonnell, F. (2003). *Threads of Hope: Learning to Live with Depression*. London: Short Books.

McManamy, J. (2006). *Living Well with Depression and Bipolar Disorder: What Your Doctor Doesn't Tell You*. New York: Collins.

Miklowitz, D.J., and Goldstein, M.J. (2006). *Bipolar Disorder: A Family-Focused Treatment Approach*. New York: Guilford Press.

Milligan, S., and Clare, A. (1993). *Depression and How to Survive It*. London: Ebury Press.

Mondimore, F. (2006). *Depression: Mood Disease*. Baltimore: Johns Hopkins University Press.

Mondimore, F.M. (2006). *Bipolar Disorder: A Guide for Patients and Families*. Baltimore: Johns Hopkins Press Health Book.

O'Brien, S. (2004). *The Family Silver: A Memoir of Depression and Inheritance.* Chicago: University of Chicago Press.

Papolos, D., and Papolos, J. (2006). *The Bipolar Child: The Definitive and Reassuring Guide to Childhood's Most Misunderstood Disorder.* 3rd Edition. New York: Broadway Books (a division of Random House).

Phelps, J. (2006). *Why Am I Still Depressed? Recognizing and Managing the Ups and Downs of Bipolar II and Soft Bipolar Disorder.* New York: McGraw-Hill.

Raeburn, P. (2004). *Acquainted With the Night: A Parent's Quest to Understand Depression and Bipolar Disorder in his Children.* New York: Broadway.

Rosenthal, N. (2005). *Winter Blues: Seasonal Affective Disorder: What It Is and How to Overcome It.* New York: Guilford Press.

Sheffield, A. (1999). *How You Can Survive When They're Depressed: Living and Coping with Depression Fallout.* New York: HarperCollins.

Solomon, A. (2001). *The Noonday Demon: An Anatomy of Depression.* New York: Scribner.

Styron, W. (1990). *Darkness Visible: A Memoir of Madness.* New York: Random House.

Vonnegut, M. (1975). *The Eden Express.* New York: Laurel Books.

Waltz, M. (1999). *Bipolar Disorders: A Guide to Helping Children and Adolescents.* Sebastopol, CA: O'Reilly & Associates, Inc.

Whybrow, P.C. (1997). *A Mood Apart: The Thinker's Guide to Emotion and Its Disorders.* New York: HarperCollins.

Wolpert, L. (1999). *Malignant Sadness.* New York: Free Press.

Wyatt, R.J., and Chew, R.H. (2005). *Wyatt's Practical Psychiatric Practice.* Washington, DC: American Psychiatric Publishing.

CHAPTER 1

Abrams, R., and Taylor, M.A. (1974). Unipolar mania: A preliminary report. *Arch Gen Psychiatry, 30,* 441–443.

Abrams, R., and Taylor, M.A. (1979). Differential EEG patterns in affective disorder and schizophrenia. *Arch Gen Psychiatry, 36,* 1355–1358.

Abrams, R., and Taylor, M.A. (1980). A comparison of unipolar and bipolar depressive illness. *Am J Psychiatry, 137,* 1084–1087.

Abrams, R., Taylor, M.A., Hayman, M.A., and Krishna, N.R. (1979). Unipolar mania revisited. *J Affect Disord, 1,* 59–68.

Ackerknecht, E.H. (1959). *A Short History of Psychiatry.* New York: Hafner Publishing Co.

Ackerknecht, E.H. (1982). *A Short History of Medicine.* Revised edition. Baltimore: Johns Hopkins University Press.

Agosti, V., and Stewart, J.W. (2001). Atypical and non-atypical subtypes of depression: Comparison of social functioning, symptoms, course of illness, co-morbidity and demographic features. *J Affect Disord, 65*(1), 75–79.

Akiskal, H.S. (1981). Subaffective disorders: Dysthymic, cyclothymic and bipolar II disorders in the "borderline" realm. *Psychiatr Clin North Am, 4,* 25–46.

Akiskal, H.S. (1983a). Dysthymic and cyclothymic disorders: A paradigm for high-risk research in psychiatry. In J.M. Davis and J.W. Mass (Eds.), *The Affective Disorders* (pp. 211–231). Washington, DC: The American Psychiatric Press.

Akiskal, H.S. (1983b). Diagnosis and classification of affective disorders: New insights from clinical and laboratory approaches. *Psychiatr Dev, 2,* 123–160.

Akiskal, H.S. (1983c). Dysthymic disorder: Psychopathology of proposed chronic depressive subtypes. *Am J Psychiatry, 140,* 11–20.

Akiskal, H.S. (1994). The temperamental borders of affective disorders. *Acta Psychiatr Scand Suppl, 379),* 32–37.

Akiskal, H.S. (1995). Toward a temperament-based approach to depression: Implications for neurobiologic research. *Adv Biochem Psychopharmacol, 49,* 99–112.

Akiskal, H.S. (1998). Toward a definition of generalized anxiety disorder as an anxious temperament type. *Acta Psychiatr Scand, 98*(Suppl. 393), 66–73.

Akiskal, H.S. (2000). *Mood Disorders: Clinical Features in Sadock & Sadock in Kaplan's Comprehensive Textbook of Psychiatry* (Edition VII). Baltimore: Williams & Wilkins, pp. 1338–1377.

Akiskal, H.S. (2001). Dysthymia and cyclothymia in psychiatric practice a century after Kraepelin. *J Affect Disord, 62,* 17–31.

Akiskal, H.S. (2003). Validating "hard" and "soft" phenotypes within the bipolar spectrum: Continuity or discontinuity? *J Affect Disord, 73:*1–5.

Akiskal, H.S., and Akiskal, K. (1988). Reassessing the prevalence of bipolar disorders: Clinical significance and artistic creativity. *Psychiatr Psychobiol, 3,* 29s–36s.

Akiskal, K.K., and Akiskal, H.S. (2005). The theoretical underpinnings of affective temperaments: Implications for evolutionary foundations of bipolar disorder and human nature. *J Affect Disord, 85*(1-2), 231–239.

Akiskal, H.S., and Benazzi, F. (2004). Validating Kraepelin's two types of depressive mixed states: "Depression with flight of ideas" and "excited depression." *World J Biol Psychiatry, 5*(2), 107–113.

Akiskal, H.S., and Benazzi F. (2005). Atypical depression: A variant of bipolar II or a bridge between unipolar and bipolar II? *J Affect Disord, 84*(2-3), 209–217.

Akiskal, H.S., and Benazzi, F. (2006). The DSM-IV and ICD-10 categories of recurrent (major) depressive and bipolar II disorders: Evidence that they lie on a dimensional spectrum. *J Affect Disord, 92*(1), 45–54.

Akiskal, H.S., and Mallya, G. (1987). Criteria for the "soft" bipolar spectrum: Treatment implications. *Psychopharmacol Bull, 23,* 68–73.

Akiskal, H.S., and Pinto, O. (1999). The evolving bipolar spectrum: Prototypes I, II, III, IV. *Psychiatr Clin North Am, 22,* 517–534.

Akiskal, H.S., Djenderedjian, A.H., Rosenthal, R.H., and Khani, M.K. (1977). Cyclothymic disorder: Validating criteria for inclusion in the bipolar affective group. *Am J Psychiatry*, 134, 1227–1233.

Akiskal, H.S., Bitar, A.H., Puzantian, V.R., Rosenthal, T.L., and Walker, P.W. (1978). The nosological status of neurotic depression: A prospective three-to-four-year follow-up examination in light of the primary–secondary and unipolar–bipolar dichotomies. *Arch Gen Psychiatry*, 35, 756–766.

Akiskal, H.S., Khani, M.K., and Scott-Strauss, A. (1979a). Cyclothymic temperamental disorders. *Psychiatr Clin North Am*, 2, 527–554.

Akiskal, H.S., Rosenthal, R.H., Rosenthal, T.L., Kashgarian, M., Khani, M.K., and Puzantian, V.R. (1979b). Differentiation of primary affective illness from situational, symptomatic, and secondary depressions. *Arch Gen Psychiatry*, 36, 635–643.

Akiskal, H.S., Walker, P., Puzantian, V.R., King, D., Rosenthal, T.L., and Dranon, M. (1983). Bipolar outcome in the course of depressive illness: Phenomenologic, familial, and pharmacologic predictors. *J Affect Disord*, 5, 115–128.

Akiskal, H.S., Downs, J., Jordan, P., Watson, S., Daugherty, D., and Pruitt, D.B. (1985). Affective disorders in referred children and younger siblings of manic-depressives: Mode of onset and prospective course. *Arch Gen Psychiatry*, 42, 996–1003.

Akiskal, H.S., Maser, J.D., Zeller, P.J., Endicott, J., Coryell, W., Keller, M., Warshaw, M., Clayton, P., and Goodwin, F.K. (1995). Switching from 'unipolar' to bipolar II. *Arch Gen Psychiatry*, 52, 114–123.

Akiskal, H.S., Hantouche, E., Bourgeois, M., Azorin, J.M., Sechter, D., Allilaire, J.F., Lancrenon, S., Fraud, J.P., and Chatenet-Duchene, L. (1998a). Gender, temperament and the clinical picture in dysphoric mixed mania: Findings from a French national study (EPIMAN). *J Affect Disord*, 50, 175–186.

Akiskal, H.S., Placidi, G.F., Signoretta, S., Liguori, A., Gervasi, R., Maremmani, I., Mallya, G., and Puzantian, V.R. (1998b). TEMPS-I: Delineating the most discriminant traits of cyclothymic, depressive, irritable and hyperthymic temperaments in a nonpatient population. *J Affect Disord*, 51, 7–19.

Akiskal, H.S., Bourgeois, M.L., Angst, J., Post, R., Moller, H.J., and Hirschfeld, R.M.A. (2000). Re-evaluating the prevalence of and diagnostic composition within the broad clinical spectrum of bipolar disorders. *J Affect Disord*, 59(Suppl. 1), 5s–30s.

Akiskal, H.S., Hantouche, E.G., Allilaire, J.F., Sechter, D., Bourgeois, M.L., Azorin, J.M., Chatenet-Duchene, L., and Lancrenon, S. (2003a). Validating antidepressant-associated hypomania (bipolar III): A systematic comparison with spontaneous hypomania (bipolar II). *J Affect Disord*, 73, 65–74.

Akiskal, H.S., Hantouche, E.G., and Lancrenon, S. (2003b). Bipolar II with and without cyclothymic temperament: "Dark" and "sunny" expressions of soft bipolarity. *J Affect Disord*, 73, 49–57.

Akiskal, H.S., Hantouche, E.G., and Allilaire J.F. (2003c). Bipolar II with and without cyclothymic temperament: "Dark" and "sunny" expressions of soft bipolarity. *J Affect Disord*, 73(1-2), 49–57.

Akiskal, H.S., Mendlowicz, M.V., Jean-Louis, G., Rapaport, M.H., Kelsoe, J.R., Gillin, J.C., and Smith, T.L. (2005). TEMPS-A: Validation of a short version of a self-rated instrument designed to measure variations in temperament. *J Affect Disord*, 85(1-2), 45–52.

Alda, M. (2004). The phenotypic spectra of bipolar disorder. *Eur Neuropsychopharmacol*, 14 (Suppl. 2), s94–s99.

Alexander, F.G., and Selesnick, S.T. (1966). *The History of Psychiatry: An Evaluation of Psychiatric Thought and Practice from Prehistoric Times to the Present*. New York: Harper & Row.

Altshuler, L.L., Gitlin, M.J., Mintz, J., Leight, K.L., and Frye, M.A. (2002). Subsyndromal depression is associated with functional impairment in patients with bipolar disorder. *J Clin Psychiatry*, 63, 807–811.

Andreasen, N.C., Grove, W.M., Shapiro, R.W., Keller, M.B., Hirschfeld, R.M.A., and McDonald-Scott, P. (1981). Reliability of lifetime diagnosis: A multicultural collaborative perspective. *Arch Gen Psychiatry*, 38, 400–405.

Andreasen, N.C., Grove, W.M., Coryell, W.H., Endicott, J., and Clayton, P.J. (1988). Bipolar versus unipolar and primary versus secondary affective disorder: Which diagnosis takes precedence? *J Affect Disord*, 15, 69–80.

Angst, J. (1966). *Zur Atiologie und Nosologie endogener depressiver Psychnose*. Berlin: Springer-Verlag.

Angst, J. (1978). The course of affective disorders: II. Typology of bipolar manic-depressive illness. *Arch Psychiatr Nervenkr*, 226, 65–73.

Angst, J. (1998). The emerging epidemiology of hypomania and bipolar II disorder. *J Affect Disord*, 50, 143–151.

Angst, J., and Marneros, A. (2001). Bipolarity from ancient to modern times: Conception, birth and rebirth. *J Affect Disord*, 67, 3–19.

Angst, J., Felder, W., Frey, R., and Stassen, H.H. (1978). The course of affective disorders: I. Change of diagnosis of monopolar, unipolar, and bipolar illness. *Arch Psychiatr Nervenkr*, 226, 57–64.

Angst, F., Stassen, H.H., Clayton, P.J., and Angst, J. (2002). Mortality of patients with mood disorders: Follow-up over 34–38 years. *J Affect Disord*, 68(2-3), 167–181.

Angst, J., Gamma, A., Benazzi, F., Ajdacic, V., Eich, D., and Rossler, W. (2003). Toward a re-definition of subthreshold bipolarity: Epidemiology and proposed criteria for bipolar-II, minor bipolar disorders and hypomania. *J Affect Disord*, 73, 133–146.

Angst, J., Gerber-Werder, R., Zuberbuhler, H.U., and Gamma, A. (2004). Is bipolar I disorder heterogeneous? *Eur Arch Psychiatry Clin Neurosci*, 254(2), 82–91.

Angst, J., Sellaro, R., Stassen, H., and Gamma, A. (2005). Diagnostic conversion from depression to bipolar disorders: Results of a long-term prospective study of hospital admissions. *J Affect Disord*, 84(2-3), 149–157.

Arato, M., Demeter, E., Rihmer, Z., and Somogyi, E. (1988). Retrospective psychiatric assessment of 200 suicides in Budapest. *Acta Psychiatr Scand*, 77(4), 454–456.

Baillarger, J. (1854). De la folie a double forme. *Annales Medico-Psychologiques*, 6, 369–391.

Baldessarini, R.J. (2000). A plea for integrity of the bipolar disorder concept. *Bipolar Disord*, 2(1), 3–7.

Baldessarini, R.J., Tondo, L., Floris, G., and Hennen, J. (2000). Effects of rapid cycling on response to lithium maintenance treatment in 360 bipolar I and II disorder patients. *J Affect Disord*, 61(1-2), 13–22.

Bauer, M.S., Simon, G.E., Ludman, E., and Unutzer, J. (2005). 'Bipolarity' in bipolar disorder: Distribution of manic and depressive symptoms in a treated population. *Br J Psychiatry*, 187, 87–88.

Beigel, A., and Murphy, D.L. (1971a). Assessing clinical characteristics of the manic state. *Am J Psychiatry*, 128, 688–694.

Beigel, A., and Murphy, D.L. (1971b). Unipolar and bipolar affective illness: Differences in clinical characteristics accompanying depression. *Arch Gen Psychiatry*, 24, 215–220.

Benazzi, F. (1997). Prevalence of bipolar II disorder in outpatient depression: A 203-case study in private practice. *J Affect Disord*, 46, 73–77.

Benazzi, F. (1999). A comparison of the age of onset of bipolar I and bipolar II outpatients. *J Affect Disord*, 54(3), 249–253.

Benazzi, F. (2001). Is 4 days the minimum duration of hypomania in bipolar II disorder? *Eur Arch Psychiatry Clin Neurosci*, 251, 32–34.

Benazzi, F. (2003a). Major depressive disorder with anger: A bipolar spectrum disorder? *Psychother Psychosom*, 72, 300–306.

Benazzi, F. (2003b). Unipolar depression with bipolar family history: Links with the bipolar spectrum. *Psychiatry Clin Neurosci*, 57(5), 497–503.

Benazzi, F., and Akiskal, H.S. (2001). Delineating bipolar II mixed states in the Ravenna–San Diego collaborative study: The relative prevalence and diagnostic significance of hypomanic features during major depressive episodes. *J Affect Disord*, 67, 115–122.

Benazzi, F., and Akiskal, H.S. (2003). Refining the evaluation of bipolar II: Beyond the strict SCID-CV guidelines for hypomania. *J Affect Disord*, 73, 33–38.

Benazzi, F., and Akiskal, H.S. (2005). A downscaled practical measure of mood lability as a screening tool for bipolar II. *J Affect Disord*, 84, 225–232.

Berrios, G.E., and Hauser, R. (1988). The early development of Kraepelin's ideas on classification: A conceptual history. *Psychol Med*, 18, 813–821.

Biondi, M., Picardi, A., Pasquini, M., Gaetano, P., and Pancheri, P. (2005). Dimensional psychopathology of depression: Detection of an 'activation' dimension in unipolar depressed outpatients. *J Affect Disord*, 84(2-3), 133–139.

Bleuler, E. (1924). *Textbook of Psychiatry* (4th German Edition). English edited by A.A. Brill. New York: Macmillan.

Brockington, I.F., Altman, E., Hillier, V., Meltzer, H.Y., and Nand, S. (1982). The clinical picture of bipolar affective disorder in its depressed phase: A report from London and Chicago. *Br J Psychiatry*, 141, 558–562.

Cantor, N., and Genero, N. (1986). Psychiatric diagnosis and natural categorization: A close analogy. In T. Millon and G.L. Klerman (Eds.), *Contemporary Directions in Psychopathology: Toward the DSM-IV* (pp. 233–256). New York: Guilford Press.

Cassano, G.B., Musetti, L., Perugi, G., Soriani, A., Mignani, V., McNair, D.M., and Akiskal, H.S. (1988). A proposed new approach to the clinical subclassification of depressive illness. *Pharmacopsychiatry*, 21, 19–23.

Cassano, G.B., Akiskal, H.S., Savino, M., Musetti, L., Perugi, G., and Soriani, A. (1992). Proposed subtypes of bipolar II and related disorders: With hypomanic episodes (or cyclothymia) and with hyperthymic temperament. *J Affect Disord*, 26, 127–140.

Cassano, G.B., Dell'Osso, L., Frank, E., Miniati, M., Fagiolini, A., Shear, K., Pini, S., and Maser, J. (1999). The bipolar spectrum: A clinical reality in search of diagnostic criteria and an assessment methodology. *J Affect Disord*, 54(3), 319–328.

Cassano, G.B., Frank, E., Miniati, M., Rucci, P., Fagiolini, A., Pini, S., Shear, M.K., and Maser, J.D. (2002). Conceptual underpinnings and empirical support for the mood spectrum. *Psychiatr Clin North Am*, 25(4), 699–712.

Cassano, G.B., Rucci, P., Frank, E., Fagiolini, A., Dell'Osso, L., Shear, M.K., and Kupfer, D.J. (2004). The mood spectrum in unipolar and bipolar disorder: Arguments for a unitary approach. *Am J Psychiatry*, 161(7), 1264–1269.

Coryell, W., Endicott, J., Reich, T., Andreasen, N., and Keller, M. (1984). A family study of bipolar II disorder. *Br J Psychiatry*, 145, 49–54.

Coryell, W., Endicott, J., Andreasen, N., and Keller, M. (1985). Bipolar I, bipolar II, and nonbipolar major depression among the relatives of affectively ill probands. *Am J Psychiatry*, 142, 817–821.

Coryell, W., Endicott, J., and Keller, M. (1992). Rapidly cycling affective disorder. Demographics, diagnosis, family history, and course. *Arch Gen Psychiatry*, 49(2), 126–131.

Coryell, W., Endicott, J., Maser, J.D., Keller, M.B., Leon, A.C., and Akiskal, H.S. (1995). Long-term stability of polarity distinctions in the affective disorders. *Am J Psychiatry*, 152, 385–390.

Coryell, W., Solomon, D., Turvey, C., Keller, M., Leon, A.C., Endicott, J., Schettler, P., Judd, L., and Mueller, T. (2003). The long-term course of rapid cycling bipolar disorder. *Arch Gen Psychiatry*, 60, 914–920.

Cutting, J. (1990). Relationship between cycloid psychosis and typical affective psychosis. *Psychopathology*, 23(4), 212–219.

Davenport, Y.B., Adland, M.L., Gold, P.W., and Goodwin, F.K. (1979). Manic-depressive illness: Psychodynamic features of multigenerational families. *Am J Orthopsychiatry*, 49, 24–35.

Davis, G.C., and Buchsbaum, B.S. (1981). Pain sensitivity and endorphins in functional psychoses. *Mod Probl Pharmacopsychiatry*, 17, 97–108.

Deckersbach, T., Perlis, R.H., Frankle, W.G., Gray, S.M., Grandin, L., Dougherty, D.D., Nierenberg, A.A., and Sachs, G.S. (2004). Presence of irritability during depressive episodes in bipolar disorder. *CNS Spectr*, 9, 227–231.

Deltito, J., Martin, L., Riefkohl, J., Austria, B., Kissilenko, A., Corless, C., and Morse, P. (2001). Do patients with borderline personality disorder belong to the bipolar spectrum? *J Affect Disord*, 67, 221–228.

Depue, R.A., and Klein, D.N. (1988). Identification of unipolar and bipolar affective conditions in nonclinical and clinical populations by the General Behavior Inventory. In D.L. Dunner, E.S. Gershon, and J.E. Barrett (Eds.), *Relatives at Risk for Mental Disorder* (pp. 179–204). New York: Raven Press.

Depue, R.A., Kleiman, R.M., Davis, P., Hutchinson, M., and Kraussm, S.O. (1981). The behavioral high risk paradigm and bipolar affective disorder: A conceptual framework with five validation studies. *J Abnorm Psychol Monograph*, 90, 381–437.

Depue, R.A., Krauss, S., Spoont, M.R., and Arbisi, P. (1989). General behavior inventory identification of unipolar and bipolar affective conditions in a nonclinical university population. *J Abnorm Psychol*, 98, 117–126.

Dilsaver, S.C., and Akiskal, H.S. (2005). High rate of unrecognized bipolar mixed states among destitute Hispanic adolescents referred for "major depressive disorder." *J Affect Disord*, 84(2-3), 179–186.

Duncan, W.C., Pettigrew, K.D., and Gillen, J.C. (1979). REM architecture changes in bipolar and unipolar depression. *Am J Psychiatry*, 136, 1424–1427.

Dunner, D.L. (1980). Unipolar and bipolar depression: Recent findings from clinical and biologic studies. In *The Psychobiology of Affective Disorders* (pp. 11–24). Pfizer Symposium Depression. Basel, Switzerland: Karger.

Dunner, D.L. (1987). Stability of bipolar II affective disorder as a diagnostic entity. *Psychiatr Ann*, 17, 18–20.

Dunner, D.L., and Tay, L.K. (1993). Diagnostic reliability of the history of hypomania in bipolar II patients and patients with major depression. *Compr Psychiatry*, 34(5), 303–307.

Dunner, D.L., Fleiss, J.L., and Fieve, R.R. (1976a). Depressive symptoms in patients with unipolar and bipolar affective disorder. *Compr Psychiatry*, 17, 447–451.

Dunner, D.L., Gershon, E.S., and Goodwin, F.K. (1976b). Heritable factors in the severity of affective illness. *Biol Psychiatry*, 11, 31–42.

Dunner, D.L., Hensel, B.M., and Fieve, R.R. (1979). Bipolar illness: Factors in drinking behavior. *Am J Psychiatry*, 136, 583–585.

Dunner, D.L., Murphy, D., Stallone, F., and Fieve, R.R. (1980). Affective episode frequency and lithium therapy. *Psychopharmacol Bull*, 16, 49–50.

Ebert, D., Barocka, A., Kalb, R., and Ott, G. (1993). Atypical depression as a bipolar spectrum disease: Evidence from a longitudinal study: The early course of atypical depression. *Psychiatria Danubina*, 5, 133–136.

Egeland, J.A., and Hotstetter, A.M. (1983). Amish study, I: Affective disorders among the Amish, 1976–1980. *Am J Psychiatry*, 140, 56–61.

Endicott, N.A. (1989). Psychophysiological correlates of 'bipolarity.' *J Affect Disord*, 17, 47–56.

Endicott, J., Nee, J., Andeason, N., Clayton P., Keller, M., and Coryell, W. (1985). Bipolar II: Combine or separate. *J Affect Disord*, 8, 17–28.

Fava, M., and Rosenbaum, J.F. (1999). Anger attacks in patients with depression. *J Clin Psychiatry*, 60(Suppl. 15), s21–S24.

Ferrier, I.N., MacMillan, I.C., and Young, A.H. (2001). The search for the wandering thymostat: A review of some developments in bipolar disorder research. *Br J Psychiatry*, 178(Suppl. 41), s103–s106.

Fieve, R.R., Go, R., Dunner, D.L., and Elston, R. (1984). Search for biological/genetic markers in a long-term epidemiological and morbid risk study of affective disorders. *J Psychiatr Res*, 18(4), 425–445.

Geller, B., Zimerman, B., Williams, M., Bolhofner, K., and Craney, J.L. (2001). Bipolar disorder at prospective follow-up of adults who had prepubertal major depressive disorder. *Am J Psychiatry*, 58(1), 125–127.

Gershon, E.S., Hamovit, J., Guroff, J.J., Dibble, E., Leckman, J.F., Sceery, W., Targum, S.D., Nurnberger, J.I., Goldin, L.R., and Bunney, W.E. (1982). A family study of schizoaffective, bipolar I, bipolar II, unipolar and normal control probands. *Arch Gen Psychiatry*, 39, 1157–1167.

Ghaemi, S.N., Sachs, G.S., Chiou, A.M., Pandurangi, A.K., and Goodwin, K. (1999). Is bipolar disorder still underdiagnosed? Are antidepressants overutilized? *J Affect Disord*, 52(1), 135–144.

Ghaemi, S.N., Ko, J.Y., and Goodwin, F.K. (2002). Cade's disease and beyond: Misdiagnosis, antidepressant use, and a proposed definition for bipolar spectrum disorder. *Can J Psychiatry*, 47, 125–134.

Ghaemi, S.N., Hsu, D.J., Ko, J.Y., Baldassano, C.F., Kontos, N.J., and Goodwin, F.K. (2004). Bipolar spectrum disorder: A pilot study. *Psychopathology*, 37(5), 222–226.

Goldberg, J.F., Harrow, M., and Whiteside, J.E. (2001). Risk for bipolar illness in patients initially hospitalized for unipolar depression. *Am J Psychiatry*, 158, 1265–1270.

Goodwin, F.K. (1977). Diagnosis of affective disorders. In M.E. Jarvik (Ed.), *Psychopharmacology in the Practice of Medicine* (pp. 219–228). New York: Appleton-Century-Crofts.

Goodwin, F.K., and Ghaemi, S.N. (2000). An introduction to and history of affective disorders. In M. Gelder, J. Lopez-Ibor, and N. Andreasen (Eds.), *New Oxford Textbook of Psychiatry*. New York: Oxford University Press, pp. 677–682.

Grayson, D.A. (1987). Can categorical and dimensional views of psychiatric illness be distinguished? *Br J Psychiatry*, 151, 355–361.

Greenhouse, S.W., and Geisser, S. (1959). On methods in the analysis of profile data. *Psychometrika*, 24, 95–112.

Griesinger, W. (1867). *Mental Pathology and Therapeutics*. Translated by C.L. Robertson and J. Rutherford. London: New Sydenhem Society.

Guze, S.B., Woodruff, R.A. Jr., and Clayton, P.J. (1975). The significance of psychotic affective disorders. *Arch Gen Psychiatry*, 32, 1147–1150.

Hantouche, E.G., and Akiskal, H.S. (2005). Bipolar II vs. unipolar depression: Psychopathologic differentiation by dimensional measures. *J Affect Disord*, 84(2-3), 127–132.

Hantouche, E.G., Akisakal, H.S., Lancrenon, S., Allilaire, J.F., Sechrer, D., Azorin, J.M., Bourgeois, M., Fraudm, J.P., and Chalenet-Duchene, L. (1998). Systemic clinical methodology for validating bipolar disorder data in mid stream from a French national multi-cite study (EPIDEP). *J Affect Disorder*, 50, 163–173.

Hantouche, E.G., Angst, J., and Akiskal, H.S. (2003a). Factor structure of hypomania: Interrelationships with cyclothymia and the soft bipolar spectrum. *J Affect Disord*, 73, 39–47.

Hantouche, E.G., Angst, J., Demonfaucon, C., Perugi, G., Lancrenon, S., and Akiskal, H.S. (2003b). Cyclothymic OCD: A distinct form? *J Affect Disord*, 75(1), 1–10.

Hartmann, E. (1968). Longitudinal studies of sleep and dream patterns in manic depressive patients. *Arch Gen Psychiatry*, 19, 312–329.

Heun, R., and Maier, W. (1993) The distinction of bipolar II disorder from bipolar I and recurrent unipolar depression: Results of a controlled family study. *Acta Psychiatr Scand*, 87(4), 279–284.

Himmelhoch, J.M., Detre, T., Kupfer, D.J., Swartzburg, M., and Byck, R. (1972). Treatment of previously intractable depressions with tranylcypromine and lithium. *J Nerv Mental Dis*, 155, 216–220.

Himmelhoch, J.M., Thase, M.E., Mallinger, A.G., and Houck, P. (1991). Tranylcypromine versus imipramine in anergic bipolar depression. *Am J Psychiatry*, 148(7), 910–916.

Horwath, E., Johnson, J., Weissman, M.M., and Hornig, C.D. (1992). The validity of major depression with atypical features based on a community study. *J Affect Disord*, 26(2), 117–125.

Jackson, S.W. (1986). *Melancholia and Depression: From Hippocratic Times to Modern Times*. New Haven, CT: Yale University Press.

Jamison, K.R. (2005). *Exuberance: The Passion for Life*. New York: Vintage Books.

Jelliffe, S.E. (1931). Some historical phases of the manic-depressive synthesis. *Research Publications Association for Research in Nervous and Mental Diseases*, 11, 3–47.

Joffe, R.T., Young, L.T., and MacQueen, G.M. (1999). A two-illness model of bipolar disorder. *Bipolar Disord*, 1(1), 25–30.

Judd, L.L., and Akiskal, H.S. (2000). Delineating the longitudinal structure of depressive illness: Beyond clinical subtypes and duration thresholds. *Pharmacopsychiatry*, 33, 3–7.

Judd, L.L., Akiskal, H.S., Schettler, P.J., Endicott, J., Maser, J., Solomon, D.A., Leon, A.C., Rice, J.A., and Keller, M.B. (2002). The long-term natural history of the weekly symptomatic status of bipolar I disorder. *Arch Gen Psychiatry*, 59, 530–537.

Judd, L.L., Akiskal, H.S., Coryell, W., Schettler, P., Maser, J., Rice, J., Solomon, D., and Keller, M. (2003a). The comparative clinical phenotype and long term longitudinal episode course of bipolar I and II: A clinical spectrum or distinct disorders? *J Affect Disord*, 73, 19–32.

Judd, L.L., Akiskal, H.S., Schettler, P., Endicott, J., Maser, J., Solomon, D., Leon, A., Coryell, W., and Keller, M. (2003b). A prospective naturalistic investigation of the long-term weekly symptomatic status of bipolar II disorder. *Arch Gen Psychiatry*, 60, 261–269.

Judd, L.L., Schettler, P.J., Akiskal, H.S., Maser, J., Coryell, W., Solomon, D., Endicott, J., and Keller, M. (2003c). Long-term symptomatic status of bipolar I vs. bipolar II disorders. *Int J Neuropsychopharmacol*, 6(2), 127–137.

Kadrmas, A., Winokur, G., and Crowe, R. (1979). Postpartum mania. *Br J Psychiatry*, 135, 551–554.

Kahlbaum, K.L. (1882). Uber cyclisches Irresein. *Der Irrenfreund*, 10, 145–157.

Katz, M.M., Robins, E., Croughan, J., Secunda, S., and Swann, A. (1982). Behavioral measurement and drug response characteristics of unipolar and bipolar depression. *Psychol Med*, 12, 25–36.

Kendell, R.E. (1968). *The Classification of Depressive Illness*. London: Oxford University Press.

Klein, D.N., Depue, R.A., and Slater, J.F. (1986). Inventory identification of cyclothymia: IX. Validation in offspring of bipolar I patients. *Arch General Psychiatry*, 43, 441–445.

Klerman, G.L. (1981). The spectrum of mania. *Compr Psychiatry*, 22, 11–20.

Kotin, J., and Goodwin, F.K. (1972). Depression during mania: Clinical observations and theoretical implications. *Am J Psychiatry*, 129, 679–686.

Koukopoulos, A. (2003). Ewald Hecker's description of cyclothymia as a cyclical mood disorder: Its relevance to the modern concept of bipolar II. *J Affect Disord*, 73, 199–205.

Koukopoulos, A. (2006). The primacy of mania. In H. Akiskal and M. Tohen (Eds.), *Bipolar Psychopharmacotherapy: Caring for the Patient*. New York: John Wiley and Sons.

Koukopoulos, A., and Koukopoulos, A. (1999). Agitated depression as a mixed state and the problem of melancholia. In H.S. Akiskal (Ed.), *Bipolarity: Beyond Classic Mania. Psychiatr Clin North Am*, 22, 547–564.

Koukopoulos, A., Caliari, B., Tundo, A., Minnai, G., Floris, G., Reginaldi, D., and Tondo, L. (1983). Rapid cyclers, temperament, and antidepressants. *Compr Psychiatry*, 24, 249–258.

Kovacs, M., Akiskal, H.S., Gatsonis, C., and Parrone, P.L. (1994). Childhood-onset dysthymic disorder: Clinical features and prospective naturalistic outcome. *Arch Gen Psychiatry*, 51, 365–374.

Kraemer, H., Noda, A., and O'Hara, R. (2004). Categorical versus dimensional approaches to diagnosis: Methodological challenges. *J Psychiatr Res*, 38, 17–25.

Kraepelin, E. (1899). *Manic Depressive Insanity and Paranoia*. Edinburgh: E. & S. Livingstone.

Kraepelin, E. (1921). *Manic-Depressive Insanity and Paranoia*. Edinburgh: E. & S. Livingstone. Originally published as *Psychiatrie. Ein Lehrbuch fur Studierende und Arzte. ed. 2. Klinische Psychiatrie. II.* Leipzig: Johann Ambrosius Barth, 1899.

Kupfer, D.J., Himmelhoch, J.M., Swartzburg, M., Anderson, C., Byck, R., and Detre, T.P. (1972). Hyperinsomnia in manic-depressive disease (a preliminary report). *Dis Nerv Syst*, 33, 720–724.

Kupfer, D.J., Weiss, B.L., Foster, F.G., Detre, T.P., Delgado, J., and McPartland, R. (1974). Psychomotor activity in affective states. *Arch Gen Psychiatry*, 30, 765–768.

Kupfer, D.J., Pakar, D., Himmelhoch, J.M., and Detre, T.P. (1975). Are there two types of unipolar depression? *Arch Gen Psychiatry*, 32, 866–871.

Leff, J. (1977). International variations in the diagnosis of psychiatric illness. *Br J Psychiatry*, 131, 329–338.

Leonhard, K. (1957). Pathogenesis of manic-depressive disease. *Nervenarzt*, 28(6), 271–272.

Leonhard, K. (1979). *The Classification of Endogenous Psychoses*, 5th edition. E. Robins (Ed.), R. Berman (Trans.). New York: Irvington Publishers, Inc., (pp. 3–4). Originally published as *Aufteilung der Endogenen Psychosen*, 1st edition. Berlin: Akademie-Verlag, 1957.

Levitan, R.D., Lesage, A., Parikh, S.V., Goering, P., and Kennedy, S.H. (1997). Reversed neurovegetative symptoms of depression: A community study of Ontario. *Am J Psychiatry*, 154(7), 934–940.

Lewis, A.J. (1936). Prognosis in the manic depressive psychosis. *Lancet*, 2, 997–999.

Mainia, G., Albert, U., Ceregato, A., and Bogetto, F. (2002). *Re-evaluating the prevalence of bipolar spectrum disorders in a clinical sample referred to a mood disorder unit: From DSM-IV criteria to a broad clinical spectrum of bipolar disorder* (Abstract). Philadelphia: American Psychiatric Association, p. 123.

Maj, M., Pirozzi, R, Formicola, A.M., and Tortorella, A. (1999). Reliability and validity of four alternative definitions of rapid cycling bipolar disorder. *Am J Psychiatry*, 156, 1421–1424.

Maj, M., Pirozzi, R., Magliano, L., and Bartoli, L. (2003). Agitated depression in bipolar I disorder: Prevalence, phenomenology, and outcome. *Am J Psychiatry*, 160(12), 2134–2140.

Manning, J.S., Haykal, R.F., Connor, P.D., and Akiskal, H.S. (1997). On the nature of depressive and anxious states in a family practice setting: The high prevalence of bipolar II and related disorders in a cohort followed longitudinally. *Compr Psychiatry*, 38, 102–108.

Marneros, A. (2001). Origin and development of concepts of bipolar mixed states. *J Affect Disord*, 67(1-3), 229–240.

Maser, J.D., and Akiskal, H.S. (2002). Spectrum concepts in major mental disorders. *Psychiatr Clin North Am*, 25(4), 685–885.

Mayer-Gross, W., Slater, E., and Roth, M. (1955). *Clinical Psychiatry*. Baltimore: Williams and Wilkens.

Mendel, E. (1881). *Die Manie*. Vienna: Urban and Schwazenberg.

Mendels, J. (1976). Lithium in the treatment of depression. *Am J Psychiatry*, 133, 373–378.

Mendelson, W.B., Sack, D.A., James, S.P., Martin, J.V., Wagner, R., Garnett, D., Milton, J., and Wehr, T.A. (1987). Frequency analysis of the sleep EEG in depression. *Psychiatry Res*, 21, 89–94.

Meyer, A. (1866–1950). *Collected Papers of Adolf Myer*. E.E. Winters (Ed.). Baltimore: Johns Hopkins University Press.

Mitchell, P.B., Parker, G., Jamieson, K., Wilhelm, K., Hickie, I., Brodaty, H., Boyce, P., Hadzi-Pavlovic, D., and Roy, K. (1992). Are there any differences between bipolar and unipolar melancholia? *J Affect Disord*, 25, 97–105.

Mitchell, P.B., Wilhelm, K., Parker, G., Austin, M.P., Ritgers, P., and Malhi, G.S. (2001). The clinical features of bipolar depression: A comparison with matched major depressive disorder patients. *J Clin Psychiatry*, 62, 212–216.

Moorhead, S.R., and Young, A.H. (2003). Evidence for a late onset bipolar-I disorder sub-group from 50 years. *J Affect Disord*, 73, 271–277.

Nurnberger, J. Jr., Roose, S.P., Dunner, D.L., and Fieve, R.R. (1979). Unipolar mania: A distinct clinical entity? *Am J Psychiatry*, 136(11), 1420–1423.

Papadimitriou, G.N., Dikeos, D.G., Daskalopoulou, E.G., and Soldatos, C.R. (2002). Co-occurrence of disturbed sleep and appetite loss differentiates between unipolar and bipolar depressive episodes. *Prog Neuropsychopharmacol Biol Psychiatry*, 26, 1041–1045.

Parker, G., Roy, K., Wilhelm, K., Mitchell, P., and Hadzi-Pavlovic, D. (2000). The nature of bipolar depression: Implications for the definition of melancholia. *J Affect Disord*, 59, 217–224.

Perlis, R.H., Smoller, J.W., Fava, M., Rosenbaum, J.F., Nierenberg, A.A., and Sachs, G.S. (2004). The prevalence and clinical correlates of anger attacks during depressive episodes in bipolar disorder. *J Affect Disord*, 79, 291–295.

Perlis, R.H., Brown, E., Baker, R.W., and Nierenberg, A.A. (2006). Clinical features of bipolar depression versus major depressive disorder in large multicenter trials. *Am J Psychiatry*, 163(2), 175–176.

Perris, C. (Ed.). (1966). A study of bipolar (manic-depressive) and unipolar recurrent depressive psychoses. *Acta Psychiatr Scand*, 42(Suppl. 194).

Perris, C. (1968). The course of depressive psychoses. *Acta Psychiatr Scand*, 44, 238–248.

Perris, C. (1971). The course of depressive psychoses. *Acta Psychiatr Scand*, (Suppl. 221), 43–51.

Perugi, G., Akiskal, H.S., Lattanzi, L., Cecconi, D., Mastrocinque, C., Patronelli, A., and Vignoli, S. (1998a). The high prevalence of soft bipolar (II) features in atypical depression. *Compr Psychiatry*, 39, 63–71.

Perugi, G., Akiskal, H.S., Rossi, L., Paiano, A., Quilici, C., Madaro, D., Musetti, L., and Cassano, G.B. (1998b). Chronic mania: Family history, prior course, clinical picture and social consequences. *Br J Psychiatry*, 173, 514–518.

Perugi, G., Akiskal, H.S., Ramacciotti, S., Nassini, S., Toni, C., Milanfranchi, A., and Musetti, L. (1999). Depressive comorbidity of panic, social phobic and obsessive-compulsive disorders: Is there a bipolar II connection? *J Psychiatr Res*, 33, 53–61.

Perugi, G., Akiskal, H.S., Toni, C., Simonini, E., and Gemignani A. (2001). The temporal relationship between anxiety disorders and (hypo)mania: A retrospective examination of 63 panic, social phobic and obsessive-compulsive patients with comorbid bipolar disorder. *J Affect Disord*, 67, 199–206.

Perugi, G., Toni, C., Travierso, M.C., and Akiskal, H.S. (2003). The role of cyclothymia in atypical depression: Toward a data-based reconceptualization of the borderline-bipolar II connection. *J Affect Disord*, 73, 87–98.

Pichot, P. (1988). European perspectives on the classification of depression. *Br J Psyciatry*, 153(Suppl. 3), 11–15.

Pichot, P. (1995). The birth of the bipolar disorder. *Eur Psychiatry*, 10, 1–10.

Pirozzi, M.M., Magliano, L., Fiorillo, A., and Bartoli, L. (2006). Agitated "unipolar" major depression: Prevalence, phenomenology, and outcome. *J Clin Psychiatry*, 67(5), 712–719.

Placidi, G.F., Signoretta, S., Liguori, A., Gervasi, R., Maremmani, I., and Akiskal, H.S. (1998). The semi-structured affective temperament interview (TEMPS-I): Reliability and psychometric properties in 1010 14–26 year students. *J Affect Disord*, 47, 1–10.

Popescu, C., Ionescu, R., Jipescu, I., and Popa, S. (1991). Psychomotor functioning in unipolar and bipolar affective disorders. *Rom J Neurol Psychiatry*, 29(1-2), 17–33.

Posternak, M.A., and Zimmerman, M. (2002). Lack of association between seasonality and psychopathology in psychiatric outpatients. *Psychiatry Res*, 112(3), 187–194.

Rao, U., Ryan, N.D., Birmaher, B., Dahl, R., Williamson, D., Kaufman, J., Rao, R., and Nelson, B. (1995). Unipolar depression in adolescents: Clinical outcome in adulthood. *J Am Acad Child Adolesc Psychiatry*, 34(5), 566–578.

Rao, U., Dahl, R.E., Ryan, N.D., Birmaher, B., Williamson, D.E., Rao, R., and Kaufman, J. (2002). Heterogeneity in EEG sleep findings in adolescent depression: Unipolar versus bipolar clinical course. *J Affect Disord*, 70(3), 273–280.

Raskin, A., and Crook, T.H. (1976). The endogenous-neurotic distribution as a predictor of response to antidepressant drug. *Psychol Med*, 6, 59–70.

Regier, D.A., Farmer, M.E., Rae, D.S., Locke, B.Z., Keith, S.J., Judd, L.L., and Goodwin, F.K. (1990). Comorbidity of mental disorders with alcohol and other drug abuse. Results from the Epidemiologic Catchment Area (ECA) Study. *JAMA*, 264(19), 2511–2518.

Reich, T., and Winokur, G. (1970). Postpartum psychoses in patients with manic depressive disease. *J Nerv Ment Dis*, 151, 60–68.

Rice, J.P., McDonald-Scott, P., Endocott, J., Coryell, W., Grove, W.M., Keller, M.B., and Altis, D. (1986). The stability of diagnosis with an application to bipolar II disorder. *Psychiatry Res*, 19, 285–296.

Rihmer, Z., and Pestality, P. (1999). Bipolar II disorder and suicidal behavior. *Psychiatr Clin North Am*, 22(3), 667–673.

Ritti, A. (1892). Circular insanity. In D. Hack Tuke (Ed.), *A Dictionary of Psychological Medicine Giving the Definition, Etymology and Synonyms of Terms Used in Medical Psychology, with the Symptoms, Treatment and Pathology of Insanity and the Law of Lunacy in Great Britain and Ireland* (p. 214), 2 volumes. Philadelphia: P. Blakiston.

Robertson, H.A., Lam, R.W., Stewart, J.N., Yatham, L.N., Tam, E.M., and Zis, A.P. (1996). Atypical depressive symptoms and clusters in unipolar and bipolar depression. *Acta Psychiatr Scand*, 94, 421–427.

Roccatagliata, G. (1986). *A History of Ancient Psychiatry*. New York: Greenwood Press.

Roth, M. (1983). Depression and affective disorder in later life. In J. Angst (Ed.), *The Origins of Depression: Current Concepts and Approaches* (pp. 39–75). Berlin: Springer-Verlag.

Rybakowski, J.K., Suwalska, A., Lojko, D., Rymaszewska, J., and Kiejna, A. (2005). Bipolar mood disorders among Polish psychiatric outpatients treated for major depression. *J Affect Disord*, 84(2-3), 141–147.

Sass, H., Herpertz, S., and Steinmeyer, E.M. (1993). Subaffective personality disorders. *Int Clin Psychopharmacol*, 8(Suppl. 1), 39–46.

Sato, T., Bottlender, R., Schroter, A., and Moller, H.J. (2003). Frequency of manic symptoms during a depressive episode and unipolar 'depressive mixed state' as bipolar spectrum. *Acta Psychiatr Scand*, 107, 268–274.

Sato, T., Bottlender, R., Kleindienst, N., and Moller, H.J. (2005). Irritable psychomotor elation in depressed inpatients: A factor validation of mixed depression. *J Affect Disord*, 84(2-3), 187–196.

Serretti, A., and Olgiati, P. (2005). Profiles of "manic" symptoms in bipolar I, bipolar II and major depressive disorders. *J Affect Disord*, 84(2-3), 159–166.

Sharma, V., Khan, M., and Smith, A. (2005). A closer look at treatment resistant depression: Is it due to a bipolar diathesis? *J Affect Disord*, 84(2-3), 251–257.

Serretti, A., Lattuada, E., Cusin, C., Macciardi, F., and Smeraldi, E. (1998). Analysis of depressive symptomatology in mood disorders. *Depress Anxiety*, 8(2), 80–85.

Shulman, K., and Post, F. (1980). Bipolar affective disorder in old age. *Br J Psychiatry*, 136, 26–32.

Shulman, K.I., and Tohen, M. (1994). Unipolar mania reconsidered: Evidence from an elderly cohort. *Br J Psychiatry*, 164(4), 547–549.

Signoretta, S., Maremmani, I., Liguori, A., Perugi, G., and Akiskal, H.S. (2005). Affective temperament traits measured by TEMPS-I and emotional-behavioral problems in clinically-well children, adolescents, and young adults. *J Affect Disord*, 85, 169–180.

Simpson, S.G., Folstein, S.E., Meyers, D.A., McMahon, F.J., Brusco, D.M., and DePaulo, J.R. (1993). Bipolar II: The most common bipolar phenotype? *Am J Psychiatry*, 150, 901–903.

Simpson, S.G., McMahon, F.J., McInnis, M.G., MacKinnon, D.F., Edwin, D., Folstein, S.E., and DePaulo, J.R. (2002). Diagnostic reliability of bipolar II disorder. *Arch Gen Psychiatry*, 59, 736–740.

Smith, D.J., Harrison, N., Muir, W., and Blackwood, D.H. (2005). The high prevalence of bipolar spectrum disorders in young adults with recurrent depression: Toward an innovative diagnostic framework. *J Affect Disord*, 84(2-3), 167–178.

Solomon, D.A., Leon, A.C., Endicott, J., Coryell, W.H., Mueller, T.I., Posternak, M.A., and Keller, M. (2003). Unipolar mania over the course of a 20-year follow-up study. *Am J Psychiatry*, 60(11), 2049–2051.

Sullivan, P.F., Prescott, C.A., and Candler, K.S. (2002). Subtypes of major depression in a twin registry. *J Affect Disorder*, 68, 273–284.

Toni, C., Perugi, G., Mata, B., Madaro, D., Maremmani, I., and Akiskal, H.S. (2001). Is mood-incongruent manic psychosis a distinct subtype? *Eur Arch Psychiatry Clin Neurosci*, 251, 12–17.

Tsuang, M.T., Faraone, S.V., and Fleming, J.A. (1985). Familial transmission of major affective disorders: Is there evidence supporting the distinction between unipolar and bipolar disorders? *Br J Psychiatry*, 146, 268–271.

Vahip, S., Kesebir, S., Alkan, M., Yazici, O., Akiskal, K.K., and Akiskal, H.S. (2005). Affective temperaments in clinically-well subjects in Turkey: Initial psychometric data on the TEMPS-A. *J Affect Disord*, 85, 113–125.

VanEerdewegh, M.M., Van Eerdewegh, P., Coryell, W., Clayton, P.J., Endicott, J., Koepke, J., and Rochberg, N. (1987). Schizoaffective disorders: Bipolar-unipolar subtyping. Natural history variables: A discriminant analysis approach. *J Affect Disord*, 12, 223–232.

van Praag, H.M. (1993). What is self-evident but does not occur as a matter-of-course; observations on the report about biological psychiatry. *Ned Tijdschr Geneeskd*, 13, 137(7), 366–368.

Vieta, E., and Barcia, D. (2000). *El trastorno bipolar en el siglo XVIII*. Burdeos, Spain: Mra ediciones.

Vieta, E., Gasto, C., Otero, A., Nieto, E., and Vallejo, J. (1997). Differential features between bipolar I and bipolar II disorder. *Compr Psychiatry*, 38(2), 98–101.

Waters, B.G.H. (1979). Early symptoms of bipolar affective psychosis: Research and clinical implications. *Can Psychiatr Assoc J*, 2, 55–60.

Weissman, M.M., Bland, R.C., Canino, G.J., Faravelli, C., Greenwald, S., Hwu, H.G., Joyce, P.R., Karam, E.G., Lee, C.K., Lellouch, J., Lepine, J.P., Newman, S.C., Rubio-Stipec, M., Wells, J.E., Wickramaratne, P.J., Wittchen, H., and Yeh, E.K. (1996). Cross-national epidemiology of major depression and bipolar disorder. *JAMA*, 276(4), 293–299.

Whitwell, J.R. (1936). *Historical Notes on Psychiatry (Early Times–End of the 16th Century)*. London: HK Lewis & Co.

Wicki, W., and Angst, J. (1991). The Zurich study. X. Hypomania in a 28- to 30-year-old cohort. *EurArch Psychiatr Clin Neurosci*, 40, 339–348.

Wightman, W.P.D. (1971). *The Emergence of Scientific Medicine*. Edinburgh: Oliver and Boyd.

Winokur. G. (1979). Unipolar depression: Is it divisible into autonomous subtypes? *Arch Gen Psychiatry*, 36, 47–52.

Winokur, G. (1980). Is there a common genetic factor in bipolar and unipolar affective disorder? *Compr Psychiatry*, 21, 460–468.

Winokur, G., and Clayton, P. (1967). Family history studies: I. Two types of affective disorders separated according to genetic and clinical factors. In J. Worris (Ed.), *Recent Advances in Biological Psychiatry* (Vol. 10) (pp. 35–50). New York: Plenum Press.

Winokur, G., Clayton, P.J., and Reich, T. (1969). *Manic Depressive Illness*. St. Louis: C.V. Mosby.

Winokur, G., Coryell, W., Endicott, J., and Akiskal, H. (1993). Further distinctions between manic-depressive illness (bipolar disorder) and primary depressive disorder (unipolar depression). *Am J Psychiatry*, 150, 1176–1181.

Winokur, G., Coryell, W., Akiskal, H.S., Endicott, J., Keller, M., and Mueller, T. (1994). Manic-depressive illness: The course in light of a prospective ten-year follow-up. *Acta Psychiatr Scand*, 89, 102–110.

Winokur, G., Coryell, W., Keller, M., Endicott, J., and Leon, A. (1995). A family study of manic-depressive (bipolar I) disease. Is it a distinct illness separable from primary unipolar depression? *Arch Gen Psychiatry*, 52, 367–373.

Winokur, G., Turvey, C., Akiskal, H., Coryell, W., Solomon, D., Leon, A., Mueller, T., Endicott, J., Maser, J., and Keller, M. (1998). Alcoholism and drug abuse in three groups—bipolar I, unipolars and their acquaintances. *J Affect Disord*, 50(2-3), 81–89.

Yazici, O., Kora, K., Ucok, A., Saylan, M., Ozdemir, O., Kiziltan, E., and Ozpulat, T. (2002). Unipolar mania: A distinct disorder? *J Affect Disord*, 71(1-3), 97–103.

Zilboorg, G. (1941). *A History of Medical Psychology*. New York: W.W. Norton.

Chapter 2

Abrams, R., and Taylor, M.A. (1976). Mania and schizoaffective disorder, manic type: A comparison. *Am J Psychiatry*, 133, 1445–1447.

Abrams, R., and Taylor, M.A. (1981). Importance of schizophrenic symptoms in the diagnosis of mania. *Am J Psychiatry*, 138, 658–661.

Abrams, R., and Taylor, M.A. (1983) The importance of mood-incongruent psychotic symptoms in melancholia. *J Affect Disord*, 5, 179–181.

Adler, D., and Harrow, M. (1974). Idiosyncratic thinking and personally overinvolved thinking in schizophrenic patients during partial recovery. *Compr Psychiatry*, 15, 57–67.

Akiskal, H.S. (1992a). Delineating irritable-choleric and hyperthymic temperaments as variants of cyclothymia. *J Person Disord*, 6, 326–342.

Akiskal, H.S. (1992b). The distinctive mixed states of bipolar I, II and III. *Clin Neuropharmacol*, 15(Suppl 1A), 632–633.

Akiskal, H.S. (Ed). (1999). Bipolarity: Beyond classic mania. *Psychiatr Clin North Am*, 22(3), 517–703.

Akiskal, H.S., and Mallya, G. (1987). Criteria for the "soft" bipolar spectrum: Treatment implications. *Psychopharmacol Bull*, 23, 68–73.

Akiskal, H.S., and Puzantian, V.R. (1979). Psychotic forms of depression and mania. *Psychiatr Clin North Am, 2*, 419–439.

Akiskal, H.S., Djenderedjian, A.H., Rosenthal, R.H., and Khani, M.K. (1977). Cyclothymic disorder: Validating criteria for inclusion in the bipolar affective group. *Am J Psychiatry*, 134, 1227–1233.

Akiskal, H.S., Khani, M.K., and Scott-Strauss, A. (1979a). Cyclothymic temperament disorders. *Psychiatr Clin North Am*, 2, 527–554.

Akiskal, H.S., Rosenthal, R.H., Rosenthal, T.L., Kashgarian, M., Khani, M.K., and Puzantian, V.R. (1979b). Differentiation of primary affective illness from situational, symptonmatic, and secondary depressions. *Arch Gen Psychiatry*, 36, 635–643.

Akiskal, H.S., Waker, P., Puzantian, V.R., King, D., Rosenthal, T.L., and Dranon, M. (1983). Bipolar outcome in the course of depressive illness: Phenomenologic, familial, and pharmacologic predictors. *J Affect Disord*, 5, 115–128.

Akiskal, H.S., Hantouche, E., Bourgeois, M., Azorin, J.M., Sechter, D., Allilaire, J.F., Lancrenon, S., Fraud, J.P., and Chatenet-Duchene, L. (1998a). Gender, temperament and the clinical picture in dysphoric mixed mania: Findings from a French national study (EPIMAN). *J Affect Disord*, 50, 175–186.

Akiskal, H.S., Placidi, G.F., Maremmani, I., Signoretta, S., Liguori, A., Gervasi, R., Mallya, G., and Puzantian, V.R. (1998b). TEMPS-I: Delineating the most discriminant traits of the cyclothymic, depressive, hyperthymic and irritable temperaments in a nonpatient population. *J Affect Disord*, 51, 7–19.

Akiskal, H.S., Bourgeois, M.L., Angst, J., Post, R., Moller, H.J., and Hirschfeld, R.M.A. (2000). Re-evaluating the prevalence of and diagnostic composition within the broad clinical spectrum of bipolar disorders. *J Affect Disord*, 59(Suppl 1), 5s–30s.

Akiskal, H.S., Hantouche, E.G., Bourgeois, M.L., Azorin, J.M., Sechter, D., Allilair, J.F., Chatenet-Duchene, L., and Lancrenon, S. (2001). Toward a refined phenomenology of DSM-IV mania: Combining clinician-assessment and self-report in the French EPIMAN study. *J Affect Disord*, 67, 89–96.

Akiskal, H.S., Azorin, J.F., and Hantouche, E.G. (2003a). A proposed multidimensional structure of mania: Beyond the euphoric–dysphoric dichotomy. *J Affect Disord*, 73, 7–18.

Akiskal, H.S., Hantouche, E.G., Allilaire, J.F., Sechter, D., Bourgeois, M.L., Azorin, J.M., Chatenet-Duchene, L., and Lancrenon, S. (2003b). Validating antidepressant-associated hypomania (bipolar III): A systematic comparison with spontaneous hypomania (bipolar II). *J Affect Disord*, 73, 65–74.

Allison, J.B., and Wilson, W.P. (1960). Sexual behaviors of manic patients: A preliminary report. *South Med J*, 53, 870–874.

Andreasen, N.C. (1979a). Thought, language, and communication disorders: I. Clinical assessment, definition of terms, and evaluation of their reliability. *Arch Gen Psychiatry*, 36, 1315–1321.

Andreasen, N.C. (1979b). Thought, language, and communication disorders: II. Diagnostic significance. *Arch Gen Psychiatry*, 36, 1325–1330.

Andreasen, N.C. (1984). *The clinical significance of "thought disorder."* Hibbs Award Lecture, 137th Annual Meeting of the American Psychiatric Association, May.

Andreasen, N.C., and Pfohl, B. (1976). Linguistic analysis of speech in affective disorders. *Arch Gen Psychiatry*, 33, 1361–1367.

Andreasen, N.C., and Powers, P.S. (1975). Creativity and psychosis: An examination of conceptual style. *Arch Gen Psychiatry*, 32, 70–73.

Aretaeus. (1856). *The Extant Works of Aretaeus, the Cappadocian.* London: Sydenham Society.

Aronson, T.A., Shukla, S., Hoff, A., and Cook, B. (1988). Proposed delusional depression subtypes: Preliminary evidence from a retrospective study of phenomenology and treatment course. *J Affect Disord*, 14, 69–74.

Astrup, C., Fossum, A., and Holmboe, R. (1959). A follow–up study of 270 patients with acute affective psychoses. *Acta Psychiatr Neurol Scand*, 34(Suppl 135), 11–65.

Azorin, J.M. (2000) Acute phase of schizophrenia: Impact of atypical antipsychotics. *Int Clin Psychopharmacol*, 15, S5–S9.

Baethge, C., Baldessarini, R.J., Freudenthal, K., Streetuwitz, A., Bauer, M., and Bschor, T. (2005). Hallucinations in bipolar disorder: Characteristics and comparison to unipolar depression and schizophrenia. *Bipolar Disord*, 7, 136–145.

Bauer, M.S., Whybrow, P.C., Gyulai, L., Gonnel, J., and Yeh, H.S. (1994). Testing definitions of dysphoric mania and hypomania: Prevalence, clinical characteristics and inter-episode stability. *J Affect Disord*, 32, 201–211.

Bauer, M.S., Simon, G.E., Ludman, E., and Unützer, J. (2005). 'Bipolarity' in bipolar disorder: Distribution of manic and depressive symptoms in a treated population. *Br J Psychiatry*, 187, 87–88.

Beck, A.T. (1967). *Depression: Causes and Treatment.* Philadelphia: University of Pennsylvania Press.

Beigel, A., and Murphy, D.L. (1971a). Assessing clinical characteristics of the manic state. *Am J Psychiatry*, 128, 688–694.

Beigel, A., and Murphy, D.L. (1971b). Unipolar and bipolar affective illness: Differences in clinical characteristics accompanying depression. *Arch Gen Psychiatry*, 24, 215–220.

Beigel, A., Murphy, D.L., and Bunney, W.E. (1971). The manic–state rating scale: Scale construction, reliability, and validity. *Arch Gen Psychiatry*, 25, 256–262.

Bell, L. (1849). On a form of disease resembling some advanced stages of mania and fever, but so contradistinguished from any ordinarily observed or described combination of symptoms as to render it probable that it may be an overlooked and hitherto unrecorded malady. *Am J Insanity*, 6, 97–127.

Benazzi, F. (2000a). Depression with DSM-IV atypical features: A marker for bipolar II disorder. *Eur Arch Psychiatry Clin Neurosci*, 250, 53–55.

Benazzi, F. (2000b). Depressive mixed states: Unipolar and bipolar II. *Eur Arch Psychiatry Clin Neurosci*, 250, 249–253.

Benazzi, F. (2001). Is 4 days the minimum duration of hypomania in bipolar II disorder? *Eur Arch Psychiatry Clin Neurosci*, 251, 32–34.

Benazzi F. (2003). Depression with racing thoughts. *Psychiatry Res*, 15, 273–282.

Benazzi F. (2004). Is depressive mixed state a transition between depression and hypomania? *Eur Arch Psychiatry Clin Neurosci*, 254, 69–75.

Benazzi, F. (2005). A. Marneros, and F. Goodwin (Eds.), *Bipolar Disorders: Mixed States, Rapid Cycling and Atypical Forms.* New York: Cambridge University Press.

Benazzi, F. (2006). Symptoms of depression as possible markers for bipolar II disorder. *Prog Neuropsychopharmacol Biol Psychiatry*, 30, 471–477.

Benazzi, F. (2007). Is overactivity the core feature of hypomania in bipolar II disorder? *Psychopathology*, 40, 54–60.

Benazzi, F., and Akiskal, H.S. (2001). Delineating bipolar II mixed states in the Ravenna–San Diego collaborative study: The relative prevalence and diagnostic significance of hypomanic features during major depressive episodes. *J Affect Disord*, 67, 115–122.

Benazzi, F., and Akiskal, H.S. (2003). Refining the evaluation of bipolar II: Beyond the strict SCID-CV guidelines for hypomania. *J Affect Disord*, 73, 33–38.

Benazzi, F., and Akiskal, H.S. (2005). Irritable-hostile depression: Further validation as a bipolar depressive mixed state. *J Affect Dis*, 84, 197–207.

Berlioz, H.L. (1966). *Memoirs of Hector Berlioz from 1803 to 1865.* Paris: Michel Lévy Bros, Annotated and translated by E. Newman. New York: Dover.

Berlioz, H.L. (1969). *Memoirs.* Translated by D. Cairns. London: Granada.

Berner, P., Gabriel, E., Katsching, H., Kieffer, W., Koehler, K., Lenz, G., Nutzinger, D., Schanda, H., and Simhandl, C. (1992). *Diagnostic Criteria for Functional Psychoses* (2nd Edition). Cambridge, England: Cambridge University Press.

Biondi, M., Picardi, A., Pasquini, M., Gaetano, P., and Pancheri, P. (2005). Dimensional psychopathology of depression: Detection of an 'activation' dimension in unipolar depressed outpatients. *J Affect Disord*, 84, 133–139.

Black, D.W., and Nasrallah, A. (1989). Hallucinations and delusions in 1,715 patients with unipolar and bipolar affective disorders. *Psychopathology*, 22, 28–34.

Bleuler, E. (1924). *Textbook of Psychiatry* (4th German Edition). A.A. Brill (Ed.). New York: The Macmillan Co.

Bond, T.C. (1980). Recognition of acute delirious mania. *Arch Gen Psychiatry*, 37, 553–554.

Bowman, K.M., and Raymond, A.F. (1931–1932a). A statistical study of delusions in the manic–depressive psychoses. *Am J Psychiatry*, 88, 111–121.

Bowman, K.M., and Raymond, A.F. (1931–1932b). A statistical study of hallucinations in the manic–depressive psychoses. *Am J Psychiatry*, 88, 299–309.

Braden, W., and Ho, C.K. (1981). Racing thoughts in psychiatric inpatients. *Arch Gen Psychiatry*, 38, 71–75.

Braden, W., and Qualls, C.B. (1979). Racing thoughts in depressed patients. *J Clin Psychiatry*, 40, 336–339.

Braunig, P., Kruger, S., and Shugar, G. (1998). Prevalence and clinical significance of catatonic symptoms in mania. *Compr Psychiatry*, 39(1), 35–46.

Breakey, W.R., and Goodell, H. (1972). Thought disorder in mania and schizophrenia evaluated by Bannister's Grid Test for schizophrenic thought disorder. *Br J Psychiatry*, 120, 391–395.

Brieger, P. (2000). Comorbidity in bipolar disorder. In A. Marneros and J. Angst (Eds.), *Bipolar Disorders: 100 Years after Manic-Depressive Insanity.* Dordrecht: Kluwer Academic Publishers, pp. 215–229.

Brieger, P., Roettig, S., Ehrt, U., Wenzel, A., Bloink, R., and Marneros, A. (2003). TEMPS-A scale in 'mixed' and 'pure' manic episodes: New data and methodological considerations on the relevance of joint anxious–depressive temperament traits. *J Affect Disord*, 73(1-2), 99–104.

Brockington, I.F., Wainwright, S., and Kendell, R.E. (1980). Manic patients with schizophrenic or paranoid symptoms. *Psychol Med*, 10, 73–83.

Brockington, I.F., Hillier, V.F., Francis, A.F., Helzer, J.E., and Wainwright, S. (1983). Definitions of mania: Concordance and prediction of outcome. *Am J Psychiatry*, 140, 435–439.

Bunney, W.E. Jr., Murphy, D., Goodwin, F.K., and Borge, G.F. (1972a). The "switch process" in manic depressive illness: I. A systematic study of sequential behavior change. *Arch Gen Psychiatry*, 27, 295–302.

Bunney, W.E. Jr., Goodwin, F.K., Murphy, D.L., House, K.M., and Gordon, E.K. (1972b). The "switch process" in manic–depressive illness: II. Relationship to catecholamines, REM sleep, and drugs. *Arch Gen Psychiatry*, 27, 304–309.

Bunney, W.E. Jr., Goodwin, F.K., and Murphy, D.L. (1972c). The "switch process" in manic–depressive illness: III. Theoretical implications. *Arch Gen Psychiatry*, 27, 312–317.

Burns, R. (1985). *The Letters of Robert Burns* (Volume 2, 1790–1796). G.R. Roy (Ed.). Letter to Mrs. W. Riddell, December, 1793. Oxford, England: Oxford University Press.

Byron, G.G. (1819, August 23). Letter to John Cam Hobhouse. In *Byron's Letters and Journals* (p. 214), Vol. 6. L. Marchand (Ed.). London: John Murray.

Calev, A., Nigal, D., and Chazan, S. (1989). Retrieval from semantic memory using meaningful and meaningless constructs by depressed, stable bipolar and manic patients. *Br J Clin Psychol*, 28, 67–73.

Campbell, J.D. (1953). *Manic–Depressive Disease: Clinical and Psychiatric Significance.* Philadelphia: Lippincott.

Carlson, G.A., and Goodwin, F.K. (1973). The stages of mania: A longitudinal analysis of the manic episode. *Arch Gen Psychiatry*, 28, 221–228.

Carlson, G., and Strober, M. (1979). Affective disorders in adolescence. *Psychiatr Clin North Am*, 2, 511–526.

Carpenter, W.T., Strauss, J.S., and Mulch, S. (1973). Are there pathognomonic symptoms in schizophrenia? An empiric investigation of Schneider's first rank symptoms. *Arch Gen Psychiatry*, 28, 847–852.

Casper, R.C., Redmond, E. Jr., Katz, M.M., Schaffer, C.B., Davis, J.M., and Koslow, S.H. (1985). Somatic symptoms in primary affective disorder: Presence and relationship to the classification of depression. *Arch Gen Psychiatry*, 42, 1098–1104.

Cassidy, F., and Carroll, B.J. (2002). Hypocholesterolemia during mixed manic episodes. *Eur Arch Psychiatry Clin Neurosci*, 252, 110–114.

Cassidy, F., Murry, E., Forest, K., and Carroll, B.J. (1998). Signs and symptoms of mania in pure and mixed episodes. *J Affect Disord*, 50, 187–201.

Cassidy, F., McEvoy, J.P., Yang, Y.K., and Wilson, W.H. (2001a). Insight is greater in mixed than in pure manic episodes of bipolar I disorder. *J Nerv Ment Dis*, 180, 398–399.

Cassidy, F., Ahearn, E., and Carroll, B.J. (2001b). A prospective study of inter-episode consistency of manic and mixed subtypes of bipolar disorder. *J Affect Disord*, 67, 181–185.

Cassidy, F., Ahearn, E.P., and Carrol, B.J. (2001c). Substance abuse in bipolar disorder. *Bipolar Disord*, 3, 181–188.

Cassidy, F., Ahearn, E.P., and Carroll, B.J. (2002). Symptom profile consistency in recurrent manic episodes. *Compr Psychiatr*, 43(3), 179–181.

Charney, D.S., and Nelson, J.C. (1981). Delusional and nondelusional unipolar depression: Further evidence for distinct subtypes. *Am J Psychiatry*, 138, 328–333.

Chiaroni, P., Hantouche, E.G., Gouvernet, J., Azorin, J.M., and Akiskal, H.S. (2005). The cyclothymic temperament in healthy controls and familially at risk individuals for mood disorder: Endophenotype for genetic studies? *J Affect Dis*, 85, 135–145.

Clayton, P., Pitts, F.N. Jr., and Winokur, G. (1965). Affective disorder: IV. Mania. *Compr Psychiatry*, 6, 313–322.

Cloninger, C.R. (1987). *The tridimensional personality questionnaire* (Version IV). St. Louis: Washington University School of Medicine.

Coate, M. (1964). *Beyond All Reason*. London: Constable & Co.

Coryell, W., and Tsuang, M.T. (1982). Primary unipolar depression and the prognostic importance of delusions. *Arch Gen Psychiatry*, 39, 1181–1184.

Coryell, W., Keller, M., Lavori, P., Endicott, J. (1990). Affective syndromes, psychotic features, and prognosis. II. Mania. *Arch Gen Psychiatry*, 47, 658–662.

Coryell, W., Leon, A.C., Turvey, C., Akiskal, H.S., Mueller, T., and Endicott, J. (2001). The significance of psychotic features in manic episodes: A report from the NIMH collaborative study. *J Affect Disord*, 67, 79–88.

Custance, J. (1952). *Wisdom, Madness, and Folly: The Philosophy of a Lunatic*. New York: Farrar, Straus & Cudahy.

Deckersbach, T., Perlis, R.H., Frankle, W.G., Gray, S.M., Grandin, L., Dougherty, D.D., Nierenberg, A.A., and Sachs, G.S. (2004). Presence of irritability during depressive episodes in bipolar disorder. *CNS Spectr*, 9, 227–231.

Dell'Osso, L., Nassi, R., Freer, P., Placidi, G.F., Cassano, G.B., and Akiskal, H.S. (1991). The manic-depressive mixed state: Familial, temperamental and psychopathologic characteristics in 108 female inpatients. *Eur Arch Psychiatry Clin Neurosci*, 240, 234–239.

Dell'Osso, L., Pini, S., Tundo, A., Sarno, N., Musetti, L., and Cassano, G.B. (2000). Clinical characteristics of mania, mixed mania, and bipolar depression with psychotic features. Compr Psychiatry, 41, 242–247.

Depue, R.A., Slater, J.F., Wolfstetter–Kausch, H., Klein, D., Goplerud, E., and Farr, D. (1981). A behavioral paradigm for identifying persons at risk for bipolar depressive disorder: A conceptual framework and five validation studies. *J Abnorm Psychol Monograph*, 90, 381–437.

Dewhurst, K. (1962). A seventeenth–century symposium on manic–depressive psychosis. *Br J Med Psychol*, 35, 113–125.

Dilsaver, S.C., Chen, R., Shoaib, A.M., and Swann, A.C. (1999). Phenomenology of mania: Evidence for distinct depressed, dysphoric, and euphoric presentations. *Am J Psychiatry*, 156, 426–430.

Dilsaver, S.C., Benazzi, F., Rihmer, Z., Akiskal, K.K., and Akiskal, H.S. (2005). Gender, suicidality and bipolar mixed states in adolescents. *J Affect Disord*, 87, 11–16.

Docherty, N.M., DeRosa, M., and Andreasen, N.C. (1996). Communication disturbances in schizophrenia and mania. *Arch Gen Psychiatry*, 53, 358–364.

Double. D. B. (1990). The factor structure of manic rating scales. *J Affect Disord*, 18, 113–119.

Double, D.B. (1991). A cluster analysis of manic states. *Compr Psychiatry*, 32, 187–194.

Endicott, J., Nee, J., Coryell, W., Keller, M., Andreasen, N., and Croughan, J. (1986). Schizoaffective, psychotic, and non–psychotic depression: Differential familial association. *Compr Psychiatry*, 27, 1–13.

Esquirol, J.E.D. (1838). *Des maladies mentales*. Paris: Balliére. Translated by E.K. Hunt as *Mental Maladies: A Treatise on Insanity*. Philadelphia: Lea and Blachard, 1845 (facsimile edition London, England: Hafner, 1966).

Falret, J.P. (1854). Mémoire sur la folie circulaire, forme de maladie mentale caractérisée par la reproduction successive et régulière de l' état maniaque, de l' état mélancolique, e d'un intervalle lucide plus ou moins prolongé. *Bulletin de l'Académie de Médecine*, 19, 382–415.

Fava, M., and Rosenbaum, J.F. (1999). Anger attacks in patients with depression. *J Clin Psychiatry*, 60(Suppl 15), 21–24.

Fennig, S., Bromet, E.J., Karant, M.T., Ram, R., and Jandorf, L. (1996). Mood-congruent versus mood-incongruent psychotic symptoms in first-admission patients with affective disorder. *J Affect Disord*, 37, 23–29.

Fink, M. (1999). Delirious mania. *Bipolar Disord*, 1, 54–60.

Fitzgerald, F.S. (1956). *The Crack–Up*. New York: New Directions (essays first published in 1936).

Fox, N.A., Henderson, H.A., Rubin, K.H., Calkins, S.D., and Schmidt, L.A. (2001). Continuity and discontinuity of behavioral inhibition and exuberance: Psychophysiological and behavioral influences across the first four years of life. *Child Dev*, 72, 1–21.

Frances, A., Brown, R.P., Kocsis, J.H., and Mann, J.J. (1981). Psychotic depression: A separate entity? *Am J Psychiatry*, 138, 831–833.

Francis, A., Divadeenam, K.M., Bush, G., and Petrides, G. (1997). Consistency of symptoms in recurrent catatonia. *Compr Psychiatry*, 38, 56–60.

Frangos, E., Athanassenas, G., Tsitourides, S., Psilolignos, P., and Katsanou, N. (1983). Psychotic depressive disorder: A separate entity? *J Affect Disord*, 5, 259–265.

Fraser, W.I., King, K.M., Thomas, P., and Kendell, R.E. (1986). The diagnosis of schizophrenia by language analysis. *Br J Psychiatry*, 148, 275–278.

Garety, P. (1985). Delusions: Problems in definition and measurement. *Br J Med Psychol*, 58, 25–34.

Garner, A. (1997). *The Voice that Thunders: Essays and Lectures*. London: Harvill Press.

Ghaemi, S.N., Stoll, A.L., and Pope, H.G. (1995). Lack of insight in bipolar disorder: The acute manic episode. *J Nerv Ment Dis*, 183, 464–467.

Glassman, A.H., and Roose, S.P. (1981). Delusional depression: A distinct clinical entity? *Arch Gen Psychiatry*, 38, 424–427.

Goes, F.S., Sadler, B., Toolan, J., Zamoiski, R.D., Mondimore, F.M., MacKinnon, D.F., Schweizer, B., Bipolar Disorder Phenome Group, DePaulo, J.R., and Potash, J.B. (in press). Psychotic features in bipolar and unipolar depression. *J Bipolar Disord*.

Goldberg, J.F., Harrow, M., and Grossman, L.S. (1995). Recurrent affective syndromes in bipolar and unipolar mood disorders at follow-up. *Br J Psychiatry*, 166, 382–385.

Goldberg, J.F., Garno, J.L., Leon, A.C., Kocsis, J.H., and Portera, L. (1999). A history of substance abuse complicates remission from acute mania in bipolar disorder. *J Clin Psychiatry*, 60, 733–740.

González-Pinto, A., Ballesteros, J., Aldama, A., Pérez de Heredia, J.L., Gutierrez, M., Mosquera, F., and González-Pinto, A. (2003). Principal components of mania. *J Affect Disord*, 76, 95–102.

Goodwin, F.K., Murphy, D.L., and Bunney, W.F. Jr. (1969). Lithium carbonate treatment in depression and mania: A longitudinal double-blind study. *Arch Gen Psychiatry*, 21, 486–496.

Goodwin, D.W., Alderson, P., and Rosenthal, R. (1971) Clinical significance of hallucinations in psychiatric disorders: A study of 116 hallucinatory patients. *Arch. Gen. Psychiatry*, 24, 76–80.

Griesinger, W. (1845). *Pathologie und Therapie der psychischen Krankheiten*. Stuttgart: Adolf Krabbe Verlag.

Griesinger, W. (1867). *Mental Pathology and Therapeutics*. Translated by C.L. Robertson and J. Rutherford. London: New Sydenham Society.

Grossman, L.S., Harrow, M., Lazar, B., Kettering, R., Meltzer, H.Y., and Lechert, J. (1981). *Do thought disorders persist in manic patients?* Abstract of paper presented at the 134th Annual Meeting of the American Psychiatric Association, May.

Grossman, L.S., Harrow, M., and Sands, J.R. (1986). Features associated with thought disorder in manic patients at 2–4 year follow–up. *Am J Psychiatry*, 143, 306–311.

Grunebaum, M.F., Oquendo, M.A., Harkavy-Friedman, J.M., Ellis, S.P., Li, S., and Haas, G.L. (2001). Delusions and suicidality. *Am J Psychiatry*, 158, 743–747.

Guze, S.B., Woodruff, R.A. Jr., and Clayton, P.J. (1975). The significance of psychotic affective disorders. *Arch Gen Psychiatry*, 32, 1147–1150.

Hantouche, E.G., Akiskal, H.S., Lancrenon, S., Allilaire, J.F., Sechter, D., Azorin, J.M., Bourgeois, M., Fraud, J.P., and Châtenet-Duchêne, L. (1998). Systematic clinical methodology for validating bipolar-II disorder: Data in mid-stream from a French national multisite study (EPIDEP). *J Affect Disord*, 50, 63–173.

Hantouche, E.G., Angst, J., and Akiskal, H.S. (2003). Factor structure of hypomania: Interrelationships with cyclothymia and the soft bipolar spectrum. *J Affect Disord*, 73, 39–47.

Hare, E. (1981). The two manias: A study of the evolution of the modern concept of mania. *Br J Psychiatry*, 138, 89–99.

Harrow, M., and Prosen, M. (1978). Intermingling and disordered logic as influences on schizophrenic thought disorders. *Arch Gen Psychiatry*, 35, 1213–1218.

Harrow, M., and Quinlan, D. (1977). Is disordered thinking unique to schizophrenia? *Arch Gen Psychiatry*, 34, 15–21.

Harrow, M., Himmelhoch, J., Tucker, G., Hersh, J., and Quinlan, D. (1972a). Overinclusive thinking in acute schizophrenic patients. *J Abnorm Psychol*, 79, 161–168.

Harrow, M., Tucker, G.J., and Adler, D. (1972b). Concrete and idiosyncratic thinking in acute schizophrenic patients. *Arch Gen Psychiatry*, 26, 433–439.

Harrow, M., Grossman, L.S., Silverstein, M.L., and Meltzer, H.Y. (1982). Thought pathology in manic and schizophrenic patients: Its occurrence at hospital admission and seven weeks later. *Arch Gen Psychiatry*, 39, 665–671.

Harrow, M., Lanin-Kettering, I., Prosen, M., and Miller, J.G. (1983). Disordered thinking in schizophrenia: Intermingling and loss of set. *Schizophr Bull*, 9, 354–367.

Harrow, M., Grossman, L.S., Silverstein, M.L., Meltzer, H.Y., and Kettering, R.L. (1986). A longitudinal study of thought disorder in manic patients. *Arch Gen Psychiatry*, 43, 781–785.

Harrow, M., Goldberg, J.F., Grossman, L.S., and Meltzer, H.Y. (1990). Outcome in manic disorders: A naturalistic follow–up study. *Arch Gen Psychiatry*, 47, 665–671.

Harvey, P.D. (1983). Speech competence in manic and schizophrenic psychoses: The association between clinically rated thought disorder and cohesion and reference performance. *J Abnorm Psychol*, 92, 368–377.

Hawton, K., Sutton, L., Haw, C., Sinclair, J., and Harris, L. (2005). Suicide and attempted suicide in bipolar disorder: A systematic review of risk factors. *J Clin Psychiatry*, 66, 693–704.

Heckers, S. (2002). How many bipolar mixed states are there? *Harvard Rev Psychiatry*, 10, 276–279.

Heinroth, J.C.A. (1818). *Lehrbuch der Stoerungen des Seelenlebens*. Leipzig: Vogel.

Helms, P.M., and Smith, R.E. (1983). Recurrent psychotic depression: Evidence of diagnostic stability. *J Affect Disord*, 5, 51–54.

Henderson, D., and Gillespie, R.D. (1956). *A Text–book of Psychiatry for Students and Practitioners* (8th Edition). London: Oxford University Press.

Himmelhoch, J.M. (1979). Mixed states, manic-depressive illness, and the nature of mood. *Psychiatr Clin North Am*, 2, 449–459.

Himmelhoch, J.M., Harrow, M., Hersh, J., and Tucker, G.J. (1973). *Manual for Assessment of Selected Aspects of Thinking: Object Sorting Test*. ASIS/NAPS #02206, New York: Microfiche Publications.

Himmelhoch, J.M., Mulla, D., Neil, J.F., Detre, T.P., and Kupfer, D.J. (1976a). Incidence and significance of mixed affective states in a bipolar population. *Arch Gen Psychiatry*, 33, 1062–1066.

Himmelhoch, J.M., Coble, P., Kupfer, D.J., and Ingenito, J. (1976b). Agitated psychotic depression associated with severe hypomanic episodes: A rare syndrome. *Am J Psychiatry*, 133, 765–771.

Hoffman, R.E., Stopek, S., and Andreasen, N.C. (1986). A comparative study of manic vs schizophrenic speech disorganization. *Arch Gen Psychiatry*, 43, 831–835.

Holzman, P.S., Solovay, M.R., and Shenton, M.E. (1985). Thought disorder specificity in functional psychoses. In M. Alpert (Ed.), *Controversies in Schizophrenia: Changes and Constancies* (pp. 228–252). New York: Guilford Press.

Ianzito, B.M., Cadoret, R.J., and Pugh, D.D. (1974). Thought disorder in depression. *Am J Psychiatry*, 131, 703–707.

James, W. (1902). *The Varieties of Religious Experience: A Study in Human Nature*. Middlesex, England: Penguin.

Jamison, K.R. (1993). *Touched with Fire: Manic-Depressive Illness and the Artistic Temperament*. New York: Free Press.

Jamison, K.R. (1995). *An Unquiet Mind: A Memoir of Moods and Madness*. New York: Alfred A. Knopf.

Jamison, K.R. (2004). *Exuberance: The Passion for Life*. New York: Alfred A. Knopf.

Jamison, K.R., Gerner, R.H., Hammen, C., and Padesky, C. (1980). Clouds and silver linings: Positive experiences associated with primary affective disorders. *Am J Psychiatry*, 137, 198–202.

Jampala, V.C., Taylor, M.A., and Abrams, R. (1989). The diagnostic implications of formal thought disorder in mania and schizophrenia: A reassessment. *Am J Psychiatry*, 146, 459–463.

Jaspers, K. (1913). *General Psychopathology*. Translated by J. Hoenig and M.W. Hamilton. Chicago: University of Chicago Press.

Jaspers, K. (1997). *General Psychopathology.* Translated by J. Hoenig and M.W. Hamilton. Chicago: University of Chicago Press, 1968. Republished by Johns Hopkins University Press, 1997.

Jelliffe, S.E. (1931). Some historical phases of the manic–depressive synthesis. *Research Publications Association for Research in Nervous and Mental Diseases,* 11, 3–47.

Johnston, M.H., and Holzman, P.S. (1979). *Assessing Schizophrenic Thinking.* San Francisco: Josey–Bass.

Juruena, M.F., Weingarthner, N., Marquardt, A.R., Fleig, S.S., Machado Viera, R., Busnello, E.A., and Broilo, L. (submitted). Bipolar II vs. bipolar I: More differences than previously thought.

Kagan, J. (1989). Temperamental contributions to social behavior. *Am Psychologist,* 44, 688–674.

Kagan, D.L., and Oltmanns, T.F. (1981). Matched tasks for measuring single–word, referent communication: The performance of patients with schizophrenic and affective disorders. *J Abnorm Psychol,* 90, 204–212.

Kagan, J., and Snidman, N. (1991). Infant predictors of inhibited and uninhibited profiles. *Psychol Sci,* 2, 40–44.

Kagan, J., Resnick, J.S., and Snidman, N. (1988). Biological basis of childhood shyness. *Science,* 240, 167–171.

Kagan, J., Snidman, N., and Arcus, D.M. (1992). Initial reactions to unfamiliarity. *Current Directions in Psychological Science,* 1, 171–174.

Kawa, I., Carter, J.D., Joyce, P.R., Doughty, C.J., Frampton, C.M., Wells, J.E., Walsh, A.E.S., and Olds, R.J. (2005). Gender differences in bipolar disorder: Age of onset, course, comorbidity, and symptom presentation. *Bipolar Disord,* 7, 119–125.

Keck, P.E., McElroy, S.L., Havens, J.R., Altshuler, L., Nolen, W.A., Frye, M.A., Suppes, T., Denicoff, K.D., Kupka, R., Leverich, G.S., Rush, J.A., and Post, R.M. (2003). Psychosis in bipolar disorder: Phenomenology and impact on morbidity and course of illness. *Compr Psychiatry,* 44, 263–269.

Kochman, F.J., Hantouche, E.G., Ferrari, P., Lancrenon, S., Bayart, D., and Akiskal, H.S. (2005). Cyclothymic temperament as a prospective predictor of bipolarity and suicidality in children and adolescents with major depressive disorder. *J Affect Disord,* 85, 181–189.

Kotin, J., and Goodwin, F.K. (1972). Depression during mania: Clinical observations and theoretical implications. *Am J Psychiatry,* 129, 679–686.

Koukopoulos, A. (2003). Ewald Hecker's description of cyclothymia as a cyclical mood disorder: Its relevance to the modern concept of bipolar II. *J Affect Disord,* 73, 199–205.

Koukopoulos, A. (2005). The primacy of mania. In H. Akiskal and M. Tohen (Eds.), *Bipolar Psychopharmacotherapy: Caring for the Patient.* New York: John Wiley.

Koukopoulos, A., and Koukopoulos, A. (1999). Agitated depression as a mixed state and the problem of melancholia. In: H.S. Akiskal (Ed.), *Bipolarity: Beyond Classic Mania. Psychiatr Clin North Am,* 22, 547–564.

Koukopoulos, A., Faedda, G., Proietti, R., D'Amico, S., De Pisa, E., and Simonetto, C. (1992). A mixed depressive syndrome. *Encéphale,* 18, 19–21.

Kraepelin, E. (1921). *Manic-Depressive Insanity and Paranoia.* Edinburgh: E & S Livingstone.

Kretschmer, E. (1936). *Physique and Character.* New York: Macmillan.

Krüger, S., Cooke, R.G., Spegg, C.C., and Bräunig, P. (2003). Relevance of the catatonic syndrome to the mixed manic episode. *J Affect Disord,* 74, 279–285.

Lange, J. (1922). *Katatonische Erscheinungen im Rahmen manischer Erkrankungen* Berlin: Julius Springer.

Leff, J.P., Fischer, M., and Bertelsen, A.C. (1976). A cross–national epidemiological study of mania. *Br J Psychiatry,* 129, 428–442.

Lerner, Y. (1980). The subjective experience of mania. In R.H. Belmaker and H.M. Van Praag (Eds.), *Mania: An Evolving Concept* (pp. 77–88). New York: Spectrum Publications.

Lewis, A.J. (1934). Melancholia: A clinical survey of depressive states. *J Ment Sci,* 80, 277–378.

Lott, P.R., Guggenbühl, S., Schneeberer, A., Pulver, A.E., and Stassen, H.H. (2002). Linguistic analysis of the speech output of schizophrenic, bipolar, and depressive patients. *Psychopathology,* 35, 220–227.

Loudon, J.B., Blackburn, I.M., and Ashworth, C.M. (1977). A study of the symptomatology and course of manic illness using a new scale. *Psychol Med,* 7, 723–729.

Lowe, G.R. (1973). The phenomenology of hallucinations as an aid to differential diagnosis. *Br J Psychiatry,* 123, 621–633.

Lundquist, G. (1945). Prognosis and course in manic–depressive psychoses: A follow–up study of 319 first admissions. *Acta Psychiatr Neurol,* (Suppl 35), 1–96.

Lykouras, E., Christodoulou, G.N., and Malliaras D. (1985). Type and content of delusions in unipolar psychotic depression. *J Affect Disord,* 9, 249–252.

Mammen, O.K., Pilkonis, P.A., Chengappa, K.N.R., and Kupfer, D.J. (2004). Anger attacks in bipolar depression: Predictors and response to citalopram added to mood stabilizers. *J Clin Psychiatry,* 65, 627–633.

Mann, S.C., Caroff, S.N., Bleier, H.R., Welz, W.K., Kling, M.A., and Hayashida, M. (1986). Lethal catatonia. *Am J Psychiatry,* 143, 1374–1381.

Mantere, O., Suominen, K., Leppämäki, S., Valtonen, H., Arvilommi, P., and Isometsä, E. (2004). The clinical characteristics of DSM-IV bipolar I and II disorders: Baseline findings from the Jorvi Bipolar Study (JoBS). *Bipolar Disord,* 6(5), 395–405.

Mantere, O., Suominen, K., Avrilommi, P., Valtonen, H., Leppämäki, S., and Isometsä, E. (2006). Clinical predictors of unrecognized bipolar I and II disorders. *J Affect Disord,* 91S, S42, S72, S73.

Maremmani, I., Akiskal, H.S., Signoretta, S., Liguori, A., Perugi, G., and Cloninger, R. (2005). The relationship of Kraepelinian affective temperaments (as measured by TEMPS-I) to the tridimensional personality questionnaire (TPQ). *J Affect Disord,* 85, 17–27.

Markov, V. (1975). *The Longer Poems of Velimir Khlebnikov.* Westport, CT: Greenwood Press.

Marneros, A. (2001). Expanding the group of bipolar disorders. *J Affect Disord,* 62, 39–44.

Marneros, A., and Angst, J. (Eds.). (2000). *Bipolar Disorders: 100 Years after Manic-Depressive Insanity.* London: Kluwer Academic Publishers.

Marneros, A., and Goodwin, F. (Eds). (2003). *Mixed States, Rapid Cycling and Atypical Bipolar Disorders.* London: Cambridge University Press.

Marneros, A., Deister, A., and Rohde, A. (1991a). *Affektive, schizoaffective und schizophrene Psychosen. Eine vergleichende Langzeitstudie.* Berlin: Springer-Verlag.

Marneros, A., Röttig, S., Wenzel, A., Blöink, R., and Brieger, P. (2004). Affective and schizoaffective mixed states. *Eur Arch Psychiatry Clin Neurosci*, 254, 76–81.

Mayer-Gross, W., Slater, E., and Roth, M. (1960). *Clinical Psychiatry* (2nd Edition). London: Cassell & Co.

McElroy, S.L., Keck, P.E., Pope, H.G., Hudson, J.I., Faedda, G.L., and Swann, A.C. (1992). Clinical and research implications of the diagnosis of dysphoric or mixed mania or hypomania. *Am J Psychiatry*, 149, 1633–1644.

McElroy, S.L., Strakowski, S.M., Keck, P.E., Tugrul, K.L., West, S.A., and Lonczak, H.S. (1995). Differences and similarities in mixed and pure mania. *Compr Psychiatry*, 36, 184–194.

McElroy, S.L., Strakowski, S.M., West, S.A., Keck, P.E., and McConville, B.S. (1997). Phenomenology of adolescent and adult mania in hospitalized patients with bipolar disorder. *Am J Psychiatry*, 154, 44–49.

Miklowitz, D. (1992). Longitudinal outcome and medication noncompliance among manic patients with and without mood-incongruent features. *J Nerv Ment Dis*, 180, 703–711.

Mitchell, P.B., Wilhelm, K., Parker, G., Austin, M.P., Rutgers, P., and Malhi, G.S. (2001). The clinical features of bipolar depression: a comparison with matched major depressive disorder patients. *J Clin Psychiatry*, 62(3), 212–216.

Morice, R.D., and Ingram, J.C. (1983). Language complexity and age of onset of schizophrenia. *Psychol Res*, 9, 233–242.

Morice, R.D., and McNicol, D. (1986). Language changes in schizophrenia: A limited replication. *Schizophr Bull*, 12, 239–251.

Murphy, D.L., and Beigel, A. (1974). Depression, elation, and lithium carbonate responses in manic patient subgroups. *Arch Gen Psychiatry*, 31, 643–648.

Nelson, W.H., Khan, A., and Orr, W.W. (1984). Delusional depression: Phenomenology, neuroendocrine function, and tricyclic antidepressant response. *J Affect Disord*, 6, 297–306.

Niecks, F. (1925). *Robert Schumann: A Supplementary and Corrective Biography*. London: JM Dent & Sons.

Nunn, C.M.H. (1979). Mixed affective states and the natural history of manic-depressive psychosis. *Br J Psychiatry*, 134, 153–160.

Orvaschel, H., Thompson, W.D., Belanger, A., Prusoff, B.A., and Kidd, K.K. (1982). Comparison of the family history method to direct interview: Factors affecting the diagnosis of depression. *J Affect Disord*, 4, 45–59.

Othmer, E., DeSouza, C.M., Penick, E.C., Nickel, E.J., Hunter, E.E., Othmer, S.C., Gabrielli, W.F., Read, M.F., Krambeer, L.L., and Powell, B.J. (in press). Psychotic features in major depressive disorder are associated with mania.

Pease, E. (1912). A note on the prognostic value of hallucinations in the manic-depressive psychosis. *Am J Insanity*, 69, 1–36.

Perlis, R.H., Smoller, J.W., Fava, M., Rosenbaum, J.F., Nierenberg, A.A., and Sachs, G.S. (2004). The prevalence and clinical correlates of anger attacks during depressive episodes in bipolar disorder. *J Affect Disord*, 79, 291–295.

Perugi, G., and Akiskal, H.S. (2002). The soft bipolar spectrum redefined: Focus on the anxious-senstivite, impulse-dyscontrol and binge-eating connection in bipolar II and related conditions. *Psychiatr Clin North Am*, 25, 713–737.

Perugi, G., Akiskal, H.S., Micheli, C., Musetti, L., Paiano, A., Quilici, C., Rossi, L., and Cassano, G.B. (1997). Clinical subtypes of bipolar mixed states: Validating a broader European definition in 143 cases. *J Affect Disord*, 43, 169–180.

Perugi, G., Akiskal, H.S., Lattanzi, L., Cecconi, D., Mastrocinque, C., Patronelli, A., and Vignoli, S. (1998a). The high prevalence of soft bipolar (II) features in atypical depression. *Compr Psychiatry*, 39, 63–71.

Perugi, G., Akiskal, H.S., Rossi, L., Paiano, A., Quilici, C., Madaro, D., Musetti, L., and Cassano, G.B. (1998b). Chronic mania: Family history, prior course, clinical picture and social consequences. *Br J Psychiatry*, 173, 514–518.

Perugi, G., Akiskal, H.S., Ramacciotti, S., Nassini, S., Toni, C., Milanfranchi, A., and Musetti, L. (1999). Depressive comorbidity of panic, social phobic and obsessive-compulsive disorders: Is there a bipolar II connection? *J Psychiatr Res*, 33, 53–61.

Perugi, G., Micheli, C., Akiskal, H.S., Modaro, D., Socci, C., Quilci, C., and Musetti, L. (2000). Polarity and course of manic-depressive illness: A retrospective analysis of 320 bipolar I patients. *Compr Psychiatry*, 41, 13–18.

Perugi, G., Akiskal, H.S., Micheli, C., Toni, C., and Madaro, D. (2001a). Clinical characterization of depressive mixed state in bipolar-I patients: Pisa–San Diego collaboration. *J Affect Disord*, 67, 105–114.

Perugi, G., Maremmani, I., Toni, C., Madaro, D., Mata, B., and Akiskal, H.S. (2001b). The contrasting influence of depressive and hyperthymic temperaments on psychometrically derived manic subtypes. *Psychiatry Res*, 101, 249–258.

Pinel, P. (1801). *Traité médico–philosophique sur l'aliénation mentale, ou La manie*. Paris: Brosson. Translated by D.D. Davis as *A Treatise on Insanity*. Sheffield, United Kingdom: Cadell and Davis (facsimile edition, New York: Hafner, 1962).

Placidi, G.F., Maremmani, I., Signoretta, S., Liguori, A., and Akiskal, H.S. (1998). The semi-structured affective temperament interview (TEMPS-I). Reliability and psychometric properties in 1010 14–26-year old students. *J Affect Disord*, 51, 199–208.

Plath, S. (1971). *The Bell Jar*. New York: Harper & Row, 1971.

Plath, S. (1982). *The Journals of Sylvia Plath*. T. Hughes and F. McCullough (Eds.). New York: Dial Press.

Pope, H.G. Jr., and Lipinski, J.S. Jr. (1978). Diagnosis in schizophrenia and manic–depressive illness: A reassessment of the specificity of "schizophrenic" symptoms in light of current research. *Arch Gen Psychiatry*, 35, 811–828.

Post, R.M., Rubinow, D.R., Uhde, T.W., Roy–Byrne, P.P., Linnoila, M., Rosoff, A., and Cowdry, R. (1989). Dysphoric mania: Clinical and biological correlates. *Arch Gen Psychiatry*, 46, 353–358.

Price, L.H., Nelson, J.C., Charney, D.S., and Quinlan, D.M. (1984). Family history in delusional depression. *J Affect Disord*, 6, 109–114.

Prien, R.F., Himmelhoch, J.M., and Kupfer, D.J. (1988). Treatment of mixed mania. *J Affect Disord*, 15, 9–15.

Ragin, A.B., and Oltmanns, T.F. (1983). Predictability as an index of impaired verbal communication in schizophrenic and affective disorders. *Br J Psychiatry*, 143, 578–583.

Ragin, A.B., and Oltmanns, T.F. (1987). Communicability and thought disorder in schizophrenics and other diagnostic groups. A follow–up study. *Br J Psychiatry*, 150, 494–500.

Rapaport, D., Gill, M.M., and Schafer, R. (1968). *Diagnostic Psychological Testing*. New York: International Universities Press.

Reiss, E. (1910). *Konstitutionelle Verstimmung und manisch–depressives Irresein: Klinische Untersuchungen über den Zusammenhang von Veranlagung und Psychose*. Berlin: J. Springer.

Rennie, T.A.C. (1942). Prognosis in manic-depressive psychoses. *Am J Psychiatry*, 98, 801–814.

Resnick, H.S., and Oltmanns, T.F. (1984). Hesitation patterns in the speech of thought-disordered schizophrenic and manic patients. *J Abnorm Psychol*, 93, 80–86.

Robertson, H.A., Lam, R.W., Stewart, J.N., Yatham, L.N., Tam, E.M., and Zis, A.P. (1996). Atypical depressive symptoms and clusters in unipolar and bipolar depression. *Acta Psychiatr Scand*, 94, 421–427.

Roccatagliata, G. (1986). *A History of Ancient Psychiatry*. New York: Greenwood Press.

Roose, S.P., and Glassman, A.H. (1988). Delusional depression. In A. Georgotas and R. Cancro (Eds.), *Depression and Mania* (pp. 76–85). New York: Elsevier.

Rosen, L.N., Rosenthal, N.E., Dunner, D.L., and Fieve, R.R. (1983a). Social outcome compared in psychotic and nonpsychotic bipolar I patients. *J Nerv Ment Dis*, 171, 272–275.

Rosen, L.N., Rosenthal, N.E., VanDusen, P.H., Dunner, D.L., and Fieve, R.R. (1983b). Age at onset and number of psychotic symptoms in bipolar I and schizoaffective disorder. *Am J Psychiatry*, 140, 1523–1524.

Rosenberg, J.D. (1986). *The Darkening Glass: A Portrait of Ruskin's Genius*. New York: Columbia University Press.

Rosenthal, N.E., Rosenthal, L.N., Stallone, F., Fleiss, J., Dunner, D.L., and Fieve, R.R. (1979). Psychosis as a predictor of response to lithium maintenance treatment in bipolar affective disorder. *J Affect Disord*, 1, 237–245.

Rosenthal, N.E., Rosenthal, L.N., Stallone, F., Dunner, D.L., and Fieve, R.R. (1980). Toward the validation of RDC schizoaffective disorder. *Arch Gen Psychiatry*, 37, 804–810.

Rush, B. (1812). *Medical Inquiries and Observations upon the Diseases of the Mind*. Philadelphia: Kimber and Richardson.

Sato, T., Bottlender, R., Kleindienst, N., and Möller, H.J. (2002). Syndromes and phenomenological subtypes underlying acute mania: A factor analytic study of 576 manic patients. *Am J Psychiatry*, 159, 968–974.

Sato, T., Bottlender, R., Schroter, A., and Möller, H.J. (2003). Frequency of manic symptoms during a depressive episode and unipolar 'depressive mixed state' as bipolar spectrum. *Acta Psychiatr Scand*, 107, 268–274.

Sato, T., Bottlender, R., Sievers, M., Schröter, A., and Möller, H.J. (2004). Evaluating the inter-episode stability of depressive mixed states. *J Affect Disord*, 81, 103–113.

Sato, T., Bottlender, R., Sievers, M., and Möller, H.-J. (2006). Distinct seasonality of depressive episodes differentiates unipolar depressive patients with and without depressive mixed states. *J Affect Disord*, 90, 1–5.

Schneider, K. (1959). *Clinical Psychopathology*. Translated by M.W. Hamilton. New York: Grune and Stratton.

Schott, A. (1904). Klinischer Beitrag zur Lehre von der chronischen Manie. *Monatschrift für Psychiatrie und Neurologie*, 15, 1–19.

Schwartz, R.C., Reynolds, C.A., Austin, J.F., and Petersen, S. (2003). Homicidality in schizophrenia: A replication study. *Am J Orthopsychiatry*, 73, 74–77.

Seager, A. (1991). *The Glass House: The Life of Theodore Roethke*. Ann Arbor, MI: University of Michigan Press.

Sedler, M.J. (1983). Falret's discovery: The origin of the concept of bipolar affective illness. *Am J Psychiatry*, 140, 1127–1133.

Serretti, A., and Olgiati, P. (2005). Profiles of "manic" symptoms in bipolar I, bipolar II and major depressive disorders. *J Affect Disord*, 84, 159–166.

Serretti, A., Mandelli, L., Lattuada, E., Cusin, C., and Smeraldi, E. (2002). Clinical and demographic features of mood disorder subtypes. *Psychiatry Res*, 15, 195–210.

Sharma, V., Khan, M., and Smith, A. (2005). A closer look at treatment resistant depression: Is it due to a bipolar diathesis? *J Affect Disord*, 84, 251–257.

Shenton, M.E., Solovay, M.R., and Holzman, P. (1987). Comparative studies of thought disorders: II. Schizoaffective disorder. *Arch Gen Psychiatry*, 44, 21–30.

Signoretta, S., Maremmani, I., Liguori, A., Perugi, G., and Akiskal, H.S. (2005). Affective temperament traits measured by TEMPS-I and emotional-behavioral problems in clinically-well children, adolescents, and young adults. *J Affect Disord* 85, 169–180.

Silberman, E.K., Post, R.M., Nurnberger, J., Theodore, W., and Boulenger, J.P. (1985). Transient sensory, cognitive and affective phenomena in affective illness: A comparison with complex partial epilepsy. *Br J Psychiatry*, 146, 81–89.

Simpson, D.M., and Davis, G.C. (1985). Measuring thought disorder with clinical rating scales in schizophrenic and non-schizophrenic patients. *Psychiatry Res*, 15, 313–318.

Slater, E., and Roth, M. (1969). *Clinical Psychiatry* (3rd Edition). Baltimore: Williams and Wilkins.

Solovay, M.R., Shenton, M.E., and Holzman, P.S. (1987). Comparative studies of thought disorders: I. Mania and schizophrenia. *Arch Gen Psychiatry*, 44, 13–20.

Sonne, S.C., Brady, K.T., and Morton, W.A. (1994). Substance abuse and bipolar affective disorder. *J Nerv Ment Dis*, 182, 349–352.

Spiker, D.G., Weiss, J.C., Dealy, R.S., Griffin, S.J., Hanin, I., Neil, J.F., Perel, J.M., Rossi, A.J., and Soloff, P.H. (1985). The pharmacological treatment of delusional depression. *Am J Psychiatry*, 142, 430–436.

Strakowski, S.M., McElroy, S.L., Keck, P.E., and West, S.A. (1996). Suicidality among patients with mixed and manic bipolar disorder. *Am J Psychiatry*, 153, 674–676.

Strakowski, S.M., Williams, J.R., Sax, K.W., Fleck, D.E., DelBello, M.P., and Bourne, M.L. (2000). Is impaired outcome following a first manic episode due to mood-incongruent psychosis? *J Affect Disord*, 61, 87–94.

Suppes, T., Leverich, G.S., Keck, P.E., Nolen, W.A., Denicoff, K.D., Altshuler, L.L., McElroy, S.L., Rush, A.J., Kupka, R., Frye, M.A., Bickel, M., and Post, R.M. (2001). The Stanley Foundation Bipolar Treatment Outcome Network II. Demographics and illness characteristics of the first 261 patients. *J Affect Disord*, 67, 45–49.

Suppes, T., Mintz, J., McElroy, S.L., Altshulet, L.L., Kupka, R.W., Frye, M.A., Keck, P.E., Nolen, W.A., Leverich, G.S., Grunze, H., Rush, A.J., and Post, R.M. (2005). Mixed hypomania in 908 patients with bipolar disorder evaluated prospectively in the Stanley Foundation Bipolar Treatment Network. *Arch Gen Psychiatry*, 62, 1089–1096.

Swann, A., Janicak, P., Calabrese, J., Bowden, C., Dilsaver, S., Morris, D., Petty, F., and Davis, J. (2001). Structure of mania: Depressive, irritable and psychotic clusters with different retrospectively assessed course patterns of illness in randomized clinical trial participants. *J Affect Disord*, 67, 123–132.

Taylor, M.A., and Abrams, R. (1973). The phenomenology of mania: A new look at some old patients. *Arch Gen Psychiatry*, 29, 520–522.

Taylor, M.A., and Abrams, R. (1975). Acute mania: Clinical and genetic study of responders and nonresponders to treatment. *Arch Gen Psychiatry*, 32, 863–865.

Taylor, M.A., and Abrams, R. (1977). Catatonia: Prevalence and importance in the manic phase of manic-depressive illness. *Arch Gen Psychiatry*, 34, 1223–1225.

Taylor, M.A., and Abrams, R. (1983). Schizo-affective disorder, manic type. A clinical, laboratory, and genetic study. *Psychiatr Clin (Basel)*, 16, 234–244.

Tetsuya, S., Bottlender, R., Sievers, M., and Möller, H.-J. (2006). Distinct seasonality of depressive episodes differentiates unipolar depressive patients with and without depressive mixed states. *J Affect Disord*, 90, 1–5.

Thomas, P., Kearney, G., Napier, E., Ellis, E., Leuder, I., and Johnson, M. (1996). Speech and language in first onset psychosis differences between people with schizophrenia, mania, and controls. *Br J Psychiatry*, 168, 337–343.

Tohen, M., Waternaux, C.M., and Tsuang, M.T. (1990). Outcome in mania. A 4-year prospective follow-up of 75 patients utilizing survival analysis. *Arch Gen Psychiatry*, 47, 1106–1111.

Tohen, M., Tsuang, M.T., and Goodwin, D.C. (1992). Prediction of outcome in mania by mood-congruent or mood-incongruent psychotic features. *Am J Psychiatry*, 149, 1580–1581.

Toni, C., Perugi, G., Mata, B., Madaro, D., Maremmani, I., and Akiskal, H.S. (2001). Is mood-incongruent manic psychosis a distinct subtype? *Eur Arch Psychiatry Clin Neurosci*, 251, 12–17.

Tuke, D.H. (1892). *A Dictionary of Psychological Medicine*. Philadelphia: P. Blakiston, Son & Co.

Vieta, E., Gasto, C., Otero, A., Nieto, E., and Vallejo, J. (1997). Differential features between bipolar I and bipolar II disorder. *Compr Psychiatry*, 38, 98–101.

Walker, F. (1968). *Hugo Wolf: A Biography*. London: JM Dent & Sons.

Waters, B.G.H. (1979). Early symptoms of bipolar affective psychosis: Research and clinical implications. *Can Psychiatr Assoc J*, 2, 55–60.

Watkins, J.G., and Stauffacher, J.C. (1952). An index of pathological thinking in the Rorschach. *J Projective Techniques*, 16, 276–286.

Wellner, J., and Marstal, H.B. (1964). Symptoms in mania, an analysis of 279 attacks of manic depressive elation. In B. Jansson (Ed.), Report on the Fourteenth Congress of Scandinavian Psychiatrist. *Acta Psychiatr Scand*, 40(Suppl 180), 175–176.

Wertham, F.I. (1929). A group of benign psychoses: Prolonged manic excitements: With a statistical study of age, duration and frequency in 2000 manic attacks. *Am J Psychiatry*, 9, 17–78.

Weygandt, W. (1899). *Uber die Mischzustande des manisch-depressiven Irreseins*. Munich: J.F. Lehmann.

Winokur, G. (1984). Psychosis in bipolar and unipolar affective illness with special reference to schizo-affective disorder. *Br J Psychiatry*, 145, 236–242.

Winokur, G., and Kadrmas, A. (1989). A polyepisodic course in bipolar illness: Possible clinical relationships. *Compr Psychiatry*, 30, 121–127.

Winokur, G., and Tsuang, M.T. (1975). Elation versus irritability in mania. *Compr Psychiatry*, 16, 435–436.

Winokur, G., Clayton, P.J., and Reich T. (1969). *Manic Depressive Illness*. St. Louis: CV Mosby.

Winokur, G., Scharfetter, C., and Angst, J. (1985). Stability of psychotic symptomatology (delusions, hallucinations), affective syndromes, and schizophrenic symptoms (thought disorder, incongruent affect) over episodes in remitting psychoses. *Eur Arch Psychiatry Neurol Sci*, 234, 303–307.

Winokur, G., Crowe, R., and Kadrmas, A. (1986). Genetic approach to heterogeneity in psychoses: Relationship of a family history of mania or depression to course in bipolar illness. *Psychopathology*, 19, 80–84.

Woods, S.W., Money, R., and Baker, C.B. (2001). Does the manic/mixed episode distinction in bipolar disorder patients run true over time? *Am J Psychiatry*, 158, 1324–1326.

Young, R.C., and Klerman, G.L. (1992) Mania in late life: focus on age at onset. *Am J Psychiatry*, 149, 867–876.

Young, R.C., Schreiber, M.T., and Nysewander, R.W. (1983). Psychotic mania. *Biol Psychiatry*, 18, 1167–1173.

CHAPTER 3

Akiskal, H.S. (1996). The prevalent clinical spectrum of bipolar disorders: Beyond DSM-IV. *J Clin Psychopharmacol*, 16(2 Suppl. 1), 4S–14S.

Akiskal, H.S. (2002). The bipolar spectrum: The shaping of a new paradigm in psychiatry. *Curr Psychiatry Rep*, 4(1), 1–3.

Akiskal, H.S. (2005). Searching for behavioral indicators of bipolar II in patients presenting with major depressive episodes: The "red sign," the "rule of three" and other biographic signs of temperamental extravagance, activism, and hypomania. *J Affect Disord*, 84, 279–290.

Akiskal, H.S., and Benazzi, F. (2003). Family history validation of the bipolar nature of depressive mixed states. *J Affect Disord*, 73(1-2), 113–122.

Akiskal, H.S., and Benazzi, F. (2005). Atypical depression: A variant of bipolar II or a bridge between unipolar and bipolar II? *J Affect Disord*, 84(2-3), 209–217.

Akiskal, H.S., Maser, J.D., Zeller, P.J., Endicott, J., Coryell, W., Keller, M., Warshaw, M., Clayton, P., and Goodwin, F. (1995). Switching from 'unipolar' to bipolar II. An 11-year prospective study of clinical and temperamental predictors in 559 patients. *Arch Gen Psychiatry*, 52(2), 114–123.

Akiskal, H.S., Hantouche, E.G., Allilaire, J.F., Sechter, D., Bourgeois, M.L., Azorin, J.M., Chatenet-Duchene, L., and Lancrenon, S. (2003). Validating antidepressant-associated hypomania (bipolar III): A systematic comparison with spontaneous hypomania (bipolar II). *J Affect Disord*, 73(1-2), 65–74.

Amador, X.F., Flaum, M., Andreasen, N.C., Strauss, D.H., Yale, S.A., Clark, S.C., and Gorman, J.M. (1994). Awareness of illness in schizophrenia and schizoaffective and mood disorders. *Arch Gen Psychiatry*, 51(10), 826–836.

American Psychiatric Association. (2005). *DSM-V prelude project: Research and outreach*. Available: http://www.dsm5.org/ [July 1, 2005].

Amin, S., Singh, S.P., Brewin, J., Jones, P.B., Medley, I., and Harrison, G. (1999). Diagnostic stability of first-episode psychosis. Comparison of ICD-10 and DSM-III-R systems. *Br J Psychiatry*, 175, 537–543.

Andreasen, N.C. (1982). Negative symptoms in schizophrenia: Definition and reliability. *Arch Gen Psychiatry*, 39, 784–788.

Andreasen, N.C., and Grove, W.M. (1982). The classification of depression: Traditional versus mathematical approaches. *Am J Psychiatry*, 139, 45–52.

Andreasen, N.C., Grove, W.M., Shapiro, R.W., Keller, M.B., Hirschfeld, R.M.A., and McDonald-Scott, P. (1981). Reliability of lifetime diagnosis: A multicenter collaborative perspective. *Arch Gen Psychiatry*, 38, 400–405.

Angst, J. (1980). Verlauf unipolar depressiver, bipolar manisch-depressiver und schizo-affektiver Erkrankungen und Psychosen: Ergebnisse einer prospektiven Studie. *Fortschr Neurol Psychiatr*, 48, 3–30.

Angst, J. (1998). The emerging epidemiology of hypomania and bipolar II disorder. *J Affect Disord*, 50(2-3), 143–151.

Angst, J., and Cassano, G. (2005). The mood spectrum: Improving the diasnosis of bipilor disorder. *Bipolar Disord*, 7 (Suppl 4), 4–12.

Angst, J., Gamma, A., Benazzi, F., Ajacic, V., Eich, D., and Rossler, W. (2003). Toward a re-definition of subthreshold bipolarity: Epidemiology and proposed criteria for bipolar-II, minor bipolar disorders and hypomania. *J Affect Disord*, 73(1-2), 133–146.

Angst, J., Sellaro, R., Stassen, H.H., and Gamma, A. (2005). Diagnostic conversion from depression to bipolar disorders: Results of a long-term prospective study of hospital admissions. *J Affect Disord*, 84, 149–157.

Atre-Vaidya, N., and Hussain, S.M. (1999). Borderline personality disorder and bipolar mood disorder: Two distinct disorders or a continuum? *J Nerv Ment Dis*, 187, 313–315.

Benazzi, F. (1999). Bipolar II disorder is common among depressed outpatients. *Psychiatry Clin Neurosci*, 53, 607–609.

Benazzi, F. (2000a). Borderline personality disorder and bipolar II disorder in private practice depressed outpatients. *Compr Psychiatry*, 41(2), 106–110.

Benazzi, F. (2000b). Depression with DSM-IV atypical features: A marker for bipolar II disorder. *Eur Arch Psychiatry Clin Neurosci*, 250(1), 53–55.

Benazzi, F. (2001). Is the minimum duration of hypomania in bipolar II disorder 4 days? *Can J Psychiatry*, 46, 86.

Benazzi, F., and Akiskal, H.S. (2005). A downscaled practical measure of mood lability as a screening tool for bipolar II. *J Affect Disord*, 84, 225–232.

Benazzi, F., and Rihmer, Z. (2000). Sensitivity and specificity of DSM-IV atypical features for bipolar II disorder diagnosis. *Psychiatry Res*, 93(3), 257–262.

Berns, S., Jaeger, J., Iannuzzo, R., et al. (2003). *A comparison of medical chart diagnosis with SCID consensus diagnosis among bipolar disorder patients* (abstract). Presented at the 5th International Conference on Bipolar Disorder, Pittsburgh, PA.

Blacker, D., and Tsuang, M.T. (1992). Contested boundaries of bipolar disorder and the limits of categorical diagnosis in psychiatry. *Am J Psychiatry*, 149, 1473–1483.

Bleuler, E. (1911). *Dementia Praecox or the Group of Schizophrenias.* Translated by J. Zinkin. New York: International Universities Press, 1950. (Originally published in German as a volume of *Aschaffenburg's Handbuch, Dementia Praecox oder die Gruppe der Schizophrenien.*)

Bleuler, M. (1968). Significance of the current theory of depression in general practice. *Ther Umsch*, 25(1), 3–4.

Bridge, T.P., Mirsky, A.F., and Goodwin, F.K. (Eds.). (1988). *Psychological, Neuropsychiatric and Substance Abuse Aspects in AIDS: Advances in Biochemical Psychopharmacology.* Vol. 44. New York: Raven Press.

Brockington, I.F., and Jeff, J.P. (1979). Schizo-affective psychoses: Definitions and incidence. *Psychol Med*, 9, 91–99.

Brockington, I.F., Kendell, R.E., and Wainwright, S. (1980). Depressed patients with schizophrenic or paranoid symptoms. *Psychol Med*, 10(4), 665–675.

Cantor, N., Smith, E.E., French, R.S., and Mezzich, J. (1980). Psychiatric diagnosis as prototype categorization. *J Abnorm Psychol*, 89(2), 181–193.

Carlson, G.A., and Goodwin, F.K. (1973). The stages of mania. A longitudinal analysis of the manic episode. *Arch Gen Psychiatry*, 28(2), 221–228.

Cassidy, F., Murry, E., Forest, K., and Carroll, B.J. (1998). Signs and symptoms of mania in pure and mixed episodes. *J Affect Disord*, 50(2-3), 187–201.

Cassidy, F., Ahearn, E., and Carroll, B.J. (2001a). A prospective study of inter-episode consistency of manic and mixed subtypes of bipolar disorder. *J Affect Disord*, 67, 181–185.

Cassidy, F., Pieper, C.F., and Carroll, B.J. (2001b). Subtypes of mania determined by grade of membership analysis. *Neuropsychopharmacology*, 25(3), 373–383.

Cassidy, F., Ahearn, E.P., and Carroll, B.J. (2002). Symptom profile consistency in recurrent manic episodes. *Compr Psychiatry*, 43(3), 179–181.

Citrome, L., and Goldberg, J.F. (2005). The many faces of bipolar disorder. How to tell them part. *Postgrad Med*, 117(2), 15–16, 19–23.

Cluss, P.A., Marcus, S.C., Kelleher, K.J., Thase, M.E., Arvay, L.A., and Kupfer, D.J. (1999). Diagnostic certainty of a voluntary bipolar disorder case registry. *J Affect Disord*, 52, 93–99.

Copper, J.E., Kendell, R.E., Gurland, B.J., Sharpe, L., Copeland, J.R.M., and Simon, R. (1972). Psychiatric diagnosis in New York and London: A comparative study of mental hospital admissions. Maudsley Monograph No. 20. London: Oxford University Press.

Coryell, W., Keller, M., Endicott, J., Andreasen, N., Clayton, P., and Hirschfeld, R. (1989). Bipolar II illness: Course and outcome over a five-year period. *Psychol Med*, 19(1), 129–141.

Coryell, W., Keller, M., Lavori, P., and Endicott, J. (1990). Affective syndromes, psychotic features, and prognosis. II. Mania. *Arch Gen Psychiatry*, 47(7), 658–662.

Craddock, N., and Owen, M.J. (2005). The beginning of the end for the Kraepelinian dichotomy. *Br J Psychiatry*, 186, 364–366.

Crow, T.J. (1990). The continuum of psychosis and its genetic origins. The sixty-fifth Maudsley lecture. *Br J Psychiatry*, 156, 788–797.

Crow, T.J. (1998). From Kraepelin to Kretschmer leavened by Schneider: The transition from categories of psychosis to dimensions of variation intrinsic to Homo sapiens. *Arch Gen Psychiatry*, 55(6), 502–504.

Cutting, J. (1990). Relationship between cycloid psychosis and typical affective psychosis. *Psychopathology*, 23(4-6), 212–219.

Danielson, C.K., Youngstrom, E.A., Findling, R.L., and Calabrese, J.R. (2003). Discriminative validity of the general behavior inventory using youth report. *J Abnorm Child Psychol*, 31(1), 29–39.

DeBattista, C., Sofuoglu, M., and Schatzberg, A.F. (1998). Serotonergic synergism: The risks and benefits of combining the selective serotonin reuptake inhibitors with other serotonergic drugs. *Biol Psychiatry*, 44(5), 341–347.

Dikeos, D.G., Wickham, H., McDonald, C., Walshe, M., Sigmundsson, T., Bramon, E., Grech, A., Toulopoulou, T., Murray, R., and Sham, P.C. (2006). Distribution of symptom dimensions across Kraepelinian divisions. *Br J Psychiatry*, 189, 346–353.

Dunner, D.L. (1992). Differential diagnosis of bipolar disorder. *J Clin Psychopharmacol*, 12(Suppl. 1), 7S–12S.

Dunner, D.L. (1998). Diagnostic revisions for DSM-IV. In P.J. Goodnick (Ed.), *Mania. Clinical and Research Perspectives* (pp. 3–10). Washington, DC: American Psychiatric Press.

Dunner, D.L., and Tay, L.K. (1993). Diagnostic reliability of the history of hypomania in bipolar II patients and patients with major depression. *Compr Psychiatry,* 34(5), 303–307.

Evans, J.D., Heaton, R.K., Paulsen, J.S., McAdams, L.A., Heaton, S.C., and Jeste, D.V. (1999). Schizoaffective disorder: A form of schizophrenia or affective disorder? *J Clin Psychiatry,* 60(12), 874–882.

Feighner, J.P., Robins, E., Guze, S.B., Woodruff, R.A., Jr., Winokur, G., and Munoz, R. (1972). Diagnostic criteria for use in psychiatric research. *Arch Gen Psychiatry,* 26(1), 57–63.

Fennig, S., Kovasznay, C., Rich, R., Ram, C., Pato, A., Miller, J., Rubinstein, G., Carlson, J.E., Schwartz, and Phelan, J. (1994). Six-month stability of psychiatric diagnoses in first-admission patients with psychosis. *Am J Psychiatry,* 151, 1200–1208.

Fergus, E.L., Miller, R.B., Luckenbaugh, D.A., Leverich, G.S., Findling, R.L., Speer, A.M., and Post, R.M. (2003). Is there progression from irritability/dyscontrol to major depressive and manic symptoms? A retrospective community survey of parents of bipolar children. *J Affect Disord,* 77(1), 71–78.

Fink, M. (1999). Delirious mania. *Bipolar Disord,* 1(1), 54–60.

Flor-Henry, P. (1969). Schizophrenic-like reactions and affective psychoses associated with temporal lobe epilepsy: Etiological factors. *Am J Psychiatry,* 126(3), 400–404.

Gabel, R.H., Barnard, N., Norko, M., and O'Connell, R.A. (1986). AIDS presenting as mania. *Compr Psychiatry,* 27(3), 251–254.

Gershon, E.S., Hamovit, J., Guroff, J.J., Dibble, E., Leckman, J.F., Sceery, W., Targum, S.D., Nurnberger, J.I., Jr., Goldin, L.R., and Bunney, W.E., Jr. (1982). A family study of schizoaffective, bipolar I, bipolar II, unipolar, and normal control probands. *Arch Gen Psychiatry,* 39(10), 1157–1167.

Ghaemi, S.N., Stoll, A.L., and Pope, H.G., Jr. (1995). Lack of insight in bipolar disorder. The acute manic episode. *J Nerv Ment Dis,* 183(7), 464–467.

Ghaemi, S.N., Sachs, G.S., Chiou, A.M., Pandurangi, A.K., and Goodwin, K. (1999). Is bipolar disorder still underdiagnosed? Are antidepressants overutilized? *J Affect Disord,* 52(1-3), 135–144.

Ghaemi, S.N., Boiman, E.E., and Goodwin, F.K. (2000). Diagnosing bipolar disorder and the effect of antidepressants: A naturalistic study. *J Clin Psychiatry,* 61(10), 804–808; quiz 809.

Ghaemi, S.N., Ko, J.Y., and Goodwin, F.K. (2002). Cade's disease and beyond: Misdiagnosis, antidepressant use, and a proposed definition for bipolar spectrum disorder. *Can J Psychiatry,* 47(2), 125–134.

Ghaemi, S.N., Hsu, D.J., Ko, J.Y., Baldassano, C.F., Kontos, N.J., and Goodwin, F.K. (2004). Bipolar spectrum disorder: A pilot study. *Psychopathology,* 37(5), 222–226.

Gibbs, F.A., and Gibbs, E.L. (1952). *Atlas of Electroencephalography.* Vol. 2, Epilepsy. Cambridge, MA: Addison-Wesley Press.

Goldberg, J.F., Harrow, M., and Grossman, L. (1995). Course and outcome in bipolar affective disorder: A longitudinal follow-up study. *Am J Psychiatry,* 152(3), 379–384.

Goldberg, J.F., Harrow, M., and Whiteside, J.E. (2001). Risk for bipolar illness in patients initially hospitalized for unipolar depression. *Am J Psychiatry,* 158, 1265–1270.

Goodwin, F.K., and Bunney, W.E., Jr. (1971). Depressions following reserpine: A reevaluation. *Semin Psychiatry,* 3, 435–448.

Goodwin, F.K., and Ghaemi, S.N. (1998). Understanding manic-depressive illness. *Arch Gen Psychiatry,* 55, 23–25.

Guy, W., and Ban, T.A. (Eds.). (1982). *The AMDP System: Manual for the Assessment and Documentation of Psychopathology.* Berlin: Springer-Verlag.

Hantouche, E.G., Allilaire, J.P., Bourgeois, M.L., Azorin, J.M., Sechter, D., Chatenet-Duchene, L., Lancrenon, S., and Akiskal, H.S. (2001). The feasibility of self-assessment of dysphoric mania in the French national EPIMAN study. *J Affect Disord,* 67(1-3), 97–103.

Hirschfeld, R.M., Williams, J.B., Spitzer, R.L., Calabrese, J.R., Flynn, L., Keck, P.E., Jr., Lewis, L., McElroy, S.L., Post, R.M., Rapport, D.J., Russell, J.M., Sachs, G.S., and Zajecka, J. (2000). Development and validation of a screening instrument for bipolar spectrum disorder: The Mood Disorder Questionnaire. *Am J Psychiatry,* 157(11), 1873–1875.

Hirschfeld, R.M., Lewis, L., and Vornik, L.A. (2003). Perceptions and impact of bipolar disorder: How far have we really come? Results of the national depressive and manic-depressive association 2000 survey of individuals with bipolar disorder. *J Clin Psychiatry,* 64(2), 161–174.

Jampala, V.C., Abrams, R., and Taylor, M.A. (1985). Mania with emotional blunting: Affective disorder or schizophrenia? *Am J Psychiatry,* 142(5), 608–612.

Jampala, V.C., Taylor, M.A., and Abrams, R. (1989). The diagnostic implications of formal thought disorder in mania and schizophrenia: A reassessment. *Am J Psychiatry,* 146, 459–463.

Jaspers, K. (1913). *General Psychology.* Translated by J. Hoenig and M.W. Hamilton. Baltimore: Johns Hopkins University Press, 1997.

Jorm, A.F. (2000). Is depression a risk factor for dementia or cognitive decline? A review. *Gerontology,* 46(4), 219–227.

Kanner, A.M. (2004). Recognition of the various expressions of anxiety, psychosis, and aggression in epilepsy. *Epilepsia,* 45(Suppl. 2), 22–27.

Kasanin, J. (1933). The acute schizoaffective psychoses. *Am J Psychiatry,* 17, 877–883.

Keitner, G.I., Solomon, D.A., Ryan, C.E., Miller, I.W., Mallinger, A., Kupfer, D.J., and Frank, E. (1996). Prodromal and residual symptoms in bipolar I disorder. *Compr Psychiatry,* 37(5), 362–367.

Keller, M.B., and Baker, L.A. (1991). Bipolar disorder: Epidemiology, course, diagnosis, and treatment. *Bull Menninger Clin,* 55(2), 172–181.

Keller, M.B., Lavori, P.W., McDonald-Scott, P., Scheftner, W.A., Andreasen, N.C., Shapiro, R.W., and Croughan, J. (1981). Reliability of lifetime diagnosis and symptoms in patients with a current psychiatric disorder. *J Psychiatr Res,* 4, 229–240.

Kendler, K.S. (1986). Kraepelin and the differential diagnosis of dementia praecox and manic-depressive insanity. *Compr Psychiatry,* 27, 549–558.

Kendler, K.S., Gruenberg, A.M., and Tsuang, M.T. (1986). A DSM-III family study of nonschizophrenic psychotic disorders. *Am J Psychiatry,* 143, 1098–1105.

Kendler, K.S., McGuire, M., Gruenberg, A.M., O'Hare, A., Spellman, M., and Walsh, D. (1993). The Roscommon family study. I. Methods, diagnosis of probands, and risk of schizophrenia in relatives. *Arch Gen Psychiatry,* 50(7), 527–540.

Kendler, K.S., Gallagher, T.J., Abelson, J.M., and Kessler, R.C. (1996). Lifetime prevalence, demographic risk factors, and diagnostic validity of nonaffective psychosis as assessed in a U.S. community sample. The National Comorbidity Survey. *Arch Gen Psychiatry*, 53(11), 1022–1031.

Kendler, K.S., Karkowski, L.M., and Walsh, D. (1998). The structure of psychosis: Latent class analysis of probands from the Roscommon Family Study. *Arch Gen Psychiatry*, 55(6), 492–499.

Keri, S., Kelemen, O., Benedek, G., and Janka, Z. (2001). Different trait markers for schizophrenia and bipolar disorder: A neurocognitive approach. *Psychol Med*, 31(5), 915–922.

Kessing, L. (2005). Diagnostic stability in bipolar disorder in clinical practice as according to ICD-10. *J Affect Disord*, 85(3), 293–299.

Kessler, R.C., Adler, L., Barkley, R., Biederman, J., Conners, C.K., Demler, O., Faraone, S.V., Greenhill, L.L., Howes, M.J., Secnik, K., Spencer, T., Ustun, T.B., Walters, E.E., and Zaslavsky, A.M. (2006). The prevalence and correlates of adult ADHD in the United States: Results from the National Comorbidity Survey Replication. *Am J Psychiatry*, 163(4), 716–723.

Ketter, T.A., Wang, P.W., Becker, O.V., Nowakowska, C., and Yang, Y.S. (2003). The diverse roles of anticonvulsants in bipolar disorders. *Ann Clin Psychiatry*, 15(2), 95–108.

Ketter, T.A., Wang, P.W., Becker, O.V., Nowakowska, C., and Yang, Y. (2004). Psychotic bipolar disorders: Dimensionally similar to or categorically different from schizophrenia? *J Psychiatr Res*, 38(1), 47–61.

Koukopoulos, A. (2001). *Treating the complex patient* (abstract). Presented at 4th Annual International Conference on Bipolar Disorder, Pittsburgh, PA.

Koukopoulos, A., Faedda, G., Proietti, R., D'Amico, S., de Pisa, E., and Simonetto, C. (1992). Mixed depressive syndrome. *Encephale*, 18 Spec(1), 19–21.

Koukopoulos, A., Albert, M.J., Sani, G., Koukopoulos, A.E., and Girardi, P. (2005). Mixed depressive states: Nosologic and therapeutic issues. *Int Rev Psychiatry*, 17(1), 12–37.

Kraepelin, E. (1896). *Ein Lehrbuch fur Studirende und Aerzte. Psychiatrie*. Leipzig: J.A. Barth, 8th ed. published in 1913. Reprinted in 1976, New York: Arno Press.

Kraepelin, E. (1913). *Psychiatrie. Ein Lehrbuch fur Studirende und Aerzte*, 8th edition. (Leipzig: JA Barth, 1896). Reprinted New York: Arno Press, 1976.

Kraepelin, E. (1921). *Manic-Depressive Insanity and Paranoia*. Edinburgh: E & S Livingstone.

Krauthammer, C., and Klerman, G.L. (1978). Secondary mania: Manic syndromes associated with antecedent physical illness or drugs. *Arch Gen Psychiatry*, 35(11), 1333–1339.

Kudo, T., Ishida, S., Kubota, H., and Yagi, K. (2001). Manic episode in epilepsy and bipolar I disorder: A comparative analysis of 13 patients. *Epilepsia*, 42(8), 1036–1042.

Leonhard, K. (1957). *Aufteilung der Endogenen Psychosen*, 1st edition. Berlin: Akademie-Verlag. Translated by R. Berman as *The Classification of Endogenous Psychoses*, 5th edition. Edited by E. Robins. New York: Irvington Publishers, 1979.

Lewis, L. (2001). *The use of surveys as an advocacy tool* (abstract). Presented at 4th International Conference for Bipolar Disorder, Pittsburgh, PA.

Lish, J.D., Dime-Meenan, S., Whybrow, P.C., Price, R.A., and Hirschfeld, R.M. (1994). The National Depressive and Manic-Depressive Association (DMDA) survey of bipolar members. *J Affect Disord*, 31(4), 281–294.

Lyketsos, C.G., Schwartz, J., Fishman, M., and Treisman, G. (1997). AIDS mania. *J Neuropsychiatry Clin Neurosci*, 9(2), 277–279.

Maj, M., Pirozzi, R., and Starace, F. (1989). Previous pattern of course of the illness as a predictor of response to lithium prophylaxis in bipolar patients. *J Affect Disord*, 17, 237–241.

Manning, J.S., Haykal, R.F., Connor, P.D., and Akiskal, H.S. (1997). On the nature of depressive and anxious states in a family practice setting: The high prevalence of bipolar II and related disorders in a cohort followed longitudinally. *Compr Psychiatry*, 38(2), 102–108.

Marneros, A. (2001). Origin and development of concepts of bipolar mixed states. *J Affect Disord*, 67(1-3), 229–240.

Marneros, A., Deister, A., Rohde, A., Junemann, H., and Fimmers, R. (1988). Long-term course of schizoaffective disorders. Part I: Definitions, methods, frequency of episodes and cycles. *Eur Arch Psychiatry Neurol Sci*, 237(5), 264–275.

Marneros, A., Rohde, A., Deister, A., and Steinmeyer, E.M. (1989). Premorbid and social markers of patients with schizoaffective psychoses. *Fortschr Neurol Psychiatr*, 57(5), 205–212.

Marneros, A., Deister, A., and Rohde, A. (1991). Stability of diagnoses in affective, schizoaffective and schizophrenic disorders. Cross-sectional versus longitudinal diagnosis. *Eur Arch Psychiatry Clin Neurosci*, 241(3), 187–192.

Marneros, A., Pillmann, F., Haring, A., and Balzuweit, S. (2000). Acute and transient psychotic disorders. *Fortschr Neurol Psychiatr*, 68(Suppl. 1), S22–S25.

McElroy, S.L., Keck, P.E., Jr., Pope, H.G., Jr., Hudson, J.I., Faedda, G.L., and Swann, A.C. (1992). Clinical and research implications of the diagnosis of dysphoric or mixed mania or hypomania. *Am J Psychiatry*, 149(12), 1633–1644.

McKenna, P.J., Kane, J.M., and Parrish, K. (1985). Psychotic syndromes in epilepsy. *Am J Psychiatry*, 142(8), 895–904.

Melton, S.T., Kirkwood, C.K., and Ghaemi, S.N. (1997). Pharmacotherapy of HIV dementia. *Ann Pharmacother*, 31(4), 457–473.

Miller, A., Fox, N.A., Cohn, J.F., Forbes, E.E., Sherrill, J.T., and Kovacs, M. (2002). Regional patterns of brain activity in adults with a history of childhood-onset depression: Gender differences and clinical variability. *Am J Psychiatry*, 159(6), 934–940.

Miller, C.J., Klugman, J., Berv, D.A., Rosenquist, K.J., and Ghaemi, S.N. (2004). Sensitivity and specificity of mood disorder questionnaire for detecting bipolar disorder. *J Affect Disord*, 81(2), 167–171.

Mitchell, P., Parker, G., Jamieson, K., Wilhelm, K., Hickie, I., Brodaty, H., Boyce, P., Hadzi-Pavlovic, D., and Roy, K. (1992). Are there any differences between bipolar and unipolar melancholia? *J Affect Disord*, 25(2), 97–105.

Mitsuda, H. (1965). The concept of "atypical psychoses" from the aspect of clinical genetics. *Acta Psychiatr Scand*, 41, 372–377.

Nierenberg, A.A., Miyahara, S., Spencer, T., Wisniewski, S.R., Otto, M.W., Simon, N., Pollack, M.H., Ostacher, M.J., Yan, L., Siegel, R., Sachs, G.S., and STEP-BD Investigators (2005). Clinical and diagnostic implications of lifetime attention-deficit/hyperactivity disorder comorbidity in adults with bipolar disorder. *Biol Psychiatry*, 57(11), 146–1473.

Parker, G., Parker, K., Malhi, G., Wilhelm, K., and Mitchell, P. (2004). Studying personality characteristics in bipolar depressed subjects: How comparator group selection can dictate results. *Acta Psychiatr Scand*, 109(5), 376–382.

Perris, C. (1988). The concept of cycloid psychotic disorder. *Psychiatr Dev*, 6(1), 37–56.

Perris, C. (1990). The importance of Karl Leonhard's classification of endogenous psychoses. *Psychopathology*, 23(4-6), 282–290.

Perugi, G., Akiskal, H.S., Micheli, C., Musetti, L., Paiano, A., Quilici, C., Rossi, L., and Cassano, G.B. (1997). Clinical subtypes of bipolar mixed states: Validating a broader European definition in 143 cases. *J Affect Disord*, 43(3), 169–180.

Perugi, G., Akiskal, H.S., Micheli, C., Toni, C., and Madaro, D. (2001). Clinical characterization of depressive mixed state in bipolar-I patients: Pisa–San Diego collaboration. *J Affect Disord*, 67(1-3), 105–114.

Pfuhlmann, B., Jabs, B., Althaus, G., Schmidtke, A., Bartsch, A., Stober, G., Beckmann, H., and Franzek, E. (2004). Cycloid psychoses are not part of a bipolar affective spectrum: Results of a controlled family study. *J Affect Disord*, 83(1), 11–19.

Phelps, J.R., and Ghaemi, S.N. (2006). Improving the diagnosis of bipolar disorder: Predictive value of screening tests. *J Affect Disord,* 92(2-3), 141–148.

Pope, H.G. (1983). Distinguishing bipolar disorder from schizophrenia in clinical practice: Guidelines and case reports. *Hosp Community Psychiatry*, 34, 322–328.

Pope, H.G., Jr., and Lipinski, J.F., Jr. (1978). Diagnosis in schizophrenia and manic-depressive illness: A reassessment of the specificity of 'schizophrenic' symptoms in the light of current research. *Arch Gen Psychiatry*, 35(7), 811–828.

Post, R.M., and Weiss, S.R. (2004). Convergences in course of illness and treatments of the epilepsies and recurrent affective disorders. *Clin EEG Neurosci*, 35(1), 14–24.

Price, L.H., Charney, D.S., Rubin, A.L., and Heninger, G.R. (1986). Alpha 2-adrenergic receptor function in depression: The cortisol response to yohimbine. *Arch Gen Psychiatry*, 43, 849–858.

Prien, R.F., Himmelhoch, J.M., and Kupfer, D.J. (1988). Treatment of mixed mania. *J Affect Disord*, 15(1), 9–15.

Rice, J.P., Rochberg, N., Endicott, J., Lavori, P.W., and Miller, C. (1992). Stability of psychiatric diagnoses. An application to the affective disorders. *Arch Gen Psychiatry*, 49, 824–830.

Sachs, G.S., Baldassano, C.F., Truman, C.J., and Guille, C. (2000). Comorbidity of attention deficit hyperactivity disorder with early- and late-onset bipolar disorder. *Am J Psychiatry*, 157(3), 466–468.

Salvatore, P., Baldessarini, R.J., Centorrino, F., Egli, S., Albert, M., Gerhard, A., and Maggini, C. (2002). Weygandt's on the mixed states of manic-depressive insanity: A translation and commentary on its significance in the evolution of the concept of bipolar disorder. *Harv Rev Psychiatry*, 10(5), 255–275.

Sato, T., Bottlender, R., Kleindienst, N., Tanabe, A., and Moller, H.J. (2002). The boundary between mixed and manic episodes in the ICD-10 classification. *Acta Psychiatr Scand*, 106(2), 109–116.

Schatzberg, A.F., and Rothschild, A.J. (1992). Psychotic (delusional) major depression: Should it be included as a distinct syndrome in DSM-IV? *Am J Psychiatry*, 149(6), 733–745.

Scheffer, R.E., and Niskala Apps, J.A. (2004). The diagnosis of preschool bipolar disorder presenting with mania: Open pharmacological treatment. *J Affect Disord*, 82(Suppl. 1), S25–S34.

Schneider, K. (1959). *Clinical Psychopathology*. Translated by M.W. Hamilton. New York: Grune and Stratton.

Serretti, A., Rietschel, M., Lattuada, E., Krauss, H., Schulze, T.G., Muller, D.J., Maier, W., and Smeraldi, E. (2001). Major psychoses symptomatology: Factor analysis of 2241 psychotic subjects. *Eur Arch Psychiatry Clin Neurosci*, 251(4), 193–198.

Smith, D., Harrison, N., Muir, W., and Blackwood D. (2005). The high prevalence of bipolar spectrum in young adults with recurrent depression: Toward an innovative diagnostic framework. *J Affect Disord*, 84, 167–178.

Spitzer, R.L., Endicott, J., Robins, E. (1978). Research diagnostic criteria: Rationale and reliability. *Arch Gen Psychiatry*, 35(6), 773–782.

Sprock, J. (1988). Classification of schizoaffective disorder. *Compr Psychiatry*, 29(1), 55–71.

Stoll, A.L., Banov, M., Kolbrener, M., Mayer, P.V., Tohen, M., Strakowski, S.M., Castillo, J., Suppes, T., and Cohen, B.M. (1994). Neurologic factors predict a favorable valproate response in bipolar and schizoaffective disorders. *J Clin Psychopharmacol*, 14(5), 311–313.

Surtees, P.G., and Kendell, R.E. (1979). The hierarchy model of psychiatric symptomatology: An investigation based on present state examination ratings. *Br J Psychiatry*, 135, 43–443.

Swann, A.C. (2000). Depression, mania, and feeling bad: The role of dysphoria in mixed states. *Bipolar Disord*, 2(4), 325–327.

Swann, A.C., Secunda, S.K., Katz, M.M., Croughan, J., Bowden, C.L., Koslow, S.H., Berman, N., and Stokes, P.E. (1993). Specificity of mixed affective states: Clinical comparison of dysphoric mania and agitated depression. *J Affect Disord*, 28(2), 81–89.

Swann, A.C., Bowden, C.L., Morris, D., Calabrese, J.R., Petty, F., Small, J., Dilsaver, S.C., and Davis, J.M. (1997). Depression during mania. Treatment response to lithium or divalproex. *Arch Gen Psychiatry*, 54(1), 37–42.

Swann, A.C., Janicak, P.L., Calabrese, J.R., Bowden, C.L., Dilsaver, S.C., Morris, D.D., Petty, F., and Davis, J.M. (2001). Structure of mania: Depressive, irritable, and psychotic clusters with different retrospectively-assessed course patterns of illness in randomized clinical trial participants. *J Affect Disord*, 67(1-3), 123–132.

Swann, A.C., Pazzaglia, P., Nicholls, A., Dougherty, D.M., and Moeller, F.G. (2003). Impulsivity and phase of illness in bipolar disorder. *J Affect Disord*, 73(1-2), 105–111.

Toomey, R., Faraone, S.V., Simpson, J.C., and Tsuang, M.T. (1998). Negative, positive, and disorganized symptom dimensions in schizophrenia, major depression, and bipolar disorder. *J Nerv Ment Dis*, 186(6), 470–476.

Tsuang, D., and Coryell, W. (1993). An 8-year follow-up of patients with DSM-III-R psychotic depression, schizoaffective disorder, and schizophrenia. *Am J Psychiatry*, 150(8), 1182–1188.

Tsuang, M.T., and Simpson, J.C. (1984). Schizoaffective disorder: Concept and reality. *Schizophr Bull*, 10(1), 14–25.

Tsuang, M.T., Winokur, G., and Crowe, R.R. (1980). Morbidity risks of schizophrenia and affective disorders among first-degree relatives of patients with schizophrenia, mania, depression and surgical conditions. *Br J Psychiatry*, 137, 497–504.

Tsuang, M.T., Woolson, R.F., and Simpson, J.C. (1981). An evaluation of the Feighner criteria for schizophrenia and affective disorders using long-term outcome data. *Psychol Med*, 11, 281–287.

Van Os, J., Castle, D.J., Takei, N., Der, G., and Murray, R.M. (1996). Psychotic illness in ethnic minorities: Clarification from the 1991 census. *Psychol Med*, 26(1), 203–208.

Van Os, J., Jones, P., Sham, P., Bebbington, P., and Murray, R.M. (1998). Risk factors for inset and persistence of psychosis. *Soc Psychiatry Psychiatr Epidemiol*, 33(12), 596–605.

van Praag, H.M. (1993). *Make-Believes in Psychiatry: Or the Perils of Progress*. New York: Brunner/Mazel.

Ventura, J., Nuechterlein, K.H., Subotnik, K.L., Gutkind, D., and Gilbert, E.A. (2000). Symptom dimensions in recent-onset schizophrenia and mania: A principal components analysis of the 24-item Brief Psychiatric Rating Scale. *Psychiatry Res, 97*(2-3), 129–135.

Vieta, E., and Salva, J. (1997). Diagnostico diferencial de los trastornos bipolares. In E. Vieta, and C. Gasto (Eds.), *Trastornos Bipolares* (pp. 175–193). Barcelona: Springer.

Vieta, E., Gasto, C., Otero, A., Nieto, E., and Vallejo, J. (1997). Differential features between bipolar I and bipolar II disorder. *Compr Psychiatry, 38*(2), 98–101.

Viguera, A.C., and Cohen, L.S. (1998). The course and management of bipolar disorder during pregnancy. *Psychopharmacol Bull, 34*(3), 339–346.

Whyte, E.M., and Mulsant, B.H. (2002). Post-stroke depression: Epidemiology, pathophysiology, and biological treatment. *Biol Psychiatry, 52*(3), 253–264.

Wilens, T.E., Biederman, J., Wozniak, J., Gunawardene, S., Wong, J., and Monuteaux, M. (2003). Can adults with attention-deficit/hyperactivity disorder be distinguished from those with comorbid bipolar disorder? Findings from a sample of clinically referred adults. *Biol Psychiatry, 54*(1), 1–8.

Wing, J., and Nixon, J. (1975). Discriminating symptoms in schizophrenia. A report from the international pilot study of schizophrenia. *Arch Gen Psychiatry, 32*(7), 853–859.

Yang, C.Y., Su, T.P., Wong, W.W., Guo, W.Y., and Su, Y.L. (2005). Association of AIDS and bipolar mania with rapid progression to dementia and death. *J Chin Med Assoc, 68*(2), 92–95.

Zimmerman, M., Posternak, M.A., Chelminski, I., and Solomon, D.A. (2004). Using questionnaires to screen for psychiatric disorders: A comment on a study of screening for bipolar disorder in the community. *J Clin Psychiatry, 65*(5), 605–610.

CHAPTER 4

Ahrens, B., Berghofer, A., Wolf, T., and Muller-Oerlinghausen, B. (1995). Suicide attempts, age and duration of illness in recurrent affective disorders. *J Affect Disord, 36*(1-2), 43–49.

Akdeniz, F., Vahip, S., Pirildar, S., Vahip, I., Doganer, I., and Bulut, I. (2003). Risk factors associated with childbearing-related episodes in women with bipolar disorder. *Psychopathology, 36*(5), 234–238.

Akiskal, H.S., Maser, J.D., Zeller, P.J., Endicott, J., Coryell, W., Keller, M., Warshaw, M., Clayton, P., and Goodwin, F. (1995). Switching from "unipolar" to bipolar II: An 11-year prospective study of clinical and temperamental predictors in 559 patients. *Arch Gen Psychiatry, 52*(2), 114–123.

Akiskal, H.S., Hantouche, E.G., Bourgeois, M.L., Azorin, J.M., Sechter, D., Allilaire, J.F., Lancrenon, S., Fraud, J.P., and Chatenet-Duchene, L. (1998). Gender, temperament, and the clinical picture in dysphoric mixed mania: Findings from a French national study (EPIMAN). *J Affect Disord, 50*(2–3), 175–186.

Almeida, O.P., and Fenner, S. (2002). Bipolar disorder: Similarities and differences between patients with illness onset before and after 65 year of age. *Int Psychogeriatr, 14*(3), 311–322.

Altshuler, L.L., Conrad, A., Hauser, P., Li, X.M., Guze, B.H., Denikoff, K., Tourtellotte, W., and Post, R. (1991). Reduction of temporal lobe volume in bipolar disorder: A preliminary report of magnetic resonance imaging. *Arch Gen Psychiatry, 48*(5), 482–483.

Altshuler, L.L., Post, R.M., Leverich, G.S., Mikalauskas, K., Rosoff, A., and Ackerman, L. (1995). Antidepressant-induced mania and cycle acceleration: A controversy revisited. *Am J Psychiatry, 152*, 1130–1138.

Altshuler, L.L., Kiriakos, L., Calcagno, J., Goodman, R., Gitlin, M., Frye, M., and Mintz, J. (2001). The impact of antidepressant discontinuation versus antidepressant continuation on 1-year risk for relapse of bipolar depression: A retrospective chart review. *J Clin Psychiatry, 62*, 612–616.

Altshuler, L.L., Gitlin, M.J., Mintz, J., Leight, K.L., and Frye, M.A. (2002). Subsyndromal depression is associated with functional impairment in patients with bipolar disorder. *J Clin Psychiatry, 63*(9), 807–811.

Ambelas, A. (1979). Psychologically stressful events in the precipitation of manic episodes. *Br J Psychiatry, 135*, 15–21.

Angst, F., Stassen, H.H., Clayton, P.J., Angst J. (2002). Mortality of patients with mood disorders: Follow-up over 34–38 years. *Affect Disord, 68*, 167–181.

Angst, J. (1978). The course of affective disorders: II. Typology of bipolar manic-depressive illness. *Arch Psychiatr Nervenkr, 226*, 65–73.

Angst, J. (1980). Verlauf unipolar depressiver, bipolar manisch-depressiver und schizo-affektiver Erkrankungen and Psychosen: Ergebnisse einer prospektiven Studie. *Fortschr Neurol Psychiatr, 48*, 3–30.

Angst, J. (1981a). Clinical indications for a prophylactic treatment of depression. *Adv Biol Psychiatry, 7*, 218–229.

Angst, J. (1981b). Course of affective disorders. In H.M. Van Praag, M.H. Lader, O.J. Rafaelsen, E.J. Sachar (Eds.), *Handbook of Biological Psychiatry* (pp. 225–242). New York: Marcel Dekker.

Angst, J. (1985). Switch from depression to mania: A record study over decades between 1920 and 1982. *Psychopathology, 18*, 140–154.

Angst, J. (1986c). The course of schizoaffective disorders. In M.T. Tsuang, A. Maneros (Eds.), *Schizoaffective Psychoses.* Berlin-Heidelberg: Springer-Verlag.

Angst, J. (1986d). The course of affective disorders. *Psychopath, 19*(Suppl. 2), 47–52.

Angst, J. (1988). *Suicides among depressive and bipolar patients.* Abstract of paper presented at the 141st annual meeting of the American Psychiatric Association, May 7–12, Montreal, Canada.

Angst, J., and Preisig, M. (1995). Course of a clinical cohort of unipolar, bipolar and schizoaffective patients: Results of a prospective study from 1959 to 1985. *Schweiz Arch Neurol Psychiatr, 146*, 5–16.

Angst, J., and Sellaro, R. (2000). Historical perspectives and natural history of bipolar disorder. *Biological Psychiatry, 48*, 445–457.

Angst, J., and Weis, P. (1967). Periodicity of depressive psychoses. In H. Brill, J.O. Cole, P. Deniker (Eds.), *Neuropsychopharmacology: Proceedings of the Fifth Internal Congress of the Collegium Internationale Neuro-pscyho-pharmalogicum* (pp. 703–710). Amsterdam: Excerpta Medica.

Angst, J., Weis, P., Grof, P., Baastrup, P.C., and Schou, M. (1970). Lithium prophylaxis in recurrent affective disorders. *Br J Psychiatry, 116*, 604–614.

Angst, J., Baastrup, P., Grof, P., Hippius, H., Poldinger, W., and Weis, P. (1973). The course of monopolar depression and bipolar psychoses. *Psychiatr Neurol Neurochir, 76*, 489–500.

Angst, J., Felder, W., Frey, R., and Stassen, H.H. (1978). The course of affective disorders: I. Change of diagnosis of monopolar, unipolar, and bipolar illness. *Arch Psychiatr Nervenkr, 226*(1), 57–64.

Angst, J., Felder, W., and Frey, R. (1979). The course of unipolar and bipolar affective disorders. In: M. Schou and E. Strömgren (Eds.), *Origin, Prevention and Treatment of Affective Disorders.* New York: Academic Press, pp. 215–226.

Angst, J., Angst, F., and Stassen, H.H. (1999). Suicide risk in patients with major depressive disorder. *J Clin Psychiatry,* 60(Suppl 2), 57–62; discussion 75–76, 113–116.

Angst, J., Gamma, A., Neuenschwander, M., Ajdacic-Gross, V., Eich, D., Rossler, W., and Merikangas, K.R. (2005). Prevalence of mental disorders in the Zurich Cohort Study: A twenty year prospective study. *Epidemiol Psichiatr Soc,* 14(2), 68–76.

Aronson, T.A., and Shukla, S. (1987). Life events and relapse in bipolar disorder: The impact of a catastrophic event. *Acta Psychiatr Scand,* 75, 571–576.

Baethge, C., Baldessarini, R.J., Freudenthal, K., Streeruwitz, A., Bauer, M., and Bschor, T. (2005). Hallucinations in bipolar disorder: Characteristics and comparison to unipolar depression and schizophrenia. *Bipolar Disord,* 7(2), 136–145.

Baldassano et al. (2002). *Gender differences in bipolar disorder.* Systematic Treatment Enhancement Program First 500 (STEP-BD), 155th annual meeting of the American Psychiatric Association, May 18–23, Philadelphia, PA.

Baldessarini, R.J., Tondo, L., Hennen, J., and Floris, G. (1999). Latency and episodes before treatment: Response to lithium maintenance in bipolar I and II disorders. *Bipolar Disorders,* 2, 91–97.

Baldessarini, R.J., Tondo, L., Floris, G., and Hennen, J. (2000). Effects of rapid cycling on response to lithium maintenance treatment in 360 bipolar I and II disorder patients. *J Affect Disord,* 61, 13–22.

Baron, M., Mendlewicz, J., and Klotz, J. (1981). Age-of-onset and genetic transmission in affective disorders. *Acta Psychiatr Scand,* 64(5), 373–380.

Bauer, M., and Whybrow, P. (1988). Thyroid hormones and the central nervous system in affective illness: Interactions that may have clinical significance. *Integrative Psychiatry,* 6, 75–100.

Bauer, M.S., Calabrese, J., Dunner, D.L., Post, R., Whybrow, P.C., Gyulai, L., Tay, L.K., Younkin, S.R., Bynum, D., and Lavori, P. (1994). Multisite data reanalysis of the validity of rapid cycling as a course modifier for bipolar disorder in DSM-IV. *Am J Psychiatry,* 151(4), 506–515.

Bellivier, F., Golmard, J.L., Henry, C., Leboyer, M., and Schurhoff, F. (2001). Admixture analysis of age at onset in bipolar I affective disorder. *Arch Gen Psychiatry,* 58(5), 510–512.

Bellivier, F., Leroux, M., Henry, C., Rayah, F., Rouillon, F., Laplanche, J.L., and Leboyer, M. (2002). Serotonin transporter gene polymorphism influences age at onset in patients with bipolar affective disorder. *Neurosci Lett,* 334(1), 17–20.

Bellivier, F., Golmard, J.L., Rietschel, M., Schulze, T.G., Malafosse, A., Preisig, M., McKeon, P., Mynett-Johnson, L., Henry, C., and Leboyer, M. (2003). Age at onset in bipolar I affective disorder: Further evidence for three subgroups. *Am J Psychiatry,* 160(5), 999–1001.

Benazzi, F. (1999). A comparison of the age of onset of bipolar I and bipolar II outpatients. *J Affect Disord,* 54, 249–253.

Benedetti, F., Lucca, A., Brambilla, F., Colombo, C., and Smeraldi, E. (2002). Interleukin-6 serum levels correlate with response to antidepressant sleep deprivation and sleep phase advance. *Prog Neuropsychopharmacol Biol Psychiatry,* 26(6), 1167–1170.

Berghofer, A., Wolf, T., and Muller-Oerlinghausen, B. (1995). Suicide attempts, age and duration of illness in recurrent affective disorders. *J Affect Disord,* 36(1–2), 43–49.

Bidzinska, E.J. (1984). Stress factors in affective diseases. *Br J Psychiatry,* 144, 161–166.

Black, D.W., Winokur, G., and Nasrallah, A. (1987a). Is death from natural causes still excessive in psychiatric patients? A follow-up of 1593 patients with major affective disorder. *J Nerv Ment Dis,* 175, 674–680.

Black, K.J., and Perlmutter, J.S. (1997). Septuagenarian Sydenham's with secondary hypomania. *Neuropsychiatry Neuropsychol Behav Neurol,* 10(2), 147–150.

Blumenthal, R.L., Egeland, J.A., Sharpe, L., Nee, J., and Endicott, J. (1987). Age of onset in bipolar and unipolar illness with and without delusions or hallucinations. *Compr Psychiatry,* 28(6), 547–554.

Bourgeois, M., and Campagne, A. (1967). Maniaco-depressive et syndrome de Garcin. *Ann Med Psychol,* 125(Suppl. 2), 451–460.

Bratfos, O., and Haug, J.O. (1968). The course of manic-depressive psychosis: A follow up investigation of 215 patients. *Acta Psychiatr Scand,* 44, 89–112.

Bratfos, O., Eitinger, L., and Tau, T. (1968). Mental illness and crime in adopted children and adoptive parents. *Acta Psychiatr Scand,* 44, 376–384.

Brieger, P., Roettig, S., Ehrt, U., Wenzel, A., Bloink, R., and Marneros, A. (2003). TEMPS-A scale in "mixed" and "pure" manic episodes: New data and methodological considerations on the relevance of joint anxious-depressive temperament traits. *J Affect Disord,* 73(1–2), 99–104.

Brody, E.B. (1973). *The lost ones.* New York: International Universities Press.

Bromet, E.J., Jandorf, L., Fennig, S., Lavelle, J., Kovasznay, B., Ram, R., Tanenberg-Karant, M., and Craig, T. (1996). The Suffolk County Mental Health Project: Demographic, premorbid and clinical correlates of 6-month outcome. *Psychol Med,* 26(5), 953–962.

Burke, K.C., Burke, J.D., Regier, D.A., and Rae, D.S. (1990). Age at onset of selected mental disorders in five community populations. *Arch Gen Psychiatry,* 47(6), 511–518.

Cannon, M., Jones, P., Gilvarry, C., Rifkin, L., McKenzie, K., Foerster, A., and Murray, R.M. (1997). Premorbid social functioning in schizophrenia and bipolar disorder: Similarities and differences. *Am J Psychiatry,* 154(11), 1544–1550.

Carlson, G.A., Kotin, J., Davenport, Y.B., and Adland, M. (1974). Follow-up of 53 bipolar manic-depressive patients. *Br J Psychiatry,* 124(579), 134–139.

Carlson, G.A., Davenport, Y.B., and Jamison, K. (1977). A comparison of outcome in adolescent- and late-onset bipolar manic-depressive illness. *Am J Psychiatry,* 134, 919–922.

Carlson, G.A., Bromet, E.J., and Sievers, S. (2000). Phenomenology and outcome of subjects with early- and adult-onset psychotic mania. *Am J Psychiatry,* 157, 213–219.

Carlson, G.A., Bromet, E.J., Driessons, C., Mojtabai, R., and Schwartz, J.E. (2002). Age at onset, childhood psychopathology, and 2-year outcome in psychotic bipolar disorder. *Am J Psychiatry,* 159(2), 307–309.

Carter, T.D., Mundo, E., Parikh, S.V., and Kennedy, J.L. (2003). Early age at onset as a risk factor for poor outcome of bipolar disorder. *J Psychiatr Res,* 37(4), 297–303.

Casanova, M.F., Kruesi, M., and Mannheim, G. (1996). Multiple sclerosis and bipolar disorder: A case report with autopsy findings. *J Neuropsychiatry Clin Neurosci,* 8(2), 206–208.

Chase, T.N., Holden, E.M., and Brody, J.A. (1973). Levodopa-induced dyskinesias. Comparison in Parkinsonism-dementia and amyotrophic lateral sclerosis. *Arch Neurol*, 29(5), 328–333.

Chaturvedi, S.K., and Upadhyaya, M. (1988). Secondary mania in a patient receiving isonicotinic acid hydrazide and pyridoxine: Case report. *Can J Psychiatry*, 33, 675–676.

Chengappa, R., Kupfer, D.J., Frank, E., Houck, P.R., Grochocinski, V.J., Cluss, P.A., and Stapf, D.A. (2003). Relationship of birth cohort and early age at onset of illness in a bipolar disorder case registry. *Am J Psychiatry*, 160, 1636–1642.

Cicero, D., El-Mallakh, R.S., Holman, J., and Robertson, J. (2003). Antidepressant exposure in bipolar children. *Psychiatry*, 66, 317–322.

Cooper, A.J. (1967). Hypomanic psychosis precipitated by hemodialysis. *Compr Psychiatry*, 8, 168–172.

Corn, T.H., and Checkley, S.A. (1983). A case of recurrent mania with recurrent hyperthyroidism. *Br J Psychiatry*, 143, 74–76.

Coryell, W., and Norten, S.G. (1980). Mania during adolescence: The pathoplastic significance of age. *J Nerv Ment Dis*, 168(10), 611–613.

Coryell, W., Keller, M., Endicott, J., Andreasen, N., Clayton, P., and Hirschfeld, R. (1989). Bipolar II illness: Course and outcome over a five-year period. *Psychol Med*, 19, 129–141.

Coryell, W., Endicott, J., and Keller, M. (1990). Outcome of patients with chronic affective disorder: A five-year follow-up. *Am J Psychiatry*, 147(12), 1627–1633.

Coryell, W., Endicott, J., and Keller, M. (1992). Rapid cycling affective disorder: Demographics, diagnosis, family history, and course. *Arch Gen Psychiatry*, 49, 126–131.

Coryell, W., Scheftner, W., Keller, M., Endicott, J., Maser, J., and Klerman, G.L. (1993). The enduring psychosocial consequences of mania and depression. *Am J Psychiatry*, 150, 720–727.

Coryell, W., Winokur, G., Maser, J.D., Akiskal, H.S., Keller, M.B., and Endicott, J. (1994). Recurrently situational (reactive) depression: A study of course, phenomenology and familial psychopathology. *J Affect Disord*, 31(3), 203–210.

Coryell, W., Endicott, J., Maser, J.D., Keller, M.B., Leon, A.C., and Akiskal, H.S. (1995). Long-term stability of polarity distinctions in the affective disorders. *Am J Psychiatry*, 152(3), 385–390.

Coryell, W., Leon, A.C., Turvey, C., Akiskal, H.S., Mueller, T., and Endicott, J. (2001). The significance of psychotic features in manic episodes: A report from the NIMH collaborative study. *J Affect Disord*, 67(1–3), 79–88.

Crane, G.E. (1956). The psychiatric side effects of iproniazid. *Am J Psychiatry*, 112, 494–501.

Cummings, J.L., and Mendez, M.F. (1984). Secondary mania with focal cerebrovascular lesions. *Am J Psychiatry*, 141, 1084–1087.

Cusin, C., Serretti, A., Lattuada, E., Mandelli, L., and Smeraldi, E. (2000). Impact of clinical variables on illness time course in mood disorders. *Psychiatry Res*, 97, 217–227.

Cutler, N.R., and Post, R.M. (1982a). Life course of illness in untreated manic-depressive patients. *Comp Psychiatry*, 23, 101–115.

Dauncey, K. (1988). Mania in the early stages of AIDS. *Br J Psychiatry*, 152, 716–717.

Deister, A., and Marneros, A. (1993). Predicting the long-term outcome of affective disorders. *Acta Psychiatr Scand*, 88(3), 174–177.

Dell'Osso, L., Akiskal, H.S., Freer, P., Barberi, M., Placidi, G.F., and Cassano, G.B. (1993). Psychotic and nonpsychotic bipolar mixed states: Comparisons with manic and schizoaffective disorders. *Eur Arch Psychiatry Clin Neurosci*, 243(2), 75–81.

Depue, R.A., Slater, J.F., Wolfstetter-Kausch, H., Klein, D., Goplerud, E., and Farr, D. (1981). A behavioral paradigm for identifying persons at risk for bipolar depressive disorder: A conceptual framework and five validation studies. *J Abnorm Psychol Monograph*, 90, 381–437.

Derby, I.M. (1933). Manic-depressive "exhaustion" deaths: An analysis of "exhaustion" case histories. *Psychiatr Q*, 7, 435–449.

Dittmann, S., Biedermann, N.C., Grunze, H., Hummel, B., Scharer, L.O., Kleindienst, N., Forsthoff, A., Matzner, N., Walser, S., and Walden, J. (2002). The Stanley Foundation Bipolar Network: Results of the naturalistic follow-up study after 2.5 years of follow-up in the German centres. *Neuropsychobiology*, 46(Suppl. 1), 2–9.

Donaldson, S., Goldstein, L.H., Landau, S., Raymont, V., and Frangou, S. (2003). The Maudsley Bipolar Disorder Project: The effect of medication, family history, and duration of illness on IQ and memory in bipolar I disorder. *J Clin Psychiatry*, 64(1), 86–93.

Dunner, D.L., Fleiss, J.L., and Fieve, R.R. (1976b). The course of development of mania in patients with recurrent depression. *Am J Psychiatry*, 133, 905–908.

Dunner, D.L., Murphy, D., Stallone, F., and Fieve, R.R. (1979b). Episode frequency prior to lithium treatment in bipolar manic-depressive patients. *Compr Psychiatry*, 20, 511–515.

Dunner, D.L., Murphy, D., Stallone, F., and Fieve, R.R. (1980). Affective episode frequency and lithium therapy. *Psychopharmacol Bull*, 16, 49–50.

Eaton, W.W., Anthony, J.C., Gallo, J., Cai, G., Tien, A., Romanoski, A., Lyketsos, C., and Chen L.S. (1997). Natural history of Diagnostic Interview Schedule/DSM-IV major depression. The Baltimore Epidemiologic Catchment Area follow-up. *Arch Gen Psychiatry*, 54, 993–999.

Egeland, J.A., Blumenthal, R.L., Nee, J., Sharpe, L., and Endicott, J. (1987a). Reliability and relationship of various ages of onset criteria for major affective disorder. *J Affect Disord*, 12(2), 159–165.

Ellicott, A.G. (1988). *A prospective study of stressful life events and bipolar illness.* Unpublished doctoral dissertation, University of California, Los Angeles.

Engstrom, C., Brandstrom, S., Sigvardsson, S., Cloninger, R., and Nylander, P.O. (2003). Bipolar disorder: II. Personality and age of onset. *Bipolar Disord*, 5(5), 340–348.

Ernst, C.L., and Goldberg, J.F. (2004). Clinical features related to age at onset in bipolar disorder. *J Affect Disord*, 82(1), 21–27.

Faedda, G.L., Tondo, L., Baldessarini, R.J., Suppes, T., and Tohen, M. (1993). Outcome after rapid vs. gradual discontinuation of lithium treatment in bipolar disorders. *Arch Gen Psychiatry*, 50(6), 448–455.

Faraone, S.V., Glatt, S.J., Su, J., and Tsuang, M.T. (2004). Three potential susceptibility loci shown by a genomic-wide scan for regions influencing the age at onset of mania. *Am J Psychiatry*, 161, 625–630.

Fisfalen, M.E., Schulze, T.G., DePaulo, J.R., DeGroot, L.J., Badner, J.A., and McMahon, F.J. (2005). Familial variation in episode frequency in bipolar affective disorder. *Am J Psychiatry*, 162(7), 1266–1272.

Fogarty, F., Russell, J.M., Newman, S.C., and Bland, R.C. (1994). Epidemiology of psychiatric disorders in Edmonton mania. *Acta Psychiatr Scand Suppl*, 376, 16–23.

France, R.D., and Krishnan, K.R. (1984). Alprazolam-induced manic reaction. *Am J Psychiatry*, 1127–1128.

Freinhar, J.P., and Alvarez, W.H. (1985b). Androgen-induced hypomania. Letter. *J Clin Psychiatry*, 46, 354–355.

Fujikawa, T., Yamawaki, S., and Touhouda, Y. (1995). Silent cerebral infarctions in patients with late-onset mania. *Stroke*, 26(6), 946–949.

Fukuda, K., Etoh, T., Iwadate, T., and Ishii, A. (1983). The course and prognosis of manic-depressive psychosis: A quantitative analysis of episodes and intervals. *Tohoku J Exp Med*, 139, 299–307.

Gabel, R.H., Barnard, N., Norko, M., and O'Connell, R.A. (1986). AIDS presenting as mania. *Compr Psychiatry*, 27, 251–254.

Geller, B., and Cook, E.H. Jr. (2000). Ultradian rapid cycling in prepubertal and early adolescent bipolarity is not in transmission disequilibrium with val/met COMT alleles. *Biol Psychiatry*, 47, 605–609.

Geller, B., Zimerman, B., Williams, M., Bolhofner, K., and Craney, J.L. (2001). Bipolar disorder at prospective follow-up of adults who had prepubertal major depressive disorder. *Am J Psychiatry*, 158, 125–127.

Geller, B., Tillman, R., Craney, J.L., and Bolhofner, K. (2004). Four-year prospective outcome and natural history of mania in children with a prepubertal and early adolescent bipolar disorder phenotype. *Arch Gen Psychiatry*, 61, 459–467.

Gershon, E.S., Hamovit, J., Guroff, J.J., Dibble, E., Leckman, J.F., Sceery, W., Targum, S.D., Nurnberger, J.I., Goldin, L.R., and Bunney, W.E. (1982). A family study of schizoaffective, bipolar I, bipolar II, unipolar, and normal control probands. *Arch Gen Psychiatry*, 39(10), 1157–1167.

Ghaemi, S.N., Sachs, G.S., Chiou, A.M., Pandurangi, A.K., and Goodwin, F.K. (1999). Is bipolar disorder still underdiagnosed? Are antidepressants overutilized? *J Affect Dis*, 52, 135–144.

Ghaemi, S.N., Boiman, E.E., and Goodwin, F.K. (2000). Diagnosing bipolar disorder and the effect of antidepressants: A naturalistic study. *J Clin Psychiatry*, 61, 804–808.

Gitlin, M.J., Swendsen, J., Heller, T.L., and Hammen, C. (1995). Relapse and impairment in bipolar disorder. *Am J Psychiatry*, 152(11), 1635–1640.

Gitlin, M., Boerlin, H., Fairbanks, L., and Hammen, C. (2003). The effect of previous mood states on switch rates: A naturalistic study. *Bipolar Disord*, 5(2), 150–152.

Glaser, G.H. (1953). Psychotic reactions induced by corticotropin (ACTH) and cortisone. *Psychosom Med*, 15, 280–291.

Glassner, B., and Haldipur, C.V. (1983). Life events and early and late onset of bipolar disorder. *Am J Psychiatry*, 140, 215–217.

Goggans, F.C. (1984). A case of mania secondary to vitamin B12 deficiency. *Am J Psychiatry*, 141, 300–301.

Goldberg, J.F. (2001). Spontaneous depression versus biphasic cycling. Letter to the editor. *Am J Psychiatry*, 158(2), 325–326.

Goldberg, J.F., and Harrow, M. (1994). Kindling in bipolar disorders: A longitudinal follow-up study. *Biol Psychiatry*, 35, 70–72.

Goldberg, J.F., and Harrow, M. (1999). *Bipolar disorders: Clinical course and outcome*. Washington, DC: American Psychiatric Press.

Goldberg, J.F., Harrow, M., and Grossman, L.S. (1995). Course and outcome in bipolar affective disorder: A longitudinal follow-up study. *American Journal of Psychiatry*, 152, 379–384.

Goldberg, J.F., Harrow, M., and Whiteside, J.E. (2001). Risk for bipolar illness in patients initially hospitalized for unipolar depression. *Am J Psychiatry*, 158, 1265–1270.

Goldberg, T.E., Gold, J.M., Greenberg, R., Griffin, S., Schulz, S.C., Pickar, D., Kleinman, J.E., and Weinberger, D.R. (1993).

Contrasts between patients with affective disorders and patients with schizophrenia on a neuropsychological test battery. *Am J Psychiatry*, 150, 1355–1362.

Goldstein, B.I., and Levitt, A.J. (2006). Further evidence for a developmental subtype of bipolar disorder defined by age at onset: Results from the national epidemiologic survey on alcohol and related conditions. *Am J Psychiatry*, 163(9), 1633–1636.

Goldstein, E.T., and Preskorn, S.H. (1989). Mania triggered by a steroid nasal spray in a patient with stable bipolar disorder. *Am J Psychiatry*, 146, 1076–1077.

Goodwin, F.K., and Ghaemi, S.N. (1998). Understanding manic-depressive illness. *Arch Gen Psychiatry*, 55(1), 23–25.

Goodwin, F.K., and Jamison, K.R. (1984). The natural course of manic-depressive illness. In R.M. Post, J.C. Ballenger (Eds.), *Neurobiology of mood disorders* (pp. 20–37). Baltimore: Williams & Wilkins.

Goolker, P., and Schein, J. (1953). Psychic effects of ACTH and cortisone. *Psychosom Med*, 15, 589–597.

Greenberg, D.B., and Brown, G.L. (1985). Mania resulting from brainstem tumor. *J Nerv Ment Dis*, 173, 434–436.

Grigoroiu-Serbanescu, M., Martinez, M., Nothen, M.M., Grinberg, M., Sima, D., Propping, P., Marinescu, E., and Hrestic, M. (2001). Different familial transmission patterns in bipolar I disorder with onset before and after age 25. *Am J Med. Genet*, 105, 765–773.

Grof, P., Alda, M., and Ahrens, B. (1995). Clinical course of affective disorders: Were Emil Kraepelin and Jules Angst wrong? *Psychopathology*, 28, 73–80.

Guttman, E., and Hermann, K. (1932). Ueber psychische Storungen bei Hirnstammerkrankungen und das Automatosesyndrom. *Z Ges Neurol Pscyhiatr*, 140, 439–472.

Guze, S.B., and Robins, E. (1970). Suicide and primary affective disorders. *Br J Psychiatry*, 117, 437–438.

Haghighat, R. (1996). Lifelong development of risk of recurrence in depressive disorders. *J Affect Disord*, 41(2), 141–147.

Harrow, M., Goldberg, J.F., Grossman, L.S., and Meltzer, H.Y. (1990). Outcome in manic disorders: A naturalistic follow-up study. *Arch Gen Psychiatry*, 47, 665–671.

Heila, H., Turpeinen, P., and Erkinjuntti, T. (1995). Case study: Mania associated with multiple sclerosis. *J Am Acad Child Adolesc Psychiatry*, 34(12), 1591–1595.

Hendrick, V., Altshuler, L.L., Gitlin, M.J., Delrahim, S., and Hammen, C. (2000). Gender and bipolar illness. *J Clin Psychiatry*, 61(5), 93–96; quiz 397.

Henry, C., Lacoste, J., Bellivier, F., Verdoux, H., Bourgeois, M.L., and Leboyer, M. (1999). Temperament in bipolar illness: Impact on prognosis. *J Affect Disord*, 56, 103–108.

Hlastala, S.A., Frank, E., Kowalski, J., Sherrill, J.T., Tu, X.M., Anderson, B., and Kupfer, D.J. (2000). Stressful life events, bipolar disorder, and the "kindling model." *J Abnorm Psychol*, 109, 777–786.

Honig, A., Hendriks, C.H., Akkerhuis, G.W., and Nolen, W.A. (2001). Usefulness of the retrospective Life-Chart method manual in outpatients with a mood disorder: A feasibility study. *Patient Educ Couns*, 43(1), 43–48.

Horrigan, J.P., and Barnhill, L.J. (1999). Guanfacine and secondary mania in children. *J Affect Disord*, 54(3), 309–314.

Hoyer, E.H., Mortensen, P.B., and Olesen, A.V. (2000). Mortality and causes of death in a total national sample of patients with affective disorders admitted for the first time between 1973 and 1993. *Br J Psychiatry*, 176, 76–82.

Hubain, P.P., Sobolski, J., and Mendlewicz, J. (1982). Cimetidine-induced mania. *Neuropsychobiology*, 8, 223–224.

Huber, M.T., Braun, H.A., and Krieg, J.C. (2001). On the impact of episode sensitization on the course of recurrent affective disorders. *J Psychiatr Res*, 35, 49–57.

Hunt, N., Bruce-Jones, W., and Silverstone, T. (1992). Life events and relapse in bipolar affective disorder. *J Affect Disord*, 25(1), 13–20.

Hyun, M., Friedman, S.D., and Dunner, D.L. (2000). Relationship of childhood physical and sexual abuse to adult bipolar disorder. *Bipolar Disord*, 2, 131–135.

Jackson, A., Cavanagh, J., and Scott, J. (2003). A systematic review of manic and depressive prodromes. *J Affect Disord*, 74(3), 209–217.

Jackson, S.L. (1957). Psychosis due to isoniazid. *Br Med J*, 2, 743–746.

Jacobson, J.E. (1965). The hypomanic alert: A program designed for greater therapeutic control. *Am J Psychiatry*, 122, 295–299.

Jampala, V.C., and Abrams, R. (1983). Mania secondary to left and right hemisphere damage. *Am J Psychiatry*, 140, 1197–1199.

Johnson, F.Y., and Naraqi, S. (1993). Manic episode secondary to cryptococcal meningitis in a previously healthy adult. *P N G Med J*, 36(1), 59–62.

Johnson, L., Andersson-Lundman, G., Aberg-Wistedt, A., and Mathe, A.A. (2000). Age of onset in affective disorder: Its correlation with hereditary and psychosocial factors. *J Affect Disord*, 59, 139–148.

Johnson, S.L., and Miller, I. (1997). Negative life events and time to recovery from episodes of bipolar disorder. *J Abnorm Psychol*, 106, 449–457.

Jorge, R.E., Robinson, R.G., Starkstein, S.E., Arndt, S.V., Forrester, A.W., and Geisler, F.H. (1993). Secondary mania following traumatic brain injury. *Am J Psychiatry*, 150(6), 916–921.

Judd, L.L., Akiskal, H.S., Maser, J.D., Zeller, P.J., Endicott, J., Coryell, W., Paulus, M.P., Kunovac, J.L., Leon, A.C., Mueller, T.I., Rice, J.A., and Keller, M.B. (1998). A prospective 12-year study of subsyndromal and syndromal depressive symptoms in unipolar major depressive disorders. *Arch Gen Psychiatry*, 55(8), 694–700.

Judd, L.L., Akiskal, H.S., Schettler, P.J., Endicott, J., Maser, J., Solomon, D.A., Leon, A.C., Rice, J.A., and Keller, M.B. (2002). The long-term natural history of the weekly symptomatic status of bipolar I disorder. *Arch Gen Psychiatry*, 59(6), 530–537.

Judd, L.L., Akiskal, H.S., Schettler, P.J., Coryell, W., Maser, J., Rice, J.A., Solomon, D.A., and Keller, M.B. (2003). The comparative clinical phenotype and long term longitudinal episode course of bipolar I and II: A clinical spectrum or distinct disorders? *J Affect Disord*, 73(1–2), 19–32.

Kadrmas, A., Winokur, G., and Crowe, R. (1979). Postpartum mania. *Br J Psychiatry*, 135, 551–554.

Kallner, G., Lindelius, R., Petterson, U., Stockman, O., and Tham, A. (2000). Mortality in 497 patients with affective disorders attending a lithium clinic or after having left it. *Pharmacopsychiatry*, 33, 8–13.

Kanai, T., Takeuchi, H., Furukawa, T.A., Yoshimura, R., Imaizumi, T., Kitamura, T., and Takahashi, K. (2003). Time to recurrence after recovery from major depressive episodes and its predictors. *Psychol Med*, 33(5), 839–845.

Kane, F.J., and Taylor, T.W. (1963). Mania associated with the use of INH and cocaine. *Am J Psychiatry*, 119, 1098–1099.

Kay, J.H., Altshuler, L.L., Ventura, J., and Mintz, J. (2002). Impact of axis II comorbidity on the course of bipolar illness in men: A retrospective chart review. *Bipolar Disord*, 4(4), 237–242.

Keck, P.E. Jr., McElroy, S.L., Strakowski, S.M., West, S.A., Hawkins, J.M., Huber, T.J., Newman, R.M., and DePriest, M. (1995). Outcome and comorbidity in first- compared with multiple-episode mania. *J Nerv Ment Dis*, 183, 320–324.

Keck, P.E. Jr., McElroy, S.L., Strakowski, S.M., West, S.A., Sax, K.W., Hawkins, J.M., Bourne, M.L., and Haggard, P. (1998). 12-Month outcome of patients with bipolar disorder following hospitalization for a manic or mixed episode. *Am J Psychiatry*, 155, 646–652.

Keck, P.E. Jr., McElroy, S.L., Havens, J.R., Altshuler, L.L., Nolen, W.A., Frye, M.A., Suppes, T., Denicoff, K.D., Kupka, R., Leverich, G.S., Rush, A.J., and Post, R.M. (2003). Psychosis in bipolar disorder: Phenomenology and impact on morbidity and course of illness. *Compr Psychiatry*, 44, 263–269.

Keitner, G.I., Solomon, D.A., Ryan, C.E., Miller, I.W., Mallinger, A., Kupfer, D.J., and Frank, E. (1996). Prodromal and residual symptoms in bipolar I disorder. *Comprehensive Psychiatry*, 37, 362–367.

Keller, M.B., and Boland, R.J. (1998). Implications of failing to achieve successful long-term maintenance treatment of recurrent unipolar major depression. *Biol Psychiatry*, 44(5), 348–360.

Keller, M.B., Shapiro, R.W., Lavori, P.W., and Wolfe, N. (1982). Relapse in major depressive disorder: Analysis with the life table. *Arch Gen Psychiatry*, 39, 911–915.

Keller, M.B., Lavori, P.W., Endicott, J., Coryell, W., and Klerman, G.L. (1983). "Double-depression": Two-year follow-up. *Am J Psychiatry*, 140, 689–694.

Keller, M.B., Lavori, P.W., Friedman, B., Nielsen, E., Endicott, J., McDonald-Scott, P., and Andreasen, N.C. (1987). The longitudinal interval follow-up evaluation: A comprehensive method for assessing outcome in prospective longitudinal studies. *Arch Gen Psychiatry*, 44(6), 540–548.

Keller, M.B., Lavori, P.W., Coryell, W., Endicott, J., and Mueller, T.I. (1993). Bipolar I: A five-year prospective follow-up. *J Nerv Ment Dis*, 181(4), 238–245.

Kendell, R.E., Wainwright, S., Hailey, A., and Shannon, B. (1976). Influence of childbirth on psychiatric morbidity. *Psychol Med*, 6, 297–302.

Kendell, R.E., Chalmers, J.C., and Platz, C. (1987). Epidemiology of puerperal psychoses. *Br J Psychiatry*, 150, 662–673.

Kendler, K.S., and Karkowski-Shuman, L. (1997). Stressful life events and genetic liability to major depression: Genetic control of exposure to the environment? *Psychol Med*, 27, 539–547.

Kendler, K.S., Thornton, L.M., and Gardner, C.O. (2000). Stressful life events and previous episodes in the etiology of major depression in women: An evaluation of the "kindling" hypothesis. *Am J Psychiatry*, 157(8), 1243–1251.

Kennedy, S., Thompson, R., Stancer, H.C., Roy, A., and Persad, E. (1983). Life events precipitating mania. *Br J Psychiatry*, 142, 398–403.

Kermani, E.J., Borod, J.C., Brown, P.H., and Tunnell, G. (1985). New psychopathologic findings in AIDS: Case report. *J Clin Psychiatry*, 46, 240–241.

Kessing, L.V. (1999). The effect of the first manic episode in affective disorder: A case register study of hospitalised episodes. *J Affect Disord*, 53, 233–239.

Kessing, L.V. (2006). Gender differences in subtypes of late-onset depression and mania. *Int Psychogeriatr*, 18, 727–738.

Kessing, L.V., and Andersen, P.K. (1999). The effect of episodes on recurrence in affective disorder: A case register study. *J Affect Disord*, 53, 225–231.

Kessing, L.V., Andersen, P.K., Mortensen, P.B., and Bolwig, T.G. (1998a). Recurrence in affective disorder: I. Case register study. *Br J Psychiatry*, 172, 23–28.

Kessing, L.V., Mortensen, P.B., and Bolwig, T.G. (1998b). Clinical consequences of sensitisation in affective disorder: A case register study. *J Affect Disord*, 47, 41–47.

Kessing, L.V., Andersen, P.K., and Mortensen, P.B. (1998c). Predictors of recurrence in affective disorder. A case register study. *J Affect Disord*, 49(2), 101–108.

Kessing, L.V., Hansen, M.G., Andersen, P.K., and Angst, J. (2004). The predictive effect of episodes on the risk of recurrence in depressive and bipolar disorders: A life-long perspective. *Acta Psychiatr Scand*, 109(5), 339–344.

Kessler, R.C., McGonagle, K.A., Swartz, M., Blazer, D.G., and Nelson, C.B. (1993). Sex and depression in the National Comorbidity Survey. I: Lifetime prevalence, chronicity and recurrence. *J Affect Disord*, 29(2-3), 85–96.

Khanna, R., Gupta, N., and Shanker, S. (1992). Course of bipolar disorder in eastern India. *J Affect Disord*, 24(1), 35–41.

Kirov, G., Murphy, K.C., Arranz, M.J., Jones, I., McCandles, F., Kunugi, H., Murray, R.M., McGuffin, P., Collier, D.A., Owen, M.J., and Craddock, N. (1998). Low activity allele of catechol-O-methyltransferase gene associated with rapid cycling bipolar disorder. *Mol Psychiatry*, 3(4), 342–345.

Klein, D.N., Taylor, E.B., Harding, K., and Dickstein, S. (1988). Double depression and episodic major depression: Demographic, clinical, familial, personality, and socioenvironmental characteristics and short-term outcome. *Am J Psychiatry*, 145(10), 1226–1231.

Koehler-Troy, C., Strober, M., and Malenbaum, R. (1986). Methylphenidate-induced mania in a prepubertal child. *J Clin Psychiatry*, 47, 566–567.

Kogan, J.N., Otto, M.W., Bauer, M.S., Dennehy, E.B., Miklowitz, D.J., Zhang, H.W., Ketter, T., Rudorfer, M.V., Wisniewski, S.R., Thase, M.E., Calabrese, J., Sachs, G.S., and STEP-BD Investigators (2004). Demographic and diagnostic characteristics of the first 1000 patients enrolled in the Systematic Treatment Enhancement Program for Bipolar Disorder (STEP-BD). *Bipolar Disord*, 6(6), 460–469.

Koukopoulos, A., and Reginaldi, D. (1973). Does lithium prevent depressions by suppressing manias? *Int Pharmacopsychiatry*, 8, 152–158.

Koukopoulos, A., Reginaldi, D., Laddomada, P., Floris, G., Serra, G., and Tondo, L. (1980). Course of the manic-depressive cycle and changes caused by treatments. *Pharmakopsychiatr Neuropsychopharmakol*, 13, 156–167.

Koukopoulos, A., Caliari, B., Tundo, A., Minnai, G., Floris, G., Reginaldi, D., and Tondo, L. (1983). Rapid cyclers, temperament, and antidepressants. *Compr Psychiatry*, 24, 249–258.

Koukopoulos, A., Sni, G., Koukopoulos, A., and Girardi, P. (2000). Cyclicity and manic-depressive illness. In A. Marneros, J. Angst (Eds.), *Bipolar Disorders: 100 Years after Manic-depressive Insanity* (pp. 315–334). London, England: Kluwer Academic Publishers.

Kraepelin, E. (1921). *Manic-depressive Insanity and Paranoia.* Translated by R. M. Barclay. Edinburgh, Scotland: E & S Livingstone.

Krauthammer, C., and Klerman, G.L. (1978). Secondary mania: Manic syndromes associated with antecedent physical illness or drugs. *Arch Gen Psychiatry*, 35, 1333–1339.

Krishnan, K.R.R., Swartz, M.S., Larson, M.J., and Santoliquido, G. (1984). Funeral mania in recurrent bipolar affective disorders: Reports on three cases. *J Clin Psychiatry*, 45, 310–311.

Kulisevsky, J., Berthier, M.L., and Pujol, J. (1993). Hemiballismus and secondary mania following a right thalamic infarction. *Neurology*, 43(7), 1422–1424.

Kupfer, D.J., Frank, E., Grochocinski, V.J., Cluss, P.A., Houck, P.R., and Stapf, D.A. (2002). Demographic and clinical characteristics of individuals in a bipolar disorder case registry. *J Clin Psychiatry*, 63(2), 120–125.

Kupka, R.W., Luckenbaugh, D.A., Post, R.M., Suppes, T., Altshuler, L.L., Keck, P.E., Frye, M.A., Denicoff, K.D., Grunze, H., Leverich, G.S., McElroy, S.L., Walden, J., and Nolen, W.A. (2005). Comparison of rapid-cycling and non-rapid-cycling bipolar disorder based on prospective mood ratings in 539 outpatients. *Am J Psychiatry*, 162(7), 1273–1280.

Kwentus, J.A., Silverman, J.J., and Sprague, M. (1984). Manic syndrome after metrizamide myelography. *Am J Psychiatry*, 141, 700–702.

Labbate, L.A., and Holzgang, A.J. (1989). Manic syndrome after discontinuation of methyldopa. *Am J Psychiatry*, 146, 1075–1076.

Lat, J. (1973). The analysis of habituation. *Acta Neurobiol Exp (Warsz)*, 33(4), 771–789.

Lazare, A. (1979). Manic behavior. In A. Lazare (Ed.), *Outpatient Psychiatry: Diagnosis and Treatment* (pp. 261–264). Baltimore: Williams & Wilkins.

Leboyer, M., Henry, C., Paillere-Martinot, M.L., and Bellivier, F. (2005). Age at onset in bipolar affective disorders: A review. *Bipolar Disord*, 7(2), 111–118.

Lee, H.J., Kim, L., Joe, S.H., and Suh, K.Y. (2002). Effects of season and climate on the first manic episode of bipolar affective disorder in Korea. *Psychiatry Res*, 113(1–2), 151–159.

Lendvai, I., Saravay, S.M., and Steinberg, M.D. (1999). Creutzfeldt-Jakob disease presenting as secondary mania. *Psychosomatics*, 40(6), 524–525.

Leverich, G.S., Nolen, W.A., Rush, A.J., McElroy, S.L., Keck, P.E., Denicoff, K.D., Suppes, T., Altshuler, L.L., Kupka, R., Kramlinger, K.G., and Post, R.M. (2001). The Stanley Foundation Bipolar Treatment Outcome Network: I. Longitudinal methodology, *J Affect Disord*, 67(1–3), 33–44.

Liegghio, N.E., and Yeragani, Y.K. (1988). Buspirone-induced hypomania. *J Clin Psychopharmacol*, 8, 226–227.

Lin, P.I., McInnis, M.G., Potash, J.B., Willour, V., MacKinnon, D.F., DePaulo, J.R., and Zandi, P.P. (2006). Clinical correlates and familial aggregation of age at onset in bipolar disorder. *Am J Psychiatry*, 163(2), 240–246.

Lish, J.D., Gyulai, L., Resnick, S.M., Kirtland, A., Amsterdam, J.D., Whybrow, P.C., and Price, R.A. (1993). A family history study of rapid-cycling bipolar disorder. *Psychiatry Res*, 48(1), 37–46.

Lish, J.D., Dime-Meenan, S., Whybrow, P.C., Price, R.A., and Hirschfeld, R.M. (1994). The National Depressive and Manic-depressive Association (DMDA) survey of bipolar members. *J Affect Disord*, 31, 281–294.

Loranger, A.W., and Levine, P.M. (1978). Age at onset of bipolar affective illness. *Arch Gen Psychiatry*, 35(11), 1345–1348.

Lundquist, G. (1945). Prognosis and course in manic-depressive psychoses: A follow-up study of 319 first admissions. *Acta Psychiatr Neurol* (Suppl. 35), 1–96.

MacDonald, J.B. (1918). Prognosis in manic-depressive insanity. *J Nerv Ment Dis*, 17, 20–30.

Maj, M., Pirozzi, R., and Starace, F. (1989). Previous pattern of course of the illness as a predictor of response to lithium prophylaxis in bipolar patients. *J Affective Disord*, 17, 237–241.

Maj, M., Magliano, L., Pirozzi, R., Marasco, C., and Guarneri, M. (1994). Validity of rapid cycling as a course specifier for bipolar disorder. *Am J Psychiatry*, 151(7), 1015–1019.

Maj, M., Pirozzi, R., and Magliano, L. (1995). Nonresponse to re-instituted lithium prophylaxis in previously responsive bipolar patients: Prevalence and predictors. *Am J Psychiatry*, 152(12), 1810–1811.

Maj, M., Pirozzi, R., Magliano, L., and Bartoli, L. (2002). The prognostic significance of "switching" in patients with bipolar disorder: A 10-year prospective follow-up study. *Am J Psychiatry*, 159(10), 1711–1717.

Maj, M., Pirozzi, R., Magliano, L., and Bartoli, L. (2003). Agitated depression in bipolar I disorder: Prevalence, phenomenology, and outcome. *Am J Psychiatry*, 160(12), 2134–2140.

Mann, A.M., and Hutchinson, J.L. (1967). Manic reaction associated with procarbazine hydrochloride therapy of Hodgkin's disease. *Can Med Assoc J*, 97, 1350–1353.

Mantere, O., Suominen, K., Leppamaki, S., Valtonen, H., Arvilommi, P., and Isometa, E. (2004). The clinical characteristics of DSM-IV bipolar I and II disorders: Baseline findings from the Jorvi Bipolar Study (JoBS). *Bipolar Disorders*, 6, 395–405.

Marneros, A., Deister, A., and Rohde, A. (1990). The concept of distinct but voluminous groups of bipolar and unipolar diseases: III. Bipolar and unipolar comparison. *Eur Arch Psychiatry Clin Neurosci*, 240(2), 90–95.

Maurizi, C.P. (1985). Influenza and mania: A possible connection with the locus ceruleus. *South Med J*, 78, 207–209.

Maxwell, S., Scheftner, W.A., Kessler, H.A., and Busch, K. (1988). Manic syndrome associated with zidovudine. *JAMA*, 259, 3406–3407.

McClellan, J., Breiger, D., McCurry, C., and Hlastala, S.A. (2003). Premorbid functioning in early-onset psychotic disorders. *J Am Acad Child Adolesc Psychiatry*, 42, 666–672.

McElroy, S.L., Strakowski, S.M., Keck, P.E. Jr., Tugrul, K.L., West, S.A., and Lonczak, H.S. (1995). Differences and similarities in mixed and pure mania. *Compr Psychiatry*, 36(3), 187–194.

McElroy, S.L., Strakowski, S.M., West, S.A., Keck, P.E., and McConville, B.J. (1997). Phenomenology of adolescent and adult mania in hospitalized patients with bipolar disorder. *Am J Psychiatry*, 154(1), 44–49.

McElroy, S.L., Altshuler, L.L., Suppes, T., Keck, P.E. Jr., Frye, M.A., Denicoff, K.D., Nolen, W.A., Kupka, R.W., Leverich, G.S., Rochussen, J.R., Rush, A.J., and Post, R.M. (2001). Axis I psychiatric comorbidity and its relationship to historical illness variables in 288 patients with bipolar disorder. *Am J Psychiatry*, 158(3), 420–426.

McGlashan, T.H. (1988). Adolescent versus adult onset of mania. *Am J Psychiatry*, 145(2), 221–223.

McKeown, S.P., and Jani, C.J. (1987). Mania following head injury. *Br J Pscyhiatry*, 151, 867–868.

McMahon, F.J., Stine, O.C., Chase, G.A., Meyers, D.A., Simpson, S.G., and DePaulo, J.R. (1994). Influence of clinical subtype, sex, and lineality on age at onset of major affective disorder in a family sample. *Am J Psychiatry*, 151(2), 210–215.

Mebane, A.H. (1984). L-Glutamine and mania. *Am J Psychiatry*, 141, 1302–1303.

Meeks, S. (1999). Bipolar disorder in the latter half of life: Symptom presentation, global functioning and age of onset. *J Affect Disord*, 52(1–3), 161–167.

Mendlewicz, J., Fieve, R.R., Rainer, J., and Fleiss, J.L. (1972a). Manic-depressive illness: A comparative study of patients with and without a family history. *Br J Psychiatry*, 120, 523–530.

Meyer, S.E., Carlson, G.A., Wiggs, E.A., Ronsaville, D.S., Martinez, P.E., Klimes-Dougan, B., Gold, P.W., and Radke-Yarrow, M. (2006). A prospective high-risk study of the association among maternal negativity, apparent frontal lobe dysfunction, and the development of bipolar disorder. *Dev Psychopathol*, 18(2), 573–589.

Mick, E., Biederman, J., Faraone, S.V., Murray, K., and Wozniak, J. (2003). Defining a developmental subtype of bipolar disorder in a sample of nonreferred adults by age at onset. *J Child Adolesc Psychopharmacol*, 13, 453–462.

Mijch, A.M., Judd, F.K., Lyketsos, C.G., Ellen, S., and Cockram, A. (1999). Secondary mania in patients with HIV infection: Are antiretrovirals protective? *J Neuropsychiatry Clin Neurosci*, 11(4), 475–480.

Molnar, G.J., Feeney, M.G., and Fava, G.A. (1988). Duration and symptoms of bipolar prodromes. *Am J Psychiatry*, 145, 1576–1578.

Moore, G.J., Bebchuk, J.M., Wilds, I.B., Chen, G., and Manji, H.K. (2000). Lithium-induced increase in human brain grey matter. Letter. *Lancet*, 356(9237), 1241–1242.

Morris, R. (2002). Clinical importance of inter-episode symptoms in patients with bipolar affective disorder. *J Affect Disord*, 72(Suppl. 1), S3–S13.

Morselli, P.L., Elgie, R., and Cesana, B.M. (2004). GAMIAN-Europe/BEAM survey II: Cross-national analysis of unemployment, family history, treatment satisfaction and impact of the bipolar disorder on life style. *Bipolar Disord*, 6(6), 487–497.

Mueller, T.I., Leon, A.C., Keller, M.B., Solomon, D.A., Endicott, J., Coryell, W., Warshaw, M., and Maser, J.D. (1999). Recurrence after recovery from major depressive disorder during 15 years of observational follow-up. *Am J Psychiatry*, 156, 1000–1006.

Muller-Oerlinghausen, B., Wolf, T., Ahrens, B., Glaenz, T., Schou, M., Grof, E., Grof, P., Lenz, G., Simhandl, C., Thau, K., Vestergaard, P., and Wolf R. (1996). Mortality of patients who dropped out from regular lithium prophylaxis: A collaborative study by the International Group for the Study of Lithium-treated patients (IGSLI). *Acta Psychiatr Scand*, 94, 344–347.

Muncie, W. (1934). Postoperative states of excitement. *Arch Neurol Psychiatry*, 34, 681–703.

Nierenberg, A.A., Miyahara, S., Spencer, T., Wisniewski, S.R., Otto, M.W., Simon, N., Pollack, M.H., Ostacher, M.J., Yan, L., Siegel, R., and Sachs, G.S. (2005). Clinical and diagnostic implications of lifetime attention-deficit/hyperactivity disorder comorbidity in adults with bipolar disorder: Data from the first 1000 STEP-BD participants. *Biol Psychiatry*, 57(11), 1467–1473.

Nolen, W.A., Luckenbaugh, D.A., Altshuler, L.L., Suppes, T., McElroy, S.L., Frye, M.A., Kupka, R.W., Keck, P.E. Jr., Leverich, G.S., and Post, R.M. (2004). Correlates of 1-year prospective outcome in bipolar disorder: Results from the Stanley Foundation Bipolar Network. *Am J Psychiatry*, 161(8), 1447–1454.

Nurnberger, J.I. Jr., Guroff, J.J., Hamovit, J., Berrettini, W., and Gershon, E.S. (1988b). A family study of rapid-cycling bipolar illness. *J Affective Disord*, 15, 87–91.

O'Brien, C.P., DiGiacomo, J.N., and Fahn, S. (1971). Mental effects of high-dosage levodopa. *Arch Gen Psychiatry*, 24, 61–64.

O'Connell, R.A., Mayo, J.A., Flatow, L., Cuthbertson, B., and O'Brien, B.E. (1991). Outcome of bipolar disorder on long-term treatment with lithium. *Br J Psychiatry*, 159, 123–129.

O'Dowd, M.A., and McKegney, F.P. (1988). Manic syndrome associated with zidovudine. *JAMA*, 260, 3587.

Oepen, G., Baldessarini, R.J., Salvatore, P., and Slater, E. (2004). On the periodicity of manic-depressive insanity, by Eliot Slater (1938): Translated excerpts and commentary. *J Affect Disord*, 78(1), 1–9.

Okuma, T., and Shimoyama, N. (1972). Course of endogenous manic-depressive psychosis, precipitating factors and premorbid personality: A statistical study. *Folia Psychiatr Neurol Japonica*, 26, 19–33.

Oppler, W. (1950). Manic psychosis in a case of parasagittal meningioma. *Arch Neurol Psychiatry*, 64, 417–430.

Osby, U., Brandt, L., Correia, N., Ekbom, A., Sparen, P. (2001). Excess mortality in bipolar and unipolar disorder in Sweden. *Arch Gen Psychiatry*, 8, 44–50.

Papolos, D.F., Veit, S., Faedda, G.L., Saito, T., and Lachman, H.M. (1998). Ultra-ultra rapid cycling bipolar disorder is associated with the low activity catecholamine-O-methyltransferase allele. *Mol Psychiatry*, 3(4), 346–349.

Patel, N.C., Delbello, M.P., and Strakowski, S.M. (2006). Ethnic differences in symptom presentation of youths with bipolar disorder. *Bipolar Disord*, 8(1), 95–99.

Perlis, R.H., Miyahara, S., Marangell, L.B., Wisniewski, S.R., Ostacher, M., DelBello, M.P., Bowden, C.L., Sachs, G.S., Nierenberg, A.A., and STEP-BD Investigators. (2004). Long-term implications of early onset in bipolar disorder: Data from the first 1000 participants in the Systematic Treatment Enhancement Program for Bipolar Disorder (STEP-BD). *Biol Psychiatry*, 55, 875–881.

Perris, C. (1968). The course of depressive psychoses. *Acta Psychiatr Scand*, 44, 238–248.

Perris, C., and d'Elia, G. (1966). A study of bipolar (manic-depressive) and unipolar recurrent depressive psychoses: X. Mortality, suicide, and life cycles. *Acta Psychiatr Scand*, 42(Suppl. 194), 172–183.

Perris, C., Eisemann, M., von Knorring, L., and Perris, H. (1984). Presentation of a subscale for the rating of depression and some additional items to the Comprehensive Psychopathological Rating Scale. *Acta Psychiatr Scand*, 70(3), 261–274.

Perugi, G., Micheli, C., Akiskal, H.S., Madaro, D., Socci, C., Quilici, C., and Musetti, L. (2000). Polarity of the first episode, clinical characteristics, and course of manic depressive illness: A systematic retrospective investigation of 320 bipolar I patients. *Compr Psychiatry*, 41, 13–18.

Pollock, H.M. (1931). Recurrence of attacks in manic-depressive psychoses. *Am J Psychiatry*, 11, 568–573.

Pope, H.G., and Katz, D.L. (1988). Affective and psychotic symptoms associated with anabolic steroid use. *Am J Psychiatry*, 145, 487–490.

Post, R.M. (1990). Sensitization and kindling perspectives for the course of affective illness: Toward a new treatment with the anticonvulsant carbamazepine. *Pharmacopsychiatry*, 23, 3–17.

Post, R.M., and Weiss, S.R. (1989). Sensitization, kindling, and anticonvulsants in mania. *J Clin Psychiatry*, 50(Suppl.), 23–30; discussion 45–47.

Post, R.M., Rubinow, D.R., Ballenger, J.C. (1986a). Conditioning and sensitisation in the longitudinal course of affective illness. *Br J Psychiatry*, 149, 191–201.

Post, R.M., Roy-Byrne, P.P., and Uhde, T.W. (1988). Graphic representation of the life course of illness in patients with affective disorder. *Am J Psychiatry*, 145(7), 844–848.

Post, R.M., Weiss, S.R., Smith, M., Rosen, J., and Frye, M. (1995). Stress, conditioning, and the temporal aspects of affective disorders. *Ann N Y Acad Sci*, 771, 677–696.

Post, R.M., Leverich, G.S., Xing, G., and Weiss, R.B. (2001). Developmental vulnerabilities to the onset and course of bipolar disorder. *Dev Psychopathol*, 13(3), 581–598.

Post, R.M., Leverich, G.S., Altshuler, L.L., Frye, M.A., Suppes, T.M., Keck, P.E. Jr., McElroy, S.L., Kupka, R., Nolen, W.A., Grunze, H., and Walden, J. (2003). An overview of recent findings of the Stanley Foundation Bipolar Network (Part I). *Bipolar Disord*, 5(5), 310–319.

Price, W.A., and Bielefeld, M. (1989). Buspirone-induced mania. *J Clin Psychopharmacol*, 9, 150–151.

Rego, M.D., and Giller, E.L. (1989). Mania secondary to amantadine treatment of neuroleptic-induced hyperprolactinemia. *J Clin Psychiatry*, 50, 143–144.

Reich, T., and Winokur, G. (1970). Postpartum psychoses in patients with manic depressive disease. *J Nerv Ment Dis*, 151, 60–68.

Reichart, C.G., van der Ende, J., Wals, M., Hillegers, M.H., Ormel, J., Nolen, W.A., and Verhulst, F.C. (2004). The use of the GBI in a population of adolescent offspring of parents with a bipolar disorder. *J Affect Disord*, 80(2–3), 263–267.

Reichenberg, A., Weiser, M., Rabinowitz, J., Caspi, A., Schmeidler, J., Mark, M., Kaplan, Z., and Davidson, M. (2002). A population-based cohort study of premorbid intellectual, language, and behavioral functioning in patients with schizophrenia, schizoaffective disorder, and nonpsychotic bipolar disorder. *Am J Psychiatry*, 159(12), 2027–2035.

Rennie, T.A.C. (1942). Prognosis in manic-depressive psychoses. *Am J Psychiatry*, 98, 801–814.

Revicki, D.A., Matza, L.S., Flood, E., and Lloyd, A. (2005). Bipolar disorder and health-related quality of life: Review of burden of disease and clinical trials. *Pharmacoeconomics*, 23(6), 583–594.

Rigby, J., Harvey, M., and Davies, D.R. (1989). Mania precipitated by benzodiazepine withdrawal. *Acta Psychiatr Scan*, 79, 406–407.

Rosenbaum, A.H., and Barry, M.J. (1975). Positive therapeutic response to lithium in hypomania secondary to organic brain syndrome. *Am J Psychiatry*, 132, 1072–1073.

Rousseva, A., Henry, C., van den Bulke, D., Fournier, G., Laplanche, J.L., Leboyer, M., Bellivier, F., Aubry, J.M., Baud, P., Boucherie, M., Buresi, C., Ferrero, F., and Malafosse, A. (2003). Antidepressant-induced mania, rapid cycling and the serotonin transporter gene polymorphism. *Pharmacogenomics J*, 3(2), 101–104.

Roy-Byrne, P., Post, R., Uhde, T., Porcu, T., and Davis, D. (1985a). The longitudinal course of recurrent affective illness: Life chart data from research patients at the NIMH. *Acta Psychiatr Scand*, 71, 1–34.

Ryback, R.S., and Schwab, R.S. (1971). Manic response to levodopa therapy: Report of a case. *N Engl J Med*, 285, 788–789.

Salazar-Calderon Perriggo, V.H., Oommen, K.J., and Sobonya, R.E. (1993). Silent solitary right parietal chondroma resulting in secondary mania. *Clin Neuropathol*, 12(6), 325–329.

Saran, B.M. (1970). The course of recurrent depressive illness in selected patients from a defined population. *Int Pharmacopsychiatry*, 5, 119–131.

Sax, K.W., Strakowski, S.M., Keck, P.E., McElroy, S.L., West, S.A., Bourne, M.L., and Larson, E.R. (1997). Comparison of patients with early-, typical-, and late-onset affective psychosis. *Am J Psychiatry*, 154(9), 1299–1301.

Sayed, A.J. (1976). Mania and bromism: A case report and a look to the future. *Am J Psychiatry*, 133, 228–229.

Schaerf, F.W., Miller, R., Pearlson, G.D., Kaminsky, M.J., and Weaver, D. (1988). Manic syndrome associated with zidovudine. *JAMA*, 260, 3587–3588.

Schulze, T.G., Muller, D.J., Krauss, H., Gross, M., Fangerau-Lefevre, H., Illes, F., Ohlraun, S., Cichon, S., Held, T., Propping, P., Nothen, M.M., Maier, W., and Rietschel, M. (2002). Further evidence for age of onset being an indicator for severity in bipolar disorder. *J Affect Disord*, 68(2–3), 343–345.

Schurhoff, F., Bellivier, F., Jouvent, R., Mouren-Simeoni, M.C., Bouvard, M., Allilaire, J.F., and Leboyer, M. (2000). Early and late onset bipolar disorders: Two different forms of manic-depressive illness? *J Affect Disord*, 58(3), 215–221.

Schwartz, R.B. (1974). Manic psychosis in connection with Q-fever. *Br J Psychiatry*, 124, 140–143.

Sharma, R., and Markar, H.R. (1994). Mortality in affective disorder. *J Affect Disord*, 31(2), 91–96.

Shulman, K., and Post, F. (1980). Bipolar affective disorder in old age. *Br J Psychiatry*, 136, 26–32.

Sierra, P., Livianos, L., and Rojo, L. (2005). Quality of life for patients with bipolar disorder: Relationship with clinical and demographic variables. *Bipolar Disord*, 7(2), 159–165.

Skop, B.P., and Masterson, B.J. (1995). Mania secondary to lisinopril therapy. *Psychosomatics*, 36(5), 508–509.

Slater, E. (1938a). Zur periodik des manische-depressiven irreseins. *Ztschr Neurol Psychiatr*, 162, 794–801.

Smeraldi, E., Gasperini, M., Macciardi, F., Bussoleni, C., and Morabito, A. (1982–1983). Factors affecting the distribution of age at onset in patients with affective disorders. *J Psychiatr Res*, 17(3), 309–317.

Sotsky, S.M., and Tossell, J.W. (1984). Tolmetin induction of mania. *Psychosomatics*, 25, 626–628.

Spencer, T.J., Biederman, J., Wozniak, J., Faraone, S.V., Wilens, T.E., and Mick, E. (2001). Parsing pediatric bipolar disorder from its associated comorbidity with the disruptive behavior disorder. *Biol Psychiatry*, 49(12), 1062–1070.

Spicer, C.C., Hare, E.H., and Slater, E. (1973). Neurotic and psychotic forms of depressive illness: Evidence from age-incidence in a national sample. *Br J Psychiatry*, 123, 535–541.

Staner, L., Tracy, A., Dramaix, M., Genevrois, C., Vanderelst, M., Vilane, A., Bauwens, F., Pardoen, D., and Mendlewicz, J. (1997). Clinical and psychosocial predictors of recurrence in recovered bipolar and unipolar depressives: A one-year controlled prospective study. *Psychiatry Res*, 69, 39–51.

Steinberg, D., Hirsch, S.R., Marston, S.D., Reynolds, K., and Sutton, R.N. (1972). Influenza infection causing manic psychosis. *Br J Psychiatry*, 120, 531–535.

Stenstedt, Å. (1952). A study in manic-depressive psychosis: Clinical, social, and genetic investigations. *Acta Psychiatr et Neurol* (Suppl. 79), 1–111.

Stephens, J.H., and McHugh, P.R. (1991). Characteristics and long-term follow-up of patients hospitalized for mood disorders in the Phipps Clinic, 1913–1940. *J Nerv Ment Dis*, 179, 64–73.

Stern, K., and Dancey, T. (1942). Glioma of the diencephalon in a manic patient. *Am J Psychiatry*, 98, 716.

Stone, K. (1989). Mania in the elderly. *Br J Psychiatry*, 155, 220–224.

Strakowski, S.M., Sax, K.W., McElroy, S.L., Keck, P.E. Jr., Hawkins, J.M., and West, S.A. (1998). Course of psychiatric and substance abuse syndromes co-occurring with bipolar disorder after a first psychiatric hospitalization. *J Clin Psychiatry*, 59(9), 465–471.

Strakowski, S.M., DelBello, M.P., Adler, C., Cecil, D.M., and Sax, K.W. (2000). Neuroimaging in bipolar disorder. *Bipolar Disord*, 2(3 Pt. 1), 148–164.

Strakowski, S.M., DelBello, M.P., Zimmerman, M.E., Getz, G.E., Mills, N.P., Ret, J., Shear, P., and Adler, C.M. (2002). Ventricular and periventricular structural volumes in first- versus multiple-episode bipolar disorder. *Am J Psychiatry*, 159(11), 1841–1847.

Sultzer, D.L., and Cummings, J.L. (1989). Drug-induced mania—Causative agents, clinical characteristics and management: A retrospective analysis of the literature. *Med Toxicol Adverse Drug Exper*, 4, 127–143.

Suppes, T., Leverich, G.S., Keck, P.E., Nolen, W.A., Denicoff, K.D., Altshuler, L.L., McElroy, S.L., Rush, A.J., Kupka, R., Frye, M.A., Bickel, M., and Post R.M. (2001). The Stanley Foundation Bipolar Treatment Outcome Network: II. Demographics and illness characteristics of the first 261 patients. *J Affect Disord*, 67(1–3), 45–59.

Swann, A.C., Secunda, S.K., Stokes, P.E., Croughan, J., Davis, J.M., Koslow, S.H., Maas, J.W. (1990). Stress, depression, and mania: Relationship between perceived role of stressful events and clinical and biochemical characteristics. *Acta Psychiatr Scand*, 81(4), 389–397.

Swann, A.C., Janicak, P.L., Calabrese, J.R., Bowden, C.L., Dilsaver, S.C., Morris, D.D., Petty, F., and Davis, J.M. (2001). Structure of mania: Depressive, irritable, and psychotic clusters with different retrospectively-assessed course patterns of illness in randomized clinical trial participants. *J Affect Disord*, 67(1–3), 123–132.

Swift, H.M. (1907). The prognosis of recurrent insanity of manic-depressive type. *Am J Insanity*, 64, 311–326.

Taschev, T. (1974). The course and prognosis of depression on the basis of 652 patients deceased. In J. Angst (Ed.), *Classification and Prediction of Outcome of Depression* (pp. 157–172). Symposium Schloss Reinhartshausen/Rhein. Symposia Medica Hoeschst 8. Stuttgart: FK Schattauer.

Taylor, M.A., and Abrams, R. (1973a). Manic states: A genetic study of early and late onset affective disorders. *Arch Gen Psychiatry*, 28, 656–658.

Tham, A., Engelbrektson, K., Mathe, A.A., Johnson, L., Olsson, E., and Aberg-Wistedt, A. (1997). Impaired neuropsychological performance in euthymic patients with recurring mood disorders. *J Clin Psychiatry*, 58, 26–29.

Tohen, M., Waternaux, C.M., and Tsuang, M. (1990). Outcome in mania: A 4-year prospective follow-up of 75 patients utilizing survival analysis. *Arch Gen Psychiatry*, 47, 1106–1111.

Tohen, M., Stoll, A.L., Strakowski, S.M., Faedda, G.L., Mayer, P.V., Goodwin, D.C., Kolbrener, M.L., and Madigan, A.M. (1992). The McLean First-Episode Psychosis Project: Six-month recovery and recurrence outcome. *Schizophr Bull*, 18(2), 273–282.

Tohen, M., Shulman, K.I., and Satlin, A. (1994). First-episode mania in late life. *Am J Psychiatry*, 151(1), 130–132.

Tohen, M., Hennen, J., Zarate, C.J., Baldessarini, R., Strakowski, S., Stoll, A., Faedda, G., Suppes, T., Gebre-Medhin, A., and Cohen, B. (2000). The McLean first episode project: Two-year syndromal and functional recovery in 219 cases of major affective disorders with psychotic features. *Am J Psychiatry*, 157(2), 220–228.

Tohen, M., Zarate, C., Hennen, J., Khalsa, H.M., Strakowski, S.M., Gebre-Medhin, P., Salvatore, P., and Baldessarini, R.J. (2003). The McLean-Harvard First-Episode Mania Study: Prediction of recovery and first recurrence. *Am J Psychiatry*, 160(12), 2099–2107.

Tondo, L., Ghiani, C., and Albert, M. (2001). Pharmacologic interventions in suicide prevention. *J Clin Psychiatry*, 62(Suppl. 25), 51–55.

Tsai, S.J., Wang, Y.C., and Hong, C.J. (2001). Association study between cannabinoid receptor gene (CNR1) and pathogenesis and psychotic symptoms of mood disorders. *Am J Med Genet*, 105, 219–221.

Tsuang, M.T. (1978). Suicide in schizophrenics, manics, depressives and surgical controls: A comparison with general suicide mortality. *Arch Gen Psychiatry*, 35, 153–155.

Tsuang, M.T., Woolson, R., and Fleming, J.A. (1979). Long-term outcome of major psychoses: I. Schizophrenia and affective disorders compared with psychiatrically symptom-free surgical conditions. *Arch Gen Psychiatry*, 36, 1295–1301.

Tsuang, M.T., Woolson, R.F., and Fleming, J.A. (1980). Causes of death in schizophrenia and manic-depression. *Br J Psychiatry*, 136, 239–242.

Turvey, C.L., Coryell, W.H., Solomon, D.A., Leon, A.C., Endicott, J., Mueller, T., Keller, M., and Akiskal, H. (1999). Long-term prognosis of bipolar I disorder. *Acta Psychiatr Scand*, 99, 110–119.

van Gorp, W.G., Altshuler, L., Theberge, D.C., Wilkins, J., and Dixon, W. (1998). Cognitive impairment in euthymic bipolar patients with and without prior alcohol dependence: A preliminary study. *Arch Gen Psychiatry*, 55(1), 41–46.

van Os, J., Takei, N., Castle, D.J., Wessely, S., Der, G., and Murray, R.M. (1995). Premorbid abnormalities in mania, schizomania, acute schizophrenia and chronic schizophrenia. *Soc Psychiatry Psychiatr Epidemiol*, 30(6), 274–278.

Van Woert, M.H., Ambani, L.M., and Weintraub, M.I. (1971). Manic behavior and levodopa. *N Engl J Med*, 285, 1326.

Venkatarangam, S.H.M., Kutcher, S.P., and Notkin, R.M. (1988). Secondary mania with steroid withdrawal. *Can J Psychiatry*, 33, 631–632.

Verdoux, H., and Bourgeois, M. (1993). A comparison of manic patient subgroups. *J Affect Disord*, 27(4), 267–272.

Vieta, E., Gasto, C., Otero, A., Nieto, E., and Vallejo, J. (1997). Differential features between bipolar I and bipolar II disorder. *Compr Psychiatry*, 38(2), 98–101.

Viguera, A.C., and Cohen, L.S. (1998). The course and management of bipolar disorder during pregnancy. *Psychopharmacol Bull*, 34, 339–346.

Viguera, A.C., Cohen, L.S., Baldessarini, R.J., and Nonacs, R. (2002). Managing bipolar disorder during pregnancy: Weighing the risks and benefits. *Can J Psychiatry*, 47, 426–436.

Viswanathan, R., and Glickman, L. (1989). Clonazepam in the treatment of steroid-induced mania in a patient after renal transplantation. *N Engl J Med*, 320, 319–320.

Vocisano, C., Klein, D.N., Keefe, R., Dienst, E.R., and Kincaid, M.M. (1996). Demographics, family history, premorbid functioning, developmental characteristics, and course of patients with deteriorated affective disorder. *Am J Psychiatry*, 153(2), 248–255.

Vuilleumier, P., Ghika-Schmid, F., Bogousslavsky, J., Assal, G., and Regli, F. (1998). Persistent recurrence of hypomania and prosopoaffective agnosia in a patient with right thalamic infarct. *Neuropsychiatry Neuropsychol Behav Neurol*, 11(1), 40–44.

Walton, R.G. (1986). Seizure and mania after high intake of aspartame. *Psychosomatics*, 27, 218–220.

Waters, B.G.H., and Lapierre, Y.D. (1981). Secondary mania associated with sympathomimetic drug use. *Am J Psychiatry*, 138, 837–838.

Wehr, T.A., and Goodwin, F.K. (1979). Rapid cycling in manic-depressives induced by tricyclic antidepressants. *Arch Gen Psychiatry*, 36, 555–559.

Wehr, T.A., and Goodwin, F.K. (1987). Can antidepressants cause mania and worsen the course of affective illness? *Am J Psychiatry*, 144, 1403–1411.

Wehr, T.A., Sack, D.A., and Rosenthal, N.E. (1987a). Sleep reduction as a final common pathway in the genesis of mania. *Am J Psychiatry*, 144, 201–204.

Wehr, T.A., Sack, D.A., Rosenthal, N.E., and Cowdry, R.W. (1988). Rapid cycling affective disorder: Contributing factors and treatment responses in 51 patients. *Am J Psychiatry*, 145, 179–184.

Weilburg, J.B., Sachs, G., and Falk, W.E. (1987). Triazolam-induced brief episodes of secondary mania in a depressed patient. *J Clin Psychiatry*, 48, 492–493.

Weisert, K.N., and Hendrie, H.C. (1977). Secondary mania? A case report. *Am J Psychiatry*, 134, 929–930.

Weiss, R.D., Ostacher, M.J., Otto, M.W., Calabrese, J.R., Fossey, M., Wisniewski, S.R., Bowden, C.L., Nierenberg, A.A., Pollack, M.H., Salloum, I.M., Simon, N.M., Thase, M.E., and Sachs, G.S. (2005). Does recovery from substance use disorder matter in patients with bipolar disorder? *J Clin Psychiatry*, 66(6), 730–735.

Weiss, S.R., Post, R.M., Costello, M., Nutt, D.J., and Tandeciarz, S. (1990). Carbamazepine retards the development of cocaine-kindled seizures but not sensitization to cocaine-induced hyperactivity. *Neuropsychopharmacology*, 3, 273–281.

Weissman, M.M., Bland, R.C., Canino, G.J., Faravelli, C., Greenwald, S., Hwu, H.G., Joyce, P.R., Karam, E.G., Lee, C.K., Lellouch, J., Lepine, J.P., Newman, S.C., Rubio-Stipec, M., Wells, J.E., Wickramaratne, P.J., Wittchen, H., and Yeh, E.K. (1996). Cross-national epidemiology of major depression and bipolar disorder. *JAMA*, 276(4), 293–299.

Winokur, G. (1974). Genetic and clinical factors associated with course in depression. Contributions to genetic aspects. *Pharmakopsychiatr Neuropsychopharmakol*, 7(2), 122–126.

Winokur, G. (1975). The Iowa 500: Heterogeneity and course of manic-depressive illness (bipolar). *Compr Psychiatry*, 16, 125–131.

Winokur, G. (1976). Duration of illness prior to hospitalization (onset) in the affective disorders. *Neuropsychobiology*, 2, 87–93.

Winokur, G., and Kadrmas, A. (1989). A polyepisodic course in bipolar illness: Possible clinical relationships. *Compr Psychiatry*, 30, 121–127.

Winokur, G., and Tsuang, M. (1975b). The Iowa 500: Suicide in mania, depression, and schizophrenia. *Am J Psychiatry*, 132, 650–651.

Winokur, G., Clayton, P.J., and Reich, T. (1969). *Manic depressive illness*. St. Louis: CV Mosby.

Winokur, G., Coryell, W., Keller, M., Endicott, J., and Akiskal, H. (1993). A prospective follow-up of patients with bipolar and primary unipolar affective disorder. *Arch Gen Psychiatry*, 50(6), 457–465.

Wright, J.M., Sachdev, P.S., Perkins, R.J., and Rodriguez, P. (1989). Zidovudine-related mania. *Med J Aust*, 150, 339–341.

Wylie, M.E., Mulsant, B.H., Pollock, B.G., Sweet, R.A., Zubenko, G.S., Begley, A.E., Gregor, M., Frank, E., Reynolds, C.F., and Kupfer, D.J. (1999). Age at onset in geriatric bipolar disorder. Effects on clinical presentation and treatment outcomes in an inpatient sample. *Am J Psychiatry*, 7(1), 77–83.

Yassa, R., Nair, V., Nastase, C., Camille, Y., and Belzile, L. (1988a). Prevalence of bipolar disorder in a psychogeriatric population. *J Affect Disord*, 14(3), 197–201.

Yatham, L.N., Lecrubier, Y., Fieve, R.R., Davis, K.H., Harris, S.D., and Krishnan, A.A. (2004). Quality of life in patients with bipolar I depression: Data from 920 patients. *Bipolar Disord*, 6(5), 379–385.

Zis, A.P., and Goodwin, F.K. (1979). Major affective disorder as a recurrent illness: A critical review. *Arch Gen Psychiatry*, 36, 835–839.

Zis, A.P., Grof, P., and Goodwin, F.K. (1979). The natural course of affective disorders: Implications for lithium prophylaxis. In T.B. Cooper, S. Gershon, N.S. Kline, and M. Schou (Eds.), *Lithium: Controversies and Unresolved Issues* (pp. 381–398). Amsterdam: Exerpta Medica.

Zis, A.P., Grof, P., Webster, M., and Goodwin, F.K. (1980). Prediction of relapse in recurrent affective disorder. *Psychopharmacol Bull*, 16, 47–49.

CHAPTER 5

Aalto-Setälä, T., Marttunen, M., Tuulio-Henriksson, A., Poikolainen, K., and Lönnqvist, J. (2001). One-month prevalence of depression and other DSM-IV disorders among young adults. *Psychol Med*, 31, 791–801.

Abood, Z., Sharkey, A., Webb, M., Kelly, A., and Gill, M. (2002). Are patients with bipolar affective disorder socially disadvantaged? A comparison with a control group. *Bipolar Disorders*, 4, 243–248.

Achenbach, T.M. (1991a). *Manual for the Child Behavior Checklist/4-18 and 1991 Profile*. Burlington, MA: University of Vermont Department of Psychiatry.

Achenbach, T.M. (1991b). *Integrative Guide for the 1991 CBCL/8-14, YSR and TRF profile*. Burlington, MA: University of Vermont Department of Psychiatry.

Ahrens, B., Berghofer, A., Wolf, T., and Muller-Oerlinghausen, B. (1995). Suicide attempts, age and duration of illness in recurrent affective disorders. *J Affect Disord*, 36(1–2), 43–49.

Akiskal, H.S. (1995). Developmental pathways to bipolarity: Are juvenile onset depressions pre-bipolar? *J Am Acad Child Adolesc Psychiatry*, 34, 754–763.

Akiskal, H.S. (1996). The prevalent clinical spectrum of bipolar disorders: Beyond DSM-IV. *J Clin Psychopharmacol*, 16, 4S–14S.

Akiskal, H.S., Bourgeois, M.L., Angst, J., Post, R., Möller, H-J., and Hirschfeld, R. (2000). Re-evaluating the prevalence of and diagnostic composition within the broad clinical spectrum of bipolar disorders. *J Affect Disord*, 59, S5–S30.

American Psychiatric Association. (1980). *Diagnostic and Statistical Manual of Mental Disorders*. 3rd ed. Washington, DC: American Psychiatric Association.

American Psychiatric Association. (1986). *Diagnostic and Statistical Manual of Mental Disorders*. 3rd ed., revised. Washington, DC: American Psychiatric Association.

American Psychiatric Association. (1994). *Diagnostic and Statistical Manual of Mental Disorders*. 4th ed. Washington, DC: American Psychiatric Association.

Andrade, L., Walters, E.E., Gentil, V., and Laurenti, R. (2002). Prevalence of ICD-10 mental disorders in a catchment area in the city of São Paulo, Brazil. *Soc Psychiat Psychiatric Epidemiol*, 37, 316–325.

Andreason, N.C. (1982). Negative symptoms in schizophrenia. *Arch Gen Psychiatry*, 39, 784–788.

Andrews, G., Sanderson, K., and Beard, J. (1998). Burden of disease: Methods of calculating disability from mental disorder. *Brit J Psychiatry*, 173, 123–131.

Angold, A. (1988). Childhood and adolescent depression: II. Research in clinical populations. *Br J Psychiatry*, 153, 476–492.

Angold, A., Costello, E.J., Worthman, C.M. (1998). Puberty and depression: The roles of age, pubertal status and pubertal timing. *Psychol Med*, 28, 51–61.

Angold, A., Costello, E.J., Erkanli, A., and Worthman, C.M. (1999). Pubertal changes in hormone levels and depression in girls. *Psychol Med*, 29, 1043–1053.

Angst, J. (1978). The course of affective disorders: II. Typology of bipolar manic-depressive illness. *Arch Psychiatr Nervenkr*, 226, 65–73.

Angst, J. (1995). Epidemiologie du spectre bipolarie. *L'Encephale*, 6, 37–42.

Angst, J. (1998). The emerging epidemiology of hypomania and bipolar II disorder. *J Affect Disord*, 50, 143–151.

Angst, J., and Gamma, A. (2002). Prevalence of bipolar disorders: Traditional and novel approaches. *Clinical Approaches in Bipolar Disorders*, 1, 10–14.

Angst, J., and Merikangas, K.R. (1992). Headache and personality. *Clin Neuropharmacol*, 15 (Suppl. 1, Pt. A), 273A–274A.

Angst, J., Dobler-Mikola, A., and Binder, A. (1984). The Zurich study: A prospective epidemiologic study of depressive, neurotic and psychomatic symptoms. I: Problem, methodology. *Eur Arch Psychiatry Neurol Sci*, 234, 13–20.

Angst, J., Degonda, M., and Ernst, C. (1992). The Zurich study: XV. Suicide attempts in a cohort from age 20–30. *Eur Arch Psychiatr Clin Neurosci*, 242, 135–141.

Angst, J., Gamma, A., and Lewinsohn, P. (2002). The evolving epidemiology of bipolar disorder. *World Psychiatry*, 1(3), 146–148.

Anthony, J.C., Folstein, M., Romanoski, A.J., Von Korff, M.R., Nestadt, G.R., Chahal, R., Merchant, A., Brown, C.H., Shapiro, S., Kramer, M., and Gruenberg, E.M. (1985). Comparison of the lay Diagnostic Interview Schedule and a standardized psychiatric diagnosis. *Arch Gen Psychiatry*, 42, 667–675.

Arce, A.A., and Vergare, M.J. (1984). Identifying and characterizing the mentally ill among the homeless. In H.R. Lamb (Ed.), *The Homeless Mentally ill: A Task Force Report of the American Psychiatric Association* (pp. 75–89). Washington, DC: American Psychiatric Association.

Babidge, N.C., Buhrich, N., and Butler, T. (2002). Mortality among homeless people with schizophrenia in Sydney, Australia: A 10-year follow-up. *Acta Psychiatr Scand*, 103, 105–110.

Badawi, M.A., Eaton, W.W., Myllyluoma, J., Weimer, L.G., and Gallo, J. (1999). Psychopathology and attrition in the Baltimore ECA 15-year follow-up 1981–1996. *Soc Psychiat Psychiatric Epidemiol*, 34, 91–98.

Bagley, C. (1973). Occupational status and symptoms of depression. *Soc Sci Med*, 7, 327–339.

Baldwin, P.A., Scully, P.J., Quinn, J.F., Morgan, M.G., Kinsella, A., O'Callaghan, E., Owens, J.M., and Waddington, J.L. (2002). First episode bipolar disorder: Systematic comparison of incidence with other affective and non-affective psychoses among an epidemiologically complete, rural population. *Bipolar Disorders*, 4(Suppl. 1), 39–40.

Benazzi, F. (1997). Prevalence of bipolar II disorder in outpatient depression: A 203 case study in private practice. *J Affect Dis*, 43, 163–166.

Biederman, J. (1995). Developmental subtypes of juvenile bipolar disorder. *Harvard Rev Psychiatry*, 327–330.

Biederman, J., Wozniak, J., Kiely, K., Ablon, S., Faraone, S., Mick, E., Mundy, E., and Kraus, I. (1995). CBCL clinical scales discriminate prepubertal children with structured-interview derived diagnosis of mania from those with ADHD. *J Am Acad Child Adolesc Psychiatry*, 34, 464–471.

Biederman, J., Farone, S.V., Wozniak, J., Mick, E., Kwon, A., and Aleardi, M. (2004). Further evidence of unique developmental phenotypic correlates of pediatric bipolar disorder: Findings from a large sample of clinically referred preadolescent children assessed over the last 7 years. *J Affect Dis*, 82(Suppl. 1), 517–523.

Bijl, R.V., de Graaf, R., Ravelli, A., Smit, F., and Vollebergh, W.A.M. (2002). Gender and age-specific first incidence of DSM-III-R psychiatric disorders in the general population. *Soc Psychiatry Psychiatr Epidemiol*, 37, 372–379.

Blazer, D. (1985). The epidemiology of psychiatric disorders in the elderly. Editorial. *J Am Geriatr Soc*, 33, 226–227.

Blehar, M.C., DePaulo, J., Gershon, E.S., Reich, T., Simpson, S.G., and Nurnberger, J.J. (1998). Women with bipolar disorder: Findings from the NIMH Genetics Initiative sample. *Psychopharmacol Bulletin*, 34, 239–243.

Breslow, N.E., and Day, N.E. (1987). *Statistical Methods in Cancer Research. Volume II: The Design and Analysis of Cohort Studies.* Lyon, France: International Agency for Research on Cancer.

Brewin, J., Cantwell, R., Dalkin, T., Fox, R., Medley, I., Glazebrook, C., Kwiecinski, R., and Harrison, G. (1997). Incidence of schizophrenia in Nottingham: A comparison of two cohorts, 1978–80 and 1992–94. *Br J Psychiatry*, 71, 140–144.

Buhrich, N., Hodder, T., and Teesson, M. (2000). Prevalence of cognitive impairment among homeless people in inner Sydney. *Psychiatry Services*, 51, 520–521.

Calabrese, J.R., Hirschfeld, R.M.A., Reed, M., Davies, M.A., Frye, M.A., Keck, P.E., Lewis, L., McElroy, S.L., McNulty, J.P., and Wagner, K.D. (2002). Impact of bipolar disorders on a U.S. community sample. *J Clin Psychiatry*.

Canino, G.J., Bird, H.R., Shrout, P.E., Rubio-Stipec, M., Bravo, M., Martinez, R., Sesman, M., and Guevara, L.M. (1987). The prevalence of specific psychiatric disorders in Puerto Rico. *Arch Gen Psychiatry*, 44, 727–735.

Carlson, G.A. (1996). Clinical features and pathogenesis of child and adolescent mania. In K.I. Schulman, M. Tohen (Eds.), *Mood Disorders across the Lifespan*. New York: Wiley-Liss.

Carney, P.A., Fitzgerald, C.T., and Monaghan, C.E. (1988). Influence of climate on the prevalence of mania. *Br J Psychiatry*, 152, 820–823.

Cassano, G.B., McElroy, S.L., Brady, K., Nolen, W.A., and Placidi, G.F. (2000). Current issues in the identification and management of bipolar spectrum disorders in "special populations." *J Affect Disord*, 59, S69–S79.

Chambers, W.J., Puig-Antich, J., Hirsch, M., Paez, P., Ambrosini, P., Tabrizi, M., and Davies, M. (1985). The assessment of affective disorders in children and adolescents by semi-structured interviews. *Arch Gen Psychiatry*, 42, 696–702.

Chen, C.N., Wong, J., Lee, N., Chan-Ho, M.W., Lau, T.F., and Fung, M. (1993). The Shatin community mental health survey in Hong Kong. *Arch Gen Psychiatry*, 50, 125–133.

Coryell, W., Endicott, J., Keller, M., Andreason, N., Grove, W., Hirschfeld, R.M.A., and Scheftner, W. (1989). Bipolar affective disorder and high achievement: A familial association. *Am J Psychiatry*, 146, 983–988.

Coryell, W., Endicott, J., Maser, J.D., Keller, M.B., Leon, A.C., and Akiskal, H.S. (1995). Long-term stability of polarity distinctions in the affective disorders. *Am J Psychiatry*, 152, 385–390.

Cowley, P., and Wyatt, J.R. (1993). Schizophrenia and manic-depressive illness. In D.T. Jamison, W.H. Mosley, A.R. Measham, J.L. Bobadilla (Eds.), *Disease Control Priorities in Developing Countries* (pp. 661–670). Oxford: Oxford University Press.

Cross-National Collaborative Group. (1992). The changing rate of major depression: Cross-national comparisons. *J Am Med Assoc*, 268, 3098–3106.

de Graaf, R., Bijl, R.V., Smit, F., Vollebergh, W.A.M., and Spijker, J. (2002). Risk factors for 12-month comorbidity of mood, anxiety and substance use disorders: Findings from the Netherlands Mental Health Survey and Incidence study. *Am J Psychiatry*, 159(4), 620–629.

Dilling, H., and Weyerer, S. (1984). Prevalence of mental disorders in the smalltown-rural region of Traunstein (Upper Bavaria). *Acta Psychiatr Scand*, 69, 60–79.

Dilsaver, S.C., and Akiskal, H.S. (2005). High rate of unrecognized bipolar mixed states among destitute Hispanic adolescents referred for "major depressive disorder." *J Affect Disord*, 84, 179–186.

Dunner, D.L., and Tay, L.K. (1993). Diagnostic reliability of the history of hypomania in bipolar II patients and patients with major depression. *Compr Psychiatry*, 34, 303–307.

Dunner, D.L., Russek, F.D., Russek, B., and Fieve, R.R. (1982). Classification of bipolar affective disorder subtypes. *Compr Psychiatry*, 23, 186–189.

Eaton, W.W., Kramer, M., Anthony, A., Dryman, S., Shapiro, S., and Locke, B.Z. (1989). The incidence of specific DIS/DSM-III mental health disorders: Data from the NIMH Epidemiologic Catchment Area Program. *Acta Psychiatr Scand*, 79, 163–178.

Egeland, J.A., and Hostetter, A.M. (1983). Amish study: I. Affective disorder among the Amish, 1976–1980. *Am J Psychiatry*, 140, 56–61.

Egeland, J.A., Hostetter, A.M., and Eshleman, S.K. III. (1983). Amish Study: III. The impact of cultural factors on diagnosis of bipolar illness. *Am J Psychiatry*, 140, 67–71.

Endicott, J., and Spitzer, R.L. (1978). A diagnostic interview: The Schedule for Affective Disorders and Schizophrenia. *Arch Gen Psychiatry*, 35, 837–844.

Faraone, S.V., Biederman, J., Mennin, D., Wozniak, J., and Spencer, T. (1997). Attention-deficit hyperactivity disorder with bipolar disorder: A familial subtype. *J Am Acad Child Adolesc Psychiatry*, 36, 1378–1387.

Faravelli, C., and Incerpi, G. (1985). Epidemiology of affective disorders in Florence. *Acta Psychiatr Scand*, 72, 331–333.

Faravelli, C., Degl'Innocenti, B.G., Aiazzi, L., Incerpi, G., and Pallanti, S. (1990). Epidemiology of mood disorders: A community survey in Florence. *J Affect Disord*, 20, 135–141.

Faravelli, C., Rosi, S., Scarpato, M.A., Lampronti, L., Amedei, S.G., and Rana, N. (2006). Threshold and subthreshold bipolar disorders in the Sesto Fiorentino Study. *J Affect Disord*, 94, 111–119.

Faris, R.E.L., and Dunham, H.W. (1939). *Mental Disorders in Urban Areas: An Ecological Study of Schizophrenia and Other Psychoses*. Chicago: University of Chicago Press.

Feinman, J.A., and Dunner, D.L. (1996). The effect of alcohol and substance abuse on the course of bipolar affective disorder. *J Affect Disord*, 12, 37(1), 43–49.

Fichter, M.M., and Quadflieg, N. (2001). Prevalence of mental illness in homeless men in Munich, Germany: Results from a representative sample. *Acta Psychiatr Scand*, 103, 94–104.

Gagrat, D.D., and Spiro, H.R. (1980). Social, cultural, and epidemiological aspects of mania. In R.H. Belmaker, H.M. van Praag (Eds.), *Mania: An Evolving Concept* (pp. 291–307). Jamaica, NY: Spectrum Publications.

Geller, B., Warner, K., Williams, M., and Zimmerman, B. (1998). Prepubertal and young adolescent bipolarity versus ADHD: Assessment and validity using the WASH-U-KSADS, CBCL, and TRF. *J Affect Disord*, 51, 93–100.

Geller, B., Zimmerman, B., Williams, M., Del Bello, M.P., Frazier, J., and Beringer, L. (2002). Phenomenology of prepubertal and early adolescent bipolar disorder: Examples of elated mood, grandiose behaviors, decreased need for sleep, racing thoughts, and hypersexuality. *J Child Adolesc Psychopharm*, 12, 3–9.

Gershon, E.S. (2000). Bipolar illness and schizophrenia as oliogenic diseases: Implications for the future. *Biol Psychiatry*, 47, 240–244.

Gershon, E.S., and Liebowitz, J.H. (1975). Sociocultural and demographic correlates of affective disorder in Jerusalem. *J Psychiatr Res*, 12, 37–50.

Gershon, E.S., Hamovit, J.H., Guroff, J.J., and Nurnberger, J.I. (1987). Birth-cohort changes in manic and depressive disorders in relatives of bipolar and schizoaffective patients. *Arch Gen Psychiatry*, 44, 314–319.

Gershon, E.S., Badner, J.A., Goldin, L.R., Sanders, A.R., Cravchik, A., and Detera-Wadleigh, S.D. (1998). Closing in on genes for manic-depressive illness and schizophrenia. *Neuropsychopharmacology*, 18, 233–242.

Glassman, A.H. (1993). Cigarette smoking: Implications for psychiatric illness. *Am J Psychiatry*, 150(4), 546–553.

Gonzalez-Pinto, A., Gutierrex, M., Ezcurra, J., Aizpuru, F., Nosquera, F., Lopez, P., and deLeon, J. (1998). Tobacco smoking and bipolar disorder. *J Clin Psychiatr*, 59, 225–228.

Gould, M.S., King, R., Greenwald, S., Fisher, P., Schwab-Stone, M., Kramer, R., Flisher, A.J., Goodman, S., Canino, G., and Shaffer, D. (1998). Psychopathology associated with suicidal ideation and attempts among children and adolescents. *J Am Acad Child Adolesc Psychiatry*, 37, 915–923.

Hare, E.H. (1968). *Bethlem Royal Hospital and the Maudsley Hospital Triennial Statistical Report: 1964–1966*. Triennial Statistical Reports. Stat Soc Ser A.

Helzer, J.E. (1975). Bipolar affective disorder in black and white men: A comparison of symptoms and familial illness. *Arch Gen Psychiatry*, 32, 1140–1143.

Helzer, J.E., and Pryzbeck, T.R. (1988). The co-occurrence of alcoholism with other psychiatric disorders in the general population and its impact on treatment. *J Stud Alcohol*, 49, 219–224.

Helzer, J.E., Robins, L.N., McEvoy, L.T., Spitznagel, E.L., Stoltzman, R.K., Farmer, A., and Brockington, I.F. (1985). A comparison of clinical and Diagnostic Interview Schedule diagnoses. *Arch Gen Psychiatry*, 42, 657–666.

Henderson, S., Andrews, G.H., and Hall, W. (2000). Australia's mental health: An overview of the general population survey. *Aust N Z J Psychiatry*, 34, 197–205.

Heun, R., and Maier, W. (1993). The distinction of bipolar II disorder from bipolar I and recurrent unipolar depression: Results of a controlled family study. *Acta Psychiatr Scand*, 87(4), 279–284.

Hibbeln, J.R. (1998). Fish consumption and major depression. *The Lancet*, 351, 1213.

Hirschfeld, R.M.A., Calabrese, J.R., Weissman, M.M., Reed, M., Davies, M.A., Frye, M.A., Keck, P.E., Lewis, L., McElroy, S.L., McNulty, J.P., and Wagner, K.D. (2001). Lifetime prevalence of bipolar spectrum disorder in the United States. Submitted. Hirschfeld, R.M.A., Calabrese, J.R., Weissman, M.M., Frye, M.A., Keck, P.E., Jr., and Wagner, K.D. *Lifetime prevalence of bipolar I & II disorders in United States*. American Psychiatric Association Annual Meeting, New Research Abstract 247, Philadelphia, PA, May 18–23, 2002.

Hirschfeld, R.M.A., Calabrese, J.R., Weissman, M.M., Reed, M., Davies, M.A., Frye, M.A., Keck, P.E., Lewis, L., McElroy, S.L., McNulty, J.P., and Wagner, K.D. (2003a). Screening for bipolar disorder in the community. *J Clin Psychiatry*, 64, 53–59.

Hirschfeld, R.M.A., Holzer, C., Calabrese, J.R., Weissman, M.M., Reed, M., Davies, M.A., Frye, M.A., Keck, P.E., McElroy, S., Lewis, L., Tierce, J., Wagner, K.D., and Hazard, E. (2003b). Validity of the Mood Disorder Questionnaire: A general population study. *Am J Psychiatry*, 160, 178–180.

Hollingshead, A.B., and Redlich, F.C. (1958). *Social Class and Mental Illness: A Community Study*. New York: J. Wiley & Sons.

Hostetter, A.M., Egeland, J.A., and Endicott, J. (1983). Amish study: II. Consensus diagnosis and reliability results. *Am J Psychiatry*, 140, 62–66.

Hwu, H.G., Yeh, E.K., and Chang, L.Y. (1989). Prevalence of psychiatric disorders in Taiwan defined by the Chinese Diagnostic Interview Schedule. *Acta Psychiatr Scand*, 79, 136–147.

Isometsa, E., Henriksson, M., Aro, H., Heikkinen, M., Kuoppasalmi, K., and Lonnqvist, J. (1994). Suicide in psychotic major depression. *J Affect Disord*, 31, 187–191.

Jenkins, R., Lewis, G., Bebbington, P., Brugha, T., Farrell, M., Gill, B., and Meltzer, H. (2003). The National Psychiatry Morbidity Surveys of Great Britian: Initial findings from the household survey. *Int Rev Psychiatry*, 15, 29–42.

Judd, L.L., and Akiskal, H.S. (2003). The prevalence and disability of bipolar spectrum disorders in the US population: Reanalysis of the ECA database taking into account subthreshold cases. *J Affect Disord*, 73(1-2), 123–131.

Karam, E.G. (1992). Depression et Guerres du Liban: Methodologies d'une Recherche. *Annales de Psychologie et des Sciences de l'Education*. Beyrouth, Lebanon: Université St. Joseph.

Keller, M.B., Lavori, P.W., Friedman, B., Nielsen, E., Endicott, J., and McDonald-Scott, P.A. (1987). The Longitudinal Enterval Follow-up Evaluation: A comprehensive method for assessing outcome in prospective longitudinal studies. *Arch Gen Psychiatry*, 44, 540–548.

Kelsoe, J.R. (2000). Mood disorders: Genetic. In B.J. Sadock, V.A. Sadock (Eds.), *Comprehensive Textbook of Psychiatry*. 7th ed. New York: Lippincott Williams & Wilkins.

Kennedy, N., Boydell, J., van Os, J., and Murray, R.M. (2004). Ethnic differences in first clinical presentation of bipolar disorder: Results from an epidemiological study. *J Affec Dis*, 83, 161–168.

Kessler, R. (1995). Development of modifications for the Composite International Diagnostic Interview (UM-CIDI) and prevalence estimates from its use in the National Comorbidity Survey (NCS). Presented at the World Psychiatric Association on May 17, New York, NY.

Kessler, R.C., McGonagle, K.A., Zhao, S., Nelson, C.B., Hughes, M., Eshleman, S., Wittchen, H.U., and Kendler, K.S. (1994). Lifetime and 12-month prevalence of DSM-III-R psychiatric disorders in the United States: Results from the National Comorbidity Study. *Arch Gen Psychiatry*, 51, 8–19.

Kessler, R.C., Rubinow, D.R., Holmes, C., Abelson, J.M., and Zhao, S. (1997). The epidemiology of DSM-III-R bipolar I disorder in a general population survey. *Psychol Med*, 27, 1079–1089.

Kessler, R.C., Berglund, P., Demler, O., Jin, R., and Walters, E.E. (2005a). Lifetime prevalence and age-of-onset distributions of DSM-IV disorders in the National Comorbidity Survey Replication. *Arch Gen Psychiatry*, 62, 593–602.

Kessler, R.C., Chiu, W.T., Demler, O., and Walters, E.E. (2005b). Prevalence, severity, and comorbidity of 12-month DSM-IV disorders in the National Comorbidity Survey Replication. *Arch Gen Psychiatry*, 62, 617–627.

Klerman, G.L. (1981). The spectrum of mania. *Compr Psychiatry*, 22, 11–20.

Klerman, G.L., and Weissman, M.M. (1989). Increasing rates of depression. *JAMA*, 261, 2229–2235.

Koegel, P., Burnam, M.A., and Farr, R.K. (1988). The prevalence of specific psychiatric disorders among homeless individuals in the inner city of Los Angeles. *Arch Gen Psychiatry*, 45, 1085–1092.

Koukopoulos, A., and Koukopoulos, A. (1999). Agitated depression as a mixed state and the problem of melancholia. *Psychiatr Clin North Am*, 22(3), 547–564.

Kovess, V., and Lazarus, C.M. (1999). The prevalence of psychiatric disorders and use of care by homeless people in Paris. *Soc Psychiatry Psychiatr Epidemiol*, 34, 580–587.

Kramer, M., von Korff, M., and Kessler, L. (1980). The lifetime prevalence of mental disorders: Estimation, uses, and limitations. *Psychol Med*, 10, 429.

Krauthammer, C., and Klerman, G.L. (1979). The epidemiology of mania. In B. Shopsin (Ed.), *Manic Illness* (pp. 11–28). New York: Raven Press.

Kringlen, E., Torgersen, S., and Cramer, V. (2001). A norwegian psychiatric epidemiological study. *Am J Psychiatry*, 158, 1091–1098.

Lahey, B.B., Flagg, E.W., Bird, H.R., Schwab-Stone, M.E., Canino, G., Dulcan, M.K., Leaf, P.J., Davies, M., Brogan, D., Bourdon, K., Horwitz, S.M., Rubio-Stipec, M., Freeman, D.H., Lichtman, J.H., Shaffer, D., Goodman, S.H., Narrow, W.E., Weissman, M.M., Kandel, D.B., Jensen, P.S., Richters, J.E., and Regier, D.A. (1996). The NIMH Methods for the Epidemiology of Child and Adolescent Mental Disorders (MECA) study: Background and methodology. *J Am Acad Child Adolesc Psychiatry*, 35, 855–864.

Lasch, K., Weissman, M., Wickramaratne, P., and Bruce, M.L. (1990). Birth-cohort changes in the rates of mania. *Psychiatry Res*, 33, 31–37.

Lasser, K., Boyd, J.W., Woolhandler, S., Himmelstein, D.U., McCormick, D., and Bor, D.H. (2000). Smoking and mental illness: A population-based prevalence study. *JAMA*, 284(20), 2606–2610.

Lee, C.K., Kwak Y.S., Yamamoto, J., Rhee, H., Kim, Y.S., Han, J.H., Choi, J.O., and Lee, Y.H. (1990a). Psychiatric epidemiology in Korea: Part I. Gender and age differences in Seoul. *J Nerv Ment Disord*, 178, 242–246.

Lee, C.K., Kwak, Y.S., Yamamoto, J., Rhee, H., Kim, Y.S., Han, J.H., Choi, J.O., and Lee, Y.H. (1990b). Psychiatric epidemiology in Korea: Part II. Urban and rural differences in Seoul. *J Nerv Ment Disord*, 178, 247–252.

Leibenluft, E. (1996). Women with bipolar illness: Clinical and research issues. *Am J Psychiatry*, 153, 163–173.

Lépine, J.P., Lellouch, J., Lovell, A., Teherani, M., Ha, C., Verdier-Taillefer, M.H., Rambourg, N., and Lemperiere, T. (1989). Anxiety and depressive disorders in a French population: Methodology and preliminary results. *Psychiatr Psychobiol*, 4, 267–274.

Lester, D. (1993). Suicidal behavior in bipolar and unipolar affective disorders: A meta-analysis. *J Affect Disord*, 27, 117–121.

Levav, J., Kohn, R., Dohrenwend, B.P., Shrout, P.E., Skodol, A.E., Schwartz, S., Link, B.G., and Naveh, G. (1993). An epidemiological study of mental disorders in a 10-year cohort of young adults in Israel. *Psychol Med*, 23, 691–707.

Lewinsohn, P.M., Klein, D.N., and Seeley, M.S. (1995). Bipolar disorders in a community sample of older adolescents: Prevalence, phenomenology, comorbidity and course. *J Am Acad Child Adolesc Psychiatry*, 34, 454–463.

Lewinsohn, P.M., Klein, D.N., and Seeley, M.S. (2000). Bipolar disorder during adolescence and young adulthood in a community sample. *Bipolar Disorders*, 2, 281–293.

Lewinsohn, P.M., Seeley, J.R., and Klein, D.N. (2003). Bipolar disorder during adolescence. *Acta Psychiatr Scand*, 108(Suppl. 418), 47–50.

Lewis, N.D., and Hubbard, L.D. (1931). Manic-depressive reactions in Negroes. *Res Pub Assoc Res Nerv Ment Dis*, 11, 779–817.

Link, B.G., Susser, E., Stueve, A., Phelan, J., Moore, R.E., and Struening, E. (1994). Lifetime and five-year prevalence of homelessness in the United States. *Am J Publ Health*, 84, 1907–1912.

MacKinnon, D.F., Jianfeng, X., McMahon, F.J., Simpson, S.G., Stine, O.C., McInnis, M.G., and DePaulo, J.R. (1998). Bipolar disorder and panic disorder in families: An analysis of chromosome 18 data. *Am J Psychiatry*, 155, 829–831.

Mathers, C.D., Lopez, A.D., and Murray, C.J.L. (2006). The burden of disease and mortality by condition: Data, methods, and results for 2001. In A.D. Lopez, C.D. Mathers, M. Ezzati, D.T. Jamison, and C.J.L. Murray (Eds.), *Global Burden of Disease and Risk Factors*. New York: Oxford University Press.

Melse, J.M., Essink-Bot, M.L., Kramers, P.G., and Hoeymans, N. on behalf of the Dutch Burden of Disease Group. (2000). A national burden of disease calculation: Dutch disability-adjusted life-years. *Am J Public Health*, 90, 1241–1247.

Merikangas, K.R., and Angst, J. (1992). Migraine and psychopathology: Epidemiologic and genetic aspects. *Clin Neuropharmacol*, 15(Suppl. 1, Pt. A), 275A–276A.

Mino, Y., Oshima, I., and Okagami, K. (2000). Seasonality of birth in patients with mood disorders in Japan. *J Affect Disord*, 59, 41–46.

Mitchell, P.B., Slade, T., and Andrews, G. (2004). Twelve-month prevalence and disability of DSM-IV bipolar disorder in an Australian population survey. *Psychol Med*, 34, 777–785.

Morens, D.H., and Andrade, L.H. (2005). The lifetime prevalence, health services utilization and risk of suicide of bipolar spectrum subjects, including subthreshold categories in the São Paulo ECA study. *J Affect Dis*, 87, 231–241.

Muñoz, M., Vázquez, C., Koegel, P., Sanz, J., and Burnam, M.A. (1998). Differential patterns of mental disorders among the homeless in Madrid (Spain) and Los Angeles (USA). *Soc Psychiatry Psychiatr Epidemiol*, 33, 514–520.

Murphy, J.M., Laird, N.M., Monson, R.R., Sobol, A.M., and Leighton, A.H. (2000). A 40-year perspective on the prevalence of depression: The Stirling County Study. *Arch Gen Psychiatry*, 57, 209–215.

Murray, C.J.L., and Lopez, A.D. (1996). *The Global Burden of Disease: Summary*. Geneva: World Health Organization.

Murray, C.J., and Lopez, A.D. (2000). Progress and directions in refining the global burden of disease approach: A response to Williams. *Health Econ*, 9(1), 69–82.

Murray, C.J.L., Lopez, A.D., and Jamison, D.T. (1994). The global burden of disease in 1990: Summary, results, sensitivity analyses, and future directions. *Bull World Health Organ*, 72, 495–508.

Nair, S.R.N., O'Reardon, J.P., Sethi, S.S., and Amsterdam, J.D. (2000). Bipolar disorder: For women a mixed picture. *Psychiatr Ann*, 30, 463–471.

Narrow, W.E., Regier, D.A., Rae, D.S., Manderscheid, M., and Locke, B.Z. (1993). Use of services by persons with mental and addictive disorders. Findings from the National Institute of Mental Health Epidemiologic Catchment Area Program. *Arch Gen Psychiatry*, 50, 95–107.

Narrow, W.E., Rae, D.S., Robins, L.N., and Regier, D.A. (2002). Revised prevalence estimates of mental disorders in the United States. *Arch Gen Psychiatry*, 59, 115–123.

Negash, A., Alem, A., Kebede, D., Deyessa, N., Shibre, T., and Kullgren, G. (2005). Prevalence and clinical characteristics of bipolar I disorder in Butajira, Ethiopia: A community-based study. *J Affect Dis*, 87, 193–201.

Nurnberger, J.I., Blehar, M.C., Kaufmann, C.A., York-Cooler, C., Simpson, S.G., Harkavy-Friedman, J., Severe, J.B., Malaspina, D., and Reich, T. (1994). Diagnostic Interview for Genetic Studies: Rationale, unique features and training. *Arch Gen Psychiatry*, 51, 849–859.

Oliver, J.M., and Simmons, M.E. (1985). Affective disorders and depression as measured by the Diagnostic Interview Schedule and the Beck Depression Inventory in an unselected adult population. *J Clin Psychol*, 41(4), 469–477.

Orn, H., Newman, S.C., and Bland, R.C. (1988). Design and field methods of the Edmonton survey of psychiatric disorders. *Acta Psychiatr Scand Suppl*, 338, 17–23.

Parker, J.B., Spielberger, C.D., Wallace, D.K., and Becker, J. (1959). Factors in manic-depressive reactions. *Dis Nerv Syst*, 20, 505–511.

Petterson, U. (1977). Manic-depressive illness: A clinical, social and genetic study. *Acta Psychiatr Scand*, 9(Suppl. 269), 1–93.

Phelan, J.C., and Link, B.G. (1999). Who are "the homeless"? Reconsidering the stability and composition of the homeless population. *Am J Public Health*, 89(9), 1334–1338.

Rao, M.S.S. (1966). Socio-economic groups and mental disorders. *Psychiatr Q*, 40, 677–691.

Rao, U., Ryan, N.D., Birmaher, B., Dahl, R.E., Williamson, D.E., Kaufman, J., Rao, R., and Nelson, B. (1995). Unipolar depression in adolescents: Clinical outcome in adulthood. *J Am Acad Child Adolesc Psychiatry*, 34, 566–578.

Regeer, E.J., Rosso, M.L., Have, M., Vollebergh, W., and Nolen, W.A. (2002). Prevalence of bipolar disorder: A further study in the Netherlands. *Bipolar Disorders*, 4(Suppl. 1), 37–38.

Regier, D.A., and Burke, J.D. (2000). Epidemiology. In B.J. Sadock, V.A. Sadock (Eds.), *Kaplan and Sadock's Comprehensive Textbook of Psychiatry*. 7th ed. New York: Lippincott Williams & Wilkins.

Regier, D.A., Meyers, J.M., Kramer, M., Robins, L.N., Blazer, D.G., Hough, R.L., Eaton, W.W., and Locke, B.Z. (1984). The NIMH Epidemiologic Catchment Area Program. *Arch Gen Psychiatry*, 41, 934–941.

Regier, D.A., Narrow, W.E., Rae, D.S., Manderscheid, R.W., Locke, B.Z., and Goodwin, F.K. (1993). The de facto U.S. mental and addictive disorders service system: Epidemiologic Catchment Area prospective 1-year prevalence rates of disorders and services. *Arch Gen Psychiatry*, 50, 85–94.

Regier, D.A., Kaelber, C.T., Rae, D.S., Farmer, M.E., Knauper, B., Kessler, R.C., Norquist, G.S. (1998). Limitations of diagnostic criteria and assessment instruments for mental disorders. *Arch Gen Psychiatry*, 55, 109–115.

Robbins, D.R., Alessi, N.E., Cook, S.C., Poznanski, E.O., and Yanchyshyn, G.W. (1982). The use of the Research Diagnostic Criteria (RDC) for depression in adolescent psychiatric inpatients. *J Am Acad Child Psychiatry*, 21(3), 251–255.

Robins, L.N., and Regier, D.A. (1991). *Psychiatric Disorders in America: The Epidemiologic Catchment Area Study*. New York: Free Press.

Robins, L.N., Helzer, J.E., Croughan, J., and Ratcliff, K. (1981). National Institute of Mental Health Diagnostic Interview Schedule: Its history, characteristics, and validity. *Arch Gen Psychiatry*, 38, 381–389.

Rothman, K.J., and Greenland, S. (1998). *Modern Epidemiology*. 2nd ed. Philadelphia: Lippincott-Raven.

Rowitz, L., and Levy, L. (1968). Ecological analysis of treated mental disorders in Chicago. *Arch Gen Psychiatry*, 19(5), 571–579.

Rybakowski, J.K., Suwalska, A., Lojko, D., Rymaszewska, J., and Kiejna, A. (2005). Bipolar mood disorders among Polish psychiatric outpatients treated for major depression. *J Affect Dis*, 84, 141–147.

Sanchez, L., Hagino, O., Weller, E., and Weller, R. (1999). Bipolarity in children. *Psychiatr Clin North Am*, 22, 629–648.

Scully, P.J., Owens, J.M., Kinsella, A., and Waddington, J.L. (2000). Small area variation in the rate of schizophrenia vs. bipolar disorder by place of birth vs. place at onset within an Irish rural catchment area population. *Schizophr Res*, 41, 64.

Scully, P.J., Owens, J.M., Kinsella, A., and Waddington, J.L. (2002a). Dimensions of psychopathology in bipolar disorder versus other affective and non-affective psychoses among an epidemiologically complete population. *Bipolar Disorders*, 4(Suppl. 1), 43–44.

Scully, P.J., Quinn, J.F., Morgan, M.G., Kinsella, A., O'Callaghan, E., Owen, J.M., and Waddington, J.L. (2002b). First-episode schizophrenia, bipolar disorder and other psychoses in a rural Irish catchment area: Incidence and gender in the Cavan-Monaghan study at 5 years. *Br J Psychiatry*, 181(Suppl. 43), S3–S9.

Sharma, V., Khan, M., and Smith, A. (2005). A closer look at treatment resistant depression: Is it due to a bipolar diathesis? *J Affect Disord*, 84, 251–257.

Shulman, K.I., and Hermann, N. (1999). The nature and management of mania in old age. *Psychiatr Clin North Am*, 22, 649–665.

Simpson, S.G., Folstein, S.E., Meyers, D.A., McMahon, F.J., Brusco, D.M., and DePaulo, J.R. Jr. (1993). Bipolar II: The most common bipolar phenotype? *Am J Psychiatry*, 150, 901–903.

Snowdon, J. (1991). A retrospective case-note study of bipolar disorder in old age. *Br J Psychiatry*, 158, 485–490.

Soldani, F., Sullivan, P.F., and Pedersen, N.L. (2005). Mania in the Swedish Twin Registry: Criterion validity and prevalence. *Aust N Z J Psychiatry*, 39, 235–243.

Spitzer, R.L., Endicott, J., and Robins, E. (1978). Research Diagnostic Criteria: Rationale and reliability. *Arch Gen Psychiatry*, 35, 773–782.

Stefansson, E., Lindal, E., Bjornsson, J.K., and Gudmundsdottir, A. (1991). Lifetime prevalence of specific mental disorders among people born in Iceland in 1931. *Acta Psychiatr Scand*, 84, 142–149.

Stoll, A.L., Severus, W.E., Freeman, M.P., Rueter, S., Zboyan, H.A., Diamond, E., Cress, K.K., and Marangell, L.B. (1999). Omega 3 fatty acids in bipolar disorder: A preliminary double-blind, placebo-controlled trial. *Arch Gen Psychiatry*, 56(5), 407–412.

Strober, M., Lampert, C., Schmidt, S., and Morrell, W. (1993). The course of major depressive disorder in adolescents: I. Recovery and risk of manic switching in a follow-up of psychotic and nonspsychotic subtypes. *J Am Acad Child Adolesc Psychiatry*, 32, 34–42.

Szadoczky, E., Papp, Z.S., Vitrai, J., Rihmer, Z., and Furedi, J. (1998). The prevalence of major depressive and bipolar disorders in Hungary: Results from a national epidemiologic survey. *J Affect Disord*, 50, 153–162.

Tanskanen, A., Hibbeln, J.R., Tuomilehto, J., Uutela, A., Viinamäki, H., Lehtonen, J., and Vartianen, E. (2001). Fish consumption and depressive symptoms in the general population in Finland. *Psychiatr Serv*, 52(4), 529–531.

Thayer, W.S. (1920). Osler, the teacher. In H.M. Thomas (Ed.), *Sir William Osler, Bart.* Baltimore: Johns Hopkins University Press.

Torrey, E.F., Miller, J., Rawlings, R., and Yolken, R.H. (1997). Seasonality of births in schizophrenia and bipolar disorder: A review of the literature. *Schizophr Res*, 28, 1–38.

Tsai, S.Y., Chen, C.C., and Yeh, E.K. (1997). Alcohol problems and long-term psychosocial outcome in Chinese patients with bipolar disorder. *J Affect Disord*, 46, 143–150.

Tsuang, M.T., Tohen, M., and Zahner, G.E.P. (1995). *Textbook in Psychiatric Epidemiology*. New York: Wiley-Liss.

Tsuchiya, K.J., Agerbo, E., Byrne, M., and Mortensen, P.B. (2004). Higher socio-economic status of parents may increase risk for bipolar disorder in the offspring. *Psychol Med*, 34, 787–793.

U.S. Department of Health and Human Services. (1992). *National Health Interview Survey, 1992*. Hyattsville, MD: Centers for Disease Control and Prevention.

U.S. Department of Health and Human Services. (1996). *National Health Interview Survey, 1996*. Data File (CD-ROM Series 10, No. 11A). Hyattsville, MD: Centers for Disease Control and Prevention.

U.S. Department of Health and Human Services. (1998). *Third National Health and Nutrition Examination Survey*, 1988–1994. NHANES III Second Laboratory Data File (CD-ROM Series II, No. 2A). Hyattsville, MD: Centers for Disease Control and Prevention.

U.S. Department of Health and Human Services. (1999). *National Household Survey on Drug Abuse, 1997*. [Computer file]. ICPSR version. Research Triangle Park, NC, and Ann Arbor, MI: Research Triangle Institute [producer] and Interuniversity Consortium for Political and Social Research [distributor].

Varanka, T.M., Weller, E.B., Weller, R.A., and Fristad, M.A. (1988). Lithium treatment of psychotic features in prepubertal children. *Am J Psychiatry*, 145, 1557–1559.

Vázquez, C., Muñoz, M., and Sanz, J. (1997). Lifetime and 12-month prevalence of DSM-III-R mental disorders among the homeless in Madrid: A European study using the CIDI. *Acta Psychiatr Scand*, 95, 523–530.

Verdoux, H., and Bourgeois, M. (1995). Social class in unipolar and bipolar probands and relatives. *J Affect Disord*, 33, 181–187.

Vicente, B., Kohn, R., Rioseco, P., Saldivia, S., Levav, I., and Torres, S. (2006). Lifetime and 12-month prevalence of DSM-III-R disorders in the Chile Psychiatric Prevalence Study. *Am J Psychiatry*, 163, 1362–1370.

Vos, T., and Mathers, C.D. (2000). The burden of mental disorders: A comparison of methods between the Australian Burden of Disease study and the Global Burden of Disease study. *Bul World Health Organ*, 78, 427–438.

Wakefield, J.C., and Spitzer, R.L. (2002). Lowered estimates—but of what? *Arch Gen Psychiatry*, 59, 129–130.

Weissman, M.M., and Klerman, G.L. (1978). Epidemiology of mental disorders: Emerging trends in the United States. *Arch Gen Psychiatry*, 35, 705–712.

Weissman, M.M., and Myers, J.K. (1978). Affective disorders in a U.S. urban community: The use of Research Diagnostic Criteria in an epidemiological survey. *Arch Gen Psychiatry*, 35, 1304–1311.

Weissman, M.M., Bland, R., Canino, G., Faravelli, C., Greenwald, S., Hwu, H.G., Joyce, P.R., Karam, E.G., Lee, C.K., Lellouch, J., Lepine, J.P., Newman, S., Rubio-Stipec, M., Wells, J.E., Wickramaratne, P., Wittchen, H.U., and Yeh, E.K. (1996). Cross national epidemiology of major depression and bipolar disorder. *JAMA*, 276, 293–299.

Weissman, M.M., Wolk, S., Goldstein, B., Moreau, D., Adams, P., Greenwald, S., Klier, C.M., Ryan, N.D., Dahl, R.E., and Wickramaratne, P. (1999a). Depressed adolescents grown up. *JAMA*, 281, 1707–1713.

Weissman, M.M., Wolk, S., Wickramaratne, P., Goldstein, B., Adams, P., Greenwald, S., Ryan, N., Dahl, R.E., and Steinberg, D. (1999b). Children with prepubertal-onset major depressive disorder and anxiety grown up. *Arch Gen Psychiatry*, 56, 794–801.

Wells, J.E., Bushnell, J.A., Hornblow, A.R., Joyce, P.R., and Oakley-Brown, M.A. (1989). Christchurch Psychiatric Epidemiology Study, part I: Methodology and lifetime prevalence for specific psychiatric disorders. *Aust N Z J Psychiatry*, 23, 315–326.

Winokur, G., Coryell, W., Akiskal, H.S., Endicott, J., Keller M., and Mueller T. (1994). Manic-depressive (bipolar) disorder: The course in light of a prospective ten-year follow-up of 131 patients. *Acta Psychiatr Scand*, 89, 102–110.

Wittchen, H.U., Essau, C.A., von Zeressen, D., Krieg, J.D., and Zaudig, M. (1992). Lifetime and six-month prevalence of mental disorders in the Munich Follow-Up Study. *Eur Arch Psychiatry Clin Neurosci*, 241, 247–258.

Wittchen, H.U., Lachner, G., Wunderlich, U., and Pfister, H. (1998a). Test-retest reliability of the computerized DSM-IV version of the Munich-Composite International Diagnostic Interview (M-CIDI). *Soc Psychiatry Psychiatr Epidemiol*, 33, 568–578.

Wittchen, H.U., Nelson, C.B., and Lachner, G. (1998b). Prevalence of mental disorders and psychosocial impairments in adolescents and young adults. *Psychol Med*, 28, 109–126.

Wittkower, E.D., and Rin, H. (1965). Transcultural psychiatry. *Arch Gen Psychiatry*, 13, 387–398.

World Bank, and Reich, M.R. (1993a). *World Development Report 1993: Investing in Health*. New York: Oxford University Press.

World Bank, Jamison, D.T., Mosley, W.H., Measham, A.R., Bobadilla, J.L. (Eds.). (1993b). *Disease Control Priorities in Developing Countries*. New York: Oxford University Press.

World Health Organization. (1990). *Composite International Diagnostic Interview (CIDI)*. Version 1.0. Geneva: World Health Organization.

World Health Organization. (1991). Mental health and behavioural disorders (including disorders of psychological development). In *International Classification of Diseases*. 10th revision. Geneva: World Health Organization.

World Health Organization. (1994). *Schedule for Clinical Assessment in Neuropsychiatry* (Version 2). Geneva: World Health Organization.

World Health Organization International Consortium of Psychiatric Epidemiology. (2000). Cross-national comparisons of mental disorders. *Bull World Health Organ*, 78, 414–426.

Wozniak, J., Biederman, J., Kiely, S., Ablon, J.S., Faraone, S.V., Mundy, W., and Mennin, D. (1995). Mania-like symptoms suggestive of childhood-onset bipolar disorder in clinically referred children. *J Am Acad Child Adolesc Psychiatry*, 34, 867–876.

Yassa, R., Nair, V., Nastase, C., Camille, Y., and Belzile, L. (1988). Prevalence of bipolar disorder in a psychogeriatric population. *J Affect Disord*, 14, 197–201.

CHAPTER 6

Achenbach, T.M. (1991). *Manual for the Child Behavior Checklist/4–18 and 1991 Profile*. Burlington, VT: University of Vermont Department of Psychiatry.

Akiskal, H.S., Downs, J., Jordan, P., Watson, S., Daugherty, D., and Pruitt, D.B. (1985). Affective disorders in referred children and younger siblings of manic-depressives. *Arch Gen Psychiatry*, 42, 996–1003.

Anderson, C.A., and Hammen, C.L. (1993). Psychosocial outcomes of children of unipolar depressed, bipolar, medically ill, and normal women: A longitudinal study. *J Consult Clin Psychol*, 61, 448–454.

Anthony, E.J., and Scott, P. (1960). Manic-depressive psychosis in childhood. *J Child Psychol Psychiatry*, 1, 53–72.

Angst, J., Gamma, A., Sellaro, A., Zhang, H., and Merikangas, K. (2003). Toward validation of atypical depression in the community: Results of the Zurich cohort study. *J Affect Disord*, 73, 133–146.

Axelson, D., Birmaher, B., Strober, M., Gill, M.K., Valeri, S., Chiappetta, L., Ryan, N., Leonard, H., Hunt, J., Iyengar, S., Bridge, J., and Keller, M. (2006). Phenomenology of children and adolescents with bipolar spectrum disorders. *Arch Gen Psychiatry*, 63, 1139–1148.

Benes, F. (1999). Neurodevelopmental approach to the study of mental illness. *Dev Neuropsychol*, 16, 359–360.

Biederman, J. (1998). Resolved: Mania is mistaken for ADHD in prepubertal children. *J Am Acad Child Adolesc Psychiatry*, 37, 1091–1093.

Biederman, J., Faraone, S., Mick, E., Wozniak, J., Chen, L., Ouellette, C., Marrs, A., Moore, P., Garcia, J., Mennin, D., and Lelon, E. (1996). Attention-deficit hyperactivity disorder and juvenile mania: An overlooked comorbidity? *J Am Acad Child Adolesc Psychiatry*, 35, 997–1008.

Biederman, J., Russell, R., Soriano, J., Wozniak, J., and Faraone, S.V. (1998). Clinical features of children with both ADHD and mania: Does ascertainment source make a difference? *J Affect Disord*, 51, 101–112.

Biederman, J., Faraone, S.V., Wozniak, J., and Monuteaux, M.C. (2000a). Parsing the association between bipolar, conduct, and substance use disorders: A familial risk analysis. *Biol Psychiatry*, 48, 1037–1044.

Biederman, J., Mick, E., Faraone, S., Spencer, T., Wilens, T., and Wozniak, J. (2000b). Pediatric mania: A developmental subtype of bipolar disorder? *Biol Psychiatry*, 48, 458–466.

Biederman, J., Spencer, T.J., Wozniak, J., Faraone, S.V., and Mick, E. (2001). Attention-deficit/hyperactivity disorder and pediatric-onset bipolar disorder. *TEN: Economics of Neuroscience*, 3, 45–48.

Biederman, J., Faraone, S.V., Woniak, J., Mick, E., Kwon, A., and Aleardi, M. (2004a). Further evidence of unique developmental phenotypic correlates of pediatric bipolar disorder: Findings from a large sample of clinically referred preadolescent children assessed over the last 7 years. *J Affect Disord*, 82(Suppl. 1), S45–S58.

Biederman, J., Kwon, A., Wozniak, J., Mick, E., Markowitz, S., Fazio, V., and Faraone, S.V. (2004b). Absence of gender differences in pediatric bipolar disorder: Findings from a large sample of referred youth. *J Affect Disord*, 83, 207–214.

Biederman, J., Mick, E., Faraone, S.V., and Wozniak, J. (2004c). Pediatric bipolar disorder or disruptive behavior disorder? *Primary Psychiatry*, 11, 36–41.

Biederman, J., Mick, E., Faraone, S.V., Van Patten, S., Burback, M., and Wozniak, J. (2004d). A prospective follow-up study of pediatric bipolar disorder in boys with attention-deficit/hyperactivity disorder. *J Affect Disord*, 82(Suppl. 1), S17–S23.

Birmaher, B., Kennah, A., Brent, D., Ehmann, M., Bridge, J., and Axelson, D. (2002). Is bipolar disorder specifically associated with panic disorder in youths? *J Clin Psychiatry*, 63, 414–419.

Birmaher, B., Axelson, D., Monk, K., Kalas, C., Ehmann, M., Pan, R., Bridge, J., Iyengar, S., Kupfer, D., and Brent, D. (2003). Psychiatric disorders in children of bipolar parents. Child and Adolescent Program of the 43rd Annual National Institutes of Health Boca Raton, FL, Mayo

Birmaher, B., Axelson, D., Strober, M., Gill, M.K., Valeri, S., Chiappetta, L., Ryan, N., Leonard, H., Hunt, J., Iyengar, S., and Keller, M. (2006). Clinical course of children and adolescents with bipolar spectrum disorders. *Arch Gen Psychiatry*, 63, 175–183.

Blumberg, H.P., Kaufman, J., Martin, A., Whiteman, R., Zhang, J.H., Gore, J.C., Charney, D.S., Krystal, J.H., and Peterson, B.S. (2003a). Amygdala and hippocampal volumes in adolescents and adults with bipolar disorder. *Arch Gen Psychiatry*, 60, 1201–1208.

Blumberg, H.P., Martin, A., Kaufman, J., Leung, H-C., Skudlarski, P., Lacadie, C., Fulbright, R.K., Gore, J.C., Charney, D.S., Krystal, J.H., and Peterson, B.S. (2003b). Frontostriatal abnormalities in adolescents with bipolar disorder: Preliminary observations from functional MRI. *Am J Psychiatry*, 160, 1345–1347.

Botteron, K., Vannier, M., Geller, B., Todd, R., and Lee, B. (1995). Preliminary study of magnetic resonance imaging characteristics in 8- to 16-year-olds with mania. *J Am Acad Child Adolesc Psychiatry*, 34, 742–749.

Breslau, N. (1987). Inquiring about the bizarre: False positives in Diagnostic Interview Schedule for Children (DISC) ascertainment of obsessions, compulsions, and psychotic symptoms. *J Am Acad Child Adolesc Psychiatry*, 26, 639–644.

Carlson, G.A. (1998). Mania and ADHD: Comorbidity or confusion. *J Affect Disord*, 51, 177–187.

Carlson, G.A. (1999). Juvenile mania vs. ADHD [Letter to the editor]. *J Am Acad Child Adolesc Psychiatry*, 38, 353.

Carlson, G.A. (2005). Early onset bipolar disorder: Clinical and research considerations. *J Clinical Child Adolescent Psychology*, 34, 333–343.

Carlson, G.A., and Goodwin, F.K. (1973). The stages of mania: A longitudinal analysis of the manic episode. *Arch Gen Psychiatry*, 28, 221–228.

Carlson, G.A., and Kelley, K.L. (1998). Manic symptoms in psychiatrically hospitalized children: What do they mean? *J Affect Disord*, 51, 123–135.

Carlson, G.A., and Mick, E. (2003). Drug-induced disinhibition in psychiatrically hospitalized children. *J Child Adolesc Psychopharmacol*, 13, 153–163.

Carlson, G., and Strober, M. (1979). Affective disorders in adolescence. *Psychiatr Clin North Am*, 2, 511–526.

Carlson, G.A., and Weintraub, S. (1993). Childhood behavior problems and bipolar disorder: Relationship or coincidence? *J Affect Disord*, 28, 143–153.

Carlson, G.A., and Youngstrom, E.A. (2003). Clinical implications of pervasive manic symptoms in children. *Bio Psychiatry*, 53, 1050–1058.

Carlson, G.A., Loney, J., Salisbury, H., and Volpe, R.J. (1998). Young referred boys with DICA-P manic symptoms vs. two comparison groups. *J Affect Disord*, 121, 113–121.

Carlson, G.A., Bromet, E.J., and Sievers, S. (2000). Phenomenology and outcome of subjects with early- and adult-onset psychotic mania. *Am J Psychiatry*, 157, 213–219.

Carlson, G.A., Bromet, E.J., Driessens, C., Mojtabai, R., and Schwartz, J.E. (2002). Age at onset, childhood psychopathology, and 2-year outcome in psychotic bipolar disorder. *Am J Psychiatry*, 159, 307–309.

Cecil, K.M., DelBello, M.P., Sellars, M.C., and Strakowski, S.M. (2003). Proton magnetic resonance spectroscopy of the frontal lobe and cerebellar vermis in children with a mood disorder and a familial risk for bipolar disorders. *J Child Adolesc Psychopharmacol*, 13, 545–555.

Chambers, C.A., Smith, A.H., and Naylor, G.J. (1982). The effect of digoxin on the response to lithium therapy in mania. *Psychol Med*, 12, 57–60.

Chang, K.D., Steiner, H., and Ketter, T. (2000). Psychiatric phenomenology of child and adolescent bipolar offspring. *J Am Acad Child Adolesc Psychiatry*, 39, 453–460.

Chang, K.D., Blasey, C.M., Ketter, T.A., and Steiner, H. (2003). Temperament characteristics of child and adolescent. *J Affect Disord*, 77, 11–19.

Chengappa, K.N.R., Kupfer, D.J., Frank, E., Houck, P.R., Grochocinski, V.J., Cluss, P.A., and Stapf, D.A. (2003). Relationship of birth cohort and early age of onset of illness in a bipolar disorder case registry. *Am J Psychiatry*, 160, 1636–1642.

Conners, C.K., Himmelhoch, J., Goyette, C.H., Ulrich, R., and Neil, J.F. (1979). Children of parents with affective illness. *J Am Acad Child Psychiatry*, 18, 503–504.

Correll, C.U., Penzer, J., Kafantaris, V., Nakayama, E., Auther, A., Lencz, T., and Cornblatt, B. (2005). Searching for prodromal symptoms in early-onset bipolar disorder. Poster presented at the American Psychiatric Association. Annual Meeting, Atlanta, GA, May.

Coyle, J., Pine, D., Charney, D., Lewis, L., Nemeroff, C., Carlson, G., and The Depression and Bipolar Support Alliance Consensus Development Panel. (2003). Depression and Bipolar Support Alliance consensus statement on the unmet needs in diagnosis and treatment of mood disorders in children and adolescents. *J Am Acad Child Adolesc Psychiatry*, 42, 1494–1503.

Craney, J.L., and Geller, B. (2003). A prepubertal and early adolescent bipolar disorder-I phenotype: Review of phenomenology and longitudinal course. *Bipolar Disord*, 5, 243–256. *J Affect Disord*, 77, 11–19.

Cytryn, L., McKnew, D.H., Bartko, J.J., Lamour, M., and Hamovit, J. (1982). Offspring of patients with affective disorders: Part 2. *J Am Acad Child Psychiatry*, 21, 389–391.

Davanzo, P., Yue, K., Thomas, M.A., Belin, T., Mintz, J., Venkatraman, T.N., Santoro, E., Barnett, S., and McCracken, J. (2003). Proton magnetic resonance spectroscopy of bipolar disorder versus intermittent explosive disorder in children and adolescents. *Am J Psychiatry*, 160, 1442–1452.

Decina, P., Kestenbaum, C.J., Farber, S., Kron, L., Gargan, M., Sackeim, H.A., and Fieve, R.R. (1983). Clinical and psychological assessment of children of bipolar probands. *Am J Psychiatry*, 140, 548–553.

DelBello, M.P., Soutullo, C.A., Hendricks, W., Niemeier, R.T., McElroy, S.L., and Strakowski, S.M. (2001). Prior stimulant treatment in adolescents with bipolar disorder: Association with age at onset. *Bipolar Disord*, 3, 53–57.

DelBello, M.P., Carlson, G., Tohen, M., Bromet, E., Schwiers, M., and Strakowski, S. (2003). Rates and predictors of developing a manic or hypomanic episode 1 to 2 years following a first hospitalization for major depression with psychotic features. *J Child Adolesc Psychopharmacol*, 13, 173–185.

DelBello, M.P., Zimmerman, M.E., Mills, N.P., Getz, G.E., and Strakowski, S.M. (2004). Magnetic resonance imaging analysis of amygdala and other subcortical brain regions in adolescents with bipolar disorder. *Bipolar Disord*, 6, 43–52.

Dickstein, D.P., Treland, J.E., Snow, J., McClure, E.B., Mehta, M.S., Towbin, K.E., Pine, D.S., and Leibenluft, E. (2004). Neuropsychological performance in pediatric bipolar disorder. *Biol Psychiatry*, 55, 32–39.

Doyle, A., Wilens, T., Kwon, A., Seidman, L., Faraone, S.V., Fried, R., Swezey, A., Snyder L., and Biederman, J. (2005). Neuropsychological functioning in youth with bipolar disorder. *Biol Psychiatry*, 58, 540–548.

Duffy, A., Alda, M., Kutcher, S., Fusee, C., and Grof, P. (1998). Psychiatric symptoms and syndromes among adolescent children of parents with lithium-responsive or lithium-nonresponsive bipolar disorder. *Am J Psychiatry*, 155, 431–433.

Duffy, A., Alda, M., Kutcher, S., Cavazzoni, P., Robertson, C., Grof, E., and Grof, P. (2002). A prospective study of the offspring of bipolar parents responsive and nonresponsive to lithium treatment. *J Clin Psychiatry*, 63(12), 1171–1178.

Dupont, R.M., Jernigan, T.L., Butters, N., Delis, D.C., Hesselink, J.R., Heindel, W., and Gillin, J.C. (1990). Subcortical abnormalities detected in bipolar affective disorder using magnetic resonance imaging: Clinical and neuropsychological significance. *Arch Gen Psychiatry*, 47, 55–59.

Eaton, W.E., Mortensen, P.B., Thomsen, P.H., and Frydenberg, M. (2001). Obstetric complications and risk for severe psychopathology in childhood. *J Autism Dev Disord*, 31, 279–285.

Egeland, J.A., Shaw, J.A., Endicott, J., Pauls, D.L., Allen, C.R., Hostetter, A.M., and Sussex, J.N. (2003). Prospective study of prodromal features for bipolarity in well Amish children. *J Am Acad Child Adolesc Psychiatry*, 42, 786–796.

Faedda, G.L., Baldessarini, R., Suppes, T., Tondo, L., Becker, I., and Lipschitz, D. (1995). Pediatric-onset bipolar disorder: A neglected clinical and public health problem. *Harvard Rev Psychiatry*, 3, 171–195.

Faedda, G.L., Baldessarini, R.J., Glovinsky, I.P., and Austin, N.B. (2004). Pediatric bipolar disorder: Phenomenology and course of illness. *Bipolar Disorders*, 6, 305–313.

Faraone, S.V., Biederman, J., Mennin, D., Wozniak, J., and Spencer, T. (1997a). Attention-deficit hyperactivity disorder with bipolar disorder: A familial subtype? *J Am Acad Child Adolesc Psychiatry*, 36, 1378–1387.

Faraone, S.V., Biederman, J., Wozniak, J., Mundy, E., Mennin, D., and O'Donnell, D. (1997b). Is comorbidity with ADHD a marker for juvenile-onset mania? *J Am Acad Child Adolesc Psychiatry*, 36, 1046–1055.

Fergus, E.L., Miller, R.B., Luckenbaugh, D.A., Leverich, G.S., Findling, R.L., Speer, A.M., and Post, R.M. (2003). Is there progression from irritability/dyscontrol to major depressive and manic symptoms? A retrospective community survey of parents of bipolar children. *J Affect Disord*, 77, 71–78.

Findling, R.L., Gracious, B.L., McNamara, N.K., Youngstrom, E.A., Demeter, C.A., Branicky, L.A., and Calabrese, J.R. (2001). Rapid, continuous cycling and psychiatric co-morbidity in pediatric bipolar-I disorder. *Bipolar Disord*, 3, 202–210.

Findling, R.L., Youngstrom, E.A., Danielson, C.K., DelPorto-Bedoya, D., Papish-David, R., Townsend, L., and Calabrese, J.R. (2002). Clinical decision-making using the General Behavior Inventory in juvenile bipolarity. *Bipolar Disord*, 4, 34–42.

Frazier, J.A., Biederman, J., Tohen, M., Feldman, P.D., Jacobs, T.G., Toma, V., Rater, M.A., Tarazi, R.A., Kim, G.S., Garfield, S.B., Sohma, M., Gonzalez-Heydrich, J., Risser, R.C., and Nowlin, Z.M. (2001). A prospective open-label treatment trial of olanzapine monotherapy in children and adolescents with bipolar disorder. *J Child Psychopharmacol*, 11(3), 239–250.

Friedman, R.C., Hurt, S.W., Clarken, J.F., and Corn, R. (1983). Primary and secondary affective disorders in adolescents and young adults. *Acta Psychiatr Scand*, 67(4), 226–235.

Friedman, L., Findling, R.L., Kenny, J.T., Swales, T.P., Stuve, T.A., Jesberger, J.A., Lewin, J.S., and Schulz, S.C. (1999). An MRI study of adolescent patients with either schizophrenia or bipolar disorder as compared to healthy control subjects. *Biol Psychiatry*, 46, 77–88.

Geller, B., and Luby, J. (1997). Child and adolescent bipolar disorder: Review of the past 10 years. *J Am Acad Child Adolesc Psychiatry*, 36, 1168–1176.

Geller, B., Fox, L.W., and Clark, K.A. (1994). Rate and predictors of prepubertal bipolarity during follow-up of 6- to 12-year-old depressed children. *J Am Acad Child Adolesc Psychiatry*, 33, 461–468.

Geller, B., Warner, K., Williams, M., and Zimerman, B. (1998a). Prepubertal and young adolescent bipolarity versus ADHD: Assessment and validity using the WASH-U-KSADs, CBCL and TRF. *J Affect Disord*, 51, 93–100.

Geller, B., Williams, M., Zimerman, B., Frazier, J., Beringer, L., and Warner, K. (1998b). Prepubertal and early adolescent bipolarity differentiate from ADHD by manic symptoms, grandiose delusions, ultra-rapid or ultradian cycling. *J Affect Disord*, 51, 81–91.

Geller, B., Bolhofner, K., Craney, J.L., Williams, M., DelBello, M.P., and Gundersen, K. (2000a). Psychosocial functioning in a prepubertal and early adolescent bipolar disorder phenotype. *J Am Acad Child Adolesc Psychiatry*, 39, 1543–1548.

Geller, B., Zimerman, B., Williams, M., Bolhofner, K., Craney, J.L., DelBello, M.P., and Soutullo, C. (2000b). Diagnostic characteristics of 93 cases of a prepubertal and early adolescent bipolar disorder phenotype by gender, puberty and co-morbid attention deficit hyperactivity disorder. *J Child Adolesc Psychopharmacol*, 10, 157–164.

Geller, B., Craney, J.L., Bolhofner, K., DelBello, M.P., Williams, M., and Zimerman, B. (2001a). One-year recovery and relapse rates of children with a prepubertal and early adolescent bipolar disorder phenotype. *Am J Psychiatry*, 158, 303–305.

Geller, B., Zimerman, B., Williams, M., Bolhofner, K., and Craney, J. (2001b). Bipolar disorder at prospective follow-up of adults who had prepubertal major depressive disorder. *Am J Psychiatry*, 158, 125–127.

Geller, B., Zimerman, B., Williams, M., Bolhofner, K., Craney, J.L., DelBello, M.P., and Soutullo, C. (2001c). Reliability of the Washington University in St. Louis Kiddie Schedule for Affective Disorders and Schizophrenia (WASH-U-KSADS) mania and rapid cycling sections. *J Am Acad Child Adolesc Psychiatry*, 40, 450–455.

Geller, B., Craney, J.L., Bolhofner, K., Nickelsburg, M.J., Williams, M., and Zimerman, B. (2002a). Two-year prospective follow-up of children with a prepubertal and early adolescent bipolar disorder phenotype. *Am J Psychiatry*, 159, 927–933.

Geller, B., Zimerman, B., Williams, M., DelBello, M., Bolhofner, K., Craney, J.L., Frazier, J., Beringer, L., and Nickelsburg, M.J. (2002b). DSM-IV mania symptoms in a prepubertal and early adolescent bipolar disorder phenotype compared to attention-deficit hyperactive and normal controls. *J Child Adolesc Psychopharmacol*, 12, 11–25.

Geller, B., Zimerman, B., Williams, M., DelBello, M.P., Frazier, J., and Beringer, L. (2002c). Phenomenology of prepubertal and early adolescent bipolar disorder: Examples of elated mood, grandiose behaviors, decreased need for sleep, racing thoughts and hypersexuality. *J Child Adolesc Psychopharmacol*, 12, 3–9.

Geller, B., Tillman, R., Craney, J.L., and Bolhofner, K. (2004). Four-year prospective and natural history of mania in children with a prepubertal and early adolescent bipolar disorder phenotype. *Arch Gen Psychiatry*, 61, 459–467.

Geller, B., Tillman, R., Bolhofner, K., Zimerman, B., Strauss, N.A., and Kaufmann, P. (2006). Controlled, blindly rated, direct-interview family study of a prepubertal and early-adolescent bipolar I disorder phenotype. *Arch Gen Psychiatry*, 63, 1139–1138.

Gershon, E.S., McKnew, D., Cytryn, L., Hamovit, J., Schreiber, J., Hibbs, E., and Pellegrini, D. (1985). Diagnoses in school-age children of bipolar affective disorder patients and normal controls. *J Affect Disord*, 8, 283–291.

Goldberg, J.F., Harrow, M., and Whiteside, J.E. (2001). Risk for bipolar illness in patients initially hospitalized for unipolar depression. *Am J Psychiatry*, 158, 1265–1270.

Goldstein, T.R., Miklowitz, D.J., and Mullen, K.L. (2006). Social skills knowledge and performance among adolescents with bipolar disorder. *Bipolar Disord*, 8, 350–361.

Greenhill, L.L., Shopsin, B., and Temple, H. (1980). Children of affectively ill parents: Psychiatric status determined by structured interview. *Psychopharmacol Bull*, 16, 23–24.

Grigoroiu-Serbanescu, M., Christodorescu, D., Jipescu, I., Totoescu, A., Marinescu, E., and Ardelean, V. (1989). Psychopathology in children aged 10–17 of bipolar parents: Psychopathology rate and correlates of the severity of the psychopathology. *J Affect Disord*, 16, 167–179.

Grigoroiu-Serbanescu, M., Christodorescu, D., Totoescu, A., and Jipescu, I. (1991). Depressive disorders and depressive personality traits in offspring aged 10–17 of bipolar and of normal parents. *J Youth Adolescence*, 20, 135–148.

Hammen, C. (1991). *Depression Runs in Families: The Social Context of Risk and Resilience in Children of Depressed Mothers.* New York: Springer-Verlag.

Hammen, C., Gordon, D., Burge, D., Adrian, C., Jaenicke, C., and Hiroto, D. (1987). Maternal affective disorders, illness, and stress: Risk for children's psychopathology. *Am J Psychiatry*, 144(6), 736–741.

Hammen, C., Burge, D., Burney, E., and Adrian, C. (1990). Longitudinal study of diagnoses in children of women with unipolar and bipolar affective disorder. *Arch Gen Psychiatry*, 47, 1112–1117.

Hammersley, P., Dias, A., Todd, G., Bowen-Jones, K., Reilly, B., and Bentall, R.P. (2003). Childhood trauma and hallucinations in bipolar affective disorder: Preliminary investigation. *Br J Psychiatry*, 182, 543–547.

Harpold, T.L., Wozniak, J., Kwon, A., Gilbert, J., Wood, J., Smith, L., and Biederman, J. (2005). Examining the association between pediatric bipolar disorder and anxiety disorders in psychiatrically referred children and adolescents. *J Affect Disord*, 88, 19–26.

Harrington, R., and Myatt, T. (2003). Is preadolescent mania the same condition as adolescent mania? A British perspective. *Biol Psychiatry*, 53, 961–969.

Hazell, P.L., Carr, V., Lewin, T.J., and Sly, K. (2003). Manic symptoms in young males with ADHD predict functioning but not diagnosis after 6 years. *J Am Acad Child Adolesc Psychiatry*, 42, 552–560.

Hellender, M. (2003). Pediatric bipolar disorder: The parent advocacy perspective. *Biol Psychiatry*, 53(11), 935–937.

Hellander, M.E., and Burke, T. (1999). Children with bipolar disorder [Letter to the editor]. *J Am Acad Child Adolesc Psychiatry*, 38, 495–496.

Hillegers, M.H.J., Reichart, G.G., Wals, M., Verhulst, F.C., Ormel, J., and Nolen, W.A. (2005). Five year prospective outcome of psychopathology in the adolescent offspring of bipolar patients. *Bipolar Disord*, 7, 344–350.

Hirshfeld-Becker, D.R., Biederman, J., Henin, A., Faraone, S.V., Cayton, G.A., and Rosenbaum, J.F. (2006). Laboratory-observed behavioral disinhibition in the young offspring of parents with bipolar disorder: A high-risk pilot study. *Am J Psychiatry*, 163, 265–271.

Hodgins, S., Faucher, B., Zarac, A., and Ellenbogen, M. (2002). Children of parents with bipolar disorder: A population at high risk for major affective disorders. *Child Adolesc Psychiatr Clin North Am*, 11, 533–553.

Hyun, M., Friedman, S.D., and Dunner, D.L. (2000). Relationship of childhood physical and sexual abuse to adult bipolar disorder. *Bipolar Disord*, 2, 131–135.

Jaideep, T., Reddy, Y.C.J., and Srinath, S. (2006). Comorbidity of attention deficit hyperactivity disorder in juvenile bipolar disorder. *Bipolar Disord*, 8, 182–187.

Jamison, K.R. (1995). *An Unquiet Mind: A Memoir of Moods and Madness.* New York: Alfred A. Knopf.

Jones, S.H., Tai, S., Evershed, K., Knowles, R., and Bentall, R. (2006). Early detection of bipolar disorder: A pilot familial high-risk study of parents with bipolar disorder and their adolescent children. *Bipolar Disord*, 8, 362–372.

Judd, L.J., and Akiskal, H.S. (2003). The prevalence and disability of bipolar spectrum disorders in the U.S. population: Re-analysis of the ECA database taking into account subthreshold cases. *J Affect Disord*, 73, 123–131.

Kafantaris, V., Coletti, D.J., Dicker, R., Padula, G., and Pollack S. (1998). Are childhood psychiatric histories of bipolar adolescents associated with family history, psychosis, and response to lithium treatment? *J Affect Disord*, 51, 153–164.

Kent, L., and Craddock, N. (2003). Is there a relationship between attention deficit hyperactivity disorder and bipolar disorder? *J Affect Disord*, 73, 211–221.

Kessler, R.C., Berglund, P., Demler, O., Jin, R., Merikangas, K.R., and Walters, E.E. (2005). Lifetime prevalence and age-of-onset distributions of DSM-IV disorders in the National Comorbidity Survey Replication. *Arch Gen Psychiatry*, 62, 593–602.

Kestenbaum, C.J. (1997). Children at risk for manic-depressive illness: Possible predictors. *Am J Psychiatry*, 136, 1206–1208.

Kim, E.Y., and Miklowitz, D.J. (2002). Childhood mania, attention deficit hyperactivity disorder and conduct disorder: A critical review of diagnostic dilemmas. *Bipolar Disord*, 4, 215–225.

Kirov, G., and Murray, R.M. (1999). Ethnic differences in the presentation of bipolar disorder. *Eur Psychiatry*, 14, 199–204.

Klein, D.N., Depue, R.A., and Slater, J.F. (1985). Cyclothymia in the adolescent offspring of parents with bipolar affective disorder. *J Abnorm Psychol*, 94, 115–127.

Klein, D.N., Lewinsohn, P.M., and Seeley, J.R. (1996). Hypomanic personality traits in a community sample of adolescents. *J Affect Disord*, 38, 135–143.

Klimes-Dougan, B., Ronsaville, D., Wiggs, E.A., and Martinez, P.E., (2006). Neuropsychological functioning in adolescent children of mothers with a history of bipolar or major depressive disorders. *Biol Psychiatry*, 60, 957–965.

Kovacs, M. (1996). Presentation and course of major depressive disorder during childhood and later years of the life span. *J Am Acad Child Adolesc Psychiatry*, 35, 705–715.

Kowatch, R.A., Suppes, T., Carmody, T.J., Bucci, J.P., Hume, J.H., Kromelis, M., Emslie, G.J., Weinberg, W.A., and Rush, A.J. (2000). Effect size of lithium, divalproex sodium, and carbamazepine in children and adolescents with bipolar disorder. *J Am Acad Child Adolesc Psychiatry*, 39(6), 713–720.

Kowatch, R.A., Fristad, M., Birmaher, B., Wagner, K.D., Findling, R.L., Hellander, M., and the Child Psychiatric Workgroup on Bipolar Disorder. (2005). Treatment guidelines for children and adolescents with bipolar disorder. *J Am Acad Child Adolesc Psychiatry*, 44, 213–235.

Kraepelin, E. (1921). *Manic-Depressive Insanity and Paranoia.* Translated by R.M. Barclay. Edinburgh: E. & S. Livingstone. Originally published as *Psychiatrie. Ein Lehrbuch fur Studierende und Ärzte.* ed. 2. *Klinische Psychiatrie.* II. Leipzig: Johann Ambrosius Barth, 1899.

Kron, L., Decina, P., Kestenbaum, C.J., Farber, S., Gargan, M., and Fieve, R. (1982). The offspring of bipolar manic-depressives: Clinical features. *Adolesc Psychiatry*, 10, 273–291.

Kutcher, S.P. (2000). Adolescent-onset bipolar illness. In A. Marneros and J. Angst (Eds.), *Bipolar Disorders: 100 Years after Manic-Depressive Insanity* (pp. 139–152). London: Kluwer Academic Publishers.

Kutcher, S.P., Marton, P., and Korenblum, M. (1990). Adolescent bipolar illness and personality disorder. *J Am Acad Child Adolesc Psychiatry*, 29, 355–358.

Kutcher, S.P., Robertson, H.A., and Bird, D. (1998). Premorbid functioning in adolescent onset bipolar I disorder: A preliminary report from an ongoing study. *J Affect Disord*, 51, 137–144.

Kuyler, P.L., Rosenthal, L., Igel, G., Dunner, D.L., and Fieve, R.R. (1980). Psychopathology among children of manic-depressive patients. *Biol Psychiatry*, 15, 589–597.

Lapalme, M., Hodgins, S., and LaRoche, C. (1997). Children of parents with bipolar disorder: A meta-analysis of risk for mental disorders. *Can J Psychiatry*, 42, 623–631.

Laroche, C., Sheiner, R., Lester, E., Benierakis, C., Marrache, M., Engelsmann, F., and Cheifetz, P. (1987). Children of parents with manic-depressive illness: A follow-up study. *Can J Psychiatry*, 32, 563–569.

Leibenluft, E., Charney, D.S., and Pine, D.S. (2003a). Researching the pathophysiology of pediatric bipolar disorder. *Biol Psychiatry*, 53, 1009–1020.

Leibenluft, E., Charney, D.S., Towbin, K.E., Bhangoo, R.K., and Pine, D.S. (2003b). Defining clinical phenotypes of juvenile mania. *Am J Psychiatry*, 160, 430–437.

Lenzenweger, M.F., and Dworkin, R.H. (Eds.). (1998). *Origins and Development of Schizophrenia*. Washington, DC: American Psychological Association Press.

Leverich, G.S., McElroy, S.L., Suppes, T., Keck, P.E., Denicoff, K.D., Nolen, W.A., Altshuler, L.A., Rush, A.J., Kupka, R., Frye, M.A., Autio, K.A., and Post, R.M. (2002). Early physical and sexual abuse associated with an adverse course of bipolar illness. *Biol Psychiatry*, 51, 288–297.

Lewinsohn, P.M., Klein, D.N., and Seeley, J.R. (1995). Bipolar disorders in a community sample of older adolescents: Prevalence, phenomenology, comorbidity, and course. *J Am Acad Child Adolesc Psychiatry*, 34, 454–463.

Lewinsohn, P.M., Klein, D.N., and Seeley, J.R. (2000). Bipolar disorder during adolescence and young adulthood in a community sample. *Bipolar Disord*, 2, 281–293.

Lewinsohn P.M., Seeley, J.R., and Klein, D.N. (2003). Bipolar disorders during adolescence. *Acta Psychiatr Scand*, 108(Suppl. 418), 47–50.

Lish, J.D., Dime-Meenan, S., Whybrow, P.C., Price, R.A., and Hirschfeld, R.M.A. (1994). The National Depressive and Manic-Depressive Association (DMDA) survey of bipolar members. *J Affect Disord*, 31, 281–294.

Luby, J., and Mrakotsky, C. (2003). Depressed preschoolers with bipolar family history: A group at high risk for later switching to mania? *J Child Adolesc Psychopharmacol*, 13, 187–197.

Masi, G., Toni, C., Perugi, G., Mucci, M., Millepiedi, S., and Akiskal, H.S. (2001). Anxiety disorders in children and adolescents with bipolar disorder: A neglected comorbidity. *Can J Psychiatry*, 46, 797–802.

Masi, G., Toni, C., Perugi, G., Travierso, M.C., Millepiedi, S., Mucci, M., Akiskal, H.S. (2003). Externalizing disorders in consecutively referred children and adolescents with bipolar disorder. *Compr Psychiatry*, 44, 184–189.

Masi, G., Perugi, G., Toni, C., Millepiedi, S., Mucci, M., Bertini, N., and Pfanner, C. (2006). Attention-deficit hyperactivity disorder—Bipolar cormobidity in children and adolescents. *Bipolar Disord*, 8, 373–381.

McClellan, J., and Werry, J.S. (1997). Practice parameters for the assessment and treatment of children and adolescents with bipolar disorder. *J Am Acad Child Adolesc Psychiatry*, 36(Suppl. 10), 157s–176s.

McClellan, J., McCurry, C., Snell, J., and DuBose, A. (1999). Early-onset psychotic disorders: Course and outcome over a 2-year period. *J Am Acad Child Adolesc Psychiatry*, 38, 1380–1388.

McClure, E.B., Treland, J.E., Snow, J., Dickstein, D.P., Towbin, K.E., Charney, D.S., Pine, D.S., and Leibenluft, E. (2005). Memory and learning in pediatric bipolar disorder. *J Am Acad Child Adolesc Psychiatry*, 44, 461–469.

McElroy, S.L., Strakowski, S.M., West, S.A., Keck, P.E., and McConville, B.J. (1997). Phenomenology of adolescent and adult mania in hospitalized patients with bipolar disorder. *Am J Psychiatry*, 154, 44–49.

McKnew, D.H., Cytryn, L., Efron, A.M., Gershon, E.S., and Bunney, W.E. (1979). Offspring of patients with affective disorders. *Br J Psychiatry*, 134, 148–152.

Miklowitz, D.J., Goldstein, M.J., Nuechterlein, K.H., Snyder, K.S., and Mintz, J. (1988). Family factors and the course of bipolar affective disorder. *Arch Gen Psychiatry*, 45(3), 225–231.

Meyer, S., Ronsaville, D.S., Gold, P.W., Radke-Yarrow, M., and Martinez, P.E. (2001). A prospective study of children at risk for mood disorder. In G.A. Carlson (Chair), *Juvenile Bipolar Disorder*. Symposium conducted at the meeting of the International Society for Research on Child and Adolescent Psychopathology, Vancouver, B.C.

Meyer, S., Carlson, G., Wiggs, E., Martinez, P., Ronsaville, D., Klimes-Dougan, B., Gold, P., and Radke-Yarrow, M. (2004a). Predictors of apparent frontal lobe dysfunction among adolescents at risk for bipolar disorders. Manuscript under review.

Meyer, S., Carlson, G., Wiggs, E., Martinez, P., Ronsaville, D., Klimes-Dougan, B., Gold, P., and Radke-Yarrow, M. (2004). A prospective study of the association among impaired executive functioning, childhood attentional problems, and the development of bipolar disorder. *Dev Psychopathol*, 16, 416–476.

Milberger, S., Biederman, J., Faraone, S.V., Murphy, J., and Tsuang, M.T. (1995). Attention deficit hyperactivity disorder and comorbid disorders: Issues of overlapping symptoms. *Am J Psychiatry*, 152, 1793–1799.

National Institute of Mental Health Research Roundtable on Prepubertal Bipolar Disorder. (2001). *J Am Acad Child Adolesc Psychiatry*, 40, 871–878.

Nurnberger, J.I., Hamovit, J., Hibbs, E.D., Pellegrini, D., Guroff, J.J., Maxwell, M.E., Smith, A., and Gershon, E.S. (1988). A high-risk study of primary affective disorder: Selection of subjects, initial assessment, and 1- to 2-year follow-up. In D.L. Dunner, E.S. Gershon, and J.E. Barrett (Eds.), *Relatives at Risk for Mental Disorder* (pp. 161–177). New York: Raven Press.

Osher, Y., Mandel, B., Shapiro, E., and Belmaker, R. (2000). Rorschach markers in offspring of manic-depressive patients. *J Affect Disord*, 59, 231–236.

Papolos, D.F. (2003). Bipolar disorder and comorbid disorders: The case for a dimensional nosology. In B. Geller and M. DelBello (Eds.), *Child and Early Adolescent Bipolar Disorder: Theory, Assessment, and Treatment*. New York: Guilford Publications.

Papolos, D., and Papolos, J. (2002). *The Bipolar Child: The Definitive and Reassuring Guide to Childhood's Most Misunderstood Disorder*. New York: Broadway Books.

Patel, N.C., DelBello, M.P., and Strakowski, S.M. (2006). Ethnic differences in symptom presentation of youths with bipolar disorder. *Bipolar Disord*, 8, 95–99.

Pavuluri, M.N., Herbener, E.S., and Sweeney, J.A. (2004). Psychotic symptoms in pediatric bipolar disorder. *J Affect Disord*, 80(1), 19–28.

Pavuluri, M.N., O'Connor, M.M., Harral, E.M., Moss, M., and Sweeney, J.A. (2006). Impact of neurocognitive function on academic difficulties in pediatric bipolar disorder: A clinical translation. *Biol Psychiatry*, 60, 951–956.

Pellegrini, D., Kosisky, S., Nackman, D., Cytryn, L., McKnew, D.H., Gershon, E., Hamovit, J., and Cammuso, K. (1986). Personal and social resources in children of patients with bipolar affective disorder and children of normal control subjects. *Am J Psychiatry*, 143, 856–861.

Post, R.M., Leverich, G.S., Fergus, E., Miller, R., and Luckenbaugh, D. (2002). Parental attitudes towards early intervention in children at high risk for affective disorders. *J Affect Disord*, 70(2), 117–124.

Quackenbush, D., Kutcher, S., Roberson, H.A., Boulos, C., and Chaban, P. (1996). Premorbid and postmorbid school functioning in bipolar adolescent description and suggested academic interventions. *Can J Psychiatry*, 41, 16–22.

Radke-Yarrow, M. (1998). *Children of Depressed Mothers: From Early Childhood to Maturity*. Cambridge, England: Cambridge University Press.

Radke-Yarrow, M., Nottelmann, E., Martinez, P., Fox, M.B., and Belmont, B. (1992). Young children of affectively ill parents: A longitudinal study of psychosocial development. *J Am Acad Child Adolesc Psychiatry*, 31, 68–77.

Rajeev, J., Srinath, S., Reddy, Y.C.J., Shashikiran, M.G., Girimaji, S.C., Seshadri, S.P., and Subbakrishna, D.K. (2003). The index manic episode in juvenile-onset bipolar disorder: The pattern of recovery. *Can J Psychiatry*, 48, 52–55.

Reichart, C.G., van der Ende, J., Wals, M., Hillegers, M.H.J., Nolen, W.A., Ormel, J., and Verhulst, F.C. (2005). The use of GBI as predictor of bipolar disorder in a population of adolescent offspring of parents with a bipolar disorder. *J Affect Disord*, 89(1-3), 147–155.

Rucklidge, J.J. (2006). Impact of ADHD on the neurocognitive functioning of adolescents with bipolar disorder. *Biol Psychiatry*, 60, 921–928.

Sachs, G.S., Baldassano, C.F., Truman, C.J., and Guille, C. (2000). Comorbidity of attention deficit hyperactivity disorder with early- and late-onset bipolar disorder. *Am J Psychiatry*, 157, 466–468.

Schneck, C.D., Miklowitz, D.J., Calabrese, J.R., Allen, M.H., Thomas, M.R., Wisniewski, S.R., Miyahara, S., Shelton, M.D., Ketter, T.A., Goldberg, J.F., Bowden, C.L., and Sachs, G.S. (2004). Phenomenology of rapid-cycling bipolar disorder: Data from the first 500 participants in the systematic treatment enhancement program. *Am J Psychiatry*, 161, 1902–1908.

Schurhoff, F., Bellivier, F., Jouvent, R., Mouren-Simeoni, M.-C., Bouvard, M., Allilaire, J.-F., and Leboyer, M. (2000). Early and late onset bipolar disorders: Two different forms of manic-depressive illness? *J Affect Disord*, 58, 215–221.

Shaffer, D. (2002). *Juvenile Mania: Newly Observed? Newly Invited? The Challenge of Adapting Adult Mood Disorder Criteria for Children*. Yokohama, Japan: World Congress of Psychiatry.

Sigurdsson, E., Fombonne, E., Sayal, K., and Checkley, S. (1999). Neurodevelopmental antecedents of early-onset bipolar affective disorder. *Br J Psychiatry*, 174, 121–127.

Smith, D.J., Harrison, N., Muir, W., and Blackwood, D.H.R. (2005). The high prevalence of bipolar spectrum disorders in young adults with recurrent depression: Toward an innovative diagnostic framework. *J Affect Disord*, 84, 167–178.

Soutullo, C.A., DelBello, M.P., Ochsner, J.E., McElroy, S.L., Taylor, S.A., Strakowski, S.M., and Keck, P.E. Jr. (2002). Severity of bipolarity in hospitalized manic adolescents with history of stimulant or antidepressant treatment. *J Affect Disord*, 70(3), 323–327.

State, R.C., Altshuler, L.L., and Frye, M.A. (2002). Mania and attention deficit hyperactivity disorder in a prepubertal child: Diagnostic and treatment challenges. *Am J Psychiatry*, 159, 918–925.

Staton, D., and Lysne, D. (1999, May). Children with bipolar disorder [Letter to the editor]. *J Am Acad Child Adolesc Psychiatry*, 38, 496.

Strakowski, S.M., McElroy, S.L., Keck, P.E., and West, S.A. (1996). Racial influence on diagnosis in psychotic manis. *J Affect Disord*, 39, 157–162.

Strober, M., and Carlson, G. (1982). Bipolar illness in adolescents with major depression: Clinical, genetic, and psychopharmacologic predictors in a three- to four-year prospective follow-up investigation. *Arch Gen Psychiatry*, 39, 549–555.

Strober, M., Schmidt-Lackner, S., Freeman, R., Bower, S., Lampert, C., and DeAntonio, M. (1995). Recovery and relapse in adolescents with bipolar affective illness: A five-year naturalistic, prospective follow-up. *J Am Acad Child Adolesc Psychiatry*, 34, 724–731.

Strober, M., DeAntonio, M., Schmidt-Lackner, S., Freeman, R., Lampert, C., and Diamond, J. (1998). Early childhood attention deficit hyperactivity disorder predicts poorer response to acute lithium therapy in adolescent mania. *J Affect Disord*, 51, 145–151.

Tillman, R., and Geller, B. (2003). Definitions of rapid, ultrarapid, and ultradian cycling and of episode duration in pediatric and adult bipolar disorders: A proposal to distinguish episodes from cycles. *J Child Adolesc Psychopharmacol*, 13, 267–271.

Tillman, R., Geller, B., Bolhofner, K., Craney, J.L., Williams, M., and Zimerman, B. (2003). Ages of onset and rates of syndromal and subsyndromal comorbid DSM-IV diagnoses in a prepubertal and early adolescent bipolar disorder phenotype. *J Am Acad Child Psychiatry*, 42(12), 1486–1493.

Tillman, R., Geller, B., Craney, J.L., Bolhofner, K., Williams, M., and Zimerman, B. (2004). Relationship of parent and child informants to prevalence of mania symptoms in children with a prepubertal and early adolescent bipolar disorder phenotype. *Am J Psychiatry*, 161, 1278–1284.

Todd, R.D., and Botteron, K.N. (2002). Etiology and genetics of early-onset mood disorders. *Child Adolesc Psychiatr Clin North Am*, 11, 499–518.

Todd, R.D., Reich, W., Petti, T.A., Joshi, P., DePaulo, J.R., Nurnberger, J., and Reich, T. (1996). Psychiatric diagnoses in the child and adolescent members of extended families identified through adult bipolar affective disorder probands. *J Am Acad Child Adolesc Psychiatry*, 35, 664–671.

Tohen, M., Greenfield, S.F., Weiss, R.D., Zarate, C.A., and Vagge, L.M. (1998). The effect of comorbid substance use disorders on the course of bipolar disorder: A review. *Harvard Rev Psychiatry, 6,* 133–141.

Walker, E.F. (2002). Adolescent neurodevelopment and psychopathology. *Curr Dir Psychol Sci,* 11, 24–28.

Wals, M., Hillegers, M.H.J., Reichart, C.G., Ormel, J., Nolen, W.A., and Verhulst, F.C. (2001). Prevalence of psychopathology in children of a bipolar parent. *J Am Acad Child Adolesc Psychiatry, 40,* 1094–1102.

Wals, M., Reichart, C.G., Hillegers, M.H.J., Van Os, J., Verhulst, F.C., Nolen, W.A., and Ormel, J. (2003). Impact of birth weight and genetic liability on psychopathology in children of bipolar parents. *J Am Acad Child Adolesc Psychiatry, 42,* 1116–1121.

Wals, M., Hillegers, M.H.J., Reichart, C.G., Verhulst, F.C., Nolen, W.A., and Ormel, J. (2005). Stressful life events and onset of mood disorders in children of bipolar parents during 14-month follow-up. *J Affect Disord, 87,* 253–263.

Waters, B.G.H., Marchenko, I., and Smiley, D. (1983). Affective disorder, paranatal, and educational factors in the offspring of bipolar manic-depressives. *Can J Psychiatry, 28,* 527–531.

Weintraub, S. (1987). Risk factors in schizophrenia: The Stony Brook High-Risk Project. *Schizophrenia Bull,* 13, 439–450.

Weintraub, S., and Neale, J.M. (1984). The Stony Brook High-Risk Project. In N.F. Watt, and J. Anthony (Eds.), *Children at Risk for Schizophrenia* (pp. 243–263). Cambridge, England: Cambridge University Press.

Weissman, M.M., Wolk, S., Goldstein, R.B., Moreau, D., Adams, P., Greenwald, S., Klier, C.M., Ryan, N.D., Dahl, R.E., and Wickramaratne, P. (1999a). Depressed adolescents grown up. *JAMA,* 281, 1707–1713.

Weissman, M.M., Wolk, S., Wickramaratne, P., Goldstein, R., Adams, P., Greenwald, S., Ryan, N., Dahl, R., and Steinberg, D. (1999b). Children with prepubertal-onset major depressive disorder and anxiety grown up. *Arch Gen Psychiatry,* 56, 794–801.

Worland, J., Lander, H., and Hesselbrock, V. (1979). Psychological evaluation of clinical disturbance in children at risk for psychopathology. *J Abnorm Psychol,* 88, 13–26.

Wozniak, J., Biederman, J., Kiely, K., Ablon, J. S., Faraone, S.V., Mundy, E., and Mennin, D. (1995). Mania-like symptoms suggestive of childhood-onset bipolar disorder in clinically referred children. *J Am Acad Child Adolesc Psychiatry,* 34, 867–876.

Wozniak, J., Biederman, J., Faraone, S.V., Blier, H., and Monuteaux, M.C. (2001). Heterogeneity of childhood conduct disorder: Further evidence of a subtype of conduct disorder linked to bipolar disorder. *J Affect Disord,* 64, 121–131.

Wozniak, J., Biederman, J., Monuteaux, M.C., Richards, J., and Faraone, S.V. (2002). Parsing the comorbidity between bipolar disorder and anxiety disorders: A familial risk analysis. *J Child Adolesc Psychopharmacol,* 12, 101–111.

Wozniak, J., Spencer, T., Biederman, J., Kwon, A., Monuteaux, M., Rettew, J., and Lail, K. (2004). The clinical characteristics of unipolar vs. bipolar major depression in ADHD youth. *J Affect Disord,* 82(Suppl. 1), S59–S69.

Youngstrom, E.A., Findling, R.L., Danielson, C.K., and Calabrese, J.R. (2001). Discriminative validity of parent report of hypomanic and depressive symptoms on the General Behavioral Inventory. *Psychol Assess,* 13, 267–276.

Youngstrom, E.A., Gracious, B.L., Danielson, C.K., Findling, R.L., and Calabrese, J.R. (2003). Toward an integration of parent and clinician report on the Young Mania Rating Scale. *J Affect Disord,* 77, 179–190.

Youngstrom, E., Findling, R.L., and Calabrese, J.R. (2004). Effects of adolescent manic symptoms on agreement between youth, parent, and teacher ratings of behavior problems. *J Affect Disord,* 825, S5–S16.

Zahn-Waxler, C., Cummings, E.M., McKnew, D.H., and Radke-Yarrow, M. (1984a). Altruism, aggression, and social interactions in young children with a manic-depressive parent. *Child Dev,* 55, 112–122.

Zahn-Waxler, C., McKnew, D.H., Cummings, E.M., Davenport, Y.B., and Radke-Yarrow, M. (1984b). Problem behaviors and peer interactions of young children with a manic-depressive parent. *Am J Psychiatry,* 141, 236–240.

Zahn-Waxler, C., Chapman, M., and Cummings, E.M. (1984c). Cognitive and social development in infants and toddlers with a bipolar parent. *Child Psychiatry Hum Dev,* 15, 75–85.

Zahn-Waxler, C., Mayfield, A., Radke-Yarrow, M., McKnew, D.H., Cytryn, L., and Davenport, Y.B. (1988). A follow-up investigation of offspring of parents with bipolar disorder. *Am J Psychiatry,* 145, 506–509.

Zito, J.M., Safer, D.J., dosReis, S., Gardner, J.F., Soeken, K., Boles, M., and Lynch, F. (2002). Rising prevalence of antidepressants among U.S. youths. *Pediatrics,* 109, 721–727.

Chapter 7

Ackerknecht, E.A. (1959). *A Short History of Psychiatry.* New York: Hafner.

American Diabetes Association, American Psychiatric Association, American Association of Clinical Endocrinologists, and North American Association for the Study of Obesity. (2004). Consensus development conference on antipsychotic drugs and obesity and diabetes. *Diabetes Care,* 27, 596–601.

Angst, F., Stassen, H.H., Clayton, P.J., and Angst, J. (2002). Mortality of patients with mood disorders: Follow-up over 34–38 years. *J Affect Disord,* 68, 167–181.

Angst, J. (1998). The emerging epidemiology of hypomania and bipolar II disorder. *J Affect Disord,* 50, 143–151.

Baldassano, C.F., Marangell, L.B., Gyulai, L., Ghaemi, S.N., Joffe, H., Kim, D.R., Sagduyu, K., Truman, C.J., Wisniewski, S.R., Sachs, G.S., and Cohen, L.S. (2005). Gender differences in bipolar disorder: Retrospective data from the first 500 STEP-BD participants. *Bipolar Disord,* 7, 465–470.

Bandelow, B., Sengos, G., Wedekind, D., Huether, G., Pilz, J., Broocks, A., Hajak, G., and Ruther, E. (1997). Urinary excretion of cortisol, norepinephrine, testosterone, and melatonin in panic disorder. *Pharmacopsychiatry,* 30, 113–117.

Bauer, M.S., Whybrow, P.C., and Winokur, A. (1990). Rapid cycling bipolar affective disorder: I. Association with grade I hypothyroidism. *Arch Gen Psychiatry,* 47, 427–432.

Bauer, M.S., Altshuler, L., Evans, D.R., Beresford, T., Williford, W.O., and Hauger, R. (2005). Prevalence and distinct correlates of anxiety, substance, and combined comorbidity in a multi-site public sector sample with bipolar disorder. *J Affect Disord,* 85, 301–315.

Bernadt, M.W., and Murray, R.M. (1986). Psychiatric disorder, drinking and alcoholism: What are the links? *Br J Psychiatry,* 148, 393–400.

Berrettini, W.H., Nurnberger, J.I., Jr., Scheinin, M., Seppala, T., Linnoila, M., Narrow, W., Simmons-Alling, S., and Gershon, E.S. (1985). Cerebrospinal fluid and plasma monoamines and their metabolites in euthymic bipolar patients. *Biol Psychiatry*, 20, 257–269.

Blehar, M.C., DePaulo, J.R., Gershon, E.S., Reich, T., Simpson, S.G., and Nurnberger, J.I. (1998). Women with bipolar disorder: Findings from the NIMH Genetics Initiative sample. *Psychopharmacol Bull*, 34(3), 239–243.

Bovasso, G.B. (2001). Cannabis abuse as a risk factor for depressive symptoms. *Am J Psychiatry*, 158, 2033–2037.

Bowen, R., South, M., and Hawkes, J. (1994). Mood swings in patients with panic disorder. *Can J Psychiatry*, 39, 91–94.

Bowers, M.B. Jr. (1977). Psychoses precipitated by psychotomimetic drugs: A follow-up study. *Arch Gen Psychiatry*, 34, 832–835.

Brieger, P. (2005). Comorbidity in mixed states and rapid-cycling forms of bipolar disorders. In A. Marneros and F.K. Goodwin (Eds.), *Bipolar Disorders: Mixed States, Rapid Cycling, and Atypical Forms*. Cambridge, UK: Cambridge University Press, pp. 263–276.

Brown, E.S., Beard, L., Dobbs, L., and Rush, A.J. (2006). Naltrexone in patients with bipolar disorder and alcohol dependence. *Depress Anxiety*, 23, 492–495.

Brownlie, B.E., Rae, A.M., Walshe, J.W., and Wells, J.E. (2000). Psychoses associated with thyrotoxicosis—"thyrotoxic psychosis": A report of 18 cases, with statistical analysis of incidence. *Eur J Endocrinol*, 142, 438–444.

Cade, J.F. (1979). *Mending the Mind: A Short History of Twentieth Century Psychiatry*. Melbourne, FL: Sun.

Calabrese, J.R., and Delucchi, G.A. (1990). Spectrum of efficacy of valproate in 55 patients with rapid-cycling bipolar disorder. *Am J Psychiatry*, 147, 431–434.

Calabrese, J.R., Hirschfeld, R.M., Reed, M., Davies, M.A., Frye, M.A., Keck, P.E., Lewis, L., McElroy, S.L., McNulty, J.P., and Wagner, K.D. (2003). Impact of bipolar disorder on a U.S. community sample. *J Clin Psychiatry*, 64(4), 425–432.

Carpenter, K.M., Hasin, D.S., Allison, D.B., and Faith, M.S. (2000). Relationships between obesity and DSM-IV major depressive disorder, suicide ideation, and suicide attempts: Results from a general population study. *Am J Public Health*, 90, 251–257.

Cassano, G.B., Pini, S., Saettoni, M., Rucci, P., and Dell'Osso, L. (1998). Occurrence and clinical correlates of psychiatric comorbidity in patients with psychotic disorders. *J Clin Psychiatry*, 59(2), 60–68.

Cassidy, F., Murry, E., Forest, K., and Carroll, B.J. (1998). Signs and symptoms of mania in pure and mixed episodes. *J Affect Disord*, 50, 187–201.

Cassidy, F., Ahearn, E., and Carroll, B.J. (1999). Elevated frequency of diabetes mellitus in hospitalized manic-depressive patients. *Am J Psychiatry*, 156, 1417–1420.

Cassidy, F., Ahearn, E.P., and Carroll, B.J. (2001). Substance abuse in bipolar disorder. *Bipolar Disord*, 3, 181–188.

Cassidy, F., Ahearn, E.P., and Carroll, B.J. (2002). Thyroid function in mixed and pure manic episodes. *Bipolar Disord*, 4(6), 393–397.

Castaneda, R., Galanter, M., and Franco, H. (1989). Self-medication among addicts with primary psychiatric disorders. *Compr Psychiatry*, 30, 80–83.

Chen, Y.W., and Dilsaver, S.C. (1995a). Comorbidity for obsessive-compulsive disorder in bipolar and unipolar disorders. *Psychiatry Res*, 59, 57–64.

Chen, Y.W., and Dilsaver, S.C. (1995b). Comorbidity of panic disorder in bipolar illness: Evidence from the Epidemiologic Catchment Area Survey. *Am J Psychiatry*, 152, 280–282.

Chengappa, K.N., Levine, J., Gershon, S., and Kupfer, D.J. (2000). Lifetime prevalence of substance or alcohol abuse and dependence among subjects with bipolar I and II disorders in a voluntary registry. *Bipolar Disord*, 2, 191–195.

Cole, D.P., Thase, M.E., Mallinger, A.G., Soares, J.C., Luther, J.F., Kupfer, D.J., and Frank, E. (2002). Slower treatment response in bipolar depression predicted by lower pretreatment thyroid function. *Am J Psychiatry*, 159, 116–121.

Davidson, J.R., Rothbaum, B.O., van der Kolk, B.A., Sikes, C.R., and Farfel, G.M. (2001). Multicenter, double-blind comparison of sertraline and placebo in the treatment of posttraumatic stress disorder. *Arch Gen Psychiatry*, 58, 485–492.

de Graaf, R., Bijl, R.V., Smit, F., Vollebergh, W.A., and Spijker, J. (2002). Risk factors for 12-month comorbidity of mood, anxiety, and substance use disorders: Findings from the Netherlands Mental Health Survey and Incidence Study. *Am J Psychiatry*, 159, 620–629.

Derby, I.M. (1933). Manic-depressive "exhaustion" deaths: An analysis of "exhaustion" case histories. *Psychiatr Q*, 7, 435–449.

Dilsaver, S.C., Chen, Y.W., Swann, A.C., Shoaib, A.M., Tsai-Dilsaver, Y., and Krajewski, K.J. (1997). Suicidality, panic disorder and psychosis in bipolar depression, depressive-mania and pure-mania. *Psychiatry Res*, 73, 47–56.

Donahue, R.P., Abbott, R.D., Bloom, E., Reed, D.M., and Yano, K. (1987). Central obesity and coronary heart disease in men. *Lancet*, 1, 821–824.

Doughty, C.J., Elisabeth Wells, J., Joyce, P.R., Olds, R.J., and Walsh, A.E. (2004). Bipolar-panic disorder comorbidity within bipolar disorder families: A study of siblings. *Bipolar Disord*, 6, 245–252.

Edmonds, L.K., Mosley, B.J., Admiraal, A.J., Olds, R.J., Romans, S.E., Silverstone, T., and Walsh, A.E. (1998). Familial bipolar disorder: Preliminary results from the Otago Familial Bipolar Genetic Study. *Aust N Z J Psychiatry*, 32(6), 823–829.

El-Guebaly, N. (1975). Manic-depressive psychosis and drug abuse. *Can Psychiatr Assoc J*, 20, 595–598.

Ellinwood, E.H., and Petrie, W.M. (1979). Drug-induced psychoses. In R.W. Pickens, L.L. Heston (Eds.), *Psychiatric Factors in Drug Abuse* (pp. 301–336). New York: Grune and Stratton.

Elmslie, J.L., Silverstone, J.T., and Mann, J.I. (2000). Prevalence of overweight and obesity in bipolar patients. *J Clin Psychiatry*, 61, 179–184.

Elmslie, J.L., Mann, J.I., and Silverstone, J.T. (2001). Determinants of overweight and obesity in patients with bipolar disorders. *J Clin Psychiatry*, 62, 486–491.

Engum, A., Bjoro, T., Mykletun, A., and Dahl, A.A. (2002). An association between depression, anxiety and thyroid function: A clinical fact or an artifact? *Acta Psychiatr Scand*, 106, 27–34.

Erard, R., Luisada, P.V., and Peele, R. (1980). The PCP psychosis: Prolonged intoxication or drug-precipitated functional illness? *J Psychedelic Drugs*, 12, 235–251.

Estroff, T.W., Dackis, C.A., Gold, M.S., and Pottash, A.L. (1985). Drug abuse and bipolar disorders. *Int J Psychiatry Med*, 15, 37–40.

Fagiolini, A., Frank, E., Houck, P.R., Mallinger, A.G., Swartz, H.A., Buysse, D.J., Ombao, H., and Kupfer, D.J. (2002). Prevalence of obesity and weight change during treatment in patients with bipolar I disorder. *J Clin Psychiatry*, 63, 528–533.

Fasmer, O.B. (2001). The prevalence of migraine in patients with bipolar and unipolar affective disorders. *Cephalalgia*, 21(9), 894–899.

Fava, M., Labbate, L.A., Abraham, M.E., and Rosenbaum, J.F. (1995). Hypothyroidism and hyperthyroidism in major depression revisited. *J Clin Psychiatry*, 56(5), 186–192.

Feinman, J.A., and Dunner, D.L. (1996). The effect of alcohol and substance abuse on the course of bipolar affective disorder. *J Affect Disord*, 37, 43–49.

Findling, R.L., Gracious, B.L., McNamara, N.K., Youngstrom, E.A., Demeter, C.A., Branicky, L.A., and Calabrese, J.R. (2001). Rapid, continuous cycling and psychiatric co-morbidity in pediatric bipolar I disorder. *Bipolar Disord*, 3, 202–210.

Flegal, K.M., Carroll, M.D., Ogden, C.L., and Johnson, C.L. (2002). Prevalence and trends in obesity among US adults, 1999–2000. *JAMA*, 288, 1723–1727.

Flynn, R.W., MacDonald, T.M., Morris, A.D., Jung, R.T., and Leese, G.P. (2004). The thyroid epidemiology, audit, and research study: Thyroid dysfunction in the general population. *J Clin Endocrinol Metab*, 89, 3879–3884.

Fogarty, F., Russell, J.M., Newman, S.C., and Bland, R.C. (1994). Epidemiology of psychiatric disorders in Edmonton: Mania. *Acta Psychiatr Scand Suppl*, 376, 16–23.

Frank, E., Cyranowski, J.M., Rucci, P., Shear, M.K., Fagiolini, A., Thase, M.E., Cassano, G.B., Grochocinski, V.J., Kostelnik, B., and Kupfer, D.J. (2002). Clinical significance of lifetime panic spectrum symptoms in the treatment of patients with bipolar I disorder. *Arch Gen Psychiatry*, 59, 905–911.

Freed, E.X. (1969). Alcohol abuse by manic patients. *Psychol Rep*, 25, 280.

Freeman, M.P., Freeman, S.A., and McElroy, S.L. (2002). The co-morbidity of bipolar and anxiety disorders: Prevalence, psychobiology, and treatment issues. *J Affect Disord*, 68, 1–23.

Frye, M.A., Denicoff, K.D., Bryan, A.L., Smith-Jackson, E.E., Ali, S.O., Luckenbaugh, D., Leverich, G.S., and Post, R.M. (1999). Association between lower serum free T4 and greater mood instability and depression in lithium-maintained bipolar patients. *Am J Psychiatry*, 156, 1909–1914.

Frye, M.A., Altshuler, L.L., McElroy, S.L., Suppes, T., Keck, P.E., Denicoff, K., Nolen, W.A., Kupka, R., Leverich, G.S., Pollio, C., Grunze, H., Walden, J., Post, R.M. (2003). Gender differences in prevalence, risk, and clinical correlates of alcoholism comorbidity in bipolar disorder. *Am J Psychiatry*, 160, 883–889.

Gawin, F.H., and Kleber, H.D. (1986). Abstinence symptomatology and psychiatric diagnosis in cocaine abusers: Clinical observations. *Arch Gen Psychiatry*, 43, 107–113.

Gaziano, J.M., Gaziano, T.A., Glynn, R.J., Sesso, H.D., Ajani, U.A., Stampfer, M.J., Manson, J.E., Hennekens, C.H., and Buring, J.E. (2000). Light-to-moderate alcohol consumption and mortality in the Physicians' Health Study enrollment cohort. *J Am Coll Cardiol*, 35, 96–105.

Gibb, B., Coles, M., and Heimberg, R. (2005). Differentiating symptoms of social anxiety and depression in adults with social anxiety disorder. *J Behav Ther Exp Psychol*, 36, 99–109.

Gijsman, H.J., Geddes, J.R., Rendell, J.M., Nolen, W.A., and Goodwin, G.M. (2004). Antidepressants for bipolar depression: A systematic review of randomized, controlled trials. *Am J Psychiatry*, 161, 1537–1547.

Gold, P.W., Goodwin, F.K., Wehr, T., and Rebar, R. (1977). Pituitary thyrotropin response to thyrotropin-releasing hormone in affective illness: Relationship to spinal fluid amine metabolites. *Am J Psychiatry*, 134, 1028–1031.

Goldberg, J.F., and Whiteside, J.E. (2002). The association between substance abuse and antidepressant-induced mania in bipolar disorder: A preliminary study. *J Clin Psychiatry*, 63, 791–795.

Goldberg, J.F., Garno, J.L., Leon, A.C., Kocsis, J.H., and Portera, L. (1999). A history of substance abuse complicates remission from acute mania in bipolar disorder. *J Clin Psychiatry*, 60, 733–740.

Goldstein, B.I., and Levitt, A.J. (2006). Factors associated with temporal priority in comorbid bipolar I disorder and alcohol use disorders: Results from the National Epidemiologic Survey on Alcohol and Related Conditions. *J Clin Psychiatry*, 67, 643–649.

Goldstein, B.I., Velyvis, V.P., and Parikh, S.V. (2005). *Does Moderate Alcohol Use in Bipolar Disorder Impact Course and Symptom Burden?* Presented at the annual meeting of the American Psychiatric Association, Atlanta.

Goldstein, B.I., Herrmann, N., and Shulman, K.I. (2006). Comorbidity in bipolar disorder among the elderly: Results from an epidemiological community sample. *Am J Psychiatry*, 163, 319–321.

Goodwin, R.D., and Hoven, C.W. (2002). Bipolar-panic comorbidity in the general population: Prevalence and associated morbidity. *J Affect Disord*, 70, 27–33.

Gortmaker, S.L., Must, A., Perrin, J.M., Sobol, A.M., and Dietz, W.H. (1993). Social and economic consequences of overweight in adolescence and young adulthood. *N Engl J Med*, 329, 1008–1012.

Gould, T.D., Chen, G., and Manji, H.K. (2004). In vivo evidence in the brain for lithium inhibition of glycogen synthase kinase-3. *Neuropsychopharmacology*, 29, 32–38.

Guo, J.J., Keck, P.E., Jang, R., Li, H., Corey Lisle, P., and Jiang, D. (2005). *Prevalence and Key Comorbidities among Patients with Bipolar Disorders in a Large Managed Care Population*. Presented at the annual meeting of the American Psychiatric Association, Atlanta.

Haggerty, J.J. Jr., Stern, R.A., Mason, G.A., Beckwith, J., Morey, C.E., and Prange, A.J. Jr. (1993). Subclinical hypothyroidism: A modifiable risk factor for depression? *Am J Psychiatry*, 150, 508–510.

Harris, E.C., and Barraclough, B. (1997). Suicide as an outcome for mental disorders: A meta analysis. *Br J Psychiatry*, 170, 205–228.

Haywood, T.W., Kravitz, H.M., Grossman, L.S., Cavanaugh, J.L. Jr., Davis, J.M., and Lewis, D.A. (1995). Predicting the "revolving door" phenomenon among patients with schizophrenic, schizoaffective, and affective disorders. *Am J Psychiatry*, 152, 856–861.

Helzer, J.E., and Pryzbeck, T.R. (1988). The co-occurrence of alcoholism with other psychiatric disorders in the general population and its impact on treatment. *J Stud Alcohol*, 49, 219–224.

Henderson, D.C., Cagliero, E., Copeland, P.M., Borba, C.P., Evins, E., Hayden, D., Weber, M.T., Anderson, E.J., Allison, D.B., Daley, T.B., Schoenfeld, D., and Goff, D.C. (2005). Glucose metabolism in patients with schizophrenia treated with atypical antipsychotic agents: A frequently sampled intravenous glucose tolerance test and minimal model analysis. *Arch Gen Psychiatry*, 62, 19–28.

Henquet, C., Krabbendam, L., de Graaf, R., ten Have, M., and van Os, J. (2006). Cannabis use and expression of mania in the general population. *J Affect Disord*, 95, 103–110.

Henry, C., Van den Bulke, D., Bellivier, F., Etain, B., Rouillon, F., and Leboyer, M. (2003). Anxiety disorders in 318 bipolar patients: Prevalence and impact on illness severity and response to mood stabilizer. *J Clin Psychiatry*, 64, 331–335.

Hensel, B., Dunner, D.L., and Fieve, R.R. (1979). The relationship of family history of alcoholism to primary affective disorder. *J Affect Disord*, 1, 105–113.

Hesselbrock, M.N., Meyer, R.E., and Keener, J.J. (1985). Psychopathology in hospitalized alcoholics. *Arch Gen Psychiatry*, 42, 1050–1055.

Hetman, M., Cavanaugh, J.E., Kimelman, D., and Xia, Z. (2000). Role of glycogen synthase kinase-3β in neuronal apoptosis induced by trophic withdrawal. *J Neurosci*, 20, 2567–2574.

Hides, L., Dawe, S., Kavanagh, D.J., and Young, R. (2006). Psychotic symptom and cannabis relapse in recent-onset psychosis. *Br J Psychiatry*, 189, 137–143.

Himmelhoch, J.M. (1998). Social anxiety, hypomania and the bipolar spectrum: Data, theory and clinical issues. *J Affect Disord*, 50, 203–213.

Himmelhoch, J.M., and Garfinkel, M.E. (1986). Sources of lithium resistance in mixed mania. *Psychopharmacol Bull*, 22, 613–620.

Himmelhoch, J.M., Mulla, D., Neil, J.F., Detre, T.P., and Kupfer, D.J. (1976). Incidence and significance of mixed affective states in a bipolar population. *Arch Gen Psychiatry*, 33, 1062–1066.

Himmelhoch, J.M., Hill, S., Steinberg, B., and May, S. (1983). Lithium, alcoholism, and psychiatric diagnosis. *J Psychiatr Treat Eval*, 5, 83–88.

Howland, R.H. (1993). Thyroid dysfunction in refractory depression: Implications for pathophysiology and treatment. *J Clin Psychiatry*, 54, 47–54.

Hu, M., Wu, H., and Chao, C. (1997). Assisting effects of lithium on hypoglycemic treatment in patients with diabetes. *Biol Trace Elem Res*, 60, 131–137.

Hudson, J.I., Pope, H.G. Jr., Wurtman, J., Yurgelun-Todd, D., Mark, S., and Rosenthal, N.E. (1988). Bulimia in obese individuals: Relationship to normal-weight bulimia. *J Nerv Ment Dis*, 176, 144–152.

Institute of Medicine (IOM). (2002). *Reducing Suicide: A National Imperative*. Washington, DC: National Academy Press.

Isojarvi, J.I., Pakarinen, A.J., and Myllyla, V.V. (1989). Thyroid function in epileptic patients treated with carbamazepine. *Arch Neurol*, 46, 1175–1178.

Jamison, K.R. (2004). *Exuberance: The Passion for Life*. New York: Alfred A. Knopf.

Johannessen, L., Strudsholm, U., Foldager, L., and Munk-Jorgensen, P. (2006). Increased risk of hypertension in patients with bipolar disorder and patients with anxiety compared to background population and patients with schizophrenia. *J Affect Disord*, 95(1–3), 13–17.

Johnson, S.L., Winett, C.A., Meyer, B., Greenhouse, W.J., and Miller, I. (1999). Social support and the course of bipolar disorder. *J Abnorm Psychol*, 108, 558–566.

Judd, L.L., Akiskal, H.S., Schettler, P.J., Coryell, W., Maser, J., Rice, J.A., Solomon, D.A., and Keller, M.B. (2003a). The comparative clinical phenotype and long term longitudinal episode course of bipolar I and II: A clinical spectrum or distinct disorders? *J Affect Disord*, 73, 19–32.

Judd, L.L., Schettler, P.J., Akiskal, H.S., Maser, J., Coryell, W., Solomon, D., Endicott, J., and Keller, M. (2003b). Long-term symptomatic status of bipolar I vs. bipolar II disorders. *Int J Neuropsychopharmacol*, 6, 127–137.

Kathol, R.G., Turner, R., and Delahunt, J. (1986). Depression and anxiety associated with hyperthyroidism: Response to antithyroid therapy. *Psychosomatics*, 27, 501–505.

Kawa, I., Carterm, J., Joyce, P., Doughty, C., Frampton, C., Well, E.J., Walsh, A., and Olds, R. (2005). Gender differences in bipolar disorder: Age of onset, course, comorbidity, and symptom presentation. *Bipolar Disord*, 7, 119–125.

Keck, P.E. Jr., McElroy, S.L., Strakowski, S.M., West, S.A., Hawkins, J.M., Huber, T.J., Newman, R.M., and DePriest, M. (1995). Outcome and comorbidity in first- compared with multiple-episode mania. *J Nerv Ment Dis*, 183, 320–324.

Keck, P.E. Jr., McElroy, S.L., Strakowski, S.M., Bourne, M.L., and West, S.A. (1997). Compliance with maintenance treatment in bipolar disorder. *Psychopharmacol Bull*, 33, 87–91.

Keeler, M.H., Taylor, C.I., and Miller, W.C. (1979). Are all recently detoxified alcoholics depressed? *Am J Psychiatry*, 136, 586–588.

Kessler, R. (2004). *Prevalence of adult ADHD in the United States: Results from the National Comorbidity Survey Replication (NCS)*. Presented at the annual meeting of the American Psychiatric Association, New York.

Kessler, R.C., McGonagle, K.A., Zhao, S., Nelson, C.B., Hughes, M., Eshleman, S., Wittchen, H.U., and Kendler, K.S. (1994). Lifetime and 12-month prevalence of DSM-III-R psychiatric disorders in the United States: Results from the National Comorbidity Survey. *Arch Gen Psychiatry*, 51, 8–19.

Kessler, R.C., Sonnega, A., Bromet, E., Hughes, M., and Nelson, C.B. (1995). Posttraumatic stress disorder in the National Comorbidity Survey. *Arch Gen Psychiatry*, 52, 1048–1060.

Kessler, R.C., Nelson, C.B., McGonagle, K.A., Edlund, M.J., Frank, R.G., and Leaf, P.J. (1996). The epidemiology of co-occurring addictive and mental disorders: Implications for prevention and service utilization. *Am J Orthopsychiatry*, 66, 17–31.

Kessler, R.C., Rubinow, D.R., Holmes, C., Abelson, J.M., and Zhao, S. (1997). The epidemiology of DSM-III-R bipolar I disorder in a general population survey. *Psychol Med*, 27, 1079–1089.

Khantzian, E.J. (1974). Opiate addiction: A critique of theory and some implications for treatment. *Am J Psychother*, 28, 59–70.

Khantzian, E.J. (1985). The self-medication hypothesis of addictive disorders: Focus on heroin and cocaine dependence. *Am J Psychiatry*, 142, 1259–1264.

Kogan, J.N., Otto, M.W., Bauer, M.S., Dennehy, E.B., Miklowitz, D.J., Zhang, H.W., Ketter, T., Rudorfer, M.V., Wisniewski, S.R., Thase, M.E., Calabrese, J., Sachs, G.S., and STEP-BD Investigators. (2004). Demographic and diagnostic characteristics of the first 1000 patients enrolled in the Systematic Treatment Enhancement Program for Bipolar Disorder (STEP-BD). *Bipolar Disord*, 6, 460–469.

Kosten, T.R., and Rounsaville, B.J. (1986). Psychopathology in opioid addicts. *Psychiatr Clin North Am*, 9, 515–532.

Kosten, T.R., Mason, J.W., Giller, E.L., Ostroff, R.B., and Harkness, L. (1987). Sustained urinary norepinephrine and epinephrine elevation in post-traumatic stress disorder. *Psychoneuroendocrinology*, 12, 13–20.

Kraepelin, E. (1921). *Manic-depressive insanity and paranoia*. Edinburgh, Scotland: E & S Livingstone.

Krüger, S., Cooke, R.G., Hasey, G.M., Jorna, T., and Persad, E. (1995). Comorbidity of obsessive compulsive disorder in bipolar disorder. *J Affect Disord*, 34, 117–120.

Krüger, S., Shugar, G., and Cooke, R.G. (1996). Comorbidity of binge eating disorder and the partial binge eating syndrome with bipolar disorder. *Int J Eat Disord*, 19, 45–52.

Krüger, S., Braunig, P., and Cooke, R.G. (2000). Comorbidity of obsessive-compulsive disorder in recovered inpatients with bipolar disorder. *Bipolar Disord*, 2, 71–74.

Kusalic, M. (1992). Grade II and grade III hypothyroidism in rapid-cycling bipolar patients. *Neuropsychobiology*, 25, 177–181.

Lazarus, J.H. (1998). The effects of lithium therapy on thyroid and thyrotropin-releasing hormone. *Thyroid*, 8, 909–913.

Leino-Arjas, P., Liira, J., Mutanen, P., Malmivaara, A., and Matikainen, E. (1999). Predictors and consequences of unemployment among construction workers: Prospective cohort study. *BMJ*, 319, 600–605.

Lensi, P., Cassano, G.B., Correddu, G., Ravagli, S., Kunovac, J.L., and Akiskal, H.S. (1996). Obsessive-compulsive disorder: Familial-developmental history, symptomatology, comorbidity and course with special reference to gender-related differences. *Br J Psychiatry*, 169, 101–107.

Lewinsohn, P.M., Striegel-Moore, R.H., Seeley, J.R. (2000). Epidemiology and natural course of eating disorders in young women from adolescence to young adulthood. *J Am Acad Child Adolesc Psychiatry*, 39, 1284–1292.

Lewis, A. (1936). Prognosis in the manic-depressive psychosis. *Lancet*, 997–999.

Liskow, B., Mayfield, D., and Thiele, J. (1982). Alcohol and affective disorder: Assessment and treatment. *J Clin Psychiatry*, 43, 144–147.

MacKinnon, D.F., McMahon, F.J., Simpson, S.G., McInnis, M.G., and DePaulo, J.R. (1997). Panic disorder with familial bipolar disorder. *Biol Psychiatry*, 42, 90–95.

MacKinnon, D.F., Zandi, P.P., Cooper, J., Potash, J.B., Simpson, S.G., Gershon, E., Nurnberger, J., Reich, T., and DePaulo, J.R. (2002). Comorbid bipolar disorder and panic disorder in families with a high prevalence of bipolar disorder. *Am J Psychiatry*, 159, 30–35.

MacKinnon, D.F., Zandi, P.P., Gershon, E., Nurnberger, J.I. Jr., Reich, T., and DePaulo, J.R. (2003). Rapid switching of mood in families with multiple cases of bipolar disorder. *Arch Gen Psychiatry*, 60, 921–928.

MacQueen, G.M., Marriott, M., Begin, H., Robb, J., Joffe, R.T., and Young, L.T. (2003). Subsyndromal symptoms assessed in longitudinal, prospective follow-up of a cohort of patients with bipolar disorder. *Bipolar Disord*, 5(5), 349–355.

Maes, M., Lin, A.H., Verkerk, R., Delmeire, L., Van Gastel, A., Van der Planken, M., and Scharpe, S. (1999). Serotonergic and noradrenergic markers of post-traumatic stress disorder with and without major depression. *Neuropsychopharmacology*, 20, 188–197.

Mahmood, T., Romans, S., and Silverstone, T. (1999). Prevalence of migraine in bipolar disorder. *J Affect Disord*, 52(1–3), 239–241.

Mantere, O., Melartin, T.R., Suominen, K., Rytsala, H.J., Valtonen, H.M., Arvilommi, P., Leppamaki, S., and Isometsa, E.T. (2006). Differences in axis-I and -II comorbidity between bipolar I and II disorders and major depressive disorder. *J Clin Psychiatry*, 67, 584–593.

Maremmani, I., Perugi, G., Pacini, M., and Akiskal, H.S. (2006). Toward a unitary perspective on the bipolar spectrum and substance abuse: Opiate addiction as a paradigm. *J Affect Disord*, 93(1-3), 1–12.

Marneros, A., and Goodwin, F.K. (Eds.). (2005). *Mixed States, Rapid Cycling and Atypical Forms*. Cambridge, MA: Cambridge University Press.

Mayfield, D.G., and Coleman, L.L. (1968). Alcohol use and affective disorder. *Dis Nerv Syst* 29, 467–474.

McElroy, S.L., Strakowski, S.M., Keck, J., Paul, E., Tugrul, K.L., West, S.A., and Lonczak, H.S. (1995). Differences and similarities in mixed and pure mania. *Compr Psychiatry*, 36, 187–194.

McElroy, S.L., Altshuler, L.L., Suppes, T., Keck, P.E. Jr., Frye, M.A., Denicoff, K.D., Nolen, W.A., Kupka, R.W., Leverich, G.S., Rochussen, J.R., Rush, A.J., and Post, R.M. (2001). Axis I psychiatric comorbidity and its relationship to historical illness variables in 288 patients with bipolar disorder. *Am J Psychiatry*, 158, 420–426.

McElroy, S.L., Frye, M.A., Suppes, T., Dhavale, D., Keck, P.E. Jr, Leverich, G.S., Altshuler, L., Denicoff, K.D., Nolen, W.A., Kupka, R., Grunze, H., Walden, J., and Post, R.M. (2002). Correlates of overweight and obesity in 644 patients with bipolar disorder. *J Clin Psychiatry*, 63, 207–213.

McElroy, S.L., Kotwal, R., Keck, P.E., and Akiskal, H.S. (2005). Comorbidity of bipolar and eating disorders: Distinct or related disorders with shared dysregulations? *J Affect Dis*, 86, 107–127.

McIntyre, R., Konarski, J., Wilkins, K., Bouffard, B., Soczynska, J.D., and Kennedy, S. (2006). The prevalence and impact of migraine headache in bipolar disorder: Results from the Canadian Community Health Survey. *Headache*, 6, 973–982.

Milkman, H., and Frosch, W.A. (1973). On the preferential abuse of heroin and amphetamine. *J Nerv Ment Dis*. 156, 242–248.

Miller, F.T., Busch, F, and Tanenbaum, J.H. (1989). Drug abuse in schizophrenia and bipolar disorder. *Am J Drug Alcohol Abuse*, 15, 291–295.

Minski, L. (1938). Psychopathology and psychoses associated with alcohol. *J Mental Sci*, 84, 985–990.

Mirin, S.M., Weiss, R.D., Sollogub, A., and Michael, J. (1984). Affective illness in substance abusers. In S.M. Mirin (Ed.), *Substance Abuse and Psychopathology* (pp. 57–78). Washington, DC: American Psychiatric Press.

Morrison, J.R. (1974). Bipolar affective disorder and alcoholism. *Am J Psychiatry*, 131, 1130–1133.

Mueser, K.T., Goodman, L.B., Trumbetta, S.L., Rosenberg, S.D., Osher, C., Vidaver, R., Auciello, P., and Foy, D.W. (1998). Trauma and posttraumatic stress disorder in severe mental illness. *J Consult Clin Psychol*, 66, 493–499.

Musselman, D.L., Tomer, A., Manatunga, A.K., Knight, B.T., Porter, M.R., Kasey, S., Marzec, U., Harker, L.A., and Nemeroff, C.B. (1996). Exaggerated platelet reactivity in major depression. *Am J Psychiatry*, 153, 1313–1317.

Narrow, W.E., Rae, D.S., Robins, L.N., and Regier, D.A. (2002). Revised prevalence estimates of mental disorders in the United States: Using a clinical significance criterion to reconcile 2 surveys' estimates. *Arch Gen Psychiatry*, 59, 115–123.

Neria, Y., Bromet, E.J., Sievers, S., Lavelle, J., and Fochtmann, L.J. (2002). Trauma exposure and posttraumatic stress disorder in psychosis: Findings from a first-admission cohort. *J Consult Clin Psychol*, 70, 246–251.

Norton, B., and Whalley, L.J. (1984). Mortality of a lithium-treated population. *Br J Psychiatry*, 145, 277–282.

Oedegaard, K.J., and Fasmer, O.B. (2005). Is migraine in unipolar depressed patients a bipolar spectrum trait? *J Affect Disord*, 84(2-3), 233–242.

Oedegaard, K.J., Neckelmann, D., and Fasmer, O.B. (2005). Type A behavior differentiates bipolar II from unipolar depressed patients. *J Affect Disord*, 90, 7–13.

Office of Applied Studies. (2001). *Summary of Findings from the 2000 National Household Survey on Drug Abuse*. Rockville, MD: Substance Abuse and Mental Health Services Administration.

Olfson, M., Guardino, M., Struening, E., Schneier, F.R., Hellman, F., and Klein, D.F. (2000). Barriers to the treatment of social anxiety. *Am J Psychiatry*, 157, 521–527.

Orena, S.J., Torchia, A.J., and Garofalo, R.S. (2000). Inhibition of glycogen-synthase kinase 3 stimulates glycogen synthase and glucose transport by distinct mechanisms in 3T3-L1 adipocytes. *J Biol Chem*, 275, 15765–15772.

Osby, U., Brandt, L., Correia, N., Ekbom. A., and Sparen, P. (2001). Excess mortality in bipolar and unipolar disorder in Sweden. *Arch Gen Psychiatry* 58(9), 844–850.

Otto, M.W., Perlman, C.A., Wernicke, R., Reese, H.E., Bauer, M.S., and Pollack, M.H. (2004). Posttraumatic stress disorder in patients with bipolar disorder: A review of prevalence, correlates, and treatment strategies. *Bipolar Disord*, 6, 470–479.

Otto, M.W., Simon, N.M., Wisniewski, S.R.., Miklowitz, D.J., Kogan, J.N.., Reilly-Harrington, N.A., Frank, E., Nierenberg, A.A., Marangell, L.B., Sagduyu, K., Weiss, R.D., Miyahara, S., Thase, M.E., Sachs, G.S., and Pollack, M.H. (2006). Prospective 12-month course of bipolar disorder in outpatients with and without comorbid anxiety disorders. *Br J Psychiatry*, 189, 20–25.

Perlick, D.A., Rosenheck, R.A., Kaczynski, R., and Kozma, L. (2004). Medication non-adherence in bipolar disorder: A patient-centered review of research findings. *Clinical Approaches in Bipolar Disorders*, 3, 56–64.

Perlis, R.H., Miyahara, S., Marangell, L.B., Wisniewski, S.R., Ostacher, M., DelBello, M.P., Bowden, C.L., Sachs, G.S., Nierenberg, A.A., and STEP-BD Investigators. (2004). Long-term implications of early onset in bipolar disorder: Data from the first 1000 participants in the Systematic Treatment Enhancement Program for Bipolar Disorder (STEP-BD). *Biol Psychiatry*, 55, 875–881.

Perry, C.G., Spiers, A., Cleland, S.J., Lowe, G.D., Petrie, J.R., and Connell, J.M. (2003). Glucocorticoids and insulin sensitivity: Dissociation of insulin's metabolic and vascular actions. *J Clin Endocrinol Metab*, 88, 6008–6014.

Perugi, G., Akiskal, H.S., Pfanner, C., Presta, S., Gemignani, A., Milanfranchi, A., Lensi, P., Ravagli, S., and Cassano, G.B. (1997). The clinical impact of bipolar and unipolar affective comorbidity on obsessive-compulsive disorder. *J Affect Disord*, 46, 15–23.

Perugi, G., Akiskal, H.S., Ramacciotti, S., Nassini, S., Toni, C., Milanfranchi, A., and Musetti, L. (1999). Depressive comorbidity of panic, social phobic, and obsessive-compulsive disorders re-examined: Is there a bipolar II connection? *J Psychiatr Res*, 33, 53–61.

Perugi, G., Akiskal, H.S., Toni, C., Simonini, E., and Gemignani, A. (2001). The temporal relationship between anxiety disorders and (hypo)mania: A retrospective examination of 63 panic, social phobic and obsessive-compulsive patients with comorbid bipolar disorder. *J Affect Disord*, 67, 199–206.

Perugi, G., Toni, C., Frare, F., Travierso, M.C., Hantouche, E., and Akiskal, H.S. (2002). Obsessive-compulsive–bipolar comorbidity: A systematic exploration of clinical features and treatment outcome. *J Clin Psychiatry*, 63(12), 1129–1134.

Pine, D.S., Goldstein, R.B., Wolk, S., and Weissman, M.M. (2001). The association between childhood depression and adulthood body mass index. *Pediatrics*, 107, 1049–1056.

Pini, S., Cassano, G.B., Simonini, E., Savino, M., Russo, A., and Montgomery, S.A. (1997). Prevalence of anxiety disorders comorbidity in bipolar depression, unipolar depression and dysthymia. *J Affect Disord*, 42, 145–153.

Pini, S., Dell'Osso, L., Mastrocinque, C., Marcacci, G., Papasogli, A., Vignoli, S., Pallanti, S., and Cassano, G. (1999). Axis I comorbidity in bipolar disorder with psychotic features. *Br J Psychiatry*, 175, 467–471.

Placidi, G.P., Boldrini, M., Patronelli, A., Fiore, E., Chiovato, L., Perugi, G., and Marazziti, D. (1998). Prevalence of psychiatric disorders in thyroid diseased patients. *Neuropsychobiology*, 38, 222–225.

Poe, E.A. (1848). *The Letters of Edgar Allan Poe* (Vol. 2, p. 356). J. Wand Ostrom (Ed.). Cambridge, MA: Harvard University Press.

Post, R.M., Kotin, J., and Goodwin, F.K. (1974). The effects of cocaine on depressed patients. *Am J Psychiatry*, 131, 511–517.

Post, R.M., Rubinow, D.R., and Ballenger, J.C. (1984). Conditioning, sensitization and kindling: Implications for the course of affective illness. In R.M. Post, J.C. Ballenger (Eds.), *The Neurobiology of Mood Disorders* (pp. 432–466). New York: Williams & Wilkins.

Post, R.M., Kramlinger, K.G., Joffe, R.T., Roy-Byrne, P.P., Rosoff, A., Frye, M.A., and Huggins, T. (1997). Rapid cycling bipolar affective disorder: Lack of relation to hypothyroidism. *Psychiatry Res*, 72, 1–7.

Potash, J.B., Willour, V.L., Chiu, Y.F., Simpson, S.G., MacKinnon, D.F., Pearlson, G.D., DePaulo, J.R. Jr., and McInnis, M.G. (2001). The familial aggregation of psychotic symptoms in bipolar disorder pedigrees. *Am J Psychiatry*, 158, 1258–1264.

Prien, R.F., Klett, C.J., and Caffey, E.M. Jr. (1973). Lithium carbonate and imipramine in prevention of affective episodes: A comparison in recurrent affective illness. *Arch Gen Psychiatry*, 29, 420–425.

Reed, C., Goetz, I., van Os, J., and Tohen, M. (2005). Comorbid Cannabis Use in Patients with Acute Mania: Functional Status. Presented at the annual meeting of the American Psychiatric Association, Atlanta.

Regier, D.A., Boyd, J.H., Burke, J.D., Jr., Rae, D.S., Myers, J.K., Kramer, M., Robins, L.N., George, L.K., Karno, M., and Locke, B.Z. (1988). One-month prevalence of mental disorders in the United States: Based on five Epidemiologic Catchment Area sites. *Arch Gen Psychiatry*, 45, 977–986.

Regier, D.A., Farmer, M.E., Rae, D.S., Locke, B.Z., Keith, S.J., Judd, L.L., and Goodwin, F.K. (1990). Comorbidity of mental disorders with alcohol and other drug abuse: Results from the Epidemiologic Catchment Area (ECA) Study. *JAMA*, 264, 2511–2518.

Reich, L.H., Davies, R.K., and Himmelhoch, J.M. (1974). Excessive alcohol use in manic-depressive illness. *Am J Psychiatry*, 131, 83–86.

Robins, L.N., and Regier, D.A. (1991). *Psychiatric Disorders in America: The Epidemiologic Catchment Area Study*. New York: Free Press.

Rounsaville, B.J., Weissman, M.M., Kleber, H., and Wilber, C. (1982). Heterogeneity of psychiatric diagnosis in treated opiate addicts. *Arch Gen Psychiatry*, 39, 161–166.

Ruzickova, M., Slaney, C., Garnham, J., and Alda, M. (2003). Clinical features of bipolar disorder with and without comorbid diabetes mellitus. *Can J Psychiatry*, 48, 458–461.

Salloum, I.M., Cornelius, J.R., Douaihy, A., Kirisci, L., Daley, D., Kelly, T. (2005). Patient characteristic and treatment implications of marijuana abuse among bipolar alcoholics: Results from a double blind, placebo-controlled study. *Addict Behav* 30(9), 1702–1708.

Sasson, Y., Chopra, M., Harrari, E., Amitai, K., and Zohar, J. (2003). Bipolar comorbidity: From diagnostic dilemmas to therapeutic challenge. *Int J Neuropsychopharmacol*, 6, 139–144.

Savino, M., Perugi, G., Simonini, E., Soriani, A., Cassano, G.B., and Akiskal, H.S. (1993). Affective comorbidity in panic disorder: Is there a bipolar connection? *J Affect Disord*, 28, 155–163.

Schneck, C.D., Miklowitz, D.J., Calabrese, J.R., Allen, M.H., Thomas, M.R., Wisniewski, S.R., Miyahara, S., Shelton, M.D., Ketter, T.A., Goldberg, J.F., Bowden, C.L., and Sachs, G.S. (2004). Phenomenology of rapid-cycling bipolar disorder: Data from the first 500 participants in the Systematic Treatment Enhancement Program. *Am J Psychiatry*, 161, 1902–1908.

Schnurr, P.P., Friedman, M.J., and Rosenberg, S.D. (1993). Premilitary MMPI scores as predictors of combat-related PTSD symptoms. *Am J Psychiatry*, 150, 479–483.

Schuckit, M.A. (1986). Genetic and clinical implications of alcoholism and affective disorder. *Am J Psychiatry*, 143, 140–147.

Schuckit, M.A., Tipp, J.E., Anthenelli, R.M., Bucholz, K.K., Hesselbrock, V.M., and Nurnberger, J.I. Jr. (1996). Anorexia nervosa and bulimia nervosa in alcohol-dependent men and women and their relatives. *Am J Psychiatry*, 153(1), 74–82.

Secnik, K., Swensen, A., and Lage, M.J. (2005). Comorbidities and costs of adult patients diagnosed with attention-deficit hyperactivity disorder. *Pharmacoeconomics*, 23, 93–102.

Sharma, R., and Markar, H.R. (1994). Mortality in affective disorder. *J Affect Disord*, 31, 91–96.

Silberman, E.K., Reus, V.I., Jimerson, D.C., Lynott, A.M., and Post, R.M. (1981). Heterogeneity of amphetamine response in depressed patients. *Am J Psychiatry*, 138, 1302–1307.

Simon, N.M., Smoller, J.W., Fava, M., Sachs, G., Racette, S.R., Perlis, R., Sonawalla, S., and Rosenbaum, J.F. (2003). Comparing anxiety disorders and anxiety-related traits in bipolar disorder and unipolar depression. *J Psychiatr Res*, 37, 187–192.

Simon, N.M., Otto, M.W., Weiss, R.D., Bauer, M.S., Miyahara, S., Wisniewski, S.R., Thase, M.E., Kogan, J., Frank, E., Nierenberg, A.A., Calabrese, J.R., Sachs, G.S., Pollack, M.H., and STEP-BD Investigators. (2004a). Pharmacotherapy for bipolar disorder and comorbid conditions: Baseline data from STEP-BD. *J Clin Psychopharmacol*, 24, 512–520.

Simon, N.M., Otto, M.W., Wisniewski, S.R., Fossey, M., Sagduyu, K., Frank, E., Sachs, G.S., Nierenberg, A.A., Thase, M.E., and Pollack, M.H. (2004b). Anxiety disorder comorbidity in bipolar disorder patients: Data from the first 500 participants in the Systematic Treatment Enhancement Program for Bipolar Disorder (STEP-BD). *Am J Psychiatry*, 161, 2222–2229.

Simpson, S.G., al-Mufti, R., Andersen, A.E., and DePaulo, J.R. Jr. (1992). Bipolar II affective disorder in eating disorder inpatients. *J Nerv Ment Dis*, 180, 719–722.

Spitzer, R.L., Yanovski, S., Wadden, T., Wing, R., Marcus, M.D., Stunkard, A., Devlin, M., Mitchell, J., Hasin, D., and Horne, R.L. (1993). Binge eating disorder: Its further validation in a multisite study. *Int J Eat Disord*, 13, 137–153.

Strakowski, S.M., Tohen, M., Stoll, A.L., Faedda, G.L., and Goodwin, D.C. (1992). Comorbidity in mania at first hospitalization. *Am J Psychiatry*, 149(4), 554–556.

Strakowski, S.M., Stoll, A.L., Tohen, M., Faedda, G.L., and Goodwin, D.C. (1993). The Tridimensional Personality Questionnaire as a predictor of six-month outcome in first episode mania. *Psychiatry Res*, 48(1), 1–8.

Strakowski, S.M., Sax, K.W., McElroy, S.L., Keck, P.E. Jr., Hawkins, J.M., and West, S.A. (1998). Course of psychiatric and substance abuse syndromes co-occurring with bipolar disorder after a first psychiatric hospitalization. *J Clin Psychiatry*, 59, 465–471.

Strakowski, S.M., DelBello, M.P., Fleck, D.E., and Arndt, S. (2000). The impact of substance abuse on the course of bipolar disorder. *Biol Psychiatry*, 48, 477–485.

Strakowski, S.M., DelBello, M.P., and Fleck, D.E. (2005). Effects of co-occurring alcohol abuse on the course of bipolar disorder following a first hospitalization for mania. *Arch Gen Psychiatry*, 62, 851–858.

Swann, A.C., Secunda, S., Davis, J.M., Robins, E., Hanin, I., Koslow, S.H., and Maas, J.W. (1983). CSF monoamine metabolites in mania. *Am J Psychiatry*, 140, 396–400.

Swartz, K.L., Pratt, L.A., Armenian, H.K., Lee, L.C., and Eaton, W.W. (2000). Mental disorders and the incidence of migraine headaches in a community sample: Results from the Baltimore Epidemiologic Catchment Area Follow-Up Study. *Arch Gen Psychiatry*, 57(10), 945–950.

Swartz, M.S., Swanson, J.W., Hiday, V.A., Borum, R., Wagner, R., and Burns, B.J. (1998). Taking the wrong drugs: The role of substance abuse and medication noncompliance in violence among severely mentally ill individuals. *Soc Psychiatry Psychiatr Epidemiol*, 33(Suppl 1), S75–S80.

Szadoczky, E., Papp, Z., Vitrai, J., Rihmer, Z., and Furedi, J. (1998). The prevalence of major depressive and bipolar disorders in Hungary: Results from a national epidemiologic survey. *J Affect Disord*, 50, 153–162.

Tabata, I., Schluter, J., Gulve, E.A., and Holloszy, J.O. (1994). Lithium increases susceptibility of muscle glucose transport to stimulation by various agents. *Diabetes*, 43, 903–907.

Thomsen, A.F., and Kessing, L.V. (2005). Increased risk of hyperthyroidism among patients hospitalized with bipolar disorder. *Bipolar Disord*, 7, 351–357.

Toalson, P., Ahmed, S., Hardy, T., and Kabinoff, G. (2004). The metabolic syndrome in patients with severe mental illnesses. *J Clin Psychiatry*, 6, 152–158.

Trzepacz, P.T., McCue, M., Klein, I., Levey, G.S., and Greenhouse, J. (1988). A psychiatric and neuropsychological study of patients with untreated Graves' disease. *Gen Hosp Psychiatry*, 10, 49–55.

Tucker, P., Zaninelli, R., Yehuda, R., Ruggiero, L., Dillingham, K., and Pitts, C.D. (2001). Paroxetine in the treatment of chronic posttraumatic stress disorder: Results of a placebo-controlled, flexible-dosage trial. *J Clin Psychiatry*, 62, 860–868.

Valle, J., Ayuso-Gutierrez, J.L., Abril, A., and Ayuso-Mateos, J.L. (1999). Evaluation of thyroid function in lithium-naive bipolar patients. *Eur Psychiatry*, 14, 341–345.

Vieta, E., Colom, F., Corbella, B., Martinez-Aran, A., Reinares, M., Benabarre, A., and Gasto, C. (2001). Clinical correlates of psychiatric comorbidity in bipolar I patients. *Bipolar Disord,* 3(5), 253–258.

Weber-Hamann, B., Hentschel, F., Kniest, A., Deuschle, M., Colla, M., Lederbogen, F., Heuser, I. (2002). Hypercortisolemic depression is associated with increased intra-abdominal fat. *Psychosom Med,* 64, 274–277.

Weeke, A. (1979). Causes of death in manic-depressives. In M. Schou, E. Strömgren (Eds.), *Origin, Prevention and Treatment of Affective Disorders.* London: Academic Press.

Weiller, E., Bisserbe, J.C., Boyer, P., Lepine, J.P., and Lecrubier, Y. (1996). Social phobia in general health care: An unrecognised undertreated disabling disorder. *Br J Psychiatry,* 168, 169–174.

Weiss, R.D., and Mirin, S.M. (1984). Drug, host, and environmental factors in the development of chronic cocaine abuse. In S.M. Mirin (Ed.), *Substance Abuse and Psychopathology* (pp. 41–56). Washington, DC: American Psychiatric Press.

Weiss, R.D., and Mirin, S.M. (1986). Subtypes of cocaine abusers. *Psychiatr Clin North Am,* 9, 491–501.

Weiss, R.D., and Mirin, S.M. (1987). Substance abuse as an attempt at self-medication. *Psychiatr Med,* 3, 357–367.

Weiss, R.D., Mirin, S.M., Michael, J.L., and Sollogub, A.C. (1986). Psychopathology in chronic cocaine abusers. *Am J Drug Alcohol Abuse,* 12, 17–29.

Weiss, R.D., Mirin, S.M., Griffin, M.L., and Michael, J.L. (1988). Psychopathology in cocaine abusers: Changing trends. *J Nerv Ment Dis,* 176, 719–725.

Weiss, R.D., Kolodziej, M., Griffin, M.L., Najavits, L.M., Jacobson, L.M., and Greenfield, S.F. (2004). Substance use and perceived symptom improvement among patients with bipolar disorder and substance dependence. *J Affect Disord,* 79, 279–283.

Wenzel, K.W., Meinhold, H., Raffenberg, M., Adlkofer, F., and Schleusener, H. (1974). Classification of hypothyroidism in evaluating patients after radioiodine therapy by serum cholesterol, T3-uptake, total T4, FT4-index, total T3, basal TSH and TRH-test. *Eur J Clin Invest,* 4, 141–148.

Whitwell, J.R. (1936). *Historical Notes on Psychiatry (Early times–End of 16th Century).* London: H.K. Lewis.

Wilens, T.E., Biederman, J., Wozniak, J., Gunawardene, S., Wong, J., and Monuteaux, M. (2003). Can adults with attention-deficit/hyperactivity disorder be distinguished from those with comorbid bipolar disorder? Findings from a sample of clinically referred adults. *Biol Psychiatry,* 54, 1–8.

Winokur, G., Clayton, P.J., and Reich, T. (1969). *Manic Depressive Illness.* St. Louis: C.V. Mosby.

Winokur, G., Coryell, W., Akiskal, H.S., Maser, J.D., Keller, M.B., Endicott, J., and Mueller, T. (1995). Alcoholism in manic-depressive (bipolar) illness: Familial illness, course of illness, and the primary-secondary distinction. *Am J Psychiatry,* 152, 365–372.

Winokur, G., Turvey, C., Akiskal, H., Coryell, W., Solomon, D., and Leon, A. (1998). Alcoholism and drug abuse in three groups: Bipolar I, unipolars, and their acquaintances. *J Affect Dis,* 50, 81–89.

Wise, T., and Fernandez, F. (1979). Psychological profiles of candidates seeking surgical correction for obesity. *Obesity/Bariatric Med,* 8, 83–86.

Wurmser, L. (1974). Pscyhoanalytic considerations of the etiology of compulsive drug use. *J Am Psychoanal Assoc,* 22, 820–843.

Yates, W.R., and Wallace, R. (1987). Cardiovascular risk factors in affective disorder. *J Affect Disord,* 12, 129–134.

Young, L.T., Cooke, R.G., Robb, J.C., Levitt, A.J., and Joffe, R.T. (1993). Anxious and non-anxious bipolar disorder. *J Affect Disord,* 29, 49–52.

Young, L.T., Warsh, J.J., Kish, S.J., Shannak, K., and Hornykeiwicz, O. (1994). Reduced brain 5-HT and elevated NE turnover and metabolites in bipolar affective disorder. *Biol Psychiatry,* 35, 121–127.

Zilboorg, G. (1941). *A History of Medical Psychology.* New York: W.W. Norton.

Zisook, S., and Schuckit, M.A. (1987). Male primary alcoholics with and without family histories of affective disorder. *J Stud Alcohol,* 48, 337–344.

CHAPTER 8

Alvarez, J.C., Cremniter, D., Bluck, N., Quintin, P., Leboyer, M., Berlin, I., Therond, P., and Spreuz-Varoquaux, O. (2000). Low serum cholesterol in violent but not in non-violent suicide attempters. *Psychiatry Res,* 21, 95(2), 103–108.

Angst, F., Strassen, H.H., Clayton, P.J., and Angst, J. (2002). Mortality of patients with mood disorders: Follow-up over 34–38 years. *J Affect Disord,* 68(2–3), 167–181.

Angst, J., Sellaro, R., and Angst, F. (1998). Long-term outcome and mortality of treated versus untreated bipolar and depressed patients: A preliminary report. *Int J Psychiatry Clin,* Practice 2, 115–119.

Angst, J., Angst, F., and Strassen, H.H. (1999). Suicide risk in patients with major depressive disorder. *J Clin Psychiatry,* 60(Suppl 2), 57–62; discussion 75–76, 113–116.

Appleby, L., Shaw, J., Amos, T., McDonnell, R., Harris, C., McCann, K., Kiernan, K., Davies, S., Bickley, H., and Parsons, R. (1999). Suicide within 12 months of contact with mental health services: National clinical survey. *BMJ,* 318(7193), 1235–1239.

Arango, V., Underwood, M.D., Gubbi, A.V., and Mann, J.J. (1995). Localized alterations in pre- and postsynaptic serotonin binding sites in the ventrolateral prefrontal cortex of suicide victims. *Brain Res,* 688(1–2), 121–133.

Arango, V., Underwood, M.D., and Mann, J.J. (1997). Postmortem findings in suicide victims: Implications for in vivo imaging studies. *Ann N Y Acad Sci,* 836, 269–287.

Arato, M., Banki, C.M., Bissette, G., and Nemeroff, C.B. (1989). Elevated CSF-CRF in suicide victims. *Biol Psychiatry,* 25(3), 355–359.

Asberg, M., Bertilisson, L., Cronholm, B., Harfast, A., Sjoqvist, F., and Tuck, D. (1972). Studies of indolamine metabolites in cerebrospinal fluid in depression. *Nord Psykiatr Tidsskr,* 26(6), 351–357.

Aschoff, J. (1981). Annual rhythms in man. In J. Aschoff (Ed.), *Handbook of Behavioral Neurobiology.* Vol. 4: *Biological Rhythms* (pp. 475–487). New York: Plenum Press.

Baca-Garcia, E., Vaquero, C., Diaz-Sastre, C., Ceverino, A., Saiz-Ruiz, J., Fernandez-Piquera, J., and de Leon, J. (2003). A pilot study on a gene-hormone interaction in female suicide attempts. *Eur Arch Psychiatry Clin Neurosci,* 253(6), 281.

Baca-Garcia, E., Vaquero, C., Diaz-Sastre, C., Garcia-Resa, E., Saiz-Ruiz, J., Fernandez-Piqueras, J., and De Leon, J. (2004). Lack of association between the serotonin transporter promoter gene polymorphism and impulsivity or aggressive behavior among suicide attempters and healthy volunteers. *Psychiatry Res,* 126(2), 99–106.

Balazs, J., Lecrubier, Y., Csiszer, N., Kosztak, J., and Bitter, L. (2003). Prevalence and comorbidity of affective disorders in persons making suicide attempts in Hungary: Importance of the first depressive episodes and of bipolar II diagnoses. *J Affect Disord*, 76(1–3), 113–119.

Baldessarini, R.J., and Hennen, J. (2004). Genetics of suicide: An overview. *Harv Rev Psychiatry*, 12(1), 1–13.

Ballenger, J.C., Goodwin, F.K., Major, F.L., and Brown, G.L. (1979). Alcohol and central serotonin metabolism in man. *Arch Gen Psychiatry*, 36, 224–227.

Barner-Rasmussen, P. (1986). Suicide in psychiatric patients in Denmark, 1971–1981. II: Hospital utilization and risk groups. *Acta Psychiatr Scand*, 73(4), 449–455.

Barraclough, B. (1970). The diagnostic classification and psychiatric treatment of 100 suicides. In R. Fox (Ed.), *Proceedings of the Fifth International Conference for Suicide Prevention* (pp. 129–132). Vienna, Austria: IASP.

Barraclough, B., Bunch, J., Nelson, B., and Sainsbury, P. (1974). A hundred cases of suicide: Clinical aspects. *Br J Psychiatry*, 125, 355–373.

Bauer, M.S., Calabrese, J., Dunner, D.L., Post, R., Whybrow, P.C., Gyulai, L., Tay, L.K., Younkin, S.R., Bynum, D., and Lavori, P. (1994). Multisite data reanalysis of the validity of rapid cycling as a course modifier for bipolar disorder in DSM-IV. *Am J Psychiatry*, 151(4), 506–515.

Beck, A.T., Brown, G.K., Steer, R.A., Dahlsgaard, K.K., and Grisham, J.R. (1999). Suicide ideation at its worst point: A predictor of eventual suicide in psychiatric outpatients. *Suicide Life Threat Behav*, 29(1), 1–9.

Behall, K.M., Scholfield, D.J., Hallfrisch, J.G., Kelsay, J.L., and Reiser, S. (1984). Seasonal variation in plasma glucose and hormone levels in adult men and women. *Am J Clin Nutr*, 40, 1352–1356.

Bertolote, J.M., and Fleischmann, A. (2002). Suicide rates in China. *Lancet*, 359(9325), 2274.

Black, D.W., Winokur, G., and Nassrallah, A. (1988). Effects of psychosis on suicide risk in 1593 patients with unipolar and bipolar affective disorders. *Am J Psychiatry*, 145, 849–852.

Bocchetta, A., Chillotti, C., Carboni, G., Oi, A., Ponti, M., and Del Zompo, M. (2001). Association of personal and familial suicide risk with low serum cholesterol concentration in male lithium patients. *Acta Psychiatr Scand*, 104(1), 37–41.

Bondy, B., Erfurth, A., de Jonge, S., Kruger, M., and Meyer, H. (2000). Possible association of the short allele of the serotonin transporter promoter gene polymorphism (5-HTTLPR) with violent suicide. *Mol Psychiatry*, 5(2), 193–195.

Bonnier, B., Garwood, P., Harmon, M., Surfeit, Y., Bony, C., and Hardy-Bale, M.C. (2002). Association of 5-HT(2A) receptor gene polymorphism with major affective disorders: The case of a subgroup of bipolar disorder with low suicide risk. *Biol Psychiatry*, 51(9), 762–765.

Boston, P.F., Durson, S.M., and Reveley, M.A. (1996). Cholesterol and mental disorder. *Br J Psychiatry*, 169, 682–689.

Bostwick, J.M., and Pankratz, V.S. (2000). Affective disorders and suicide risk: A reexamination. *Am J Psychiatry*, 157(12), 1925–1932.

Bottlender, R., Jager, M., Strauss, A., and Moller, H.J. (2000). Suicidality in bipolar compared to unipolar depressed inpatients. *Eur Arch Psychiatry Clin Neurosci*, 250(5), 257–261.

Brent, D.A., Bridge, J., Johnson, B.A., Connolly, J. (1996). Suicidal behavior runs in families: A controlled family study of adolescent suicide victims. *Arch Gen Psychiatry*, 53(2), 1145–1152.

Brent, D.A., Oquendo, M., Birmaher, B., Greenhill, L., Kolko, D., Stanley, B., Zelazny, J., Brodsky, B., Firinciogullari, S., Ellis, S.P., and Mann, J.J. (2003). Peripubertal suicide attempts in offspring of suicide attempters siblings concordant for suicidal behavior. *Am J Psychiatry*, 160(8), 1486–1493.

Brodersen, A., Licht, R.W., Vestergaard, P., Olesen, A.V., and Mortensen, P.B. (2000). *Br J Psychiatry*, 176, 429–433.

Brown, G.K., Beck, A.T., Steer, R.A., and Grisham, J.R, (2000). Risk factors for suicide in psychiatric outpatients: A 20-year prospective study. *J Consult Clin Psychol*, 68(3), 371–377.

Brown, R.P., Mason, B., Stoll, P., Brizer, D., Kocsis, J., Stokes, P.E., and Mann, J.J. (1986). Consistency of pituitary-adrenocortical function across multiple psychiatric hospitalizations. *Psychiatry Research*. 17, 317–323.

Brunner, J., and Bronisch, T. (1999). Neurobiological correlates of suicidal behavior. *Fortschr Neurol Psychiatr*, 67(9), 391–412.

Bulik, C.M., Carpenter, L.L., Kupfer, D.J., and Frank, E. (1990). Features associated with suicide attempts in recurrent major depression. *J Affect Disord*, 18(1), 29–37.

Bunney, W.E., and Fawcett, J.A. (1965). Possibility of a biochemical test for suicidal potential: An analysis of endocrine findings prior to three studies. *Arch Gen Psychiatry* 13, 232–239.

Bunney, W.E. Jr., Fawcett, J.A., Davis, J.M., and Gifford, S. (1969). Further evaluation of urinary 17-hydroxycorticosteroids in suicidal patients. *Arch Gen Psychiatry*, 21(2), 138–150.

Busch, K.A., Fawcett, J., and Jacobs, D.G. (2003). Clinical correlates of inpatient suicide. *J Clin Psychiatry*, 64(1), 14–19.

Caetano, S.C., Olvera, R.L., Hunter, K., Hatch, J.P., Najt, P., Bowden, C., Pliszka, S., and Soares, J.C. (2006). Association of psychosis with suicidality in pediatric bipolar I, II and bipolar NOS patients. *J Affect Disord*, 91, 33–37.

Carlsson, A., Svennerholm, L., and Winblad, B. (1979). Seasonal and circadian monoamine variations in human brains examined postmorten. *Acta Psychiatr Scand*, 280, 75–83.

Caspi, A., Sugden, K., Moffitt, T.E., Taylor, A., Craig, I.W., Harrington, H., McClay, J., Mill, J., Martin, J., Braithwaite, A., and Poulton, R. (2003). Influence of life stress on depression: Moderation by a polymorphism in the 5-HTT gene. *Science*, 301(5631), 386–389.

Cassano, G.B., Akiskal, H.S., Savino, M., Musetti, S.M., and Perugi, G. (1992). Proposed subtypes of bipolar II and related disorders: With hypomanic episodes (or cyclothymia) and with hyperthymic temperament. *J Affect Disord*, 26(2), 127–140.

Cassidy, F., and Carroll, B.J. (2002a). Hypocholesterolemia during mixed manic episodes. *Eur Arch Psychiatry Clin Neurosci*, 252(3), 110–114.

Cassidy, F., and Carroll, B.J. (2002b). Seasonal variation of mixed and pure episodes of bipolar disorder. *J Affect Disord*, 68(1), 25–31.

Cheng, A.T., Chen, T.H., Chen, C.C., and Jenkins, R. (2000). Psychosocial and psychiatric risk factors for suicide: Case-control psychological autopsy study. *Br J Psychiatry*, 177, 360–365.

Chew, K.S., and McCleary, R. (1995). The spring peak in suicides: A cross-national analysis. *Soc Sci Med*, 40(2), 223–230.

Clark, D.A. (1991). *Crisis Intervention and Suicide Prevention from a Rural Perspective*. New York: NLN. NLN Publication 21-2408, pp. 165–172.

Cloninger, C.R. (2000). A practical way to diagnose personality disorder: A proposal. *J Personal Disord*, 14(2), 99–108.

Cloninger, C.R., Svrakic, D.M., and Przybeck, T.R. (1993). A psychobiological model of temperament and character. *Arch Gen Psychiatry*, 50(12), 975–990.

Cloninger, C.R., Van Eerdewegh, P., Goate, A., Edenberg, H.J., Blangero, J., Hesselbrock, V., Reich, T., Nurnberger, J. Jr., Schuckit, M., Porjesz, B., Crowe, R., Rice, J.P., Foroud, T., Przybeck, T.R., Almasy, L., Bucholz, K., Wu, W., Shears, S., Carr, K., Crose, C., Willig, C., Zhao, J., Tischfield, J.A., Li, T.K., and Conneally, P.M. (1998). Anxiety proneness linked to epistatic loci in genome scan of human personality traits. *Am J Med Genet*, 81(4), 313–317.

Cornelius, J.R., Salloum, I.M., Mezzich, J., Cornelius, M.D., Fabrega, H. Jr., Ehler, J.G., Ulrich, R.F., Thast, M.E., and Mann, J.J. (1995). Disproportionate suicidality in patients with comorbid major depression and alcoholism. *Am J Psychiatry*, 152(3), 358–364.

Coryell, W. (1990). DST abnormality as a predictor of course in major depression. *J Affect Disord*, 19(3), 163–169.

Coryell, W., and Schlesser, M. (2001). The dexamethasone suppression test and suicide prediction. *Am J Psychiatry*, 158(5), 748–753.

Coryell, W., and Tsuang, M.T. (1982). Primary unipolar depression and the prognostic importance of delusions. *Arch Gen Psychiatry*, 39, 1181–1184.

Coryell, W., Andreasen, N.C., Endicott, J., and Keller, M. (1987). The significance of past mania or hypomania in the course and outcome of major depression. *Am J Psychiatry*, 144(3), 309–315.

Coryell, W., Solomon, D., Turvey, C., Keller, M., Leon, A.C., Endicott, J., Schettler, P., Judd, L., and Mueller, T. (2003). The long-term course of rapid-cycling bipolar disorder. *Arch Gen Psychiatry*, 60(9), 914–920.

Courtet, P., Picot, M.C., Bellivier, F., Torres, S., Jollant, F., Michelon, C., Castelnau, D., Astruc, B., Buresi, C., and Malafosse, A. (2004). Serotonin transporter gene may be involved in short-term risk of subsequent suicide attempts. *Biol Psychiatry*, 55(1), 46–51.

D'Hondt, P., Maes, M., Leysen, J.E., Gommeren, W., Scharpe, S., and Cosyns, P. (1994). Binding of [3H]paroxetine to platelets of depressed patients: Seasonal differences and effects of diagnostic classification. *J Affect Disord*, 32(1), 27–35.

D'Mello, D.A., McNeil, J.A., and Msibi, B. (1995). Seasons and bipolar disorder. *Ann Clin Psychiatry*, 7(1), 11–18.

De Vriese, S.R., Christophe, A.B., and Maes, M. (2004). In humans, the seasonal variation in poly-unsaturated fatty acids is related to the seasonal variation in violent suicide and serotonergic markers of violent suicide. *Prostaglandins Leukot Essent Fatty Acids*, 71(1), 13–18.

Desai, R.A., Dausey, D.J., and Rosenheck, R.A. (2005). Mental health service delivery and suicide risk: The role of individual patient and facility factors. *Am J Psychiatry*, 162(2), 311–318.

Dilsaver, S.C., and Chen, Y.W. (2003). Social phobia, panic disorder and suicidality in subjects with pure and depressive mania. *J Affect Disord*, 77(2), 173–177.

Dilsaver, S.C., Chen, Y.W., Swann, A.C., Shoaib, A.M., and Krajewski, K.J. (1994). Suicidality in patients with pure and depressive mania. *Am J Psychiatry*, 151(9), 1312–1315.

Dilsaver, S.C., Chen, Y.W., Swann, A.C., Shoaib, A.M., Tsai-Dilsaver, Y., and Krajewski, K.J. (1997). Suicidality, panic disorder and psychosis in bipolar depression, depressive-mania and pure-mania. *Psychiatry Res*, 73(1-2), 47–56.

Dilsaver, S.C., Benazzi, F., Rihmer, Z., Akiskal, K.K., and Akiskal, H.S. (2005). Gender, suicidality and bipolar mixed states in adolescents. *J Affect Disord*, 87, 11–16.

Dorovini-Zis, K., and Zis, A.P. (1987). Increased adrenal weight in victims of violent suicide. *Am J Psychiatry*, 144(9), 1214–1215.

Dorpat, T.L., and Ripley, H.S. (1960). A study of suicide in the Seattle area. *Compr Psychiatry*, 1, 349–359.

Dunner, D.L., Gershon, E.S., and Goodwin, F.K. (1976). Heritable factors in the severity of affective illness. *Biol Psychiatry*, 11(1), 31–42.

Egeland, J.A., and Sussex, J.N. (1985). Suicide and family loading for affective disorders. *JAMA*, 254(7), 915–918.

Ellison, L.F., and Morrison, H.I. (2001). Low serum cholesterol concentration and risk of suicide. *Epidemiology*, 12(2), 168–172.

Endicott, J., Nee, J., Andreasen, N., Clayton, P., Keller, M., and Coryell, W. (1985). Bipolar II: Combine or keep separate? *J Affect Disord*, 8(1), 17–28.

Engstrom, C., Brandstrom, S., Sigvardsson, S., Cloninger, R., and Nylander, P.O. (2003). Bipolar disorder II: Personality and age of onset. *Bipolar Disord*, 5(5), 340–348.

Fawcett, J., and Bunney, W.E. (1967). Pituitary adrenal function and depression: An outline for research. *Arch Gen Psychiatry*, 16, 517–535.

Fawcett, J., Edwards, J.H., Kravitz, H.M., and Jeffriess, H. (1987). Alprazolam: An antidepressant? Alprazolam, desipramine, and an alprazolam-desipramine combination in the treatment of adult depressed outpatients. *J Clin Psychopharmacol*, 7(5), 295–310.

Fawcett, J., Scheftner, W.A., Fogg, L., Clark, D.C., Young, M.A., Hedeker, D. (1990). Gibbons, R. Time-related predictors of suicide in major affective disorder. *Am J Psychiatry*, 147(9), 1189–1194.

Fawcett, J., Busch, K.A., Jacobs, D., Kravitz, H.M., and Fogg, L. (1997). Suicide: A four-pathway clinical-biochemical model. *Ann N Y Acad Sci*, 836, 288–301.

Fisher, A.J., Parry, C.D., Bradshaw, D., and Juritz, J.M. (1997). Seasonal variation of suicide in South Africa. *Psychiatry Res*, 66(1), 13–22.

Fitch, D., Lesage, A., Seguin, M., Trousignant, M., Bankelfat, C., Rouleau, G.A., and Turecki, G. (2001). Suicide and the serotonin transporter gene. *Mol Psychiatry*, 6(2), 127–128.

Foster, T., Gillespie, K., McClelland, R., and Patterson, C. (1999). Risk factors for suicide independent of DSM-III-R Axis I disorder: Case-control psychological autopsy study in Northern Ireland. *Br J Psychiatry*, 175, 175–179.

Frangos, E., Athanassenas, G., Tsitourides, S., Psilolignos, P., and Katsanou, N. (1983). Psychotic depressive disorder: A separate entity? *J Affective Disord*, 5, 259–265.

Frank, J.D., and Frank, J.B. (1991). *Persuasion and Healing: A Comparative Study of Psychotherapy*, 3rd ed. Baltimore: Johns Hopkins University Press.

Fruehwald, S., Frottler, P., Matschnig, T., Loenig, F., Lehr, S., and Eher, R. (2004). Do monthly or seasonal variations exist in suicides in a high-risk setting? *Psychiatry Res*, 121(3), 301–302.

Fu, Q., Heath, A., Bucholz, K.K., Nelson, E.C., Glowinski, A., Goldberg, J., Lyons, M.J., Tsuang, M.T., Jacob, T., True, M.R., and Eisen, S.A. (2002). A twin study of genetic and environmental influences on suicidality in men. *Psychol Med*, 32, 11–24.

Galfalvy, H., Oquendo, M.A., Carballo, J.J., Sher, L., Grunebaum, M.F., Burke, A., and Mann, J.J. (2006). Clinical predictors of suicidal acts after major depression in bipolar disorder: A prospective study. *Bipolar Disord*, 8, 586–595.

Geddes, J.R., and Juszczak, E. (1995). Period trends in rate of suicide in first 28 days after discharge from psychiatric hospital in Scotland, 1968–1992. *BMJ*, 311(7001), 357–360.

Geddes, J.R., Juszczak, E., O'Brien, F., and Kendrick, S. (1997). Suicide in the 12 months after discharge from psychiatric inpatient care, Scotland 1968–1992. *J Epidemiol Community Health*, 51(4), 430–434.

Geijer, T., Frisch, A., Persson, M.L., Wasserman, D., Rockah, R., Michaelovsky, E., Apter, A., Jonsson, E.G., Nothen, M.M., and Weizman, A. (2000). Search for association between suicide attempt and serotonergic polymorphisms. *Psychiatr Genet*, 10(1), 19–26.

Glowinski, A.L., Bucholtz, K.K., Nelson, E.C., Fu, Q., Madden, P.A., Reich, W., Heath, A.C. (2001). Suicide attempts in an adolescent female twin sample. *J Am Acad Child Adolesc Psychiatry*, 40(11), 1300–1307.

Goldberg, J.F., and Ernst, C.L. (2004). Clinical correlates of childhood and adolescent adjustment in adult patients with bipolar disorder. *J Nerv Ment Dis*, 192(3), 187–192.

Goldberg, J.F., Garno, J.L., Leon, A.C., Kocsis, J.H., and Portera, L. (1998). Association of recurrent suicidal ideation with nonremission from acute mixed mania. *Am J Psychiatry*, 155(12), 1753–1755.

Goldberg, J.F., Garno, J.L., Portera, L., Leon, A.C., Kocsis, J.H., Whiteside, J.E. (1999). Correlates of suicidal ideation in dysphoric mania. *J Affect Disord*, 56(1), 75–81.

Goldstein, R.B., Black, D.W., Nasrallah, A., and Winokur, G. (1991). The prediction of suicide: Sensitivity, specificity, and predictive value of a multivariate model applied to suicide among 1906 patients with affective disorders. *Arch Gen Psychiatry*, 48(5), 418–422.

Golomb, B.A., Tenkanen, L., Alikoski, T., Niskanen, T., Manninen, V., Huttunen, M., and Mednick, S.A. (2002). Insulin sensitivity markers: Predictors of accidents and suicides in Helsinki Heart Study screenees. *J Clin Epidemiol*, 55(8), 767–773.

Gonzalez-Maeso, J., Rodriguez-Puertas, R., Meana, J.J., Garcia-Sevilla, J.A., and Guimon, J. (2002). Neurotransmitter receptor-mediated activation of G-proteins in brains of suicide victims with mood disorders: Selective supersensitivity of alpha (2A)-adrenoceptors. *Mol Psychiatry*, 7(7), 755–767.

Gonzalez-Pinto, A., Mosquera, F., Alonso, M., Lopez, P., Ramirez, F., Vieta, E., and Baldessarini, R.J. (2006). Suicidal risk in bipolar I disorder patients and adherence to long-term lithium treatment. *Bipolar Disord*, 8, 618–624.

Gordon, D.J., Trost, D.C., Hyde, J., Whaley, F.S., Hannan, P.J., Jacobs, D.R., and Ekelund, L.-G. (1987). Seasonal cholesterol cycles: The lipid research clinics coronary primary prevention trial placebo group. *Circulation*, 76, 1224–1231.

Granberg, D., and Westerberg, C. (1999). On abandoning life when it is least difficult. *Soc Biol*, 46(1–2), 154–162.

Greening, L., and Stoppelbein, L. (2002). Religiosity, attributional style, and social support as psychosocial buffers for African American and white adolescents' perceived risk for suicide. *Suicide Life Threat Behav*, 32(4), 404–417.

Grunebaum, M.F., Galfalvy, H.C., Oquendo, M.A., Burke, A.K., and Mann, J.J. (2004). Melancholia and the probability and lethality of suicide attempt. *Br J Psychiatry*, 184, 534–535.

Grunebaum, M.F., Ramsay, S.R., Galfalvy, H.C., Ellis, S.P., Burke, A.K., Sher, L., Printz, D.J., Kahn, D.A., Mann, J.J., and

Oquendo, M.A. (2006). Correlates of suicide attempt history in bipolar disorder: A stress-diathesis perspective. *Bipolar Disord*, 8, 551–557.

Guze, S.B., and Robins, E. (1970). Suicide and primary affective disorders. *Br J Psychiatry*, 117(539), 437–439.

Haberlandt, W.F. (1967). Contribution to the genetics of suicide. Data in twins and familial findings. *Folia Clin Int (Barc)*, 17(6), 319–322.

Hagnell, O., Lanke, J., and Rorsman, B. (1981). Suicide rates in the Lundby Study: Mental illness as a risk factor for suicide. *Neuropsychobiology*, 7, 248–253.

Hakko, H., Rasanen, P., and Tiihonen, J. (1998). Seasonal variation in suicide occurrence in Finland. *Acta Psychiatr Scand*, 98(2), 92–97.

Hall, R.C., Platt, D.E., and Hall, R.C. (1999). Suicide risk assessment: A review of risk factors for suicide in 100 patients who made severe suicide attempts. Evaluation of suicide risk in a time of managed care. *Psychosomatics*, 40(1), 18–27.

Harris, E.C., and Barraclough, B. (1997). Suicide as an outcome for mental disorders. A meta-analysis. *Br J Psychiatry*, 170, 205–228.

Hawton, K., Sutton, L., Haw, C., Sinclair, J., and Harriss, L. (2005). Suicide and attempted suicide in bipolar disorder: A system review of risk factors. *J Clin Psychiatry*, 66, 693–704.

Heikkinen, M.E., Henriksson, M.M., Isometsa, E.T., Marttunen, M.H., Aro, H.M., and Lonnqvist, J.K. (1997). Recent life events and suicide in personality disorders. *J Nerv Ment Dis*, 185(6), 373–381.

Heim, C., and Nemeroff, C.B. (1999). The impact of early adverse experiences on brain systems involved in the pathophysiology of anxiety and affective disorders. *Biol Psychiatry*, 46(11), 1509–1522.

Heim, C., and Nemeroff, C.B. (2002). Neurobiology of early life stress: Clinical studies. *Semin Clin Neuropsychiatry*, 7(2), 147–159.

Henriksson, M.M., Aro, H.M., Marttunen, M.J., Heikkinen, M.E., Isometsa, E.T., Kuoppasalmi, K.I., and Lonnqvist, J.K. (1993). Mental disorders and comorbidity in suicide. *Am J Psychiatry*, 150(6), 935–940.

Hibbeln, J.R. (1998). Fish consumption and major depression. *Lancet*, 351, 1213.

Hillbrand, M., and Spitz, R.T. (Eds.) (1992). *Lipids, Health, and Behavior*. Washington, DC: American Psychiatric Association.

Hiroi, N., Wong, M.L., Licino, J., Park, C., Young, M., Gold, P.W., Chrousos, G.P., and Bornstein, S.R. (2001). Expression of corticotropin releasing hormone receptors type I and type II mRNA in suicide victims and controls. *Mol Psychiatry*, 6(5), 540–546.

Hucks, D., Lowther, S., Cromptom, M.R., Katona, C.L., and Horton, R.W. (1997). Corticotropin-releasing factor binding sites in cortex of depressed suicides. *Psychopharmacology (Berl)*, 134(2), 174–178.

Inskip, H.M., Harris, E.C., and Barraclough, B. (1998). Lifetime risk of suicide for affective disorder, alcoholism and schizophrenia. *Br J Psychiatry*, 172, 35–37.

Institute of Medicine (IOM). (2002). *Reducing Suicide: A National Imperative*. Washington, DC: National Academy Press.

Isometsa, E.T., Henriksson, M.M., Aro, H.M., and Lonnqvist, J.K. (1994a). Suicide in bipolar disorder in Finland. *Am J Psychiatry*, 151(7), 1020–1024.

Isometsa, E.T., Henriksson, M.M., Aro, H.M., Heikkinen, M.E., Kuoppasalmi, K.I., and Lönnqvist, J.K. (1994b). Suicide in major depression. *Am J Psychiatry*, 151, 530–536.

Jacobs, D.G., Baldessarini, R.J., Conwell, Y., Fawcett, J., Horton, L., Meltzer, H., Pfeffer, C.R., and Simon, R.L. (2003). Practice guideline for the assessment and treatment of patients with suicide behaviors. American Psychiatric Association. Available: http://www.psych.org/psych_pract/treatg/pg/suicidalbehaviors_05-15-06.pdf (accessed 12/1/06).

Jameison, G.R. (1936). Suicide and mental disease: A clinical analysis of one hundred cases. *Arch Neurol Psychiatry*, 36, 1–12.

Jameison, G.R., and Wall, J.H. (1933). Some psychiatric aspects of suicide. *Psychiatr Q*, 7, 211–229.

Jamison, K.R. (1999). *Night Falls Fast: Understanding Suicide.* New York: Alfred A. Knopf.

Johnson, B.A., Brent, D.A., Bridge, J., and Connolly, J. (1998). The familial aggregation of adolescent suicide attempts. *Acta Psychiatr Scan*, 97(1), 18–24.

Johnson, G.F., and Hunt, G. (1979). Suicidal behavior in bipolar manic-depressive patients and their families. *Compr Psychiatry*, 20, 159–164.

Johnson, J.L., and Cameron, M.C. (2001). Barriers to providing effective mental health services to American Indians. *Ment Health Serv Res*, 3(4), 215–223.

Joiner, T.E., Jr., Conwell, Y., Fitzpatrick, K.K., Witte, T.K., Schmidt, N.B., Berlim, M.T., Fleck, M.P.A., and Rudd, M.D. (2005). Four studies on how past and current suicidology relate even when "everything but the kitchen sink" is covaried. *J Abnorm Psychol*, 114, 291–303.

Juurlink, D.N., Herrmann, N., Szalai, J.P., Kopp, A., and Redelmeier, D.A. (2004). Medical illness and the risk of suicide in the elderly. *Arch Intern Med*, 164(11), 1179–1184.

Kaslow, N.J., Thompson, M.P., Meadows, L., Chance, S., Puett, R., Hollins, L., Jessee, S., and Kellermann A. (2000). Risk factors for suicide attempts among African American women. *Depress Anxiety*, 12(1), 13–20.

Kaslow, N.J., Price, A.W., Wyckoff, S., Bender Grall, M., Sherry, A., Young, S., Scholl, L., Millington Upshaw, V., Rashid, A., Jackson, E.B., and Bethea, K. (2004). Person factors associated with suicidal behavior among African American women and men. *Cultur Divers Ethnic Minor Psychol*, 10(1), 5–22.

Keilp, J.G., Sackeim, H.A., Brodsky, B.S., Oquendo, M.A., Malone, K.M., and Mann, J.J. (2001). Neuropsychological dysfunction in depressed suicide attempters. *Am J Psychiatry*, 158(5), 735–741.

Keith-Spiegel, P., and Spiegel, D.E. (1967). Affective states of patients immediately preceding suicide. *J Psychiatr Res*, 5(2), 89–93.

Keith-Spiegel, P., and Spiegel, D.E. (1979). Affective states of patients immediately preceding suicide. *J Psychiatr Res*, 5, 89–93.

Kety, S.S. (1987). The significance of genetic factors in the etiology of schizophrenia: Results from the national study of adoptees in Denmark. *J Psychiart Res*, 21(4), 423–429.

Kety, S.S., Rosenthal, D., Wender, P.H., and Schulsinger, F. (1968). The types and prevalence of mental illness in the biological and adoptive families of adopted schizophrenics. *J Psychiatr Res*, 6, 345–362.

Kim, C., Lesage, A., Seguin, M., Chawky, N., Vanier, C., Lipp, O., and Turecki, G. (2003). Patterns of co-morbidity in male suicide completers. *Psychol Med*, 33(7), 1299–1309.

Kotin, J., and Goodwin, F.K. (1972). Depression during mania: Clinical observations and theoretical implications. *Am J Psychiatry*, 129, 679–686.

Koukopoulos, A., and Koukopoulos, A. (1999). Agitated depression as a mixed state and the problem of melancholia. *Psychiatr Clin North Am*, 22(3), 547–564.

Kraepelin, E. (1921). *Manic-Depressive Insanity and Paranoia.* Translated by R.M. Barclay. Edinburgh, Scotland: E & S Livingstone.

Krieger, G. (1970). Biochemical predictors of suicide. *Dis Nerv Syst*, 31(7), 478–482.

Kunugi, H., Ishida, S., Kato, T., Sakai, T., Tatsumi, M., Hirose, T., and Nanko, S. (1999). No evidence for an association of polymorphisms of the tryptophan hydroxylase gene with affective disorders or attempted suicide among Japanese patients. *Am J Psychiatry*, 156(5), 774–776.

Lacoste, V., and Wirz-Justice, A. (1989). Seasonal variation in normal subjects: An update of variables current in depression research. In N. Rosenthal, M. Blehar (Eds.), *Seasonal Affective Disorders and Phototherapy* (pp. 167–229). New York: Guilford Press.

Lalovic, A., Sequeira, A., DeGuzman, R., Chawky, N., Lesage, A., Seguin, M., and Turecki, G. (2004). Investigation of completed suicide and genes involved in cholesterol metabolism. *J Affect Disord*, 79(1–3), 25–32.

Lee, H.-C., Lin, H.-C., Tsai, S.-Y., Li, C.-Y., Chen, C.-C., and Huang, C.-C. (2006). Suicide rates and the association with climate: A population-based study. *J Affect Disord*, 92, 221–226.

Lesch, K.P., Bengel, D., Heils, A., Sabol, S.Z., Greenberg, B.D., Petri, S., Benjamin, J., Muller, C.R., Hamer, D.H., Murphy, D.L. (1996). Association of anxiety-related traits with a polymorphism in the serotonin transporter gene regulatory region. *Science*, 274(5292), 1527–1531.

Lester, D. (1992). The dexamethasone suppression test as an indicator of suicide: A meta-analysis. *Pharmacopsychiatry*, 25(6), 265–270.

Lester, D. (1995). The concentration of neurotransmitter metabolites in the cerebrospinal fluid of suicidal individuals: A meta-analysis. *Pharmacopsychiatry*, 28(2), 45–50.

Lester, D. (2002). Serum cholesterol levels and suicide: A meta-analysis. *Suicide Life Threat Behav*, 32(3), 333–346.

Leverich, G.S., McElroy, S.L., Suppes, T., Keck, P.E. Jr., Denicoff, K.D., Nolen, W.A., Altshuler, L.L., Rush, A.J., Kupka, R., Frye, M.A., Autio, K.A., and Post, R.M. (2002). Early physical and sexual abuse associated with an adverse course of bipolar illness. *Biol Psychiatry*, 51(4), 288–297.

Leverich, G.S., Altshuler, L.L., Frye, M.A., Suppes, T., Keck, P.E. Jr., McElroy, S.L., Denicoff, K.D., Obrocea, G., Nolen, W.A., Kupka, R., Walden, J., Grunze, H., Perez, S., Luckenbaugh, D.A., and Post, R.M. (2003). Factors associated with suicide attempts in 648 patients with bipolar disorder in the Stanley Foundation Bipolar Network. *J Clin Psychiatry*, 64(5), 506–515.

Levy, B., and Hansen, E. (1969). Failure of the urinary test for suicide potential: Analysis of urinary 17-OHCS steroid findings prior to suicide in two patients. *Arch Gen Psychiatry*, 20(4), 415–418.

Lin, P.Y., and Tsai, G. (2004). Association between serotonin transporter gene promoter polymorphism and suicide: Results of a meta-analysis. *Biol Psychiatry*, 55(10), 1023–1030.

Linkowski, P., Martin, F., and De Maertelaer, V. (1992). Effect of some climatic factors on violent and non-violent suicides in Belgium. *J Affect Disord*, 25(3), 161–166.

Linnoila, V.M., and Virkkunen, M. (1992). Aggression, suicidality, and serotonin. *J Clin Psychiatry*, 53(Suppl), 46–51.

Losonczy, M.F., Mohs, R.C., and Davis, K.L. (1984). Seasonal variations of human lumbar CSF neurotransmitter metabolite concentrations. *Psychiatry Res*, 12, 79–87.

Luoma, J.B., Martin, C.E., and Pearson, J.L. (2002). Contact with mental health and primary care providers before suicide: A review of the evidence. *Am J Psychiatry*, 159(6), 909–916.

MacKinnon, D.F., Potash, J.B., McMahon, F.J., Simpson, S.G., and DePaulo, R. (2005). Rapid moon switching and suicidality in familial bipolar disorder. *Bipolar Disord, 7*, 441–448.

MacQueen, G.M., and Young, L.T. (2001). Bipolar II disorder: Symptoms, course, and response to treatment. *Psychiatr Serv*, 52(3), 358–361.

Maes, M., Cosyns, P., Meltzer, H.Y., De Meyer, F., and Peeters, D. (1993a). Seasonality in violent suicide but not in nonviolent suicide or homicide. *Am J Psychiatry*, 150(9), 1380–1385.

Maes, M., Meltzer, H.Y., Suy, E., De Meyer, F. (1993b). Seasonality in severity of depression: Relationships to suicide and homicide occurrence. *Acta Psychiatr Scand*, 88(3), 156–161.

Maes, M., De Meyer, F., Thompson, P., Peeters, D., and Cosyns, P. (1994). Synchronized annual rhythms in violent suicide rate, ambient temperature and the light-dark span. *Acta Psychiatr Scand*, 90(5), 391–396.

Maes, M., Scharpe, S., Verkerk, R., D'Hondt, P., Peeters, D., Cosyns, P., Thompson, P., De Meyer, F., Wauters, A., and Neels, H. (1995). Seasonal variation in plasma L-tryptophan availability in healthy volunteers: Relationships to violent suicide occurrence. *Arch Gen Psychiatry*, 52(11), 937–946.

Maj, M., Magliano, L., Pirozzi, R., Marasco, C., and Guarneri, M. (1994). Validity of rapid cycling as a course specifier for bipolar disorder. *Am J Psychiatry*, 151(7), 1015–1019.

Maldonado, G., and Kraus, J.F. (1991). Variation in suicide occurrence by time of day, day of the week, month, and lunar phase. *Suicide Life Threat Behav*, 21(2), 174–187.

Manfredini, R., Caracciolo, S., Salmi, R., Boari, B., Tomelli, A., and Gallerani, M. (2000). The association of low serum cholesterol with depression and suicidal behaviors: New hypotheses for the missing link. *J Int Med Res*, 28(6), 247–257.

Mann, J.J. (1998). The neurobiology of suicide. *Nat Med*, 4(1), 25–30.

Mann, J.J. (2002). A current perspective of suicide and attempted suicide. *Ann Intern Med* 136(4), 302–311.

Mann, J.J., McBride, P.A., Brown, R.P., Linnoila, M., Leon, A.C., DeMeo, M., Mieczkowski, T., Myers, J.E., and Stanley, M. (1992). Relationship between central and peripheral serotonin indexes in depressed and suicidal psychiatric inpatients. *Arch Gen Psychiatry*, 49(6), 442–446.

Mann, J.J., Waternaux, C., Haas, G.L., and Malone, K.M. (1999). Toward a clinical model of suicidal behavior in psychiatric patients. *Am J Psychiatry*, 156(2), 181–189.

Mann, J.J., Huang, Y.Y., Underwood, M.D., Kassir, S.A., Oppenheim, S., Kelly, T.M., Dwork, A.J., and Arango, V. (2000). A serotonin transporter gene promoter polymorphism (5-HTTLPR) and prefrontal cortical binding in major depression and suicide. *Arch Gen Psychiatry*, 57(8), 729–738.

Marangell, L.B., Bauer, M.S., Dennehy, E.B., Wisniewski, S.R., Allen, M.H., Miklowitz, D.J., Oquendo, M.A., Frank, E., Perlis, R.H., Martinez, J.M., Fagiolini, A., Otto, M.W., Chessick, C.A., Zboyan, H.A., Miyahara, S., Sachs, G., and Thase, M.E. (2006). Prospective predictors of suicide and suicide attempts in 1,556 patients with bipolar disorders followed for up to 2 years. *Bipolar Disord*, 8, 566–575.

Marion, S.A., Agbayewa, M.O., and Wiggins, S. (1999). The effect of season and weather on suicide rates in the elderly in British Columbia. *Can J Public Health*, 90(6), 418–422.

Martin, S.J., Kelly, I.W., and Saklofske, D.H. (1992). Suicide and lunar cycles: A critical review over 28 years. *Psychol Rep*, 71(3, Pt 1), 787–795.

Mathers, C.D., Lopez, A.D., and Murray, C.J.L. (2006). The burden of disease and mortality by condition: Data, methods, and results for 2001. In A.D. Lopez, C.D. Mathers, M. Ezzate, D.T. Jamison, and C.J.L. Murral (Eds.), *Global Burden of Disease and Risk Factors*. New York: Oxford University Press.

McElroy, S.L., Keck, P.E. Jr., Pope, H.G. Jr., Hudson, J.I., Faedda, G.L., and Swann, A. (1992). Clinical and research implications of the diagnosis of dysphoric mixed mania or hypomania. *Am J Psychiatry*, 149(12), 1633–1644.

McElroy, S.L., Strakowski, S.M., Keck, P.E. Jr., Tugrul, K.L., West, S.A., and Loneza, H.S. (1995). Differences and similarities in mixed and pure mania. *Compr Psychiatry*, 36(3), 187–194.

McElroy, S.L., Altshuler, L.L., Suppes, T., Keck, P.E. Jr., Frye, M.A., Denicoff, K.D., Nolen, W.A., Kupka, R.W., Leverich, G.S., Rochussen, J.R., Rush, A.J., and Post, R.M. (2001). Axis I psychiatric comorbidity and its relationship to historical illness variables in 288 patients with bipolar disorder. *Am J Psychiatry*, 158(3), 420–426.

Micciolo, R., Zimmermann-Tansella, C., Williams, P., and Tansella, M. (1989). Seasonal variation in suicide: Is there a sex difference? *Psychol Med*, 19(1), 199–203.

Micciolo, R., Williams, P., Zimmermann-Tansella, C., and Tansella, M. (1991). Geographical and urban-rural variation in the seasonality of suicide: Some further evidence. *J Affect Disord*, 21(1), 39–43.

Michaelis, B.H., Goldberg, J.F., Davis, G.P., Singer, T.M., Garno, J.L., and Wenze, S.J. (2004). Dimensions of impulsivity and aggression associated with suicide attempts among bipolar patients: A preliminary study. *Suicide Life Threat Behav*, 34, 172–176.

Modai, I., Malmgren, R., Wetterberg, L., Eneroth, P., Valevski, A., and Asberg, M. (1992). Blood levels of melatonin, serotonin, cortisol, and prolactin in relation to the circadian rhythm of platelet serotonin uptake. *Psychiatry Res*, 43, 161–166.

Morken, G., Lilleeng, S., and Linaker, O.M. (2002). Seasonal variation in suicides and in admissions to hospital for mania and depression. *J Affect Disord*, 69(1-3), 39–45.

Morrison, J.R. (1975). The family histories of manic-depressive patients with and without alcoholism. *J Nerv Ment Dis*, 160, 227–229.

Motto, J.A. (1985). The recognition and management of the suicidal patient. In F.F. Flach, S.C. Draghi (Eds.), *The Nature and Treatment of Depression* (pp. 229–254). New York: John Wiley & Sons.

Mulder, R.T., Cosgriff, J.P., Smith, A.M., and Joyce, P.R. (1990). Seasonality of mania in New Zealand. *Aust N Z J Psychiatry*, 24(2), 187–190.

Muldoon, M.F., Manuck, S.B., Mendelsohn, A.B., Kaplan, J.R., and Belle, S.H. (2001). Cholesterol reduction and non-illness mortality: Meta-analysis of randomised clinical trials. *BMJ*, 322(7277), 11–15.

Murphy, G.E. (1988). Suicide and substance abuse. *Arch Gen Psychiatry*, 45(6), 593–594.

National Center for Injury Prevention and Control (NCIPC). (2005). Web-based injury statistics query and reporting system. Available: http://www.cdc.gov/ncipc/wisqars/ (accessed August 31, 2006).

Neeleman, J., Wessely, S., and Lewis, G. (1998). Suicide acceptability in African- and white Americans: The role of religion. *J Nerv Ment Dis*, 186(1), 12–16.

Nemeroff, C.B., Owens, M.J., Bissette, G., Andorn, A.C., and Stanley, M. (1988). Reduced corticotropin releasing factor binding sites in the frontal cortex of suicide victims. *Arc Gen Psychiatry*, 45(6), 577–579.

Nordstrom, P., Asberg, M., Aberg-Wistedt, A., and Nordin, C. (1995a). Attempted suicide predicts suicide risk in mood disorders. *Acta Psychiatr Scand*, 92, 345–350.

Nordstrom, P., Samuelsson, M., and Asberg, M. (1995b). Survival analyses of suicide risk after attempted suicide. *Acta Psychiatr Scand*, 91, 336–340.

Norman, W.H., Brown, W.A., Miller, I.W., Keitner, G.I., and Overholser, J.C. (1990). The dexamethasone suppression test and completed suicide. *Acta Psychiatr Scand*, 81(2), 120–125.

Oddie, T.H., Klein, A.H., Foley, T.P., and Fisher, D.A. (1979). Variation in values for iodothyronine hormones, thyrotropin, and thyroxine-binding globulin in normal umbilical cord serum with season and duration of storage. *Clinical Chemistry*, 25(7), 1251–1253.

Ono, H., Shirakawa, O., Nishiguchi, N., Nishimura, A., Nushida, H., Ueno, Y., Maeda, K. (2000). Tryptophan hydroxylase gene polymorphisms are not associated with suicide. *Am J Med Genet*, 96(6), 861–863.

Ono, H., Shirakawa, O., Nushida, H., Ueno, Y., and Maeda, K. (2004). Association between catechol-O-methyltransferase functional polymorphism and male suicide completers. *Neuropsychopharmacology*, 29(7), 1374–1377.

Oquendo, M.A., and Mann, J.J. (2000). The biology of impulsivity and suicidality. *Psychiatr Clin North Am*, 23(1), 11–25.

Oquendo, M.A., and Mann, J.J. (2001). Identifying and managing suicide risk in bipolar patients. *J Clin Psychiatry*, 62(Suppl 25), 31–34.

Oquendo, M.A., Placidi, G.P., Malone, K.M., Campbell, C., Keilp, J., Brodsky, B., Kegeles, L.S., Cooper, T.B., Parsey, R.V., van Heertum, R.L., and Mann, J.J. (2003). Positron emission tomography of regional brain metabolic responses to a serotonergic challenge and lethality of suicide attempts in major depression. *Arch Gen Psychiatry*, 60(1), 14–22.

Oquendo, M.A., Galfalvy, H., Russo, S., Ellis, S.P., Grunebaum, M.F., Burke, A., and Mann, J.J. (2004). Prospective study of clinical predictors of suicidal acts after a major depressive episode in patients with major depressive disorder or bipolar disorder. *Am J Psychiatry*, 161(8), 1433–1441.

Oravecz, R., Rocchi, M.B., Sisti, D., Zorko, M., Marusic, A., and Preti, A. (2006). Changes in the seasonality of suicides over time in Slovenia, 1971 to 2002. *J Affect Disord*, 95(1–3), 135–140.

Ordway, G.A. (1997). Pathophysiology of the locus coeruleus in suicide. *Ann N Y Acad Sci*, 836, 233–252.

Osby, U., Brandt, L., Correia, N., Ekbom, A., and Sparen, P. (2001). Excess mortality in bipolar and unipolar disorder in Sweden. *Arch Gen Psychiatry*, 58(9), 844–850.

Osby, U., Brandt, L., Correia, N., Ekbom, A., and Sparen, P. (2005). *Excess Mortality in Bipolar and Unipolar Disorder*. Paper presented to the annual meeting of the American Psychiatric Association, Atlanta.

Pandey, G.N., Dwivedi, Y., Rizavl, H.S., Ren, X., Pandey, S.C., Pesold, C., Robert, R.C., Conley, R.R., and Tamminga, C.A. (2002). Higher expression of serotonin 5-HT(2A) receptors in the postmortem brains of teenage suicide victims. *Am J Psychiatry*, 159(3), 419–429.

Papadopoulos, F.C., Frangakis, C.E., Skalkidou, A., Petridou, E., Stevens, R.G., and Trichopoulos, D. (2005). Exploring lag and duration effect of sunshine in triggering suicide. *J Affect Disord*, 88, 287–297.

Papolos, D., Hennen, J., and Cockerham, M.S. (2005). Factors associated with patient-reported suicide threats by children and adolescents with community-diagnosed bipolar disorder. *J Affect Dis*, 86, 267–275.

Parker, G., and Walter, S. (1982). Seasonal variation in depressive disorders and suicidal deaths in New South Wales. *Br J Psychiatry*, 140, 626–632.

Parker, G., Gao, F., and Machin, D. (2001). Seasonality of suicide in Singapore: Data from the equator. *Psychol Med*, 31(7), 1323–1325.

Partonen, T., Haukka, J., Virtamo, J., Taylor, P.R., and Lonnqvist, J. (1999). Association of low serum total cholesterol with major depression and suicide. *Br J Psychiatry*, 175, 259–262.

Perez, P.R., Lopez, J.G., Makeos, I.P., Escribano, A.D., and Sanchez, M.L.S. (1980). Seasonal variations in thyroid hormones in plasma. *Revista Clínica Española*, 156, 245–247.

Perlis, R.H., Miyahara, S., Marangell, L.B., Wisniewski, S.R., Ostacher, M., DelBello, M.P., Bowden, C.L., Sachs, G.S., and Nierenberg, A.A. (2004). STEP-BD investigators: Long-term implications of early onset in bipolar disorder. Data from the first 1000 participants in the Systematic Treatment Enhancement Program for Bipolar Disorder (STEP-BD). *Biol Psychiatry*, 55(9), 875–881.

Petridou, E., Papadopoulos, F.C., Frangakis, C.E., Skalkidou, A., and Trichopoulos, D. (2002). A role of sunshine in the triggering of suicide. *Epidemiology*, 13(1), 106–109.

Pfeffer, C.R., Normandin, L., and Kakuma, T. (1994). Suicidal children grow up: suicidal behavior and psychiatric disorders among relatives. *J Am Acad Child Adolesc Psychiatry*, 33(8), 1087–1097.

Pfeffer, C.R., Normandin, L., and Kakuma, T. (1998). Suicidal children grow up: Relations between family psychopathology and adolescents' lifetime suicidal behavior. *J Nerv Ment Dis*, 186(5), 269–275.

Pine, D.S., Trautman, P.D., Shaffer, D., Cohen, L., Davies, M., Stanley, M., and Parsons, B. (1995). Seasonal rhythm of platelet [^{3}H]imipramine binding in adolescents who attempted suicide. *Am J Psychiatry*, 152(6), 923–925.

Pini, S., Dell'Osso, L., Mastrocinque, C., Marcacci, G., Papasogli, A., Vignoli, S., Pallanti, S., and Cassano, G. (1999). Axis I comorbidity in bipolar disorder with psychotic features. *Br J Psychiatry*, 175, 467–471.

Pokorny, A.D. (1983). Prediction of suicide in psychiatric patients: Report of a prospective study. *Arch Gen Psychiatry*, 40(3), 249–257.

Pokorny, L.J. (1991). A summary measure of client level of functioning: Progress and challenges for use within mental health agencies. *J Ment Health Admin*, 18(2), 80–87.

Pooley, E.C., Houston, K., Hawton, K., and Harrison, P.J. (2003). Deliberate self-harm is associated with allelic variation in the tryptophan hydroxylase gene (TPH A779C), but not with polymorphisms in five other serotonergic genes. *Psychol Med*, 33(5), 775–783.

Potash, J.B., Kane, H.S., Chiu, Y.F., Simpson, S.G., MacKinnon, D.F., McInnis, M.G., McMahon, F.J., and DePaulo, J.R. Jr. (2000). Attempted suicide and alcoholism in bipolar disorder: Clinical and familial relationships. *Am J Psychiatry*, 157(12), 2048–2050.

Preti, A., and Miotto, P. (1998). Seasonality in suicides: The influence of suicide method, gender and age on suicide distribution in Italy. *Psychiatry Res*, 81(2), 219–231.

Preti, A., Miotto, P., and De Coppi, M. (2000). Season and suicide: Recent findings from Italy. *Crisis*, 21(2), 59–70.

Qin, P., and Nordentoft, M. (2005). Suicide risk in relation to psychiatric hospitalization: Evidence based on longitudinal registers. *Arch Gen Psychiatry*, 667, 427–432.

Qin, P., Agerbo, E., and Mortensen, P.B. (2002). Suicide risk in relation to family history of completed suicide and psychiatric disorders: A nested case-control study based on longitudinal registers. *Lancet*, 360(9340), 1126–1130.

Rasanen, P., Hakko, H., Jokelainen, J., Tihonen, J. (2002). Seasonal variation in specific methods of suicide: A national register study of 20,234 Finnish people. *J Affect Disord*, 71, 51–59.

Reich, J. (1998). The relationship of suicide attempts, borderline personality traits and major depressive disorder in a veteran outpatient population. *J Affect Disord*, 49(2), 151–156.

Retamal, P., and Humphreys, D. (1998). Occurrence of suicide and seasonal variation. *Rev Saude Publica*, 32(5), 408–412.

Rich, C.L., Ricketts, J.E., Fowler, R.C., and Young, D. (1988). Some differences between men and women who commit suicide. *Am J Psychiatry*, 145, 718–722.

Rihmer, Z., and Kiss, K. (2002). Bipolar disorders and suicidal behaviour. *Bipolar Disord*, 4(Suppl. 1), 21–25.

Rihmer, Z., and Pestality, P. (1999). Bipolar II disorder and suicidal behavior. *Psychiatr Clin North Am*, 22(3), 667–673, ix–x.

Rihmer, Z., Barsi, J., Arato, M., and Demeter, E. (1990). Suicide in subtypes of primary depression. *J Affect Disord*, 18(3), 221–225.

Rihmer, Z., Rutz, W., and Pihlgren, H. (1995). Depression and suicide on Gotland: An intensive study of all suicides before and after a depression-training programme for general practitioners. *J Affect Disord*, 35(4), 147–152.

Rihmer, Z., Rutz, W., Pihlgren, H., and Pestality, P. (1998). Decreasing tendency of seasonality in suicide may indicate lowering rate of depressive suicides in the population. *Psychiatry Res*, 81(2), 233–240.

Robins, E. (1981). *The Final Months: A Study of the Lives of 134 Persons Who Committed Suicide.* New York: Oxford University Press.

Robins, E., Murphy, G.E., Wilkinson, R.H. Jr., Gassner, S., and Kayes, J. (1959). Some clinical considerations in the prevention of suicide based on a study of 134 successful suicides. *Am J Public Health*, 49(7), 888–899.

Rock, D., Greenberg, D.M., and Hallmayer, J.F. (2003). Increasing seasonality of suicide in Australia 1970–1999. *Psychiatry Res*, 120(1), 43–51.

Roose, S.P., Glassman, A.H., Walsh, B.T., Woodring, S., Vital-Herne, J. (1983). Depression, delusions, and suicide. *Am J Psychiatry*, 140(9), 1159–1162.

Rosenthal, N.E., Davenport, Y., Cowdry, R.W., Webster, M.H., and Goodwin, F.K. (1980). Monamine metabolite in cerebrospinal fluid of depressive subgroups. *Psychiatry Research*, 2, 113–119.

Roy, A. (1994). Recent biologic studies on suicide. *Suicide Life Threat Behav*, 24(1), 10–14.

Roy, A., Segal, N.L., Centerwall, B.S., and Robinette, C.D. (1991). Suicide in twins. *Arch Gen Psychiatry*, 48(1), 29–32.

Roy, A., Nielsen, D., Rylander, G., Sarchiapone, M., and Segal, N. (1999). Genetics of suicide in depression. *J Clin Psychiatry*, 60(Suppl 2), 12–17; discussion 18–20, 113–116.

Rudd, M.D., Dahm, P.F., and Rajab, M.H. (1993). Diagnostic comorbidity in persons with suicidal ideation and behavior. *Am J Psychiatry*, 150(6), 928–934.

Runeson, B. (1989). Mental disorder in youth suicide. DSM-III-R Axes I and II. *Acta Psychiatr Scand*, 79(5), 490–497.

Rush, B. (1812). *Medical Inquiries and Observations upon the Diseases of the Mind.* Philadelphia: Kimber and Richardson.

Russ, M.J., Lachman, H.M., Kashdan, T., Saito, T., and Bajmakovic-Kacila, S. (2000). Analysis of catechol-O-methyltransferase and 5-hydroxytryptamine transporter polymorphisms in patients at risk for suicide. *Psychiatry Res*, 93(1), 73–78.

Rutter, P.A., and Behrendt, A.E. (2004). Adolescent suicide risk: Four psychosocial factors. *Adolescence*, 39, 295–302.

Salib, E. (1997). Elderly suicide and weather conditions: Is there a link? *Int J Geriatr Psychiatry*, 12(9), 937–941.

Sarrias, M.J., Artigas, F., Martinez, E., and Gelpi, E. (1989). Seasonal changes of plasma serotonin and related parameters: Correlation with environmental measures. *Biol Psychiatry*, 26, 695–706.

Sato, T., Bottlender, R., Tanabe, A., and Moller, H.J. (2004). Cincinnati criteria for mixed mania and suicidality in patients with acute mania. *Compr Psychiatry*, 45(1), 62–69.

Schmauss, C. (2003). Serotonin 2C receptors: Suicide, serotonin, and runaway RNA editing. *Neuroscientist*, 9(4), 237–242.

Schnyder, U., Valach, L., Bichsel, K., and Michel, K. (1999). Attempted suicide: Do we understand the patients' reasons? *Gen Hosp Psychiatry*, 21(1), 62–69.

Schulsinger, F., Kety, S.S., Rosenthal, D., and Wender, P.H. (1979). A family study of suicide. In M. Schou, E. Strömgren (Eds.), *Origin, Prevention, and Treatment of Affective Disorders* (pp. 277–287). London: Academic Press.

Schweizer, E., Dever, A., and Clary, C. (1988). Suicide upon recovery from depression: A clinical note. *J Nerv Ment Dis*, 176, 633–636.

Sharma, R., and Markar, H.R. (1994). Mortality in affective disorder. *J Affect Disord*, 31(2), 91–96.

Sher, L., Carballo, J.J., Grunebaum, M.F., Burke, A.K., Zalsman, G., Huang, Y.-Y., Mann, J.J., and Oquendo, M.A. (2006). A prospective study of the association of cerebrospinal fluid monoamine metabolite levels with lethality of suicide attempts in patients with bipolar disorder. *Bipolar Disord*, 8, 543–550.

Simkin, S., Hawton, K., Yip, P.S., Yam, C.H. (2003). Seasonality in suicide: A study of farming suicides in England and Wales. *Crisis*, 24(3), 93–97.

Simon, N.M., Otto, M.W., Wisniewski, S.R., Fossey, M., Sagduyu, K., Frank, E., Sachs, G.S., Nierenberg, A.A., Thase, M.E., and Pollack, M.H. (2004). Anxiety disorder comorbidity in bipolar disorder patients: Data from the first 500 participants in the Systematic Treatment Enhancement Program for Bipolar Disorder (STEP-BD). *Am J Psychiatry*, 161(12), 2222–2229.

Simpson, S.G., and Jamison, K.R. (1999). The risk of suicide in patients with bipolar disorders. *J Clin Psychiatry*, 60(Suppl 2), 53–56; discussion 75–76, 113–116.

Slater, E., and Roth, M. (1969). *Clinical Psychiatry* (3rd edition). Baltimore: Williams & Wilkins.

Sokero, T.P., Melartin, T.K., Rytsälä, H.J., Leskelä, U.S., Lestelä–Mielonen, L.A., and Isometsä, E.T. (2005). Prospective study of risk factors for attempted suicide among patients with DSM-IV major depressive disorder. *Br J Psychiat*, 186, 314–318.

Souêtre, E., Salvati, E., Belugou, J.L., Douillet, P., Braccini, T., and Darcourt, G. (1989). Seasonal variation of serotonin function in humans: Research and clinical implications. *Ann Clin Psychiatry*, 1, 153–164.

Strakowski, S.M., McElroy, S.L., Keck, P.E. Jr., West, S.A. (1996). Suicidality among patients with mixed and manic bipolar disorder. *Am J Psychiatry*, 153(5), 674–676.

Statham, D.J., Heath, A.C., Madden, P.A., Bucholz, K.K., Bierut, L., Dinwiddie, S.H., Slutske, W.S., Dunne, M.P., and Martin, N.G. (1998). Suicidal behavior: An epidemiological and genetic study. *Psychol Med*, 28(4), 839–855.

Swann, A.C., Dougherty, D.M., Pazzaglia, P.J., Pham, M., and Moeller, F.G. (2004). Impulsivity: A link between bipolar disorder and substance abuse. *Bipolar Disord*, 6(3), 204–212.

Swann, A.C., Doughery, D.M., Pazzaglia, P.J., Pham, M., Steinberg, J.L. and Moeller, F.G. (2005). Increased impulsivity associated with severity of suicide attempt history in patients with bipolar disorder. *Am J Psychiatry*, 162, 1680–1687.

Szigethy, E., Conwell, Y., Forbes, N.T., Cox, C., and Caine, E.D. (1994). Adrenal weight and morphology in victims of completed suicide. *Biol Psychiatry*, 36(6), 374–380.

Takahashi, E. (1964). Seasonal variation of conception and suicide. *Tohoku J Exp Med*, 84, 215–227.

Takei, N., O'Callaghan, E., Sham, P., Glover, G., Tamura, A., Murray, R. (1992). Seasonality of admissions in the psychoses: Effect of diagnosis, sex, and age at onset. *Br J Psychiatry*, 161, 506–511.

Tanskanen, A., Tuomilehto, J., and Vinamaki, H. (2000). Cholesterol, depression and suicide. *Br J Psychiatry*, 176, 398–399.

Tietjen, G.H., Kripke, D.F. (1994). Suicides in California (1968–1977): Absence of seasonality in Los Angeles and Sacramento counties. *Psychiatry Res*, 53(2), 161–172.

Timonen, M., Viilo, K., Hakko, H., Sarkioja, T., Meyer-Rochow, V.B., Vaisanen, E., Rasanen, P. (2004). Is seasonality of suicides stronger in victims with hospital-treated atopic disorders? *Psychiatry Res*, 126(2), 167–175.

Tondo, L., Baldessarini, R.J., Hennen, J., Minnai, G.P., Salis, P., Scamonatti, L., Masia, M., Ghiani, C., and Mannu, P. (1999). Suicide attempts in major affective disorder patients with comorbid substance use disorders. *J Clin Psychiatry*, 60(Suppl 2), 63–69, discussion 75–76, 113–116.

Tondo, L., Isacsson, G., and Baldessarini, R. (2003). Suicidal behaviour in bipolar disorder: Risk and prevention. *CNS Drugs*, 17(7), 491–511.

Tsai, S.Y., Kuo, C.J., Chen, C.C., and Lee, H.C. (2002). Risk factors for completed suicide in bipolar disorder. *J Clin Psychiatry*, 63(6), 469–476.

Tsuang, M.T. (1977). Genetic factors in suicide. *Dis Nerv Syst*, 38(7), 498–501.

Tsuang, M.T. (1983). Risk of suicide in the relatives of schizophrenics, manics, depressives, and controls. *J Clin Psychiatry*, 44(11), 396–400.

Tsuang, M.T., and Woolson, R.F. (1977). Mortality in patients with schizophrenia, mania, depression and surgical conditions. *Br J Pscyhiatry*, 130, 162–166.

Turecki, G., Zhu, Z., Tzenova, J., Lesage, A., Seguin, M., Tousignant, M., Chawky, N., Vanier, C., Lipp, O., Alda, M., Joober, R., Benkelfat, C., Rouleau, G.A. (2001). TPH and suicidal behavior: A study in suicide completers. *Mol Psychiatry*, 6(1), 98–102.

Turecki, G., Dequeira, A., Gingras, Y., Seguin, M., Lesage, A., Tousignant, M., Chawky, N., Vanier, C., Lipp, O., Benkelfat, C., Rouleau, G.A. (2003). Suicide and serotonin: Study of variation at seven serotonin receptor genes in suicide completers. *Am J Med Genet*, 118B(1), 36–40.

U.S. Department of Health and Human Services. (2000). *In Harm's Way: Suicide in America.* Washington, DC: U.S. Public Health Service.

U.S. Public Health Service. (1999). *Office of the Surgeon General: The Surgeon General's Call to Action to Prevent Suicide.* Washington, DC: U.S. Public Health Service.

Valtonen, H.M., Suominen, K., Mantere, O., Leppämäki, S., Arvilommi, P., and Isometsä, E.T. (2006). Prospective study of risk factors for attempted suicide among patients with bipolar disorder. *Bipolar Disord*, 8, 576–585.

Verkes, R.J., Kerkhof, G.A., Beld, E., Hengeveld, M.W., and van Kempen, G.M.J. (1996). Suicidality, circadian activity rhythms and platelet serotonergic measures in patients with recurrent suicidal behaviour. *Acta Psychiatr Scand*, 93, 27–34.

Vieta, E., Benabarre, A., Colom, F., Gasto, C., Nieto, E., Otero, A., Vallejo, J. (1997). Suicidal behavior in bipolar I and bipolar II disorder. *J Nerv Ment Dis*, 185(6), 407–409.

Vieta, E., Colom, F., Martinez-Aran, A., Benabarre, A., Reinares, M., and Gastro, C. (2000). Bipolar II disorder and comorbidity. *Compr Psychiatry*, 41(5), 339–343.

Vieta, E., Colom, F., Corbella, B., Martinez-Aran, A., Reinares, M., Benabarre, A., and Gasto, C. (2001). Clinical correlates of psychiatric comorbidity in bipolar I patients. *Bipolar Disord*, 3(5), 253–258.

Virkkunen, M., and Linnoila, M. (1993). Brain serotonin, type II alcoholism and impulsive violence. *J Stud Alcohol Suppl*, 11, 163–169.

Waller, S.J., Lyons, J.S., and Costantini-Ferrando, M.F. (1999). Impact of comorbid affective and alcohol use disorders on suicidal ideation and attempts. *J Clin Psychol*, 55(5), 585–595.

Weeke, A. (1979). Causes of death in manic-depressives. In M. Schou, E. Strömgren (Eds.), *Origin, Prevention and Treatment of Affective Disorders* (pp. 289–299). London: Academic Press.

Wehr, T.A. (1992). In short photoperiods, human sleep is biphasic. *J Sleep Res*, 1(2), 103–107.

Wender, P.H., Kety, S.S., Rosenthal, D., Schulsinger, F., Ortmann, J., and Lunde, I. (1986). Psychiatric disorders in the biological and adoptive families of adopted individuals with affective disorders. *Arch Gen Psychiatry*, 43(10), 923–929.

Wetterberg, L., Eriksson, D., Friberg, Y., and Vango, B. (1978). Melatonin in humans: Physiological and clinical studies. *Clin Chim Acta*, 86, 169–177.

Whitney, D.K., Sharma, V., and Kueneman, K. (1999). Seasonality of manic depressive illness in Canada. *J Affect Disord*, 55(2–3), 99–105.

Winokur, G., Clayton, P.J., and Reich, T. (1969). Manic depressive illness. St. Louis: C.V. Mosby.

World Health Organization. (2001a). *The World Report on Violence and Health.* Geneva: World Health Organization.

World Health Organization [WHO] (2001b). *Mental Health and Brain Disorders, Suicide Rates (Per 100,000).* Geneva: World Health Organization. [Online]. Available: http://www.who.int/mental_health/Topic_Suicide/ Suicide_rates.html [accessed January 7, 2002].

Wu, L.H., and Dunner, D.L. (1993). Suicide attempts in rapid cycling bipolar disorder patients. *J Affect Disord*, 29(1), 57–61.

Yip, P.S., Chao, A., and Ho, T.P. (1998). Are-examination of seasonal variation in suicides in Australia and New Zealand. *J Affect Disord*, 47(1–3), 141–150.

Young, M.A., Fogg, L.F., Scheftner, W., Fawcett, J., Akiskal, H., and Maser, J. (1996). Stable trait components of hopelessness: Baseline and sensitivity to depression. *J Abnorm Psychol*, 105(2), 155–165.

Zajicek, K.B., Price, C.S., Shoaf, S.E., Mehlman, P.T., Suomi, S.J., Linnoila, M., and Dee Higgley, J. (2000). Seasonal variation in CSF 5-HIAA concentrations in male rhesus macaques. *Neuropsychopharmacology*, 22(3), 240–250.

Chapter 9

Addington, J., and Addington, D. (1998). Facial affect recognition and information processing in schizophrenia and bipolar disorder. *Schizophr Res*, 32, 171–181.

Agarwal, A.K., Kalra, R., Natu, M.V., Dadhich, A.P., and Deswal, R.S. (2002). Psychomotor performance of psychiatric inpatients under therapy: Assessment by paper and pencil tests. *Hum Psychopharmacol*, 17(2), 91–93.

Ahearn, E.P., Steffens, D.C., Cassidy, F., Van Meter, S.A., Provenzale, J.M., Seldin, M.F., Weisler, R.H., and Krishnan, K.R. (1998). Familial leukoencephalopathy in bipolar disorder. *Am J Psychiatry*, 155, 1605–1607.

Ahn, K.H., Lyoo, I.K., Lee, H.K., Song, I.C., Oh, J.S., Hwang, J., Kwon, J., Kim, M.J., Kim, M., and Renshaw, P.F. (2004). White matter hyperintensities in subjects with bipolar disorder. *Psychiatry Clin Neurosci*, 58, 516–521.

Albus, M., Hubmann, W., Wahlheim, C., Sobizack, N., Franz, U., and Mohr, F. (1996). Contrasts in neuropsychological test profile between patients with first-episode schizophrenia and first-episode affective disorders. *Acta Psychiatr Scand*, 94, 87–93.

Alema, G., and Donini, G. (1960). On the clinical and electroencephalographic changes caused by the intracarotid administration of sodium 5-isoamyl-5-ethylbarbiturate in man. *Bollettino–Societa Italiana Biologia Sperimentale*, 36, 900–904.

Ali, S.O., Denicoff, K.D., Altshuler, L.L., Hauser, P., Li, X., Conrad, A.J., Mirsky, A.F., Smith-Jackson, E.E., and Post, R.M. (2000). A preliminary study of the relation of neuropsychological performance to neuroanatomic structures in bipolar disorder. *Neuropsychiatry Neuropsychol Behav Neurol*, 13(1), 20–28.

Alpert, M., Pouget, E.R., and Silva, R.R. (2001). Reflections of depression in acoustic measures of the patient's speech. *J Affect Disord*, 66, 59–69.

Altshuler, L.L. (1993). Bipolar disorder: Are repeated episodes associated with neuroanatomic and cognitive changes? *Biol Psychiatry*, 33, 563–565.

Altshuler, L.L., Ventura, J., van Gorp, W.G., Green, M.F., Theberge, D.C., and Mintz, J. (2004). Neurocognitive function in clinically stable men with bipolar I disorder or schizophrenia and normal control subjects. *Biol Psychiatry*, 56, 560–569.

Amminger, G.P., Edwards, J., Brewer, W.J., Harrigan, S., and McGorry, P.D. (2002). Duration of untreated psychosis and cognitive deterioration in first-episode schizophrenia. *Schizophr Res*, 54, 223–230.

Andersen, G., Vestergaard, K., and Riis, J.O. (1993). Citalopram for post-stroke pathological crying. *Lancet*, 342, 837–839.

Andreasen, N.C. (1987). Creativity and mental illness: Prevalence rates in writers and their first-degree relatives. *Am J Psychiatry*, 144, 1288–1292.

Andreasen, N.C., and Glick, I.D. (1988). Bipolar affective disorder and creativity: Implications and clinical management. *Compr Psychiatry*, 29, 207–217.

Arroyo, S., Lesser, R.P., Gordon, B., Uematsu, S., Hart, J., Schwerdt, P., Andreasson, K., and Fisher, R.S. (1993). Mirth, laughter and gelastic seizures. *Brain*, 116(Pt. 4), 757–780.

Asarnow, R.F., and MacCrimmon, D.J. (1981). Span of apprehension deficits during the postpsychotic stages of schizophrenia: A replication and extension. *Arch Gen Psychiatry*, 38, 1006–1011.

Ashton, E.A., Berg, M.J., Parker, K.J., Weisberg, J., Chen, C.W., and Ketonen, L. (1995). Segmentation and feature extraction techniques, with applications to MRI head studies. *Magn Reson Med*, 33, 670–677.

Atre-Vaidya, N., Taylor, M.A., Seidenberg, M., Reed, R., Perrine, A., and Glick-Oberwise, F. (1998). Cognitive deficits, psychopathology, and psychosocial functioning in bipolar mood disorder. *Neuropsychiatry Neuropsychol Behav Neurol*, 11, 120–126.

Austin, M.P., Mitchell, P., Hadzi-Pavlovic, D., Hickie, I., Parker, G., Chan, J., and Eyers, K. (2000). Effect of apomorphine on motor and cognitive function in melancholic patients: A preliminary report. *Psychiatry Res*, 97, 207–215.

Aylward, E.H., Roberts-Twillie, J.V., Barta, P.E., Kumar, A.J., Harris, G.J., Geer, M., Peyser, C.E., and Pearlson, G.D. (1994). Basal ganglia volumes and white matter hyperintensities in patients with bipolar disorder. *Am J Psychiatry*, 151, 687–693.

Baddeley, A. (1986). *Working Memory*. Oxford, England: Clarendon.

Baldwin, R.C., Walker, S., Simpson, S.W., Jackson, A., and Burns, A. (2000). The prognostic significance of abnormalities seen on magnetic resonance imaging in late life depression: Clinical outcome, mortality and progression to dementia at three years. *Int J Geriatr Psychiatry*, 15, 1097–1104.

Baloh, R.W., Yue, Q., Socotch, T.M., and Jacobson, K.M. (1995). White matter lesions and disequilibrium in older people: I. Case-control comparison. *Arch Neurol*, 52, 970–974.

Barona, A., Reynolds, C., and Chastain, R. (1984). A demographically based index of premorbid intelligence for the WAIS-R. *J Consult Clin Psychol*, 52, 885–887.

Bayles, K.A., Trosset, M.W., Tomoeda, C.K., Montgomery, E.B. Jr., and Wilson, J. (1993). Generative naming in Parkinson disease patients. *J Clin Exper Neuropsychol*, 15, 547–562.

Bayley, P.J., Salmon, D.P., Bondi, M.W., Bui, B.K., Olichney, J., Delis, D.C., Thomas, R.G., and Thal, L.J. (2000). Comparison of the serial position effect in very mild Alzheimer's disease, mild Alzheimer's disease, and amnesia associated with electroconvulsive therapy. *J Int Neuropsychol Soc*, 6, 290–298.

Bearden, C.E., Hoffman, K.M., and Cannon, T.D. (2001). The neuropsychology and neuroanatomy of bipolar affective disorder: A critical review. *Bipolar Disord*, 3, 106–150; discussion 151–103.

Becerra, R., Amos, A., and Jongenelis, S. (2002). Organic alexithymia: A study of acquired emotional blindness. *Brain Injury*, 16, 633–645.

Beck, A.T., Steer, R.A., and Brown, G.K. (1996). *Beck Depression Inventory Manual* (2nd edition). San Antonio, TX: Psychological Corporation.

Beck, L.H., Bransome, E.D. Jr., Mirsky, A.F., Rosvold, H.E., and Sarason, I. (1956). A continuous performance test of brain damage. *J Consult Psychol*, 20, 343–350.

Bejjani, B.P., Damier, P., Arnulf, I., Thivard, L., Bonnet, A.M., Dormont, D., Cornu, P., Pidoux, B., Samson, Y., and Agid, Y.

(1999). Transient acute depression induced by high-frequency deep-brain stimulation. *N Engl J Med*, 340, 1476–1480.

Bench, C.J., Friston, K.J., Brown, R.G., Scott, L.C., Frackowiak, R.S., and Dolan, R.J. (1992). The anatomy of melancholia: Focal abnormalities of cerebral blood flow in major depression. *Psychol Med*, 22, 607–615.

Benedek, D.M., and Peterson, K.A. (1995). Sertraline for treatment of pathological crying. *Am J Psychiatry*, 152, 953–954.

Berney, A., Vingerhoets, F., Perrin, A., Guex, P., Villemure, J.G., Burkhard, P.R., Benkelfat, C., and Ghika, J. (2002). Effect on mood of subthalamic DBS for Parkinson's disease: A consecutive series of 24 patients. *Neurology*, 59, 1427–1429.

Black, D.W. (1982). Pathological laughter: A review of the literature. *J Nerv Ment Dis*, 170, 67–71.

Blackburn, I.M. (1975). Mental and psychomotor speed in depression and mania. *Br J Psychiatry*, 132, 329–335.

Blaney, P.H. (1986). Affect and memory: A review. *Psychol Bull*, 99, 229–246.

Boone, K.B., Miller, B.L., Lesser, I.M., Mehringer, C.M., Hill-Gutierrez, E., Goldberg, M.A., and Berman, N.G. (1992). Neuropsychological correlates of white-matter lesions in healthy elderly subjects: A threshold effect. *Arch Neurol*, 49, 549–554.

Borod, J.C., Koff, E., Lorch, M.P., Nicholas, M., and Welkowitz, J. (1988). Emotional and non-emotional facial behaviour in patients with unilateral brain damage. *J Neurol Neurosurg Psychiatry*, 51, 826–832.

Botteron, K.N., Vannier, M.W., Geller, B., Todd, R.D., and Lee, B.C. (1995). Preliminary study of magnetic resonance imaging characteristics in 8- to 16-year-olds with mania. *J Am Acad Child Adolesc Psychiatry*, 34, 742–749.

Bouhuys, A.L., and Mulder-Hajonides van der Meulen, W.R. (1984). Speech timing measures of severity, psychomotor retardation, and agitation in endogenously depressed patients. *J Commun Disord*, 17, 277–288.

Bouhuys, A.L., Bloem, G.M., and Groothuis, T.G. (1995). Induction of depressed and elated mood by music influences the perception of facial emotional expressions in healthy subjects. *J Affect Disord*, 33, 215–226.

Bozikas, V.P., Tonia, T., Fokas, K., Karavatos, A., and Kosmidis, M.H. (2006). Impaired emotion processing in remitted patients with bipolar disorder. *J Affect Disord*, 91, 53–56.

Branch, C., Milner, B., and Rasmussen, T. (1964). Intracarotid sodium amytal for the lateralization of cerebral speech dominance: Observations in 123 patients. *J Neurosurg*, 21, 399–405.

Breeze, J.L., Hesdorffer, D.C., Hong, X., Frazier, J.A., and Renshaw, P.F. (2003). Clinical significance of brain white matter hyperintensities in young adults with psychiatric illness. *Harv Rev Psychiatry*, 11, 269–283.

Breslow, R., Kocsis, J., and Belkin, B. (1980). Memory deficits in depression: Evidence utilizing the Wechsler Memory Scale. *Percept Motor Skills*, 51, 541–542.

Breslow, R., Kocsis, J., and Belkin, B. (1981). Contribution of the depressive perspective to memory function in depression. *Am J Psychiatry*, 138, 227–230.

Breteler, M.M., van Swieten, J.C., Bots, M.L., Grobbee, D.E., Claus, J.J., van den Hout, J.H., van Harskamp, F., Tanghe, H.L., de Jong, P.T., and van Gijn, J. (1994). Cerebral white matter lesions, vascular risk factors, and cognitive function in a population-based study: The Rotterdam Study. *Neurology*, 44, 1246–1252.

Brown, E.S., Rush, A.J., and McEwen, B.S. (1999). Hippocampal remodeling and damage by corticosteroids: Implications for mood disorders. *Neuropsychopharmacology*, 21, 474–484.

Brown, F.W., Lewine, R.J., Hudgins, P.A., and Risch, S.C. (1992). White matter hyperintensity signals in psychiatric and nonpsychiatric subjects. *Am J Psychiatry*, 149, 620–625.

Burt, D.B., Zembar, M.J., and Niederehe, G. (1995). Depression and memory impairment: A meta-analysis of the association, its pattern, and specificity. *Psychol Bull*, 117, 285–305.

Burt, T., Prudic, J., Peyser, S., Clark, J., and Sackeim, H.A. (2000). Learning and memory in bipolar and unipolar major depression: Effects of aging. *Neuropsychiatry Neuropsychol Behav Neurol*, 13, 246–253.

Burt, T., Lisanby, S.H., and Sackeim, H.A. (2002). Neuropsychiatric applications of transcranial magnetic stimulation: A meta analysis. *Int J Neuropsychopharmacol*, 5, 73–103.

Buschke, H. (1973). Selective reminding for analysis of memory and learning. *J Verbal Learning Verbal Behav*, 12, 543–550.

Cadelo, M., Inzitari, D., Pracucci, G., and Mascalchi, M. (1991). Predictors of leukoaraiosis in elderly neurological patients. *Cerebrovasc Dis*, 1, 345–351.

Calev, A., and Erwin, P. (1985). Recall and recognition in depressives: Use of matched tasks. *Br J Clin Psychol*, 24, 127–128.

Caligiuri, M.P., and Ellwanger, J. (2000). Motor and cognitive aspects of motor retardation in depression. *J Affect Disord*, 57, 83–93.

Caligiuri, M.P., Brown, G.G., Meloy, M.J., Eberson, S.C., Kindermann, S.S., Frank, L.R., Zorrilla, L.E., and Lohr, J.B. (2003). An fMRI study of affective state and medication on cortical and subcortical brain regions during motor performance in bipolar disorder. *Psychiatry Res*, 123, 171–182.

Caligiuri, M.P., Brown, G.G., Meloy, M.J., Eyler, L.T., Kindermann, S.S., Eberson, S., Frank, L.R., and Lohr, J.B. (2004). A functional magnetic resonance imaging study of cortical asymmetry in bipolar disorder. *Bipolar Disord*, 6, 183–196.

Cannizzaro, M., Harel, B., Reilly, N., Chappell, P., and Snyder, P.J. (2004). Voice acoustical measurement of the severity of major depression. *Brain Cognition*, 56, 30–35.

Carson, A.J., MacHale, S., Allen, K., Lawrie, S.M., Dennis, M., House, A., and Sharpe, M. (2000). Depression after stroke and lesion location: A systematic review. *Lancet*, 356, 122–126.

Cavanagh, J.T., Van Beck, M., Muir, W., and Blackwood, D.H. (2002). Case-control study of neurocognitive function in euthymic patients with bipolar disorder: An association with mania. *Br J Psychiatry*, 180, 320–326.

Chamberlain, S.R., and Sahakian, B.J. (2004). Cognition in mania and depression: Psychological models and clinical implications. *Curr Psychiatry Rep*, 6, 451–458.

Chapman, L.J., and Chapman, J.P. (1973). *Disordered Thought in Schizophrenia*. Englewood Cliffs, NJ: Prentice Hall.

Christensen, H., Griffiths, K., Mackinnon, A., and Jacomb, P. (1997). A quantitative review of cognitive deficits in depression and Alzheimer-type dementia. *J Int Neuropsychol Soc*, 3, 631–651.

Christodoulou, G.N., Kokkevi, A., Lykouras, E.P., Stefanis, C.N., and Papadimitriou, G.N. (1981). Effects of lithium on memory. *Am J Psychiatry*, 138, 847–848.

Clark, D.M., and Teasdale, J.D. (1982). Diurnal variation in clinical depression and accessibility of memories of positive and negative experiences. *J Abnorm Psychology*, 91, 87–95.

Clark, L., Iversen, S.D., and Goodwin, G.M. (2001). A neuropsychological investigation of prefrontal cortex involvement in acute mania. *Am J Psychiatry,* 158, 1605–1611.

Clark, L., Iversen, S.D., Goodwin, G.M. (2002). Sustained attention deficit in bipolar disorder. *Br J Psychiatry,* 180, 313–319.

Clark, L., Kempton, M.J., Scarna, A., Grasby, P.M., and Goodwin, G.M. (2005). Sustained attention-deficit confirmed in euthymic bipolar disorder but not in first-degree relatives of bipolar patients or euthymic unipolar depression. *Biol Psychiatry,* 57, 183–187.

Coffey, C.E., Figiel, G.S., Djang, W.T., and Weiner, R.D. (1990). Subcortical hyperintensity on magnetic resonance imaging: A comparison of normal and depressed elderly subjects. *Am J Psychiatry,* 147, 187–189.

Coffey, C.E., Wilkinson, W.E., Weiner, R.D., Parashos, I.A., Djang, W.T., Webb, M.C., Figiel, G.S., and Spritzer, C.E. (1993). Quantitative cerebral anatomy in depression: A controlled magnetic resonance imaging study. *Arch Gen Psychiatry,* 50, 7–16.

Coffman, J.A., Bornstein, R.A., Olson, S.C., Schwarzkopf, S.B., and Nasrallah, H.A. (1990). Cognitive impairment and cerebral structure by MRI in bipolar disorder. *Biol Psychiatry,* 27, 1188–1196.

Cohen, N., and Squire, L. (1980). Preserved learning and retention of pattern-analyzing skill in amnesia: Dissociation of knowing how and knowing that. *Science,* 210, 207–210.

Cohen, R., Weingartner, H., Smallberg, S., Pickar, D., and Murphy, D. (1982). Effort and cognition in depression. *Arch Gen Psychiatry,* 39, 593–597.

Cohen-Gadol, A.A., Westerveld, M., Alvarez-Carilles, J., and Spencer, D.D. (2004). Intracarotid Amytal memory test and hippocampal magnetic resonance imaging volumetry: Validity of the Wada test as an indicator of hippocampal integrity among candidates for epilepsy surgery. *J Neurosurgery,* 101, 926–931.

Colvin, C.R., and Block, J. (1994). Do positive illusions foster mental health? An examination of the Taylor and Brown formulation. *Psychol Bull,* 116, 3–20.

Cools, R., and Robbins, T.W. (2004). Chemistry of the adaptive mind. *Philos Transact A Math Phys Eng Sci,* 362, 2871–2888.

Corwin, J., Peselow, E., Feenan, K., Rotrosen, J., and Fieve, R. (1990). Disorders of decision in affective disease: An effect of beta-adrenergic dysfunction? *Biol Psychiatry,* 27, 813–833.

Coryell, W., Endicott, J., Reich, T., Andreasen, N., and Keller, M. (1984). A family study of bipolar II disorder. *Br J Psychiatry,* 145, 49–54.

Coryell, W., Endicott, J., Keller, M., Andreasen, N., Grove, W., Hirschfeld, R.M., and Scheftner, W. (1989). Bipolar affective disorder and high achievement: A familial association. *Am J Psychiatry,* 146(8), 983–988.

Coyne, J.C., and Gotlib, I.H. (1983). The role of cognition in depression: A critical appraisal. *Psychol Bull,* 94, 472–505.

Craik, F.I., and Jennings, J.M. (1992). Human memory. In F.I.M. Crisk, T.A. Salthouse (Eds.), *The Handbook of Aging and Cognition* (pp. 51–110). Hillsdale, NJ: Erlbaum.

Craik, F.I., and Tulving, E. (1975). Depth of processing and the retention of words in episodic memory. *J Exp Psychol (Gen),* 1, 268–294.

Cronholm, B., and Ottosson, J.-O. (1961). Memory functions in endogenous depression: Before and after electroconvulsive therapy. *Arch Gen Psychiatry,* 5, 193–199.

Cronholm, B., and Ottosson, J.-O. (1963). The experience of memory function after electroconvulsive therapy. *Br J Psychiatry,* 109, 251–258.

Cummings, J.L., and Mendez, M.F. (1984). Secondary mania with focal cerebrovascular lesions. *Am J Psychiatry,* 141, 1084–1087.

Custance, J. (1952). *Wisdom, Madness and Folly: The Philosophy of a Lunatic.* London: Pellegrini & Cudahy.

Dahabra, S., Ashton, C.H., Bahrainian, M., Britton, P.G., Ferrier, I.N., McAllister, V.A., Marsh, V.R., and Moore, P.B. (1998). Structural and functional abnormalities in elderly patients clinically recovered from early- and late-onset depression. *Biol Psychiatry,* 44, 34–46.

Dalby J.T., and Williams, R. (1986). Preserved reading and spelling ability in psychotic disorders. *Psychol Med,* 16, 171–175.

Daly, D.D., and Mulder, D.W. (1957). Gelastic epilepsy. *Neurology,* 7, 189–192.

Daly, J.J., Prudic, J., Devanand, D.P., Nobler, M.S., Lisanby, S.H., Peyser, S., Roose, S.P., and Sackeim, H.A. (2001). ECT in bipolar and unipolar depression: Differences in speed of response. *Bipolar Disord,* 3, 95–104.

David, A.S., and Cutting, J.C. (1990). Affect, affective disorder and schizophrenia: A neuropsychological investigation of right hemisphere function. *Br J Psychiatry,* 156, 491–495.

Davidson, M. (1939). Studies in the application of mental tests to psychotic patients. *Br J Med Psychol,* 18, 44–52.

Davidson, R.J. (1995). Cerebral asymmetry, emotion, and affective style. In R.J. Davidson, K. Hugdahl (Eds.), *Brain Asymmetry* (pp. 361–387). Cambridge, MA: MIT Press.

Davison, C., and Kelman, H. (1939). Pathological laughing and crying. *Arch Neurol Psychiatry,* 42, 595–643.

Decina, P., Kestenbaum, C.J., Farber, S., Kron, L., Gargan, M., Sackeim, H.A., and Fieve, R.R. (1983). Clinical and psychological assessment of children of bipolar probands. *Am J Psychiatry,* 140, 548–553.

DelBello, M.P., Adler, C.M., Amicone, J., Mills, N.P., Shear, P.K., Warner, J., and Strakowski, S.M. (2004). Parametric neurocognitive task design: A pilot study of sustained attention in adolescents with bipolar disorder. *J Affect Disord,* 82(Suppl. 1), S79–S88.

Demers, R.G., and Heninger, G.R. (1971). Visual-motor performance during lithium treatment: A preliminary report. *J Clin Pharmacol New Drugs,* 11, 274–279.

Den Hartog, H.M., Derix, M.M., Van Bemmel, A.L., Kremer, B., and Jolles, J. (2003). Cognitive functioning in young and middle-aged unmedicated out-patients with major depression: Testing the effort and cognitive speed hypotheses. *Psychol Med,* 33, 1443–1451.

Denicoff, K.D., Ali, S.O., Mirsky, A.F., Smith-Jackson, E.E., Leverich, G.S., Duncan, C.C., Connell, E.G., and Post, R.M. (1999). Relationship between prior course of illness and neuropsychological functioning in patients with bipolar disorder. *J Affect Disord,* 56, 67–73.

Deptula, D., Manevitz, A., and Yozawitz, A. (1991). Asymmetry of recall in depression. *J Clin Exper Neuropsychol,* 13, 854–870.

Dhingra, U., and Robins, P.V. (1991). Mania in the elderly: A 5–7 year follow-up. *J Am Geriatr Soc,* 39, 581–583.

Dickstein, D.P., Treland, J.E., Snow, J., McClure, E.B., Mehta, M.S., Towbin, K.E., Pine, D.S., and Leibenluft, E. (2004). Neuropsychological performance in pediatric bipolar disorder. *Biol Psychiatry,* 55, 32–39.

Dixon, T., Kravariti, E., Frith, C., Murray, R.M., and McGuire, P.K. (2004). Effect of symptoms on executive function in bipolar illness. *Psychol Med*, 34, 811–821.

Docherty, N.M., Hawkins, K.A., Hoffman, R.E., Quinlan, D.M., Rakfeldt, J., and Sledge, W.H. (1996). Working memory, attention, and communication disturbances in schizophrenia. *J Abnorm Psychol*, 105(2), 212–219.

Dolan, R.J., Bench, C.J., Liddle, P.F., Friston, K.J., Frith, C.D., Grasby, P.M., and Frackowiak, R.S. (1993). Dorsolateral prefrontal cortex dysfunction in the major psychoses; Symptom or disease specificity? *J Neurol Neurosurg Psychiatry*, 56(12), 1290–1294.

Dolan, R.J., Bench, C.J., Brown, R.G., Scott, L.C., and Frackowiak, R.S. (1994). Neuropsychological dysfunction in depression: The relationship to regional cerebral blood flow. *Psychol Med*, 24, 849–857.

Donnelly, E.F., Murphy, D.L., Goodwin, F.K., and Waldman, I.N. (1982). Intellectual function in primary affective disorder. *Br J Psychiatry*, 140, 633–636.

Drevets, W.C., Bogers, W., and Raichle, M.E. (2002). Functional anatomical correlates of antidepressant drug treatment assessed using PET measures of regional glucose metabolism. *Eur Neuropsychopharmacol*, 12, 527–544.

Dunner, D.L., Dwyer, T., and Fieve, R.R. (1976). Depressive symptoms in patients with unipolar and bipolar affective disorder. *Compr Psychiatry*, 17, 447–451.

Dupont, R.M., Jernigan, T.L., Gillin, J.C., Butters, N., Delis, D.C., and Hesselink, J.R. (1987). Subcortical signal hyperintensities in bipolar patients detected by MRI. *Psychiatry Res*, 21, 357–358.

Dupont, R.M., Jernigan, T.L., Butters, N., Delis, D., Hesselink, J.R., Heindel, W., and Gillin, J.C. (1990). Subcortical abnormalities detected in bipolar affective disorder using magnetic resonance imaging: Clinical and neuropsychological significance [see comments]. *Arch Gen Psychiatry*, 47, 55–59.

Dupont, R.M., Butters, N., Schafer, K., Wilson, T., Hesselink, J., and Gillin, J.C. (1995). Diagnostic specificity of focal white matter abnormalities in bipolar and unipolar mood disorder. *Biol Psychiatry*, 38, 482–486.

Ebmeier, K.P., Prentice, N., Ryman, A., Halloran, E., Rimmington, J.E., Best, J.K., and Goodwin, G.M. (1997). Temporal lobe abnormalities in dementia and depression: A study using high resolution single photon emission tomography and magnetic resonance imaging. *J Neurol Neurosurg Psychiatry*, 63, 597–604.

Eisemann, M. (1986). Social class and social mobility in depressed patients. *Acta Psychiatr Scand*, 73(4), 399–402.

el Massioui, F., and Lesevre, N. (1988). Attention impairment and psychomotor retardation in depressed patients: An event-related potential study. *Electroencephalogr Clin Neurophysiol*, 70, 46–55.

El-Badri, S.M., Ashton, C.H., Moore, P.B., Marsh, V.R., and Ferrier, I.N. (2001). Electrophysiological and cognitive function in young euthymic patients with bipolar affective disorder. *Bipolar Disord*, 3, 79–87.

Ellenbogen, M.A., Young, S.N., Dean, P., Palmour, R.M., and Benkelfat, C. (1996). Mood response to acute tryptophan depletion in healthy volunteers: Sex differences and temporal stability. *Neuropsychopharmacology*, 15, 465–474.

Engel, J., Kuhl, D.E., and Phelps, M.E. (1982). Patterns of human local cerebral glucose metabolism during epileptic seizures. *Science*, 218, 64–66.

Engelsmann, F., Katz, J., Ghadirian, A.M., and Schachter, D. (1988). Lithium and memory: A long-term follow-up study. *J Clin Psychopharmacol*, 8, 207–212.

Erkinjuntti, T., Gao, F., Lee, D.H., Eliasziw, M., Merskey, H., and Hachinski, V.C. (1994). Lack of difference in brain hyperintensities between patients with early Alzheimer's disease and control subjects. *Arch Neurol*, 51, 260–268.

Ferrier, I.N., Stanton, B.R., Kelly, T.P., and Scott, J. (1999). Neuropsychological function in euthymic patients with bipolar disorder. *Br J Psychiatry*, 175, 246–251.

Ferrier, I.N., Chowdhury, R., Thompson, J.M., Watson, S., and Young, A.H. (2004). Neurocognitive function in unaffected first-degree relatives of patients with bipolar disorder: A preliminary report. *Bipolar Disord*, 6, 319–322.

Fleck, D.E., Shear, P.K., Zimmerman, M.E., Getz, G.E., Corey, K.B., Jak, A., Lebowitz, B.K., and Strakowski, S.M. (2003). Verbal memory in mania: Effects of clinical state and task requirements. *Bipolar Disord*, 5(5), 375–380.

Fleminger, J.J., Dalton, R., and Standage, K.F. (1977). Handedness in psychiatric patients. *Br J Psychiatry*, 131, 448–452.

Flor-Henry, P. (1976). Lateralized temporal-limbic dysfunction and psychopathology. *Ann N Y Acad Sci*, 280, 777–797.

Flor-Henry, P. (1979). On certain aspects of the localization of the cerebral systems regulating and determining emotion. *Biol Psychiatry*, 14, 677–698.

Flor-Henry, P. (1983). *The Cerebral Basis of Psychopathology.* Boston: John Wright.

Flor-Henry, P., and Gruzalier, J. (1983). *Laterality and Psychopathology*, Amsterdam: Elsevier.

Flor-Henry, P., and Yeudall, L.T. (1979). Neuropsychological investigation of schizophrenia and manic-depressive psychoses. In J. Gruzelier, P. Flor-Henry (Eds.), *Hemispheric Asymmetries of Function in Psychopathology* (pp. 341–362). Amsterdam: Elsevier.

Foster, F.G., and Kupfer, D.J. (1975). Psychomotor activity as a correlate of depression and sleep in acutely disturbed psychiatric inpatients. *Am J Psychiatry*, 132, 928–931.

Frangou, S., Donaldson, S., Hadjulis, M., Landau, S., and Goldstein, L.H. (2006). The Maudsley Bipolar Disorder Project: Executive dysfunction in bipolar disorder I and its clinical correlates. *Biol Psychiatry*, 58, 859–864.

Frith, C., Stevens, M., Johnstone, E., Deakin, J., Lawler, P., and Crow, T.J. (1983). Effects of ECT and depression on various aspects of memory. *Br J Psychiatry*, 142, 610–617.

Fujikawa, T., Yamawaki, S., and Touhouda, Y. (1995). Silent cerebral infarctions in patients with late-onset mania. *Stroke*, 26, 946–949.

Gainotti, G. (1970). Emotional behavior of patients with right and left brain damage in neuropsychological test conditions. *Archivio di Psicologia, Neurologia e Psichiatria*, 31, 457–480.

Gainotti, G. (1972). Emotional behavior and hemispheric side of the lesion. *Cortex*, 8, 41–55.

Gascon, G.G., and Lombroso, C.T. (1971). Epileptic (gelastic) laughter. *Epilepsia*, 12, 63–76.

Gass, C.S., and Russell, E.W. (1986). Differential impact of brain damage and depression on memory test performance. *J Consult Clin Psychol*, 54, 261–263.

Geschwind, N. (1965). Disconnexion syndromes in animals and man. *Brain*, 88, 273–294, 584–644.

Getz, G.E., Shear, P.K., and Strakowski, S.M. (2003). Facial affect recognition deficits in bipolar disorder. *J Int Neuropsychol Soc*, 9, 623–632.

Ghacibeh, G.A., and Heilman, K.M. (2003). Progressive affective aprosodia and prosoplegia. *Neurology, 60,* 1192–1194.

Ghadirian, A.M., Engelsmann, F., and Ananth, J. (1983). Memory functions during lithium therapy. *J Clin Psychopharmacol, 3,* 313–315.

Gildengers, A.G., Butters, M.A., Seligman, K., McShea, M., Miller, M.D., Mulsant, B.H., Kupfer, D.J., and Reynolds, C.F. III. (2004). Cognitive functioning in late-life bipolar disorder. *Am J Psychiatry, 161*(4), 736–738.

Godfrey, H.P., and Knight, R.G. (1984). The validity of actometer and speech activity measures in the assessment of depressed patients. *Br J Psychiatry, 145,* 159–163.

Goldman-Rakic, P.S. (1987). Circuitry of primate prefrontal cortex and regulation of behavior by representational memory. In F. Plum, V. Mountcastle (Eds.), *The Handbook of Physiology: Section 1. The Nervous System:* Vol. 5. *Higher Functions of the Brain:* Part 1 (pp. 373–417). Bethesda, MD: American Physiological Society.

Goode, D.J., Meltzer, H.Y., Moretti, R., Kupfer, D.J., and McPartland, R.J. (1979). The relationship between wrist-monitored motor activity and serum CPK activity in psychiatric inpatients. *Br J Psychiatry, 135,* 62–66.

Goswami, U., Sharma, A., Khastigir, U., Ferrier, I.N., Young, A.H., Gallagher, P., Thompson, J.M., and Moore, P.B. (2006). Neuropsychological dysfunction, soft neurological signs and social disability in euthymic patients with bipolar disorder. *Br J Psychiatry, 188,* 366–373.

Gotlib, I.H. (1981). Self-reinforcement and recall: Differential deficits in depressed and nondepressed psychiatric inpatients. *J Abnorm Psychol, 90,* 521–530.

Gotlib, I.H., and Olson, J.M. (1983). Depression, psychopathology, and self-serving attributions. *Br J Clin Psychol, 22*(Pt. 4), 309–310.

Gourovitch, M.L., Torrey, E.F., Gold, J.M., Randolph, C., Weinberger, D.R., and Goldberg, T.E. (1999). Neuropsychological performance of monozygotic twins discordant for bipolar disorder. *Biol Psychiatry, 45,* 639–646.

Greden, J.F. (1982). Biological markers of melancholia and reclassification of depressive disorders. *Encephale, 8,* 193–202.

Greden, J.F., and Carroll, B.J. (1980). Decrease in speech pause times with treatment of endogenous depression. *Biol Psychiatry, 15,* 575–587.

Greden, J.F., Albala, A.A., Smokler, I.A., Gardner, R., and Carroll, B.J. (1981). Speech pause time: A marker of psychomotor retardation among endogenous depressives. *Biol Psychiatry, 16,* 851–859.

Green, A., Nutt, D., and Cowen, P. (1982). Increased seizure threshold following convulsion. In M. Sandler (Ed.), *Psychopharmacology of Anticonvulsants* (pp. 16–26). Oxford, England: Oxford University Press.

Green, M., and Walker, E. (1986). Attentional performance in positive- and negative-symptom schizophrenia. *J Nerv Ment Dis, 174*(4), 208–213.

Greenwald, B.S., Kramer-Ginsberg, E., Krishnan, K.R., Ashtari, M., Auerbach, C., and Patel, M. (1998). Neuroanatomic localization of magnetic resonance imaging signal hyperintensities in geriatric depression. *Stroke, 29,* 613–617.

Gruzelier, J., Seymour, K., Wilson, L., Jolley, A., and Hirsch, S. (1988). Impairments on neuropsychologic tests of temporo-hippocampal and frontohippocampal functions and word fluency in remitting schizophrenia and affective disorders. *Arch Gen Psychiatry, 45*(7), 623–629.

Haldane, M., and Frangou, S. (2004). New insights help define the pathophysiology of bipolar affective disorder: Neuroimaging and neuropathology findings. *Prog Neuropsychopharmacology Biol Psychiatry, 28,* 943–960.

Hammar, A. (2003). Automatic and effortful information processing in unipolar major depression. *Scand J Psychol, 44,* 409–413.

Hammar, A., Lund, A., and Hugdahl, K. (2003a). Long-lasting cognitive impairment in unipolar major depression: A 6-month follow-up study. *Psychiatry Res, 118,* 189–196.

Hammar, A., Lund, A., and Hugdahl, K. (2003b). Selective impairment in effortful information processing in major depression. *J Int Neuropsychol Soc, 9,* 954–959.

Hardy, P., Jouvent, R., and Widlocher, D. (1984). Speech pause time and the retardation rating scale for depression (ERD): Towards a reciprocal validation. *J Affect Disord, 6,* 123–127.

Harmer, C.J., Clark, L., Grayson, L., and Goodwin, G.M. (2002). Sustained attention deficit in bipolar disorder is not a working memory impairment in disguise. *Neuropsychologia, 40,* 1586–1590.

Hartlage, S., Alloy, L.B., Vazquez, C., and Dykman, B. (1993). Automatic and effortful processing in depression. *Psycho Bul, 113,* 247–278.

Harvey, P.D., and Brault, J. (1986). Speech performance in mania and schizophrenia: The association of positive and negative thought disorders and reference failures. *J Commun Disord, 19*(3), 161–173.

Harvey, P.D., and Serper, M.R. (1990). Linguistic and cognitive failures in schizophrenia. A multivariate analysis. *J Nerv Ment Dis, 178*(8), 487–493.

Harvey, P.D., Earle-Boyer, E.A., Weilgus, M.S., and Levinson, J.C. (1986). Encoding, memory, and thought disorder in schizophrenia and mania. *Schizaphr Bull, 12*(2), 252–261.

Hasher, L., and Zacks, R. (1979). Automatic and effortful processes in memory. *J Exp Psychol (Gen), 108,* 356–388.

Hawkins, K.A., Hoffman, R.E., Quinlan, D.M., Rakfeldt, J., Docherty, N.M., and Sledge, W.H. (1997). Cognition, negative symptoms, and diagnosis: A comparison of schizophrenic, bipolar, and control samples. *J Neuropsychiatry Clin Neurosci, 9*(1), 81–89.

Head, H. (1921). Release of function in the nervous system. *Proc R Soc Lond Biol, 92,* 184–209.

Heilman, K.M., Scholes, R., and Watson, R.T. (1975). Auditory affective agnosia: Disturbed comprehension of affective speech. *J Neurol Neurosurg Psychiatry, 38,* 69–72.

Henry, M.E., Schmidt, M.E., Matochik, J.A., Stoddard, E.P., and Potter, W.Z. (2001). The effects of ECT on brain glucose: A pilot FDG PET study. *J ECT, 17,* 33–40.

Hickie, I., Parsonage, B., and Parker, G. (1990a). Prediction of response to electroconvulsive therapy: Preliminary validation of a sign-based typology of depression. *Br J Psychiatry, 157,* 65–71.

Hickie, I., Parsonage, B., and Parker, G. (1990b). Prediction of response to electroconvulsive therapy: Preliminary validation of a sign-based typology of depression. *Br J Psychiatry, 157,* 65–71.

Hickie, I., Scott, E., Mitchell, P., Wilhelm, K., Austin, M.P., and Bennett, B. (1995). Subcortical hyperintensities on magnetic resonance imaging: Clinical correlates and prognostic significance in patients with severe depression. *Biol Psychiatry, 37,* 151–160.

Hickie, I., Mason, C., Parker, G., and Brodaty, H. (1996). Prediction of ECT response: Validation of a refined sign-based

(CORE) system for defining melancholia. *Br J Psychiatry*, 169, 68–74.

Hickie, I., Scott, E., Wilhelm, K., and Brodaty, H. (1997). Subcortical hyperintensities on magnetic resonance imaging in patients with severe depression: A longitudinal evaluation. *Biol Psychiatry*, 42, 367–374.

Hoffmann, G.M., Gonze, J.C., and Mendlewicz, J. (1985). Speech pause time as a method for the evaluation of psychomotor retardation in depressive illness. *Br J Psychiatry*, 146, 535–538.

Hoffman, R.E., Quinlan, D.M., Mazure, C.M., and McGlashan, T.M. (2001). Cortical instability and the mechanism of mania: A neural network simulation and perceptual text. *Biol Psychiatry*, 49(6), 500–509.

Holtzheimer, P.E., III, Russo, J., and Avery, D.H. (2001). A meta-analysis of repetitive transcranial magnetic stimulation in the treatment of depression. *Psychopharmacol Bull*, 35, 149–169.

Hommes, O.R. (1965). Semming sanomalien als neurologisch symptoom. *Nederlands Tijdschrift Voor Geneeskunde*, 109, 588–589.

House, A.O., Hackett, M.L., Anderson, C.S., and Horrocks, J.A. (2004). Pharmaceutical interventions for emotionalism after stroke. *Cochrane Database Syst Rev* CD003690.

Hughlings Jackson, J. (1958). *Selected Writings of John Hughling Jackson*. New York: Classics of Neurology and Neurosurgery. Richmond, VA: Staples Publishing.

Iverson, G.L. (2004). Objective assessment of psychomotor retardation in primary care patients with depression. *J Behav Med*, 27, 31–37.

James, W. (1890). *The Principles of Psychology* [microform]. New York: H. Holt.

Jamison, K.R. (1993). Manic-depressive illness and creativity. *Scientific American*. Available: http://www.sciamdigital.com/index.cfm?fa=Products.ViewIssuePreview&ARTICLEID_CHAR=3C9F2798-2B35-221B-6FA853B375CBA8C4.

Jenkins, M., Malloy, P., Salloway, S., Cohen, R., Rogg, J., Tung, G., Kohn, R., Westlake, R., Johnson, E.G., and Richardson, E. (1998). Memory processes in depressed geriatric patients with and without subcortical hyperintensities on MRI. *J Neuroimaging*, 8, 20–26.

Jeret, J.S. (1997). Treatment of poststroke pathological crying. *Stroke*, 28, 2321–2322.

Joanette, I., and Goulet, P. (1986). Criterion-specific reduction of verbal fluency in right brain-damaged right handers. *Neuropsychologia*, 24, 857–879.

Joffe, R.T., MacDonald, C., and Kutcher, S.P. (1988). Lack of differential cognitive effects of lithium and carbamazapine in bipolar affective disorder. *J Clin Psychopharmacol*, 8(6), 425–428.

Jorge, R.E., Robinson, R.G., Starkstein, S.E., Arndt, S.V., Forrester, A.W., and Geisler, F.H. (1993). Secondary mania following traumatic brain injury. *Am J Psychiatry*, 150, 916–921.

Judd, L.L. (1979). Effect of lithium on mood, cognition, and personality function in normal subjects. *Arch Gen Psychiatry*, 36, 860–866.

Junqué, C., Pujol, J., Vendrell, P., Bruna, O., Jódar, M., Ribas, J.C., Viñas, J., Capdevila, A., and Marti-Vilalta, J.L. (1990). Leukoaraiosis on magnetic resonance imaging and speed of mental processing. *Arch Neurol*, 47, 151–156.

Kano, M., Fukudo, S., Gyoba, J., Kamachi, M., Tagawa, M., Mochizuki, H., Itoh, M., Hongo, M., and Yanai, K. (2003). Specific brain processing of facial expressions in people with alexithymia: An H2 15O-PET study. *Brain*, 126, 1474–1484.

Kaprinis, G., Nimatoudis, J., Karavatos, A., Kandylis, D., and Kaprinis, S. (1995). Functional brain organization in bipolar affective patients during manic phase and after recovery: A digit dichotic listening study. *Percept Motor Skills*, 80(3 Pt. 2), 1275–1282.

Karniol, I.G., Dalton, J., and Lader, M.H. (1978). Acute and chronic effects of lithium chloride on physiological and psychological measures in normals. *Psychopharmacology*, 57, 289–294.

Kaschka, W.P., Meyer, A., Schier, K.R., and Froscher, W. (2001). Treatment of pathological crying with citalopram. *Pharmacopsychiatry*, 34, 254–258.

Keilp, J.G., Sackeim, H.A., Brodsky, B.S., Oquendo, M.A., Malone, K.M., and Mann, J.J. (2001). Neuropsychological dysfunction in depressed suicide attempters. *Am J Psychiatry*, 158, 735–741.

Keri, S., Kelemen, O., Benedek, G., and Janka, Z. (2001). Different trait markers for schizophrenia and bipolar disorder: A neurocognitive approach. *Psychol Med*, 31, 915–922.

Kessing, L.V. (1998). Cognitive impairment in the euthymic phase of affective disorder. *Psychol Med*, 28, 1027–1038.

Kestenbaum, C.J. (1979). Children at risk for manic-depressive illness: Possible predictors. *Am J Psychiatry*, 136(9), 1206–1208.

Kety, S.S., Woodford, R.B., Harmel, M.H., Freyhan, F.A., Appel, K.E., and Schmidt, C.F. (1948). Cerebral blood flow and metabolism in schizophrenia. *Am J Psychiatry*, 104, 765–770.

Kimbrell, T.A., Little, J.T., Dunn, R.T., Frye, M.A., Greenberg, B.D., Wassermann, E.M., Repella, J.D., Danielson, A.L., Willis, M.W., Benson, B.E., Speer, A.M., Osuch, E., George, M.S., and Post, R.M. (1999). Frequency dependence of antidepressant response to left prefrontal repetitive transcranial magnetic stimulation (rTMS) as a function of baseline cerebral glucose metabolism. *Biol Psychiatry*, 46, 1603–1613.

Kjellman, B.F., Karlberg, B.E., and Thorell, L.H. (1980). Cognitive and affective functions in patients with affective disorders treated with lithium: An assessment by questionnaire. *Acta Psychiatr Scand*, 62, 32–46.

Klein, D., Gittelman, R., Quitkin, F., and Rifkin, A. (1980). *Diagnosis and Drug Treatment of Psychiatric Disorders: Adults and Children*. Baltimore: Williams and Wilkins.

Kluger, A., and Goldberg, E. (1990). IQ patterns in affective disorder, lateralized and diffuse brain damage. *J Clin Exper Neuropsychol*, 12, 182–194.

Kocsis, J.H., Shaw, E.D., Stokes, P.E., Wilner, P., Elliot, A.S., Sikes, C., Myers, B., Manevitz, A., and Parides, M. (1993). Neuropsychologic effects of lithium discontinuation. *J Clin Psychopharmacol*, 13, 268–275.

Kolb, B., and Milner, B. (1981). Observations on spontaneous facial expression after focal cerebral excisions and after intracarotid injection of sodium amytal. *Neuropsychologia*, 19, 505–514.

Kolur, U.S., Reddy, Y.C.J., John, J.P., Kandavel, T., and Jain, S. (2006). Sustained attention and executive functions in euthymic young people with bipolar disorder. *Br J Psychiatry*, 189, 453–458.

Kopelman, M.D. (2002). Disorders of memory. *Brain*, 125, 2152–2190.

Kotin, J., and Goodwin, F.K. (1972). Depression during mania: Clinical observations and theoretical implications. *Am J Psychiatry*, 129, 679–686.

Krabbendam, L., Honig, A., Wiersma, J., Vuurman, E.F., Hofman, P.A., Derix, M.M., Nolen, W.A., and Jolles, J. (2000).

Cognitive dysfunctions and white matter lesions in patients with bipolar disorder in remission. *Acta Psychiatr Scand,* 101, 274–280.

Kraemer, G.W., and McKinney, W.T. (1979). Interactions of pharmacological agents which alter biogenic amine metabolism and depression: An analysis of contributing factors within a primate model of depression. *J Affect Disord,* 1, 33–54.

Kraepelin, E. (1896). *Dementia Praecox and Paraphrenia.* Reprinted (1971) (Trans. R.M. Barclay). Melbourne, FL: Krieger.

Kremen, W.S., Seidman, L.J., Faraone, S.V., and Tsuang, M.T. (2003). Is there disproportionate impairment in semantic or phonemic fluency in schizophrenia? *J Int Neuropsychol Soc,* 9(1), 79–88.

Krishnan, K.R., Taylor, W.D., McQuoid, D.R., MacFall, J.R., Payne, M.E., Provenzale, J.M., and Steffens, D.C. (2004). Clinical characteristics of magnetic resonance imaging-defined subcortical ischemic depression. *Biol Psychiatry,* 55, 390–397.

Kriss, A., Blumhardt, L., Halliday, A., and Pratt, R. (1978). Neurological asymmetries immediately after unilateral ECT. *J Neurol Neurosurg Psychiatry,* 41, 1135–1144.

Kropf, D., and Muller-Oerlinghausen, B. (1979). Changes in learning, memory, and mood during lithium treatment: Approach to a research strategy. *Acta Psychiatr Scand,* 59, 97–124.

Kumar, A., Jin, Z., Bilker, W., Udupa, J., and Gottlieb, G. (1998). Late-onset minor and major depression: Early evidence for common neuroanatomical substrates detected by using MRI. *Proc Natl Acad Sci U S A,* 95, 7654–7658.

Kupfer, D.J., and Foster, F.G. (1973). Sleep and activity in a psychotic depression. *J Nerv Ment Dis,* 156, 341–348.

Kupfer, D.J., Weiss, B.L., Foster, G., Detre, T.P., and McPartland, R. (1974). Psychomotor activity in affective states. *Arch Gen Psychiatry,* 30, 765–768.

Kupfer, D.J., Foster, F.G., Detre, T.P., and Himmelhoch, J. (1975). Sleep EEG and motor activity as indicators in affective states. *Neuropsychobiology,* 1, 296–303.

Kurthen, M., Linke, D.B., Reuter, B.M., Hufnagel, A., and Elger, C.E. (1991). Severe negative emotional reactions in intracarotid sodium amytal procedures: Further evidence for hemispheric asymmetries? *Cortex,* 27, 333–337.

Kyte, Z.A., Carlson, G.A., and Goodyer, I.M. (2006). Clinical and neuropsychological characteristics of child and adolescent bipolar disorder. *Psychol Med,* 36(9), 1197–1211.

Larsen, J.K., Brand, N., Bermond, B., and Hijman, R. (2003). Cognitive and emotional characteristics of alexithymia: A review of neurobiological studies. *J Psychosom Res,* 54, 533–541.

Lesser, I.M., Hill-Gutierrez, E., Miller, B.L., and Boone, K.B. (1993). Late-onset depression with white matter lesions. *Psychosomatics,* 34, 364–367.

Lesser, I.M., Boone, K.B., Mehringer, C.M., Wohl, M.A., Miller, B.L., and Berman, N.G. (1996). Cognition and white matter hyperintensities in older depressed patients. *Am J Psychiatry,* 153, 1280–1287.

Lewis, D.A. (1983). Unrecognized chronic lithium neurotoxic reactions. *JAMA,* 250, 2029–2030.

Lezak, M.D. (1995). *Neuropsychological Assessment* (3rd edition). New York: Oxford University Press.

Lisanby, S.H., Bazil, C.W., Resor, S.R., Nobler, M.S., Finck, D.A., and Sackeim, H.A. (2001). ECT in the treatment of status epilepticus. *J ECT,* 17, 210–215.

Lishman, W.A. (1968). Brain damage in relation to psychiatric disability after head injury. *Br J Psychiatry,* 114, 373–410.

Liu, S.K., Chiu, C.H., Chang, C.J., Hwang, T.J., Hwu, H.G., and Chen, W.J. (2002). Deficits in sustained attention in schizophrenia and affective disorders: Stable versus state-dependent markers. *Am J Psychiatry,* 159, 975–982.

Lohr, J.B., and Caligiuri, M.P. (1995). Motor asymmetry, a neurobiologic abnormality in the major psychoses. *Psychiatry Res,* 57, 279–282.

Lohr, J.B., and Caligiuri, M.P. (1997). Lateralized hemispheric dysfunction in the major psychotic disorders: Historical perspectives and findings from a study of motor asymmetry in older patients. *Schizophr Res,* 27, 191–198.

Lund, Y., Nissen, M., and Rafaelsen, O.J. (1982). Long-term lithium treatment and psychological functions. *Acta Psychiatr Scand,* 65, 233–244.

Lupien, S.J., Nair, N.P., Briere, S., Maheu, F., Tu, M.T., Lemay, M., McEwen, B.S., and Meaney, M.J. (1999). Increased cortisol levels and impaired cognition in human aging: Implication for depression and dementia in later life. *Rev Neurosci,* 10, 117–139.

Lyoo, I.K., Lee, H.K., Jung, J.H., Noam, G.G., and Renshaw, P.F. (2002). White matter hyperintensities on magnetic resonance imaging of the brain in children with psychiatric disorders. *Compr Psychiatry,* 43, 361–368.

MacQueen, G.M., Campbell, S., McEwen, B.S., Macdonald, K., Amano, S., Joffe, R.T., Nahmias, C., and Young, L.T. (2003). Course of illness, hippocampal function, and hippocampal volume in major depression. *Proc Natl Acad Sci U S A,* 100, 1387–1392.

Madsen, T.M., Greisen, M.H., Nielsen, S.M., Bolwig, T.G., and Mikkelsen, J.D. (2000). Electroconvulsive stimuli enhance both neuropeptide Y receptor Y1 and Y2 messenger RNA expression and levels of binding in the rat hippocampus. *Neuroscience,* 98, 33–39.

Mandzia, J.L., Black, S.E., McAndrews, M.P., Grady, C., and Graham, S. (2004). fMRI differences in encoding and retrieval of pictures due to encoding strategy in the elderly. *Hum Brain Mapp,* 21, 1–14.

Manji, H.K., Moore, G.J., and Chen, G. (2000a). Clinical and preclinical evidence for the neurotrophic effects of mood stabilizers: Implications for the pathophysiology and treatment of manic-depressive illness. *Biol Psychiatry,* 48, 740–754.

Manji, H.K., Moore, G.J., Rajkowska, G., and Chen, G. (2000b). Neuroplasticity and cellular resilience in mood disorders. *Mol Psychiatry,* 5, 578–593.

Mann, J.J., Waternaux, C., Haas, G.L., and Malone, K.M. (1999). Toward a clinical model of suicidal behavior in psychiatric patients. *Am J Psychiatry,* 156, 181–189.

Martinez-Arán, A., Vieta, E., Colom, F., Reinares, M., Benabarre, A., Gasto, C., and Salamero, M. (2000). Cognitive dysfunctions in bipolar disorder: Evidence of neuropsychological disturbances. *Psychother Psychosom,* 69, 2–18.

Martinez-Arán, A., Penades, R., Vieta, E., Colom, F., Reinares, M., Benabarre, A., Salamero, M., and Gasto, C. (2002a). Executive function in patients with remitted bipolar disorder and schizophrenia and its relationship with functional outcome. *Psychother Psychosom,* 71, 39–46.

Martinez-Arán, A., Vieta, E., Colom, F., Reinares, M., Benabarre, A., Torrent, C., Goikolea, J.M., Corbella, B., Sanchez-Moreno, J., and Salamero, M. (2002b). Neuropsychological performance in depressed and euthymic bipolar patients. *Neuropsychobiology,* 46(Suppl. 1), 16–21.

Martinez-Arán, A., Vieta, E., Colom, F., Torrent, C., Sanchez-Moreno, J., Reinares, M., Benabarre, A., Goikolea, J.M., Brugue, E., Daban, C., and Salamero, M. (2004a). Cognitive impairment in euthymic bipolar patients: Implications for clinical and functional outcome. *Bipolar Disord*, 6, 224–232.

Martinez-Arán, A., Vieta, E., Reinares, M., Colom, F., Torrent, C., Sanchez-Moreno, J., Benabarre, A., Goikolea, J.M., Comes, M., and Salamero, M. (2004b). Cognitive function across manic or hypomanic, depressed, and euthymic states in bipolar disorder. *Am J Psychiatry*, 161, 262–270.

Marvel, C.L., and Paradiso, S. (2004). Cognitive and neurological impairment in mood disorders. *Psychiatr Clin North Am*, 27, 19–36, vii–viii.

Mason, C.F. (1956). Pre-illness intelligence of mental hospital patients. *J Consult Psychol*, 20, 297–300.

Matarazzo, J.D. (1980). Behavioral health and behavioral medicine: Frontiers for a new health psychology. *Am Psychol*, 35(9), 807–817.

Mayberg, H.S., Liotti, M., Brannan, S.K., McGinnis, S., Mahurin, R.K., Jerabek, P.A., Silva, J.A., Tekell, J.L., Martin, C.C., Lancaster, J.L., and Fox, P.T. (1999). Reciprocal limbic-cortical function and negative mood: Converging PET findings in depression and normal sadness. *Am J Psychiatry*, 156, 675–682.

McCarthy, J., Arrese, D., McGlashan, A., Rappaport, B., Kraseski, K., Conway, F., Mule, C., and Tucker, J. (2004). Sustained attention and visual processing speed in children and adolescents with bipolar disorder and other psychiatric disorders. *Psychol Rep*, 95, 39–47.

McCullagh, S., and Feinstein, A. (2000). Treatment of pathological affect: Variability of response for laughter and crying. *J Neuropsychiatry Clin Neurosci*, 12, 100–102.

McElhiney, M.C., Moody, B.J., Steif, B.L., Prudic, J., Devanand, D.P., Nobler, M.S., and Sackeim, H.A. (1995). Autobiographical memory and mood: Effects of electroconvulsive therapy. *Neuropsychology*, 9, 501–517.

McKay, A.P., Tarbuck, A.F., Shapleske, J., and McKenna, P.J. (1995). Neuropsychological function in manic-depressive psychosis: Evidence for persistent deficits in patients with chronic, severe illness. *Br J Psychiatry*, 167, 51–57.

McNamara, B., Ray, J.L., Arthurs, O.J., and Boniface, S. (2001). Transcranial magnetic stimulation for depression and other psychiatric disorders. *Psychol Med*, 31, 1141–1146.

McPartland, R.J., Kupfer, D.J., Foster, F.G., Reisler, K.L., and Matthews, G. (1975). Objective measurement of human motor activity: A preliminary normative study. *Biotelemetry*, 2, 317–323.

Merrin, E.L. (1984). Motor and sighting dominance in chronic schizophrenics: Relationship to social competence, age at first admission, and clinical course. *Br J Psychiatry*, 145, 401–406.

Mesulam, M.M. (2000). *Principles of Behavioral and Cognitive Neurology* (2nd edition). Oxford, New York: Oxford University Press.

Meyer, S., Carlson, G., Wiggs, E., Martinez, P., Ronsaville, D., Klimes-Dougan, B., Gold, P., and Radke-Yarrow, M. (2004). Predictors of apparent frontal lobe dysfunction among adolescents at risk for bipolar disorders. *Dev Psychopathol*, 16(2), 461–476.

Miller, W.R. (1975). Psychological deficit in depression. *Psychol Bull*, 82, 238–260.

Mills, C.K. (1912). The cerebral mechanisms of emoitonal expression. *Trans Coll Physicians Philadelphia*, 34, 147–185.

Mitchell, P., Parker, G., Jamieson, K., Wilhelm, K., Hickie, I., Brodaty, H., Boyce, P., Hadzi-Pavlovic, D., and Roy, K. (1992). Are there any differences between bipolar and unipolar melancholia? *J Affect Disord*, 25, 97–105.

Mitchell, P., Hadzi-Pavlovic, D., Parker, G., Hickie, I., Wilhelm, K., Brodaty, H., and Boyce, P. (1996). Depressive psychomotor disturbance, cortisol, and dexamethasone. *Biol Psychiatry*, 40, 941–950.

Mitchell, P.B., Wilhelm, K., Parker, G., Austin, M.P., Rutgers, P., and Malhi, G.S. (2001). The clinical features of bipolar depression: A comparison with matched major depressive disorder patients. *J Clin Psychiatry*, 62, 212–216; quiz 217.

Moore, G.J., Bebchuk, J.M., Wilds, I.B., Chen, G., Manji, H.K., and Menji, H.K. (2000). Lithium-induced increase in human brain grey matter. *Lancet*, 356, 1241–1242.

Morice, R. (1990). Cognitive inflexibility and pre-frontal dysfunction in schizophrenia and mania. *Br J Psychiatry*, 157, 50–54.

Moscovitch, M. (1994). Memory and working with memory: Evaluation of a component process model and comparisons with other models. In D.L. Schacter, E. Tulving (Eds.), *Memory Systems 1994* (pp. 269–310). Cambridge, MA: MIT Press.

Mukherjee, S., Sackeim, H.A., and Schnur, D.B. (1994). Electroconvulsive therapy of acute manic episodes: A review of 50 years' experience. *Am J Psychiatry*, 151, 169–176.

Murphy, F.C., and Sahakian, B.J. (2001). Neuropsychology of bipolar disorder. *Br J Psychiatry Suppl*, 41, s120–s127.

Murphy, F.C., Sahakian, B.J., Rubinsztein, J.S., Michael, A., Rogers, R.D., Robbins, T.W., and Paykel, E.S. (1999). Emotional bias and inhibitory control processes in mania and depression. *Psychol Med*, 29, 1307–1321.

Murray, L.A., Whitehouse, W.G., and Alloy, L.B. (1999). Mood congruence and depressive deficits in memory: A forced-recall analysis. *Memory*, 7, 175–196.

Narushima, K., Kosier, J.T., and Robinson, R.G. (2003). A reappraisal of poststroke depression, intra- and inter-hemispheric lesion location using meta-analysis. *J Neuropsychiatry Clin Neurosci*, 15, 422–430.

Nehra, R., Chakrabarti, S., Pradham, B.D., and Khehra, N. (2005). Comparison of cognitive functions between first- and multiepisode bipolar affective disorders. *J Affect Disord*, 93, 185–192.

Nelson, L.D., Cicchetti, D., Satz, P., Sowa, M., and Mitrushina, M. (1994). Emotional sequelae of stroke: A longitudinal perspective. *J Clin Exper Neuropsychol*, 16, 796–806.

Nelson, R.E., and Craighead, W.E. (1977). Selective recall of positive and negative feedback, self-control behaviors, and depression. *J Abnorm Psychol*, 86, 379–388.

Newell, B.R., and Andrews, S. (2004). Levels of processing effects on implicit and explicit memory tasks: Using question position to investigate the lexical-processing hypothesis. *Exp Psychol*, 51, 132–144.

Nilsonne, A. (1987). Acoustic analysis of speech variables during depression and after improvement. *Acta Psychiatr Scand*, 76, 235–245.

Nilsonne, A. (1988). Speech characteristics as indicators of depressive illness. *Acta Psychiatr Scand*, 77, 253–263.

Nobler, M.S., Sackeim, H.A., Solomou, M., Luber, B., Devanand, D.P., and Prudic, J. (1993). EEG manifestations during ECT: Effects of electrode placement and stimulus intensity. *Biol Psychiatry*, 34, 321–330.

Nobler, M.S., Sackeim, H.A., Prohovnik, I., Moeller, J.R., Mukherjee, S., Schnur, D.B., Prudic, J., and Devanand, D.P.

(1994). Regional cerebral blood flow in mood disorders: III. Treatment and clinical response. *Arch Gen Psychiatry*, 51, 884–897.

Nobler, M.S., Teneback, C.C., Nahas, Z., Bohning, D.E., Shastri, A., Kozel, F.A., and George, M.S. (2000). Structural and functional neuroimaging of electroconvulsive therapy and transcranial magnetic stimulation. *Depression Anxiety*, 12, 144–156.

Nobler, M.S., Oquendo, M.A., Kegeles, L.S., Malone, K.M., Campbell, C.C., Sackeim, H.A., and Mann, J.J. (2001). Decreased regional brain metabolism after ECT. *Am J Psychiatry*, 158, 305–308.

Norman, R.M., and Malla, A.K. (2001). Duration of untreated psychosis: A critical examination of the concept and its importance. *Psychol Med*, 31, 381–400.

Okun, M.S., Raju, D.V., Walter, B.L., Juncos, J.L., DeLong, M.R., Heilman, K., McDonald, W.M., and Vitek, J.L. (2004). Pseudobulbar crying induced by stimulation in the region of the subthalamic nucleus. *J Neurol Neurosurg Psychiatry*, 75, 921–923.

Oltmanns, T.F. (1978). Selective attention in schizophrenic and manic psychoses: The effect of distraction on information processing. *J Abnorm Psychol*, 87(2), 212–225.

Oquendo, M.A., and Mann, J.J. (2001). Identifying and managing suicide risk in bipolar patients. *J Clin Psychiatry*, 62(Suppl. 25), 31–34.

Oquendo, M.A., Galfalvy, H., Russo, S., Ellis, S.P., Grunebaum, M.F., Burke, A., and Mann, J.J. (2004). Prospective study of clinical predictors of suicidal acts after a major depressive episode in patients with major depressive disorder or bipolar disorder. *Am J Psychiatry*, 161, 1433–1441.

Paradiso, S., Lamberty, G.J., Garvey, M.J., and Robinson, R.G. (1997). Cognitive impairment in the euthymic phase of chronic unipolar depression. *J Nerv Ment Dis*, 185(12), 748–754.

Park, S. (1997). Association of an oculomotor delayed response task and the Wisconsin card sort test in schizophrenic patients. *Int J Psychophysiol*, 27(2), 147–151.

Park, S., and Holzman, P.S. (1992). Schizophrenics show spatial working memory deficits. *Arch Gen Psychiatry*, 49(12), 975–982.

Parker, G., and Hadzi-Pavlovic, D. (1993). Prediction of response to antidepressant medication by a sign-based index of melancholia. *Aust N Z J Psychiatry*, 27, 56–61.

Parker, G., Hadzi-Pavlovic, D., Brodaty, H., Boyce, P., Mitchell, P., Wilhelm, K., Hickie, I., and Eyers, K. (1993). Psychomotor disturbance in depression: Defining the constructs. *J Affect Disord*, 27(4), 255–265.

Parker, G., Hadzi-Pavlovic, D., Austin, M.P., Mitchell, P., Wilhelm, K., Hickie, I., Boyce, P., and Eyers, K. (1995a). Sub-typing depression: I. Is psychomotor disturbance necessary and sufficient to the definition of melancholia? *Psychol Med*, 25, 815–823.

Parker, G., Hadzi-Pavlovic, D., Hickie, I., Brodaty, H., Boyce, P., Mitchell, P., and Wilhelm, K. (1995b). Sub-typing depression: III. Development of a clinical algorithm for melancholia and comparison with other diagnostic measures. *Psychol Med*, 25, 833–840.

Parker, G., Roy, K., Wilhelm, K., Mitchell, P., and Hadzi-Pavlovic, D. (2000). The nature of bipolar depression: Implications for the definition of melancholia. *J Affect Disord*, 59, 217–224.

Pavuluri, M.N., Schenkel, L.S., Aryal, S., Harral, E.M., Hill, S.K., Herbener, E.S., and Sweeney, J.A. (2006). Neurocognitive function in unmedicated manic and medicated euthymic pediatric bipolar patients. *Am J Psychiatry*, 163, 286–293.

Penfield, W., and Jasper, H. (1954). *Epilepsy and the Functional Anatomy of the Human Brain*. Boston: Little, Brown.

Perera, T.D., Luber, B., Nobler, M.S., Prudic, J., Anderson, C., and Sackeim, H.A. (2004). Seizure expression during electroconvulsive therapy: Relationships with clinical outcome and cognitive side effects. *Neuropsychopharmacology*, 29(4), 813–825.

Petterson, U. (1977). Manic-depressive illness: A clinical, social and genetic study. *Acta Psychiatr Scand Suppl* (269), 1–93.

Phillips, M.L., Drevets, W.C., Rauch, S.L., and Lane, R. (2003a). Neurobiology of emotion perception: I. The neural basis of normal emotion perception. *Biol Psychiatry*, 54, 504–514.

Phillips, M.L., Drevets, W.C., Rauch, S.L., and Lane, R. (2003b). Neurobiology of emotion perception: II. Implications for major psychiatric disorders. *Biol Psychiatry*, 54, 515–528.

Pier, M.P., Hulstijn, W., and Sabbe, B.G. (2004). Psychomotor retardation in elderly depressed patients. *J Affect Disord*, 81, 73–77.

Pillai, J.J., Friedman, L., Stuve, T.A., Trinidad, S., Jesberger, J.A., Lewin, J.S., Findling, R.L., Swales, T.P., and Schulz, S.C. (2002). Increased presence of white matter hyperintensities in adolescent patients with bipolar disorder. *Psychiatr Res*, 114, 51–56.

Politis, A., Lykouras, L., Mourtzouchou, P., and Christodoulou, G.N. (2004). Attentional disturbances in patients with unipolar psychotic depression: A selective and sustained attention study. *Compr Psychiatry*, 45, 452–459.

Post, F. (1996). Verbal creativity, depression and alcoholism: An investigation of one hundred American and British writers. *Br J Psychiatry*, 168, 545–555.

Post, R.M. (1990). Sensitization and kindling perspectives for the course of affective illness: Toward a new treatment with the anticonvulsant carbamazepine. *Pharmacopsychiatry*, 23, 3–17.

Post, R.M. (2002). Do the epilepsies, pain syndromes, and affective disorders share common kindling-like mechanisms? *Epilepsy Res*, 50, 203–219.

Pratt, R., and Warrington, E. (1972). The assessment of cerebral dominance with unilateral ECT. *Br J Psychiatry*, 121, 327–328.

Pratt, R., Warrington, E., and Halliday, A. (1971). Unilateral ECT as a test for cerebral dominance, with a strategy for treating left-handers. *Br J Psychiatry*, 119, 79–83.

Quraishi, S., and Frangou, S. (2002). Neuropsychology of bipolar disorder: A review. *J Affect Disord*, 72, 209–226.

Reus, V.I., Targum, S.D., Weingarter, H., and Post, R.M. (1979). Effect of lithium carbonate on memory processes of bipolar affectively ill patients. *Psychopharmacology*, 63, 39–42.

Rey, A. (1941). L'examen psychologique dans les cas d'encephalopathie traumatique. *Archives de Psychologie*, 28, 286–340.

Richell, R.A., and Anderson, M. (2004). Reproducibility of negative mood induction: A self-referent plus musical mood induction procedure and a controllable/uncontrollable stress paradigm. *J Psychopharmacol*, 18, 94–101.

Robertson, G., and Taylor, P.J. (1985). Some cognitive correlates of affective disorders. *Psychol Med*, 15(2), 297–309.

Robinson, L.J., Thompson, J.M., Gallagher, P., Goswami, U., Young, A.H., Ferrier, I.N., and Moore, P.B. (2006). A meta-analysis of cognitive deficits in euthymic patients with bipilor disorder. *J Affect Disord*, 93, 105–115.

Robinson, R.G. (1997). Neuropsychiatric consequences of stroke. *Ann Rev Med*, 48, 217–229.

Robinson, R.G., and Szetela, B. (1981). Mood change following left hemispheric brain injury. *Ann Neurol*, 9, 447–453.

Robinson, R.G., Kubos, K.L., Starr, L.B., Rao, K., and Price, T.R. (1984). Mood disorders in stroke patients: Importance of location of lesion. *Brain,* 107(Pt. 1), 81–93.

Rogers, M.A., Bradshaw, J.L., Phillips, J.G., Chiu, E., Vaddadi, K., Presnel, I., and Mileshkin, C. (2000). Parkinsonian motor characteristics in unipolar major depression. *J Clin Exper Neuropsychol,* 22, 232–244.

Rogers, M.A., Kasai, K., Koji, M., Fukuda, R., Iwanami, A., Nakagome, K., Fukuda, M., and Kato, N. (2004). Executive and prefrontal dysfunction in unipolar depression: A review of neuropsychological and imaging evidence. *Neurosci Res,* 50, 1–11.

Rosadini, G., and Rossi, G.F. (1967). On the suggested cerebral dominance for consciousness. *Brain,* 90, 101–112.

Rosenberg, R., Vorstrup, S., Anderson, A., and Bolwig, T.G. (1988). Effect of ECT on cerebral blood flow in melancholia assessed with SPECT. *Convulsive Ther,* 4, 62–73.

Rossi, G.F., and Rosadini, G. (1967). Experimental analysis of cerebral dominance. In C.H. Millikan (Ed.), *Brain Mechanisms Underlying Speech and Language* (pp. 167–184). New York: Grune and Stratton.

Rossi, A., Arduini, L., Daneluzzo, E., Bustini, M., Prosperini, P., and Stratta, P. (2000). Cognitive function in euthymic bipolar patients, stabilized schizophrenic patients, and healthy controls. *J Psychiatr Res,* 34(4–5), 333–339.

Rothenberg, A. (2001). Bipolar illness, creativity, and treatment. *Psychiatr Q,* 72, 131–147.

Roy-Byrne, P.P., Weingartner, H., Bierer, L.M., Thompson, K., and Post, R.M. (1986). Effortful and automatic cognitive processes in depression. *Arch Gen Psychiatry,* 43, 265–267.

Royant-Parola, S., Borbely, A.A., Tobler, I., Benoit, O., and Widlocher, D. (1986). Monitoring of long-term motor activity in depressed patients. *Br J Psychiatry,* 149, 288–293.

Rubinsztein, J.S., Michael, A., Paykel, E.S., and Sahakian, B.J. (2000). Cognitive impairment in remission in bipolar affective disorder. *Psychol Med,* 30, 1025–1036.

Rush, A.J., Schlesser, M.A., Roffwarg, H.P., Giles, D.E., Orsulak, P.J., and Fairchild, C. (1983). Relationships among the TRH, REM latency, and dexamethasone suppression tests: Preliminary findings. *J Clin Psychiatry,* 44(8 Pt. 2), 23–29.

Sackeim, H.A. (1986). A neuropsychodynamic perspective on the self: Brain, thought, emotion. In L.M. Hartman and K.R. Blankstein (Eds.), *Perception of Self in Emotional Disorder and Psychotherapy* (pp. 51–83). New York: Plenum.

Sackeim, H.A. (1999). The anticonvulsant hypothesis of the mechanisms of action of ECT: Current status. *J ECT,* 15, 5–26.

Sackeim, H.A. (2000a). Memory and ECT: From polarization to reconciliation. *J ECT,* 16, 87–96.

Sackeim, H.A. (2000b). Repetitive transcranial magnetic stimulation: What are the next steps? *Biol Psychiatry,* 48, 959–961.

Sackeim, H.A. (2004). The convulsant and anticonvulsant properties of electroconvulsive therapy: Towards a focal form of brain stimulation. *Clin Neurosci Rev,* 4, 39–57.

Sackeim, H.A., and Decina, P. (1983). Lateralized neuropsychological abnormalities in bipolar adults and in children of bipolar probands. In P. Flor-Henry, J. Gruzelier (Eds.), *Laterality and Psychopathology* (pp. 103–128). New York: Elsevier.

Sackeim, H.A., and Prohovnik, I. (1993). Brain imaging studies in depressive disorders. In J.J. Mann, D. Kupfer (Eds.), *Biology of Depressive Disorders* (pp. 205–258). New York: Plenum.

Sackeim, H.A., and Wegner, A.Z. (1986). Attributional patterns in depression and euthymia. *Arch Gen Psychiatry,* 43, 553–560.

Sackeim, H.A., Gur, R.C., and Saucy, M.C. (1978). Emotions are expressed more intensely on the left side of the face. *Science,* 202, 434–436.

Sackeim, H.A., Greenberg, M.S., Weiman, A.L., Gur, R.C., Hungerbuhler, J.P., and Geschwind, N. (1982). Hemispheric asymmetry in the expression of positive and negative emotions: Neurologic evidence. *Arch Neurol,* 39, 210–218.

Sackeim, H.A., Decina, P., Prohovnik, I., Malitz, S., and Resor, S.R. (1983a). Anticonvulsant and antidepressant properties of electroconvulsive therapy: A proposed mechanism of action. *Biol Psychiatry,* 18, 1301–1310.

Sackeim, H.A., Prohovnik, I., Decina, P., Malitz, S., and Resor, S. (1983b). Anticonvulsant properties of electroconvulsive therapy: Theory and case report. In M. Baldy-Moulinier, D.H. Ingvar, B.S. Meldrum (Eds.), *Current Problems in Epilepsy: Cerebral Blood Flow, Metabolism, and Epilepsy* (pp. 370–377). London: Libbey.

Sackeim, H.A., Decina, P., Portnoy, S., Neeley, P., and Malitz, S. (1987). Studies of dosage, seizure threshold, and seizure duration in ECT. *Biol Psychiatry,* 22, 249–268.

Sackeim, H.A., Freeman, J., McElhiney, M., Coleman, E., Prudic, J., and Devanand, D.P. (1992). Effects of major depression on estimates of intelligence. *J Clin Exp Neuropsychol,* 14, 268–288.

Sackeim, H.A., Prudic, J., Devanand, D.P., Kiersky, J.E., Fitzsimons, L., Moody, B.J., McElhiney, M.C., Coleman, E.A., and Settembrino, J.M. (1993). Effects of stimulus intensity and electrode placement on the efficacy and cognitive effects of electroconvulsive therapy. *N Engl J Med,* 328, 839–846.

Sackeim, H.A., Luber, B., Katzman, G.P., Moeller, J.R., Prudic, J., Devanand, D.P., and Nobler, M.S. (1996). The effects of electroconvulsive therapy on quantitative electroencephalograms: Relationship to clinical outcome. *Arch Gen Psychiatry,* 53, 814–824.

Sackeim, H.A., Prudic, J., Devanand, D.P., Nobler, M.S., Lisanby, S.H., Peyser, S., Fitzsimons, L., Moody, B.J., and Clark, J. (2000b). A prospective, randomized, double-blind comparison of bilateral and right unilateral electroconvulsive therapy at different stimulus intensities. *Arch Gen Psychiatry,* 57, 425–434.

Salloway, S., Malloy, P., Kohn, R., Gillard, E., Duffy, J., Rogg, J., Tung, G., Richardson, E., Thomas, C., and Westlake, R. (1996). MRI and neuropsychological differences in early- and late-life-onset geriatric depression. *Neurology,* 46, 1567–1574.

Sanacora, G., Mason, G.F., Rothman, D.L., Hyder, F., Ciarcia, J.J., Ostroff, R.B., Berman, R.M., and Krystal, J.H. (2003). Increased cortical GABA concentrations in depressed patients receiving ECT. *Am J Psychiatry,* 160, 577–579.

Sapin, L.R., Berrettini, W.H., Nurnberger, J.I., and Rothblat, L.A. (1987). Mediational factors underlying cognitive changes and laterality in affective illness. *Biol Psychiatry,* 22, 979–986.

Savard, R.J., Rey, A.C., and Post, R.M. (1980). Halstead-Reitan Category Test in bipolar and unipolar affective disorders: Relationship to age and phase of illness. *J Nerv Ment Dis,* 168, 297–304.

Sax, K.W., Strakowski, S.M., Zimmerman, M.E., DelBello, M.P., Keck, P.E. Jr., and Hawkins, J.M. (1999). Frontosubcortical neuroanatomy and the continuous performance test in mania. *Am J Psychiatry,* 156(1), 139–141.

Schachter, S., and Singer, J. (1962). Cognitive, social and physiological determinants of emotional state. *Psych Review, 69,* 379–407.

Schaefer, A., Collette, F., Philippot, P., van der Linden, M., Laureys, S., Delfiore, G., Degueldre, C., Maquet, P., Luxen, A., and Salmon, E. (2003). Neural correlates of "hot" and "cold" emotional processing: A multilevel approach to the functional anatomy of emotion. *Neuroimage, 18,* 938–949.

Schlosser, R., Hutchinson, M., Joseffer, S., Rusinek, H., Saarimaki, A., Stevenson, J., Dewey, S.L., and Brodie, J.D. (1998). Functional magnetic resonance imaging of human brain activity in a verbal fluency task. *J Neurol Neurosurg Psychiatry, 64,* 492–498.

Seidman, L.J., Kremen, W.S., Koren, D., Faraone, S.V., Goldstein, J.M., and Tsuang, M.T. (2002). A comparative profile analysis of neuropsychological functioning in patients with schizophrenia and bipolar psychoses. *Schizophr Res, 53*(1–2), 31–44.

Seidman, L.J., Lanca, M., Kremen, W.S., Faraone, S.V., and Tsuang, M.T. (2003). Organizational and visual memory deficits in schizophrenia and bipolar psychoses using the Rey-Osterrieth complex figure: Effects of duration of illness. *J Clin Exp Neuropsychol, 25*(7), 949–964.

Seminowicz, D.A., Mayberg, H.S., McIntosh, A.R., Goldapple, K., Kennedy, S., Segal, Z., and Rafi-Tari, S. (2004). Limbic-frontal circuitry in major depression: A path modeling metanalysis. *Neuroimage, 22,* 409–418.

Shallice, T. (1982). Specific impairments of planning. *Philos Trans R Soc Lond B Biol Sci, 298,* 199–209.

Shansis, F.M., Busnello, J.V., Quevedo, J., Forster, L., Young, S., Izquierdo, I., and Kapczinski, F. (2000). Behavioural effects of acute tryptophan depletion in healthy male volunteers. *J Psychopharmacol, 14,* 157–163.

Shaw, E.D., Mann, J.J., Stokes, P.E., and Manevitz, A.Z. (1986). Effects of lithium carbonate on associative productivity and idiosyncrasy in bipolar outpatients. *Am J Psychiatry, 143,* 1166–1169.

Shaw, E.D., Stokes, P.E., Mann, J.J., and Manevitz, A.Z. (1987). Effects of lithium carbonate on the memory and motor speed of bipolar outpatients. *J Abnorm Psychology, 96,* 64–69.

Sheline, Y.I., Wang, P.W., Gado, M.H., Csernansky, J.G., and Vannier, M. (1996). Hippocampal atrophy in recurrent major depression. *Proc Natl Acad Sci U S A, 93*(9), 3908–3913.

Sheline, Y.I., Sanghavi, M., Mintun, M.A., and Gado, M.H. (1999). Depression duration but not age predicts hippocampal volume loss in medically healthy women with recurrent major depression. *J Neurosci, 19,* 5034–5043.

Silfverskiöld, P., and Risberg, J. (1989). Regional cerebral blood flow in depression and mania. *Arch Gen Psychiatry, 46,* 253–259.

Silverstone, T., McPherson, H., Li, Q., and Doyle, T. (2003). Deep white matter hyperintensities in patients with bipolar depression, unipolar depression and age-matched control subjects. *Bipolar Disord, 5,* 53–57.

Simpson, S., Talbot, P.R., Snowden, J.S., and Neary, D. (1997a). Subcortical vascular disease in elderly patients with treatment resistant depression [Letter]. *J Neurol Neurosurg Psychiatry, 62,* 196–197.

Simpson, S.W., Jackson, A., Baldwin, R.C., and Burns, A. (1997b). 1997 IPA/Bayer Research Awards in Psychogeriatrics. Subcortical hyperintensities in late-life depression: Acute response to treatment and neuropsychological impairment. *Int Psychogeriatr, 9,* 257–275.

Simpson, S., Baldwin, R.C., Jackson, A., and Burns, A.S. (1998). Is subcortical disease associated with a poor response to antidepressants? Neurological, neuropsychological and neuroradiological findings in late-life depression. *Psychol Med, 28,* 1015–1026.

Small, J.G., Milstein, V., Kellams, J.J., Miller, M.J., Woodham, G.C., and Small, I.F. (1993). Hemispheric components of ECT response in mood disorders and shizophrenia. In C.E. Coeffey (Ed.), *The Clinical Science of Electroconvulsive Therapy* (pp. 111–123). Washington, DC: American Psychiatric Press.

Smith, A.G., Montealegre-Orjuela, M., Douglas, J.E., and Jenkins, E.A. (2003). Venlafaxine for pathological crying after stroke. *J Clin Psychiatry, 64,* 731–732.

Snyder, P.J., and Harris, L.J. (1997). The intracarotid amobarbital procedure: An historical perspective. *Brain Cognition, 33,* 18–32.

Soares, J.C., and Mann, J.J. (1997). The functional neuroanatomy of mood disorders. *J Psychiatr Res, 31,* 393–432.

Sobczak, S., Riedel, W.J., Booij, I., Aan Het Rot, M., Deutz, N.E., and Honig, A. (2002). Cognition following acute tryptophan depletion: Difference between first-degree relatives of bipolar disorder patients and matched healthy control volunteers. *Psychol Med, 32,* 503–515.

Sobin, C., and Sackeim, H.A. (1997). Psychomotor symptoms of depression. *Am J Psychiatry, 154,* 4–17.

Souza, V.B., Muir, W.J., Walker, M.T., Glabus, M.F., Roxborough, H.M., Sharp, C.W., Dunan, J.R., and Blackwood, D.H. (1995). Auditory p300 event-related potentials and neuropsychological performance in schizophrenia and bipolar affective disorder. *Biol Psychiatry, 37*(5), 300–310.

Speer, A.M., Kimbrell, T.A., Wassermann, E.M., J, D.R., Willis, M.W., Herscovitch, P., and Post, R.M. (2000). Opposite effects of high and low frequency rTMS on regional brain activity in depressed patients. *Biol Psychiatry, 48,* 1133–1141.

Spence, S.A., Liddle, P.F., Stefan, M.D., Hellewell, J.S., Sharma, T., Friston, K.J., Hirsch, S.R., Frith, C.D., Murray, R.M., Deakin, J.F., and Grasby, P.M. (2000). Functional anatomy of verbal fluency in people with schizophrenia and those at genetic risk: Focal dysfunction and distributed disconnectivity reappraised. *Br J Psychiatry, 176,* 52–60.

Spitzer, R.L., Endicott, J., and Robins, E. (1978). Research diagnostic criteria: Rationale and reliability. *Arch Gen Psychiatry, 35,* 773–782.

Spreen, O., and Strauss, E. (1998). *A Compendium of Neuropsychological Tests: Administration, Norms, and Commentary* (2nd edition). New York: Oxford University Press.

Squire, L.R., Judd, L.L., Janowsky, D.S., and Huey, L.Y. (1980). Effects of lithium carbonate on memory and other cognitive functions. *Am J Psychiatry, 137,* 1042–1046.

Squire, L.R., Stark, C.E., and Clark, R.E. (2004). The medial temporal lobe. *Ann Rev Neurosci, 27,* 279–306.

Starkstein, S.E., Boston, J.D., and Robinson, R.G. (1988). Mechanisms of mania after brain injury: 12 case reports and review of the literature. *J Nerv Ment Dis, 176,* 87–100.

Stefurak, T., Mikulis, D., Mayberg, H., Lang, A.E., Hevenor, S., Pahapill, P., Saint-Cyr, J., and Lozano, A. (2003). Deep brain stimulation for Parkinson's disease dissociates mood and motor circuits: A functional MRI case study. *Movement Disord, 18,* 1508–1516.

Steif, B., Sackeim, H., Portnoy, S., Decina, P., and Malitz, S. (1986). Effects of depression and ECT on anterograde memory. *Biol Psychiatry, 21,* 921–930.

Steingart, A., Hachinski, V., Lau, C., Fox, A.J., Diaz, F., Cape, R., Lee, D., Inzitari, D., and Merskey, H. (1987). Cognitive and neurologic findings in subjects with diffuse white matter lucencies on computed tomographic scans (leuko-araiosis). *Arch Neurol*, 44, 32–35.

Stern, Y., and Sackeim, H.A. (2002). The neuropsychology of memory and amnesia. In S.C. Yudofsky, R.E. Hales (Eds.), *The American Psychiatric Press Textbook of Neuropsychiatry and Clinical Neurosciences* (4th edition, pp. 597–622). Washington, DC: American Psychiatric Press.

Stern, Y., Sano, M., Pauson, J., and Mayeux, R. (1987). Modified mini-mental status examination: Validity and reliability. *Neurology*, 37(Suppl. 1), 179.

Sternberg, D.E., and Jarvik, M.E. (1976). Memory function in depression: Improvement with antidepressant medication. *Arch Gen Psychiatry*, 33, 219–224.

Stoll, A.L., Locke, C.A., Vuckovic, A., and Mayer, P.V. (1996). Lithium-associated cognitive and functional deficits reduced by a switch to divalproex sodium: A case series. *J Clin Psychiatry*, 57, 356–359.

Strakowksi, S.M., Adler, C.M., Holland, S.K., Mills, N.P., DelBello, M.P., and Eliassen, J.C. (2005). Abnormal fMRI brain activation in euthymic bipolar disorder patients during a counting stroop interference task. *Am J Psychiatry*, 162, 1697–1705.

Strömgren, L. (1977). The influence of depression on memory. *Acta Psychiatr Scand*, 56, 109–128.

Suppes, T., Webb, A., Carmody, T., Gordon, E., Gutierrez-Esteinou, R., Hudson, J.I., and Pope, H.G.J. (1996). Is postictal electrical silence a predictor of response to electroconvulsive therapy? *J Affect Disord*, 41, 55–58.

Swann, A.C., Katz, M.M., Bowden, C.L., Berman, N.G., and Stokes, P.E. (1999). Psychomotor performance and monoamine function in bipolar and unipolar affective disorders. *Biol Psychiatry*, 45, 979–988.

Swann, A.C., Pazzaglia, P., Nicholls, A., Dougherty, D.M., and Moeller, F.G. (2003). Impulsivity and phase of illness in bipolar disorder. *J Affect Disord*, 73(1–2), 105–111.

Swanson, J., Castellanos, F.X., Murias, M., LaHoste, G., and Kennedy, J. (1998). Cognitive neuroscience of attention deficit hyperactivity disorder and hyperkinetic disorder. *Curr Opin Neurobiol*, 8, 263–271.

Swayze, V.W.D., Andreasen, N.C., Alliger, R.J., Ehrhardt, J.C., and Yuh, W.T. (1990). Structural brain abnormalities in bipolar affective disorder: Ventricular enlargement and focal signal hyperintensities. *Arch Gen Psychiatry*, 47, 1054–1059.

Sweeney, J.A., Kmiec, J.A., and Kupfer, D.J. (2000). Neuropsychologic impairments in bipolar and unipolar mood disorders on the CANTAB neurocognitive battery. *Biol Psychiatry*, 48, 674–684.

Szabadi, E., Bradshaw, C.M., and Besson, J.A. (1976). Elongation of pause-time in speech: A simple, objective measure of motor retardation in depression. *Br J Psychiatry*, 129, 592–597.

Takayama, M., Miyamoto, S., Ikeda, A., Mikuni, N., Takahashi, J.B., Usui, K., Satow, T., Yamamoto, J., Matsuhashi, M., Matsumoto, R., Nagamine, T., Shibasaki, H., and Hashimoto, N. (2004). Intracarotid propofol test for speech and memory dominance in man. *Neurology*, 63, 510–515.

Tanaka, M., and Sumitsuji, N. (1991). Electromyographic study of facial expressions during pathological laughing and crying. *Electromyogr Clin Neurophysiol*, 31, 399–406.

Tateno, A., Jorge, R.E., and Robinson, R.G. (2004). Pathological laughing and crying following traumatic brain injury. *J Neuropsychiatry Clin Neurosci*, 16, 426–434.

Tavares, J.V., Drevets, W.C., and Sahakian, B.J. (2003). Cognition in mania and depression. *Psychol Med*, 33, 959–967.

Taylor, M.A., and Abrams, R. (1983). Schizo-affective disorder, manic type. A clinical, laboratory, and genetic study. *Psychiatr Clin (Basel)*, 16(2–4), 234–244.

Taylor, S.E., and Brown, J.D. (1988). Illusion and well-being: A social psychological perspective on mental health. *Psychol Bull*, 103, 193–210.

Taylor, S.E., and Brown, J.D. (1994). Positive illusions and well-being revisited: Separating fact from fiction. *Psychol Bull*, 116, 21–27; discussion 28.

Teicher, M.H., Lawrence, J.M., Barber, N.I., Finklestein, S.P., Lieberman, H.R., and Baldessarini, R.J. (1988). Increased activity and phase delay in circadian motility rhythms in geriatric depression: Preliminary observations. *Arch Gen Psychiatry*, 45, 913–917.

Telford, R., and Worrall, E.P. (1978). Cognitive functions in manic-depressives: Effects of lithium and physostigmine. *Br J Psychiatry*, 133, 424–428.

Teneback, C.C., Nahas, Z., Speer, A.M., Molloy, M., Stallings, L.E., Spicer, K.M., Risch, S.C., and George, M.S. (1999). Changes in prefrontal cortex and paralimbic activity in depression following two weeks of daily left prefrontal TMS. *J Neuropsychiatry Clin Neurosci*, 11, 426–435.

Terao, Y., and Ugawa, Y. (2002). Basic mechanisms of TMS. *J Clin Neurophysiol*, 19, 322–343.

Terzian, H. (1964). Behavioural and EEG effects of intracarotid sodium amytal injection. *Acta Neurochirurgica*, 12, 230–239.

Terzian, H., and Cecotto, C. (1959). Determination and study of hemispheric dominance by means of intracarotid injection of sodium amytal in man: I. Clinical modifications. *Bollettino–Societa Italiana Biologia Sperimentale*, 35, 1623–1626.

Tham, A., Engelbrektson, K., Mathe, A.A., Johnson, L., Olsson, E., and Aberg-Wistedt, A. (1997). Impaired neuropsychological performance in euthymic patients with recurring mood disorders. *J Clin Psychiatry*, 58, 26–29.

Thomas, P., Kearney, G., Napier, E., Ellis, E., Leuder, I., and Johnson, M. (1996). Speech and language in first onset psychosis differences between people with schizophrenia, mania, and controls. *Br J Psychiatry*, 168(3), 337–343.

Thomas, P., Goudemand, M., and Rousseaux, M. (1999). Attentional resources in major depression. *Eur Arch Psychiatry Clin Neurosci*, 249, 79–85.

Tohen, M., Waternaux, C.M., and Tsuang, M.T. (1990a). Outcome in Mania: A 4-year prospective follow-up of 75 patients utilizing survival analysis. *Arch Gen Psychiatry*, 47, 1106–1111.

Tohen, M., Waternaux, C.M., Tsuang, M.T., and Hunt, A.T. (1990b). Four-year follow-up of twenty-four first-episode manic patients. *J Affect Disord*, 19, 79–86.

Tohen, M., Hennen, J., Zarate, C.M. Jr., Baldessarini, R.J., Strakowski, S.M., Stoll, A.L., Faedda, G.L., Suppes, T., Gebre-Medhin, P., and Cohen, B.M. (2000). Two-year syndromal and functional recovery in 219 cases of first-episode major affective disorder with psychotic features. *Am J Psychiatry*, 157, 220–228.

Torrent, C., Martinez-Aran, A., Daban, C., Sanchez-Moreno, J., Comes, M., Goikolea, J.M., Salamero, M., and Vieta, E. (2006). Cognitive impairment in bipolar II disorder. *Br J Psychiatry*, 189, 254–259.

Tortella, F.C., and Long, J.B. (1985). Endogenous anticonvulsant substance in rat cerebrospinal fluid after a generalized seizure. *Science*, 228, 1106–1108.

Umbricht, D., Koller, R., Schmid, L., Skrabo, A., Grubel, C., Huber, T., and Stassen, H. (2003). How specific are deficits in mismatch negativity generation to schizophrenia? *Biol Psychiatry*, 53(12), 1120–1131.

van Gorp, W.G., Altshuler, L., Theberge, D.C., Wilkins, J., and Dixon, W. (1998). Cognitive impairment in euthymic bipolar patients with and without prior alcohol dependence: A preliminary study. *Arch Gen Psychiatry*, 55, 41–46.

van Gorp, W.G., Altshuler, L., Theberge, D.C., and Mintz, J. (1999). Declarative and procedural memory in bipolar disorder. *Biol Psychiatry*, 46, 525–531.

van Vugt, J.P., Siesling, S., Piet, K.K., Zwinderman, A.H., Middelkoop, H.A., van Hilten, J.J., and Roos, R.A. (2001). Quantitative assessment of daytime motor activity provides a responsive measure of functional decline in patients with Huntington's disease. *Movement Disord*, 16, 481–488.

Velten, E. Jr. (1968). A laboratory task for induction of mood states. *Behav Res Ther*, 6, 473–482.

Videbech, P. (1997). MRI findings in patients with affective disorder: A meta-analysis. *Acta Psychiatr Scand*, 96, 157–168.

Volkers, A.C., Tulen, J.H., van den Broek, W.W., Bruijn, J.A., Passchier, J., and Pepplinkhuizen, L. (2003). Motor activity and autonomic cardiac functioning in major depressive disorder. *J Affect Disord*, 76, 23–30.

Volkow, N.D., Bellar, S., Mullani, N., Jould, L., and Dewey, S. (1988). Effects of electroconvulsive therapy on brain glucose metabolism: A preliminary study. *Convulsive Ther*, 4, 199–205.

Vuilleumier, P., Ghika-Schmid, F., Bogousslavsky, J., Assal, G., and Regli, F. (1998). Persistent recurrence of hypomania and prosopoaffective agnosia in a patient with right thalamic infarct. *Neuropsychiatry Neuropsychol Behav Neurol*, 11, 40–44.

Wada, J.A. (1997). Clinical experimental observations of carotid artery injections of sodium amytal. *Brain Cognition*, 33, 11–13.

Wassermann, E.M., Pascual-Leone, A., Valls-Sole, J., Toro, C., Cohen, L.G., and Hallett, M. (1993). Topography of the inhibitory and excitatory responses to transcranial magnetic stimulation in a hand muscle. *Electroencephalogr Clin Neurophysiol*, 89, 424–433.

Wechsler, D. (1981). *Wechsler Adult Intelligence Scale—Revised*. New York: Psychological Corporation.

Weingartner, H., Miller, H., and Murphy, D.L. (1977). Mood-state-dependent retrieval of verbal associations. *J Abnorm Psychol*, 86, 276–284.

Weingartner, H., Cohen, R.M., Murphy, D.L., Martello, J., and Gerdt, C. (1981). Cognitive processes in depression. *Arch Gen Psychiatry*, 38, 42–47.

Weiss, B.L., Foster, F.G., Reynolds, C.F. III, and Kupfer, D.J. (1974a). Psychomotor activity in mania. *Arch Gen Psychiatry*, 31, 379–383.

Weiss, B.L., Kupfer, D.J., Foster, F.G., and Delgado, J. (1974b). Psychomotor activity, sleep, and biogenic amine metabolites in depression. *Biol Psychiatry*, 9, 45–54.

Whitehead, A. (1973a). The pattern of WAIS performance in elderly psychiatric patients. *Br J Social Clin Psychol*, 12, 435–436.

Whitehead, A. (1973b). Verbal learning and memory in elderly depressives. *Br J Psychiatry*, 123, 203–208.

Wickelgren, W. (1973). The long and short of of memory. *Psychol Bull*, 80, 425–438.

Widlocher, D.J. (1983). Psychomotor retardation: Clinical, theoretical, and psychometric aspects. *Psychiatr Clin North Am*, 6, 27–40.

Wielgus, M.S., and Harvey, P.D. (1988). Dichotic listening and recall in schizophrenia and mania. *Schizophr Bull*, 14(4), 689–700.

Winter, L., Lawton, M.P., Casten, R.J., and Sando, R.L. (2000). The relationship between external events and affect states in older people. *Int J Aging Hum Dev*, 50, 85–96.

Wolfe, J., Granholm, E., Butters, N., Saunders, E., and Janowsky, D. (1987). Verbal memory deficits associated with major affective disorders: A comparison of unipolar and bipolar patients. *J Affect Disord*, 13, 83–92.

Wolff, E.A. III, Putnam, F.W., and Post, R.M. (1985). Motor activity and affective illness: The relationship of amplitude and temporal distribution to changes in affective state. *Arch Gen Psychiatry*, 42, 288–294.

Woodruff, R., Robins, L., and Winokur, G. (1968). Educational and occupational achievement in primary affective disorder. *Am J Psychiatry*, 124, 57–64.

Woodruff, R.J., Robins, L.N., Winokur, G., and Reich, T. (1971). Manic depressive illness and social achievement. *Acta Psychiatr Scand*, 47, 237–249.

Woods, D.L., Knight, R.T., and Scabini, D. (1993). Anatomical substrates of auditory selective attention: Behavioral and electrophysiological effects of posterior association cortex lesions. *Brain Res Cognitive Brain Res*, 1, 227–240.

Wu, J.C., Gillin, J.C., Buchsbaum, M.S., Hershey, T., Johnson, J.C., and Bunney, W.E.J. (1992). Effect of sleep deprivation on brain metabolism of depressed patients. *Am J Psychiatry*, 149, 538–543.

Wu, J., Buchsbaum, M.S., Gillin, J.C., Tang, C., Cadwell, S., Wiegand, M., Najafi, A., Klein, E., Hazen, K., Bunney, W.E.J., Fallon, J.H., and Keator, D. (1999). Prediction of antidepressant effects of sleep deprivation by metabolic rates in the ventral anterior cingulate and medial prefrontal cortex. *Am J Psychiatry*, 156, 1149–1158.

Wu, L., Goto, Y., Taniwaki, T., Kinukawa, N., and Tobimatsu, S. (2002). Different patterns of excitation and inhibition of the small hand and forearm muscles from magnetic brain stimulation in humans. *Clin Neurophysiol*, 113, 1286–1294.

Wyatt, R.J. (1991). Neuroleptics and the natural course of schizophrenia. *Schizophrenia Bull*, 17, 325–351.

Wyatt, R.J. (1995). Early intervention for schizophrenia: Can the course of the illness be altered? *Biol Psychiatry*, 38, 1–3.

Yan, S.M., Flor-Henry, P., Chen, D.Y., Li, T.G., Qi, S.G., and Ma, Z.X. (1985). Imbalance of hemispheric functions in the major psychoses: A study of handedness in the People's Republic of China. *Biol Psychiatry*, 20, 906–917.

Yang, J.A., and Rehm, L.P. (1993). A study of autobiographical memories in depressed and nondepressed elderly individuals. *Int J Aging Hum Devel*, 36, 39–55.

Yen, C.F., Chung, L.C., and Chen, C.S. (2002). Insight and neuropsychological functions in bipolar outpatients in remission. *J Nerv Ment Dis*, 190, 713–715.

Yovell, Y., Sackeim, H.A., Epstein, D.G., Prudic, J., Devanand, D.P., McElhiney, M.C., Settembrino, J.M., and Bruder, G.E. (1995). Hearing loss and asymmetry in major depression. *J Neuropsychiatry Clin Neurosci*, 7, 82–89.

Yu, L., Liu, C.K., Chen, J.W., Wang, S.Y., Wu, Y.H., and Yu, S.H. (2004). Relationship between post-stroke depression and lesion location: A meta-analysis. *Kaohsiung J Med Sci*, 20, 372–380.

Zakzanis, K.K., Leach, L., and Kaplan, E. (1998). On the nature and pattern of neurocognitive function in major depressive disorder. *Neuropsychiatry Neuropsychol Behav Neurol*, 11, 111–119.

Zalla, T., Joyce, C., Szoke, A., Schurhoff, F., Pillon, B., Komano, O., Perez-Diaz, F., Bellivier, F., Alter, C., Dubois, B., Rouillon, F., Houde, O., and Leboyer, M. (2004). Executive dysfunctions as potential markers of familial vulnerability to bipolar disorder and schizophrenia. *Psychiatry Res*, 121, 207–217.

Zarate, C.A. Jr., Tohen, M., Land, M., and Cavanagh, S. (2000). Functional impairment and cognition in bipolar disorder. *Psychiatr Q*, 71, 309–329.

Zubenko, G.S., Sullivan, P., Nelson, J.P., Belle, S.H., Huff, F.J., and Wolf, G.L. (1990). Brain imaging abnormalities in mental disorders of late life. *Arch Neurol*, 47, 1107–1111.

Zubieta, J.K., Huguelet, P., O'Neil, R.L., and Giordani, B.J. (2001). Cognitive function in euthymic bipolar I disorder. *Psychiatry Res*, 102, 9–20.

CHAPTER 10

Abou-Saleh, M.T., and Coppen, A. (1984). Classification of depressive illness: Clinico-psychological correlates. *J Affect Disord*, 6(1), 53–66.

Abraham, K. (1911). Notes on the psycho-analytical investigation and treatment of manic-depressive insanity and allied conditions. In D. Bryan, A. Strachey (Translators), *Selected Papers of Karl Abraham, M.D.* (pp. 137–156). London, England: Hogarth Press, 1927.

Abraham, K. (1924). A short study of the development of the libido, viewed in the light of mental disorders. In D. Bryan, A. Strachey (Translators), *Selected Papers of Karl Abraham, M.D.* (pp. 418–480). London, England: Hogarth Press, 1927.

Akiskal, H.S., Djenderedjian, A.M., Rosenthal, R.H., and Khani, M.K. (1977). Cyclothymic disorder: Validating criteria for inclusion in the bipolar affective group. *Am J Psychiatry*, 134(11), 1227–1233.

Akiskal, H.S., Hirschfeld, R.M., and Yerevanian, B.I. (1983). The relationship of personality to affective disorders. *Arch Gen Psychiatry*, 40(7), 801–810.

Akiskal, H.S., Chen, S.E., Davis, G.C., Puzantian, V.R., Kashgarian, M., and Bolinger, J.M. (1985). Borderline: An adjective in search of a noun. *J Clin Psychiatry*, 46(2), 41–48.

Akiskal, H.S., Bourgeois, M.L., Angst, J., Post, R., Moller, H., and Hirschfeld, R. (2000). Re-evaluating the prevalence of and diagnostic composition within the broad clinical spectrum of bipolar disorders. *J Affect Disord*, 59(Suppl. 1), S5–S30.

Akiskal, H.S., Kilzieh, N., Maser, J.D., Clayton, P.J., Schettler, P.J., Shea, M.T., Endicott, J., Scheftner, W., Hirschfeld, R.M.A., and Keller, M.B. (2006). The distinct temperament profiles of bipolar I, bipolar II and unipolar patients. *J Affect Disord*, 92, 19–33.

Alexander, F. (1948). *Fundamentals of Psychoanalysis*. New York: WW Norton.

Allison, J.B., and Wilson, W.P. (1960). Sexual behaviors of manic patients: A preliminary report. *South Med J*, 53, 870–874.

Allport, G.W. (1961). *Pattern and Growth in Personality*. New York: Holt, Rinehart and Winston.

Anderson, C.A., and Hammen, C.L. (1993). Psychosocial outcomes of children of unipolar depressed, bipolar, medically ill, and normal women: A longitudinal study. *J Consult Clin Psychol*, 61(3), 448–454.

Anderson, P., Beach, S.R.H., and Kaslow, N.J. (1999). Marital discord and depression: The potential of attachment theory to guide integrative clinical intervention. In T. Joiner, C.C. Coyne (Eds.), *The Interactional Nature of Depression* (pp. 271–297). Washington, DC: American Psychological Association.

Arieti, S. (1959). Manic-depressive psychoses. In S. Arieti (Ed.), *American Handbook of Psychiatry*. New York: Basic Books.

Barbato, N., and Hafner, R.J. (1998). Comorbidity of bipolar and personality disorder. *Aust N Z J Psychiatry*, 32(2), 276–280.

Bauer, M.S., Kirk, G.F., Gavin, C., and Williford, W.O. (2001). Determinants of functional outcome and healthcare costs in bipolar disorder: A high-intensity follow-up study. *J Affect Disord*, 65(3), 231–241.

Bauwens, F., Tracy, A., Pardoen, D., Vander Elst, M., and Mendlewicz, J. (1991). Social adjustment of remitted bipolar and unipolar out-patients: A comparison with age- and sex-matched controls. *Br J Psychiatry*, 159, 239–244.

Beach, S.R.H., and Jones, D. (2002). Marital and family therapy for depression in adults. In I. Gotlib, C. Hammen (Eds.), *Handbook of Depression* (pp. 422–440). New York: Guilford Press.

Beardslee, W.R., Versage, E.M., and Gladstone, T.R. (1998). Children of affectively ill parents: A review of the past 10 years. *J Am Acad Child Adolesc Psychiatry*, 37(11), 1134–1141.

Bech, P., Shapiro, R.W., Sihm, F., Nielsen, B.M., Sorensen, B., and Rafaelsen, O.J. (1980). Personality in unipolar and bipolar manic-malancholic patients. *Acta Psychiatr Scand*, 62(3), 245–257.

Beigel, A., Murphy, D.L., and Bunney, W.E. (1971). The Manic-State Rating Scale: Scale construction, reliability, and validity. *Arch Gen Psychiatry*, 25, 256–262.

Belmaker, R.H., Lehrer, R., Ebstein, R.P., Lettik, H., and Kugelmass, S. (1979). A possible cardiovascular effect of lithium. *Am J Psychiatry*, 136, 577–579.

Benazzi, F. (2000). Exploring aspects of DSM-IV interpersonal sensitivity in bipolar II. *J Affect Disord* 60(1), 43–46.

Benazzi, F., and Akiskal, H.S. (2005). A downscaled practical measure of mood lability as a screening tool for bipolar II. *J Affect Disord*, 84, 225–232.

Bieling, P.J., MacQueen, G.M., Marriot, M.J., Robb, J.C., Begin, H., Joffe, R.T., and Young, L.T. (2003). Longitudinal outcome in patients with bipolar disorder assessed by life-charting is influenced by DSM-IV personality disorder symptoms. *Bipolar Disord*, 5(1), 14–21.

Billings, A.G., and Moos, R.H. (1985). Psychosocial processes of remission in unipolar depression: Comparing depressed patients with matched community controls. *J Consult Clin Psychol*, 53(3), 314–325.

Blairy, S., Linotte, S., Souery, D., Papadimitriou, G.N., Dikeos, D., Lerer, B., Kaneva, R., Milanova, V., Serretti, A., Macciardi, F., and Mendlewicz, J. (2004). Social adjustment and self-esteem of bipolar patients: A multicenter study. *J Affect Disord*, 79, 97–103.

Blalock, J.R. (1936). Psychology of the manic phase of the manic-depressive psychoses. *Psychiatr Q*, 10, 263–344.

Bleuler, E. (1924). *Textbook of Psychiatry* (4th German Edition). A.A. Brill (Ed.). New York: Macmillan.

Bonetti, U., Johansson, F., Von Knorring, L., Perris, C., and Strandman, E. (1977). Prophylactic lithium and personality variables: An international collaborative study. *Int Pharmacopsychiatry*, 12, 14–19.

Brieger, P., Ehrt, U., and Marneros, A. (2003). Frequency of co-morbid personality disorders in bipolar and unipolar affective disorders. *Compr Psychiatry*, 44(1), 28–34.

Brodie, H.K., and Leff, M.J. (1971). Bipolar depression: A comparative study of patient characteristics. *Am J Psychiatry*, 127(8), 1086–1090.

Brown, G.W., and Harris, T. (1986). Establishing causal links: The Bedford College studies of depression. In H. Katschnig (Ed.), *Life Events and Psychiatric Disorders: Controversial Issues* (pp. 107–187). Cambridge, England: Cambridge University Press.

Campbell, J.D. (1953). *Manic-Depressive Disease: Clinical and Psychiatric Significance*. Philadelphia: JB Lippincott.

Cannon, M., Jones, P., Gilvarry, C., Rifkin, L., McKenzie, K., Foerster, A., and Murray, R.M. (1997). Premorbid social functioning in schizophrenia and bipolar disorder: Similarities and differences, *Am J Psychiatry*, 154(11), 1544–1550.

Carpenter, D., Clarkin, J.F., Glick, I.D., and Wilner, P.J. (1995). Personality pathology among married adults with bipolar disorder. *J Affect Disord*, 34(4), 269–274.

Carpenter, D., Clarkin, J.F., Isman, L., and Patten, M. (1999). The impact of neuroticism upon married bipolar patients. *J Personal Disord*, 13(1), 60–66.

Carpenter, K.M., and Hittner, J.B. (1995). Dimensional characteristics of the SCL-90-R: Evaluation of gender differences in dually diagnosed inpatients. *J Clin Psychol*, 51(3), 383–390.

Casper, R.C., Redmond, E. Jr., Katz, M.M., Schaffer, C.B., Davis, J.M., and Koslow, S.H. (1985). Somatic symptoms in primary affective disorder: Presence and relationship to the classification of depression. *Arch Gen Psychiatry*, 42, 1098–1104.

Cassano, G.B., Akiskal, H.S., Savino, M., Musetti, L., and Perugi, G. (1992). Proposed subtypes of bipolar II and related disorders; with hypomanic episodes (or cyclothymia) and with hyperthymic temperament. *J Affect Disord*, 26, 127–140.

Chakrabarti, S., and Gill, S. (2002). Coping and its correlates among caregivers of patients with bipolar disorder: A preliminary study. *Bipolar Disord*, 4(1), 50–60.

Chang, K.D., Blasey, C., Ketter, T.A., and Steiner, H. (2001). Family environment of children and adolescents with bipolar parents. *Bipolar Disord*, 3(2), 73–78.

Chang, K.D., Blascy, C.M., Ketter, T.A., and Steiner, H. (2003). Temperament characteristics of child and adolescent bipolar offspring. *J Affect Disord*, 77, 11–19.

Chodoff, P. (1972). The depressive personality: A critical review. *Arch Gen Psychiatry*, 27(5), 666–673.

Clark, L.A., Watson, D., and Mineka, S. (1994). Temperament, personality, and the mood and anxiety disorders. *J Abnorm Psychol*, 103(1), 103–116.

Clarkin, J.F., Carpenter, D., Hull, J., Wilner, P., and Glick, I. (1998). Effects of psychoeducational intervention for married patients with bipolar disorder and their spouses. *Psychiatr Serv*, 49(4), 531–533.

Clayton, P.J., Ernst, C., and Angst, J. (1994). Premorbid personality traits of men who develop unipolar or bipolar disorders. *Eur Arch Psychiatry Clin Neurosci*, 243(6), 340–346.

Cloninger, C.R. (1987). A systematic method for clinical description and classification of personality variants. A proposal. *Arch Gen Psychiatry*, 44(6), 573–588.

Cohen, A.N., Hammen, C., Henry, R.M., and Daley, S.E. (2004). Effects of stress and social support on recurrence in bipolar disorder. *J Affect Disord*, 82(1), 143–147.

Cohen, M.B., Baker, G., Cohen, R.A., Fromm-Reichmann, F., and Weigert, E.V. (1954). An intensive study of twelve cases of manic-depressive psychosis. *Psychiatry*, 17, 103–137.

Colombo, M., Cox, G., and Dunner, D.L. (1990). Assortative mating in affective and anxiety disorders: Preliminary findings. *Psychiatr Genet*, 1, 35–44.

Cooke, R.G., Robb, J.C., Young, L.T., and Joffe, R.T. (1996). Well-being and functioning in patients with bipolar disorder assessed using the MOS 20-ITEM short form (SF-20). *J Affect Disord*, 39(2), 93–97.

Coryell, W., Endicott, J., and Keller, M. (1992). Major depression in a nonclinical sample. Demographic and clinical risk factors for first onset. *Arch Gen Psychiatry*, 49(2), 117–125.

Coryell, W., Scheftner, W., Keller, M., Endicott, J., Maser, J., and Klerman, G.L. (1993). The enduring psychosocial consequences of mania and depression. *Am J Psychiatry*, 150(5), 720–727.

Coryell, W., Turvey, C., Endicott, J., Leon, A.C., Mueller, T., Solomon, D., and Keller, M. (1998). Bipolar I affective disorder: Predictors of outcome after 15 years. *J Affect Disord*, 50(2–3), 109–116.

Costa, P.T., and McCrae, R.R. (1985). *The NEO-Personality Inventory Manual*. Odessa, FL: Psychological Assessment Resources.

Costa, P.T., and McCrae, R.R. (1992). *NEO PI-R Professional Manual: Revised NEO Personality Inventory (NEO PI-R) and NEO Five-Factor Inventory (NEO-FFI)*. Odessa, FL: Psychological Assessment Resources.

Coyne, J.C. (1976). Depression and the response of others. *J Abnorm Psychol*, 85(2), 186–193.

Coyne, J.C., Kessler, R.C., Tal, M., Turnbull, J., Wortman, C.B., and Greden, J.F. (1987). Living with a depressed person. *J Consult Clin Psychol*, 55(3), 347–352.

Cronin, C., and Zuckerman, M. (1992). Sensation seeking and bipolar affective disorder. *Pers Individ Dif*, 13, 385–387.

Custance, J. (1952). *Wisdom, Madness, and Folly: The Philosophy of a Lunatic*. New York: Farrar, Straus, & Cudahy.

Dax, E.C. (1953). *Experimental Studies in Psychiatric Art*. London: Faber & Faber.

Deltito, J., Martin, L., Riefkohl, J., Austria, B., Kissilenko, A., Corless, C., and Morse, P. (2001). Do patients with borderline personality disorder belong to the bipolar spectrum? *J Affect Disord*, 67(1–3), 221–228.

Demers, R.G., and Davis, L.S. (1971). The influence of prophylactic lithium treatment on the marital adjustment of manic-depressives and their spouses. *Compr Psychiatry*, 12(4), 348–353.

DePaulo, J.R., Correa, E.I., and Folstein, M.F. (1983). Does lithium stabilize mood? *Biol Psychiatry*, 18, 1093–1097.

Depue, R.A., and Iacono, W.G. (1988). Neurobehavioral aspects of affective disorders. *Ann Rev Psychol*, 40, 457–492.

Depue, R.A., Slater, J.F., Wolfstetter-Kausch, H., Klein, D., Goplerud, E., and Farr, D. (1981). A behavioral paradigm for identifying persons at risk for bipolar depressive disorder: A conceptual framework and five validation studies. *J Abnorm Psychol*, 90(5), 381–437.

Depue, R.A., Luciana, M., Arbisi, P., Collins, P., and Leon, A. (1994). Dopamine and the structure of personality: Relation of agonist-induced dopamine activity to positive emotionality. *J Pers Soc Psychol*, 67(3), 485–498.

Dickerson, F.B., Sommerville, J., Origoni, A.E., Ringel, N.B., and Parente, F. (2001). Outpatients with schizophrenia and bipolar I disorder: Do they differ in their cognitive and social functioning? *Psychiatry Res*, 102(1), 21–27.

Donnelly, E.F., and Murphy, D.L. (1973). Primary affective disorder: MMPI differences between unipolar and bipolar depressed subjects. *J Clin Psychol*, 29(3), 303–306.

Donnelly, E.F., and Murphy, D.L. (1974). Primary affective disorder: Bender-Gestalt sequence of placement as an indicator of impulse control. *Percept Motor Skills*, 38(3), 1079–1082.

Donnelly, E.F., Murphy, D.L., and Goodwin, F.K. (1976). Cross-sectional and longitudinal comparisons of bipolar and unipolar depressed groups on the MMPI. *J Consult Clin Psychol*, 44(2), 233–237.

Dooley, L. (1921). A psychoanalytic study of manic depressive psychoses. *Psychoanal Rev*, 8, 144–167.

Dore, G., and Romans, S.E. (2001). Impact of bipolar affective disorder on family and partners. *J Affect Disord*, 67(1–3), 147–158.

Dorz, S., Borgherini, G., Cognolato, S., Conforti, D., Fiorellini, A.L., Scarso, C., and Magni, G. (2002). Social adjustment in in-patients with affective disorders: Predictive factors. *J Affect Disord*, 70(1), 49–56.

Downey, G., and Coyne, J.C. (1990). Children of depressed parents: An integrative review. *Psychol Bull*, 108(1), 50–76.

Dunayevich, E., Strakowski, S.M., Sax, K.W., Sorter, M.T., Keck, P.E. Jr., McElroy, S.L., and McConville, B.J. (1996). Personality disorders in first- and multiple-episode mania. *Psychiatry Res*, 64(1), 69–75.

Dunayevich, E., Sax, K.W., Keck, P.E. Jr., McElroy, S.L., Sorter, M.T., McConville, B.J., and Strakowski, S.M. (2000). Twelve-month outcome in bipolar patients with and without personality disorders. *J Clin Psychiatry*, 61(2), 134–139.

English, O.S. (1949). Observation of trends in manic-depressive psychosis. *Psychiatry*, 12, 125–133.

Engström, C., Brändström, S., Sigvardsson, S., Cloninger, R., Nylander, P.-O. (2003). Bipolar disorder: II. Personality and age of onset. *Bipolar Disord*, 5, 340–348.

Evans, L., Akiskal, H.S., Keck, P.E., McElroy, S.L., Sadovnick, A.D., Remick, R.A., and Kelsoe, J.R. (2005). Familialry of temperament in bipolar disorder: Support for a genetic spectrum. *J Affect Disord*, 85, 153–168.

Eysenck, H.J. (1956). The questionnaire measurement of neuroticism and extraversion. *Revista di Psicologia*, 50, 113–140.

Eysenck, H.J. (1959). *The Manual of the Maudsley Personality Inventory*. London: University of London Press.

Eysenck, H.J., and Eysenck, S.B.G. (1963a). *Eysenck Personality Inventory*. San Diego: Educational and Industrial Testing Service.

Eysenck, H.J., and Eysenck, S.B.G. (1963b). *Manual of the Eysenck Personality Inventory*. San Diego: Educational and Industrial Testing Service.

Fadden, G., Bebbington, P., and Kuipers, L. (1987). Caring and its burdens. A study of the spouses of depressed patients. *Br J Psychiatry*, 151, 660–667.

Fenichel, O. (1945). *The Psychoanalytic Theory of Neuroses*. New York: WW Norton.

Flick, S.N., Roy-Byrne, P.P., Cowley, D.S., Shores, M.M., and Dunner, D.L. (1993). DSM-III-R personality disorders in a mood and anxiety disorders clinic: Prevalence, comorbidity, and clinical correlates. *J Affect Disord*, 27(2), 71–79.

Folstein, M.F., DePaulo, J.R. Jr., and Trepp, K. (1982). Unusual mood stability in patients taking lithium. *Br J Psychiatry*, 140, 188–191.

Frank, E., Targum, S.D., Gershon, E.S., Anderson, C., Stewart, B.D., Davenport, Y., Ketchum, K.L., and Kupfer, D.J. (1981). A comparison of nonpatient and bipolar patient–well spouse couples. *Am J Psychiatry*, 138(6), 764–768.

Freud, S. (1917). Mourning and melancholia. In W. Gaylin (Ed.), *The Meaning of Despair: Psychoanalytic Contributions to the Understanding of Depression*. New York: Science House, 1968.

Frey, R. (1977). Die prämorbide Persönlichkeit von monopolar und bipolar Depressiven: Ein Vergleich aufgrund von Persönlichkeitstests. *Archiv Psychiatr Nervenkr*, 224, 161–173.

Fromm-Reichmann, F. (1949). Intensive psychotherapy of manic-depressives: A preliminary report. *Confina Neurologica*, 9, 158–165.

Garma, A. (1968). The deceiving superego and the masochistic ego in mania. *Psychoanal Q*, 37(1), 63–79.

Gelfand, D.M., and Teti, D.M. (1990). The effects of maternal depression on children. *Clin Psychol Rev*, 10, 320–354.

George, E.L., Miklowitz, D.J., Richards, J.A., Simoneau, T.L., and Taylor, D.O. (2003). The comorbidity of bipolar disorders and axis II personality disorders: Prevalence and clinical correlates. *Bipolar Disord*, 5(2), 115–122.

Gerö, G. (1936). Construction of depression. *Int J Psychoanal*, 17, 423–461.

Gershon, E.S., McKnew, D., Cytryn, L., Hamovit, J., Schreiber, J., Hibbs, E., and Pellegrini, D. (1985). Diagnoses in school-age children of bipolar affective disorder patients and normal controls. *J Affect Disord*, 8(3), 283–291.

Gibson, R.W., Cohen, M.B., and Cohen, R.A. (1959). On the dynamics of the manic-depressive personality. *Am J Psychiatry*, 115, 1101–1107.

Gitlin, M.J., Swendsen, J., Heller, T.L., and Hammen, C. (1995). Relapse and impairment in bipolar disorder. *Am J Psychiatry*, 152(11), 1635–1640.

Goodman, S.H., and Gotlib, I.H. (1999). Risk for psychopathology in the children of depressed mothers: A developmental model for understanding mechanisms of transmission. *Psychol Rev*, 106(3), 458–490.

Gordon, D., Burge, D., Hammen, C., Adrian, C., Jaenicke, C., and Hiroto, D. (1989). Observations of interactions of depressed women with their children. *Am J Psychiatry*, 146(1), 50–55.

Gotlib, I.H., and Whiffen, V.E. (1989). Depression and marital functioning: An examination of specificity and gender differences. *J Abnorm Psychol*, 98(1), 23–30.

Grant, B.F., Stinson, F.S., Hasin, D.S., Dawson, D.A., Chou, P., Ruan, W.J., and Huang, B. (2005). Prevalence, correlates, and comorbidity of bipolar I disorder and axis I and II disorders: Results from the National Epidemiologic Survey on Alcohol and Related Conditions. *J Clin Psychiatry*, 66, 1205–1215.

Gray, J.A. (1982). *The Neuropsychology of Anxiety: An Enquiry into the Functions of the Septa-Hippocampal System*. Oxford, England: Clarendon Press.

Grigoroiu-Serbanescu, M., Christodorescu, D., Jipescu, I., Totoescu, A., Marinescu, E., and Ardelean, V. (1989). Psychopathology in children aged 10–17 of bipolar parents: Psychopathology rate and correlates of the severity of the psychopathology. *J Affect Disord*, 16(2–3), 167–179.

Grigoroiu-Serbanescu, M., Christodorescu, D., Totoescu, A., and Jipescu, I. (1991). Depressive disorders and depressive personality traits in offspring aged 10–17 of bipolar and of normal parents. *Journal of Youth and Adolescence*, 20, 135–148.

Grotstein, J.S. (1986). The psychology of powerlessness: Disorders of self-regulation and interactional regulation as a newer paradigm for psychopathology. *Psychoanal Inq*, 6, 93–118.

Gunderson, J.G., Weinberg, I., Daversa, M.T., Kueppenbender, K.D., Zanarini, M.C., Shea, M.T., Skodol, A.E., Sanislow, C.A., Yen, S., Morey, L.C., Grilo, C.M., McGlashan, T.H., Stout, R.L., and Dyck, I.D. (2006). Descriptive and longitudinal observations on the relationship of borderline personality disorder and bipolar disorder. *Am J Psychiatry*, 163, 1173–1178.

Gurtman, M.B. (1986). Depression and the response of others: Reevaluating the reevaluation. *J Abnorm Psychol*, 95(1), 99–101.

Hall, C.S., and Lindzey, G. (1970). *Theories of Personality*. New York: John Wiley & Sons.

Hamilton, M. (1982). Symptoms and assessment of depression. In E.S. Paykel (Ed.), *Handbook of Affective Disorders* (pp. 3–11). Edinburgh, Scotland: Churchill Livingstone.

Hammen, C.L. (1991). *Depression Runs in Families: The Social Context of Risk and Resilience in Children of Depressed Mothers*. New York: Springer-Verlag.

Hammen, C. (1997). *Depression*. London: Psychology Press.

Hammen, C., and Brennan, P.A. (2002). Interpersonal dysfunction in depressed women: Impairments independent of depressive symptoms. *J Affect Disord*, 72(2), 145–156.

Hantouche, E.G., Akiskal, H.S., Lancrenon, S, Allilaire, J.F., Sechter, D., Azorin, J.M., Bourgeois, M., Fraud, J.P., and Chatenet-Duchene, L. (1998). Systematic clinical methodology for validating bipolar-II disorder: Data in mid-stream from a French national multi-site study. *J Affect Disord*, 50, 163–173.

Harrow, M., Goldberg, J.F., Grossman, L.S., and Meltzer, H.Y. (1990). Outcome in manic disorders: A naturalistic follow-up study. *Arch Gen Psychiatry*, 47(7), 665–671.

Hipwell, A.E., and Kumar, R. (1996). Maternal psychopathology and prediction of outcome based on mother–infant interaction ratings (BMIS). *Br J Psychiatry*, 169(5), 655–661.

Hirschfeld, R.M.A. (1985). Personality and bipolar disorder. Paper presented at the Symposium on New Results in Depression Research. Munich.

Hirschfeld, R.M.A., and Klerman, G.L. (1979). Personality attributes and affective disorders. *Am J Psychiatry*, 136, 67–70.

Hirschfeld, R.M.A., Klerman, G.L., Clayton, P.J., Keller, M.B., McDonald-Scott, P., and Larkin, B.H. (1983). Assessing personality: Effects of the depressive state on trait measurement. *Am J Psychiatry*, 140(6), 695–699.

Hirschfeld, R.M.A., Klerman, G.L., Keller, M.B., Andreasen, N.C., and Clayton, P.J. (1986). Personality of recovered patients with bipolar affective disorder. *J Affect Disord*, 11(1), 81–89.

Holinger, P.C., and Wolpert, E.A. (1979). A ten year follow-up of lithium use. *IMJ Ill Med J*, 156, 99–104.

Hooley, J.M., Richters, J.E., Weintraub, S., and Neale, J.M. (1987). Psychopathology and marital distress: The positive side of positive symptoms. *J Abnorm Psychol*, 96(1), 27–33.

Hoover, C.F., and Fitzgerald, R.G. (1981). Marital conflict of manic-depressive patients. *Arch Gen Psychiatry*, 38(1), 65–67.

Jacobson, E. (1953). Contribution of the metapsychology of cyclothymic depression. In P. Greenacre (Ed.), *Affective Disorders: Psychoanalytic Contribution to Their Study* (pp. 49–83). New York: International Universities Press.

Jamison, K.R. (2004). *Exuberance: The Passion for Life*. New York: Alfred A. Knopf.

Jamison, K.R., Gerner, R.H., Hammen, C., and Padesky, C. (1980). Clouds and silver linings: Positive experiences associated with primary affective disorders. *Am J Psychiatry*, 137, 198–202.

Jamison, K.R., Litman-Adizes, T., Gitlin, M.J., and Fieve, R.R. (Unpublished data). Personality and attitudinal patterns in affective illness.

Janowsky, D.S., Leff, M., and Epstein, R.S. (1970). Playing the manic game: Interpersonal maneuvers of the acutely manic patient. *Arch Gen Psychiatry*, 22(3), 252–261.

Janowsky, D.S., El-Yousef, M.K., and Davis, J.M. (1974). Interpersonal maneuvers of manic patients. *Am J Psychiatry*, 131, 250–255.

Janowsky, D.S., Morter, S., Hong, L., and Howe, L. (1999). Myers Briggs Type Indicator and Tridimensional Personality Questionnaire differences between bipolar patients and unipolar depressed patients. *Bipolar Disord*, 1(2), 98.

Janowsky, D.S., El-Yousef, M.K., and Davis, J.M. (2003). Interpersonal maneuvers of manic patients. *Focus*, 1, 58–63.

Jelliffe, S.E. (1931). Some historical phases of the manic-depressive synthesis. *Res Publ Assoc Res Nerv Ment Dis*, 11, 3–47.

Johnson, L., Lundstroem, O., Aberg-Wistedt, A., and Mathe, A.A. (2003). Social support in bipolar disorder: Its revelance to remission and relapse. *Bipolar Disord*, 5(2), 129–137.

Johnson, S.L., and Jacob, T. (1997). Marital interactions of depressed men and women. *J Consult Clin Psychol*, 65(1), 15–23.

Johnson, S.L., Meyer, B., Winett, C., and Small, J. (2000). Social support and self-esteem predict changes in bipolar depression but not mania. *J Affect Disord*, 58(1), 79–86.

Johnson, S.L., Winters, R., and Meyer, B. (in press). A polarity-specific model of bipolar disorder. In T. Joiner (Ed.), *A Festschrift for Jack Hokanson*. Washington, DC: American Psychological Association Press.

Joiner, T., and Coyne J.C. (1999). *The Interactional Nature of Depression: Advances in Interpersonal Approaches*. Washington, DC: American Psychological Association.

Judd, L.L., Hubbard, B., Janowsky, D.S., Huey, L.Y., and Attewell, P.A. (1977). The effect of lithium carbonate on affect, mood, and personality of normal subjects. *Arch Gen Psychiatry*, 34, 346–351.

Kay, J.H., Altshuler, L.L., Ventura, J., and Mintz, J. (1999). Prevalence of axis II comorbidity in bipolar patients with and without alcohol use disorders. *Ann Clin Psychiatry*, 11(4), 187–195.

Kay, J.H., Altshuler, L.L., Ventura, J., and Mintz, J. (2002). Impact of axis II comorbidity on the course of bipolar illness in men: A retrospective chart review. *Bipolar Disord*, 4(4), 237–242.

Keller, M.B., Lavori, P.W., Coryell, W., Endicott, J., and Mueller, T.I. (1993). Bipolar I: A five-year prospective follow-up. *J Nerv Ment Dis*, 181(4), 238–245.

Kim, E.Y., and Miklowitz, D.J. (2004). Expressed emotion as a predictor of outcome among bipolar patients undergoing family therapy. *J Affect Disord*, 82, 343–352.

Klein, D.N., and Depue, R.A. (1985). Obsessional personality traits and risk for bipolar affective disorder: An offspring study. *J Abnorm Psychol*, 94(3), 291–297.

Klein, D.N., Depue, R.A., and Krauss, S.P. (1986). Social adjustment in the offspring of parents with bipolar affective disorder. *J Psychopathol Behav Assess*, 8, 355–366.

Klerman, G.L. (1973). The relationships between personality and clinical depressions: Overcoming the obstacles to verifying psychodynamic theories. *Int J Psychiatry*, 11(2), 227–233.

Klerman, G.L., Weissman, M.M., Rounsaville, B.J., and Chevron, E.S. (1984). *Interpersonal Psychotherapy of Depression*. New York: Basic Books.

Kotin, J., and Goodwin, F.K. (1972). Depression during mania: Clinical observations and theoretical implications. *Am J Psychiatry*, 129(6), 679–686.

Kraepelin, E. (1921). *Manic-Depressive Insanity and Paranoia.* R.M. Barclay (Translator), G.M. Robertson (Ed.). Edinburgh, Scotland: E & S Livingstone.

Kretschmer, E. (1936). *Physique and Character.* New York: Macmillan.

Kron, L., Decina, P., Kestenbaum, C.J., Farber, S., Gargan, M., and Fieve, R. (1982). The offspring of bipolar manic-depressives: Clinical features. *Adolesc Psychiatry*, 10, 273–291.

Kropf, D., and Müller-Oerlinghausen, B. (1975). The influence of lithium long-term medication on personality and mood. *Pharmacopsychiatry*, 18, 104–105.

Kropf, D., and Müller-Oerlinghausen, B. (1979). Changes in learning, memory, and mood during lithium treatment: Approach to a research strategy. *Acta Psychiatr Scand*, 59, 97–124.

Kulhara, P., Basu, D., Mattoo, S.K., Sharan, P., and Chopra, R. (1999). Lithium prophylaxis of recurrent bipolar affective disorder: Long-term outcome and its psychosocial correlates. *J Affect Disord*, 54(1–2), 87–96.

Kutcher, S.P., Marton, P., and Korenblum, M. (1990). Adolescent bipolar illness and personality disorder. *J Am Acad Child Adolesc Psychiatry*, 29(3), 355–358.

Lam, D., and Wong, G. (1997). Prodromes, coping strategies, insight and social functioning in bipolar affective disorders. *Psychol Med*, 27(5), 1091–1100.

Lam, D., Donaldson, C., Brown, Y., and Malliaris, Y. (2005). Burden and marital and sexual satisfaction in the partners of bipolar patients. *Bipolar Disord*, 7, 431–440.

Leonhard, K. (1957). *Aufteilung der Endogenen Psychosen* (1st edition). Berlin: Akademie-Verlag.

Lepkifker, E., Horesh, N., and Floru, S. (1988). Life satisfaction and adjustment in lithium-treated affective patients in remission. *Acta Psychiatr Scand*, 78(3), 391–395.

Levkovitz, V., Fennig, S., Horesh, N., Barak, V., and Treves, I. (2000). Perception of ill spouse and dyadic relationship in couples with affective disorder and those without. *J Affect Disord*, 58(3), 237–240.

Lewis, N.D.C. (1931). Mental dynamisms and psychotherapeutic modifications in manic-depressive psychoses. *Res Publ Assoc Res Nerv Ment Dis*, 11, 754–776.

Liebowitz, M.R., Stallone, F., Dunner, D.L., and Fieve, R.F. (1979). Personality features of patients with primary affective disorder. *Acta Psychiatr Scand*, 60(2), 214–224.

Lion, J.R. (1975). Conceptual issues in the use of drugs for the treatment of aggression in man. *J Nerv Ment Dis*, 160, 76–82.

Lorimy, F., Lôo, H., and Deniker, P. (1977). Effets cliniques des traitements prolongés par les sels de lithium sur le sommeil, l'appétit et la sexualité. *L'Encéphale*, 3, 227–239.

Lozano, B.E., and Johnson, S.L. (2001). Can personality traits predict increases in manic and depressive symptoms? *J Affect Disord*, 63(1–3), 103–111.

Lumry, A.E., Gottesman, I.I., and Tuason, V.B. (1982). MMPI state dependency during the course of bipolar psychosis. *Psychiatry Res*, 7(1), 59–67.

MacKinnon, D.F., and Pies, R. (2006). Affective instability as rapid cycling: Theoretical and clinical implications for borderline personality and bipolar spectrum disorders. *Bipolar Disord*, 8, 1–14.

Mathews, C.A., and Reus, V.I. (2001). Assortative mating in the affective disorders: A systematic review and meta-analysis. *Compr Psychiatry*, 42(4), 257–262.

Matsumoto, S., Akiyama, T., Tsuda, H., Miyake, Y., Kawamura, Y., Noda, T., Akiskal, K.K., and Akiskal, H.S. (2005). Reliability and validity of TEMPS-A in a Japanese non-clinical population: Application to unipolar and bipolar depressives. *J Affect Disord*, 85, 83–92.

Matussek, P., and Feil, W.B. (1983). Personality attributes of depressive patients: Results of group comparisons. *Arch Gen Psychiatry*, 40, 783–790.

Mayer-Gross, W., Slater, E., and Roth, M. (1955). *Clinical Psychiatry.* Baltimore: Williams & Wilkins.

McKnight, D.L., Nelson-Grey, R.O., and Gullick, E. (1989). Interactional patterns of bipolar patients and their spouses. *J Psychopathol Behav Assess* 11, 269–289.

Mendlewicz, M.V., Jean-Louis, G., Kelsoe, J.R., and Akiskal, H.S. (2005). A comparison of recovered bipolar patients, healthy relatives of bipolar probands, and normal controls using the short TEMPS-A. *J Affect Disord*, 85(1-2), 147–151.

Merikangas, K.R., and Spiker, D.G. (1982). Assortative mating among in-patients with primary affective disorder. *Psychol Med*, 12(4), 753–764.

Miklowitz, D.J., and Goldstein, M.J. (1997). *Bipolar Disorder: A Family-Focused Treatment Approach.* New York: Guilford Press.

Miklowitz, D.J., Goldstein, M.J., Nuechterlein, K.H., Snyder, K.S., and Mintz, J. (1988). Family factors and the course of bipolar affective disorder. *Arch Gen Psychiatry*, 45(3), 225–231.

Miklowitz, D.J., George, E.L., Richards, J.A., Simoneau, T.L., and Suddath, R.L. (2003). A randomized study of family-focused psychoeducation and pharmacotherapy in the outpatient management of bipolar disorder. *Arch Gen Psychiatry*, 60, 904–912.

Millingen, J. (1831). *Memoirs of the Affairs of Greece: Containing an Account of the Military and Political Events which Occurred in 1823 and Following Years. With Various Anecdotes Relating to Lord Byron, and an Account of His Last Illness and Death.* London: John Rodwell, p. 16.

Millon, T. (1987). *Millon Clinical Multiaxial Inventory-II Manual.* Minneapolis: National Computer Systems.

Mundt, C., Kronmuller, K., and Backenstrass, M. (2000). Interactional styles in bipolar disorder. In A. Marneros, J. Angst (Eds.), *Bipolar Disorders: 100 Years after Manic-Depressive Insanity* (pp. 201–213). London: Kluwer Academic Publishers.

Murphy, D.L., Beigel, A., Weingartner, H., and Bunney, W.E. Jr. (1974). The quantitation of manic behavior. *Mod Probl Pharmacopsychiatry*, 7, 203–220.

Murray, L.G., and Blackburn, I.M. (1974). Personality differences in patients with depressive illness and anxiety neurosis. *Acta Psychiatr Scand*, 50(2), 183–191.

NICHD Early Child Care Research Network. (1999). Chronicity of maternal depressive symptoms, maternal sensitivity, and child functioning at 36 months. *Dev Psychol*, 35(5), 1297–1310.

Nowakowska, C., Strong, C.M., Santosa, C.M., Wang, P.W., and Ketter, T.A., (2005). Temperamental commonalities and differences in eurthymic mood disorder patients, creative controls, and healthy controls. *J Affect Disord*, 85, 207–215.

Nurnberger, J. Jr., Guroff, J.J., Hamovit, J., Berrettini, W., and Gershon, E. (1988). A family study of rapid-cycling bipolar illness. *J Affect Disord*, 15(1), 87–91.

O'Connell, R.A., and Mayo, J.A. (1981). A biopsychosocial perspective. *Compr Psychiatry*, 22, 87–93.

O'Connell, R.A., Mayo, J.A., Eng, L.K., Jones, J.S., and Gabel, R.H. (1985). Social support and long-term lithium outcome. *Br J Psychiatry*, 147, 272–275.

O'Connell, R.A., Mayo, J.A., Flatow, L., Cuthbertson, B., and O'Brien, B.E. (1991). Outcome of bipolar disorder on long-term treatment with lithium. *Br J Psychiatry*, 159, 123–129.

Oedegaard, K.J., Neckelmann, D., and Fasmer, O.B. (2006). Type A behaviour differentiates bipolar II from unipolar depressed patients. *J Affect Dis*, 90, 7–13.

Osher, Y., Cloninger, C.R., and Belmaker, R.H. (1996). TPQ in euthymic manic-depressive patients. *J Psychiatr Res*, 30(5), 353–357.

Parker, G., Parker, K., Malhi, G., Wilhelm, K., and Mitchell, P. (2004). Studying personality characteristics in bipolar depressed subjects: How comparator group selection can dictate results. *Acta Psychiatr Scand*, 109, 376–382.

Perlick, D., Clarkin, J.F., Sirey, J., Raue, P., Greenfield, S., Struening, E., and Rosenheck, R. (1999). Burden experienced by care-givers of persons with bipolar affective disorder. *Br J Psychiatry*, 175, 56–62.

Perlick, D.A., Rosenheck, R.R., Clarkin, J.F., Raue, P., and Sirey, J. (2001). Impact of family burden and patient symptom status on clinical outcome in bipolar affective disorder. *J Nerv Ment Dis*, 189(1), 31–37.

Perris, C. (1971). Personality patterns in patients with affective disorders. *Acta Psychiatr Scand Suppl*, 221, 43–45.

Perugi, G., Akiskal, H.S., Lattanzi, L., Cecconi, D., Mastrocinque, C., Patronelli, A., Vignoli, S., and Bemi, E. (1998). The high prevalence of "soft" bipolar (II) features in atypical depression. *Compr Psychiatry*, 39, 63–71.

Peselow, E.D., Sanfilipo, M.P., and Fieve, R.R. (1995). Relationship between hypomania and personality disorders before and after successful treatment. *Am J Psychiatry*, 152(2), 232–238.

Platman, S.R., Plutchik, R., Fieve, R.R., and Lawlor, W.G. (1969). Emotion profiles associated with mania and depression. *Arch Gen Psychiatry*, 20(2), 210–214.

Popescu, C., Totoescu, A., Christodorescu, D., and Ionescu, R. (1985). Personality attributes in unipolar and bipolar affective disorders. *Neurol Psychiatr (Bucur)*, 23(4), 231–242.

Radke-Yarrow, M. (1998). *Children of Depressed Mothers: From Early Childhood to Maturity*. Cambridge, England: Cambridge University Press.

Rado, S. (1928). The problem of melancholia. *Int J Psychoanal*, 9, 420–438.

Romans, S.E., and McPherson, H.M. (1992). The social networks of bipolar affective disorder patients. *J Affect Disord*, 25(4), 221–228.

Rossi, A., Daneluzzo, E., Arduini, L., Di Domenico, M., Pollice, R., and Petruzzi, C. (2001). A factor analysis of signs and symptoms of the manic episode with Bech-Rafaelsen Mania and Melancholia Scales. *J Affect Disord*, 64(2–3), 267–270.

Rowe, C.J., and Daggett, D.R. (1954). Prepsychotic personality traits in manic depressive disease. *J Nerv Ment Dis*, 119, 412–420.

Ruestow, P., Dunner, D.L., Bleecker, B., and Fieve, R.R. (1978). Marital adjustment in primary affective disorder. *Compr Psychiatry*, 19(6), 565–571.

Sauer, H., Richter, P., Czernik, A., Ludwig-Mayerhofer, W., Schöchlin, C., Greil, W., and von Zerssen, D. (1997). Personality differences between patients with major depression and bipolar disorder—The impact of minor symptoms on self-ratings of personality. *J Affect Disord*, 42, 169–177.

Savitz, J.B., and Ramesar, R.S. (2006). Personality: Is it a viable endophenotype for genetic studies of bipolar affective disorder? *Bipolar Disord*, 8, 322–337.

Schou, M. (1968). Lithium in psychiatric therapy and prophylaxis. *J Psychiatr Res*, 6, 67–95.

Schwartz, D.A. (1961). Some suggestions for a unitary formulation of the manic-depressive reactions. *Psychiatry*, 24, 238–245.

Sheard, M.H. (1971). Effect of lithium on human aggression. *Nature*, 230, 113–114.

Sheard, M.H. (1975). Lithium in the treatment of aggression. *J Nerv Ment Dis*, 160, 108–118.

Simoneau, T.L., Miklowitz, D.J., Richards, J.A., Saleem, R., and George, E.L. (1999). Bipolar disorder and family communication: Effects of a psychoeducational treatment program. *J Abnorm Psychol*, 108(4), 588–597.

Smith, D.J., Muir, W.J., and Blackwood, D.H.R. (2005). Borderline personality disorder characteristics in young adults with recurrent mood disorders: A comparison of bipolar and unipolar depression. *J Affect Dis*, 87, 17–23.

Smith, J.H. (1960). The metaphor of the manic-depressive. *Psychiatry*, 123, 375–383.

Solomon, D.A., Shea, M.T., Leon, A.C., Mueller, T.I., Coryell, W., Maser, J.D., Endicott, J., and Keller, M.B. (1996). Personality traits in subjects with bipolar I disorder in remission. *J Affect Disord*, 40(1–2), 41–48.

Spalt, L. (1975). Sexual behavior and affective disorders. *Dis Nerv Syst*, 36, 974–977.

Stefos, G., Bauwens, F., Staner, L., Pardoen, D., and Mendlewicz, J. (1996). Psychosocial predictors of major affective recurrences in bipolar disorder: A 4-year longitudinal study of patients on prophylactic treatment. *Acta Psychiatr Scand*, 93(6), 420–426.

Stoddard, F.J., Post, R.M., and Bunney, W.E. (1977). Slow and rapid psychobiological alterations in a manic-depressive patient: Clinical phenomenology. *Br J Psychiatry*, 130, 72–78.

Stone, M.H. (1978). Toward early detection of manic-depressive illness in psychoanalytic patients: I. Patients who later develop a manic illness. *Am J Psychother*, 32(3), 427–439.

Strakowski, S.M., Faedda, G.L., Tohen, M., Goodwin, D.C., and Stoll, A.L. (1992). Possible affective-state dependence of the Tridimensional Personality Questionnaire in first-episode psychosis. *Psychiatry Res*, 41(3), 215–226.

Strakowski, S.M., Stoll, A.L., Tohen, M., Faedda, G.L., and Goodwin, D.C. (1993). The Tridimensional Personality Questionnaire as a predictor of six-month outcome in first episode mania. *Psychiatry Res*, 48(1), 1–8.

Strandman, E. (1978). Psychogenic needs in patients with affective disorders. *Acta Psychiatr Scand*, 58(1), 16–29.

Suppes, T., Leverich, G.S., Keck, P.E., Nolen, W.A., Denicoff, K.D., Altshuler, L.L., McElroy, S.L., Rush, A.J., Kupka, R., Frye, M.A., Bickel, M., and Post, R.M. (2001). The Stanley Foundation Bipolar Treatment Outcome Network: II. Demographics and illness characteristics of the first 261 patients. *J Affect Disord*, 67(1–3), 45–59.

Targum, S.D., Dibble, E.D., Davenport, Y.B., and Gershon, E.S. (1981). The Family Attitudes Questionnaire: Patients' and spouses' views of bipolar illness. *Arch Gen Psychiatry*, 38(5), 562–568.

Tohen, M., Waternaux, C.M. and Tsuang, M.T. (1990). Outcome in mania: A 4-year prospective follow-up of 75 patients utilizing survival analysis. *Arch Gen Psychiatry*, 47(12), 1106–1111.

Tuke, D.H. (1892). *A Dictionary of Psychological Medicine.* Philadelphia: P. Blakiston, Son & Co.

Ucok, A., Karaveli, D., Kundakci, T., and Yazici, O. (1998). Comorbidity of personality disorders with bipolar mood disorders. *Compr Psychiatry*, 39(2), 72–74.

Vieta, E., Colom, F., Martinez-Aran, A., Benabarre, A., and Gasto, C. (1999). Personality disorders in bipolar II patients. *J Nerv Ment Dis*, 187(4), 245–248.

von Zerssen, D. (1977). Premorbid personality and affective psychoses. In G.D. Burrows (Ed.), *Handbook of Studies on Depression.* Amsterdam: Excerpta Medica.

Watson, D., Clark, L.A., and Harkness, A.R. (1994). Structures of personality and their relevance to psychopathology. *J Abnorm Psychol*, 103(1), 18–31.

Weissman, M.M. (1987). Advances in psychiatric epidemiology: Rates and risks for major depression. *Am J Public Health*, 77(4), 445–451.

Weissman, M.M. (1993). The epidemiology of personality disorders: A 1990 update. *J Pers Disord* 7(Suppl. 1), 44–62.

Weissman, M.M., and Paykel, E.S. (1974). *The Depressed Woman: A Study of Social Relationships.* Chicago: University of Chicago Press.

Weissman, M.M, Warner, V., Wickramaratne, P., Moreau, D., and Olfson, M. (1997). Offspring of depressed parents: 10 years later. *Arch Gen Psychiatry*, 54, 932–940.

Weissman, M.M., Markowitz, J.C., and Klerman, G.L. (2000). *Comprehensive Guide to Interpersonal Psychotherapy.* New York: Basic Books.

Wetzler, S., Khadivi, A., and Oppenheim, S. (1995). The psychological assessment of depression: Unipolars versus bipolars. *J Pers Assess*, 65(3), 557–566.

Whisman, M.A. (2001). The association between depression and marital dissatisfaction. In S.R.H. Beach (Ed.), *Marital and Family Processes in Depression: A Scientific Foundation for Clinical Practice* (pp. 3–24). Washington, DC: American Psychological Association.

White, K., Bohart, R., Whipple, K., and Boyd, J. (1979). Lithium effects on normal subjects: Relationships to plasma and RBC lithium levels. *Int Pharamacopsychiatry*, 14, 176–183.

Widiger, T., and Rogers, J.H. (1989). Prevalence and comorbidity of personality disorders. *Psychiatric Ann*, 19, 132–136.

Wilson, D.C. (1951). Families of manic depressives. *Dis Nerv Sys*, 12, 362–369.

Winokur, G., Clayton, P.J., and Reich, T. (1969). *Manic Depressive Illness.* St. Louis: CV Mosby.

Winters, K.C., and Neale, J.M. (1985). Mania and low self-esteem. *J Aborm Psychol*, 94, 282–290.

Worland, J., Lander, H., and Hesselbrock, V. (1979). Psychological evaluation of clinical disturbance in children at risk for psychopathology. *J Abnorm Psychol*, 88(1), 13–26.

Yan, L.J., Hammen, C., Cohen, A.N., Daley, S.E., and Henry, R.M. (2004). Expressed emotion versus relationship quality variables in the prediction of recurrence in bipolar patients. *J Affect Disord*, 83, 199–206.

Yazici, O., Kora, K., Ucok, A., Tunali, D., and Turan, N. (1999). Predictors of lithium prophylaxis in bipolar patients. *J Affect Disord*, 55(2–3), 133–142.

Young, L.T., Bagby, R.M., Cooke, R.G., Parker, J.D., Levitt, A.J., and Joffe, R.T. (1995). A comparison of Tridimensional Personality

Questionnaire dimensions in bipolar disorder and unipolar depression. *Psychiatry Res*, 58(2), 139–143.

CHAPTER 11

Ahearn, E.P., and Carroll, B.J. (1996). Short-term variability of mood ratings in unipolar and bipolar depressed patients. *J Affect Disord*, 36(3–4), 107–115.

Akiskal, H.S., Hantouche, E.G., Bourgeois, M.L., Azorin, J.M., Sechter, D., Allilaire, J.F., Chatenet-Duchene, L., and Lancrenon, S. (2001). Toward a refined phenomenology of mania: Combining clinician-assessment and self-report in the French EPIMAN study. *J Affect Disord*, 67(1–3), 89–96.

Akiskal, H.S., Mendlowicz, M.V., Jean-Louis, G., Rapaport, M.H., Kelsoe, J.R., Gillin, J.C., and Smith, T.L. (2005a). TEMPS-A: Validation of a short version of a self-rated instrument designed to measure variations in temperament. *J Affect Disord*, 85, 45–52.

Akiskal, H.S., Akiskal, K.K., Haykal, R.F., Manning J.S., and Connor, P.D. (2005b). TEMPS-A: Progress towards validation of a self-rated clinical version of the Temperament Evaluation of the Memphis, Pisa, Paris, and San Diego Autoquestionnaire. *J Affect Disord*, 85, 3–16.

Akiskal, H.S., Akiskal, K., Allilaire, J.-F., Azorin, J.-M., Bourgeois, M.L., Sechter, D., Fraud, J.-P., Chatenêt-Duchêne, L., Lancrenon, S., Perugi, G., and Hantouche, E.G. (2005c). Validating affective temperaments in their subaffective and socially positive attributes: Psychometric, clinical and familial data from a French national study. *J Affect Disord*, 85, 29–36.

Akiyama, T., Tsuda, H., Matsumoto, S., Miyake, Y., Kawamura, Y., Noda, T., Akiskal, K.K., and Akiskal, H.S. (2005). The proposed factor structure of temperament and personality in Japan: Combining traits from TEMPS-A and MPT. *J Affect Disord*, 85, 93–100.

Altman, E.G., Hedeker, D.R., Janicak, P.G., Peterson, J.L., and Davis, J.M. (1994). The Clinician-Administered Rating Scale for Mania (CARS-M): Development, reliability, and validity. *Biol Psychiatry*, 36(2), 124–134.

Altman, E.G., Hedeker, D., Peterson, J.L., and Davis, J.M. (1997). The Altman Self-Rating Mania Scale. *Biol Psychiatry*, 42(10), 948–955.

Altman, E., Hedeker, D., Peterson, J.L., and Davis, J.M. (2001). A comparative evaluation of three self-rating scales for acute mania. *Biol Psychiatry*, 50(6), 468–471.

Ambrosini, P.J. (2000). A review of pharmacotherapy of major depression in children and adolescents. *Psychiatr Serv*, 51(5), 627–633.

Asberg, M., Montgomery, S.A., Perris, C., Schalling, D., and Sedvall, G. (1978). A comprehensive psychopathological rating scale. *Acta Psychiatr Scand Suppl* (271), 5–27.

Baldessarini, R.J. (2003). Assessment of treatment response in mania: Commentary and new findings. *Bipolar Disord*, 5(2), 79–84.

Bauer, M.S., Crits-Christoph, P., Ball, W.A., Dewees, E., McAllister, T., Alahi, P., Cacciola, J., and Whybrow, P.C. (1991). Independent assessment of manic and depressive symptoms by self-rating: Scale characteristics and implications for the study of mania. *Arch Gen Psychiatry*, 48(9), 807–812.

Bauer, M.S., Vojta, C., Kinosian, B., Altshuler, L., and Glick, H. (2000). The Internal State Scale: Replication of its discriminating abilities in a multisite, public sector sample. *Bipolar Disord*, 2(4), 340–346.

Bech, P. (1981). Rating scales for affective disorders: Their validity and consistency. *Acta Psychiatr Scand Suppl*, 295, 1–101.

Bech, P. (2002). The Bech-Rafaelsen Mania Scale in clinical trials of therapies for bipolar disorder: A 20-year review of its use as an outcome measure. *CNS Drugs*, 16(1), 47–63.

Bech, P., and Rafaelsen, O.J. (1980). The use of rating scales exemplified by a comparison of the Hamilton and the Bech-Rafaelsen Melancholia Scale. *Acta Psychiatr Scand Suppl*, 285, 128–132.

Bech, P., Bolwig, T.G., Kramp, P., and Rafaelsen, O.J. (1979). The Bech-Rafaelsen Mania Scale and the Hamilton Depression Scale. *Acta Psychiatr Scand*, 59(4), 420–430.

Bech, P., Kastrup, M., and Rafaelsen, O.J. (1986). Mini-compendium of rating scales for states of anxiety depression mania schizophrenia with corresponding DSM-III syndromes. *Acta Psychiatr Scand Suppl*, 326, 1–37.

Bech, P., Rasmussen, N.A., Olsen, L.R., Noerholm, V., and Abildgaard, W. (2001). The sensitivity and specificity of the Major Depression Inventory, using the Present State Examination as the index of diagnostic validity. *J Affect Disord*, 66(2–3), 159–164.

Beck, A.T., Ward, C.H., Mendelsohn, M., Mock, J., and Erbaugh, J. (1961). An inventory for measuring depression. *Arch Gen Psychiatry*, 4, 561–571.

Beck, A.T., Steer, R.A., and Garbin, M.G. (1988). Psychometric properties of the Beck Depression Inventory: Twenty-five years of evaluation. *Clin Psychol Rev*, 8, 77–100.

Beck, A.T., Steer, R.A., and Brown, G.K. (1996). *Manual for the BDI-II*. San Antonio, TX: The Psychological Corporation.

Beigel, A., and Murphy, D.L. (1971). Assessing clinical characteristics of the manic state. *Am J Psychiatry*, 128(6), 688–694.

Beigel, A., Murphy, D.L., and Bunney, W.E. (1971). The Manic-State Rating Scale: Scale construction, reliability, and validity. *Arch Gen Psychiatry*, 25, 256–262.

Berk, M., Malhi, G.S., Mitchell, P.B., Cahill, C.M., Carman, A.C., Hadzi-Pavlovic, D., Hawkins, M.T., and Tohen, M. (2004). Scale matters: The need for a Bipolar Depression Rating Scale (BDRS). *Acta Psychiatr Scand*, 100(Suppl. 422), 39–45.

Blackburn, I.M., Loudon, J.B., and Ashworth, C.M. (1977). A new scale for measuring mania. *Psychol Med*, 7(3), 453–458.

Bosc, M., Dubini, A., and Polin, V. (1997). Development and validation of a social functioning scale, the Social Adaptation Self-evaluation Scale. *Eur Neuropsychopharmacol*, 7(Suppl. 1), S57–S70, discussion S71–S73.

Boyle, M.H., and Pickles, A.R. (1997). Influence of maternal depressive symptoms on ratings of childhood behavior. *J Abnorm Child Psychol*, 25(5), 399–412.

Braunig, P., Shugar, G., and Kruger, S. (1996). An investigation of the Self-Report Manic Inventory as a diagnostic and severity scale for mania. *Compr Psychiatry*, 37, 52–55.

Bunney, W.E., and Hamburg, D.A. (1963). Methods for reliable longitudinal observation of behavior. *Arch Gen Psychiatry*, 9, 280–294.

Burnam, M.A., Wells, K.B., Leake, B., and Landsverk, J. (1988). Development of a brief screening instrument for detecting depressive disorders. *Med Care*, 26, 775–789.

Carney, M.W.P., Roth, M., and Garside, R.F. (1965). The diagnosis of depressive syndromes and the prediction of E.C.T. response. *Br J Psychiatry*, 111, 659–674.

Carroll, B.J. (1991). Psychopathology and neurobiology of manic-depressive disorders. In B.J. Carroll, J.E. Barrett (Eds.), *Psychopathology and the Brain* (pp. 265–285). New York: Raven Press.

Carroll, B. (1998). *Carroll Depression Scales-Revised (CDS-R): Technical Manual*. Toronto: Multi-Health Systems.

Carroll, B.J., Feinberg, M., Smouse, P.E., Rawson, S.G., and Greden, J.F. (1981). The Carroll rating scale for depression: I. Development, reliability and validation. *Br J Psychiatry*, 138, 194–200.

Chapman, L.J., Chapman, J.P., Numbers, J.S., Edell, W.S., Carpenter, B.N., and Beckfield, D. (1984). Impulsive nonconformity as a trait contributing to the prediction of psychotic-like and schizotypal symptoms. *J Nerv Ment Dis*, 172(11), 681–691.

Cooke, R.G., Kruger, S., and Shugar, G. (1996). Comparative evaluation of two self-report Mania Rating Scales. *Biol Psychiatry*, 40(4), 279–283.

Corruble, E., Legrand, J.M., Duret, C., Charles, G., and Guelfi, J.D. (1999). IDS-C and IDS-SR: Psychometric properties in depressed in-patients. *J Affect Disord*, 56(2–3), 95–101.

Craddock, N., Jones, I., Kirov, G., and Jones, L. (2004). The Bipolar Affective Disorder Dimension Scale (BADDS): A dimensional scale for rating lifetime psychopathology in bipolar spectrum disorders. *BMC Psychiatry*, 4, 19.

Cronholm, B., and Ottosson, J.O. (1996). Experimental studies of the therapeutic action of electroconvulsive therapy in endogenous depression: The role of the electrical stimulation and of the seizure studied by variation of stimulus intensity and modification by lidocaine of seizure discharge. *Acta Psychiatr Neurol Scand Suppl*, 12 (3), 172–194.

Das, A.K., Olfson, M., Gameroff, M.J., Pilowsky, D.J., Blanco, C., Feder, A., Gross, R., Neria, Y., Lantigua, R., Shea, S., and Weissman, M.M. (2005). Screening for bipolar disorder in a primary care practice. *JAMA*, 23(293), 8.

Davidson, J., Turnbull, C.D., Strickland, R., Miller, R., and Graves, K. (1986). The Montgomery-Asberg Depression Scale: Reliability and validity. *Acta Psychiatr Scand*, 73(5), 544–548.

Denicoff, K.D., Smith-Jackson, E.E., Disney, E.R., Suddath, R.L., Leverich, G.S., and Post, R.M. (1997). Preliminary evidence of the reliability and validity of the prospective life-chart methodology (LCM-p). *J Psychiatr Res*, 31(5), 593–603.

Depue, R.A., Slater, J.F., Wolfstetter-Kausch, H., Klein, D., Goplerud, E., and Farr, D. (1981). A behavioral paradigm for identifying persons at risk for bipolar depressive disorder: A conceptual framework and five validation studies. *J Abnorm Psychol*, 90(5), 381–437.

Depue, R.A., Krauss, S., Spoont, M.R., and Arbisi, P. (1989). General behavior inventory identification of unipolar and bipolar affective conditions in a nonclinical university population. *J Abnorm Psychol*, 98(2), 117–126.

Eckblad, M., and Chapman, L.J. (1986). Development and validation of a scale for hypomanic personality. *J Abnorm Psychol*, 95(3), 214–222.

Ellicott, A., Hammen, C., Gitlin, M., Brown, G., and Jamison, K. (1990). Life events and the course of bipolar disorder. *Am J Psychiatry*, 147(9), 1194–1198.

Endicott, J., Spitzer, R.L., Fleiss, J.L., and Cohen, J. (1976). The global assessment scale: A procedure for measuring overall severity of psychiatric disturbance. *Arch Gen Psychiatry*, 33(6), 766–771.

Erfurth, A., Gerlach, A.L., Michael, N., Boenigk, I., Hellweg, I., Signoretta, S., Akiskal, K., and Akiskal, H.S. (2005a). Distribution and gender effects of the subscales of a German version of the temperament autoquestionnaire brief TEMPS-M in a university student population. *J Affect Disord*, 85, 71–76.

Erfurth, A., Gerlach, A.L., Hellweg, I., Boenigk, I., Michael, N., and Akiskal, H.S. (2005b). Studies on a German (Münster) version of the temperament auto-questionnaire TEMPS-A: Construction and validation of the brief TEMPS-M. *J Affect Disord*, 85, 53–69.

Feighner, J.P., Meredith, C.H., Stern, W.C., Hendrickson, G., and Miller, L.L. (1984). A double-blind study of bupropion and placebo in depression. *Am J Psychiatry*, 141(4), 525–529.

Feinberg, M., Carroll, B.J., Smouse, P.E., and Rawson, S.G. (1981). The Carroll rating scale for depression: III. Comparison with other rating instruments. *Br J Psychiatry*, 138, 205–209.

Fergusson, D.M., Lynskey, M.T., and Horwood, L.J. (1993). The effect of maternal depression on maternal ratings of child behavior. *J Abnorm Child Psychol*, 21(3), 245–269.

Findling, R.L., Youngstrom, E.A., Danielson, C.K., DelPorto-Bedoya, D., Papish-David, R., Townsend, L., and Calabrese, J.R. (2002). Clinical decision-making using the General Behavior Inventory in juvenile bipolarity. *Bipolar Disord*, 4(1), 34–42.

Folstein, M.F., and Luria, R. (1973). Reliability, validity, and clinical application of the Visual Analogue Mood Scale. *Psychol Med*, 3(4), 479–486.

Frank, E., Swartz, H.A., Mallinger, A.G., Thase, M.E., Weaver, E.V., and Kupfer, D.J. (1999). Adjunctive psychotherapy for bipolar disorder: Effects of changing treatment modality. *J Abnorm Psychol*, 108(4), 579–587.

Furukawa, T., Anraku, K., Hiroe, T., Takahashi, K., Kitamura, T., Hirai, T., and Iida, M. (1997). Screening for depression among first-visit psychiatric patients: Comparison of different scoring methods for the Center for Epidemiologic Studies Depression Scale using receiver operating characteristic analyses. *Psychiatry Clin Neurosci*, 51(2), 71–78.

Geller, B., Zimerman, B., Williams, M., Bolhofner, K., Craney, J.L., DelBello, M.P., and Soutullo, C. (2001). Reliability of the Washington University in St. Louis Kiddie Schedule for Affective Disorders and Schizophrenia (WASH-U-KSADS) mania and rapid cycling sections. *J Am Acad Child Adolesc Psychiatry*, 40(4), 450–455.

Ghaemi, S.N., Miller, C.J., Berv, D.A., Klugman, J., Rosenquist, K.J., and Pies, R.W. (2005). Sensitivity and specificity of a new bipolar spectrum diagnostic scale. *J Affect Disord*, 84, 273–277.

Gitlin, M.J., Swendsen, J., Heller, T.L., and Hammen, C. (1995). Relapse and impairment in bipolar disorder. *Am J Psychiatry*, 152(11), 1635–1640.

Glick, H.A., McBride, L., and Bauer, M.S. (2003). A manic-depressive symptom self-report in optical scanable format. *Bipolar Disorders*, 5(5), 366–369.

Gracious, B., Youngstrom, E., Findling, R., and Calabrese, J. (2002). Discriminative validity of a parent version of the Young Mania Rating Scale. *J Am Acad Child Adolesc Psychiatry*, 41, 1350–1359.

Hamilton, M. (1960). A rating scale for depression. *J Neurol Neurosurg Psychiatry*, 12, 56–62.

Hamilton, M. (1976). Clinical evaluation of depressions: Clinical criteria and rating scales, including a Guttman Scale. In D.M. Gallant, G.M. Simpson (Eds.), *Depression: Behavioral, Biochemical, Diagnostic and Treatment Concepts* (pp. 155–179). New York: Spectrum Publications.

Hamilton, M. (1988). Assessment of depression and mania. In A. Georgotas, R. Cancro (Eds.), *Depression and Mania* (pp. 625–637). New York: Elsevier.

Hammen, C., Ellicott, A., Gitlin, M., and Jamison, K.R. (1989). Sociotropy/autonomy and vulnerability to specific life events in patients with unipolar depression and bipolar disorders. *J Abnorm Psychol*, 98(2), 154–160.

Hammen, C., Davila, J., Brown, G., Gitlin, M., and Ellicott, A. (1992). Stress as a mediator of the effects of psychiatric history on severity of unipolar depression. *J Abnorm Psychol*, 101, 45–52.

Hammen, C., Gitlin, M., and Altshuler, L. (2000). Predictors of work adjustment in bipolar I patients: A naturalistic longitudinal follow-up. *J Consult Clin Psychol*, 68(2), 220–225.

Hantouche, E.G., Allilaire, J.P., Bourgeois, M.L., Azorin, J.M., Sechter, D., Chatenet-Duchene, L., Lancrenon, S., and Akiskal, H.S. (2001). The feasibility of self-assessment of dysphoric mania in the French national EPIMAN study. *J Affect Disord*, 67(1–3), 97–103.

Harrow, M., Goldberg, J.F., Grossman, L.S., and Meltzer, H.Y. (1990). Outcome in manic disorders: A naturalistic follow-up study. *Arch Gen Psychiatry*, 47(7), 665–671.

Hayes, M.H.S., and Patterson, D.G. (1921). Experimental development of the graphic rating method. *Psychol Bull*, 18, 98–99.

Hays, R.D., Wells, K.B., Sherbourne, C.D., Rogers, W., and Spritzer, K. (1995). Functioning and well-being outcomes of patients with depression compared with chronic general medical illnesses. *Arch Gen Psychiatry*, 52(1), 11–19.

Hedlund, J.L., and Vieweg, B.W. (1979). The Hamilton Rating Scale for Depression: A comprehensive review. *J Operational Psychiatry*, 10, 149–165.

Hett, W.S. (Transl.) (1936). *Aristotle, Problems II: Books XXII-XXXVIII*. Cambridge, MA: Harvard University Press, pp. 155–157.

Hirschfeld, R.M. (2002). The mood disorder questionnaire: A simple, patient-rated screening instrument for bipolar disorder. *Prim Care Companion J Clin Psychiatry*, 4(1), 9–11.

Hirschfeld, R.M., Williams, J.B., Spitzer, R.L., Calabrese, J.R., Flynn, L., Keck, P.E. Jr., Lewis, L., McElroy, S.L., Post, R.M., Rapport, D.J., Russell, J.M., Sachs, G.S., and Zajecka, J. (2000). Development and validation of a screening instrument for bipolar spectrum disorder: The Mood Disorder Questionnaire. *Am J Psychiatry*, 157(11), 1873–1875.

Hirschfeld, R.M., Calabrese, J.R., Weissman, M.M., Reed, M., Davies, M.A., Frye, M.A., Keck, P.E. Jr., Lewis, L., McElroy, S.L., McNulty, J.P., and Wagner, K.D. (2003a). Screening for bipolar disorder in the community. *J Clin Psychiatry*, 64(1), 53–59.

Hirschfeld, R.M., Holzer, C., Calabrese, J.R., Weissman, M., Reed, M., Davies, M., Frye, M.A., Keck, P., McElroy, S., Lewis, L., Tierce, J., Wagner, K.D., and Hazard, E. (2003b). Validity of the mood disorder questionnaire: A general population study. *Am J Psychiatry*, 160(1), 178–180.

Hofmann, B.U., and Meyer, T.D. (2006). Mood fluctuations in people putatively at risk for bipolar disorders. *Br J Clin Psychol*, 45, 105–110.

Jones, S., Mansell, W., and Waller, L. (2006). Appraisal of hypomania-relevant experiences: Development of a questionnaire to assess positive self-dispositional appraisals in bipolar and behavioural high risk samples. *J Affect Disord*, 93, 19–28.

Judd, L.L., Akiskal, H.S., Zeller, P.J., Paulus, M., Leon, A.C., Maser, J.D., Endicott, J., Coryell, W., Kunovac, J.L., Mueller, T.I., Rice, J.P., and Keller, M.B. (2000). Psychosocial disability during the long-term course of unipolar major depressive disorder. *Arch Gen Psychiatry*, 57(4), 375–380.

Katz, M.M., and Itil, T.M. (1974). Video methodology for research in psychopathology and psychopharmacology: Rationale and application. *Arch Gen Psychiatry*, 31(2), 204–210.

Keller, M.B., Lavori, P.W., Friedman, B., Nielsen, E., Endicott, J., McDonald-Scott, P., and Andreasen, N.C. (1987). The Longitudinal Interval Follow-up Evaluation: A comprehensive method for assessing outcome in prospective longitudinal studies. *Arch Gen Psychiatry*, 44(6), 540–548.

Khan, A., Brodhead, A.E., and Kolts, R.L. (2004). Relative sensitivity of the Montgomery-Asberg Depression Rating Scale, the Hamilton Depression Rating Scale and the Clinical Global Impressions Rating Scale in antidepressant clinical trials: A replication analysis. *Int Clin Psychopharmacol*, 19(3), 157–160.

Klein, D.N., and Depue, R.A. (1984). Continued impairment in persons at risk for bipolar affective disorder: Results of a 19-month follow-up study. *J Abnorm Psychol*, 93(3), 345–347.

Klein, D.N., Depue, R.A., and Slater, J.F. (1986). Inventory identification of cyclothymia: IX. Validation in offspring of bipolar I patients. *Arch Gen Psychiatry*, 43(5), 441–445.

Klein, D.N., Lewinsohn, P.M., and Seeley, J.R. (1996). Hypomanic personality traits in a community sample of adolescents. *J Affect Disord*, 38(2–3), 135–143.

Kovacs, M. (1981). Rating scales to assess depression in school-aged children. *Acta Paedopsychiatrica*, 46, 305–315.

Kraepelin, E. (1921). *Manic-Depressive Insanity and Paranoia*. R.M. Barclay (Translator), G.M. Robertson (Ed.). Edinburgh, Scotland: E & S Livingstone.

Kramlinger, K.G., and Post, R.M. (1996). Ultra-rapid and ultradian cycling in bipolar affective illness. *Br J Psychiatry*, 168(3), 314–323.

Kwapil, T.R., Miller, M.B., Zinser, M.C., Chapman, L.J., Chapman, J., and Eckblad, M. (2000). A longitudinal study of high scorers on the hypomanic personality scale. *J Abnorm Psychol*, 109(2), 222–226.

Leverich, G.S., Nolen, W.A., Rush, A.J., McElroy, S.L., Keck, P.E., Denicoff, K.D., Suppes, T., Altshuler, L.L., Kupka, R., Kramlinger, K.G., and Post, R.M. (2001). The Stanley Foundation Bipolar Treatment Outcome Network: I. Longitudinal methodology. *J Affect Disord*, 67(1–3), 33–44.

Licht, R.W., and Jensen, J. (1997). Validation of the Bech-Rafaelsen Mania Scale using latent structure analysis. *Acta Psychiatr Scand*, 96, 67–72.

Livianos-Aldana, L., and Rojo-Moreno, L. (2001). Rating and quantification of manic syndromes. *Acta Psychiatr Scand Suppl*, (409), 2–33.

Lorr, M. (1974). Assessing psychotic behavior by the IMPS. *Mod Probl Pharmacopsychiatry*, 7(0), 50–63.

Loudon, J.B., Blackburn, I.M., and Ashworth, C.M. (1977). A study of the symptomatology and course of manic illness using a new scale. *Psychol Med*, 7(4), 723–729.

Lubin, B. (1994). *State Trait-Dependent Adjective Check Lists: Professional Manual*. Odessa, FL: Psychological Assessment Resources.

Luria, R.E. (1975). The validity and reliability of the visual analogue mood scale. *J Psychiatr Res*, 12(1), 51–57.

Mansell, W., and Jones, S.H. (2006). The Brief-HAPPI: A questionnaire to assess cognitions that distinguish between individuals with a diagnosis of bipolar disorder and non-clinical controls. *J Affect Disord*, 93, 29–34.

Matsumoto, S., Akiyama, T., Tsuda, H., Miyake, Y., Kawamura, Y., Noda, T., Akiskal, K.K., and Akiskal, H.S. (2005). Reliability and validity of TEMPS-A in a Japanese non-clinical population: Application to unipolar and bipolar depressives. *J Affect Disord*, 85, 85–92.

Mendels, J., Weinstein, N., and Cochrane, C. (1972). The relationship between depression and anxiety. *Arch Gen Psychiatry*, 27(5), 649–653.

Mendlowicz, M.V., Akiskal, H.S., Kelsoe, J.R., Rapaport, M.H., Jean-Louis, G., and Gillin, J.C. (2005). Temperament in the clinical differentiation of depressed bipolar and unipolar major depressive patients. *J Affect Disord*, 84, 219–223.

Meyer, T.D., and Hautzinger, M. (2003). Screening for bipolar disorders using the Hypomanic Personality Scale. *J Affect Disord*, 75, 149–154.

Mintz, J., Mintz, L.I., Arruda, M.J., and Hwang, S.S. (1992). Treatments of depression and the functional capacity to work. *Arch Gen Psychiatry*, 49(10), 761–768.

Montgomery, S.A., and Asberg, M. (1979). A new depression scale designed to be sensitive to change. *Br J Psychiatry*, 134, 382–389.

Montgomery, S., Asberg, M., Jornestedt, L., Thoren, P., Traskman, L., McAuley, R., Montgomery, D., and Shaw, P. (1978a). Reliability of the CPRS between the disciplines of psychiatry, general practice, nursing and psychology in depressed patients. *Acta Psychiatr Scand Suppl*, 271, 29–32.

Montgomery, S., Asberg, M., Traskman, L., and Montgomery, D. (1978b). Cross cultural studies on the use of CPRS in English and Swedish depressed patients. *Acta Psychiatr Scand Suppl*, (271), 33–37.

Murphy, D.L., Beigel, A., Weingartner, H., Bunney, W.E. Jr. (1974). The quantitation of manic behavior. *Mod Probl Pharmacopsychiatry*, 7(0), 203–220.

Murphy D.L., Pickar D., and Alterman, I.S. (1982). Methods for the quantitative assessment of depressive and manic behavior. In E.I. Burdock, A. Sudilovsky, S. Gershon (Eds.), *The Behavior of Psychiatric Patients: Quantitative Techniques for Evaluation* (pp. 355–392). New York: Marcel Dekker.

Nezu, A.M., Ronan, G.F., Meadows, E.A., and McClure, K.S. (2000). *Practitioner's Guide to Empirically Based Measures of Depression*. New York: Kluwer Academic/Plenum Publishers.

Paykel, E.S., and Prusoff, B.A. (1973). Response set and observer set in the assessment of depressed patients. *Psychol Med*, 3(2), 209–216.

Paykel, E.S., and Weissman, M.M. (1973). Social adjustment and depression: A longitudinal study. *Arch Gen Psychiatry*, 28(5), 659–663.

Paykel, E.S., Prusoff, B.A., Klerman, G.L., and DiMascio, A. (1973). Self-report and clinical interview ratings in depression. *J Nerv Ment Dis*, 156(3), 166–182.

Perris, C. (1979). Reliability and validity studies of the comprehensive Psychopathological Rating Scale (CPRS). *Prog Neuropsychopharmacol*, 3(4), 413–421.

Petterson, U., Fyro, B., and Sedvall, G. (1973). A new scale for the longitudinal rating of manic states. *Acta Psychiatr Scand*, 49(3), 248–256.

Phelps, J.R., and Ghaemi, S.N. (2006). Improving the diagnosis of bipolar disorder: Predictive value of screening tests. *J Affect Disord*, 92, 141–148.

Pinard, G., and Tetreault, L. (1974). Concerning semantic problems in psychological evaluation. *Mod Probl Pharmacopsychiatry*, 7(0), 8–22.

Platman, S.R., Plutchik, R., Fieve, R.R., and Lawlor, W.G. (1969). Emotion profiles associated with mania and depression. *Arch Gen Psychiatry*, 20(2), 210–214.

Plutchik, R., Platman, S.R., Tilles, R., and Fieve, R.R. (1970). Construction and evaluation of a test for measuring mania and depression. *J Clin Psychol*, 26(4), 499–503.

Prusoff, B.A., Klerman, G.L., and Paykel, E.S. (1972a). Pitfalls in the self-report assessment of depression. *Can Psychiatr Assoc J*, 17(2), SS101.

Prusoff, B.A., Klerman, G.L., and Paykel, E.S. (1972b). Concordance between clinical assessments and patients' self-report in depression. *Arch Gen Psychiatry*, 26(6), 546–552.

Radloff, L.S. (1977). The CED-D Scale: A self-report depression scale for research in the general population. *Appl Psychol Measure*, 1, 385–401.

Rafaelsen, O.J., Bech, P., Bolwig, T.G., Kramp P., and Gjerris, A. (1980). The Bech-Rafaelsen combined rating scale for mania and melancholia. In K. Achte, V. Aalberg, J. Lonnqvist (Eds.), *Psychopathology of Depression: Proceedings of the Symposium by the Section of Clinical Psychopathology of the World Psychiatric Association* (pp. 327–331). Helsinki: Psychiatric Fennica.

Raskin, A., Schulterbrandt, J.G., Reatig, N., and McKeon, J.J. (1970). Differential response to chlorpromazine, imipramine, and placebo: A study of subgroups of hospitalized depressed patients. *Arch Gen Psychiatry*, 23(2), 164–173.

Reichart, C.G., van der Ende, J., Wals, M., Hillegers, M.H.J., Nolen, W.A., Ormel, J., and Verhulst, F.C. (2005). The use of the GBI as predictor of bipolar disorder in a population of adolescent offspring of parents with a bipolar disorder. *J Affect Disord*, 89, 147–155.

Renouf, A.G., and Kovacs, M. (1994). Concordance between mothers' reports and children's self-reports of depressive symptoms: A longitudinal study. *J Am Acad Child Adolesc Psychiatry*, 33(2), 208–216.

Reynolds, W.M., and Kobak, K.A. (1995). *Hamilton Depression Inventory (HDI): Professional Manual*. Odessa, FL: Psychological Assessment Resources.

Reynolds, W.M., and Kobak, K.A. (1998). *Reynolds Depression Screening Inventory: Professional Manual*. Odessa, FL: Psychological Assessment Resources.

Richters, J.E. (1992). Depressed mothers as informants about their children: A critical review of the evidence for distortion. *Psychol Bull*, 112(3), 485–499.

Rickels, K., Gordon, P.E., Mecklenburg, R., Sablosky, L., Whalen, E.M., and Dion, H. (1968). Iprindole in neurotic depressed general practice patients: A controlled study. *Psychosomatics*, 9(4), 208–214.

Ronan, G.F., Dreer, L.E., and Dollard, K.M. (2000). Measuring patient symptom change on rural psychiatric units: Utility of the symptom checklist-90 revised. *J Clin Psychiatry*, 61(7), 493–497.

Rossi, A., Daneluzzo, E., Arduini, L., Di Domenico, M., Pollice, R., and Petruzzi, C. (2001). A factor analysis of signs and symptoms of the manic episode with Bech-Rafaelsen Mania and Melancholia Scales, *J Affect Disord* 64(2–3): 267–270.

Roth, M., Gurney, C., and Mountjoy, C.Q. (1983). The newcastle rating scales. *Acta Psychiatr Scand Suppl*, 310, 42–54.

Rouget, W.B., Gervasoni, N., Dubuis, V., Gex-Fabry, M., Bondolfi, G., and Aubry, J.M. (2005). Screening for bipolar disorders using a French version of the Mood Disorder Questionnaire (MDQ). *J Affect Disord*, 88, 103–108.

Roy-Byrne, P., Post, R.M., Uhde, T.W., Porcu, T., and Davis, D. (1985). The longitudinal course of recurrent affective illness: Life chart data from research patients at the NIMH. *Acta Psychiatr Scand Suppl*, 317, 1–34.

Rush, A.J., Giles, D.E., Schlesser, M.A., Fulton, C.L., Weissenburger, J., and Burns, C. (1986). The Inventory for Depressive Symptomatology (IDS): Preliminary findings. *Psychiatry Res*, 18(1), 65–87.

Rush, A.J., Giles, D.E., Schlesser, M.A., Orsulak, P.J., Parker, C.R. Jr., Weissenburger, J.E., Crowley, G.T., Khatami, M., and Vasavada, N. (1996a). The dexamethasone suppression test in patients with mood disorders. *J Clin Psychiatry*, 57(10), 470–484.

Rush, A.J., Gullion, C.M., Basco, M.R., Jarrett, R.B., and Trivedi, M.H. (1996b). The Inventory of Depressive Symptomatology (IDS): Psychometric properties. *Psychol Med*, 26(3), 477–486.

Rush, A.J., Trivedi, M.H., Ibrahim, H.M., Carmody, T.J., Arnow, B., Klein, D.N., Markowitz, J.C., Ninan, P.T., Kornstein, S., Manber, R., Thase, M.E., Kocsis, J.H., and Keller, M.B. (2003). The 16-item Quick Inventory of Depressive Symptomatology (QIDS), clinician rating (QIDS-C), and self-report (QIDS-SR): A psychometric evaluation in patients with chronic major depression. *Biol Psychiatry*, 54(5), 573–583.

Scharer, L.O., Hartweg, V., Valerius, G., Graf, M., Hoern, M., Biedermann, C., Walser, S., Boensch, A., Dittmann, S., Forsthoff, A., Hummel, B., Grunze, H., and Walden, J. (2002). Life charts on a palmtop computer: First results of a feasibility study with an electronic diary for bipolar patients. *Bipolar Disord*, 4(Suppl. 1), 107–108.

Schou, M. (1979). Artistic productivity and lithium prophylaxis in manic-depressive illness. *Br J Psychiatry*, 135, 97–103.

Secunda, S.K., Katz, M.M., Swann, A., Koslow, S.H., Maas, J.W., Chuang, S., and Croughan, J. (1985). Mania: Diagnosis, state measurement and prediction of treatment response. *J Affect Disord*, 8(2), 113–121.

Shaffer, D., Fisher, P., Lucas, C.P., Dulcan, M.K., and Schwab-Stone, M.E. (2000). NIMH Diagnostic Interview Schedule for Children Version IV (NIMH DISC-IV): Description, differences from previous versions, and reliability of some common diagnoses. *J Am Acad Child Adolesc Psychiatry*, 39(1), 28–38.

Shugar, G., Schertzer, S., Toner, B., and DiGasbarro, I. (1992). Development, use, and factor analysis of a self-report inventory for mania. *Comprehensive Psychiatry*, 33(5), 325–331.

Smouse, P.E., Feinberg, M., Carroll, B.J., Park, M.H., and Rawson, S.G. (1981). The Carroll rating scale for depression: II. Factor analyses of the feature profiles. *Br J Psychiatry*, 138, 201–204.

Snaith, P. (1993). What do depression rating scales measure? *Br J Psychiatry*, 163, 293–298.

Snaith, R.P. (1981). Rating scales. *Br J Psychiatry*, 138, 512–514.

Solomon, D.A., Keller, M.B., Leon, A.C., Mueller, T.I., Lavori, P.W., Shea, M.T., Coryell, W., Warshaw, M., Turvey, C., Maser, J.D., and Endicott, J. (2000). Multiple recurrences of major depressive disorder. *Am J Psychiatry*, 157(2), 229–233.

Solomon, D.A., Leon, A.C., Maser, J.D., Truman, C.J., Coryell, W., Endicott, J., Teres, J.J., and Keller, M.B. (2006). Distinguishing bipolar major depression from unipolar major depression with the Screening Assessment of Depression-Polarity (SAD-P). *J Clin Psychiatry*, 67, 434–442.

Spearing, M.K., Post, R.M., Leverich, G.S., Brandt, D., and Nolen, W. (1997). Modification of the Clinical Global Impressions (CGI) Scale for use in bipolar illness (BP): The CGI-BP. *Psychiatry Res*, 73(3), 159–171.

Spitzer, R.L., and Endicott, J. (1978). *Schedule for Affective Disorders and Schizophrenia*. New York, NY: Biometrics Research, Evaluation Section, New York State Psychiatric Institute.

Squillace, K., Post, R.M., Savard, R., and Erwin-Gorman, M. (1984). Life charting of the longitudinal course of recurrent affective illness. In R.M. Post, J.C. Ballenger (Eds.), *Neurobiology of Mood Disorders* (pp. 38–59). Baltimore: Williams & Wilkins.

Svanborg, P., and Asberg, M. (2001). A comparison between the Beck Depression Inventory (BDI) and the self-rating version of the Montgomery Asberg Depression Rating Scale (MADRS). *J Affect Disord*, 64(2–3), 203–216.

Tandon, R., Flegel, P., and Greden, J.F. (1986). *Carroll and Hamilton Rating Scales for Depression* (Abstract). Washington, DC: American Psychiatric Association.

Thalbourne, M.A., and Bassett, D.L. (1998). The Manic Depressiveness Scale: A preliminary effort at replication and extension. *Psychol Rep*, 83(1), 75–80.

Thalbourne, M.A., Delin, P.S., and Bassett, D.L. (1994). An attempt to construct short scales measuring manic-depressive-like experience and behaviour. *Br J Clin Psychol*, 33(Pt. 2), 205–207.

Thase, M.E., Hersen, M., Bellack, A.S., Himmelhoch, J.M., and Kupfer, D.J. (1983). Validation of a Hamilton subscale for endogenomorphic depression. *J Affect Disord*, 5(3), 267–278.

Tillman, R., and Geller, B. (2005). A brief screening tool for a prepubertal and early adolescent bipolar disorder phenotype. *Am J Psychiatry*, 162, 1214–1216.

Tillman, R., Geller, B., Craney, J.L., Bolhofner, K., Williams, M., and Zimerman, B. (2004). Relationship of parent and child informants to prevalence of mania symptoms in children with a prepubertal and early adolescent bipolar disorder phenotype. *Am J Psychiatry*, 151, 1278–1284.

Tohen, M., Jacobs, T.G., Grundy, S.L., McElroy, S.L., Banov, M.C., Janicak, P.G., Sanger, T., Risser, R., Zhang, F., Toma, V., Francis, J., Tollefson, G.D., and Breier, A. (2000). Efficacy of olanzapine in acute bipolar mania: A double-blind, placebo-controlled study. The Olanzipine HGGW Study Group. *Arch Gen Psychiatry*, 57(9), 841–849.

Trivedi, M.H., Rush, A.J., Ibrahim, H.M., Carmody, T.J., Biggs, M.M., Suppes, T., Crismon, M.L., Shores-Wilson, K., Toprac, M.G., Dennehy, E.B., Witte, B., and Kashner, T.M. (2004). The Inventory of Depressive Symptomatology, Clinician Rating (IDS-C) and Self-Report (IDS-SR), and the Quick Inventory of Depressive Symptomatology, Clinician Rating (QIDS-C) and Self-Report (QIDS-SR) in public sector patients with mood disorders: A psychometric evaluation. *Psychol Med*, 34(1), 73–82.

Tyrer, S.P., and Shopsin, B. (1982). Symptoms and assessment of mania. In E.S. Paykel (Ed.), *Handbook of Affective Disorders* (pp. 12–23). Edinburgh, Scotland: Churchill Livingstone.

Vojta, C., Kinosian, B., Glick, H., Altshuler, L., and Bauer, M.S. (2001). Self-reported quality of life across mood states in bipolar disorder. *Compr Psychiatry*, 42(3), 190–195.

von Zerssen, D., and Cording, C. (1978). The measurement of change in endogenous affective disorders. *Arch Psychiatr Nervenkr*, 226(2), 95–112.

Ware, J.E. Jr., and Sherbourne, C.D. (1992). The MOS 36-item short-form health survey (SF-36): I. Conceptual framework and item selection. *Med Care*, 30(6), 473–483.

Warren, W.L. (1994). *Revised Hamilton Rating Scale for Depression (RHRSD): Manual*. Los Angeles: Western Psychological Services.

Warshaw, M.G., Keller, M.B., and Stout, R.L. (1994). Reliability and validity of the longitudinal interval follow-up evaluation for assessing outcome of anxiety disorders. *J Psychiatr Res*, 28(6), 531–545.

Weissman, M.M. (1997). Beyond symptoms: Social functioning and the new antidepressants. *J Psychopharmacol*, 11(Suppl. 4), S5–S8.

Weissman, M.M., and Bothwell, S. (1976). Assessment of social adjustment by patient self-report. *Arch Gen Psychiatry*, 33(9), 1111–1115.

Weissman, M.M., Sholomskas, D., Pottenger, M., Prusoff, B.A., and Locke, B.Z. (1977). Assessing depressive symptoms in five psychiatric populations: A validation study. *Am J Epidemiol*, 106(3), 203–214.

Weissman, M.M., Prusoff, B.A., Thompson, W.D., Harding, P.S., and Myers, J.K. (1978). Social adjustment by self-report in a community sample and in psychiatric outpatients. *J Nerv Ment Dis*, 166(5), 317–326.

Weissman, M.M., Sholomskas, D., and John, K. (1981). The assessment of social adjustment: An update. *Arch Gen Psychiatry*, 38(11), 1250–1258.

Wells, K.B., Stewart, A., Hays, R.D., Burnam, M.A., Rogers, W., Daniels, M., Berry, S., Greenfield, S., and Ware, J. (1989). The functioning and well-being of depressed patients: Results from the Medical Outcomes Study. *JAMA*, 262(7), 914–919.

Whybrow, P.C., Grof, P., Gyalai, L., Rasgon, N., Glenn, T., and Bauer, M. (2003). The electronic assessment of the longitudinal course of bipolar disorder: The ChronoRecord software. *Pharmaco*, 36(Suppl. 3), S244–S249.

Williams, J.B.W. (2000). Mental health status, functioning, and disabilities measures. In *Handbook of Psychiatric Measures* (pp. 93–115). Washington, DC: American Psychiatric Association.

Williamson, D., Brown, E., Perlis, R.H., Ahl, J., Baker, R.W., and Tohen, M. (2006). Clinical relevance of depressive symptom improvement in bipolar I depressed patients. *J Affect Disord*, 92, 261–266.

Young, R.C., Biggs, J.T., Ziegler, V.E., and Meyer, D.A. (1978). A rating scale for mania: Reliability, validity and sensitivity. *Br J Psychiatry*, 133, 429–435.

Youngstrom, E.A., Findling, R.L., Danielson, C.K., and Calabrese, J.R. (2001). Discriminative validity of parent report of hypomanic and depressive symptoms on the General Behavior Inventory. *Psychol Assess*, 13(2), 267–276.

Youngstrom, E., Danielson, C., Findling, R., Gracious, B., and Calabrese, J. (2002). Factor structure of the Young Mania Rating Scale for use with youths aged 5 to 17 years. *J Clin Child Adolesc Psychol*, 31, 567–572.

Youngstrom, E., Gracious, B., Danielson, C., Findling, R., and Calabrese, J. (2003). Toward an integration of parent and clinician report on the Young Mania Rating Scale. *J Affect Disord*, 77, 179–190.

Youngstrom, E.A., Findling, R.L., and Calabrese, J.R. (2004). Effects of adolescent manic symptoms on agreement between youth, parent, and teacher ratings of behavior problems. *J Affect Disord*, 828, S5–S16.

Zealley, A.K., and Aitken, R.C. (1969). Measurement of mood. *Proc R Soc Med*, 62(10), 993–996.

Zimmerman, M., Coryell, W., Corenthal, C., and Wilson, S. (1986). A self-report scale to diagnose major depressive disorder. *Arch Gen Psychiatry*, 43(11), 1076–1081.

Zimmerman, M., Sheeran, T., and Young, D. (2004a). The diagnostic inventory for depression: A self-report scale to diagnose

DSM-IV major depressive disorder. *J Clin Psychol*, 60(1), 87–110.

Zimmerman, M., Posternak, M.A., Chelminski, I., and Solomon, D.A. (2004b). *Using Questionnaires to Screen for Psychiatric Disorders: A Comment on a Study of Screening for Bipolar Disorder in the Community*. Providence, RI: Physicians Postgraduate Press.

Zung, W.W. (1974). The measurement of affects: Depression and anxiety. *Mod Probl Pharmacopsychiatry*, 7(0), 170–188.

Zung, W.W., Richards, C.B., and Short, M.J. (1965). Self-rating depression scale in an outpatient clinic: Further validation of the SDS. *Arch Gen Psychiatry*, 13(6), 508–515.

CHAPTER 12

Akiskal, K.K., Savino, M., and Akiskal, H.S. (2005). Temperament profiles in physicians, lawyers, managers, industrialists, architects, journalists, and artists: A study in psychiatric outpatients. *J Affect Disord*, 85, 201–206.

Andreasen, N.C. (1980). Mania and creativity. In R.H. Belmaker and H.M. Praag (Eds.), *Mania: An Evolving Concept*. New York: Spectrum, pp. 377–386.

Andreasen, N.C. (1987). Creativity and mental illness: Prevalence rates in writers and their first-degree relatives. *Am J Psychiatry*, 144, 1288–1292.

Andreasen, N.C., and Canter, A. (1974). The creative writer: Psychiatric symptoms and family history. *Compr Psychiatry*, 15, 123–131.

Andreasen, N.C., and Glick, I.D. (1988). Bipolar affective disorder and creativity: Implications and clinical management. *Compr Psychiatry*, 29(3), 207–217.

Andreasen, N.C., and Powers, P.S. (1975). Creativity and psychosis: An examination of conceptual style. *Arch Gen Psychiatry*, 32, 70–73.

Aristotle. (1936). *Problems II: Books XXII–XXXVIII*. Translated by W.S. Hett. Cambridge, MA: Harvard University Press.

Babcock, W.L. (1895). On the morbid heredity and predisposition to insanity of the Man of Genius. *J Ment Nerv Disorders*, 20, 749–769.

Berryman, J. (1976). *Writers at Work: The Paris Review Interviews*. G. Plimpton (Ed.). New York: Viking Press, p. 322.

Bett, W.R. (1952). *The Infirmities of Genius*. London: Johnson.

Bleuler, E. (1924). *Textbook of Psychiatry*. A.A. Brill (Transl.). New York: Macmillan.

Bold, A. (1983). *Byron: Wrath and Rhyme*. London: Vision Press.

Brody, J.F. (2001). Evolutionary recasting: ADHD, mania and its variants. *J Affect Disord*, 65, 197–215.

Carson, S.H., Peterson, J.B., and Higgins, D.M. (2003). Decreased latent inhibition is associated with increased creative achievement in high-functioning individuals. *J Pers Soc Psychol*, 85, 499–506.

Collins, F. (1990, September 17). Tracking down killer genes. *Time*. p. 12.

Coryell, W., Endicott, J., Keller, M., Andreasen, N., Grove, W., Hirschfeld, R.M.A., and Scheftner, W. (1989). Bipolar affective disorder and high achievement: A familial association. *Am J Psychiatry*, 146, 983–988.

Czeizel, E. (2001). Aki költo akar lenni, pokolra kell annak menni? Magyar költo-géniuszok testi és lelki betegségei. GMR Reklámügynökség, Budapest.

Dax, E.C. (1953). *Experimental Studies in Psychiatric Art*. London: Faber & Faber.

Donnelly, E.F., Murphy, D.L., Goodwin, F.K., and Waldman, I.N. (1982). Intellectual function in primary affective disorder. *Br J Psychiatry*, 140, 633–636.

Enâchescu, C. (1971). Aspects of pictorial creation in manic-depressive psychosis. *Confin Psychiatr*, 14, 133–142.

Fodor, E.M. (1999). Subclinical inclination toward manic-depression and creative performance on the Remote Associates Test. *Person Individual Differences*, 27, 1273–1283.

Fodor, E.M., and Laird, B.A. (2004). Therapeutic intervention, bipolar inclination, and literary creativity. *Creativity Res J*, 16, 149–161.

Folley, B.S., Doop, M.L., and Park. S. (2003). Psychoses and creativity: Is the missing link a biological mechanism related to phospholipids turnover? *Prostoglandins Leukot Essent Fatty Acids*, 69, 467–476.

Galton, F. (1892). *Hereditary Genius*. London: Walter Scott.

Gardner, H. (1993). *Creating Minds*. New York: Basic Books.

Gardner, R. Jr. (1982). Mechanisms in manic-depressive disorder: An evolutionary model. *Arch Gen Psychiatry*, 39(12), 1436–1441.

George, M.S., Melvin, J.A., and Mossman, D. (1988). Mental illness and creativity. *Am J Psychiatry*, 145, 908.

Getzels, J.W., and Jackson, P.W. (1963). The highly intelligent and the highly creative adolescent: A summary of some research findings. In C.W. Taylor and F. Barron (Eds.), *Scientific Creativity: Its Recognition and Development*. New York: John Wiley & Sons, pp. 161–172.

Ghacibeh, G.A., Shenker, J.I., Shenal, B., Uthman, B.M., and Heilman, K.M. (2006). Effect of vagus nerve stimulation on creativity and cognitive flexibility. *Epilepsy Behav*, 8, 720–725.

Gilbert, P. (2004). Depression: A biopsychosocial, integrative and evolutionary approach. In M. Power (Ed.), *Mood Disorders: A Handbook of Science and Practice*. Chichester: John Wiley, pp. 99–142.

Gilbert, P. (2006). Evolution and depression: Issues and implications. *Psychol Med*, 36, 287–297.

Giroux, R. (Ed.). (1987). *Robert Lowell: Collected Prose*. New York: Farrar, Straus, Giroux.

Greene, T.R., and Noice, H. (1988). Influence of positive affect upon creative thinking and problem solving in children. *Psychol Rep*, 63, 895–898.

Guilford, J.P. (1957). A revised structure of intellect. *Report of the Psychological Laboratory, University of Southern California* (No. 19).

Guilford, J.P. (1959). Traits of creativity. In H.H. Anderson (Ed.), *Creativity and Its Cultivation*. New York: Harper, pp. 142–161.

Henry, G.M., Weingartner, H., and Murphy, D.L. (1971). Idiosyncratic patterns of learning and word association during mania. *Am J Psychiatry*, 128, 564–574.

Hoffman, R.E., Quinlan, D.M., Mazure, C.M., and McGlashan, T.M. (2001). Cortical instability and the mechanism of mania: A neural network simulation and perceptual test. *Soc Biol Psychiatry*, 49, 500–509.

Hudson, L. (1966). *Contrary Imaginations: A Psychological Study of the English Schoolboy*. Middlesex, England: Penguin Books.

Isen, A.M. (1999). On creative problem solving. In S. Russ (Ed.), *Affect, Creative Experience, and Psychological Adjustment*. Philadelphia: Taylor and Francis, pp. 3–17.

Isen, A.M., and Daubman, K.A. (1984). The influence of affect on categorization. *J Pers Soc Psychol*, 47, 1206–1217.

Isen, A.M., Johnson, M.S., Mertz, E., and Robinson, G.F. (1985). The influence of positive affect on the unusualness of word associations. *J Pers Soc Psychol*, 48, 1413–1426.

Isen, A.M., Daubman, K.A., and Nowicki, G.P. (1987). Positive affect facilitates creative problem solving. *J Pers Soc Psychol*, 52, 1122–1131.

Jacobson, A.C. (1912). Literary genius and manic depressive insanity. *Med Rec*, 82, 937–939.

James, W. (1902). *The Varieties of Religious Experience: A Study in Human Nature.*

Jamison, K.R. (1989). Mood disorders and seasonal patterns in British writers and artists. *Psychiatry*, 52, 125–134.

Jamison, K.R. (1993). *Touched with Fire: Manic-Depressive Illness and the Artistic Temperament.* New York: Free Press.

Jamison, K.R. (2004). *Exuberance: The Passion for Life.* New York: Alfred A. Knopf.

Juda, A. (1949). The relationship between highest mental capacity and psychic abnormalities. *Am J Psychiatry*, 106, 296–307.

Judd, L.L., Hubbard, B., Janowsky, D.S., Huey, L.Y., and Takahashi, K.I. (1977). The effect of lithium carbonate on the cognitive functions of normal subjects. *Arch Gen Psychiatry*, 34, 355–357.

Karlsson, J.L. (1970). Genetic association of giftedness and creativity with schizophrenia. *Hereditas*, 66, 177–182.

Keller, M.C., and Miller G. (2006). Resolving the paradox of common harmful, heritable mental disorders: Which evolution genetic models work best? *Behavioral and Brain Sciences*, 29, 385–452.

Keller, M.C., and Nesse, R.M. (2005). Is low mood an adaptation? Evidence for subtypes with symptoms that match precipitants. *J Affect Disord*, 86, 27–35.

Kocsis, J.H., Shaw, E.D., Stokes, P.E., Wilner, P., Elliot, A.S., Sikes, C., Myers, B., Manevitz, A., and Parides, M. (1993). Neuropsycholic effects of lithium discontinuation. *J Clin Psychopharmacol*, 13, 268–276.

Koukopoulos, A., and Koukopoulos, A. (1999). Agitated depression as a mixed state and the problem of melancholia. *Psychiatr Clin North Am*, 22(3), 547–564.

Kraepelin E. (1921). *Manic-Depressive Insanity and Paranoia*. R.M. Barclay (Ed.), G.M. Robertson (Transl.). Edinburgh: E & S Livingstone. Reprinted New York: Arno Press, 1976.

Lamb, C. (1987). *Elia and the Last Essays of Elia.* New York: Oxford University Press, pp. 212–213.

Lange-Eichbaum, W. (1932). *The Problem of Genius.* Translated by E. Paul and C. Paul. New York: Macmillan.

Larsen, R.J., Diener E., and Cropanzano, R.S. (1987). Cognitive operations associated with the characteristic of Intense Emotional Responsiveness. *J Pers Soc Psychol*, 53, 767–774.

Levine, J., Schild, K., Kimhi, R., and Schreiber, G. (1996). Word associative production in affective versus schizophrenic psychoses. *Psychopathology*, 29, 7–13.

Lombroso, C. (1891). *The Man of Genius,* 2nd Edition. London: Walter Scott. New York: Charles Scribners Sons (1905).

Ludwig, A.M. (1992). Creative achievement and psychopathology: Comparison among professions. *Am J Psychother*, 46(3), 330–356.

Ludwig, A.M. (1994). Mental illness and creative activity in female writers. *Am J Psychiatry*, 151, 1650–1656.

Ludwig, A.M. (1995). *The Price of Greatness: Resolving the Creativity and Madness Controversy.* New York: Guilford Press.

Luxenburger, H. (1933). Berufsgliederun und soziale Schichtung in den Familien erblich Geisteskranker. *Eugenik*, 3, 34–40.

MacKinnon, D.W. (1962). The personality correlates of creativity: A study of American architects. *Proceedings of the Fourteenth Congress on Applied Psychology*, 2, 11–39.

Marshall, M.H., Neumann, C.P., and Robinson, M. (1970). Lithium, creativity, and manic-depressive illness: Review and prospectus. *Psychosomatics*, 11, 406–488.

Martindale, C. (1972). Father's absence, psychopathology, and poetic eminence. *Psychol Rep*, 31(3), 843–847.

McNeil, T.F. (1971). Prebirth and postbirth influence on the relationship between creative ability and recorded mental illness. *J Pers*, 39, 391–406.

Moore, T. (1832). *The Works of Lord Byron: With His Letters and Journals and His Life.* R.H. Stoddard (Ed.). (Reprint, London: Francis A. Nicholls, 1900), Vol. 16, p. 237.

Murphy, G. (1923). Types of word-association in dementia praecox, manic-depressives, and normal persons. *Am J Psychiatry*, 79, 539–571.

Myerson, A., and Boyle, R. (1941). The incidence of manic-depressive psychosis in certain socially important families. *Am J Psychiatry*, 98, 11–21.

Nowakowska, C., Strong, C.M., Santosa, C.M., Wang, P.W., and Ketter, T.A. (2005). Temperamental commonalities and differences in euthymic mood disorder patients, creative controls, and healthy controls. *J Affect Disord*, 85, 207–215.

Ochse, R. (1990). *Before the Gates of Excellence: The Determinants of Creative Genius.* Cambridge, UK: Cambridge University Press.

Piirto, J. (1994). *Talented Children and Adults: Their Development and Education.* New York: Macmillan.

Plato. (1974). *Phaedrus and the Seventh and Eighth Letters.* Translated by W. Hamilton. Middlesex, England: Penguin.

Plokker, J.J. (1965). *Art from the Mentally Disturbed, the Scattered Vision of Schizophrenics.* Boston: Little Brown.

Polatin, P., and Fieve, R.R. (1971). Patient rejection of lithium carbonate prophylaxis. *JAMA*, 218, 864–866.

Pons, L., Nurberger, J.I. Jr., and Murphy, D.L. (1985). Mood-independent aberrancies in associative processes in bipolar affective disorder: An apparent stabilizing effect of lithium. *Psychiatry Res*, 14, 315–322.

Post, F. (1994). Creativity and psychopathology: A study of 291 world-famous men. *Br J Psychiatry*, 165, 22–34.

Post, F. (1996). Verbal creativity, depression and alcoholism: An investigation of one hundred American and British writers. *Br J Psychiatry*, 168, 545–555.

Price, J.S. (1967). Hypothesis: The dominance hierarchy and the evolution of mental illness. *Lancet*, ii, 243–246.

Price, J.S. (1972). Genetic and phylogenetic aspects of mood variation. *Int J Ment Health*, 1, 124–144.

Price, J., Sloman, L., Gardner, R., Gilbert, P., and Rohde, P. (1994). The social competition hypothesis of depression. *Br J Psychiatry*, 164, 309–315.

Reid, E.C. (1912). Manifestations of manic-depressive insanity in literary genius. *Am J Insanity*, 68, 595–632.

Reitman, F. (1950). *Psychotic Art.* London: Rutledge and Kegan Paul.

Richards, R.L. (1981). Relationships between creativity and psychopathology: An evaluation and interpretation of the evidence. *Genet Psychol Monogr*, 103, 261–324.

Richards, R., and Kinney, D.K. (1990). Mood swings and creativity. *Creativity Res J*, 3, 202–217.

Richards, R.L., Kinney, D.K., Lunde, I., Benet, M., and Merzel, A.P. (1988). Creativity in manic-depressives, cyclothymes, their normal relatives, and control subjects. *J Abnorm Psychol*, 97, 281–288.

Robins, L.N., Helzer, J.E., Weissman, M.M., Orvaschel, H., Gruenberg, E., Burk, J.D. Jr., and Regier, D.A. (1984). Lifetime prevalence of specific psychiatric disorders in three sites. *Arch Gen Psychiatry*, 41, 949–958.

Roe, A. (1946). The personality of artists. *Educat Psychol Measurement*, 6, 401–408.

Roe, A. (1951). A psychological study of eminent biologists. *Psychol Monogr*, 65, 1–68.

Roe, A. (1952). A psychologist examines sixty-four eminent scientists. *Sci Am*, 187, 21–25.

Rush, B. (1812). *Medical Inquiries and Observations upon the Diseases of the Mind*. Philadelphia: Kimber and Richardson, pp. 153–154.

Schildkraut, J.J., and Hirshfeld, A.J. (1995). Mind and mood in modern art I: Miro and "Melancolie." *Creativity Res J*, 8, 139–156.

Schildkraut, J.J., Hirshfeld, A.J., and Murphy, J.M. (1994). Mind and mood in modern art, II: Depressive disorders, spirituality, and early deaths in the Abstract Expressionist Artists of the New York School. *Am J Psychiatry*, 151, 482–488.

Schou, M. (1968). Lithium in psychiatric therapy and prophylaxis. *J Psychiatr Res*, 6, 67–95.

Schou, M. (1979). Artistic productivity and lithium prophylaxis in manic-depressive illness. *Br J Psychiatry*, 135, 97–103.

Schuldberg, D. (1990). Schizotypal and hypomanic traits, creativity, and psychological health. *Creativity Res J*, 3, 218–230.

Sexton, L.G., and Ames, L. (Eds). (1977). *Anne Sexton: A Self-Portrait in Letters*. Boston: Houghton Mifflin.

Shaw, E.D., Mann, J.J., Stokes, P.E., and Manevitz, A.Z. (1986). Effects of lithium carbonate on associative productivity and idiosyncrasy in bipolar outpatients. *Am J Psychiatry*, 143, 1166–1169.

Shenton, M.E., Solovay, M.R., and Holzman, P. (1987). Comparative studies of thought disorders: II. Schizoaffective disorder. *Arch Gen Psychiatry*, 44, 21–30.

Simeonova, D.I., Chang, K.D., Strong, C., and Ketter, T.A. (2005). Creativity in familial bipolar disorder. *J Psychiatr Res*, 39, 623–631.

Simonton, D.K. (1994). *Greatness: Who Makes History and Why*. New York: Guilford Press.

Solovay, M.R., Shenton, M.E., and Holzman, P.S. (1987). Comparative studies of thought disorders: I. Mania and schizophrenia. *Arch Gen Psychiatry*, 44, 13–20.

Steffan, T.G. (1971). *Byron's Don Juan: The Making of a Masterpiece*. Austin, TX: University of Texas Press, p. 345.

Stoll, A.L., Locke, C.A., Vuckovic, A., and Mayer, P.V. (1996). Lithium-associated cognitive and functional deficits reduced by a switch to divalproex sodium: A case series. *J Clin Psychiatry*, 57, 356–359.

Trethowan, W.H. (1977). Music and mental disorder. In M. Critchley and R.E. Henson (Eds.), *Music and the Brain*. London: Heinemann, pp. 398–442.

Wadeson, H.S., and Carpenter, W.T. Jr. (1976). A comparative study of art expression of schizophrenic, unipolar depressive, and bipolar manic-depressive patients. *J Nerv Ment Dis*, 162, 334–344.

Watson, P.J., and Andrews, P.W. (2002). Toward a revised evolutionary adaptationist analysis of depression: The social navigation hypothesis. *J Affect Disord*, 72, 1–14.

Welch, L., Diethelm, O., and Long, L. (1946). Measurement of hyper-associative activity during elation. *J Psychol*, 21, 113–126.

Welsh, G.S. (1977). Personality correlates of intelligence and creativity in gifted adolescents. In J.C. Stanley, W.C. George, and C.H. Solano (Eds.), *The Gifted and the Creative: A Fifty-Year Perspective*. Baltimore: Johns Hopkins University Press, pp. 197–221.

White, R.K. (1930). Note on the psychopathology of genius. *J Soc Psychol*, I, 311–315.

Wills, G.I. (2003). Forty lives in the bebop business: Mental health in a group of eminent jazz musicians. *Br J Psychiatry*, 183, 255–259.

Wilson, D.R. (1993). Evolutionary epidemiology: Darwinian theory in the service of medicine and psychiatry. *Acta Biotheoretica*, 41, 205–218.

Winner, E. (1996). *Gifted Children: Myths and Realities*. New York: Basic Books.

Woodruff, R.A. Jr., Robins, L.N., Winokur, G., and Reich, T. (1971). Manic depressive illness and social achievement. *Acta Psychiatry*, 119, 33–38.

Zimmerman, J., and Garfinkle, L. (1942). Preliminary study of the art productions of the adult psychotic. *Psychiatr Q*, 16, 313–318.

CHAPTER 13

Abkevich, V., Camp, N.J., Hensel, C.H., Neff, C.D., Russell, D.L., Hughes, D.C., Plenk, A.M., Lowry, M.R., Richards, R.L., Carter, C., Frech, G.C., Stone, S., Rowe, K., Chau, C.A., Cortado, K., Hunt, A., Luce, K., O'Neil, G., Poarch, J., Potter, J., Poulsen, G.H., Saxton, H., Bernat-Sestak, M., Thompson, V., Gutin, A., Skolnick, M.H., Shattuck, D., and Cannon-Albright, L. (2003). Predisposition locus for major depression at chromosome 12q22-12q23.2. *Am J Hum Genet*, 73(6), 1271–1281.

Abrams, R., and Taylor, M.A. (1980). A comparison of unipolar and bipolar depressive illness. *Am J Psychiatry*, 137, 658–661.

Adams, L.J., Mitchell, P.B., Fielder, S.L., Rosso, A., Donald, J.A., and Schofield, P.R. (1998). A susceptibility locus for bipolar affective disorder on chromosome 4q35. *Am J Hum Genet*, 62(5), 1084–1091.

Ahearn, E.P., Speer, M.C., Chen, Y.T., Steffens, D.C., Cassidy, F., Van Meter, S., Provenzale, J.M., Weisler, R.H., and Krishnan, K.R. (2002). Investigation of Notch3 as a candidate gene for bipolar disorder using brain hyperintensities as an endophenotype. *Am J Med Genet*, 114(6), 652–658.

Albrecht, U., Sutcliffe, J.S., Cattanach, B.M., Beechey, C.V., Armstrong, D., Eichele, G., and Beaudet, A.L. (1997). Imprinted expression of the murine Angelman syndrome gene, *Ube3a*, in hippocampal and Purkinje neurons. *Nat Genet*, 17(1), 75–78.

Alda, M., Turecki, G., Grof, P., Cavazzoni, P., Duffy, A., Grof, E., Ahrens, B., Berghofer, A., Muller-Oerlinghausen, B., Dvorakova, M., Libigerova, E., Vojtechovsky, M., Zvolsky, P., Joober, R., Nilsson, A., Prochazka, H., Licht, R.W., Rasmussen, N.A., Schou, M., Vestergaard, P., Holzinger, A., Schumann, C., Thau, K., and Rouleau, G.A. (2000). Association and linkage studies of CRH and PENK genes in bipolar disorder: A collaborative IGSLI study. *Am J Med Genet*, 96(2), 178–181.

Andreasen, N.C., Grove, W.M., Shapiro, R.W., Keller, M.B., Hirschfeld, R.M., and McDonald-Scott, P. (1981). Reliability of lifetime diagnosis: A multicenter collaborative perspective. *Arch Gen Psychiatry*, 38(4), 400–405.

Andreasen, N.C., Hoffman, R.E., and Grove, W.M. (1985). Mapping abnormalities in language and cognition. In M. Alpert (Ed.), *Controversies in Schizophrenia: Changes and Constancies* (pp. 199–227). New York: Guilford Press.

Andreasen, N.C., Rice, J., Endicott, J., Reich, T., and Coryell, W. (1986). The family history approach to diagnosis. How useful is it? *Arch Gen Psychiatry*, 43(5), 421–429.

Andreasen, N.C., Rice, J., Endicott, J., Coryell, W., Grove, W.M., and Reich, T. (1987). Familial rates of affective disorder. A report from the national institute of mental health collaborative study. *Arch Gen Psychiatry*, 44(5), 461–469.

Andrews, G., Stewart, G., Allen, R., and Henderson, A.S. (1990) The genetics of six neurotic disorders: A twin study. *J Affect Disord*, 19(1), 23–29.

Angst, J. (1961). A clinical analysis of the effects of tranfranil in depression. Longitudinal and follow-up studies. Treatment of blood relations. *Psychopharmacologia*, 2, 381–407.

Angst, J. (1964). Antidepressive Effekt und genetische Faktoren. *Arzneimittelforschung*, 14(Suppl.), 496–500.

Arai, M., Itokawa, M., Yamada, K., Toyota, T., Arai, M., Haga, S., Ujike, H., Sora, I., Ikeda, K., and Yoshikawa, T. (2004). Association of neural cell adhesion molecule 1 gene polymorphisms with bipolar affective disorder in Japanese individuals. *Biol Psychiatry*, 55(8), 804–810.

Arinami, T., Itokawa, M., Aoki, J., Shibuya, H., Ookubo, Y., Iwawaki, A., Ota, K., Shimizu, H., Hamaguchi, H., and Toru, M. (1996). Further association study on dopamine D2 receptor variant S311C in schizophrenia and affective disorders. *Am J Med Genet*, 67(2), 133–138.

Arranz, M.J., Erdmann, J., Kirov, G., Rietschel, M., Sodhi, M., Albus, M., Ball, D., Maier, W., Davies, N., Franzek, E., Abusaad, I., Weigelt, B., Murray, R., Shimron-Abarbanell, D., Kerwin, R., Propping, P., Sham, P., Nothen, M.M., and Collier, D.A. (1997). 5-HT2A receptor and bipolar affective disorder: Association studies in affected patients. *Neurosci Lett*, 224(2), 95–98.

Asghari, V., Sanyal, S., Buchwaldt, S., Paterson, A., Jovanovic, V., and Van Tol, H.H. (1995). Modulation of intracellular cyclic AMP levels by different human dopamine D4 receptor variants. *J Neurochem*, 65(3), 1157–1165.

Asherson, P., Mant, R., Williams, N., Cardno, A., Jones, L., Murphy, K., Collier, D.A., Nanko, S., Craddock, N., Morris, S., Muir, W., Blackwood, B., McGuffin, P., and Owen, M.J. (1998). A study of chromosome 4p markers and dopamine D5 receptor gene in schizophrenia and bipolar disorder. *Mol Psychiatry*, 3(4), 310–320.

Avramopoulos, D., Willour, V.L., Zandi, P.P., Huo, Y., MacKinnon, D.F., Potash, J.B., DePaulo, J.R. Jr., and McInnis, M.G. (2004). Linkage of bipolar affective disorder on chromosome 8q24: Follow-up and parametric analysis. *Mol Psychiatry*, 9(2), 191–196.

Badenhop, R.F., Moses, M.J., Scimone, A., Mitchell, P.B., Ewen-White, K.R., Rosso, A., Donald, J.A., Adams, L.J., and Schofield, P.R. (2002). A genome screen of 13 bipolar affective disorder pedigrees provides evidence for susceptibility loci on chromosome 3 as well as chromosomes 9, 13 and 19. *Mol Psychiatry*, 7(8), 851–859.

Badner, J.A., and Gershon, E.S. (2002). Meta-analysis of whole-genome linkage scans of bipolar disorder and schizophrenia. *Mol Psychiatry*, 7(4):405–411.

Banse, D. (1929). Zum Problem der Erbprognosebestimmung. Die Erkrankungsaussuchten der Vettern und Basen von Manisch-Depressiven. [The problem of empirical hereditary risk. The morbidity risk of cousins of manic depressive patients]. *Z Ges Neurol Psychiatrie*, 119, 576–612.

Baron, M., Mendlewicz, J., and Klotz, J. (1981). Age-of-onset and genetic transmission in affective disorders. *Acta Psychiatr Scand*, 64(5), 373–380.

Baron, M., Barkai, A., Asnis, L., and Kane, J. (1982). Schizoaffective illness, schizophrenia and affective disorders: Morbidity risk and genetic transmission. *Acta Psychiatr Scand*, 65, 253–262.

Baron, M., Risch, N., Hamburger, R., Mandel, B., Kushner, S., Newman, M., Drumer, D., and Belmaker, R.H. (1987). Genetic linkage between X-chromosome markers and bipolar affective illness. *Nature*, 326(6110), 289–292.

Baron, M., Freimer, N.F., Risch, N., Lerer, B., Alexander, J.R., Straub, R.E., Asokan, S., Das, K., Peterson, A., and Amos, J. (1993). Diminished support for linkage between manic depressive illness and X-chromosome markers in three Israeli pedigrees [see comments]. *Nat Genet*, 3(1), 49–55.

Battersby, S., Ogilvie, A.D., Smith, C.A., Blackwood, D.H., Muir, W.J., Quinn, J.P., Fink, G., Goodwin, G.M., and Harmar, A.J. (1996). Structure of a variable number tandem repeat of the serotonin transporter gene and association with affective disorder. *Psychiatr Genet*, 6(4), 177–181.

Bellivier, F., Henry, C., Szoke, A., Schurhoff, F., Nosten-Bertrand, M., Feingold, J., Launay, J.M., Leboyer, M., and Laplanche, J.L. (1998a). Serotonin transporter gene polymorphisms in patients with unipolar or bipolar depression. *Neurosci Lett*, 255(3), 143–146.

Bellivier, F., Leboyer, M., Courtet, P., Buresi, C., Beaufils, B., Samolyk, D., Allilaire, J.F., Feingold, J., Mallet, J., and Malafosse, A. (1998b). Association between the tryptophan hydroxylase gene and manic-depressive illness. *Arch Gen Psychiatry*, 55(1), 33–37.

Bellivier, F., Szoke, A., Henry, C., Lacoste, J., Bottos, C., Nosten-Bertrand, M., Hardy, P., Rouillon, F., Launay, J.M., Laplanche, J.L., and Leboyer, M. (2000). Possible association between serotonin transporter gene polymorphism and violent suicidal behavior in mood disorders. *Biol Psychiatry*, 48(4), 319–322.

Belmaker, R.H., Henry, C., Szoke, A., Schurhoff, F., Nosten-Bertrand, M., Feingold, J., Launay, J.M., Leboyer, M., and Laplanche, J.L. (2002). Reduced inositol content in lymphocyte-derived cell lines from bipolar patients. *Bipolar Disord*, 4(1), 67–69.

Bennett, P., Segurado, R., Jones, I., Bort, S., McCandless, F., Lambert, D., Heron, J., Comerford, C., Middle, F., Corvin, A., Pelios, G., Kirov, G., Larsen, B., Mulcahy, T., Williams, N., O'Connell, R., O'Mahony, E., Payne, A., Owen, M., Holmans, P., Craddock, N., and Gill, M. (2002). The Wellcome trust UK-Irish bipolar affective disorder sibling-pair genome screen: First stage report. *Mol Psychiatry*, 7(2), 189–200.

Berrettini, W.H. (2000). Are schizophrenic and bipolar disorders related? A review of family and molecular studies. *Biol Psychiatry*, 48(6), 531–538.

Berrettini, W.H., Goldin, L.R., Gelernter, J., Gejman, P.V., Gershon, E.S., and Detera-Wadleigh, S. (1990). X-chromosome markers and manic-depressive illness. Rejection of linkage to Xq28 in nine bipolar pedigrees [see comments]. *Arch Gen Psychiatry*, 47(4), 366–373.

Berrettini, W.H., Ferraro, T.N., Goldin, L.R., Weeks, D.E., Detera-Wadleigh, S., Nurnberger, J.I. Jr., and Gershon, E.S. (1994). Chromosome 18 DNA markers and manic-depressive illness: evidence for a susceptibility gene. *Proc Natl Acad Sci USA*, 91(13), 5918–5921.

Bertelsen, A., Harvald, B., and Hauge, M. (1977). A Danish twin study of manic-depressive disorders. *Br J Psychiatry*, 130, 330–351.

Bezchlibnyk, Y.B., Wang, J.F., McQueen, G.M., and Young, L.T. (2001). Gene expression differences in bipolar disorder revealed by cDNA array analysis of post-mortem frontal cortex. *J Neurochem*, 79(4), 826–834.

Bierut, L.J., Heath, A.C., Bucholz, K.K., Dinwiddie, S.H., Madden, P.A., Statham, D.J., Dunne, M.P., and Martin, N.G. (1999). Major depressive disorder in a community-based twin sample: Are there different genetic and environmental contributions for men and women? *Arch Gen Psychiatry*, 56(6), 557–563.

Billings, P.R., Hubbard, R., and Newman, S.A. (1999). Human germline gene modification: A dissent. *Lancet*, 353(9167), 1873–1875.

Biomed European Bipolar Collaborative Group. (1997). No association between bipolar disorder and alleles at a functional polymorphism in the COMT gene. *Br J Psychiatry*, 170, 526–528.

Blackwood, D.H., He, L., Morris, S.W., McLean, A., Whitton, C., Thomson, M., Walker, M.T., Woodburn, K., Sharp, C.M., Wright, A.F., Shibasaki, Y., St. Clair, D.M., Porteous, D.J., and Muir, W.J. (1996). A locus for bipolar affective disorder on chromosome 4p. *Nat Genet*, 12(4), 427–430.

Blackwood, D.H., Fordyce, A., Walker, M.T., St. Clair, D.M., Porteous, D.J., and Muir, W.J. (2001). Schizophrenia and affective disorders—cosegregation with a translocation at chromosome 1q42 that directly disrupts brain-expressed genes: Clinical and P300 findings in a family. *Am J Hum Genet*, 69(2), 428–433.

Bland, R.C., Newman, S.C., and Orn, H. (1986). Recurrent and nonrecurrent depression. A family study. *Arch Gen Psychiatry*, 43(11), 1085–1089.

Blouin, J.L., Dombroski, B.A., Nath, S.K., Lasseter, V.K., Wolyniec, P.S., Nestadt, G., Thornquist, M., Ullrich, G., McGrath, J., Kasch, L., Lamacz, M., Thomas, M.G., Gehrig, C., Radhakrishna, U., Snyder, S.E., Balk, K.G., Neufeld, K., Swartz, K.L., DeMarchi, N., Papadimitriou, G.N., Dikeos, D.G., Stefanis, C.N., Chakravarti, A., Childs, B., Housman, D.E., Kazazian, H.H., Antonarakis, S., and Pulver, A.E. (1998). Schizophrenia susceptibility loci on chromosomes 13q32 and 8p21. *Nat Genet*, 20(1), 70–73.

Bocchetta, A., Piccardi, M.P., Palmas, M.A., Chillotti, C., Oi, A., Del Zompo, M. (1999). Family-based association study between bipolar disorder and DRD2, DRD4, DAT, and SERT in Sardinia. *Am J Med Genet*, 88(5), 522–526.

Bondy, B., Erfurth, A., de Jonge, S., Kruger, M., and Meyer, H. (2000). Possible association of the short allele of the serotonin transporter promoter gene polymorphism (5-HTTLPR) with violent suicide. *Mol Psychiatry*, 5(2), 193–195.

Borglum, A.D., Bruun, T.G., Kjeldsen, T.E., Ewald, H., Mors, O., Kirov, G., Russ, C., Freeman, B., Collier, D.A., and Kruse, T.A. (1999). Two novel variants in the DOPA decarboxylase gene: Association with bipolar affective disorder. *Mol Psychiatry*, 4(6), 545–551.

Borglum, A.D., Kirov, G., Craddock, N., Mors, O., Muir, W., Murray, V., McKee, I., Collier, D.A., Ewald, H., Owen, M.J., Blackwood, D., and Kruse, T.A. (2003). Possible parent-of-origin effect of Dopa decarboxylase in susceptibility to bipolar affective disorder. *Am J Med Genet*, 117B(1), 18–22.

Botstein, D., and Risch, N. (2003). Discovering genotypes underlying human phenotypes: Past successes for mendelian disease, future approaches for complex disease. *Nat Genet*, 33(Suppl.), 228–237.

Botstein, D., White, R.L., Skolnick, M., and Davis, R.W. (1980). Construction of a genetic linkage map in man using restriction fragment length polymorphisms. *Am J Hum Genet*, 32(3), 314–331.

Bowen, T., Ashworth, L., Kirov, G., Guy, C.A., Jones, I.R., McCandless, F., Craddock, N., O'Donovan, M.C., and Owen, M.J. (2000). No evidence of association from transmission disequilibrium analysis of the hKCa3 gene in bipolar disorder. *Bipolar Disord*, 2(4), 328–331.

Brunner, H.G., Nelen, M., Breakefield, X.O., Ropers, H.H., and van Oost, B.A. (1993). Abnormal behavior associated with a point mutation in the structural gene for monoamine oxidase A. *Science*, 262(5133), 578–580.

Brzustowicz, L.M., Honer, W.G., Chow, E.W., Little, D., Hogan, J., Hodgkinson, K., and Bassett, A.S. (1999). Linkage of familial schizophrenia to chromosome 13q32. *Am J Hum Genet*, 65(4), 1096–1103.

Bucher, K.D., Elston, R.C., Green, R., Whybrow, P., Helzer, J., Reich, T., Clayton, P., and Winokur, G. (1981). The transmission of manic depressive illness: II. Segregation analysis of three sets of family data. *J Psychiatr Res*, 16(1), 65–78.

Bunzel, R., Blumcke, I., Cichon, S., Normann, S., Schramm, J., Propping, P., and Nothen, M.M. (1998). Polymorphic imprinting of the serotonin-2A (5-HT2A) receptor gene in human adult brain. *Brain Res Mol Brain Res*, 59(1), 90–92.

Burgert, E., Crocq, M.A., Bausch, E., Macher, J.P., and Morris-Rosendahl, D.J. (1998). No association between the tyrosine hydroxylase microsatellite marker HUMTH01 and schizophrenia or bipolar I disorder. *Psychiatr Genet*, 8(2), 45–48.

Burton, R. (1621). *The Anatomy of Melancholy*. Republished 2001, New York: New York Review of Books.

Caberlotto, L., Jimenez, P., Overstreet, D.H., Hurd, Y.L., Mathe, A.A., and Fuxe, K. (1999). Alterations in neuropeptide Y levels and Y1 binding sites in the Flinders Sensitive Line rats, a genetic animal model of depression. *Neurosci Lett*, 265(3), 191–194.

Cadoret, R.J., O'Gorman, T.W., Heywood, E., and Troughton, E. (1985). Genetic and environmental factors in major depression. *J Affect Disord*, 9(2), 155–164.

Cardno, A.G., Marshall, E.J., Coid, B., Macdonald, A.M., Ribchester, T.R., Davies, N.J., Venturi, P., Jones, L.A., Lewis, S.W., Sham, P.C., Gottesman, I.I., Farmer, A.E., McGuffin, P., Reveley, A.M., and Murray, R.M. (1999). Heritability estimates for psychotic disorders: The Maudsley twin psychosis series. *Arch Gen Psychiatry*, 56(2), 162–168.

Cardno, A.G., Rijsdijk, F.V., Sham, P.C., Murray, R.M., and McGuffin, P. (2002). A twin study of genetic relationships between psychotic symptoms. *Am J Psychiatry*, 159(4), 539–545.

Carmelli, D., DeCarli, C., Swan, G.E., Jack, L.M., Reed, T., Wolf, P.A., and Miller, B.L. (1998). Evidence for genetic variance in white matter hyperintensity volume in normal elderly male twins. *Stroke*, 29(6), 1177–1181.

Carrasquillo, M.M., McCallion, A.S., Puffenberger, E.G., Kashuk, C.S., Nouri, N., and Chakravarti, A. (2002). Genome-wide association study and mouse model identify interaction between RET and EDNRB pathways in Hirschsprung disease. *Nat Genet*, 32(2), 237–244.

Caspi, A., Sugden, K., Moffitt, T.E., Taylor, A., Craig, I.W., Harrington, H., McClay, J., Mill, J., Martin, J., Braithwaite, A., and Poulton, R. (2003). Influence of life stress on depression: Moderation by a polymorphism in the 5-HTT gene. *Science*, 301(5631), 386–389.

Cavazzoni, P., Alda, M., Turecki, G., Rouleau, G., Grof, E., Martin, R., Duffy, A., and Grof, P. (1996). Lithium-responsive affective disorders: no association with the tyrosine hydroxylase gene. *Psychiatry Res*, 64(2), 91–96.

Chakravarti, A. (1999). Population genetics: Making sense out of sequence. *Nat Genet*, 21(Suppl. 1), 56–60.

Chandy, K.G., Fantino, E., Wittekindt, O., Kalman, K., Tong, L.L., Ho, T.H., Gutman, G.A., Crocq, M.A., Ganguli, R., Nimgaonkar, V., Morris-Rosendahl, D.J., and Gargus, J.J. (1998). Isolation of a novel potassium channel gene hSKCa3 containing a polymorphic CAG repeat: A candidate for schizophrenia and bipolar disorder? *Mol Psychiatry*, 3(1), 32–37.

Chang, K.D., Steiner, H., and Ketter, T.A. (2000). Psychiatric phenomenology of child and adolescent bipolar offspring. *J Am Acad Child Adolesc Psychiatry*, 39(4), 453–460.

Chee, I.S., Lee, S.W., Kim, J.L., Wang, S.K., Shin, Y.O., Shin, S.C., Lee, Y.H., Hwang, H.M., and Lim, M.R. (2001). 5-HT2A receptor gene promoter polymorphism-1438A/G and bipolar disorder. *Psychiatr Genet*, 11(3), 111–114.

Chen, Y.S., Akula, N., Detera-Wadleigh, S.D., Schulze, T.G., Thomas, J., Potash, J.B., DePaulo, J.R., McInnis, M.G., Cox, N.J., and McMahon, F.J. (2004). Findings in an independent sample support an association between bipolar affective disorder and the G72/G30 locus on chromosome 13q33. *Mol Psychiatry*, 9(1), 87–92; image 5.

Cheung, V.G., Conlin, L.K., Weber, T.M., Arcaro, M., Jen, K.Y., Morley, M., and Spielman, R.S. (2003). Natural variation in human gene expression assessed in lymphoblastoid cells. *Nat Genet*, 33(3), 422–425.

Chumakov, I., Blumenfeld, M., Guerassimenko, O., Cavarec, L., Palicio, M., Abderrahim, H., Bougueleret, L., Barry, C., Tanaka, H., La Rosa, P., Puech, A., Tahri, N., Cohen-Akenine, A., Delabrosse, S., Lissarrague, S., Picard, F.P., Maurice, K., Essioux, L., Millasseau, P., Grel, P., Debailleul, V., Simon, A.M., Caterina, D., Dufaure, I., Malekzadeh, K., Belova, M., Luan, J.J., Bouillot, M., Sambucy, J.L., Primas, G., Saumier, M., Boubkiri, N., Martin-Saumier, S., Nasroune, M., Peixoto, H., Delaye, A., Pinchot, V., Bastucci, M., Guillou, S., Chevillon, M., Sainz-Fuertes, R., Meguenni, S., Aurich-Costa, J., Cherif, D., Gimalac, A., Van Duijn, C., Gauvreau, D., Ouellette, G., Fortier, I., Raelson, J., Sherbatich, T., Riazanskaia, N., Rogaev, E., Raeymaekers, P., Aerssens, J., Konings, F., Luyten, W., Macciardi, F., Sham, P.C., Straub, R.E., Weinberger, D.R., Cohen, N., and Cohen, D. (2002). Genetic and physiological data implicating the new human gene G72 and the gene for D-amino acid oxidase in schizophrenia. *Proc Natl Acad Sci USA*, 99(21), 13675–13680.

Cichon, S., Nothen, M.M., Rietschel, M., Korner, J., and Propping, P. (1994). Single-strand conformation analysis (SSCA) of the dopamine D1 receptor gene (DRD1) reveals no significant mutation in patients with schizophrenia and manic depression. *Biol Psychiatry*, 36(12), 850–853.

Cichon, S., Nothen, M.M., Stober, G., Schroers, R., Albus, M., Maier, W., Rietschel, M., Korner, J., Weigelt, B., Franzek, E., Wildenauer, D., Fimmers, R., and Propping, P. (1996). Systematic screening for mutations in the 5'-regulatory region of the human dopamine D1 receptor (DRD1) gene in patients with schizophrenia and bipolar affective disorder. *Am J Med Genet*, 67(4), 424–428.

Cichon, S., Schumacher, J., Muller, D.J., Hurter, M., Windemuth, C., Strauch, K., Hemmer, S., Schulze, T.G., Schmidt-Wolf, G., Albus, M., Borrmann-Hassenbach, M., Franzek, E., Lanczik, M., Fritze, J., Kreiner, R., Reuner, U., Weigelt, B., Minges, J., Lichtermann, D., Lerer, B., Kanyas, K., Baur, M.P., Wienker, T.F., Maier, W., Rietschel, M., Propping, P., and Nothen, M.M. (2001). A genome screen for genes predisposing to bipolar affective disorder detects a new susceptibility locus on 8q. *Hum Mol Genet*, 10(25), 2933–2944.

Cichon, S., Buervenich, S., Kirov, G., Akula, N., Dimitrova, A., Green, E., Schumacher, J., Klopp, N., Becker, T., Ohlraun, S., Schulze, T.G., Tullius, M., Gross, M.M., Jones, L., Krastev, S., Nikolov, I., Hamshere, M., Jones, I., Czerski, P.M., Leszczynska-Rodziewicz, A., Kapelski, P., Bogaert, A.V., Illig, T., Hauser, J., Maier, W., Berrettini, W., Byerley, W., Coryell, W., Gershon, E.S., Kelsoe, J.R., McInnis, M.G., Murphy, D.L., Nurnberger, J.I., Reich, T., Scheftner, W., O'Donovan, M.C., Propping, P., Owen, M.J., Rietschel, M., Nothen, M.M., McMahon, F.J., and Craddock, N. (2004). Lack of support for a genetic association of the XBP1 promoter polymorphism with bipolar disorder in probands of European origin. *Nat Genet*, 36(8), 783–784.

Collier, D.A., Arranz, M.J., Sham, P., Battersby, S., Vallada, H., Gill, P., Aitchison, K.J., Sodhi, M., Li, T., Roberts, G.W., Smith, B., Morton, J., Murray, R.M., Smith, D., and Kirov, G. (1996a). The serotonin transporter is a potential susceptibility factor for bipolar affective disorder. *Neuroreport*, 7(10), 1675–1679.

Collier, D.A., Stober, G., Li, T., Heils, A., Catalano, M., Di Bella, D., Arranz, M.J., Murray, R.M., Vallada, H.P., Bengel, D., Muller, C.R., Roberts, G.W., Smeraldi, E., Kirov, G., Sham, P., and Lesch, K.P. (1996b). A novel functional polymorphism within the promoter of the serotonin transporter gene: Possible role in susceptibility to affective disorders. *Mol Psychiatry*, 1(6), 453–460.

Coon, H., Jensen, S., Hoff, M., Holik, J., Plaetke, R., Reimherr, F., Wender, P., Leppert, M., and Byerley, W. (1993). A genome-wide search for genes predisposing to manic-depression, assuming autosomal dominant inheritance. *Am J Hum Genet*, 52(6), 1234–1249.

Coon, H., Hoff, M., Holik, J., Hadley, D., Fang, N., Reimherr, F., Wender, P., and Byerley, W. (1996). Analysis of chromosome 18 DNA markers in multiplex pedigrees with manic depression. *Biol Psychiatry*, 39(8), 689–696.

Coryell, W., Endicott, J., and Keller, M. (1992). Rapidly cycling affective disorder. Demographics, diagnosis, family history, and course. *Arch Gen Psychiatry*, 49(2), 126–131.

Coryell, W., Akiskal, H., Leon, A.C., Turvey, C., Solomon, D., and Endicott, J. (2000). Family history and symptom levels during treatment for bipolar I affective disorder. *Biol Psychiatry*, 47(12), 1034–1042.

Coryell, W., Leon, A.C., Turvey, C., Akiskal, H.S., Mueller, T., and Endicott, J. (2001). The significance of psychotic features in manic episodes. *J Affect Disord*, 67, 79–88.

Courtet, P., Baud, P., Abbar, M., Boulenger, J.P., Castelnau, D., Mouthon, D., Malafosse, A., and Buresi, C. (2001). Association between violent suicidal behavior and the low activity allele of the serotonin transporter gene. *Mol Psychiatry*, 6(3), 338–341.

Craddock, N., Owen, M., Burge, S., Kurian, B., Thomas, P., and McGuffin, P. (1994). Familial cosegregation of major affective disorder and Darier's disease (keratosis follicularis) [see comments]. *Br J Psychiatry*, 164(3), 355–358.

Craddock, N., Daniels, J., Roberts, E., Rees, M., McGuffin, P., and Owen, M.J. (1995a). No evidence for allelic association between bipolar disorder and monoamine oxidase A gene polymorphisms. *Am J Med Genet, 60*(4), 322–324.

Craddock, N., Khodel, V., Van Eerdewegh, P., and Reich, T. (1995b). Mathematical limits of multilocus models: The genetic transmission of bipolar disorder. *Am J Hum Genet, 57*(3), 690–702.

Craddock, N., Roberts, Q., Williams, N., McGuffin, P., and Owen, M.J. (1995c). Association study of bipolar disorder using a functional polymorphism (Ser311→Cys) in the dopamine D2 receptor gene. *Psychiatr Genet, 5*(2), 63–65.

Craddock, N., Dave, S., and Greening, J. (2001). Association studies of bipolar disorder. *Bipolar Disord, 3*(6), 284–298.

Curtis, D., Kalsi, G., Brynjolfsson, J., McInnis, M., O'Neill, J., Smyth, C., Moloney, E., Murphy, P., McQuillin, A., Petursson, H., and Gurling, H. (2003). Genome scan of pedigrees multiply affected with bipolar disorder provides further support for the presence of a susceptibility locus on chromosome 12q23-q24, and suggests the presence of additional loci on 1p and 1q. *Psychiatr Genet, 13*(2), 77–84.

da Fonseca A. (1959). Analise Heredo-Clinca Das Perturbacoes Afectivas (Estudio De 60 Pares De Gemeos, e Sues Conganguin Neos). Proto: Impresna Protuguesa.

Dawson, E., Gill, M., Curtis, D., Castle, D., Hunt, N., Murray, R., and Powell, J. (1995). Genetic association between alleles of pancreatic phospholipase A2 gene and bipolar affective disorder. *Psychiatr Genet, 5*(4), 177–180.

DeBaun, M.R., Niemitz, E.L., and Feinberg, A.P. (2003). Association of in vitro fertilization with Beckwith-Wiedemann syndrome and epigenetic alterations of LIT1 and H19. *Am J Hum Genet, 72*(1), 156–160.

de Bruyn, A., Mendelbaum, K., Sandkuijl, L.A., Delvenne, V., Hirsch, D., Staner, L., Mendlewicz, J., and Van Broeckhoven, C. (1994). Nonlinkage of bipolar illness to tyrosine hydroxylase, tyrosinase, and D2 and D4 dopamine receptor genes on chromosome 11. *Am J Psychiatry, 151*(1), 102–106.

de Bruyn, A., Souery, D., Mendelbaum, K., Mendlewicz, J., and Van Broeckhoven, C. (1996). Linkage analysis of families with bipolar illness and chromosome 18 markers. *Biol Psychiatry, 39*(8), 679–688.

Decina, P., Kestenbaum, C.J., Farber, S., Kron, L., Gargan, M., Sackeim, H.A., and Fieve, R.R. (1983). Clinical and psychological assessment of children of bipolar probands. *Am J Psychiatry, 140*(5), 548–553.

Deckert, J., Nothen, M.M., Albus, M., Franzek, E., Rietschel, M., Ren, H., Stiles, G.L., Knapp, M., Weigelt, B., Maier, W., Beckmann, H., and Propping, P. (1998). Adenosine A1 receptor and bipolar affective disorder: Systematic screening of the gene and association studies. *Am J Med Genet, 81*(1), 18–23.

Del Favero, J., Gestel, S.V., Borglum, A.D., Muir, W., Ewald, H., Mors, O., Ivezic, S., Oruc, L., Adolfsson, R., Blackwood, D., Kruse, T., Mendlewicz, J., Schalling, M., and Van Broeckhoven, C. (2002). European combined analysis of the CTG18.1 and the ERDA1 CAG/CTG repeats in bipolar disorder. *Eur J Hum Genet, 10*(4), 276–280.

DeLisi, L.E., Goldin, L.R., Maxwell, M.E., Kazuba, D.M., and Gershon, E.S. (1987). Clinical features of illness in siblings with schizophrenia or schizoaffective disorder. *Arch Gen Psychiatry, 44*(10), 891–896.

Detera-Wadleigh, S.D., Berrettini, W.H., Goldin, L.R., Boorman, D., Anderson, S., and Gershon, E.S. (1987). Close linkage of c-Harvey-ras-1 and the insulin gene to affective disorder is ruled out in three North American pedigrees. *Nature, 325*(6107), 806–808.

Detera-Wadleigh, S.D., Badner, J.A., Goldin, L.R., Berrettini, W.H., Sanders, A.R., Rollins, D.Y., Turner, G., Moses, T., Haerian, H., Muniec, D., Nurnberger, J.I. Jr., and Gershon, E.S. (1996). Affected-sib-pair analyses reveal support of prior evidence for a susceptibility locus for bipolar disorder, on 21q. *Am J Hum Genet, 58*(6), 1279–1285.

Detera-Wadleigh, S.D., Badner, J.A., Yoshikawa, T., Sanders, A.R., Goldin, L.R., Turner, G., Rollins, D.Y., Moses, T., Guroff, J.J., Kazuba, D., Maxwell, M.E., Edenberg, H.J., Foroud, T., Lahiri, D., Nurnberger, J.I. Jr., Stine, O.C., McMahon, F., Meyers, D.A., MacKinnon, D., Simpson, S., McInnis, M., DePaulo, J.R., Rice, J., Goate, A., and Gershon, E.S. (1997). Initial genome scan of the NIMH genetics initiative bipolar pedigrees: chromosomes 4, 7, 9, 18, 19, 20, and 21q. *Am J Med Genet, 74*(3), 254–262.

Detera-Wadleigh, S.D., Badner, J.A., Berrettini, W.H., Yoshikawa, T., Goldin, L.R., Turner, G., Rollins, D.Y., Moses, T., Sanders, A.R., Karkera, J.D., Esterling, L.E., Zeng, J., Ferraro, T.N., Guroff, J.J., Kazuba, D., Maxwell, M.E., Nurnberger, J.I. Jr., and Gershon, E.S. (1999). A high-density genome scan detects evidence for a bipolar-disorder susceptibility locus on 13q32 and other potential loci on 1q32 and 18p11.2. *Proc Natl Acad Sci USA, 96*(10), 5604–5609.

Di Bella, D., Catalano, M., Cichon, S., and Nothen, M.M. (1996). Association study of a null mutation in the dopamine D4 receptor gene in Italian patients with obsessive-compulsive disorder, bipolar mood disorder and schizophrenia. *Psychiatr Genet, 6*(3), 119–121.

Dick, D.M., Foroud, T., Edenberg, H.J., Miller, M., Bowman, E., Rau, N.L., DePaulo, J.R., McInnis, M., Gershon, E., McMahon, F., Rice, J.P., Bierut, L.J., Reich, T., and Nurnberger, J. Jr. (2002). Apparent replication of suggestive linkage on chromosome 16 in the NIMH genetics initiative bipolar pedigrees. *Am J Med Genet, 114*(4), 407–412.

Dick, D.M., Foroud, T., Flury, L., Bowman, E.S., Miller, M.J., Rau, N.L., Moe, P.R., Samavedy, N., El-Mallakh, R., Manji, H., Glitz, D.A., Meyer, E.T., Smiley, C., Hahn, R., Widmark, C., McKinney, R., Sutton, L., Ballas, C., Grice, D., Berrettini, W., Byerley, W., Coryell, W., DePaulo, R., MacKinnon, D.F., Gershon, E.S., Kelsoe, J.R., McMahon, F.J., McInnis, M., Murphy, D.L., Reich, T., Scheftner, W., and Nurnberger, J.I. Jr. (2003). Genomewide linkage analyses of bipolar disorder: A new sample of 250 pedigrees from the National Institute of Mental Health Genetics Initiative. *Am J Hum Genet, 73*(1), 107–114. Erratum in: *Am J Hum Genet, 73*(4), 979.

Dimitrova, A., Georgieva, L., Nikolov, I., Poriazova, N., Krastev, S., Toncheva, D., Owen, M.J., and Kirov, G. (2002). Major psychiatric disorders and the serotonin transporter gene (SLC6A4): Family-based association studies. *Psychiatr Genet, 12*(3), 137–141.

Duffy, A., Turecki, G., Grof, P., Cavazzoni, P., Grof, E., Joober, R., Ahrens, B., Berghofer, A., Muller-Oerlinghausen, B., Dvorakova, M., Libigerova, E., Vojtechovsky, M., Zvolsky, P., Nilsson, A., Licht, R.W., Rasmussen, N.A., Schou, M., Vestergaard, P., Holzinger, A., Schumann, C., Thau, K., Robertson, C., Rouleau, G.A., and Alda, M. (2000). Association and linkage studies of candidate genes involved in GABAergic neurotransmission in lithium-responsive bipolar disorder. *J Psychiatry Neurosci, 25*(4), 353–358.

Eastwood, S.L., Burnet, P.W., and Harrison, P.J. (2000). Expression of complexin I and II mRNAs and their regulation by antipsychotic drugs in the rat forebrain. *Synapse*, 36(3), 167–177.

Edenberg, H.J., Foroud, T., Conneally, P.M., Sorbel, J.J., Carr, K., Crose, C., Willig, C., Zhao, J., Miller, M., Bowman, E., Mayeda, A., Rau, N.L., Smiley, C., Rice, J.P., Goate, A., Reich, T., Stine, O.C., McMahon, F., DePaulo, J.R., Meyers, D., Detera-Wadleigh, S.D., Goldin, L.R., Gershon, E.S., Blehar, M.C., and Nurnberger, J.I. Jr. (1997). Initial genomic scan of the NIMH genetics initiative bipolar pedigrees: Chromosomes 3, 5, 15, 16, 17, and 22. *Am J Med Genet*, 74(3), 238–246.

Egeland, J.A., Gerhard, D.S., Pauls, D.L., Sussex, J.N., Kidd, K.K., Allen, C.R., Hostetter, A.M., and Housman, D.E. (1987). Bipolar affective disorders linked to DNA markers on chromosome 11. *Nature*, 325(6107), 783–787.

Ekholm, J.M., Kieseppa, T., Hiekkalinna, T., Partonen, T., Paunio, T., Perola, M., Ekelund, J., Lonnqvist, J., Pekkarinen-Ijas, P., and Peltonen, L. (2003). Evidence of susceptibility loci on 4q32 and 16p12 for bipolar disorder. *Hum Mol Genet*, 12(15), 1907–1915.

Endicott, J., and Spitzer, R.L. (1978). A diagnostic interview: the schedule for affective disorders and schizophrenia. *Arch Gen Psychiatry*, 35(7), 837–844.

Erdmann, J., Shimron-Abarbanell, D., Cichon, S., Albus, M., Maier, W., Lichtermann, D., Minges, J., Reuner, U., Franzek, E., and Ertl, M.A. (1995). Systematic screening for mutations in the promoter and the coding region of the 5-HT1A gene. *Am J Med Genet*, 60(5), 393–399.

Erdmann, J., Nothen, M.M., Shimron-Abarbanell, D., Rietschel, M., Albus, M., Borrmann, M., Maier, W., Franzek, E., Korner, J., Weigelt, B., Fimmers, R., and Propping, P. (1996). The human serotonin 7 (5-HT7) receptor gene: Genomic organization and systematic mutation screening in schizophrenia and bipolar affective disorder. *Mol Psychiatry*, 1(5), 392–397.

Erlenmeyer-Kimling, L., and Cornblatt, B.A. (1992). A summary of attentional findings in the New York High-Risk Project. *J Psychiatr Res*, 26(4), 405–426.

Erlenmeyer-Kimling, L., Adamo, U.H., Rock, D., Roberts, S.A., Bassett, A.S., Squires-Wheeler, E., Cornblatt, B.A., Endicott, J., Pape, S., and Gottesman, I.I. (1997). The New York High-Risk Project. Prevalence and comorbidity of axis I disorders in offspring of schizophrenic parents at 25-year follow-up. *Arch Gen Psychiatry*, 54(12), 1096–1102.

Esterling, L.E., Yoshikawa, T., Turner, G., Badner, J.A., Bengel, D., Gershon, E.S., Berrettini, W.H., and Detera-Wadleigh, S.D. (1998). Serotonin transporter (5-HTT) gene and bipolar affective disorder. *Am J Med Genet*, 81(1), 37–40.

Etain, B., Rousseva, A., Roy, I., Henry, C., Malafosse, A., Buresi, C., Preisig, M., Rayah, F., Leboyer, M., and Bellivier, F. (2004). Lack of association between 5HT2A receptor gene haplotype, bipolar disorder and its clinical subtypes in a West European sample. *Am J Med Genet B Neuropsychiatr Genet*, 129(1), 29–33.

Evans, K.L., Le Hellard, S., Morris, S.W., Lawson, D., Whitton, C., Semple, C.A., Fantes, J.A., Torrance, H.S., Malloy, M.P., Maule, J.C., Humphray, S.J., Ross, M.T., Bentley, D.R., Muir, W.J., Blackwood, D.H., and Porteous, D.J. (2001). A 6.9-Mb high-resolution BAC/PAC contig of human 4p15.3-p16.1, a candidate region for bipolar affective disorder. *Genomics*, 71(3), 315–323.

Ewald, H., Mors, O., Flint, T., Koed, K., Eiberg, H., and Kruse, T.A. (1995a). A possible locus for manic depressive illness on chromosome 16p13. *Psychiatr Genet*, 5(2), 71–81.

Ewald, H., Mors, O., Flint, T., Friedrich, U., Eiberg, H., and Kruse, T.A. (1995b). Linkage analysis between manic-depressive illness and markers on the long arm of chromosome 11. *Am J Med Genet*, 60(5), 386–392.

Ewald, H., Mors, O., Koed, K., Eiberg, H., and Kruse, T.A. (1997). Susceptibility loci for bipolar affective disorder on chromosome 18? A review and a study of Danish families. *Psychiatr Genet*, 7(1), 1–12.

Ewald, H., Degn, B., Mors, O., and Kruse, T.A. (1998). Significant linkage between bipolar affective disorder and chromosome 12q24. *Psychiatr Genet*, 8(3), 131–140.

Falconer, D.S. (1965). The inheritance of liability to certain diseases, estimated from the incidence among relatives. *Ann Hum Genet*, 29, 51–76.

Fallin, M.D., Lasseter, V.K., Wolyniec, P.S., McGrath, J.A., Nestadt, G., Valle, D., Liang, K.Y., and Pulver, A.E. (2004). Genomewide linkage scan for bipolar-disorder susceptibility loci among Ashkenazi Jewish families. *Am J Hum Genet*, 75(2), 204–219.

Faraone, S.V., Tsuang, M.T., and Gutierrez, J.M. (1987). Long-term outcome and family psychiatric illness in unipolar and bipolar disorders. *Psychopharmacol Bull*, 23(3), 465–467.

Faraone, S.V., Biederman, J., Mennin, D., Wozniak, J., and Spencer, T. (1997), Attention-deficit hyperactivity disorder with bipolar disorder: a familial subtype? *J Am Acad Child Adolesc Psychiatry*, 36(10), 1378–1387.

Faraone, S.V., Matise, T., Svrakic, D., Pepple, J., Malaspina, D., Suarez, B., Hampe, C., Zambuto, C.T., Schmitt, K., Meyer, J., Markel, P., Lee, H., Harkavy Friedman, J., Kaufmann, C., Cloninger, C.R., and Tsuang, M.T. (1998). Genome scan of European-American schizophrenia pedigrees: Results of the NIMH Genetics Initiative and Millennium Consortium. *Am J Med Genet*, 81(4), 290–295.

Faraone, S.V., Doyle, A.E., Mick, E., and Biederman, J. (2001a). Meta-analysis of the association between the 7-repeat allele of the dopamine D(4) receptor gene and attention deficit hyperactivity disorder. *Am J Psychiatry*, 158(7), 1052–1057.

Faraone, S.V., Biederman, J., and Monuteaux, M.C. (2001b). Attention deficit hyperactivity disorder with bipolar disorder in girls: Further evidence for a familial subtype? *J Affect Disord*, 64(1), 19–26.

Faraone, S.V., Glatt, S.J., Su, J., and Tsuang, M.T. (2004). Three potential susceptibility loci shown by a genome-wide scan for regions influencing the age at onset of mania. *Am J Psychiatry*, 161(4), 625–630.

Farmer, A.E., McGuffin, P., and Gottesman, I.I. (1987). Twin concordance for DSM-III schizophrenia. Scrutinizing the validity of the definition. *Arch Gen Psychiatry*, 44(7), 634–641.

Farmer, A., Breen, G., Brewster, S., Craddock, N., Gill, M., Korszun, A., Maier, W., Middleton, L., Mors, O., Owen, M., Perry, J., Preisig, M., Rietschel, M., Reich, T., Jones, L., Jones, I., and McGuffin, P. (2004). The Depression Network (DeNT) Study: Methodology and sociodemographic characteristics of the first 470 affected sibling pairs from a large multi-site linkage genetic study. *BMC Psychiatry*, 4(1), 42.

Ferrier, I.N., and Thompson, J.M. (2002). Cognitive impairment in bipolar affective disorder: Implications for the bipolar diathesis. *Br J Psychiatry*, 180, 293–295.

Foroud, T., Castelluccio, P.F., Koller, D.L., Edenberg, H.J., Miller, M., Bowman, E., Rau, N.L., Smiley, C., Rice, J.P., Goate, A., Armstrong, C., Bierut, L.J., Reich, T., Detera-Wadleigh, S.D., Goldin, L.R., Badner, J.A., Guroff, J.J., Gershon, E.S., McMahon, F.J.,

Simpson, S., MacKinnon, D., McInnis, M., Stine, O.C., De-Paulo, J.R., Blehar, M.C., and Nurnberger, J.I. Jr. (2000). Suggestive evidence of a locus on chromosome 10p using the NIMH genetics initiative bipolar affective disorder pedigrees. *Am J Med Genet*, 96(1), 18–23.

Franks, E., Guy, C., Jacobsen, N., Bowen, T., Owen, M.J., O'Donovan, M.C., and Craddock, N. (1999). Eleven trinucleotide repeat loci that map to chromosome 12 excluded from involvement in the pathogenesis of bipolar disorder. *Am J Med Genet*, 88(1), 67–70.

Freimer, N.B., Reus, V.I., Escamilla, M.A., McInnes, L.A., Spesny, M., Leon, P., Service, S.K., Smith, L.B., Silva, S., Rojas, E., Gallegos, A., Meza, L., Fournier, E., Baharloo, S., Blankenship, K., Tyler, D.J., Batki, S., Vinogradov, S., Weissenbach, J., Barondes, S.H., and Sandkuijl, L.A. (1996). Genetic mapping using haplotype, association and linkage methods suggests a locus for severe bipolar disorder (BPI) at 18q22–q23. *Nat Genet*, 12(4), 436–441.

Friddle, C., Koskela, R., Ranade, K., Hebert, J., Cargill, M., Clark, C.D., McInnis, M., Simpson, S., McMahon, F., Stine, O.C., Meyers, D., Xu, J., MacKinnon, D., Swift-Scanlan, T., Jamison, K., Folstein, S., Daly, M., Kruglyak, L., Marr, T., DePaulo, J.R., and Botstein, D. (2000). Full-genome scan for linkage in 50 families segregating the bipolar affective disease phenotype. *Am J Hum Genet*, 66(1), 205–215.

Furlong, R.A., Coleman, T.A., Ho, L., Rubinsztein, J.S., Walsh, C., Paykel, E.S., and Rubinsztein, D.C. (1998a). No association of a functional polymorphism in the dopamine D2 receptor promoter region with bipolar or unipolar affective disorders. *Am J Med Genet*, 81(5), 385–387.

Furlong, R.A., Ho, L., Rubinsztein, J.S., Walsh, C., Paykel, E.S., and Rubinsztein, D.C. (1998b). No association of the tryptophan hydroxylase gene with bipolar affective disorder, unipolar affective disorder, or suicidal behaviour in major affective disorder. *Am J Med Genet*, 81(3), 245–247.

Furlong, R.A., Ho, L., Walsh, C., Rubinsztein, J.S., Jain, S., Paykel, E.S., Easton, D.F., and Rubinsztein, D.C. (1998c). Analysis and meta-analysis of two serotonin transporter gene polymorphisms in bipolar and unipolar affective disorders. *Am J Med Genet*, 81(1), 58–63.

Furlong, R.A., Ho, L., Rubinsztein, J.S., Walsh, C., Paykel, E.S., and Rubinsztein, D.C. (1999a). Analysis of the monoamine oxidase A (MAOA) gene in bipolar affective disorder by association studies, meta-analyses, and sequencing of the promoter. *Am J Med Genet*, 88(4), 398–406.

Furlong, R.A., Rubinsztein, J.S., Ho, L., Walsh, C., Coleman, T.A., Muir, W.J., Paykel, E.S., Blackwood, D.H., and Rubinsztein, D.C. (1999b). Analysis and metaanalysis of two polymorphisms within the tyrosine hydroxylase gene in bipolar and unipolar affective disorders. *Am J Med Genet*, 88(1), 88–94.

Gabriel, S.B., Schaffner, S.F., Nguyen, H., Moore, J.M., Roy, J., Blumenstiel, B., Higgins, J., DeFelice, M., Lochner, A., Faggart, M., Liu-Cordero, S.N., Rotimi, C., Adeyemo, A., Cooper, R., Ward, R., Lander, E.S., Daly, M.J., and Altshuler, D. (2002). The structure of haplotype blocks in the human genome. *Science*, 296(5576), 2225–2229.

Gass, P., Reichardt, H.M., Strekalova, T., Henn, F., and Tronche, F. (2001). Mice with targeted mutations of glucocorticoid and mineralocorticoid receptors: Models for depression and anxiety? *Physiol Behav*, 73(5), 811–825.

Geller, B., and Cook, E.H. Jr. (2000). Ultradian rapid cycling in prepubertal and early adolescent bipolarity is not in transmission disequilibrium with val/met COMT alleles. *Biol Psychiatry*, 47(7), 605–609.

Geller, B., Badner, J.A., Tillman, R., Christian, S.L., Bolhofner, K., and Cook, E.H. Jr. (2004). Linkage disequilibrium of the brain-derived neurotrophic factor Val66Met polymorphism in children with a prepubertal and early adolescent bipolar disorder phenotype. *Am J Psychiatry*, 161(9), 1698–1700.

Georgieva, L., Dimitrova, A., Nikolov, I., Koleva, S., Tsvetkova, R., Owen, M.J., Toncheva, D., and Kirov, G. (2002). Dopamine transporter gene (DAT1) VNTR polymorphism in major psychiatric disorders: Family-based association study in the Bulgarian population. *Acta Psychiatr Scand*, 105(5), 396–399.

Gershon, E.S., and Goldin, L.R. (1989). Linkage data on affective disorders in an epidemiologic context. *Genet Epidemiol*, 6(1), 201–209.

Gershon, E.S., Hamovit, J., Guroff, J.J., Dibble, E., Leckman, J.F., Sceery, W., Targum, S.D., Nurnberger, J.I. Jr., Goldin, L.R., and Bunney, W.E. Jr. (1982). A family study of schizoaffective, bipolar I, bipolar II, unipolar, and normal control probands. *Arch Gen Psychiatry*, 39(10), 1157–1167.

Gershon, E.S., McKnew, D., Cytryn, L., Hamovit, J., Schreiber, J., Hibbs, E., and Pellegrini, D. (1985). Diagnoses in school-age children of bipolar affective disorder patients and normal controls. *J Affect Disord*, 8(3), 283–291.

Gershon, E.S., Weissman, M.M., Guroff, J.J., Prusoff, B.A., and Leckman, J.F. (1986). Validation of criteria for major depression through controlled family study. *J Affect Disord*, 11(2), 125–131.

Gershon, E.S., DeLisi, L.E., Hamovit, J., Nurnberger, J.I. Jr., Maxwell, M.E., Schreiber, J., Dauphinais, D., Dingman, C.W. II, and Guroff, J.J. (1988). A controlled family study of chronic psychoses. Schizophrenia and schizoaffective disorder. *Arch Gen Psychiatry*, 45(4), 328–336.

Gershon, E.S., Goldin, L.R., Guroff, J.J., and Hamovit, J.R. (1989). Description of the National Institute of Mental Health family study of affective disorders. *Genet Epidemiol*, 6(1), 183–185.

Gill, M., Castle, D., Hunt, N., Clements, A., Sham, P., and Murray, R.M. (1991). Tyrosine hydroxylase polymorphisms and bipolar affective disorder. *J Psychiatr Res*, 25(4), 179–184.

Gill, M., Vallada, H., Collier, D., Sham, P., Holmans, P., Murray, R., McGuffin, P., Nanko, S., Owen, M., Antonarakis, S., Housman, D., Kazazian, H., Nestadt, G., Pulver, A.E., Straub, R.E., MacLean, C.J., Walsh, D., Kendler, K.S., DeLisi, L., Polymeropoulos, M., Coon, H., Byerley, W., Lofthouse, R., Gershon, E., and Read, C.M. (1996). A combined analysis of D22S278 marker alleles in affected sib-pairs: Support for a susceptibility locus for schizophrenia at chromosome 22q12. Schizophrenia Collaborative Linkage Group (Chromosome 22). *Am J Med Genet*, 67(1), 40–45.

Ginns, E.I., St. Jean, P., Philibert, R.A., Galdzicka, M., Damschroder-Williams, P., Thiel, B., Long, R.T., Ingraham, L.J., Dalwaldi, H., Murray, M.A., Ehlert, M., Paul, S., Remortel, B.G., Patel, A.P., Anderson, M.C., Shaio, C., Lau, E., Dymarskaia, I., Martin, B.M., Stubblefield, B., Falls, K.M., Carulli, J.P., Keith, T.P., Fann, C.S., Lacy, L.G., Allen, C.R., Hostetter, A.M., Elston, R.C., Schork, N.J., Egeland, J.A., and Paul, S.M. (1998). A genome-wide search for chromosomal loci linked to mental health wellness in relatives at high risk for bipolar affective disorder among the Old Order Amish. *Proc Natl Acad Sci USA*, 95(26), 15531–15536.

Goldin, L.R., Gershon, E.S., Targum, S.D., Sparkes, R.S., and McGinniss, M. (1983). Segregation and linkage analyses in families of patients with bipolar, unipolar, and schizoaffective mood disorders. *Am J Hum Genet,* 35(2), 274–287.

Goldstein, J.M., Faraone, S.V., Chen, W.J., and Tsuang, M.T. (1993). The role of gender in understanding the familial transmission of schizoaffective disorder. *Br J Psychiatry,* 163, 763–768.

Gomez-Casero, E., Perez de Castro, I., Saiz-Ruiz, J., Llinares, C., and Fernandez-Piqueras, J. (1996). No association between particular DRD3 and DAT gene polymorphisms and manic-depressive illness in a Spanish sample. *Psychiatr Genet,* 6(4), 209–212.

Goossens, D., Del Favero, J., and Van Broeckhoven, C. (2001). Trinucleotide repeat expansions: Do they contribute to bipolar disorder? *Brain Res Bull,* 56(3–4), 243–257.

Gourovitch, M.L., Torrey, E.F., Gold, J.M., Randolph, C., Weinberger, D.R., and Goldberg, T.E. (1999). Neuropsychological performance of monozygotic twins discordant for bipolar disorder. *Biol Psychiatry,* 45(5), 639–646.

Griffith, A.J., and Friedman, T.B. (1999). Making sense out of sound [news]. *Nat Genet,* 21(4), 347–349.

Grigoroiu-Serbanescu, M., Wickramaratne, P.J., Hodge, S.E., Milea, S., and Mihailescu, R. (1997). Genetic anticipation and imprinting in bipolar I illness. *Br J Psychiatry,* 170, 162–166.

Grigoroiu-Serbanescu, M., Martinez, M., Nothen, M.M., Grinberg, M., Sima, D., Propping, P., Marinescu, E., and Hrestic, M. (2001). Different familial transmission patterns in bipolar I disorder with onset before and after age 25. *Am J Med Genet,* 105(8), 765–773.

Grof, P., Duffy, A., Cavazzoni, P., Grof, E., Garnham, J., MacDougall, M., O'Donovan, C., and Alda, M. (2002). Is response to prophylactic lithium a familial trait? *J Clin Psychiatry,* 63(10), 942–947.

Guidotti, A., Auta, J., Davis, J.M., Di-Giorgi-Gerevini, V., Dwivedi, Y., Grayson, D.R., Impagnatiello, F., Pandey, G., Pesold, C., Sharma, R., Uzunov, D., and Costa, E. (2000). Decrease in reelin and glutamic acid decarboxylase67 (GAD67) expression in schizophrenia and bipolar disorder: A postmortem brain study. *Arch Gen Psychiatry,* 57(11), 1061–1069. Erratum in: Arch Gen Psychiatry, 2002, 59(1), 12.

Gutierrez, B., Arranz, M., Fananas, L., Valles, V., Guillamat, R., van Os, J., and Collier, D. (1995). 5HT2A receptor gene and bipolar affective disorder [letter]. *Lancet,* 346(8980), 969.

Gutierrez, B., Fananas, L., Arranz, M.J., Valles, V., Guillamat, R., van Os, J., and Collier, D. (1996). Allelic association analysis of the 5-HT2C receptor gene in bipolar affective disorder. *Neurosci Lett,* 212(1), 65–67.

Gutierrez, B., Bertranpetit, J., Guillamat, R., Valles, V., Arranz, M.J., Kerwin, R., and Fananas, L. (1997). Association analysis of the catechol-O-methyltransferase gene and bipolar affective disorder. *Am J Psychiatry,* 154(1), 113–115.

Gutierrez, B., Arranz, M.J., Collier, D.A., Valles, V., Guillamat, R., Bertranpetit, J., Murray, R.M., and Fanas, L. (1998). Serotonin transporter gene and risk for bipolar affective disorder: An association study in Spanish population. *Biol Psychiatry,* 43(11), 843–847.

Gutierrez, B., Arias, B., Papiol, S., Rosa, A., and Fananas, L. (2001). Association study between novel promoter variants at the 5-HT2C receptor gene and human patients with bipolar affective disorder. *Neurosci Lett,* 309(2), 135–137.

Guy, C.A., Bowen, T., Williams, N., Jones, I.R., McCandless, F., McGuffin, P., Owen, M.J., Craddock, N., and O'Donovan,

M.C. (1999). No association between a polymorphic CAG repeat in the human potassium channel gene hKCa3 and bipolar disorder. *Am J Med Genet,* 88(1), 57–60.

Haines, J.L., and Pericak-Vance, M.A. (1998). Overview of mapping common and genetically complex human disease traits. In J.L. Haines and M.A. Pericak-Vance (Eds.), *Approaches to Gene Mapping in Complex Human Diseases.* New York: John Wiley and Sons.

Hariri, A.R., Mattay, V.S., Tessitore, A., Kolachana, B., Fera, F., Goldman, D., Egan, M.F., and Weinberger, D.R. (2002). Serotonin transporter genetic variation and the response of the human amygdala. *Science,* 297(5580), 400–403.

Hashimoto, K., Maruyama, H., Nishiyama, M., Asaba, K., Ikeda, Y., Takao, T., Iwasaki, Y., Kumon, Y., Suehiro, T., Tanimoto, N., Mizobuchi, M., and Nakamura, T. (2005). Susceptibility alleles and haplotypes of human leukocyte antigen DRB1, DQA1, and DQB1 in autoimmune polyglandular syndrome type III in Japanese population. *Horm Res,* 64(5), 253–260.

Hattori, E., Yamada, K., Ebihara, M., Toyota, T., Nankai, M., Shibuya, H., and Yoshikawa, T. (2002). Association study of the short tandem repeat in the 5' upstream region of the cholecystokinin gene with mood disorders in the Japanese population. *Am J Med Genet,* 114(5), 523–526.

Hattori, E., Liu, C., Badner, J.A., Bonner, T.I., Christian, S.L., Maheshwari, M., Detera-Wadleigh, S.D., Gibbs, R.A., and Gershon, E.S. (2003). Polymorphisms at the G72/G30 gene locus, on 13q33, are associated with bipolar disorder in two independent pedigree series. *Am J Hum Genet,* 72(5), 1131–1140.

Hauser, E.R., Boehnke, M., Guo, S.W., and Risch, N. (1996). Affected-sib-pair interval mapping and exclusion for complex genetic traits: sampling considerations. *Genet Epidemiol,* 13(2), 117–137.

Hawi, Z., Mynett-Johnson, L., Murphy, V., Straub, R.E., Kendler, K.S., Walsh, D., McKeon, P., and Gill, M. (1999). No evidence to support the association of the potassium channel gene hSKCa3 CAG repeat with schizophrenia or bipolar disorder in the Irish population. *Mol Psychiatry,* 4(5), 488–491.

Hayward, B.E., Moran, V., Strain, L., and Bonthron, D.T. (1998). Bidirectional imprinting of a single gene: GNAS1 encodes maternally, paternally, and biallelically derived proteins. *Proc Natl Acad Sci USA,* 95(26), 15475–15480.

Heath, A.C., Berg, K., Eaves, L.J., Solaas, M.H., Corey, L.A., Sundet, J., Magnus, P., and Nance, W.E. (1985). Education policy and the heritability of educational attainment. *Nature,* 314(6013), 734–736.

Heckers, S., Stone, D., Walsh, J., Shick, J., Koul, P., and Benes, F.M. (2002). Differential hippocampal expression of glutamic acid decarboxylase 65 and 67 messenger RNA in bipolar disorder and schizophrenia. *Arch Gen Psychiatry,* 59(6), 521–529.

Heiden, A., Schussler, P., Itzlinger, U., Leisch, F., Scharfetter, J., Gebhardt, C., Fuchs, K., Willeit, M., Nilsson, L., Miller-Reiter, E., Stompe, T., Meszaros, K., Sieghart, W., Hornik, K., Kasper, S., and Aschauer, H.N. (2000). Association studies of candidate genes in bipolar disorders. *Neuropsychobiology,* 42(Suppl. 1), 18–21.

Hettema, J.M., Neale, M.C., and Kendler, K.S. (1995). Physical similarity and the equal-environment assumption in twin studies of psychiatric disorders. *Behav Genet,* 25(4), 327–335.

Heun, R., and Maier, W. (1993). The distinction of bipolar II disorder from bipolar I and recurrent unipolar depression: Results of a controlled family study. *Acta Psychiatr Scand,* 87(4), 279–284.

Hodgkinson, S., Gurling, H.M., Marchbanks, R.H., McInnis, M., and Petursson, H. (1987a). Minisatellite mapping in manic depression. *J Psychiatr Res*, 21(4), 589–596.

Hodgkinson, S., Sherrington, R., Gurling, H., Marchbanks, R., Reeders, S., Mallet, J., McInnis, M., Petursson, H., and Brynjolfsson, J. (1987b). Molecular genetic evidence for heterogeneity in manic depression. *Nature*, 325(6107), 805–806.

Hodgkinson, C.A., Goldman, D., Jaeger, J., Persaud S., Kane, J.M., Lipsky, R.H., and Malhotra, A.K. (2004). Disrupted in schizophrenia 1 (DISC1): Association with schizophrenia, schizoaffective disorder, and bipolar disorder. *Am J Hum Genet*, 75(5), 862–872.

Hoehe, M.R., Wendel, B., Grunewald, I., Chiaroni, P., Levy, N., Morris-Rosendahl, D., Macher, J.P., Sander, T., and Crocq, M.A. (1998). Serotonin transporter (5-HTT) gene polymorphisms are not associated with susceptibility to mood disorders. *Am J Med Genet*, 81(1), 1–3

Hoffmann, H. (1921). *Die Nachkommenschaft bei endogenen Psychosen.* Berlin: Springer-Verlag.

Holmans, P., Zubenko, G.S., Crowe, R.R., DePaulo, J.R. Jr., Scheftner, W.A., Weissman, M.M., Zubenko, W.N., Boutelle, S., Murphy-Eberenz, K., MacKinnon, D., McInnis, M.G., Marta, D.H., Adams, P., Knowles, J.A., Gladis, M., Thomas, J., Chellis, J., Miller, E., and Levinson, D.F. (2004). Genomewide significant linkage to recurrent, early-onset major depressive disorder on chromosome 15q. *Am J Hum Genet*, 74(6), 1154–1167.

Holmes, A., Yang, R.J., Murphy, D.L., and Crawley, J.N. (2002). Evaluation of antidepressant-related behavioral responses in mice lacking the serotonin transporter. *Neuropsychopharmacology*, 27(6), 914–923.

Hong, C.J., Tsai, S.J., Cheng, C.Y., Liao, W.Y., Song, H.L., and Lai, H.C. (1999). Association analysis of the 5-HT(6) receptor polymorphism (C267T) in mood disorders. *Am J Med Genet*, 88(6), 601–602.

Hong, C.J., Liu, H.C., Liu, T.Y., Lin, C.H., Cheng, C.Y., and Tsai, S.J. (2003). Brain-derived neurotrophic factor (BDNF) Val66Met polymorphisms in Parkinson's disease and age of onset. *Neurosci Lett*, 353(1), 75–77.

Horikawa, Y., Oda, N., Cox, N.J., Li, X., Orho-Melander, M., Hara, M., Hinokio, Y., Lindner, T.H., Mashima, H., Schwarz, P.E., del Bosque-Plata, L., Horikawa, Y., Oda, Y., Yoshiuchi, I., Colilla, S., Polonsky, K.S., Wei, S., Concannon, P., Iwasaki, N., Schulze, J., Baier, L.J., Bogardus, C., Groop, L., Boerwinkle, E., Hanis, C.L., and Bell, G.I. (2000). Genetic variation in the gene encoding calpain-10 is associated with type 2 diabetes mellitus. *Nat Genet*, 26(2), 163–175.

Horikawa, Y., Oda, N., Yu, L., Imamura, S., Fujiwara, K., Makino, M., Seino, Y., Itoh, M., and Takeda, J. (2003). Genetic variations in calpain-10 gene are not a major factor in the occurrence of type 2 diabetes in Japanese. *J Clin Endocrinol Metab*, 88(1), 244–247.

Horiuchi, Y., Nakayama, J., Ishiguro, H., Ohtsuki, T., Detera-Wadleigh, S.D., Toyota, T., Yamada, K., Nankai, M., Shibuya, H., Yoshikawa, T., and Arinami, T. (2004). Possible association between a haplotype of the GABA-A receptor alpha 1 subunit gene (GABRA1) and mood disorders. *Biol Psychiatry*, 55(1), 40–45.

Hou, S.J., Yen, F.C., Cheng, C.Y., Tsai, S.J., and Hong, C.J. (2004). X-box binding protein 1 (XBP1) C—116G polymorphisms in bipolar disorders and age of onset. *Neurosci Lett*, 367(2), 232–234.

Huang, Y.Y., Oquendo, M.A., Friedman, J.M., Greenhill, L.L., Brodsky, B., Malone, K.M., Khait, V., and Mann, J.J. (2003). Substance abuse disorder and major depression are associated with the human 5-HT1B receptor gene (HTR1B) G861C polymorphism. *Neuropsychopharmacology*, 28(1), 163–169.

Humm, D.G. (1932). Mental disorders in siblings. *Am J Psychiatry*, 89, 239–284.

Hurd, Y.L. (2002). Subjects with major depression or bipolar disorder show reduction of prodynorphin mRNA expression in discrete nuclei of the amygdaloid complex. *Mol Psychiatry*, 7(1), 75–81.

Inayama, Y., Yoneda, H., Sakai, T., Ishida, T., Kobayashi, S., Nonomura, Y., Kono, Y., Koh, J., and Asaba, H. (1993). Lack of association between bipolar affective disorder and tyrosine hydroxylase DNA marker. *Am J Med Genet*, 48(2), 87–89.

Ishiguro, H., Ohtsuki, T., Okubo, Y., Kurumaji, A., and Arinami, T. (2001). Association analysis of the pituitary adenyl cyclase activating peptide gene (PACAP) on chromosome 18p11 with schizophrenia and bipolar disorders. *J Neural Transm*, 108(7), 849–854.

Itokawa, M., Yamada, K., Iwayama-Shigeno, Y., Ishitsuka, Y., Detera-Wadleigh, S., and Yoshikawa, T. (2003). Genetic analysis of a functional GRIN2A promoter (GT)n repeat in bipolar disorder pedigrees in humans. *Neurosci Lett*, 345(1), 53–56.

Iwamoto, K., Kakiuchi, C., Bundo, M., Ikeda, K., and Kato T. (2004). Molecular characterization of bipolar disorder by comparing gene expression profiles of postmortem brains of major mental disorders. *Mol Psychiatry*, 9(4), 406–416.

Iwamoto, K., Bundo, M., and Kato, T. (2005). Altered expression of mitochondria-related genes in postmortem brains of patients with bipolar disorder or schizophrenia, as revealed by large-scale DNA microarray analysis. *Hum Mol Genet*, 14(2), 241–253.

Jacobsen, N., Daniels, J., Moorhead, S., Harrison, D., Feldman, E., McGuffin, P., Owen, M.J., and Craddock, N. (1996). Association study of bipolar disorder at the phospholipase A2 gene (PLA2A) in the Darier's disease (DAR) region of chromosome 12q23-q24.1. *Psychiatr Genet*, 6(4), 195–199.

Jahnes, E., Muller, D.J., Schulze, T.G., Windemuth, C., Cichon, S., Ohlraun, S., Fangerau, H., Held, T., Maier, W., Propping, P., Nothen, M.M., and Rietschel, M. (2002). Association study between two variants in the DOPA decarboxylase gene in bipolar and unipolar affective disorder. *Am J Med Genet*, 114(5), 519–522.

Jakimow-Venulet, B. (1981). Hereditary factors in the pathogenesis of affective illnesses. *Br J Psychiatry*, 139, 450–456.

James, N.M., and Chapman, C.J. (1975). A genetic study of bipolar affective disorder. *Br J Psychiatry*, 126, 449–456.

Jamison, K.R. (1993). *Touched with Fire: Manic-Depressive Illness and the Artistic Temperament.* New York: The Free Press.

Jin, D.K., Hwang, H.Z., Oh, M.R., Kim, J.S., Lee, M., Kim, S., Lim, S.W., Seo, M.Y., Kim, J.H., and Kim, D.K. (2001). CAG repeats of CTG18.1 and KCNN3 in Korean patients with bipolar affective disorder. *J Affect Disord*, 66(1), 19–24.

Johnson, G.F., and Leeman, M.M. (1977). Analysis of familial factors in bipolar affective illness. *Arch Gen Psychiatry*, 34(9), 1074–1083.

Johnston, N.L., Cervenak, J., Shore, A.D., Torrey, E.F., and Yolken, R.H. (1997). Multivariate analysis of RNA levels from postmortem human brains as measured by three different methods of RT-PCR. Stanley Neuropathology Consortium. *J Neurosci Methods*, 77(1), 83–92.

Jones, I., Middle, F., McCandless, F., Coyle, N., Robertson, E., Brockington, I., Lendon, C., and Craddock, N. (2000). Molecular genetic studies of bipolar disorder and puerperal psychosis at two polymorphisms in the estrogen receptor alpha gene (ESR 1). *Am J Med Genet*, 96(6), 850–853.

Jones, I., Scourfield, J., McCandless, F., and Craddock, N. (2002). Attitudes towards future testing for bipolar disorder susceptibility genes: A preliminary investigation. *J Affect Disord*, 71(1–3), 189–193.

Jun, T.Y., Lee, K.U., Pae, C.U., Kweon, Y.S., Chae, J.H., Bahk, W.M., Kim, K.S., Lew, T.Y., and Han, H. (2004). No evidence for an association of the CTLA4 gene with bipolar I disorder. *Psychiatry Clin Neurosci*, 58(1), 21–24.

Jung, S.K., Hong, M.S., Suh, G.J., Jin, S.Y., Lee, H.J., Kim, B.S., Lim, Y.J., Kim, M.K., Park, H.K., Chung, J.H., and Yim, S.V. (2004). Association between polymorphism in intron 1 of cocaine- and amphetamine-regulated transcript gene with alcoholism, but not with bipolar disorder and schizophrenia in Korean population. *Neurosci Lett*, 365(1), 54–57.

Kakiuchi, C., Iwamoto, K., Ishiwata, M., Bundo, M., Kasahara, T., Kusumi, I., Tsujita, T., Okazaki, Y., Nanko, S., Kunugi, H., Sasaki, T., and Kato, T. (2003). Impaired feedback regulation of XBP1 as a genetic risk factor for bipolar disorder. *Nat Genet*, 35(2), 171–175.

Kallmann, F.J. (1953). *Heredity in Health and Mental Disorder*. New York: W.W. Norton and Company.

Kallmann, F.J. (1954). Genetic principles in manic-depressive psychosis. In P.H. Hoch and J. Zubin (Eds.), *Depression*. New York: Grune and Stratton.

Kato, M.V., Shimizu, T., Nagayoshi, M., Kaneko, A., Sasaki, M.S., and Ikawa, Y. (1996a). Genomic imprinting of the human serotonin-receptor (HTR2) gene involved in development of retinoblastoma. *Am J Hum Genet*, 59(5), 1084–1090.

Kato, T., Winokur, G., Coryell, W., Keller, M.B., Endicott, J., and Rice, J. (1996b). Parent-of-origin effect in transmission of bipolar disorder. *Am J Med Genet*, 67(6), 546–550.

Kato, T., Kunugi, H., Nanko, S., and Kato, N. (2000). Association of bipolar disorder with the 5178 polymorphism in mitochondrial DNA. *Am J Med Genet*, 96(2), 182–186.

Kato, T., Kunugi, H., Nanko, S., and Kato, N. (2001), Mitochondrial DNA polymorphisms in bipolar disorder. *J Affect Disord*, 62(3), 151–164.

Kato, T., Iwamoto, K., Washizuka, S., Mori, K., Tajima, O., Akiyama, T., Nanko, S., Kunugi, H., and Kato, N. (2003). No association of mutations and mRNA expression of WFS1/wolframin with bipolar disorder in humans. *Neurosci Lett*, 338(1), 21–24.

Kawada, Y., Hattori, M., Dai, X.Y., and Nanko, S. (1995a). Possible association between monoamine oxidase A gene and bipolar affective disorder [letter; comment] [see comments]. *Am J Hum Genet*, 56(1), 335–336.

Kawada, Y., Hattori, M., Fukuda, R., Arai, H., Inoue, R., and Nanko, S. (1995b). No evidence of linkage or association between tyrosine hydroxylase gene and affective disorder. *J Affect Disord*, 34(2), 89–94.

Kealey, C., Reynolds, A., Mynett-Johnson, L., Claffey, E., and McKeon, P. (2001). No evidence to support an association between the oestrogen receptor beta gene and bipolar disorder. *Psychiatr Genet*, 11(4), 223–226.

Kelsoe, J.R., Spence, M.A., Loetscher, E., Foguet, M., Sadovnick, A.D., Remick, R.A., Flodman, P., Khristich, J., Mroczkowski-Parker, Z., Brown, J.L., Masser, D., Ungerleider, S., Rapaport, M.H., Wishart, W.L., and Luebbert, H. (1989). Re-evaluation of the linkage relationship between chromosome 11p loci and the gene for bipolar affective disorder in the Old Order Amish [see comments]. *Nature*, 342(6247), 238–243.

Kelsoe, J.R., Spence, M.A., Loetscher, E., Foguet, M., Sadovnick, A.D., Remick, R.A., Flodman, P., Khristich, J., Mroczkowski-Parker, Z., Brown, J.L., Masser, D., Ungerleider, S., Rapaport, M.H., Wishart, W.L., and Luebbert, H. (2001). A genome survey indicates a possible susceptibility locus for bipolar disorder on chromosome 22. *Proc Natl Acad Sci USA*, 98(2), 585–590.

Kendler, K.S. (1986). Kraepelin and the differential diagnosis of dementia praecox and manic-depressive insanity. *Compr Psychiatry*, 27, 549–558.

Kendler, K.S. (2001). Twin studies of psychiatric illness: An update. *Arch Gen Psychiatry*, 58(11), 1005–1014.

Kendler, K.S., and Prescott, C.A. (1999). A population-based twin study of lifetime major depression in men and women. *Arch Gen Psychiatry*, 56(1), 39–44. Erratum in: *Arch Gen Psychiatry*, 57(1), 94–95.

Kendler, K.S., and Walsh, D. (1995). Gender and schizophrenia. Results of an epidemiologically based family study. *Br J Psychiatry*, 167(2), 184–192.

Kendler, K.S., Gruenberg, A.M., and Tsuang, M.T. (1985). Psychiatric illness in first-degree relatives of schizophrenic and surgical control patients. A family study using DSM-III criteria. *Arch Gen Psychiatry*, 42(8), 770–779.

Kendler, K.S., Gruenberg, A.M., and Tsuang, M.T. (1986). A DSM-III family study of the nonschizophrenic psychotic disorders. *Am J Psychiatry*, 143(9), 1098–1105.

Kendler, K.S., McGuire, M., Gruenberg, A.M., O'Hare, A., Spellman, M., and Walsh, D. (1993a). The Roscommon Family Study. I. Methods, diagnosis of probands, and risk of schizophrenia in relatives. *Arch Gen Psychiatry*, 50(7), 527–540.

Kendler, K.S., McGuire, M., Gruenberg, A.M., O'Hare, A., Spellman, M., and Walsh, D. (1993b). The Roscommon Family Study. IV. Affective illness, anxiety disorders, and alcoholism in relatives. *Arch Gen Psychiatry*, 50(12), 952–960.

Kendler, K.S., Neale, M.C., Kessler, R.C., Heath, A.C., and Eaves, L.J. (1993c). A test of the equal-environment assumption in twin studies of psychiatric illness. *Behav Genet*, 23(1), 21–27.

Kendler, K.S., Karkowski-Shuman, L., O'Neill, F.A., Straub, R.E., MacLean, C.J., and Walsh, D. (1997). Resemblance of psychotic symptoms and syndromes in affected sibling pairs from the Irish Study of High-Density Schizophrenia Families: Evidence for possible etiologic heterogeneity. *Am J Psychiatry*, 154(2), 191–198.

Kendler, K.S., Myers, J., and Prescott, C.A. (2000). Parenting and adult mood, anxiety and substance use disorders in female twins: An epidemiological, multi-informant, retrospective study. *Psychol Med*, 30(2), 281–294.

Kent, L., and Craddock, N. (2003). Is there a relationship between attention deficit hyperactivity disorder and bipolar disorder? *J Affect Disord*, 73(3), 211–221.

Keverne, E.B., Fundele, R., Narasimha, M., Barton, S.C., and Surani, M.A. (1996). Genomic imprinting and the differential roles of parental genomes in brain development. *Brain Res Dev Brain Res*, 92(1), 91–100.

Kevles, D.J. (1995). *In the Name of Eugenics: Genetics and the Uses of Human Heredity*. Cambridge, MA: Harvard University Press.

Kim, D.K., Lim, S.W., Lee, S., Sohn, S.E., Kim, S., Hahn, C.G., and, Carroll, B.J. (2000). Serotonin transporter gene polymorphism and antidepressant response. *Neuroreport,* 11(1), 215–219.

Kirk, R., Furlong, R.A., Amos, W., Cooper, G., Rubinsztein, J.S., Walsh, C., Paykel, E.S., and Rubinsztein, D.C. (1999). Mitochondrial genetic analyses suggest selection against maternal lineages in bipolar affective disorder. *Am J Hum Genet,* 65(2), 508–518.

Kirov, G., Murphy, K.C., Arranz, M.J., Jones, I., McCandles, F., Kunugi, H., Murray, R.M., McGuffin, P., Collier, D.A., Owen, M.J., and Craddock, N. (1998). Low activity allele of catechol-O-methyltransferase gene associated with rapid cycling bipolar disorder. *Mol Psychiatry,* 3(4), 342–345.

Kirov, G., Jones, I., McCandless, F., Craddock, N., and Owen, M.J. (1999a). Family-based association studies of bipolar disorder with candidate genes involved in dopamine neurotransmission: DBH, DAT1, COMT, DRD2, DRD3 and DRD5. *Mol Psychiatry,* 4(6), 558–565.

Kirov, G., Norton, N., Jones, I., McCandless, F., Craddock, N., and Owen, M.J. (1999b). A functional polymorphism in the promoter of monoamine oxidase A gene and bipolar affective disorder. *Int J Neuropsychopharmcol,* 2(4), 293–298.

Kirov, G., Rees, M., Jones, I., MacCandless, F., Owen, M.J., and Craddock, N. (1999c). Bipolar disorder and the serotonin transporter gene: A family-based association study. *Psychol Med,* 29(5), 1249–1254.

Kirov, G., Lowry, C.A., Stephens, M., Oldfield, S., O'Donovan, M.C., Lightman, S.L., and Owen, M.J. (2001). Screening ABCG1, the human homologue of the *Drosophila* white gene, for polymorphisms and association with bipolar affective disorder. *Mol Psychiatry,* 6(6), 671–677.

Koh, P.O., Undie, A.S., Kabbani, N., Levenson, R., Goldman-Rakic, P.S., and Lidow, M.S. (2003). Up-regulation of neuronal calcium sensor-1 (NCS-1) in the prefrontal cortex of schizophrenic and bipolar patients. *Proc Natl Acad Sci USA,* 100(1), 313–317.

Koido, K., Koks, S., Nikopensius, T., Maron, E., Altmae, S., Heinaste, E., Vabrit, K., Tammekivi, V., Hallast, P., Kurg, A., Shlik, J., Vasar, V., Metspalu, A., and Vasar, E. (2005). Polymorphisms in wolframin (WFS1) gene are possibly related to increased risk for mood disorders. *Int J Neuropsychopharmacol,* 8(2), 235–244.

Konradi, C., Eaton, M., MacDonald, M.L., Walsh, J., Benes, F.M., and Heckers, S. (2004). Molecular evidence for mitochondrial dysfunction in bipolar disorder. *Arch Gen Psychiatry,* 61(3), 300–308. Erratum in: *Arch Gen Psychiatry,* 2004, 61(6), 538.

Kornberg, J.R., Brown, J.L., Sadovnick, A.D., Remick, R.A., Keck, P.E. Jr., McElroy, S.L., Rapaport, M.H., Thompson, P.M., Kaul, J.B., Vrabel, C.M., Schommer, S.C., Wilson, T., Pizzuco, D., Jameson, S., Schibuk, L., and Kelsoe, J.R. (2000). Evaluating the parent-of-origin effect in bipolar affective disorder. Is a more penetrant subtype transmitted paternally? *J Affect Disord,* 59(3), 183–192.

Korner, J., Fritze, J., and Propping, P. (1990). RFLP alleles at the tyrosine hydroxylase locus: No association found to affective disorders. *Psychiatry Res,* 32(3), 275–280.

Korner, J., Rietschel, M., Hunt, N., Castle, D., Gill, M., Nothen, M.M., Craddock, N., Daniels, J., Owen, M., Fimmers, R. (1994). Association and haplotype analysis at the tyrosine hydroxylase locus in a combined German-British sample of manic depressive patients and controls. *Psychiatr Genet,* 4(3), 167–175.

Kraepelin, E. (1899). *Manic-Depressive Insanity and Paranoia.* Edinburgh: E. & S. Livingstone.

Kraepelin, E (1921). *Manic-Depressive Insanity and Paranoia.* Translated by R.M. Barclay, edited by G.M. Robertson. Edinburgh: E. & S. Livingstone. Originally published as *Psychiatrie. Ein Lehrbuch fur Studierende und Ärzte. ed. 2. Klinische Psychiatrie.* II. Leipzig: Johann Ambrosius Barth, 1899.

Kringlen, E. (1967). *Heredity and Environment in the Functional Psychoses* (Vol. 1, pp. 27–47). Oslo: Universitetsforlaget.

Kunugi, H., Hattori, M., Kato, T., Tatsumi, M., Sakai, T., Sasaki, T., Hirose, T., and Nanko, S. (1997a). Serotonin transporter gene polymorphisms: Ethnic difference and possible association with bipolar affective disorder. *Mol Psychiatry,* 2(6), 457–462.

Kunugi, H., Vallada, H.P., Hoda, F., Kirov, G., Gill, M., Aitchison, K.J., Ball, D., Arranz, M.J., Murray, R.M., and Collier, D.A. (1997b). No evidence for an association of affective disorders with high- or low- activity allele of catechol-O-methyltransferase gene. *Biol Psychiatry,* 42(4), 282–285.

Kunugi, H., Ishida, S., Kato, T., Tatsumi, M., Sakai, T., Hattori, M., Hirose, T., and Nanko, S. (1999). A functional polymorphism in the promoter region of monoamine oxidase-A gene and mood disorders. *Mol Psychiatry,* 4(4), 393–395.

Kunugi, H., Kato, T., Fukuda, R., Tatsumi, M., Sakai, T., and Nanko, S. (2002). Association study of C825T polymorphism of the G-protein b3 subunit gene with schizophrenia and mood disorders. *J Neural Transm,* 109(2), 213–218.

Kunugi, H., Iijima, Y., Tatsumi, M., Yoshida, M., Hashimoto, R., Kato, T., Sakamoto, K., Fukunaga, T., Inada, T., Suzuki, T., Iwata, N., Ozaki, N., Yamada, K., and Yoshikawa, T. (2004). No association between the Val66Met polymorphism of the brain-derived neurotrophic factor gene and bipolar disorder in a Japanese population: A multicenter study. *Biol Psychiatry,* 56(5), 376–378.

Kurumaji, A., Nomoto, H., Yamada, K., Yoshikawa, T., and Toru, M. (2001). No association of two missense variations of the benzodiazepine receptor (peripheral) gene and mood disorders in a Japanese sample. *Am J Med Genet,* 105(2), 172–175.

Lachman, H.M., Kelsoe, J., Moreno, L., Katz, S., and Papolos, D.F. (1997). Lack of association of catechol-O-methyltransferase (COMT) functional polymorphism in bipolar affective disorder. *Psychiatr Genet,* 7(1), 13–17.

Lander, E., and Kruglyak, L. (1995). Genetic dissection of complex traits: Guidelines for interpreting and reporting linkage results. *Nat Genet,* 11(3), 241–247.

Lasky-Su, J.A., Faraone, S.V., Glatt, S.J., and Tsuang, M.T. (2005). Meta-analysis of the association between two polymorphisms in the serotonin transporter gene and affective disorders. Am J Med Genet B Neuropsychiatr Genet, 133(1), 110–115.

Leboyer, M., Malafosse, A., Boularand, S., Campion, D., Gheysen, F., Samolyk, D., Henriksson, B., Denise, E., des Lauriers, A., and Lepine, J.P. (1990). Tyrosine hydroxylase polymorphisms associated with manic-depressive illness. *Lancet,* 335(8699), 1219.

Leboyer, M., Bellivier, F., McKeon, P., Albus, M., Borrman, M., Perez-Diaz, F., Mynett-Johnson, L., Feingold, J., and Maier, W. (1998). Age at onset and gender resemblance in bipolar siblings. *Psychiatry Res,* 81(2), 125–131.

Lerer, B., Macciardi, F., Segman, R.H., Adolfsson, R., Blackwood, D., Blairy, S., Del Favero, J., Dikeos, D.G., Kaneva, R., Lilli, R., Massat, I., Milanova, V., Muir, W., Noethen, M., Oruc, L., Petrova, T.,

Papadimitriou, G.N., Rietschel, M., Serretti, A., Souery, D., Van Gestel, S., Van Broeckhoven, C., and Mendlewicz, J. (2001). Variability of 5-HT2C receptor cys23ser polymorphism among European populations and vulnerability to affective disorder. *Mol Psychiatry*, 6(5), 579–585.

Lesch, K.P., Bengel, D., Heils, A., Sabol, S.Z., Greenberg, B.D., Petri, S., Benjamin, J., Muller, C.R., Hamer, D.H., and Murphy, D.L. (1996). Association of anxiety-related traits with a polymorphism in the serotonin transporter gene regulatory region. *Science*, 274(5292), 1527–1531.

Leszczynska-Rodziewicz, A., Czerski, P.M., Kapelski, P., Godlewski, S., Dmitrzak-Weglarz, M., Rybakowski, J., and Hauser, J. (2002). A polymorphism of the norepinephrine transporter gene in bipolar disorder and schizophrenia: Lack of association. *Neuropsychobiology*, 45(4), 182–185.

Levinson, D.F. (2006). The genetics of depression: A review. *Biol Psychiatry*, 60, 84–92.

Li, T., Vallada, H., Curtis, D., Arranz, M., Xu, K., Cai, G., Deng, H., Liu, J., Murray, R., Liu, X., and Collier, D.A. (1997). Catechol-O-methyltransferase Val158Met polymorphism: Frequency analysis in Han Chinese subjects and allelic association of the low activity allele with bipolar affective disorder. *Pharmacogenetics*, 7(5), 349–353.

Li, L., Keverne, E.B., Aparicio, S.A., Ishino, F., Barton, S.C., and Surani, M.A. (1999a). Regulation of maternal behavior and offspring growth by paternally expressed Peg3. *Science*, 284(5412), 330–333.

Li, T., Liu, X., Sham, P.C., Aitchison, K.J., Cai, G., Arranz, M.J., Deng, H., Liu, J., Kirov, G., Murray, R.M., and Collier, D.A. (1999b). Association analysis between dopamine receptor genes and bipolar affective disorder. *Psychiatry Res*, 86(3), 193–201.

Licinio, J., and Wong, M.L. (2002). Brain-derived neurotrophic factor (BDNF) in stress and affective disorders. *Mol Psychiatry*, 7(6), 519.

Liddell, M.B., Lovestone, S., and Owen, M.J. (2001). Genetic risk of Alzheimer's disease: Advising relatives. *Br J Psychiatry*, 178(1), 7–11.

Lim, L.C., Nothen, M.M., Korner, J., Rietschel, M., Castle, D., Hunt, N., Propping, P., Murray, R., and Gill, M. (1994). No evidence of association between dopamine D4 receptor variants and bipolar affective disorder. *Am J Med Genet*, 54(3), 259–263.

Lim, L.C., Powell, J., Sham, P., Castle, D., Hunt, N., Murray, R., and Gill, M. (1995). Evidence for a genetic association between alleles of monoamine oxidase A gene and bipolar affective disorder. *Am J Med Genet*, 60(4), 325–331.

Lin, J.P., and Bale, S.J. (1997). Parental transmission and D18S37 allele sharing in bipolar affective disorder. *Genet Epidemiol*, 14(6), 665–668.

Lin, M.W., Sham, P., Hwu, H.G., Collier, D., Murray, R., and Powell, J.F. (1997). Suggestive evidence for linkage of schizophrenia to markers on chromosome 13 in Caucasian but not Oriental populations. *Hum Genet*, 99(3), 417–420.

Lin, C.N., Tsai, S.J., and Hong, C.J. (2001). Association analysis of a functional G protein beta3 subunit gene polymorphism (C825T) in mood disorders. *Neuropsychobiology*, 44(3), 118–121.

Lin, P.-I., McInnis, M.G., Potash, J.B., Willour, V.L., MacKinnon, D.F., Miao, K., DePaulo, J.R., and Zandi, P.P. (2005). Assessment of the age at onset on linkage to bipolar disorder: Evidence on chromosomes 18p and 21q. *Am J Hum Genet*, 77, 545–555.

Lin, P.I., McInnis, M.G., Potash, J.B., Willour, V., MacKinnon, D.F., DePaulo, J.R., and Zandi, P.P. (2006). Clinical correlates and familial aggregation of age at onset in bipolar disorder. *Am J Psychiatry*, 163(2), 240–246.

Lish, J.D., Gyulai, L., Resnick, S.M., Kirtland, A., Amsterdam, J.D., Whybrow, P.C., and Price, R.A. (1993). A family history study of rapid-cycling bipolar disorder. *Psychiatry Res*, 48(1), 37–46.

Liu, W., Gu, N., Feng, G., Li, S., Bai, S., Zhang, J., Shen, T., Xue, H., Breen, G., St., Clair, D., and He, L. (1999). Tentative association of the serotonin transporter with schizophrenia and unipolar depression but not with bipolar disorder in Han Chinese. *Pharmacogenetics*, 9(4), 491–495.

Liu, C., Badner, J.A., Christian, S.L., Guroff, J.J., Detera-Wadleigh, S.D., and Gershon, E.S. (2001a). Fine mapping supports previous linkage evidence for a bipolar disorder susceptibility locus on 13q32. *Am J Med Genet*, 105(4), 375–380.

Liu, J., Juo, S.H., Terwilliger, J.D., Grunn, A., Tong, X., Brito, M., Loth, J.E., Kanyas, K., Lerer, B., Endicott, J., Penchaszadeh, G., Gilliam, T.C., and Baron, M. (2001b). A follow-up linkage study supports evidence for a bipolar affective disorder locus on chromosome 21q22. *Am J Med Genet*, 105(2), 189–194.

Liu, J., Juo, S.H., Dewan, A., Grunn, A., Tong, X., Brito, M., Park, N., Loth, J.E., Kanyas, K., Lerer, B., Endicott, J., Penchaszadeh, G., Knowles, J.A., Ott, J., Gilliam, T.C., and Baron, M. (2003). Evidence for a putative bipolar disorder locus on 2p13-16 and other potential loci on 4q31, 7q34, 8q13, 9q31, 10q21-24, 13q32, 14q21 and 17q11-12. *Mol Psychiatry*, 8(3), 333–342.

Lucotte, G., Landoulsi, A., Berriche, S., David, F., and Babron, M.C. (1992). Manic depressive illness is linked to factor IX in a French pedigree [see comments]. *Ann Genet*, 35(2), 93–95.

Luxenburger, H. (1928). Vorlaufiger Bericht uber psychiatrische Serinumtersuchungen an Zwillinger. *Z Ges Neurol Psychiatrie*, 116, 297–326.

Luxenburger, H. (1930). Psychiatrisch-neurologisch Zwillingspathologie. *Z Ges Neurol Psychiatrie*, 56, 145–180.

Luxenburger, H. (1942). *Handbuch der Erbkrankheiten*. Leipzig: Georg Thieme Verlag.

Lyons, M.J., Eisen, S.A., Goldberg, J., True, W., Lin, N., Meyer, J.M., Toomey, R., Faraone, S.V., Merla-Ramos, M., and Tsuang, M.T. (1998). A registry-based twin study of depression in men. *Arch Gen Psychiatry*, 55(5), 468–472.

Lytton, H., Martin, N.G., and Eaves, L. (1977). Environmental and genetic causes of variation in ethological aspects of behavior in two-year-old boys. *Soc Biol*, 24(3), 200–211.

Macgregor, S., Visscher, P.M., Knott, S.A., Thomson, P., Porteous, D.J., Millar, J.K., Devon, R.S., Blackwood, D., and Muir, W.J. (2004). A genome scan and follow-up study identify a bipolar disorder susceptibility locus on chromosome 1q42. *Mol Psychiatry*, 9(12), 1083–1090.

MacKenzie, A., and Quinn, J. (1999). A serotonin transporter gene intron 2 polymorphic region, correlated with affective disorders, has allele-dependent differential enhancer-like properties in the mouse embryo. *Proc Natl Acad Sci USA*, 96(26), 15251–15255.

MacKinnon, D.F., McMahon, F.J., Simpson, S.G., McInnis, M.G., and DePaulo, J.R. (1997). Panic disorder with familial bipolar disorder. *Biol Psychiatry*, 42(2), 90–95.

MacKinnon, D.F., Zandi, P.P., Cooper, J., Potash, J.B., Simpson, S.G., Gershon, E., Nurnberger, J., Reich, T., and DePaulo, J.R.

(2002). Comorbid bipolar disorder and panic disorder in families with a high prevalence of bipolar disorder. *Am J Psychiatry*, 159(1), 30–35.

MacKinnon, D.F., Zandi, P.P., Gershon, E., Nurnberger, J.I. Jr., Reich, T., and DePaulo, J.R. (2003a). Rapid switching of mood in families with multiple cases of bipolar disorder. *Arch Gen Psychiatry*, 60(9), 921–928.

MacKinnon, D.F., Zandi, P.P., Gershon, E.S., Nurnberger, J.I. Jr., and DePaulo, J.R. Jr. (2003b). Association of rapid mood switching with panic disorder and familial panic risk in familial bipolar disorder. *Am J Psychiatry*, 160(9), 1696–1698.

MacQueen, G.M., Ramakrishnan, K., Croll, S.D., Siuciak, J.A., Yu, G., Young, L.T., and Fahnestock, M. (2001). Performance of heterozygous brain-derived neurotrophic factor knockout mice on behavioral analogues of anxiety, nociception, and depression. *Behav Neurosci*, 115(5), 1145–1153.

Mahieu, B., Souery, D., Lipp, O., Mendelbaum, K., Verheyen, G., De Maertelaer, V., Van Broeckhoven, C., and Mendlewicz, J. (1997). No association between bipolar affective disorder and a serotonin receptor (5-HT2A) polymorphism. *Psychiatry Res*, 70(2), 65–69.

Maier, W., Lichtermann, D., Minges, J., Hallmayer, J., Heun, R., Benkert, O., and Levinson, D.F. (1993). Continuity and discontinuity of affective disorders and schizophrenia. Results of a controlled family study. *Arch Gen Psychiatry*, 50(11), 871–883.

Malafosse, A., Leboyer, M., d'Amato, T., Amadeo, S., Abbar, M., Campion, D., Canseil, O., Castelnau, D., Gheysen, F., Granger, B., Henrikson, B., Poirier, M.F., Sabate, O., Samolyk, D., Feingold, J., and Mallet, J. (1997). Manic-depressive illness and tyrosine hydroxylase gene: linkage heterogeneity and association. *Neurobiol Dis*, 4(5), 337–349.

Manki, H., Kanba, S., Muramatsu, T., Higuchi, S., Suzuki, E., Matsushita, S., Ono, Y., Chiba, H., Shintani, F., Nakamura, M., Yagi, G., and Asai, M. (1996). Dopamine D2, D3 and D4 receptor and transporter gene polymorphisms and mood disorders. *J Affect Disord*, 40(1–2), 7–13.

Massat, I., Souery, D., Lipp, O., Blairy, S., Papadimitriou, G., Dikeos, D., Ackenheil, M., Fuchshuber, S., Hilger, C., Kaneva, R., Milanova, V., Verheyen, G., Raeymaekers, P., Staner, L., Oruc, L., Jakovljevic, M., Serretti, A., Macciardi, F., Van Broeckhoven, C., and Mendlewicz, J. (2000). A European multicenter association study of HTR2A receptor polymorphism in bipolar affective disorder. *Am J Med Genet*, 96(2), 136–140.

Massat, I., Souery, D., Del-Favero, J., Oruc, L., Noethen, M.M., Blackwood, D., Thomson, M., Muir, W., Papadimitriou, G.N., Dikeos, D.G., Kaneva, R., Serretti, A., Lilli, R., Smeraldi, E., Jakovljevic, M., Folnegovic, V., Rietschel, M., Milanova, V., Valente, F., Van Broeckhoven, C., and Mendlewicz, J. (2002a). Excess of allele1 for alpha3 subunit GABA receptor gene (GABRA3) in bipolar patients: A multicentric association study. *Mol Psychiatry*, 7(2), 201–207.

Massat, I., Souery, D., Del-Favero, J., Van Gestel, S., Serretti, A., Macciardi, F., Smeraldi, E., Kaneva, R., Adolfsson, R., Nylander, P.O., Blackwood, D., Muir, W., Papadimitriou, G.N., Dikeos, D., Oruc, L., Segman, R.H., Ivezic, S., Aschauer, H., Ackenheil, M., Fuchshuber, S., Dam, H., Jakovljevic, M., Peltonen, L., Hilger, C., Hentges, F., Staner, L., Milanova, V., Jazin, E., Lerer, B., Van Broeckhoven, C., and Mendlewicz, J. (2002b). Positive association of dopamine D2 receptor polymorphism with bipolar affective disorder in a European Multicenter Association Study of affective disorders. *Am J Med Genet*, 114(2), 177–185.

Maziade, M., Roy, M.A., Rouillard, E., Bissonnette, L., Fournier, J.P., Roy, A., Garneau, Y., Montgrain, N., Potvin, A., Cliché, D., Dion, C., Wallot, H., Fournier, A., Nicole, L., Lavallee, J.C., and Merette, C. (2001). A search for specific and common susceptibility loci for schizophrenia and bipolar disorder: A linkage study in 13 target chromosomes. *Mol Psychiatry*, 6(6), 684–693.

Maziade, M., Roy, M.A., Chagnon, Y.C., Cliché, D., Fournier, J.P., Montgrain, N., Dion, C., Lavallee, J.C., Garneau, Y., Gingras, N., Nicole, L., Pires, A., Ponton, A.M., Potvin, A., Wallot, H., and Merette, C. (2005). Shared and specific susceptibility loci for schizophrenia and bipolar disorder: A dense genome scan in Eastern Quebec families. *Mol Psychiatry*, 10(5), 486–499.

McGuffin, P., Katz, R., and Bebbington, P. (1987). Hazard, heredity and depression. A family study. *J Psychiatr Res*, 21(4), 365–375.

McGuffin, P., Katz, R., Watkins, S., and Rutherford, J. (1996). A hospital-based twin register of the heritability of DSM-IV unipolar depression. Arch Gen Psychiatry, 53(2), 129–136.

McHugh, P.R., and Slavney, P.R. (1998). *The Perspectives of Psychiatry*, Second Edition. Baltimore: Johns Hopkins University Press.

McInnes, L.A., Escamilla, M.A., Service, S.K., Reus, V.I., Leon, P., Silva, S., Rojas, E., Spesny, M., Baharloo, S., Blankenship, K., Peterson, A., Tyler, D., Shimayoshi, N., Tobey, C., Batki, S., Vinogradov, S., Meza, L., Gallegos, A., Fournier, E., Smith, L.B., Barondes, S.H., Sandkuijl, L.A., and Freimer, N.B. (1996). A complete genome screen for genes predisposing to severe bipolar disorder in two Costa Rican pedigrees. *Proc Natl Acad Sci USA*, 93(23), 13060–13065.

McInnes, L.A., Service, S.K., Reus, V.I., Barnes, G., Charlat, O., Jawahar, S., Lewitzky, S., Yang, Q., Duong, Q., Spesny, M., Araya, C., Araya, X., Gallegos, A., Meza, L., Molina, J., Ramirez, R., Mendez, R., Silva, S., Fournier, E., Batki, S.L., Mathews, C.A., Neylan, T., Glatt, C.E., Escamilla, M.A., Luo, D., Gajiwala, P., Song, T., Crook, S., Nguyen, J.B., Roche, E., Meyer, J.M., Leon, P., Sandkuijl, L.A., Freimer, N.B., and Chen, H. (2001). Fine-scale mapping of a locus for severe bipolar mood disorder on chromosome 18p11.3 in the Costa Rican population. *Proc Natl Acad Sci USA*, 98(20), 11485–11490.

McInnis, M.G., McMahon, F.J., Chase, G.A., Simpson, S.G., Ross, C.A., and DePaulo, J.R. Jr. (1993). Anticipation in bipolar affective disorder. *Am J Hum Genet*, 53(2), 385–390.

McInnis, M.G., Breschel, T.S., Margolis, R.L., Chellis, J., MacKinnon, D.F., McMahon, F.J., Simpson, S.G., Lan, T.H., Chen, H., Ross, C.A., and DePaulo, J.R. (1999). Family-based association analysis of the hSKCa3 potassium channel gene in bipolar disorder. *Mol Psychiatry*, 4(3), 217–219.

McInnis, M.G., Swift-Scanlanl, T., Mahoney, A.T., Vincent, J., Verheyen, G., Lan, T.H., Oruc, L., Riess, O., Van Broeckhoven, C., Chen, H., Kennedy, J.L., MacKinnon, D.F., Margolis, R.L., Simpson, S.G., McMahon, F.J., Gershon, E., Nurnberger, J., Reich, T., DePaulo, J.R., and Ross, C.A. (2000). Allelic distribution of CTG18.1 in Caucasian populations: Association studies in bipolar disorder, schizophrenia, and ataxia. *Mol Psychiatry*, 5(4), 439–442.

McInnis, M.G., Lan, T.H., Willour, V.L., McMahon, F.J., Simpson, S.G., Addington, A.M., MacKinnon, D.F., Potash, J.B., Mahoney, A.T., Chellis, J., Huo, Y., Swift-Scanlan, T., Chen, H., Koskela, R., Stine, O.C., Jamison, K.R., Holmans, P., Folstein, S.E., Ranade, K., Friddle, C., Botstein, D., Marr, T., Beaty, T.H.,

Zandi, P., and DePaulo, J.R. (2003). Genome-wide scan of bipolar disorder in 65 pedigrees: Supportive evidence for linkage at 8q24, 18q22, 4q32, 2p12, and 13q12. *Mol Psychiatry*, 8(3), 288–298.

McKnew, D.H., Cytryn, L., Buchsbaum, M.S., Hamovit, J., Lamour, M., Rapoport, J.L., and Gershon, E.S. (1981). Lithium in children of lithium-responding parents. *Psychiatry Res*, 4(2), 171–180.

McMahon, F.J., Stine, O.C., Meyers, D.A., Simpson, S.G., and DePaulo, J.R. (1995). Patterns of maternal transmission in bipolar affective disorder [see comments]. *Am J Hum Genet*, 56(6), 1277–1286.

McMahon, F.J., Hopkins, P.J., Xu, J., McInnis, M.G., Shaw, S., Cardon, L., Simpson, S.G., MacKinnon, D.F., Stine, O.C., Sherrington, R., Meyers, D.A., and DePaulo, J.R. (1997). Linkage of bipolar affective disorder to chromosome 18 markers in a new pedigree series. *Am J Hum Genet*, 61(6), 1397–1404.

McMahon, F.J., Chen, Y.S., Patel, S., Kokoszka, J., Brown, M.D., Torroni, A., DePaulo, J.R., and Wallace, D.C. (2000). Mitochondrial DNA sequence diversity in bipolar affective disorder. *Am J Psychiatry*, 157(7), 1058–1064.

McMahon, F.J., Simpson, S.G., McInnis, M.G., Badner, J.A., MacKinnon, D.F., and DePaulo, J.R. (2001). Linkage of bipolar disorder to chromosome 18q and the validity of bipolar II disorder. *Arch Gen Psychiatry*, 58(11), 1025–1031.

McQueen, M.B., Devlin, B., Faraone, S.V., Nimgaonkar, V.L., Sklar, P., Smoller, J.W., Abou, J.R., Albus, M., Bacanu, S.A., Baron, M., Barrett, T.B., Berrettini, W., Blacker, D., Byerley, W., Cichon, S., Coryell, W., Craddock, N., Daly, M.J., DePaulo, J.R., Edenberg, H.J., Foroud, T., Gill, M., Gilliam, T.C., Hamshere, M., Jones, I., Jones, L., Juo, S.H., Kelsoe, J.R., Lambert, D., Lange, C., Lerer, B., Liu, J., Maier, W., Mackinnon, J.D., McInnis, M.G., McMahon, F.J., Murphy, D.L., Nothen, M.M., Nurnberger, J.I., Pato, C.N., Pato, M.T., Potash, J.B., Propping, P., Pulver, A.E., Rice, J.P., Rietschel, M., Scheftner, W., Schumacher, J., Segurado, R., Van Steen, K., Xie, W., Zandi, P.P., and Laird, N.M. (2005). Combined analysis from eleven linkage studies of bipolar disorder provides strong evidence of susceptibility loci on chromosomes 6q and 8q. *Am J Hum Genet*, 77(4), 582–595.

McQuillin, A., Lawrence, J., Curtis, D., Kalsi, G., Smyth, C., Hannesdottir, S., and Gurling, H. (1999). Adjacent genetic markers on chromosome 11p15.5 at or near the tyrosine hydroxylase locus that show population linkage disequilibrium with each other do not show allelic association with bipolar affective disorder. *Psychol Med*, 29(6), 1449–1454.

Meira-Lima, I.V., and Vallada, H. (2003). Genes related to phospholipid metabolism as risk factors related to bipolar affective disorder. *Rev Bras Psiquiatr*, 25(1), 51–55.

Meira-Lima, I.V., Pereira, A.C., Mota, G.F., Krieger, J.E., and Vallada, H. (2000). Angiotensinogen and angiotensin converting enzyme gene polymorphisms and the risk of bipolar affective disorder in humans. *Neurosci Lett*, 293(2), 103–106.

Meira-Lima, I.V., Zhao, J., Sham, P., Pereira, A.C., Krieger, J.E., and Vallada, H. (2001). Association and linkage studies between bipolar affective disorder and the polymorphic CAG/CTG repeat loci ERDA1, SEF2-1B, MAB21L and KCNN3. *Mol Psychiatry*, 6(5), 565–569.

Meira-Lima, I.V., Pereira, A.C., Mota, G.F., Floriano, M., Araujo, F., Mansur, A.J., Krieger, J.E., and Vallada, H. (2003a). Analysis of a polymorphism in the promoter region of the tumor necrosis factor alpha gene in schizophrenia and bipolar disorder: Further support for an association with schizophrenia. *Mol Psychiatry*, 8(8), 718–720.

Meira-Lima, I., Jardim, D., Junqueira, R., Ikenaga, E., Vallada, H. (2003b). Allelic association study between phospholipase A2 genes and bipolar affective disorder. *Bipolar Disord*, 5(4), 295–299.

Mellon, C.D. (1996). Hereditary Madness: The Evolution of Psychiatric Genetic Thought. Placitas, NM: Genetics Heritage Press.

Meloni, R., Leboyer, M., Bellivier, F., Barbe, B., Samolyk, D., Allilaire, J.F., and Mallet, J. (1995). Association of manic-depressive illness with tyrosine hydroxylase microsatellite marker. *Lancet*, 345(8954), 932.

Mendes de Oliveira J.R., Otto, P.A., Vallada, H., Lauriano, V., Elkis, H., Lafer, B., Vasquez, L., Gentil, V., Passos-Bueno, M.R., and Zatz, M. (1998). Analysis of a novel functional polymorphism within the promoter region of the serotonin transporter gene (5-HTT) in Brazilian patients affected by bipolar disorder and schizophrenia. *Am J Med Genet*, 81(3), 225–227.

Mendlewicz, J., and Rainer, J.D. (1974). Morbidity risk and genetic transmission in manic-depressive illness. *Am J Hum Genet*, 26(6), 692–701.

Mendlewicz, J., and Rainer, J.D. (1977). Adoption study supporting genetic transmission in manic–depressive illness. *Nature*, 268(5618), 327–329.

Mendlewicz, J., Fleiss, J.L., and Fieve, R.R. (1972). Evidence for X-linkage in the transmission of manic-depressive illness. *JAMA*, 222(13), 1624–1627.

Mendlewicz, J., Linkowski, P., Guroff, J.J., and Van Praag, H.M. (1979). Color blindness linkage to bipolar manic-depressive illness. New evidence. *Arch Gen Psychiatry*, 36(13), 1442–1447.

Mendlewicz, J., Linkowski, P., and Wilmotte, J. (1980). Linkage between glucose-6-phosphate dehydrogenase deficiency and manic-depressive psychosis. *Br J Psychiatry*, 137, 337–342.

Mendlewicz, J., Simon, P., Sevy, S., Charon, F., Brocas, H., Legros, S., and Vassart, G. (1987). Polymorphic DNA marker on X chromosome and manic depression. *Lancet*, 1(8544), 1230–1232.

Mendlewicz, J., Massat, I., Souery, D., Del-Favero, J., Oruc, L., Nothen, M.M., Blackwood, D., Muir, W., Battersby, S., Lerer, B., Segman, R.H., Kaneva, R., Serretti, A., Lilli, R., Lorenzi, C., Jakovljevic, M., Ivezic, S., Rietschel, M., Milanova, V., Van Broeckhoven, C. (2004). Serotonin transporter 5HTTLPR polymorphism and affective disorders: No evidence of association in a large european multicenter study. *Eur J Hum Genet*, 12(5), 377–382.

Merette, C., Roy-Gagnon, M.H., Ghazzali, N., Savard, F., Boutin, P., Roy, M.A., and Maziade, M. (2000). Anticipation in schizophrenia and bipolar disorder controlling for an information bias. *Am J Med Genet*, 96(1), 61–68.

Merikangas, K.R., Leckman, J.F., Prusoff, B.A., Pauls, D.L., and Weissman, M.M. (1985). Familial transmission of depression and alcoholism. *Arch Gen Psychiatry*, 42(4), 367–372.

Middle, F., Jones, I., McCandless, F., Barrett, T., Khanim, F., Owen, M.J., Lendon, C., and Craddock, N. (2000). Bipolar disorder and variation at a common polymorphism (A1832G) within exon 8 of the Wolfram gene. *Am J Med Genet*, 96(2), 154–157.

Middleton, F.A., Pato, M.T., Gentile, K.L., Morley, C.P., Zhao, X., Eisener, A.F., Brown, A., Petryshen, T.L., Kirby, A.N., Medeiros, H., Carvalho, C., Macedo, A., Dourado, A., Coelho, I., Valente, J., Soares, M.J., Ferreira, C.P., Lei, M., Azevedo, M.H., Kennedy, J.L., Daly, M.J., Sklar, P., and Pato, C.N.

(2004). Genomewide linkage analysis of bipolar disorder by use of a high-density single-nucleotide-polymorphism (SNP) genotyping assay: A comparison with microsatellite marker assays and finding of significant linkage to chromosome 6q22. *Am J Hum Genet*, 74(5), 886–897.

Miki, Y., Swensen, J., Shattuck-Eidens, D., Futreal, P.A., Harshman, K., Tavtigian, S., Liu, Q., Cochran, C., Bennett, L.M., and Ding, W. (1994). A strong candidate for the breast and ovarian cancer susceptibility gene BRCA1. *Science*, 266(5182), 66–71.

Mimmack, M.L., Ryan, M., Baba, H., Navarro-Ruiz, J., Iritani, S., Faull, R.L., McKenna, P.J., Jones, P.B., Arai, H., Starkey, M., Emson, P.C., and Bahn, S. (2002). Gene expression analysis in schizophrenia: Reproducible up-regulation of several members of the apolipoprotein L family located in a high-susceptibility locus for schizophrenia on chromosome 22. *Proc Natl Acad Sci USA*, 99(7), 4680–4685.

Montkowski, A., Barden, N., Wotjak, C., Stec, I., Ganster, J., Meaney, M., Engelmann, M., Reul, J.M., Landgraf, R., and Holsboer, F. (1995). Long-term antidepressant treatment reduces behavioural deficits in transgenic mice with impaired glucocorticoid receptor function. *J Neuroendocrinol*, 7(11), 841–845.

Morison, I.M., and Reeve, A.E. (1998). A catalogue of imprinted genes and parent-of-origin effects in humans and animals. *Hum Mol Genet*, 7(10), 1599–1609.

Morissette, J., Villeneuve, A., Bordeleau, L., Rochette, D., Laberge, C., Gagne, B., Laprise, C., Bouchard, G., Plante, M., Gobeil, L., Shink, E., Weissenbach, J., and Barden, N. (1999). Genome-wide search for linkage of bipolar affective disorders in a very large pedigree derived from a homogeneous population in Quebec points to a locus of major effect on chromosome 12q23-q24. Am J Med Genet, 88(5), 567–587.

Muglia, P., Petronis, A., Mundo, E., Lander, S., Cate, T., and Kennedy, J.L. (2002). Dopamine D4 receptor and tyrosine hydroxylase genes in bipolar disorder: Evidence for a role of DRD4. *Mol Psychiatry*, 7(8), 860–866.

Muir, W.J., Thomson, M.L., McKeon, P., Mynett-Johnson, L., Whitton, C., Evans, K.L., Porteous, D.J., and Blackwood, D.H. (2001). Markers close to the dopamine D5 receptor gene (DRD5) show significant association with schizophrenia but not bipolar disorder. *Am J Med Genet*, 105(2), 152–158.

Mundo, E., Walker, M., Tims, H., Macciardi, F., and Kennedy, J.L. (2000). Lack of linkage disequilibrium between serotonin transporter protein gene (SLC6A4) and bipolar disorder. *Am J Med Genet*, 96(3), 379–383.

Mundo, E., Walker, M., Cate, T., Macciardi, F., and Kennedy, J.L. (2001a). The role of serotonin transporter protein gene in antidepressant-induced mania in bipolar disorder: Preliminary findings. *Arch Gen Psychiatry*, 58(6), 539–544.

Mundo, E., Zai, G., Lee, L., Parikh, S.V., and Kennedy, J.L. (2001b). The 5HT1Dbeta receptor gene in bipolar disorder: A family-based association study. *Neuropsychopharmacology*, 25(4), 608–613.

Muramatsu, T., Matsushita, S., Kanba, S., Higuchi, S., Manki, H., Suzuki, E., and Asai, M. (1997). Monoamine oxidase genes polymorphisms and mood disorder. *Am J Med Genet*, 74(5), 494–496.

Murphy, V.E., Mynett-Johnson, L.A., Claffey, E., Shields, D.C., and McKeon, P. (2001). No association between 5HT-2A and bipolar disorder irrespective of genomic imprinting. *Am J Med Genet*, 105(5), 422–425.

Murphy, G.M. Jr., Hollander, S.B., Rodrigues, H.E., Kremer, C., and Schatzberg, A.F. (2004). Effects of the serotonin transporter gene promoter polymorphism on mirtazapine and paroxetine efficacy and adverse events in geriatric major depression. *Arch Gen Psychiatry*, 61(11), 1163–1169.

Mynett-Johnson, L.A., Murphy, V.E., Claffey, E., Shields, D.C., and McKeon, P. (1998). Preliminary evidence of an association between bipolar disorder in females and the catechol-O-methyltransferase gene. *Psychiatr Genet*, 8(4), 221–225.

Mynett-Johnson, L., Kealey, C., Claffey, E., Curtis, D., Bouchier-Hayes, L., Powell, C., and McKeon, P. (2000). Multimarker haplotypes within the serotonin transporter gene suggest evidence of an association with bipolar disorder. *Am J Med Genet*, 96(6), 845–849.

Nakamura, M., Ueno, S., Sano, A., and Tanabe, H. (2000). The human serotonin transporter gene linked polymorphism (5-HTTLPR) shows ten novel allelic variants. *Mol Psychiatry*, 5(1), 32–38.

Nakata, K., Ujike, H., Sakai, A., Uchida, N., Nomura, A., Imamura, T., Katsu, T., Tanaka, Y., Hamamura, T., and Kuroda, S. (2003). Association study of the brain-derived neurotrophic factor (BDNF) gene with bipolar disorder. *Neurosci Lett*, 337(1), 17–20.

Nemanov, L., Ebstein, R.P., Belmaker, R.H., Osher, Y., and Agam, G. (1999). Effect of bipolar disorder on lymphocyte inositol monophosphatase mRNA levels. *Int J Neuropsychopharmcol*, 2(1), 25–29.

Neves-Pereira, M., Mundo, E., Muglia, P., King, N., Macciardi, F., and Kennedy, J.L. (2002). The brain-derived neurotrophic factor gene confers susceptibility to bipolar disorder: Evidence from a family-based association study. *Am J Hum Genet*, 71(3), 651–655.

Ni, X., Trakalo, J.M., Mundo, E., Lee, L., Parikh, S., and Kennedy, J.L. (2002a). Family-based association study of the serotonin-2A receptor gene (5-HT2A) and bipolar disorder. *Neuromol Med*, 2(3), 251–259.

Ni, X., Trakalo, J.M., Mundo, E., Macciardi, F.M., Parikh, S., Lee, L., and Kennedy, J.L. (2002b). Linkage disequilibrium between dopamine D1 receptor gene (DRD1) and bipolar disorder. *Biol Psychiatry*, 52(12), 1144–1150.

Niculescu, A.B., III, Segal, D.S., Kuczenski, R., Barrett, T., Hauger, R.L., and Kelsoe, J.R. (2000). Identifying a series of candidate genes for mania and psychosis: A convergent functional genomics approach. *Physiol Genomics*, 4(1), 83–91.

Noga, J.T., Vladar, K., and Torrey, E.F. (2001). A volumetric magnetic resonance imaging study of monozygotic twins discordant for bipolar disorder. *Psychiatry Res*, 106(1), 25–34.

Nothen, M., Korner, J., Lanczik, M., Fritze, J., and Propping, P. (1990). Tyrosine hydroxylase polymorphisms and manic-depressive illness. *Lancet*, 336(8714), 575.

Nothen, M.M., Erdmann, J., Korner, J., Lanczik, M., Fritze, J., Fimmers, R., Grandy, D.K., O'Dowd, B., and Propping, P. (1992). Lack of association between dopamine D1 and D2 receptor genes and bipolar affective disorder. *Am J Psychiatry*, 149(2), 199–201.

Nothen, M.M., Eggermann, K., Albus, M., Borrmann, M., Rietschel, M., Korner, J., Maier, W., Minges, J., Lichtermann, D., and Franzek, E. (1995). Association analysis of the monoamine oxidase A gene in bipolar affective disorder by using family-based internal controls. *Am J Hum Genet*, 57(4), 975–978.

Nothen, M.M., Cichon, S., Rohleder, H., Hemmer, S., Franzek, E., Fritze, J., Albus, M., Borrmann-Hassenbach, M., Kreiner,

R., Weigelt, B., Minges, J., Lichtermann, D., Maier, W., Craddock, N., Fimmers, R., Holler, T., Baur, M.P., Rietschel, M., and Propping, P. (1999). Evaluation of linkage of bipolar affective disorder to chromosome 18 in a sample of 57 German families. *Mol Psychiatry*, 4(1), 76–84.

Nurnberger, J. Jr., Guroff, J.J., Hamovit, J., Berrettini, W., and Gershon, E. (1988). A family study of rapid-cycling bipolar illness. *J Affect Disord*, 15(1), 87–91.

Nyegaard, M., Borglum, A.D., Bruun, T.G., Collier, D.A., Russ, C., Mors, O., Ewald, H., and Kruse, T.A. (2002). Novel polymorphisms in the somatostatin receptor 5 (SSTR5) gene associated with bipolar affective disorder. *Mol Psychiatry*, 7(7), 745–754.

Nylander, P.O., Engstrom, C., Chotai, J., Wahlstrom, J., and Adolfsson, R. (1994). Anticipation in Swedish families with bipolar affective disorder. *J Med Genet*, 31(9), 686–689.

Ogura, Y., Bonen, D.K., Inohara, N., Nicolae, D.L., Chen, F.F., Ramos, R., Britton, H., Moran, T., Karaliuskas, R., Duerr, R.H., Achkar, J.P., Brant, S.R., Bayless, T.M., Kirschner, B.S., Hanauer, S.B., Nunez, G., and Cho, J.H. (2001). A frameshift mutation in NOD2 associated with susceptibility to Crohn's disease. *Nature*, 411(6837), 603–606.

Ohara, K., Suzuki, Y., Ushimi, Y., Yoshida, K., and Ohara, K. (1998a). Anticipation and imprinting in Japanese familial mood disorders. *Psychiatry Res*, 79(3), 191–198.

Ohara, K., Nagai, M., and Suzuki, Y. (1998b). Low activity allele of catechol-O-methyltransferase gene and Japanese unipolar depression. *Neuroreport*, 9(7), 1305–1308.

Ohtsuki, T., Ishiguro, H., Detera-Wadleigh, S.D., Toyota, T., Shimizu, H., Yamada, K., Yoshitsugu, K., Hattori, E., Yoshikawa, T., and Arinami, T. (2002). Association between serotonin 4 receptor gene polymorphisms and bipolar disorder in Japanese case-control samples and the NIMH Genetics Initiative Bipolar Pedigrees. *Mol Psychiatry*, 7(9), 954–961.

Omahony, E., Corvin, A., O'Connell, R., Comerford, C., Larsen, B., Jones, R., McCandless, F., Kirov, G., Cardno, A.G., Craddock, N., and Gill, M. (2002). Sibling pairs with affective disorders: Resemblance of demographic and clinical features. *Psychol Med*, 32(1), 55–61.

Ophoff, R.A., Escamilla, M.A., Service, S.K., Spesny, M., Meshi, D.B., Poon, W., Molina, J., Fournier, E., Gallegos, A., Mathews, C., Neylan, T., Batki, S.L., Roche, E., Ramirez, M., Silva, S., De Mille, M.C., Dong, P., Leon, P.E., Reus, V.I., Sandkuijl, L.A., and Freimer, N.B. (2002). Genomewide linkage disequilibrium mapping of severe bipolar disorder in a population isolate. *Am J Hum Genet*, 71(3), 565–574.

Oruc, L., Furac, I., Croux, C., Jakovljevic, M., Kracun, I., Folnegovic, V., and Van Broeckhoven, C. (1996). Association study between bipolar disorder and candidate genes involved in dopamine–serotonin metabolism and GABAergic neurotransmission: A preliminary report. *Psychiatr Genet*, 6(4), 213–217.

Oruc, L., Verheyen, G.R., Furac, I., Jakovljevic, M., Ivezic, S., Raeymaekers, P., and Van Broeckhoven, C. (1997a). Analysis of the tyrosine hydroxylase and dopamine D4 receptor genes in a Croatian sample of bipolar I and unipolar patients. *Am J Med Genet*, 74(2), 176–178.

Oruc, L., Verheyen, G.R., Furac, I., Jakovljevic, M., Ivezic, S., Raeymaekers, P., and Van Broeckhoven, C. (1997b). Association analysis of the 5-HT2C receptor and 5-HT transporter genes in bipolar disorder. *Am J Med Genet*, 74(5), 504–506.

Ospina-Duque, J., Duque, C., Carvajal-Carmona, L., Ortiz-Barrientos, D., Soto, I., Pineda, N., Cuartas, M., Calle, J., Lopez, C., Ochoa, L., Garcia, J., Gomez, J., Agudelo, A., Lozano, M., Montoya, G., Ospina, A., Lopez, M., Gallo, A., Miranda, A., Serna, L., Montoya, P., Palacio, C., Bedoya, G., McCarthy, M., Reus, V., Freimer, N., and Ruiz-Linares, A. (2000). An association study of bipolar mood disorder (type I) with the 5-HTTLPR serotonin transporter polymorphism in a human population isolate from Colombia. *Neurosci Lett*, 292(3), 199–202.

Oswald, P., Del-Favero, J., Massat, I., Souery, D., Claes, S., Van Broeckhoven, C., and Mendlewicz, J. (2004). Non-replication of the brain-derived neurotrophic factor (BDNF) association in bipolar affective disorder: A Belgian patient–control study. *Am J Med Genet B Neuropsychiatr Genet*, 129(1), 34–35.

Ozeki, Y., Tomoda, T., Kleiderlein, J., Kamiya, A., Bord, L., Fujii, K., Okawa, M., Yamada, N., Hatten, M.E., Snyder, S.H., Ross, C.A., and Sawa, A. (2003). Disrupted-in-Schizophrenia-1 (DISC-1): Mutant truncation prevents binding to NudE-like (NUDEL) and inhibits neurite outgrowth. *Proc Natl Acad Sci USA*, 100(1), 289–294.

Pae, C.U., Yu, H.S., Kim, T.S., Lee, C.U., Lee, S.J., Jun, T.Y., Lee, C., Serretti, A., and Paik, I.H. (2004). Monocyte chemoattractant protein-1 (MCP1) promoter-2518 polymorphism may confer a susceptibility to major depressive disorder in the Korean population. *Psychiatry Res*, 127(3), 279–281.

Papadimitriou, G.N., Dikeos, D.G., Karadima, G., Avramopoulos, D., Daskalopoulou, E.G., Vassilopoulos, D., and Stefanis, C.N. (1998). Association between the GABA(A) receptor alpha5 subunit gene locus (GABRA5) and bipolar affective disorder. *Am J Med Genet*, 81(1), 73–80.

Papadimitriou, G.N., Dikeos, D.G., Karadima, G., Avramopoulos, D., Daskalopoulou, E.G., and Stefanis, C.N. (2001). GABA-A receptor beta3 and alpha5 subunit gene cluster on chromosome 15q11-q13 and bipolar disorder: A genetic association study. *Am J Med Genet*, 105(4), 317–320.

Papolos, D.F., Veit, S., Faedda, G.L., Saito, T., and Lachman, H.M. (1998). Ultra-ultra rapid cycling bipolar disorder is associated with the low activity catecholamine-O-methyltransferase allele. *Mol Psychiatry*, 3(4), 346–349.

Pare, C.M., and Mack, J.W. (1971). Differentiation of two genetically specific types of depression by the response to antidepressant drugs. *J Med Genet*, 8(3), 306–309.

Pare, C.M., Rees, B.L., and Sainsbury, M.J. (1962). Differentiation of two genetically specific types of depression by the response to anti-depressants. Lancet, 2, 1340–1343.

Park, N., Juo, S.H., Cheng, R., Liu, J., Loth, J.E., Lilliston, B., Nee, J., Grunn, A., Kanyas, K., Lerer, B., Endicott, J., Gilliam, T.C., and Baron, M. (2004). Linkage analysis of psychosis in bipolar pedigrees suggests novel putative loci for bipolar disorder and shared susceptibility with schizophrenia. *Mol Psychiatry*, 9(12), 1091–1099.

Parsian, A., and Todd, R.D. (1997). Genetic association between monoamine oxidase and manic-depressive illness: Comparison of relative risk and haplotype relative risk data. *Am J Med Genet*, 74(5), 475–479.

Parsian, A., Chakraverty, S., and Todd, R.D. (1995). Possible association between the dopamine D3 receptor gene and bipolar affective disorder. *Am J Med Genet*, 60(3), 234–237.

Pauls, D.L., Morton, L.A., and Egeland, J.A. (1992). Risks of affective illness among first-degree relatives of bipolar I old-order Amish probands. *Arch Gen Psychiatry*, 49(9), 703–708.

Pauls, D.L., Bailey, J.N., Carter, A.S., Allen, C.R., and Egeland, J.A. (1995). Complex segregation analyses of old order Amish families ascertained through bipolar I individuals. *Am J Med Genet*, 60(4), 290–297.

Pauls, J., Bandelow, B., Ruther, E., and Kornhuber, J. (2000). Polymorphism of the gene of angiotensin converting enzyme: Lack of association with mood disorder. *J Neural Transm*, 107(11), 1361–1366.

Pekkarinen, P., Terwilliger, J., Bredbacka, P.E., Lonnqvist, J., and Peltonen, L. (1995). Evidence of a predisposing locus to bipolar disorder on Xq24-q27.1 in an extended Finnish pedigree. *Genome Res*, 5(2), 105–115.

Perez de Castro, I., Torres, P., Fernandez-Piqueras, J., Saiz-Ruiz, J., and Llinares, C. (1994). No association between dopamine D4 receptor polymorphism and manic depressive illness. *J Med Genet*, 31(11), 897–898.

Perez de Castro, I., Santos, J., Torres, P., Visedo, G., Saiz-Ruiz, J., Llinares, C., and Fernandez-Piqueras, J. (1995). A weak association between TH and DRD2 genes and bipolar affective disorder in a Spanish sample. *J Med Genet*, 32(2), 131–134.

Peters, E.J., Slager, S.L., McGrath, P.J., Knowles, J.A., and Hamilton, S.P. (2004). Investigation of serotonin-related genes in antidepressant response. *Mol Psychiatry*, 9(9), 879–889.

Petronis, A. (2001). Human morbid genetics revisited: Relevance of epigenetics. *Trends Genet*, 17(3), 142–146.

Piccardi, M.P., Severino, G., Bocchetta, A., Palmas, M.A., Ruiu, S., and Del Zompo, M. (1997). No evidence of association between dopamine D3 receptor gene and bipolar affective disorder. *Am J Med Genet*, 74(2), 137–139.

Piccardi, M.P., Ardau, R., Chillotti, C., Deleuze, J.F., Mallet, J., Meloni, R., Oi, A., Severino, G., Congiu, D., Bayorek, M., and Del Zompo, M. (2002). Manic-depressive illness: An association study with the inositol polyphosphate 1-phosphatase and serotonin transporter genes. *Psychiatr Genet*, 12(1), 23–27.

Pollock, B.G., Ferrell, R.E., Mulsant, B.H., Mazumdar, S., Miller, M., Sweet, R.A., Davis, S., Kirshner, M.A., Houck, P.R., Stack, J.A., Reynolds, C.F., and Kupfer, D.J. (2000). Allelic variation in the serotonin transporter promoter affects onset of paroxetine treatment response in late-life depression. *Neuropsychopharmacology*, 23(5), 587–590.

Pollock, H.M., Malzberg, B., and Fuller, R.G. (1939). *Hereditary and Environmental Factors in the Causation of Manic-Depressive Psychoses and Dementia Praecox*. Utica, NY: State Hospital Press.

Potash, J.B., Willour, V.L., Chiu, Y.F., Simpson, S.G., MacKinnon, D.F., Pearlson, G.D., DePaulo, J.R. Jr., and McInnis, M.G. (2001). The familial aggregation of psychotic symptoms in bipolar disorder pedigrees. *Am J Psychiatry*, 158(8), 1258–1264.

Potash, J.B., Chiu, Y.F., MacKinnon, D.F., Miller, E.B., Simpson, S.G., McMahon, F.J., McInnis, M.G., and DePaulo, J.R. Jr. (2003a). Familial aggregation of psychotic symptoms in a replication set of 69 bipolar disorder pedigrees. *Am J Med Genet*, 160, 680–686.

Potash, J.B., Zandi, P.P., Willour, V.L., Lan, T.H., Huo, Y., Avramopoulos, D., Shugart, Y.Y., MacKinnon, D.F., Simpson, S.G., McMahon, F.J., DePaulo, J.R. Jr., and McInnis, M.G. (2003b). Suggestive linkage to chromosomal regions 13q31 and 22q12 in families with psychotic bipolar disorder. *Am J Psychiatry*, 160(4), 680–686.

Prathikanti, S., Schulze, T.G., Chen, Y.S., Harr, B., Akula, N., Hennessy, K., Potluri, S., Lyons, J., Nguyen, T., and McMahon, F.J. (2004). Neither single-marker nor haplotype analyses support an association between genetic variation near NOTCH4 and bipolar disorder. *Am J Med Genet B Neuropsychiatr Genet*, 131(1), 10–15.

Preisig, M., Bellivier, F., Fenton, B.T., Baud, P., Berney, A., Courtet, P., Hardy, P., Golaz, J., Leboyer, M., Mallet, J., Matthey, M.L., Mouthon, D., Neidhart, E., Nosten-Bertrand, M., Stadelmann-Dubuis, E., Guimon, J., Ferrero, F., Buresi, C., and Malafosse, A. (2000). Association between bipolar disorder and monoamine oxidase A gene polymorphisms: Results of a multicenter study. *Am J Psychiatry*, 157(6), 948–955.

Puertollano, R., Visedo, G., Saiz-Ruiz, J., Llinares, C., and Fernandez-Piqueras, J. (1995). Lack of association between manic-depressive illness and a highly polymorphic marker from GABRA3 gene. *Am J Med Genet*, 60(5), 434–435.

Puertollano, R., Visedo, G., Zapata, C., and Fernandez-Piqueras, J. (1997). A study of genetic association between manic-depressive illness and a highly polymorphic marker from the GABRbeta-1 gene. *Am J Med Genet*, 74(3), 342–344.

Pulver, A.E., Mulle, J., Nestadt, G., Swartz, K.L., Blouin, J.L., Dombroski, B., Liang, K.Y., Housman, D.E., Kazazian, H.H., Antonarakis, S.E., Lasseter, V.K., Wolyniec, P.S., Thornquist, M.H., and McGrath, J.A. (2000). Genetic heterogeneity in schizophrenia: Stratification of genome scan data using co-segregating related phenotypes. *Mol Psychiatry*, 5(6), 650–653.

Ranade, S.S., Mansour, H., Wood, J., Chowdari, K.V., Brar, L.K., Kupfer, D.J., and Nimgaonkar, V.L. (2003). Linkage and association between serotonin 2A receptor gene polymorphisms and bipolar I disorder. *Am J Med Genet B Neuropsychiatr Genet*, 121(1), 28–34.

Rasmussen, S.K., Urhammer, S.A., Berglund, L., Jensen, J.N., Hansen, L., Echwald, S.M., Borch-Johnsen, K., Horikawa, Y., Mashima, H., Lithell, H., Cox, N.J., Hansen, T., Bell, G.I., and Pedersen, O. (2002). Variants within the calpain-10 gene on chromosome 2q37 (NIDDM1) and relationships to type 2 diabetes, insulin resistance, and impaired acute insulin secretion among Scandinavian Caucasians. *Diabetes*, 51(12), 3561–3567.

Rausch, J.L., Johnson, M.E., Fei, Y.J., Li, J.Q., Shendarkar, N., Hobby, H.M., Ganapathy, V., and Leibach, F.H. (2002). Initial conditions of serotonin transporter kinetics and genotype: Influence on SSRI treatment trial outcome. *Biol Psychiatry*, 51(9), 723–732.

Rees, M., Norton, N., Jones, I., McCandless, F., Scourfield, J., Holmans, P., Moorhead, S., Feldman, E., Sadler, S., Cole, T., Redman, K., Farmer, A., McGuffin, P., Owen, M.J., and Craddock, N. (1997). Association studies of bipolar disorder at the human serotonin transporter gene (hSERT; 5HTT). *Mol Psychiatry*, 2(5), 398–402.

Reich, D.E., and Lander, E.S. (2001). On the allelic spectrum of human disease. *Trends Genet*, 17(9), 502–510.

Reich, T., Clayton, P.J., and Winokur, G. (1969). Family history studies: V. The genetics of mania. *Am J Psychiatry*, 125(10), 1358–1369.

Reich, T., Van Eerdewegh, P., Rice, J., Mullaney, J., Endicott, J., and Klerman, G.L. (1987). The familial transmission of primary major depressive disorder. *J Psychiatr Res*, 21(4), 613–624.

Rice, J., Reich, T., Andreasen, N.C., Endicott, J., Van Eerdewegh, M., Fishman, R., Hirschfeld, R.M., and Klerman, G.L. (1987). The familial transmission of bipolar illness. *Arch Gen Psychiatry*, 44(5), 441–447.

Rice, J.P., Goate, A., Williams, J.T., Bierut, L., Dorr, D., Wu, W., Shears, S., Gopalakrishnan, G., Edenberg, H.J., Foroud, T.,

Nurnberger, J. Jr., Gershon, E.S., Detera-Wadleigh, S.D., Goldin, L.R., Guroff, J.J., McMahon, F.J., Simpson, S., MacKinnon, D., McInnis, M., Stine, O.C., DePaulo, J.R., Blehar, M.C., and Reich, T. (1997). Initial genome scan of the NIMH genetics initiative bipolar pedigrees: Chromosomes 1, 6, 8, 10, and 12. *Am J Med Genet,* 74(3), 247–253.

Rietschel, M., Nothen, M.M., Lannfelt, L., Sokoloff, P., Schwartz, J.C., Lanczik, M., Fritze, J., Cichon, S., Fimmers, R., and Korner, J. (1993). A serine to glycine substitution at position 9 in the extracellular N-terminal part of the dopamine D3 receptor protein: No role in the genetic predisposition to bipolar affective disorder. *Psychiatry Res,* 46(3), 253–259.

Rietschel, M., Schorr, A., Albus, M., Franzek, E., Kreiner, R., Held, T., Knapp, M., Muller, D.J., Schulze, T.G., Propping, P., Maier, W., and Nothen, M.M. (2000). Association study of the tryptophan hydroxylase gene and bipolar affective disorder using family-based internal controls. *Am J Med Genet,* 96(3), 310–311.

Risch, N. (1990). Linkage strategies for genetically complex traits. I. Multilocus models. *Am J Hum Genet,* 46(2), 222–228.

Risch, N.J. (2000). Searching for genetic determinants in the new millennium. *Nature,* 405(6788), 847–856.

Roberts, S.B., MacLean, C.J., Neale, M.C., Eaves, L.J., and Kendler, K.S. (1999). Replication of linkage studies of complex traits: An examination of variation in location estimates. *Am J Hum Genet,* 65(3), 876–884.

Rohrmeier, T., Putzhammer, A., Schoeler, A., Sartor, H., Dallinger, P., Nothen, M.M., Propping, P., Knapp, M., Albus, M., Borrmann, M., Knothe, K., Kreiner, R., Franzek, E., Lichtermann, D., Rietschel, M., Maier, W., Klein, H.E., and Eichhammer, P. (1999). hSKCa3: No association of the polymorphic CAG repeat with bipolar affective disorder and schizophrenia. *Psychiatr Genet,* 9(4), 169–175.

Roll, A., and Entres, J.L. (1936). Zum Problem der Erbprognosebestimmung. *Z Ges Neurol Psychiatrie,* 156, 169–202.

Rosanoff, A.J., Handy, L., and Plesset, I.R. (1935). The etiology of manic-depressive syndromes with special reference to their occurrence in twins. *Am J Psychiatry,* 91, 725–762.

Rosenthal, D. (1970). *Genetic Theory and Abnormal Behavior.* New York: McGraw-Hill.

Rotondo, A., Mazzanti, C., Dell'Osso, L., Rucci, P., Sullivan, P., Bouanani, S., Gonnelli, C., Goldman, D., and Cassano, G.B. (2002). Catechol-O-methyltransferase, serotonin transporter, and tryptophan hydroxylase gene polymorphisms in bipolar disorder patients with and without comorbid panic disorder. *Am J Psychiatry,* 159(1), 23–29.

Rubinsztein, D.C., Leggo, J., Goodburn, S., Walsh, C., Jain, S., and Paykel, E.S. (1996). Genetic association between monoamine oxidase A microsatellite and RFLP alleles and bipolar affective disorder: Analysis and meta-analysis. *Hum Mol Genet,* 5(6), 779–782.

Rujescu, D., Giegling, I., Sato, T., and Moeller, H.J. (2001). A polymorphism in the promoter of the serotonin transporter gene is not associated with suicidal behavior. *Psychiatr Genet,* 11(3), 169–172.

Saleem, Q., Ganesh, S., Vijaykumar, M., Reddy, Y.C., Brahmachari, S.K., and Jain, S. (2000a). Association analysis of 5HT transporter gene in bipolar disorder in the Indian population. *Am J Med Genet,* 96(2), 170–172.

Saleem, Q., Sreevidya, V.S., Sudhir, J., Savithri, J.V., Gowda, Y., B-Rao, C., Benegal, V., Majumder, P.P., Anand, A., Brahmachari, S.K., and Jain, S. (2000b). Association analysis of CAG repeats at the KCNN3 locus in Indian patients with bipolar disorder and schizophrenia. *Am J Med Genet,* 96(6), 744–748.

Savoye, C., Laurent, C., Amadeo, S., Gheysen, F., Leboyer, M., Lejeune, J., Zarifian, E., and Mallet, J. (1998). No association between dopamine D1, D2, and D3 receptor genes and manic-depressive illness. *Biol Psychiatry,* 44(7), 644–647.

Scharfetter, C. (1981). Subdividing the functional psychoses: A family hereditary approach. *Psychol Med,* 11(3), 637–640.

Schizophrenia Collaborative Linkage Group for Chromosome 22. (1998). A transmission disequilibrium and linkage analysis of D22S278 marker alleles in 574 families: Further support for a susceptibility locus for schizophrenia at 22q12. *Schizophr Res,* 32(2), 115–121.

Schulze, T.G., Chen, Y.S., Badner, J.A., McInnis, M.G., DePaulo, J.R. Jr., and McMahon, F.J. (2003). Additional, physically ordered markers increase linkage signal for bipolar disorder on chromosome 18q22. *Biol Psychiatry,* 53(3), 239–243.

Schulze, T.G., Buervenich, S., Badner, J.A., Steele, C.J., Detera-Wadleigh, S.D., Dick, D., Foroud, T., Cox, N.J., MacKinnon, D.F., Potash, J.B., Berrettini, W.H., Byerley, W., Coryell, W., DePaulo, J.R. Jr., Gershon, E.S., Kelsoe, J.R., McInnis, M.G., Murphy, D.L., Reich, T., Scheftner, W., Nurnberger, J.I. Jr., and McMahon, F.J. (2004). Loci on chromosomes 6q and 6p interact to increase susceptibility to bipolar affective disorder in the National Institute of Mental Health genetics initiative pedigrees. *Biol Psychiatry,* 56(1), 18–23.

Schulze, T.G., Ohlraun, S., Czerski, P.M., Schumacher, J., Kassem, L., Deschner, M., Gross, M., Tullius, M., Heidmann, V., Kovalenko, S., Jamra, R.A., Becker, T., Leszczynska-Rodziewicz, A., Hauser, J., Illig, T., Klopp, N., Wellek, S., Cichon, S., Henn, F.A., McMahon, F.J., Maier, W., Propping, P., Nothen, M.M., and Rietschel, M. (2005). Genotype–phenotype studies in bipolar disorder showing association between the DAOA/G30 locus and persecutory delusions: A first step toward a molecular genetic classification of psychiatric phenotypes. *Am J Psychiatry,* 162, 2101–2108.

Schumacher, J., Jamra, R.A., Freudenberg, J., Becker, T., Ohlraun S., Otte, A.C., Tullius, M., Kovalenko, S., Bogaert, A.V., Maier, W., Rietschel, M., Propping, P., Nothen, M.M., and Cichon, S. (2004). Examination of G72 and D-amino-acid oxidase as genetic risk factors for schizophrenia and bipolar affective disorder. *Mol Psychiatry,* 9(2), 203–207.

Schurhoff, F., Szoke, A., Meary, A., Bellivier, F., Rouillon, F., Pauls, D., and Leboyer, M. (2003). Familial aggregation of delusional proneness in schizophrenia and bipolar pedigrees. *Am J Psychiatry,* 160(7), 1313–1319.

Schwab, S.G., Hallmayer, J., Lerer, B., Albus, M., Borrmann, M., Honig, S., Strauss, M., Segman, R., Lichtermann, D., Knapp, M., Trixler, M., Maier, W., and Wildenauer, D.B. (1998). Support for a chromosome 18p locus conferring susceptibility to functional psychoses in families with schizophrenia, by association and linkage analysis. *Am J Hum Genet,* 63(4), 1139–1152.

Schwab, S.G., Hallmayer, J., Albus, M., Lerer, B., Eckstein, G.N., Borrmann, M., Segman, R.H., Hanses, C., Freymann, J., Yakir, A., Trixler, M., Falkai, P., Rietschel, M., Maier, W., and Wildenauer, D.B. (2000). A genome-wide autosomal screen for schizophrenia susceptibility loci in 71 families with affected siblings: Support for loci on chromosome 10p and 6. *Mol Psychiatry,* 5(6), 638–649.

Segman, R.H., Shapira, Y., Modai, I., Hamdan, A., Zislin, J., Heresco-Levy, U., Kanyas, K., Hirschmann, S., Karni, O., Finkel, B., Schlafman, M., Lerner, A., Shapira, B., Macciardi, F., and Lerer, B. (2002). Angiotensin converting enzyme gene insertion/deletion polymorphism: Case–control association studies in schizophrenia, major affective disorder, and tardive dyskinesia and a family-based association study in schizophrenia. *Am J Med Genet*, 114(3), 310–314.

Segurado, R., Detera-Wadleigh, S.D., Levinson, D.F., Lewis, C.M., Gill, M., Nurnberger, J.I. Jr., Craddock, N., DePaulo, J.R., Baron, M., Gershon, E.S., Ekholm, J., Cichon, S., Turecki, G., Claes, S., Kelsoe, J.R., Schofield, P.R., Badenhop, R.F., Morissette, J., Coon, H., Blackwood, D., McInnes, L.A., Foroud, T., Edenberg, H.J., Reich, T., Rice, J.P., Goate, A., McInnis, M.G., McMahon, F.J., Badner, J.A., Goldin, L.R., Bennett, P., Willour, V.L., Zandi, P.P., Liu, J., Gilliam, C., Juo, S.H., Berrettini, W.H., Yoshikawa, T., Peltonen, L., Lonnqvist, J., Nothen, M.M., Schumacher, J., Windemuth, C., Rietschel, M., Propping, P., Maier, W., Alda, M., Grof, P., Rouleau, G.A., Del-Favero, J., Van Broeckhoven, C., Mendlewicz, J., Adolfsson, R., Spence, M.A., Luebbert, H., Adams, L.J., Donald, J.A., Mitchell, P.B., Barden, N., Shink, E., Byerley, W., Muir, W., Visscher, P.M., Macgregor, S., Gurling, H., Kalsi, G., McQuillin, A., Escamilla, M.A., Reus, V.I., Leon, P., Freimer, N.B., Ewald, H., Kruse, T.A., Mors, O., Radhakrishna, U., Blouin, J.L., Antonarakis, S.E., and Akarsu, N. (2003). Genome scan meta-analysis of schizophrenia and bipolar disorder, part III: Bipolar disorder. *Am J Hum Genet*, 73(1), 49–62.

Sen, S., Nesse, R.M., Stoltenberg, S.F., Li, S., Gleiberman, L., Chakravarti, A., Weder, A.B., and Burmeister, M. (2003). A BDNF coding variant is associated with the NEO personality inventory domain neuroticism, a risk factor for depression. *Neuropsychopharmacology*, 28(2), 397–401.

Serretti, A., Macciardi, F., Cusin, C., Verga, M., Pedrini, S., and Smeraldi, E. (1998). Tyrosine hydroxylase gene in linkage disequilibrium with mood disorders. *Mol Psychiatry*, 3(2), 169–174.

Serretti, A., Lilli, R., Di Bella, D., Bertelli, S., Nobile, M., Novelli, E., Catalano, M., and Smeraldi, E. (1999a). Dopamine receptor D4 gene is not associated with major psychoses. *Am J Med Genet*, 88(5), 486–491.

Serretti, A., Lilli, R., Lorenzi, C., Gasperini, M., and Smeraldi, E. (1999b). Tryptophan hydroxylase gene and response to lithium prophylaxis in mood disorders. *J Psychiatr Res*, 33(5), 371–377.

Serretti, A., Lilli, R., Mandelli, L., Lorenzi, C., and Smeraldi, E. (2001). Serotonin transporter gene associated with lithium prophylaxis in mood disorders. *Pharmacogenomics*, J1(1), 71–77.

Serretti, A., Cristina, S., Lilli, R., Cusin, C., Lattuada, E., Lorenzi, C., Corradi, B., Grieco, G., Costa, A., Santorelli, F., Barale, F., Nappi, G., and Smeraldi, E. (2002). Family-based association study of 5-HTTLPR, TPH, MAO-A, and DRD4 polymorphisms in mood disorders. *Am J Med Genet*, 114(4), 361–369.

Serretti, A., Lilli, R., and Smeraldi, E. (2002c). Pharmacogenetics in affective disorders. *Eur J Pharmacol*, 438(3), 117–128.

Serretti, A., Cusin, C., Cristina, S., Lorenzi, C., Lilli, R., Lattuada, E., Grieco, G., Costa, A., Santorelli, F., Barale, F., Smeraldi, E., and Nappi, G. (2003). Multicentre Italian family-based association study on tyrosine hydroxylase, catechol-O-methyl transferase and Wolfram syndrome 1 polymorphisms in mood disorders. *Psychiatr Genet*, 13(2), 121–126.

Serretti, A., Cusin, C., Rossini, D., Artioli, P., Dotoli, D., and Zanardi, R. (2004). Further evidence of a combined effect of SERTPR and TPH on SSRIs response in mood disorders. *Am J Med Genet B Neuropsychiatr Genet*, 129(1), 36–40.

Shaikh, S., Ball, D., Craddock, N., Castle, D., Hunt, N., Mant, R., Owen, M., Collier, D., and Gill, M. (1993). The dopamine D3 receptor gene: no association with bipolar affective disorder. *J Med Genet*, 30(4), 308–309.

Sham, P.C., MacLean, C.J., and Kendler, K.S. (1994). A typological model of schizophrenia based on age at onset, sex and familial morbidity. *Acta Psychiatr Scand*, 89(2), 135–141.

Sham, P.C., Castle, D.J., Wessely, S., Farmer, A.E., and Murray, R.M. (1996). Further exploration of a latent class typology of schizophrenia. *Schizophr Res*, 20(1-2), 105–115.

Shimon, H., Agam, G., Belmaker, R.H., Hyde, T.M., and Kleinman, J.E. (1997). Reduced frontal cortex inositol levels in postmortem brain of suicide victims and patients with bipolar disorder. *Am J Psychiatry*, 154(8), 1148–1150.

Shorter, E. (1996). A History of Psychiatry: From the Era of the Asylum to the Age of Prozac. New York: John Wiley and Sons.

Simpson, S.G., Folstein, S.E., Meyers, D.A., McMahon, F.J., Brusco, D.M., and DePaulo, J.R. Jr. (1993). Bipolar II: The most common bipolar phenotype? *Am J Psychiatry*, 150(6), 901–903.

Simpson, S.G., McMahon, F.J., McInnis, M.G., MacKinnon, D.F., Edwin, D., Folstein, S.E., and DePaulo, J.R. (2002). Diagnostic reliability of bipolar II disorder. *Arch Gen Psychiatry*, 59(8), 736–740.

Sjögren, T. (1948). Genetic-statistical and psychiatric investigations of a West Swedish population. *Acta Psychiatr Neurol*, 24 (Suppl.), 269–271.

Sjoholt, G., Ebstein, R.P., Lie, R.T., Berle, J.O., Mallet, J., Deleuze, J.F., Levinson, D.F., Laurent, C., Mujahed, M., Bannoura, I., Murad, I., Molven, A., and Steen, V.M. (2004). Examination of IMPA1 and IMPA2 genes in manic-depressive patients: Association between IMPA2 promoter polymorphisms and bipolar disorder. *Mol Psychiatry*, 9(6), 621–629.

Sklar, P., Gabriel, S.B., McInnis, M.G., Bennett, P., Lim, Y.M., Tsan, G., Schaffner, S., Kirov, G., Jones, I., Owen, M., Craddock, N., DePaulo, J.R., and Lander, E.S. (2002). Family-based association study of 76 candidate genes in bipolar disorder: BDNF is a potential risk locus. Brain-derived neutrophic factor. *Mol Psychiatry*, 7(6), 579–593.

Skuse, D.H., James, R.S., Bishop, D.V., Coppin, B., Dalton, P., Aamodt-Leeper, G., Bacarese-Hamilton, M., Creswell, C., McGurk, R., and Jacobs, P.A. (1997). Evidence from Turner's syndrome of an imprinted X-linked locus affecting cognitive function [see comments]. *Nature*, 387(6634), 705–708.

Slater, E. (1936a). The inheritance of manic-depressive insanity. *Proc R Soc Med*, 29, 981–990.

Slater, E. (1936b). The inheritance of manic-depressive insanity and its relation to mental defect. *J Ment Sci*, 82:626–634.

Slater, E. (1938). Erbpathologie des manisch-depressiven Irreseins. Die Eltern und Kinder von Manisch-Depressiven. [Hereditary pathology of manic-depressive illness. Parents and offspring of manic-depressives]. *Z Ges Neurol Psychiatrie*, 163, 1–47.

Slater, E., and Shields, J. (1953). Psychotic and neurotic illnesses in twins. In: *Medical Research Current Special Report*, Series #ZN8. London: HMSO.

Smeraldi, E., Negri, F., and Melica, A.M. (1977). A genetic study of affective disorders. *Acta Psychiatr Scand*, 56(5), 382–398.

Smeraldi, E., Zanardi, R., Benedetti, F., Di Bella, D., Perez, J., and Catalano, M. (1998). Polymorphism within the promoter of the serotonin transporter gene and antidepressant efficacy of fluvoxamine. *Mol Psychiatry*, 3(6), 508–511.

Smith, D.J., Stevens, M.E., Sudanagunta, S.P., Bronson, R.T., Makhinson, M., Watabe, A.M., O'Dell, T.J., Fung, J., Weier, H.U., Cheng, J.F., and Rubin, E.M. (1997). Functional screening of 2 Mb of human chromosome 21q22.2 in transgenic mice implicates minibrain in learning defects associated with Down syndrome. *Nat Genet*, 16(1), 28–36.

Smith, L.B., Sapers, B., Reus, V.I., and Freimer, N.B. (1996). Attitudes towards bipolar disorder and predictive genetic testing among patients and providers. *J Med Genet*, 33(7), 544–549.

Souery, D., Lipp, O., Mahieu, B., Mendelbaum, K., De Bruyn, A., De Maertelaer, V., Van Broeckhoven, C., and Mendlewicz, J. (1996a). Excess tyrosine hydroxylase restriction fragment length polymorphism homozygosity in unipolar but not bipolar patients: A preliminary report. *Biol Psychiatry*, 40(4), 305–308.

Souery, D., Lipp, O., Mahieu, B., Mendelbaum, K., De Martelaer, V., Van Broeckhoven, C., and Mendlewicz, J. (1996b). Association study of bipolar disorder with candidate genes involved in catecholamine neurotransmission: DRD2, DRD3, DAT1, and TH genes. *Am J Med Genet*, 67(6), 551–555.

Souery, D., Lipp, O., Rivelli, S.K., Massat, I., Serretti, A., Cavallini, C., Ackenheil, M., Adolfsson, R., Aschauer, H., Blackwood, D., Dam, H., Dikeos, D., Fuchshuber, S., Heiden, M., Jakovljevic, M., Kaneva, R., Kessing, L., Lerer, B., Lonnqvist, J., Mellerup, T., Milanova, V., Muir, W., Nylander, P.O., Oruc, L., and Mendlewicz, J. (1999). Tyrosine hydroxylase polymorphism and phenotypic heterogeneity in bipolar affective disorder: A multicenter association study. *Am J Med Genet*, 88(5), 527–532.

Souery, D., Van Gestel, S., Massat, I., Blairy, S., Adolfsson, R., Blackwood, D., Del-Favero, J., Dikeos, D., Jakovljevic, M., Kaneva, R., Lattuada, E., Lerer, B., Lilli, R., Milanova, V., Muir, W., Nothen, M., Oruc, L., Papadimitriou, G., Propping, P., Schulze, T., Serretti, A., Shapira, B., Smeraldi, E., Stefanis, C., Thomson, M., Van Broeckhoven, C., and Mendlewicz, J. (2001). Tryptophan hydroxylase polymorphism and suicidality in unipolar and bipolar affective disorders: A multicenter association study. *Biol Psychiatry*, 49(5), 405–409.

Speight, G., Turic, D., Austin, J., Hoogendoorn, B., Cardno, A.G., Jones, L., Murphy, K.C., Sanders, R., McCarthy, G., Jones, I., McCandless, F., McGuffin, P., Craddock, N., Owen, M.J., Buckland, P., and O'Donovan, M.C. (2000). Comparative sequencing and association studies of aromatic L-amino acid decarboxylase in schizophrenia and bipolar disorder. *Mol Psychiatry*, 5(3), 327–331.

Spence, M.A., Flodman, P.L., Sadovnick, A.D., Bailey-Wilson, J.E., Ameli, H., and Remick, R.A. (1995). Bipolar disorder: Evidence for a major locus [see comments]. *Am J Med Genet*, 60(5), 370–376.

Spielman, R.S., McGinnis, R.E., and Ewens, W.J. (1993). Transmission test for linkage disequilibrium: The insulin gene region and insulin-dependent diabetes mellitus (IDDM). *Am J Hum Genet*, 52(3), 506–516.

Spitzer, R.L., and Endicott, J. (1975). *Research Diagnostic Criteria (RDC) for a Selected Group of Functional Disorders.* New York: New York State Psychiatric Institute, Biometrics Research.

Stenstedt, Å. (1952). A study in manic-depressive psychosis: Clinical, social, and genetic investigations. *Acta Psychiatr Neurol*, (Suppl. 79), 1–111.

St. George-Hyslop, P.H. (2000). Molecular genetics of Alzheimer's disease. *Biol Psychiatry*, 47(3), 183–199.

Stine, O.C., Xu, J., Koskela, R., McMahon, F.J., Gschwend, M., Friddle, C., Clark, C.D., McInnis, M.G., Simpson, S.G., and Breschel, T.S. (1995). Evidence for linkage of bipolar disorder to chromosome 18 with a parent-of-origin effect. *Am J Hum Genet*, 57(6), 1384–1394.

Stine, O.C., McMahon, F.J., Chen, L., Xu, J., Meyers, D.A., MacKinnon, D.F., Simpson, S., McInnis, M.G., Rice, J.P., Goate, A., Reich, T., Edenberg, H.J., Foroud, T., Nurnberger, J.I. Jr., Detera-Wadleigh, S.D., Goldin, L.R., Guroff, J., Gershon, E.S., Blehar, M.C., and DePaulo, J.R. (1997). Initial genome screen for bipolar disorder in the NIMH genetics initiative pedigrees: Chromosomes 2, 11, 13, 14, and X. *Am J Med Genet*, 74(3), 263–269.

Stober, G., Nothen, M.M., Porzgen, P., Bruss, M., Bonisch, H., Knapp, M., Beckmann, H., and Propping, P. (1996). Systematic search for variation in the human norepinephrine transporter gene: Identification of five naturally occurring missense mutations and study of association with major psychiatric disorders. *Am J Med Genet*, 67(6), 523–532.

Stober, G., Jatzke, S., Heils, A., Jungkunz, G., Knapp, M., Mossner, R., Riederer, P., and Lesch, K.P. (1998). Insertion/deletion variant (−141C Ins/Del) in the 5' regulatory region of the dopamine D2 receptor gene: Lack of association with schizophrenia and bipolar affective disorder. Short communication. *J Neural Transm*, 105(1), 101–109.

Straub, R.E., Lehner, T., Luo, Y., Loth, J.E., Shao, W., Sharpe, L., Alexander, J.R., Das, K., Simon, R., and Fieve, R.R. (1994). A possible vulnerability locus for bipolar affective disorder on chromosome 21q22.3. *Nat Genet*, 8(3), 291–296.

Straub, R.E., MacLean, C.J., Martin, R.B., Ma, Y., Myakishev, M.V., Harris-Kerr, C., Webb, B.T., O'Neill, F.A., Walsh, D., and Kendler, K.S. (1998). A schizophrenia locus may be located in region 10p15-p11. *Am J Med Genet*, 81(4), 296–301.

Strober, M., Morrell, W., Burroughs, J., Lampert, C., Danforth, H., and Freeman, R. (1988). A family study of bipolar I disorder in adolescence. Early onset of symptoms linked to increased familial loading and lithium resistance. *J Affect Disord*, 15(3), 255–268.

Strömgren, E. (1938) Beitrage zur psychiatrischen Erblehre. Copenhagen: Munksgaard.

Sullivan, P.F., Neale, M.C., and Kendler, K.S. (2000). Genetic epidemiology of major depression: Review and meta-analysis. *Am J Psychiatry*, 157(10), 1552–1562.

Sun, Y., Zhang, L., Johnston, N.L., Torrey, E.F., and Yolken, R.H. (2001). Serial analysis of gene expression in the frontal cortex of patients with bipolar disorder. *Br J Psychiatry*, (Suppl. 41), s137–s141.

Swift-Scanlan, T., Lan, T.H., Fallin, M.D., Coughlin, J.M., Potash, J.B., DePaulo, J.R., and McInnis, M.G. (2002). Genetic analysis of the (CTG)n NOTCH4 polymorphism in 65 multiplex bipolar pedigrees. *Psychiatr Genet*, 12(1), 43–47.

Syagailo, Y.V., Stober, G., Grassle, M., Reimer, E., Knapp, M., Jungkunz, G., Okladnova, O., Meyer, J., and Lesch, K.P. (2001). Association analysis of the functional monoamine oxidase A gene promoter polymorphism in psychiatric disorders. *Am J Med Genet*, 105(2), 168–171.

Tadokoro, K., Hashimoto, R., Tatsumi, M., Kamijima, K., and Kunugi, H. (2004). Analysis of enhancer activity of a dinucleotide repeat polymorphism in the neurotrophin-3 gene and its association with bipolar disorder. *Neuropsychobiology,* 50(3), 206–210.

Tanna, V.L., and Winokur, G. (1968). A study of association and linkage of ABO blood types and primary affective disorder. *Br J Psychiatry,* 114(514), 1175–1181.

Tkachev, D., Mimmack, M.L., Ryan, M.M., Wayland, M., Freeman, T., Jones, P.B., Starkey, M., Webster, M.J., Yolken, R.H., and Bahn, S. (2003). Oligodendrocyte dysfunction in schizophrenia and bipolar disorder. *Lancet,* 362(9386), 798–805.

Todd, R.D., and O'Malley, K.L. (1989). Population frequencies of tyrosine hydroxylase restriction fragment length polymorphisms in bipolar affective disorder. *Biol Psychiatry,* 25(5), 626–630.

Todd, R.D., Lobos, E.A., Parsian, A., Simpson, S., and DePaulo, J.R. (1996). Manic-depressive illness and tyrosine hydroxylase markers. Bipolar Disorder Working Group. *Lancet,* 347(9015), 1634.

Torgersen, S. (1986). Genetic factors in moderately severe and mild affective disorders. *Arch Gen Psychiatry,* 43(3), 222–226.

Toyota, T., Watanabe, A., Shibuya, H., Nankai, M., Hattori, E., Yamada, K., Kurumaji, A., Karkera, J.D., Detera-Wadleigh, S.D., and Yoshikawa, T. (2000). Association study on the DUSP6 gene, an affective disorder candidate gene on 12q23, performed by using fluorescence resonance energy transfer-based melting curve analysis on the LightCycler. *Mol Psychiatry,* 5(5), 489–494.

Toyota, T., Hattori, E., Meerabux, J., Yamada, K., Saito, K., Shibuya, H., Nankai, M., and Yoshikawa, T. (2002). Molecular analysis, mutation screening, and association study of adenylate cyclase type 9 gene (ADCY9) in mood disorders. *Am J Med Genet,* 114(1), 84–92.

Tremolizzo, L., Carboni, G., Ruzicka, W.B., Mitchell, C.P., Sugaya, I., Tueting, P., Sharma, R., Grayson, D.R., Costa, E., and Guidotti, A. (2002). An epigenetic mouse model for molecular and behavioral neuropathologies related to schizophrenia vulnerability. *Proc Natl Acad Sci USA,* 99(26), 17095–17100.

Trippitelli, C.L., Jamison, K.R., Folstein, M.F., Bartko, J.J., and DePaulo, J.R. (1998). Pilot study on patients' and spouses' attitudes toward potential genetic testing for bipolar disorder. *Am J Psychiatry,* 155(7), 899–904.

Tsai, S.J., Hong, C.J., Hsu, C.C., Cheng, C.Y., Liao, W.Y., Song, H.L., and Lai, H.C. (1999). Serotonin-2A receptor polymorphism (102T/C) in mood disorders. *Psychiatry Res,* 87(2–3), 233–237.

Tsai, S.J., Wang, Y.C., and Hong, C.J. (2001). Association study between cannabinoid receptor gene (CNR1) and pathogenesis and psychotic symptoms of mood disorders. *Am J Med Genet,* 105(3), 219–221.

Tsai, S.J., Cheng, C.Y., Yu, Y.W., Chen, T.J., and Hong, C.J. (2003). Association study of a brain-derived neurotrophic-factor genetic polymorphism and major depressive disorders, symptomatology, and antidepressant response. *Am J Med Genet B Neuropsychiatr Genet,* 123(1), 19–22.

Tsuang, M.T., and Faraone, S.V. (1990). *The Genetics of Mood Disorders.* Baltimore: Johns Hopkins University Press.

Tsuang, M.T., Woolson, R., and Fleming, J.A. (1980). Causes of death in schizophrenia and manic-depression. *Br J Psychiatry,* 136, 239–242.

Turecki, G., Alda, M., Grof, P., Martin, R., Cavazzoni, P.A., Duffy, A., Maciel, P., and Rouleau, G.A. (1996). No association between chromosome-18 markers and lithium-responsive affective disorders. *Psychiatry Res,* 63(1), 17–23.

Turecki, G., Grof, P., Cavazzoni, P., Duffy, A., Grof, E., Ahrens, B., Berghofer, A., Muller-Oerlinghausen, B., Dvorakova, M., Libigerova, E., Vojtechovsky, M., Zvolsky, P., Joober, R., Nilsson, A., Prochazka, H., Licht, R.W., Rasmussen, N.A., Schou, M., Vestergaard, P., Holzinger, A., Schumann, C., Thau, K., Rouleau, GA., and Alda, M. (1998). Evidence for a role of phospholipase C-gamma1 in the pathogenesis of bipolar disorder. *Mol Psychiatry,* 3(6), 534–538.

Turecki, G., Grof, P., Cavazzoni, P., Duffy, A., Grof, E., Ahrens, B., Berghofer, A., Muller-Oerlinghausen, B., Dvorakova, M., Libigerova, E., Vojtechovsky, M., Zvolsky, P., Joober, R., Nilsson, A., Prochazka, H., Licht, R.W., Rasmussen, N.A., Schou, M., Vestergaard, P., Holzinger, A., Schumann, C., Thau, K., Rouleau, G.A., and Alda, M. (1999). MAOA: Association and linkage studies with lithium responsive bipolar disorder. *Psychiatr Genet,* 9(1), 13–16.

Turecki, G., Grof, P., Grof, E., D'Souza, V., Lebuis, L., Marineau, C., Cavazzoni, P., Duffy, A., Betard, C., Zvolsky, P., Robertson, C., Brewer, C., Hudson, T.J., Rouleau, G.A., and Alda, M. (2001). Mapping susceptibility genes for bipolar disorder: A pharmacogenetic approach based on excellent response to lithium. *Mol Psychiatry,* 6(5), 570–578.

Tut, T.G., Wang, J.L., and Lim, C.C. (2000). Negative association between T102C polymorphism at the 5-HT2A receptor gene and bipolar affective disorders in Singaporean Chinese. *J Affect Disord,* 58(3), 211–214.

Ujike, H., Yamamoto, A., Tanaka, Y., Takehisa, Y., Takaki, M., Taked, T., Kodama, M., and Kuroda, S. (2001). Association study of CAG repeats in the KCNN3 gene in Japanese patients with schizophrenia, schizoaffective disorder and bipolar disorder. *Psychiatry Res,* 101(3), 203–207.

Van Tol, H.H., Bunzow, J.R., Guan, H.C., Sunahara, R.K., Seeman, P., Niznik, H.B., and Civelli, O. (1991). Cloning of the gene for a human dopamine D4 receptor with high affinity for the antipsychotic clozapine. *Nature,* 350(6319), 610–614.

Van Tol, H.H., Wu, C.M., Guan, H.C., Ohara, K., Bunzow, J.R., Civelli, O., Kennedy, J., Seeman, P., Niznik, H.B., and Jovanovic, V. (1992). Multiple dopamine D4 receptor variants in the human population. *Nature,* 358(6382), 149–152.

Vawter, M.P., Thatcher, L., Usen, N., Hyde, T.M., Kleinman, J.E., and Freed, W.J. (2002). Reduction of synapsin in the hippocampus of patients with bipolar disorder and schizophrenia. *Mol Psychiatry,* 7(6), 571–578.

Venken, T., Claes, S., Sluijs, S., Paterson, A.D., van Duijn, C., Adolfsson, R., Del-Favero, J., and Van Broeckhoven, C. (2005). Genomewide scan for affective disorder susceptibility Loci in families of a northern Swedish isolated population. *Am J Hum Genet,* 76(2), 237–248.

Vincent, J.B., Masellis, M., Lawrence, J., Choi, V., Gurling, H.M., Parikh, S.V., and Kennedy, J.L. (1999). Genetic association analysis of serotonin system genes in bipolar affective disorder. *Am J Psychiatry,* 156(1), 136–138.

Vogt, I.R., Shimron-Abarbanell, D., Neidt, H., Erdmann, J., Cichon, S., Schulze, T.G., Muller, D.J., Maier, W., Albus, M., Borrmann-Hassenbach, M., Knapp, M., Rietschel, M., Propping, P., and Nothen, M.M. (2000). Investigation of the human serotonin 6 [5-HT6] receptor gene in bipolar affective disorder and schizophrenia. *Am J Med Genet,* 96(2), 217–221.

von Knorring, A.L., Cloninger, C.R., Bohman, M., and Sigvardsson, S. (1983). An adoption study of depressive disorders and substance abuse. *Arch Gen Psychiatry,* 40(9), 943–950.

Waldman, I.D., Robinson, B.F., and Feigon, S.A. (1997). Linkage disequilibrium between the dopamine transporter gene (DAT1) and bipolar disorder: Extending the transmission disequilibrium test (TDT) to examine genetic heterogeneity. *Genet Epidemiol*, 14(6), 699–704.

Washizuka, S., Ikeda, A., Kato, N., and Kato, T. (2003). Possible relationship between mitochondrial DNA polymorphisms and lithium response in bipolar disorder. *Int J Neuropsychopharmacol*, 6(4), 421–424.

Weber, M.M. (1996). Ernst Rudin, 1874–1952: A German psychiatrist and geneticist. *Am J Med Genet*, 67(4), 323–331.

Weinberg, I., and Lobstein, J. (1936). Beitrag zur Vererbung des manisch-depressiven Irreseins. *Psychiatr Neurol*, 1, 337.

Weiss, J., Magert, H.J., Cieslak, A., and Forssmann, W.G. (1996). Association between different psychotic disorders and the DRD4 polymorphism, but no differences in the main ligand binding region of the DRD4 receptor protein compared to controls. *Eur J Med Res*, 1(9), 439–445.

Weissman, M.M., Gershon, E.S., Kidd, K.K., Prusoff, B.A., Leckman, J.F., Dibble, E., Hamovit, J., Thompson, W.D., Pauls, D.L., and Guroff, J.J. (1984). Psychiatric disorders in the relatives of probands with affective disorders. The Yale University–National Institute of Mental Health collaborative study. *Arch Gen Psychiatry*, 41(1), 13–21.

Weissman, M.M., Wickramaratne, P., Adams, P.B., Lish, J.D., Horwath, E., Charney, D., Woods, S.W., Leeman, E., and Frosch, E. (1993). The relationship between panic disorder and major depression. A new family study. *Arch Gen Psychiatry*, 50(10), 767–780.

Weksberg, R., Shuman, C., Caluseriu, O., Smith, A.C., Fei, Y.L., Nishikawa, J., Stockley, T.L., Best, L., Chitayat, D., Olney, A., Ives, E., Schneider, A., Bestor, T.H., Li, M., Sadowski, P., and Squire, J. (2002). Discordant KCNQ1OT1 imprinting in sets of monozygotic twins discordant for Beckwith-Wiedemann syndrome. *Hum Mol Genet*, 11(11), 1317–1325.

Wender, P.H., Kety, S.S., Rosenthal, D., Schulsinger, F., Ortmann, J., and Lunde, I. (1986). Psychiatric disorders in the biological and adoptive families of adopted individuals with affective disorders. *Arch Gen Psychiatry*, 43(10), 923–929.

Williams, R.S., Cheng, L., Mudge, A.W., and Harwood, A.J. (2002). A common mechanism of action for three mood-stabilizing drugs. *Nature*, 417(6886), 292–295.

Willour, V.L., Zandi, P.P., Huo, Y., Diggs, T.L., Chellis, J.L., MacKinnon, D.F., Simpson, S.G., McMahon, F.J., Potash, J.B., Gershon, E.S., Reich, T., Foroud, T., Nurnberger, J.I. Jr., DePaulo, J.R. Jr., and McInnis, M.G. (2003). Genome scan of the fifty-six bipolar pedigrees from the NIMH genetics initiative replication sample: Chromosomes 4, 7, 9, 18, 19, 20, and 21. *Am J Med Genet B Neuropsychiatr Genet*, 121(1), 21–27.

Winokur, G., and Clayton, P. (1967). Family history studies: I. Two types of affective disorders separated according to genetic and clinical factors. In J. Wortis (Ed.), Recent Advances in Biological Psychiatry (Vol. 10). New York: Plenum Press, pp. 35–50

Woo, T.U., Walsh, J.P., and Benes, F.M. (2004). Density of glutamic acid decarboxylase 67 messenger RNA-containing neurons that express the N-methyl-D-aspartate receptor subunit NR2A in the anterior cingulate cortex in schizophrenia and bipolar disorder. *Arch Gen Psychiatry*, 61(7), 649–657.

Wooster, R., Neuhausen, S.L., Mangion, J., Quirk, Y., Ford, D., Collins, N., Nguyen, K., Seal, S., Tran, T., Averill, D. (1994). Localization of a breast cancer susceptibility gene, BRCA2, to chromosome 13q12-13. *Science*, 265(5181), 2088–2090.

Wozniak, J., Biederman, J., Mundy, E., Mennin, D., and Faraone, S.V. (1995). A pilot family study of childhood-onset mania. *J Am Acad Child Adolesc Psychiatry*, 34 (12), 1577–1583.

Wozniak, J., Biederman, J., Monuteaux, M.C., Richards, J., and Faraone, S.V. (2002). Parsing the comorbidity between bipolar disorder and anxiety disorders: A familial risk analysis. *J Child Adolesc Psychopharmacol*, 12(2), 101–111.

Wright, A.F., Carothers, A.D., and Pirastu, M. (1999). Population choice in mapping genes for complex diseases. *Nat Genet*, 23(4), 397–404.

Xian, H., Scherrer, J.F., Eisen, S.A., True, W.R., Heath, A.C., Goldberg, J., Lyons, M.J., and Tsuang, M.T. (2000). Self-Reported zygosity and the equal-environments assumption for psychiatric disorders in the Vietnam Era Twin Registry. *Behav Genet*, 30(4), 303–310.

Xing, G., Russell, S., Hough, C., O'Grady, J., Zhang, L., Yang, S., Zhang, L.X., and Post, R. (2002). Decreased prefrontal CaMKII alpha mRNA in bipolar illness. *Neuroreport*, 13(4), 501–505.

Yamamoto, A., Lucas, J.J., and Hen, R. (2000). Reversal of neuropathology and motor dysfunction in a conditional model of Huntington's disease. *Cell*, 101(1), 57–66.

Yang, Q., Khoury, M.J., Botto, L., Friedman, J.M., and Flanders, W.D. (2003). Improving the prediction of complex diseases by testing for multiple disease-susceptibility genes. *Am J Hum Genet*, 72(3), 636–649.

Yen, F.C., Hong, C.J., Hou, S.J., Wang, J.K., and Tsai, S.J. (2003). Association study of serotonin transporter gene VNTR polymorphism and mood disorders, onset age and suicide attempts in a Chinese sample. *Neuropsychobiology*, 48(1), 5–9.

Yoon, I.S., Li, P.P., Siu, K.P., Kennedy, J.L., Macciardi, F., Cooke, R.G., Parikh, S.V., and Warsh, J.J. (2001). Altered TRPC7 gene expression in bipolar-I disorder. *Biol Psychiatry*, 50(8), 620–626.

Yoshida, K., Ito, K., Sato, K., Takahashi, H., Kamata, M., Higuchi, H., Shimizu, T., Itoh, K., Inoue, K., Tezuka, T., Suzuki, T., Ohkubo, T., Sugawara, K., and Otani, K. (2002). Influence of the serotonin transporter gene–linked polymorphic region on the antidepressant response to fluvoxamine in Japanese depressed patients. *Prog Neuropsychopharmacol Biol Psychiatry*, 26(2), 383–386.

Yoshida, K., Takahashi, H., Higuchi, H., Kamata, M., Ito, K., Sato, K., Naito, S., Shimizu, T., Itoh, K., Inoue, K., Suzuki, T., and Nemeroff, C.B. (2004). Prediction of antidepressant response to milnacipran by norepinephrine transporter gene polymorphisms. *Am J Psychiatry*, 161(9), 1575–1580.

Young, L.T., Asghari, V., Li, P.P., Kish, S.J., Fahnestock, M., and Warsh, J.J. (1996). Stimulatory G-protein alpha-subunit mRNA levels are not increased in autopsied cerebral cortex from patients with bipolar disorder. *Brain Res Mol Brain Res*, 42(1), 45–50.

Young, L.E., Sinclair, K.D., and Wilmut, I. (1998). Large offspring syndrome in cattle and sheep. *Rev Reprod*, 3(3), 155–163.

Yu, Y.W., Tsai, S.J., Chen, T.J., Lin, C.H., and Hong, C.J. (2002). Association study of the serotonin transporter promoter polymorphism and symptomatology and antidepressant response in major depressive disorders. *Mol Psychiatry*, 7(10), 1115–1119.

Zanardi, R., Benedetti, F., Di Bella, D., Catalano, M., Smeraldi, E. (2000). Efficacy of paroxetine in depression is influenced by a functional polymorphism within the promoter of the serotonin transporter gene. *J Clin Psychopharmacol*, 20(1), 105–107.

Zanardi, R., Artigas, F., Moresco, R., Colombo, C., Messa, C., Gobbo, C., Smeraldi, E., and Fazio, F. (2001). Increased 5-hydroxytryptamine-2 receptor binding in the frontal cortex of depressed patients responding to paroxetine treatment: A position emission tomography scan study. *J Clin Psychopharmacol*, 21(1), 53–58.

Zandi, P.P., Willour, V.L., Huo, Y., Chellis, J., Potash, J.B., MacKinnon, D.F., Simpson, S.G., McMahon, F.J., Gershon, E., Reich, T., Foroud, T., Nurnberger, J., Jr., DePaulo, J.R. Jr., McInnis, M.G., and National Institute of Mental Health Genetics Initiative Bipolar Group. (2003). Genome scan of a second wave of NIMH genetics initiative bipolar pedigrees: chromosomes 2, 11, 13, 14, and X. *Am J Med Genet B Neuropsychiatr Genet*, 119(1), 69–76.

Zhang, H.Y., Ishigaki, T., Tani, K., Chen, K., Shih, J.C., Miyasato, K., Ohara, K., and Ohara, K. (1997). Serotonin2A receptor gene polymorphism in mood disorders. *Biol Psychiatry*, 41(7), 768–773.

Zubenko, G.S., Hughes, H.B. III, Maher, B.S., Stiffler, J.S., Zubenko, W.N., and Marazita, M.L. (2002). Genetic linkage of region containing the CREB1 gene to depressive disorders in women from families with recurrent, early-onset, major depression. *Am J Med Genet*, 114(8), 980–987.

Zubenko, G.S., Maher, B., Hughes, H.B. III, Zubenko, W.N., Stiffler, J.S., Kaplan, B.B., and Marazita, M.L. (2003). Genome-wide linkage survey for genetic loci that influence the development of depressive disorders in families with recurrent, early-onset, major depression. *Am J Med Genet B Neuropsychiatr Genet*, 123(1), 1–18.

Chapter 14

Abarca, C., Albrecht, U., and Spanagel, R. (2002). Cocaine sensitization and reward are under the influence of circadian genes and rhythm. *Proc Natl Acad Sci USA*, 99, 9026–9030.

Aberg-Wistedt, A., Hasselmark, L., Stain-Malmgren, R., Aperia, B., Kjellman, B.F., and Mathe, A.A. (1998). Serotonergic "vulnerability" in affective disorder: a study of the tryptophan depletion test and relationships between peripheral and central serotonin indexes in citalopram-responders. *Acta Psychiatr Scand*, 97, 374–380.

Abou-Saleh, M.T., and Coppen, A. (1989). The efficacy of low-dose lithium: Clinical, psychological and biological correlates. *J Psychiatr Res*, 23, 157–162.

Adams, J.M., and Cory, S. (1998). The Bcl-2 protein family: Arbiters of cell survival. *Science*, 281, 1322–1326.

Aguiar, M.S., and Brandao, M.L. (1996). Effects of microinjections of the neuropeptide substance P in the dorsal periqueductal grey on the behaviour of rats in the plus mazetest. *Physiol Behav*, 60, 1183–1186.

Ahluwalia, P., and Singhal, R.L. (1980). Effect of low-dose lithium administration and subsequent withdrawal on biogenic amines in rat brain. *Br J Pharmacol*, 71, 601–607.

Ahluwalia, P., Grewaal, D.S., and Singhal, R.L. (1981). Brain GABA-ergic and dopaminergic systems following lithium treatment and withdrawal. *Prog Neuropsychopharmacol*, 5, 527–530.

Aigner, T., Weiss, S.R.B., and Post, R.M. (1990). Carbamazepine attenuates i.v. cocaine self-administration in rhesus monkeys. *Am Coll Neuropsychopharmacol San Juan*, 181.

Akagawa, K., Watanabe, M., and Tsukada, Y. (1980). Activity of erythrocyte Na,K-ATPase in manic patients. *J Neurochem*, 35, 258–260.

Albert, I., Cicala, G.A., and Siegel, J. (1970). The behavioral effects of REM sleep deprivation in rats. *Psychophysiology*, 6, 550–560.

Albright, P.S., and Burnham, W.M. (1980). Development of a new pharmacological seizure model: Effects of anticonvulsants on cortical- and amygdala-kindled seizures in the rat. *Epilepsia*, 21, 681–689.

Alda, M., Turecki, G., Grof, P., Cavazzoni, P., Duffy, A., Grof, E., Ahrens, B., Berghofer, A., Muller-Oerlinghausen, B., Dvorakova, M., Libigerova, E., Vojtechovsky, M., Zvolsky, P., Joober, R., Nilsson, A., Prochazka, H., Licht, R.W., Rasmussen, N.A., Schou, M., Vestergaard, P., Holzinger, A., Schumann, C., Thau, K., and Rouleau, G.A. (2000). Association and linkage studies of CRH and PENK genes in bipolar disorder: A collaborative IGSLI study. *Am J Med Genet*, 96, 178–181.

Alda, M., Keller, D., Grof, E., Turecki, G., Cavazzoni, P., Duffy, A., Rouleau, G.A., Grof, P., and Young, L.T. (2001). Is lithium response related to G(s)alpha levels in transformed lymphoblasts from subjects with bipolar disorder? *J Affect Disord*, 65(2), 117–122.

Alexander, D.R., Deeb, M., Bitar, F., and Antun, F. (1986). Sodium-potassium, magnesium, and calcium ATPase activities in erythrocyte membranes from manic-depressive patients responding to lithium. *Biol Psychiatry*, 21, 997–1007.

Allada, R., Emery, P., Takahashi, J.S., and Rosbash, M. (2001). Stopping time: The genetics of fly and mouse circadian clocks. *Annu Rev Neurosci*, 24, 1091–1119.

Allard, P., and Norlén, M. (1997). Unchanged density of caudate nucleus dopamine uptake sites in depressed suicide victims. *J Neural Transm*, 104, 1353–1360.

Allison, J.H., and Stewart, M.A. (1971). Reduced brain inositol in lithium-treated rats. *Nat New Biol*, 233, 267–268.

Alrecht, J., and Muller-Oerlinghausen, B. (1976). Clinical relevance of lithium determination in RBC: Results of a catamnestic study [in German]. *Arzneimittelforschung*, 26(6), 1145–1147.

Altamura, C.A., Mauri, M.C., Ferrara, A., Moro, A.R., D'Andrea, G., and Zamberlan, F. (1993). Plasma and platelet excitatory amino acids in psychiatric disorders. *Am J Psychiatry*, 150, 1731–1733.

Altshuler, L.L., Casanova, M.F., Goldberg, T.E., and Kleinman, J.E. (1990). The hippocampus and parahippocampus in schizophrenic, suicide, and control brains. *Arch Gen Psychiatry*, 47, 1029–1034.

Alvarez, G., Munoz-Montano, J.R., Satrustegui, J., Avila, J., Bogonez, E., and Diaz-Nido, J. (1999). Lithium protects cultured neurons against beta-amyloid-induced neurodegeneration. *FEBS Lett*, 453, 260–264.

Amsterdam, J.D. (1991). Use of high dose tranylcypromine in resistant depression. In J.D. Amsterdam (Ed.), *Advances in Neuropsychiatry and Psychopharmacology: Refractory Depression* (Vol. 2) (pp. 123–130). New York: Raven Press.

Amsterdam, J.D., Winokur, A., Caroff, S., and Mendels, J. (1981). Thyrotropin-releasing hormone's mood-elevating effects in depressed patients, anorectic patients, and normal volunteers. *Am J Psychiatry*, 138, 115–116.

Anand, A., Darnell, A., Miller, H.L., Berman, R.M., Cappiello, A., Oren, D.A., Woods, S.W., and Charney, D.S. (1999). Effect of catecholamine depletion on lithium-induced long-term remission of bipolar disorder. *Biol Psychiatry*, 45, 972–978.

Anand, A., Charney, D.S., Oren, D.A., Berman, R.M., Hu, X.S., Cappiello, A., and Krystal, J.H. (2000a). Attenuation of the neuropsychiatric effects of ketamine with lamotrigine: Support for hyperglutamatergic effects of N-methyl-D-aspartate receptor antagonists. *Arch Gen Psychiatry*, 57, 270–276.

Anand, A., Verhoeff, P., Seneca, N., Zoghbi, S.S., Seibyl, J.P., Charney, D.S., and Innis, R.B. (2000b). Brain SPECT imaging of amphetamine-induced dopamine release in euthymic bipolar disorder patients. *Am J Psychiatry*, 157, 1108–1114.

Andersen, P.H., and Geisler, A. (1984). Lithium inhibition of forskolin-stimulated adenylate cyclase. *Neuropsychobiology*, 12, 1–3.

Anderson, G.M., and Horne, W.C. (1992). Activators of protein kinase C decrease serotonin transport in human platelets. *Biochim Biophys Acta*, 1137, 331–337.

Andersson, A., Eriksson, A., and Marcusson, J. (1992). Unaltered number of brain serotonin uptake sites in suicide victims. *J Psychopharmacol*, 6, 509–513.

Angers, A., Fioravante, D., Chin, J., Cleary, L.J., Bean, A.J., and Byrne, J.H. (2002). Serotonin stimulates phosphorylation of aplysia synapsin and alters its subcellular distribution in sensory neurons. *J Neurosci*, 22, 5412–5422.

Angst, J., Autenreith, V., Brem, F., Koukkou, M., Meyer, H., Stassen, H.H., and Storck, U. (1979). Preliminary results of treatment with β-endorphin in depression. In E. Usdin, W.E., Bunney, and N.S. Kline (Eds.), *Endorphins in Mental Health Research* (pp. 518–528). New York: Oxford University Press.

Anlezark, G.M., Horton, R.W., Meldrum, B.S., Sawaya, M.C., and Stephenson, J.D. (1976). Proceedings: Gamma-aminobutyric acid metabolism and the anticonvulsant action of ethanolamine-O-sulphate and di-N-propylacetate. *Br J Pharmacol*, 56, 383P–384P.

Ansseau, M., von Frenckell, R., Cerfontaine, J.L., Papart, P., Franck, G., Timsit-Berthier, M., Geenen, V., and Legros, J.J. (1987). Neuroendocrine evaluation of catecholaminergic neurotransmission in mania. *Psychiatry Res*, 22, 193–206.

Ansseau, M., Von Frenckell, R., Cerfontaine, J.L., Papart, P., Franck, G., Timsit-Berthier, M., Geenen, V., and Legros, J.J. (1988). Blunted response of growth hormone to clonidine and apomorphine in endogenous depression. *Br J Psychiatry*, 153, 65–71.

Antelman, S.M., and Caggiula, A.R. (1996). Oscillation follows drug sensitization: Implications. *Crit Rev Neurobiol*, 10, 101–117.

Antelman, S.M., Caggiula, A.R., Kiss, S., Edwards, D.J., Kocan, D., and Stiller, R. (1995). Neurochemical and physiological effects of cocaine oscillate with sequential drug treatment: Possibly a major factor in drug variability. *Neuropsychopharmacology*, 12(4), 297–306.

Antelman, S.M., Caggiula, A.R., Kucinski, B.J., Fowler, H., Gershon, S., Edwards, D.J., Austin, M.C., Stiller, R., Kiss, S., and Kocan, D. (1998). The effects of lithium on a potential cycling model of bipolar disorder. *Prog Neuropsychopharmacol Biol Psychiatry*, 22, 495–510.

Antoniou, K., Kafetzopoulos, E., Papadopoulou-Daifoti, Z., Hyphantis, T., and Marselos, M. (1998). D-amphetamine, cocaine and caffeine: A comparative study of acute effects on locomotor activity and behavioural patterns in rats. *Neurosci Biobehav Rev*, 23, 189–196.

Apparsundaram, S., Galli, A., DeFelice, L.J., Hartzell, H.C., and Blakely, R.D. (1998). Acute regulation of norepinephrine transport: I. Protein kinase C–linked muscarinic receptors influence transport capacity and transporter density in SK-N-SH cells. *J Pharmacol Exp Ther*, 287, 733–743.

Arana, G.W., Barreira, P.J., Cohen, B.M., Lipinski, J.F., and Fogelson, D. (1983). The dexamethasone suppression test in psychotic disorders. *Am J Psychiatry*, 140, 1521–1523.

Arango, V., Ernsberger, P., Marzuk, P.M., Chen, J.S., Tierney, H., Stanley, M., Reis, D.J., and Mann, J.J. (1990). Autoradiographic demonstration of increased serotonin 5-HT$_2$ and beta-adrenergic receptor binding sites in the brain of suicide victims. *Arch Gen Psychiatry*, 47, 1038–1047.

Arango, V., Ernsberger, P., Sved, A.F., and Mann, J.J. (1993). Quantitative autoradiography of alpha 1- and alpha 2-adrenergic receptors in the cerebral cortex of controls and suicide victims. *Brain Res*, 630(1-2), 271–282.

Arango, V., Underwood, M.D., Gubbi, A.V., and Mann, J.J. (1995). Localized alterations in pre- and postsynaptic serotonin binding sites in the ventrolateral prefrontal cortex of suicide victims. *Brain Res*, 688, 121–133.

Arango, V., Underwood, M.D., and Mann, J.J. (1996a). Fewer pigmented locus coeruleus neurons in suicide victims: Preliminary results. *Biol Psychiatry*, 39(2), 112–120.

Arango, V., Underwood, M.D., Pauler, D.K., Kass, R.E., and Mann, J.J. (1996b). Differential age-related loss of pigmented locus coeruleus neurons in suicides, alcoholics, and alcoholic suicides. *Alcohol Clin Exp Res*, 20(7), 1141–1147.

Arato, M., Tekes, K., Tothfalusi, L., Magyar, K., Palkovits, M., Demeter, E., and Falus, A. (1987). Serotonergic split brain and suicide. *Psychiatry Res*, 21, 355–356.

Arato, M., Banki, C.M., Bissette, G., and Nemeroff, C.B. (1989). Elevated CSF CRF in suicide victims. *Biol Psychiatry*, 25, 355–359.

Arendt, T., Lehmann, K., Seeger, G., and Gartner, U. (1999). Synergistic effects of tetrahydroaminoacridine and lithium on cholinergic function after excitotoxic basal forebrain lesions in rat. *Pharmacopsychiatry*, 32, 242–247.

Arnsten, A.F., Mathew, R., Ubriani, R., Taylor, J.R., and Li, B.M. (1999). Alpha-1 noradrenergic receptor stimulation impairs prefrontal cortical cognitive function. *Biol Psychiatry*, 45, 26–31.

Arora, R.C., and Meltzer, H.Y. (1989a). 3H-imipramine binding in the frontal cortex of suicides. *Psychiatry Res*, 30, 125–135.

Arora, R.C., and Meltzer, H.Y. (1989b). Increased serotonin2 (5-HT$_2$) receptor binding as measured by 3H-lysergic acid diethylamide (3H-LSD) in the blood platelets of depressed patients. *Life Sci*, 44, 725–734.

Arora, R.C., and Meltzer, H.Y. (1991). Laterality and 3H-imipramine binding: Studies in the frontal cortex of normal controls and suicide victims. *Biol Psychiatry*, 29, 1016–1022.

Arora, R.C., and Meltzer, H.Y. (1993). Serotonin2 receptor binding in blood platelets of schizophrenic patients. *Psychiatry Res*, 47, 111–119.

Arranz, B., Blennow, K., Eriksson, A., Mansson, J.E., and Marcusson, J. (1997). Serotonergic, noradrenergic, and dopaminergic measures in suicide brains. *Biol Psychiatry*, 41, 1000–1009.

Artigas, F., Sarrias, M.J., Martinez, E., Gelpi, E., Alvarez, E., and Udina, C. (1989). Increased plasma free serotonin but unchanged platelet serotonin in bipolar patients treated chronically with lithium. *Psychopharmacology (Berl)*, 99, 328–332.

Arystarkhova, E., and Sweadner, K.J. (1996). Isoform-specific monoclonal antibodies to Na,K-ATPase alpha subunits. Evidence for a tissue-specific post-translational modification of the alpha subunit. *J Biol Chem*, 271, 23407–23417.

Asberg, M., Bertilsson, L., Tuck, D., Cronholm, B., and Sjoqvist, F. (1973). Indoleamine metabolites in the cerebrospinal fluid of depressed patients before and during treatment with nortriptyline. *Clin Pharmacol Ther*, 14, 277–286.

Asberg, M., Bertilsson, L., and Martensson, B. (1984). CSF monoamine metabolites, depression, and suicide. *Adv Biochem Psychopharmacol*, 39, 87–97.

Asghar, S.J., Tanay, V.A., Baker, G.B., Greenshaw, A., and Silverstone, P.H. (2003). Relationship of plasma amphetamine levels to physiological, subjective, cognitive and biochemical measures in healthy volunteers. *Hum Psychopharmacol*, 18(4), 291–299.

Ashcroft, G.W., Blackburn, I.M., Eccleston, D., Glen, A.I., Hartley, W., Kinloch, N.E., Lonergan, M., Murray, L.G., and Pullar, I.A. (1973). Changes on recovery in the concentrations of tryptophan and the biogenic amine metabolites in the cerebrospinal fluid of patients with affective illness. *Psychol Med*, 3, 319–325.

Asnis, G.M., Sachar, E.J., Halbreich, U., Nathan, R.S., Ostrow, L., and Halpern, F.S. (1981). Cortisol secretion and dexamethasone response in depression. *Am J Psychiatry*, 138, 1218–1221.

Aston, C., Jiang, L., and Sokolov, B.P. (2004). Microarray analysis of postmortem temporal cortex from patients with schizophrenia. *J Neurosci Res*, 77(6), 858–866.

Aston, C., Jiang, L., and Sokolov, B.P. (2005). Transcriptional profiling reveals evidence for signaling and oligodendroglial abnormalities in the temporal cortex from patients with major depressive disorder. *Mol Psychiatry*, 10(3), 309–322.

Atack, J.R. (1996). Inositol monophosphatase, the putative therapeutic target for lithium. *Brain Res Brain Res Rev*, 22(2), 183–190.

Atkinson, J.H., Jr., Kremer, E.F., Risch, S.C., and Janowsky, D.S. (1986). Basal and post-dexamethasone cortisol and prolactin concentrations in depressed and non-depressed patients with chronic pain syndromes. *Pain*, 25, 23–34.

Attar-Levy, D., Martinot, J.L., Blin, J., Dao-Castellana, M.H., Crouzel, C., Mazoyer, B., Poirier, M.F., Bourdel, M.C., Aymard, N., Syrota, A., and Feline, A. (1999). The cortical serotonin2 receptors studied with positron-emission tomography and [18F]-setoperone during depressive illness and antidepressant treatment with clomipramine. *Biol Psychiatry*, 45, 180–186.

Auer, D.P., Putz, B., Kraft, E., Lipinski, B., Schill, J., and Holsboer, F. (2000). Reduced glutamate in the anterior cingulate cortex in depression: An in vivo proton magnetic resonance spectroscopy study. *Biol Psychiatry*, 47, 305–313.

Aujla, H., and Beninger, R.J. (2003). Intra-accumbens protein kinase C inhibitor NPC 15437 blocks amphetamine-produced conditioned place preference in rats. *Behav Brain Res*, 147(1-2), 41–48.

Austin, J., Hoogendoorn, B., Buckland, P., Jones, I., McCandless, F., Williams, N., Middle, F., Owen, M.J., Craddock, N., and O'Donovan, M.C. (2000). Association analysis of the proneurotensin gene and bipolar disorder. *Psychiatr Genet*, 10(1), 51–54.

Avissar, S., Barki-Harrington, L., Nechamkin, Y., Roitman, G., and Schreiber, G. (1996). Reduced beta-adrenergic receptor-coupled Gs protein function and Gs alpha immunoreactivity in mononuclear leukocytes of patients with depression. *Biol Psychiatry*, 39, 755–760.

Avissar, S., Nechamkin, Y., Barki-Harrington, L., Roitman, G., and Schreiber, G. (1997). Differential G protein measures in mononuclear leukocytes of patients with bipolar mood disorder are state dependent. *J Affect Disord*, 43, 85–93.

Axelrod, J., and Reisine, T.D. (1984). Stress hormones: Their interaction and regulation. *Science*, 224, 452–459.

Azorin, J.M., Tramoni, V. (1987). Kindling models and antikindling effects of mood normalizers. *Pharmacopsychiatry*, 20, 189–191.

Bach, R.O., and Gallicchio, V.S. (1990). *Lithium and Cell Physiology* (June Edition). New York: Springer Verlag.

Bachmann, C.G., Linthorst, A.C., Holsboer, F., and Reul, J.M. (2003). Effect of chronic administration of selective glucocorticoid receptor antagonists on the rat hypothalamic–pituitary–adrenocortical axis. *Neuropsychopharmacology*, 28(6), 1056–1067.

Bachmann, R.F., Schloesser, R.J., Gould, T.D., and Manji, H.K. (2005). Mood stabilizers target cellular plasticity and resilience cascades: Implications for the development of novel therapeutics. *Mol Neurobiol*, 32(2), 173–202.

Bachus, S.E., Hyde, T.M., Akil, M., Weickert, C.S., Vawter, M.P., and Kleinman, J.E. (1997). Neuropathology of suicide. A review and an approach. *Ann NY Acad Sci*, 836, 201–219.

Backstrom, P., and Hyytia, P. (2003). Attenuation of cocaine-seeking behaviour by the AMPA/kainate receptor antagonist CNQX in rats. *Psychopharmacology (Berl)*, 166(1), 69–76.

Baghai, T.C., Schule, C., Zwanzger, P., Minov, C., Zill, P., Ella, R., Eser, D., Oezer, S., Bondy, B., and Rupprecht, R. (2002). Hypothalamic–pituitary–adrenocortical axis dysregulation in patients with major depression is influenced by the insertion/deletion polymorphism in the angiotensin I-converting enzyme gene. *Neurosci Lett*, 328, 299–303.

Bahr, B.A., Bendiske, J., Brown, Q.B., Munirathinam, S., Caba, E., Rudin M., Urwyler, S., Sauter, A., and Rogers, G. (2002). Survival signaling and selective neuroprotection through glutamatergic transmission. *Exp Neurol*, 174, 37–47.

Bakchine, S., Lacomblez, L., Benoit, N., Parisot, D., Chain, F., and Lhermitte, F. (1989). Manic-like state after bilateral orbitofrontal and right temporoparietal injury: Efficacy of clonidine. *Neurology*, 39, 777–781.

Baker, E.F. (1971). Sodium transfer to cerebrospinal fluid in functional psychiatric illness. *Can Psychiatr Assoc J*, 16, 167–170.

Baker, K.A., Hong, M., Sadi, D., and Mendez, I. (2000). Intrastriatal and intranigral grafting of hNT neurons in the 6-OHDA rat model of Parkinson's disease. *Exp Neurol*, 162, 350–360.

Ballenger, J.C., Post, R.M., Gold, P.W., Goodwin, F.K., Bunney, W.E., and Robertson, G. (1980). *Endocrine correlates of personality and cognition in normals* (pp. 144–145). 133rd Annual Meeting of the American Psychiatric Association.

Baltuch, G.H., Couldwell, W.T., Villemure, J.G., and Yong, V.W. (1993). Protein kinase C inhibitors suppress cell growth in established and low-passage glioma cell lines. A comparison between staurosporine and tamoxifen. *Neurosurgery*, 33:495–501; discussion 501.

Banay-Schwartz, M., DeGuzman, T., Faludi, G., Lajtha, A., and Palkovits, M. (1998). Alteration of protease levels in different brain areas of suicide victims. *Neurochem Res*, 23, 953–959.

Banerjee, S.P., Kung, L.S., Riggi, S.J., and Chanda, S.K. (1977). Development of beta-adrenergic receptor subsensitivity by antidepressants. *Nature*, 268, 455–456.

Banki, C.M., Bissette, G., Arato, M., O'Connor, L., and Nemeroff, C.B. (1987). CSF corticotropin-releasing factor-like immunoreactivity in depression and schizophrenia. *Am J Psychiatry*, 144, 873–877.

Banki, C.M., Bissette, G., Arato, M., and Nemeroff, C.B. (1988). Elevation of immunoreactive CSF TRH in depressed patients. *Am J Psychiatry*, 145, 1526–1531.

Banki, C.M., Karmacsi, L., Bissette, G., and Nemeroff, C.B. (1992). CSF corticotropin-releasing hormone and somatostatin in major depression: Response to antidepressant treatment and relapse. *Eur Neuropsychopharmacol*, 2, 107–113.

Baptista, T., Weiss, S.R., Post, R.M. (1993). Carbamazepine attenuates cocaine-induced increases in dopamine in the nucleus accumbens: An in vivo dialysis study. *Eur J Pharmacol*, 236, 39–42.

Barbini, B., Colombo, C., Benedetti, F., Campori, E., Bellodi, L., and Smeraldi, E. (1998). The unipolar–bipolar dichotomy and the response to sleep deprivation. *Psychiatry Res*, 79, 43–50.

Barnes, R.F., Veith, R.C., Borson, S., Verhey, J., Raskind, M.A., and Halter, J.B. (1983). High levels of plasma catecholamines in dexamethasone-resistant depressed patients. *Am J Psychiatry*, 140, 1623–1625.

Bartalena, L., Pellegrini, L., Meschi, M., Antonangeli, L., Bogazzi, F., Dell'Osso, L., Pinchera, A., and Placidi, G.F. (1990). Evaluation of thyroid function in patients with rapid-cycling and non-rapid-cycling bipolar disorder. *Psychiatry Res*, 34, 13–17.

Basturk, M., Karaaslan, F., Esel, E., Sofuoglu, S., Tutus, A., and Yabanoglu, I. (2001). Effects of short- and long-term lithium treatment on serum prolactin levels in patients with bipolar affective disorder. *Prog Neuropsychopharmacol Biol Psychiatry*, 25, 315–322.

Bauer, M.S., and Whybrow, P.C. (1988). *Rapid cycling bipolar affective disorder: Thyroid function and response to adjuvant treatment with high-dose thyroxine.* 43rd Annual meeting of the Society of Biological Psychiatry.

Bauer, M.S., and Whybrow, P.C. (1990). Rapid cycling bipolar affective disorder. II. Treatment of refractory rapid cycling with high-dose levothyroxine: A preliminary study. *Arch Gen Psychiatry*, 47, 435–440.

Bauer, M.S., Whybrow, P.C., and Winokur, A. (1990). Rapid cycling bipolar affective disorder. I. Association with grade I hypothyroidism. *Arch Gen Psychiatry*, 47(5), 427–432.

Bauer, M.S., Hellweg, R., Graf, K.J., and Baumgartner, A. (1998a). Treatment of refractory depression with high-dose thyroxine. *Neuropsychopharmacology*, 18, 444–455.

Bauer, M.S., Hellweg, R., and Baumgartner, A. (1998b). High dosage thyroxine treatment in therapy and prevention refractory patients with affective psychoses. *Nervenarzt*, 69(11), 1019–1022.

Bauman, A.L., Apparsundaram, S., Ramamoorthy, S., Wadzinski, B.E., Vaughan, R.A., and Blakely, R.D. (2000). Cocaine and antidepressant-sensitive biogenic amine transporters exist in regulated complexes with protein phosphatase 2A. *J Neurosci*, 20, 7571–7578.

Baumann, B., Danos, P., Krell, D., Diekmann, S., Wurthmann, C., Bielau, H., Bernstein, H.G., and Bogerts, B. (1999a). Unipolar–bipolar dichotomy of mood disorders is supported by noradrenergic brainstem system morphology. *J Affect Disord*, 54, 217–224.

Baumann, B., Danos, P., Krell, D., Diekmann, S., Leschinger, A., Stauch, R., Wurthmann, C., Bernstein, H.G., and Bogerts, B. (1999b). Reduced volume of limbic system–affiliated basal ganglia in mood disorders: Preliminary data from a postmortem study. *J Neuropsychiatry Clin Neurosci*, 11, 71–78.

Baumgartner, A., Graf, K. J., Kurten, I., Meinhold, H., and Scholz, P. (1990a). Neuroendocrinological investigations during sleep deprivation in depression. I. Early morning levels of thyrotropin, TH, cortisol, prolactin, LH, FSH, estradiol, and testosterone. *Biol Psychiatry*, 28(7), 556–568.

Baumgartner, A., Riemann, D., and Berger, M. (1990b). Neuroendocrinological investigations during sleep deprivation in depression. II. Longitudinal measurement of thyrotropin, TH, cortisol, prolactin, GH, and LH during sleep and sleep deprivation. *Biol Psychiatry*, 28(7), 569–587.

Baumgartner, A., Bauer, M., and Hellweg, R. (1994). Treatment of intractable non-rapid cycling bipolar affective disorder with high-dose thyroxine: An open clinical trial. *Neuropsychopharmacology*, 10, 183–189.

Bebchuk, J.M., Arfken, C.L., Dolan-Manji, S., Murphy, J., Hasanat, K., and Manji, H.K. (2000). A preliminary investigation of a protein kinase C inhibitor in the treatment of acute mania. *Arch Gen Psychiatry*, 57, 95–97.

Bech, P., Kirkegaard, C., Bock, E., Johannesen, M., and Rafaelsen, O.J. (1978). Hormones, electrolytes, and cerebrospinal fluid proteins in manic-melancholic patients. *Neuropsychobiology*, 4, 99–112.

Beckmann, H., and Jakob, H. (1991). Prenatal disturbances of nerve cell migration in the entorhinal region: A common vulnerability factor in functional psychoses? *J Neural Transm*, 84, 155–164.

Beckmann, H., St.-Laurent, J., and Goodwin, F.K. (1975). The effect of lithium on urinary MHPG in unipolar and bipolar depressed patients. *Psychopharmacologia*, 42, 277–282.

Belanoff, J.K., Kalehzan, M., Sund, B., Fleming Ficek, S.K., and Schatzberg, A.F. (2001). Cortisol activity and cognitive changes in psychotic major depression. *Am J Psychiatry*, 158(10), 1612–1616.

Belanoff, J.K., Rothschild, A.J., Cassidy, F., DeBattista, C., Baulieu, E.E., Schold, C., and Schatzberg, A.F. (2002). An open label trial of c-1073 (mifepristone) for psychotic major depression. *Biol Psychiatry*, 52(5), 386–392.

Bellivier, F., Henry, C., Szoke, A., Schurhoff, F., Nosten-Bertrand, M., Feingold, J., Launay, J.M., Leboyer, M., and Laplanche, J.L. (1998a). Serotonin transporter gene polymorphisms in patients with unipolar or bipolar depression. *Neurosci Lett*, 255, 143–146.

Bellivier, F., Leboyer, M., Courtet, P., Buresi, C., Beaufils, B., Samolyk, D., Allilaire, J.F., Feingold, J., Mallet, J., and Malafosse, A. (1998b). Association between the tryptophan hydroxylase gene and manic-depressive illness. *Arch Gen Psychiatry*, 55, 33–37.

Benazzi, F. (1998). Mania associated with donepezil. *Int J Geriatr Psychiatry*, 13, 814–815.

Benazzi, F. (1999). Mania associated with donepezil. *J Psychiatry Neurosci*, 24, 468–469.

Benedetti, F., Colombo, C., Barbini, B., Campori, E., and Smeraldi, E. (1999). Ongoing lithium treatment prevents relapse after total sleep deprivation. *J Clin Psychopharmacol*, 19, 240–245.

Benes, F.M., Kwok, E.W., Vincent, S.L., and Todtenkopf, M.S. (1998). A reduction of nonpyramidal cells in sector CA2 of schizophrenics and manic depressives. *Biol Psychiatry*, 44, 88–97.

Benes, F.M., Todtenkopf, M.S., Logiotatos, P., and Williams, M. (2000). Glutamate decarboxylase(65)-immunoreactive terminals in cingulate and prefrontal cortices of schizophrenic and bipolar brain. *J Chem Neuroanat*, 20, 259–269.

Benes, F.M., Vincent, S.L., and Todtenkopf, M. (2001). The density of pyramidal and nonpyramidal neurons in anterior cingulate cortex of schizophrenic and bipolar subjects. *Biol Psychiatry*, 50(6), 395–406.

Benes, F.M., Matzilevich, D., Burke, R.E., and Walsh, J. (2006). The expression of proapoptosis genes is increased in bipolar disorder, but not in schizophrenia. *Mol Psychiatry*, 11(3), 241–251.

Benkelfat, C., Seletti, B., Palmour, R.M., Hillel, J., Ellenbogen, M., and Young, S.N. (1995). Tryptophan depletion in stable lithium-treated patients with bipolar disorder in remission. *Arch Gen Psychiatry*, 52, 154–156.

Berger, M., Riemann, D., Hochli, D., and Spiegel, R. (1989). The cholinergic rapid eye movement sleep induction test with RS-86. State or trait marker of depression? *Arch Gen Psychiatry*, 46, 421–428.

Berger, M., Riemann, D., and Krieg, C. (1991). Cholinergic drugs as diagnostic and therapeutic tools in affective disorders. *Acta Psychiatr Scand Suppl*, 366, 52–60.

Berggren, U. (1985). Effects of chronic lithium treatment on brain monoamine metabolism and amphetamine-induced locomotor stimulation in rats. *J Neural Transm*, 64, 239–250.

Bergquist, J., Bergquist, S., Axelsson, R., and Ekman, R. (1993). Demonstration of immunoglobulin G with affinity for dopamine in cerebrospinal fluid from psychotic patients. *Clin Chim Acta*, 217, 129–142.

Bergstrom, D.A., and Kellar, K.J. (1979). Effect of electroconvulsive shock on monoaminergic receptor binding sites in rat brain. *Nature*, 278, 464–466.

Berk, M. (1999). Lamotrigine and the treatment of mania in bipolar disorder. *Eur Neuropsychopharmacol*, 9(Suppl. 4), S119–S123.

Berk, M., Bodemer, W., van Oudenhove, T., and Butkow, N. (1994). Dopamine increases platelet intracellular calcium in bipolar affective disorder and controls. *Int Clin Psychopharmacol*, 9(4), 291–293.

Berk, M., Kirchmann, N.H., and Butkow, N. (1996). Lithium blocks 45Ca^{2+} uptake into platelets in bipolar affective disorder and controls. *Clin Neuropharmacol*, 19(1), 48–51.

Berk, M., Plein, H., and Ferreira, D. (2001). Platelet glutamate receptor supersensitivity in major depressive disorder. *Clin Neuropharmacol*, 24, 129–132.

Berman, R.M., Cappiello, A., Anand, A., Oren, D.A., Heninger, G.R., Charney, D.S., and Krystal, J.H. (2000). Antidepressant effects of ketamine in depressed patients. *Biol Psychiatry*, 47, 351–354.

Bernasconi, R. (1982). The GABA hypothesis of affective illness: Influence of clinically effective antimanic drugs on GABA turnover. In H.M. Emrich, J.B. Aldenhoff, H.D., and Lux (Eds.), *Basic Mechanisms in the Action of Lithium* (pp. 183–192). Amsterdam: Excerpta Medica.

Bernstein, H.G., Stanarius, A., Baumann, B., Henning, H., Krell, D., Danos, P., Falkai, P., and Bogerts, B. (1998). Nitric oxide synthase–containing neurons in the human hypothalamus: Reduced number of immunoreactive cells in the paraventricular nucleus of depressive patients and schizophrenics. *Neuroscience*, 83, 867–875.

Berrettini, W.H., and Post, R.M. (1984). GABA in affective illness. In *Neurobiology of Mood Disorders* (pp. 673–685). Baltimore: Williams & Wilkins.

Berrettini, W.H., Umberkoman-Wiita, B., Nurnberger, J.I., Jr., Vogel, W.H., Gershon, E.S., and Post, R.M. (1982). Platelet GABA-transaminase in affective illness. *Psychiatry Res*, 7, 255–260.

Berrettini, W.H., Nurnberger, J.I. Jr., Hare, T.A., Simmons-Alling, S., Gershon, E.S., and Post, R.M. (1983). Reduced plasma and CSF gamma-aminobutyric acid in affective illness: Effect of lithium carbonate. *Biol Psychiatry*, 18, 185–194.

Berrettini, W.H., Nurnberger, J.I. Jr., Gold, P.W., Chretien, M., Chrousos, G.P., Chan, J.S., Goldin, L.R., and Gershon, E.S. (1985a). Neuropeptides in human cerebrospinal fluid. *Life Sci*, 37, 1265–1270.

Berrettini, W.H., Nurnberger, J.I. Jr., Scheinin, M., Seppala, T., Linnoila, M., Narrow, W., Simmons-Alling, S., and Gershon, E.S. (1985b). Cerebrospinal fluid and plasma monoamines and their metabolites in euthymic bipolar patients. *Biol Psychiatry*, 20, 257–269.

Berrettini, W.H., Runinow, D.R., Nurnberger, J.I., Simmons-Alling, S., Post, R.M., and Gershon, E.S. (1985c). CSF substance P immunoreactivity in affective disorders. *Biol Psychiatry*, 20(9), 965–970.

Berrettini, W.H., Nurnberger, J.I. Jr., Hare, T.A., Simmons-Alling, S., and Gershon, E.S. (1986). CSF GABA in euthymic manic-depressive patients and controls. *Biol Psychiatry*, 21, 844–846.

Berrettini, W.H., Nurnberger, J.I. Jr., Zerbe, R.L., Gold, P.W., Chrousos, G.P., and Tomai, T. (1987). CSF neuropeptides in euthymic bipolar patients and controls. *Br J Psychiatry*, 150, 208–212.

Berridge, M.J., and Irvine, R.F. (1989). Inositol phosphates and cell signalling. *Nature*, 341, 197–205.

Berridge, M.J., Downes, C.P., and Hanley, M.R. (1982). Lithium amplifies agonist-dependent phosphatidylinositol responses in brain and salivary glands. *Biochem J*, 206, 587–595.

Berridge, M.J., Downes, C.P., and Hanley, M.R. (1989). Neural and developmental actions of lithium: A unifying hypothesis. *Cell*, 59, 411–419.

Berton, O., and Nestler, E.J. (2006). New approaches to antidepressant drug discovery: Beyond monoamines. *Nat Rev Neurosci*, 7(2), 137–151.

Beskow, J., Gottfries, C.G., Roos, B.E., and Winblad, B. (1976). Determination of monoamine and monoamine metabolites in the human brain: Post mortem studies in a group of suicides and in a control group. *Acta Psychiatr Scand*, 53, 7–20.

Beyer, J.L., and Krishnan, K.R. (2002). Volumetric brain imaging findings in mood disorders. *Bipolar Disord*, 4, 89–104.

Bezchlibnyk, Y., and Young, L.T. (2002). The neurobiology of bipolar disorder: Focus on signal transduction pathways and the regulation of gene expression. *Can J Psychiatry*, 47, 135–148.

Bhalla, U.S., and Iyengar, R. (1999). Emergent properties of networks of biological signaling pathways. *Science*, 283, 381–387.

Biegon, A., and Fieldust, S. (1992). Reduced tyrosine hydroxylase immunoreactivity in locus coeruleus of suicide victims. *Synapse*, 10, 79–82.

Biegon, A., and Israeli, M. (1988). Regionally selective increases in beta-adrenergic receptor density in the brains of suicide victims. *Brain Res*, 442, 199–203.

Biegon, A., Weizman, A., Karp, L., Ram, A., Tiano, S., and Wolff, M. (1987). Serotonin 5-HT$_2$ receptor binding on blood platelets—a peripheral marker for depression? *Life Sci*, 41, 2485–2492.

Biegon, A., Essar, N., Israeli, M., Elizur, A., Bruch, S., and Bar-Nathan, A.A. (1990a). Serotonin 5-HT$_2$ receptor binding on blood platelets as a state dependent marker in major affective disorder. *Psychopharmacology (Berl)*, 102, 73–75.

Biegon, A., Grinspoon, A., Blumenfeld, B., Bleich, A., Apter, A., and Mester, R. (1990b). Increased serotonin 5-HT$_2$ receptor binding on blood platelets of suicidal men. *Psychopharmacology (Berl)*, 100, 165–167.

Biggs, C.S., Pearce, B.R., Fowler, L.J., and Whitton, P.S. (1992). Regional effects of sodium valproate on extracellular concentrations of 5-hydroxytryptamine, dopamine, and their metabolites in the rat brain: An in vivo microdialysis study. *J Neurochem, 59*, 1702–1708.

Bijur, G.N., De Sarno, P., and Jope, R.S. (2000). Glycogen synthase kinase-3β facilitates staurosporine- and heat shock-induced apoptosis. Protection by lithium. *J Biol Chem, 275*, 7583–7590.

Binder, E.B., Kinkead, B., Owens, M.J., and Nemeroff, C.B. (2001). The role of neurotensin in the pathophysiology of schizophrenia and the mechanism of action of antipsychotic drugs. *Biol Psychiatry, 50*, 856–872.

Birkett, J.T., Arranz, M.J., Munro, J., Osbourn, S., Kerwin, R.W., and Collier, D.A. (2000). Association analysis of the 5-HT5A gene in depression, psychosis and antipsychotic response. *Neuroreport, 11*, 2017–2020.

Birnbaum, S., Yuan, P.X., Wang, M., Vijayraghaven, S., Bloom, A.K., Davis, D.J., Gobeske, K.T., Sweatt, J.D., Manji, H.K., and Arnsten, A. (2004). Protein kinase C overactivity impairs prefrontal cortical regulation of working memory. *Science, 306*, 882–884.

Biver, F., Lotstra, F., Monclus, M., Dethy, S., Damhaut, P., Wikler, D., Luxen, A., and Goldman, S. (1997). In vivo binding of [18F]altanserin to rat brain 5HT2 receptors: A film and electronic autoradiographic study. *Nucl Med Biol, 24*, 357–360.

Blakely, R.D., Ramamoorthy, S., Schroeter, S., Qian, Y., Apparsundaram, S., Galli, A., and DeFelice, L.J. (1998). Regulated phosphorylation and trafficking of antidepressant-sensitive serotonin transporter proteins. *Biol Psychiatry, 44*, 169–178.

Blancquaert, J.P., Lefebvre, R.A., and Willems, J.L. (1987). Anti-aversive properties of opioids in the conditioned taste aversion test in the rat. *Pharmacol Biochem Behav, 27*, 437–441.

Blehar, M.C., DePaulo, J.R. Jr., Gershon, E.S., Reich, T., Simpson, S.G., and Nurnberger, J.I. Jr. (1998). Women with bipolar disorder: Findings from the NIMH genetics initiative sample. *Psychopharmacol Bull, 34*, 239–243.

Blier, P., and De Montigny, C. (1985). Short-term lithium administration enhances serotonergic neurotransmission: Electrophysiological evidence in the rat CNS. *Eur J Pharmacol, 113*, 69–77.

Blier, P., de Montigny, C., and Tardif, D. (1987). Short-term lithium treatment enhances responsiveness of postsynaptic 5-HT$_{1A}$ receptors without altering 5-HT autoreceptor sensitivity: An electrophysiological study in the rat brain. *Synapse, 1*, 225–232.

Bligh-Glover, W., Kolli, T.N., Shapiro-Kulnane, L., Dilley, G.E., Friedman, L., Balraj, E., Rajkowska, G., and Stockmeier, C.A. (2000). The serotonin transporter in the midbrain of suicide victims with major depression. *Biol Psychiatry, 47*, 1015–1024.

Bloch, M., Schmidt, P.J., Danaceau, M.A., Adams, L.F., and Rubinow, D.R. (1999). Dehydroepiandrosterone treatment of midlife dysthymia. *Biol Psychiatry, 45*(12), 1533–1541.

Bloom, F.E., Baetge, G., Deyo, S., Ettenberg, A., Koda, L., Magistretti, P.J., Shoemaker, W.J., and Staunton, D.A. (1983). Chemical and physiological aspects of the actions of lithium and antidepressant drugs. *Neuropharmacology, 22*(Spec No. 3), 359–365.

Board, F., Wadeson, R., and Persky, H. (1957). Depressive affect and endocrine functions; blood levels of adrenal cortex and thyroid hormones in patients suffering from depressive reactions. *AMA Arch Neurol Psychiatry, 78*, 612–620.

Bodick, N.C., Offen, W.W., Levey, A.I., Cutler, N.R., Gauthier, S.G., Satlin, A., Shannon, H.E., Tollefson, G.D., Rasmussen, K., Bymaster, F.P., Hurley, D.J., Potter, W.Z., and Paul, S.M. (1997). Effects of xanomeline, a selective muscarinic receptor agonist, on cognitive function and behavioral symptoms in Alzheimer disease. *Arch Neurol, 54*, 465–473.

Boerlin, H.L., Gitlin, M.J., Zoellner, L.A., and Hammen, C.L. (1998). Bipolar depression and antidepressant-induced mania: A naturalistic study. *J Clin Psychiatry, 59*, 374–379.

Bohus, B., Kovacs, G.L., and de Wied, D. (1978). Oxytocin, vasopressin and memory: Opposite effects on consolidation and retrieval processes. *Brain Res, 157*, 414–417.

Bond, P.A., Jenner, F.A., and Sampson, G.A. (1972). Daily variations of the urine content of 3-methoxy-4-hydroxyphenylglycol in two manic-depressive patients. *Psychol Med, 2*, 81–85.

Bonnier, B., Gorwood, P., Hamon, M., Sarfati, Y., Boni, C., and Hardy-Bayle, M.C. (2002). Association of 5-HT(2A) receptor gene polymorphism with major affective disorders: The case of a subgroup of bipolar disorder with low suicide risk. *Biol Psychiatry, 51*, 762–765.

Borglum, A.D., Bruun, T.G., Kjeldsen, T.E., Ewald, H., Mors, O., Kirov, G., Russ, C., Freeman, B., Collier, D.A., and Kruse, T.A. (1999). Two novel variants in the DOPA decarboxylase gene: Association with bipolar affective disorder. *Mol Psychiatry, 4*, 545–551.

Born, G.V., Grignani, G., and Martin, K. (1980). Long-term effect of lithium on the uptake of 5-hydroxytryptamine by human platelets. *Br J Clin Pharmacol, 9*, 321–325.

Borsini, F., and Meli, A. (1988). Is the forced swimming test a suitable model for revealing antidepressant activity? *Psychopharmacology (Berl), 94*, 147–160.

Bothwell, R.A., Eccleston, D., and Marshall, E. (1994). Platelet intracellular calcium in patients with recurrent affective disorders. *Psychopharmacology (Berl), 114*(2), 375–381.

Bottlender, R., Rudolf, D., Strauss, A., and Moller, H.J. (2000). Are low basal serum levels of the thyroid stimulating hormone (b-TSH) a risk factor for switches into states of expansive syndromes (known in Germany as "maniform syndromes") in bipolar I depression? *Pharmacopsychiatry, 33*, 75–77.

Bouras, C., Kovari, E., Hof, P.R., Riederer, B.M., and Giannakopoulos, P. (2001). Anterior cingulate cortex pathology schizophrenia and bipolar disorder. *Acta Neuopathol, 102*, 373–379.

Bourne, H.R., and Nicoll, R. (1993). Molecular machines integrate coincident synaptic signals. *Cell, 72*(Suppl.), 65–75.

Bourne, H.R., Bunney, W.E. Jr., Colburn, R.W., Davis, J.M., Davis, J.N., Shaw, D.M., and Coppen, A.J. (1968). Noradrenaline, 5-hydroxytryptamine, and 5-hydroxyindoleacetic acid in hindbrains of suicidal patients. *Lancet, 2*, 805–808.

Bousquet, P., and Feldman, J. (1987). The blood pressure effects of alpha-adrenoceptor antagonists injected in the medullary site of action of clonidine: The nucleus reticularis lateralis. *Life Sci, 40*, 1045–1052.

Bowden, C.L., Huang, L.G., Javors, M.A., Johnson, J.M., Seleshi, E., McIntyre, K., Contreras, S., and Maas, J.W. (1988). Calcium function in affective disorders and healthy controls. *Biol Psychiatry, 23*, 367–376.

Bowden, C.L., Brugger, A.M., Swann, A.C., Calabrese, J.R., Janicak, P.G., Petty, F., Dilsaver, S.C., Davis, J.M., Rush, A.J., and Small, J.G. (1994). Efficacy of divalproex vs. lithium and placebo in the treatment of mania. The Depakote Mania Study Group. *JAMA, 271*, 918–924.

Bowden, C., Cheetham, S.C., Lowther, S., Katona, C.L., Crompton, M.R., and Horton, R.W. (1997a). Dopamine uptake sites, labelled with [3H]GBR12935, in brain samples from depressed suicides and controls. *Eur Neuropsychopharmacol*, 7, 247–252.

Bowden, C., Theodorou, A.E., Cheetham, S.C., Lowther, S., Katona, C.L., Crompton, M.R., and Horton, R.W. (1997b). Dopamine D1 and D2 receptor binding sites in brain samples from depressed suicides and controls. *Brain Res*, 752, 227–233.

Bowden, C., Cheetham, S.C., Lowther, S., Katona, C.L., Crompton, M.R., and Horton, R.W. (1997c). Reduced dopamine turnover in the basal ganglia of depressed suicides. *Brain Res*, 769, 135–140.

Bowden, C.L., Davis, J., Morris, D., Swann, A., Calabrese, J., Lambert, M., and Goodnick, P. (1997d). Effect size of efficacy measures comparing divalproex, lithium and placebo in acute mania. *Depress Anxiety*, 6, 26–30.

Bowen, D.M., Najlerahim, A., Procter, A.W., Francis, P.T., and Murphy, E. (1989). Circumscribed changes of the cerebral cortex in neuropsychiatric disorders of later life. *Proc Natl Acad Sci USA*, 86, 9504–9508.

Bowers, M.B. Jr., and Heninger, G.R. (1977). Lithium: Clinical effects and cerebrospinal fluid acid monoamine metabolites. *Commun Psychopharmacol*, 1, 135–145.

Bowers, M.B. Jr., Mazure, C.M., Nelson, J.C., and Jatlow, P.I. (1992). Lithium in combination with perphenazine: Effect on plasma monoamine metabolites. *Biol Psychiatry*, 32, 1102–1107.

Boyer, P., Davila, M., Schaub, C., Kanowski, S., and Nasset, J. (1986). Growth hormone response to clonidine stimulation in depressive states. Part I. *Psychiatr Psychobiol*, 1, 189–195.

Brake, W.G., Alves, S.E., Dunlop, J.C., Lee, S.J., Bulloch, K., Allen, P.B., Greengard, P., and McEwen, B.S. (2001). Novel target sites for estrogen action in the dorsal hippocampus: An examination of synaptic proteins. *Endocrinology*, 142, 1284–1289.

Browman, K.E., Kantor, L., Richardson, S., Badiani, A., Robinson, T.E., and Gnegy, M.E. (1998). Injection of the protein kinase C inhibitor ro31-8220 into the nucleus accumbens attenuates the acute response to amphetamine: Tissue and behavioral studies. *Brain Res*, 814(1-2), 112–119.

Brown, D.W. (1993). Abnormal fluctuations of acetylcholine and serotonin. *Med Hypotheses*, 40, 309–310.

Brown, W.A., Johnston, R., and Mayfield, D. (1979). The 24-hour dexamethasone suppression test in a clinical setting: Relationship to diagnosis, symptoms, and response to treatment. *Am J Psychiatry*, 136, 543–547.

Brown, A.S., Mallinger, A.G., and Renbaum, L.C. (1993). Elevated platelet membrane phosphatidylinositol-4,5-bisphosphate in bipolar mania. *Am J Psychiatry*, 150, 1252–1254.

Brown, E.S., Rush, A.J., and McEwen, B.S. (1999). Hippocampal remodeling and damage by corticosteroids: Implications for mood disorders. *Neuropsychopharmacology*, 21(4), 474–484.

Brown, E.S., Suppes, T., Khan, D.A., and Carmody, T.J. III. (2002). Mood changes during prednisone bursts in outpatients with asthma. *J Clin Psychopharmacol*, 22(1), 55–61.

Bruckheimer, E.M., Cho, S.H., Sarkiss, M., Herrmann, J., and McDonnell, T.J. (1998). The Bcl-2 gene family and apoptosis. *Adv Biochem Eng Biotechnol*, 62, 75–105.

Bruno, V., Sortino, M.A., Scapagnini, U., Nicoletti, F., and Canonico, P.L. (1995). Antidegenerative effects of Mg(2+)-valproate in cultured cerebellar neurons. *Funct Neurol*, 10, 121–130.

Brunson, K.L., Eghbal-Ahmadi, M., Bender, R., Chen, Y., and Baram, T.Z. (2001). Long-term, progressive hippocampal cell loss and dysfunction induced by early-life administration of corticotropin-releasing hormone reproduce the effects of early-life stress. *Proc Natl Acad Sci USA*, 98, 8856–8861.

Brusov, O.S., Beliaev, B.S., Katasonov, A.B., Zlobina, G.P., Factor, M.I., and Lideman, R.R. (1989). Does platelet serotonin receptor supersensitivity accompany endogenous depression? *Biol Psychiatry*, 25, 375–381.

Bschor, T., Berghofer, A., Strohle, A., Kunz, D., Adli, M., Muller-Oerlinghausen, B., and Bauer, M. (2002). How long should the lithium augmentation strategy be maintained? A 1-year follow-up of a placebo-controlled study in unipolar refractory major depression. *J Clin Psychopharmacol*, 22(4), 427–430.

Bschor, T., Baethge, C., Adli, M., Eichmann, U., Ising, M., Uhr, M., Modell, S., Kunzel, H., Muller-Oerlinghausen, B., and Bauer, M. (2003). Association between response to lithium augmentation and the combined DEX/CRH test in major depressive disorder. *J Psychiatr Res*, 37(2), 135–143.

Buervenich, S., Carmine, A., Arvidsson, M., Xiang, F., Zhang, Z., Sydow, O., Jonsson, E.G., Sedvall, G.C., Leonard, S., Ross, R.G., Freedman, R., Chowdari, K.V., Nimgaonkar, V.L., Perlmann, T., Anvret, M., and Olson, L. (2000). NURR1 mutations in cases of schizophrenia and manic-depressive disorder. *Am J Med Genet*, 96, 808–813.

Buervenich, S., Xiang, F., Sydow, O., Jonsson, E.G., Sedvall, G.C., Anvret, M., and Olson, L. (2001). Identification of four novel polymorphisms in the calcitonin/alpha-CGRP (CALCA) gene and an investigation of their possible associations with Parkinson disease, schizophrenia, and manic depression. *Hum Mutat*, 17(5), 435–436.

Bunney, W.E. Jr., and Davis, J.M. (1965). Norepinephrine in depressive reactions. A review. *Arch Gen Psychiatry*, 13, 483–494.

Bunney, W.E. Jr., and Garland, B. (1982). A second generation catecholamine hypothesis. *Pharmacopsychiatry*, 15(4), 111–115.

Bunney, W.E. Jr., and Garland, B.L. (1983). Possible receptor effects of chronic lithium administration. *Neuropharmacology*, 22, 367–372.

Bunney, W.E. Jr., and Garland-Bunney, B.L. (1987). Mechanisms of action of lithium in affective illness: Basic and clinical implications. In H.Y. Meltzer (Ed.), *Psychopharmacology: The Third Generation of Progress* (pp. 553–565). New York: Raven Press.

Bunney, W.E. Jr., Mason, J.W., and Hamburg, D.A. (1965). Correlations between behavioral variables and urinary 17-hydroxycorticosteroids in depressed patients. *Psychosom Med*, 27, 299–308.

Bunney, W.E. Jr., Brodie, H.K.H., Murphy, D.L., and Goodwin, F.K. (1970). *Psychopharmacological differentiation between two subgroups of depressed patients*. Abstract of a paper presented at the 125th Annual Meeting of the American Psychiatric Association, May.

Bunney, W.E. Jr., Murphy, D., Goodwin, F.K., and Borge, G.F. (1972a). The "switch process" in manic-depressive illness: I. A systematic study of sequential behavior change. *Arch Gen Psychiatry*, 27, 295–302.

Bunney, W.E. Jr., Goodwin, F.K., Murphy, D.L., House, K.M., and Gordon, E.K. (1972b). The "switch process" in manic-depressive illness: II. Relationship to catecholamines, REM sleep, and drugs. *Arch Gen Psychiatry*, 27, 304–309.

Bunney, W.E. Jr., Goodwin, F.K., and Murphy, D.L. (1972c). The "switch process" in manic-depressive illness: III. Theoretical implications. *Arch Gen Psychiatry*, 27, 312–317.

Burnet, P.W., and Harrison, P.J. (2000). Substance P (NK1) receptors in the cingulate cortex in unipolar and bipolar mood disorder and schizophrenia. *Biol Psychiatry*, 47, 80–83.

Burns, G., Herz, A., and Nikolarakis, K.E. (1990). Stimulation of hypothalamic opioid peptide release by lithium is mediated by opioid autoreceptors: Evidence from a combined in vitro, ex vivo study. *Neuroscience*, 36(3), 691–697.

Burt, T., Sachs, G.S., and Demopulos, C. (1999). Donepezil in treatment-resistant bipolar disorder. *Biol Psychiatry*, 45, 959–964.

Busa, W.B., and Gimlich, R.L. (1989). Lithium-induced teratogenesis in frog embryos prevented by a polyphosphoinositide cycle intermediate or a diacylglycerol analog. *Dev Biol*, 132, 315–324.

Bylund, D.B., Ray-Prenger, C., and Murphy, T.J. (1988). Alpha-2A and alpha-2B adrenergic receptor subtypes: Antagonist binding in tissues and cell lines containing only one subtype. *J Pharmacol Exp Ther*, 245, 600–607.

Caberlotto, L., and Hurd, Y.L. (1999). Reduced neuropeptide Y mRNA expression in the prefrontal cortex of subjects with bipolar disorder. *Neuroreport*, 10, 1747–1750.

Caberlotto, L., and Hurd, Y.L. (2001). Neuropeptide Y Y(1) and Y(2) receptor mRNA expression in the prefrontal cortex of psychiatric subjects. Relationship of Y(2) subtype to suicidal behavior. *Neuropsychopharmacology*, 25, 91–97.

Caggiula, A.R., Antelman, S.M., Palmer, A.M., Kiss, S., Edwards, D.J., and Docan, D. (1996). The effects of ethanol on striatal dopamine and frontal cortical D-[3H]aspartate efflux oscillate with repeated treatment. Relevance to individual differences in drug responsiveness. *Neuropsychopharmacology*, 15, 125–132.

Caggiula, A.R., Antelman, S.M., Kucinski, B.J., Fowler, H., Edwards, D.J., Austin, M.C., Gershon, S., and Stiller, R. (1998). Oscillatory-sensitization model of repeated drug exposure: Cocaine's effects on shock-induced hypoalgesia. *Prog Neuropsychopharmacol Biol Psychiatry*, 22(3), 511–521.

Calabrese, J.R., Bowden, C.L., Sachs, G.S., Ascher, J.A., Monaghan, E., and Rudd, G.D. (1999). A double-blind placebo-controlled study of lamotrigine monotherapy in outpatients with bipolar I depression. Lamictal 602 Study Group. *J Clin Psychiatry*, 60, 79–88.

Calabresi, P., Siniscalchi, A., Pisani, A., Stefani, A., Mercuri, N.B., and Bernardi, G. (1996). A field potential analysis on the effects of lamotrigine, GP 47779, and felbamate in neocortical slices. *Neurology*, 47, 557–562.

Caldji, C., Francis, D., Sharma, S., Plotsky, P.M., and Meaney, M.J. (2000). The effects of early rearing environment on the development of GABAA and central benzodiazepine receptor levels and novelty-induced fearfulness in the rat. *Neuropsychopharmacology*, 22, 219–229.

Callado, L.F., Meana, J.J., Grijalba, B., Pazos, A., Sastre, M., and Garcia-Sevilla, J.A. (1998). Selective increase of a2A-adrenoceptor agonist binding sites in brains of depressed suicide victims. *J Neurochem*, 70, 1114–1123.

Callahan, A.M., Frye, M.A., Marangell, L.B., George, M.S., Ketter, T.A., L'Herrou, T., and Post, R.M. (1997). Comparative antidepressant effects of intravenous and intrathecal thyrotropin-releasing hormone: Confounding effects of tolerance and implications for therapeutics. *Biol Psychiatry*, 41, 264–272.

Calogero, A.E., Gallucci, W.T., Chrousos, G.P., and Gold, P.W. (1988). Interaction between GABAergic neurotransmission and rat hypothalamic corticotropin-releasing hormone secretion in vitro. *Brain Res*, 463, 28–36.

Calogero, A.E., Gallucci, W.T., Kling, M.A., Chrousos, G.P., and Gold, P.W. (1989). Cocaine stimulates rat hypothalamic corticotropin-releasing hormone secretion in vitro. *Brain Res*, 505, 7–11.

Cameron, H.A., and McKay, R.D. (1999). Restoring production of hippocampal neurons in old age. *Nat Neurosci*, 2, 894–897.

Canessa, M., Adragna, N., Solomon, H.S., Connolly, T.M., and Tosteson, D.C. (1980). Increased sodium-lithium countertransport in red cells of patients with essential hypertension. *N Engl J Med*, 302, 772–776.

Canessa, M., Brugnara, C., and Escobales, N. (1987). The Li+-Na+ exchange and Na+-K+-Cl- cotransport systems in essential hypertension. *Hypertension*, 10, I4–10.

Cappeliez, P., and Moore, E. (1990). Effects of lithium on an amphetamine animal model of bipolar disorder. *Prog Neuropsychopharmacol Biol Psychiatry*, 14, 347–358.

Cappiello, A., Malison, R.T., McDougle, C.J., Vegso, S.J., Charney, D.S., Heninger, G.R., and Price, L.H. (1996). Seasonal variation in neuroendocrine and mood responses to i.v. L-tryptophan in depressed patients and healthy subjects. *Neuropsychopharmacology*, 15, 475–483.

Cappiello, A., Sernyak, M.J., Malison, R.T., McDougle, C.J., Heninger, G.R., and Price, L.H. (1997). Effects of acute tryptophan depletion in lithium-remitted manic patients: A pilot study. *Biol Psychiatry*, 42(11), 1076–1078.

Carletti, R., Corsi, M., Melotto, S., and Caberlotto, L. (2005). Down-regulation of amygdala preprotachykinin A mRNA but not 3H-SP receptor binding sites in subjects affected by mood disorders and schizophrenia. *Eur J Neurosci*, 21(6), 1712–1718.

Carli, M., Morissette, M., Hebert, C., Di Paolo, T., and Reader, T.A. (1997). Effects of a chronic lithium treatment on central dopamine neurotransporters. *Biochem Pharmacol*, 54, 391–397.

Carlson, P.J., Singh, J.B., Zarazte, C.A., Drevets, W.C., and Manji, H.K. (2006). Neural circuitry and neuroplasticity in mood disorders: Insights for novel therapeutic targets. *Neurotherapeutics*, 3, 22–41.

Carman, J.S., Wyatt, E.S., Smith, W., Post, R.M., and Ballenger, J.C. (1984). Calcium and calcitonin in bipolar affective disorder. In R.M. Post and J.C. Ballinger (Eds.), *Neurobiology of Mood Disorders* (pp. 340–355). Baltimore: Williams & Wilkins.

Carmeliet, E.E. (1964). Influence of lithium ions on the transmembrane potential and cation content of cardiac cells. *J Gen Physiol*, 47, 501–530.

Carroll, B.J. (1972). Sodium and potassium transfer to cerebrospinal fluid in severe depression. In B. Davies, B.J. Caroll, and R.M. Mowbray (Eds.), *Depressive Illness: Some Research Studies* (pp. 247–257). Springfield, IL: Charles C. Thomas.

Carroll, B.J. (1976). Limbic system–adrenal cortex regulation in depression and schizophrenia. *Psychosom Med*, 38, 106–121.

Carroll, B.J. (1980). Dexamethasone suppression test in depression. *Lancet*, 2, 1249.

Carroll, B.J. (1982). Clinical applications of the dexamethasone suppression test for endogenous depression. *Pharmacopsychiatria*, 15, 19–25.

Carroll, B.J., Martin, F.I., and Davies, B. (1968). Resistance to suppression by dexamethasone of plasma 11-O.H.C.S. levels in severe depressive illness. *BMJ*, 3, 285–287.

Carstens, M.E., Engelbrecht, A.H., Russell, V.A., van Zyl, A.M., and Taljaard, J.J. (1988). Biological markers in juvenile depression. *Psychiatry Res*, 23, 77–88.

Casebolt, T.L., and Jope, R.S. (1989). Long-term lithium treatment selectively reduces receptor-coupled inositol phospholipid hydrolysis in rat brain. *Biol Psychiatry*, 25, 329–340.

Cassidy, F., Murry, E., and Carroll, B.J. (1998a). Tryptophan depletion in recently manic patients treated with lithium. *Biol Psychiatry*, 43, 230–232.

Cassidy, F., Ritchie, J.C., and Carroll, B.J. (1998b). Plasma dexamethasone concentration and cortisol response during manic episodes. *Biol Psychiatry*, 43, 747–754.

Castillo, M., Kwock, L., Courvoisie, H., and Hooper, S.R. (2000). Proton MR spectroscopy in children with bipolar affective disorder: Preliminary observations. *AJNR Am J Neuroradiol*, 21, 832–838.

Catherino, W.H., Jeng, M.H., and Jordan, V.C. (1993). Norgestrel and gestodene stimulate breast cancer cell growth through an oestrogen receptor mediated mechanism. *Br J Cancer*, 67(5), 945–952.

Cazzullo, C.L., Smeraldi, E., Scchetti, E., and Bottinelli, S. (1975). Letter: Intracellular lithium concentration and clinical response. *Br J Psychiatry*, 126, 298–300.

Cervantes, P., Gelber, S., Kin, F.N., Nair, V.N., and Schwartz, G. (2001). Circadian secretion of cortisol in bipolar disorder. *J Psychiatry Neurosci*, 26(5), 411–416.

Chalecka-Franaszek, E., and Chuang, D.M. (1999). Lithium activates the serine/threonine kinase Akt-1 and suppresses glutamate-induced inhibition of Akt-1 activity in neurons. *Proc Natl Acad Sci USA*, 96, 8745–8750.

Chana, G., Landau, S., Beasley, C., Everall, I.P., and Cotter, D. (2003). Two-dimensional assessment of cytoarchitecture in the anterior cingulate cortex in major depressive disorder, bipolar disorder, and schizophrenia: Evidence for decreased neuronal somal size and increased neuronal density. *Biol Psychiatry*, 53, 1086–1098.

Chang, D.C., and Reppert, S.M. (2001). The circadian clocks of mice and men. *Neuron*, 29(3), 555–558.

Chang, M.C., Grange, E., Rabin, O., Bell, J.M., Allen, D.D., and Rapoport, S.I. (1996). Lithium decreases turnover of arachidonate in several brain phospholipids. *Neurosci Lett*, 220, 171–174.

Chang, M.C., Contreras, M.A., Rosenberger, T.A., Rintala, J.J., Bell, J.M., and Rapoport, S.I. (2001). Chronic valproate treatment decreases the in vivo turnover of arachidonic acid in brain phospholipids: A possible common effect of mood stabilizers. *J Neurochem*, 77, 796–803.

Charles, H.C., Lazeyras, F., Krishnan, K.R., Boyko, O.B., Payne, M., and Moore, D. (1994). Brain choline in depression: In vivo detection of potential pharmacodynamic effects of antidepressant therapy using hydrogen localized spectroscopy. *Prog Neuropsychopharmacol Biol Psychiatry*, 18, 1121–1127.

Charlton, B.G., Leake, A., Wright, C., Gairbairn, A.F., McKeith, U.G., Candy, J.M., and Ferrier, I.N. (1988). Somatostatin content and receptors in the cerebral cortex of depressed and control subjects. *J Neurol Neurosurg Psychiatry*, 51, 719–721.

Charney, D.S., and Heninger, G.R. (1986). Abnormal regulation of noradrenergic function in panic disorders. Effects of clonidine in healthy subjects and patients with agoraphobia and panic disorder. *Arch Gen Psychiatry*, 43, 1042–1054.

Charney, D.S., and Manji, H.K. (2004). Life stress, genes, and depression: Multiple pathways lead to increased risk and new opportunities for intervention. *Sci STKE*, 2004(225), re5.

Charney, D.S., Heninger, G.R., Sternberg, D.E., Hafstad, K.M., Giddings, S., and Landis, D.H. (1982). Adrenergic receptor sensitivity in depression. Effects of clonidine in depressed patients and healthy subjects. *Arch Gen Psychiatry*, 39, 290–294.

Charney, D.S., Heninger, G.R., and Redmond, D.E. Jr. (1983). Yohimbine induced anxiety and increased noradrenergic function in humans: Effects of diazepam and clonidine. *Life Sci*, 33(1), 19–29.

Chazot, G., Claustrat, B., Brun, J., and Olivier, M. (1985). Rapid antidepressant activity of destyr gamma endorphin: Correlation with urinary melatonin. *Biol Psychiatry*, 20, 1026–1030.

Checkley, S.A., Slade, A.P., and Shur, E. (1981). Growth hormone and other responses to clonidine in patients with endogenous depression. *Br J Psychiatry*, 138, 51–55.

Checkley, S.A., Glass, I.B., Thompson, C., Corn, T., and Robinson, P. (1984). The GH response to clonidine in endogenous as compared with reactive depression. *Psychol Med*, 14, 773–777.

Checkley, S.A., Thompson, C., Burton, S., Franey, C., and Arendt, J. (1985). Clinical studies of the effect of (+) and (−) oxaprotiline upon noradrenaline uptake. *Psychopharmacology (Berl)*, 87(1), 116–118.

Chee, I.S., Lee, S.W., Kim, J.L., Wang, S.K., Shin, Y.O., Shin, S.C., Lee, Y.H., Hwang, H.M., and Lim, M.R. (2001). 5-HT2A receptor gene promoter polymorphism −1438A/G and bipolar disorder. *Psychiatr Genet*, 11, 111–114.

Cheetham, S.C., Crompton, M.R., Katona, C.L., and Horton, R.W. (1988). Brain 5-HT2 receptor binding sites in depressed suicide victims. *Brain Res*, 443, 272–280.

Cheetham, S.C., Crompton, M.R., Czudek, C., Horton, R.W., Katona, C.L., and Reynolds, G.P. (1989). Serotonin concentrations and turnover in brains of depressed suicides. *Brain Res*, 502, 332–340.

Cheetham, S.C., Crompton, M.R., Katona, C.L., and Horton, R.W. (1990). Brain 5-HT1 binding sites in depressed suicides. *Psychopharmacology*, 102, 544–548.

Chen, A.C., Shirayama, Y., Shin, K.H., Neve, R.L., and Duman, R.S. (2001). Expression of the cAMP response element binding protein (CREB) in hippocampus produces an antidepressant effect. *Biol Psychiatry*, 49, 753–762.

Chen, B., Dowlatshahi, D., MacQueen, G.M., Wang, J.F., and Young, L.T. (2001). Increased hippocampal BDNF immunoreactivity in subjects treated with antidepressant medication. *Biol Psychiatry*, 50, 260–265.

Chen, D.F., Schneider, G.E., Martinou, J.C., and Tonegawa, S. (1997). Bcl-2 promotes regeneration of severed axons in mammalian CNS. *Nature*, 385, 434–439.

Chen, G., and Manji, H.K. (2006). The extracellular signal-regulated kinase pathway: An emerging promising target for mood stabilizers. *Curr Opin Psychiatry*, 19(3), 313–323.

Chen, G., Manji, H.K., Hawver, D.B., Wright, C.B., and Potter, W.Z. (1994). Chronic sodium valproate selectively decreases protein kinase C alpha and epsilon in vitro. *J Neurochem*, 63, 2361–2364.

Chen, G., Manji, H.K., Wright, C.B., Hawver, D.B., and Potter, W.Z. (1996a). Effects of valproic acid on beta-adrenergic receptors, G-proteins, and adenylyl cyclase in rat C6 glioma cells. *Neuropsychopharmacology*, 15, 271–280.

Chen, G., Pan, B., Hawver, D.B., Wright, C.B., Potter, W.Z., and Manji, H.K. (1996b). Attenuation of cyclic AMP production by carbamazepine. *J Neurochem*, 67, 2079–2086.

Chen, G., Yuan, P.X., Jiang, Y.M., Huang, L.D., and Manji, H.K. (1998). Lithium increases tyrosine hydroxylase levels both in vivo and in vitro. *J Neurochem*, 70, 1768–1771.

Chen, G., Hasanat, K.A., Bebchuk, J.M., Moore, G.J., Glitz, D., and Manji, H.K. (1999). Regulation of signal transduction pathways and gene expression by mood stabilizers and antidepressants. *Psychosom Med*, 61, 599–617.

Chen, G., Masana, M.I., and Manji, H.K. (2000). Lithium regulates PKC-mediated intracellular cross-talk and gene expression in the CNS in vivo. *Bipolar Disord*, 2, 217–236.

Chen, G., Einat, H., Yuan, P., and Manji, H. (2002). Evidence for the involvement of the MAP/ERK signaling pathway in mood modulation. *Biol Psychiatry*, 51, 126S.

Chen, R.W., and Chuang, D.M. (1999). Long-term lithium treatment suppresses p53 and bax expression but increases bcl-2 expression. A prominent role in neuroprotection against excitotoxicity. *J Biol Chem*, 274(10), 6039–6042.

Chen, T.J., Zitter, R.N., Tao, R., Hunter, W.R., and Rife, J.C. (1995). Optical constants of lithium triborate crystals in the 55–71 ev region. *Phys Rev B Condensed Matter*, 52(19), 13703–13706.

Chi, P., Greengard, P., and Ryan, T.A. (2001). Synapsin dispersion and reclustering during synaptic activity. *Nat Neurosci*, 4, 1187–1193.

Chiaroni, P., Azorin, J.M., Dassa, D., Henry, J.M., Giudicelli, S., Malthiery, Y., and Planells, R. (2000). Possible involvement of the dopamine D3 receptor locus in subtypes of bipolar affective disorder. *Psychiatr Genet*, 10, 43–49.

Cho, J.T., Bone, S., Dunner, D.L., Colt, E., and Fieve, R.R. (1979). The effect of lithium treatment on thyroid function in patients with primary affective disorder. *Am J Psychiatry*, 136, 115–116.

Choi, S.J., Taylor, M.A., and Abrams, R. (1977). Depression, ECT, and erythrocyte adenosinetriphosphatase activity. *Biol Psychiatry*, 12, 75–81.

Choi, Y.R., and Akera, T. (1977). Kinetics studies on the interaction between ouabain and (Na+,K+)-ATPase. *Biochim Biophys Acta*, 481, 648–659.

Chouinard, G., Steinberg, S., and Steiner, W. (1987). Estrogen–progesterone combination: Another mood stabilizer? *Am J Psychiatry*, 144(6), 826.

Chronwall, B.M., and Zukowska, Z. (2004). Neuropeptide Y, ubiquitous and elusive. *Peptides*, 25(3), 359–363.

Chuang, D.M. (1989). Inositol lipids and transmembrane signalling. In M.J. Berridge and R.H. Michell (Eds.), *Inositol Lipids and Transmembrane Signalling* (pp. 40–53). London: Scholium Intl.

Cirelli, C. (2002). How sleep deprivation affects gene expression in the brain: A review of recent findings. *J Appl Physiol*, 92, 394–400.

Cirelli, C., and Tononi, G. (2000a). Differential expression of plasticity-related genes in waking and sleep and their regulation by the noradrenergic system. *J Neurosci*, 20, 9187–9194.

Cirelli, C., and Tononi, G. (2000b). On the functional significance of c-fos induction during the sleep-waking cycle. *Sleep*, 23(4), 453–469.

Cirelli, C., and Tononi, G. (2000c). Gene expression in the brain across the sleep-waking cycle. *Brain Res*, 885(2), 303–321.

Clark, L.D., Quarton, G.C., Cobb, S., and Bauer, W. (1953). Further observations on mental disturbances associated with cortisone and acth therapy. *N Engl J Med*, 249(5), 178–183.

Cochran, E., Robins, E., and Grote, S. (1976). Regional serotonin levels in brain: A comparison of depressive suicides and alcoholic suicides with controls. *Biol Psychiatry*, 11, 283–294.

Coffman, J.F., and Petty, F. (1986). Plasma GABA: A potential indicator of altered GABAergic function in psychiatric illness. In G.L. Bartholinim, P.L. Morselli, (Eds.), *GABA and Mood Disorders: Experimental and Clinical Research* (pp. 179–185). New York: Raven Press.

Cohen, P., and Frame, S. (2001). The renaissance of GSK3. *Nat Rev Mol Cell Biol*, 2, 769–776.

Cohn, C.K., Dunner, D.L., and Axelrod, J. (1970). Reduced catechol-O-methyltransferase activity in red blood cells of women with primary affective disorder. *Science*, 170, 1323–1324.

Colin, S.F., Chang, H.C., Mollner, S., Pfeuffer, T., Reed, R.R., Duman, R.S., and Nestler, E.J. (1991). Chronic lithium regulates the expression of adenylate cyclase and Gi-protein alpha subunit in rat cerebral cortex. *Proc Natl Acad Sci USA*, 88, 10634–10637.

Collard, K.J. (1978). The effect of lithium on the increase in forebrain 5-hydroxyindoleacetic acid produced by raphe stimulation. *Br J Pharmacol*, 62, 137–142.

Collard, K.J., and Roberts, M.H. (1977). Effects of lithium on the elevation of forebrain 5-hydroxyindoles by tryptophan. *Neuropharmacology*, 16, 671–673.

Collier, D.A., Arranz, M.J., Sham, P., Battersby, S., Vallada, H., Gill, P., Aitchison, K.J., Sodhi, M., Li, T., Roberts, G.W., Smith, B., Morton, J., Murray, R.M., Smith, D., and Kirov, G. (1996a). The serotonin transporter is a potential susceptibility factor for bipolar affective disorder. *Neuroreport*, 7, 1675–1679.

Collier, D.A., Stober, G., Li, T., Heils, A., Catalano, M., Di Bella, D., Arranz, M.J., Murray, R.M., Vallada, H.P., Bengel, D., Muller, C.R., Roberts, G.W., Smeraldi, E., Kirov, G., Sham, P., and Lesch, K.P. (1996b). A novel functional polymorphism within the promoter of the serotonin transporter gene: Possible role in susceptibility to affective disorders. *Mol Psychiatry*, 1, 453–460.

Conn, P., and Sweatt, J. (1994). Protein kinase C in the nervous system. In J. Kuo (Ed.), *Protein Kinase C* (pp. 199–235). New York: Oxford University Press.

Consogno, E., Racagni, G., and Popoli, M. (2001a). Modifications in brain CaM kinase II after long-term treatment with desmethylimipramine. *Neuropsychopharmacology*, 24, 21–30.

Consogno, E., Tiraboschi, E., Iuliano, E., Gennarelli, M., Racagni, G., and Popoli, M. (2001b). Long-term treatment with S-adenosylmethionine induces changes in presynaptic CaM kinase II and synapsin I. *Biol Psychiatry*, 50, 337–344.

Cooney, J.M., Lucey, J.V., and Dinan, T.G. (1997). Enhanced growth hormone responses to pyridostigmine challenge in patients with panic disorder. *Br J Psychiatry*, 170, 159–161.

Cooper, S.J., Kelly, J.G., and King, D.J. (1985). Adrenergic receptors in depression. Effects of electroconvulsive therapy. *Br J Psychiatry*, 147, 23–29.

Coppen, A. (1960). Abnormality in the blood: Cerebrospinal fluid barrier of patients suffering from a depressive illness. *J Neurol Neuroserg Psychiatry*, 23, 156–161.

Coppen, A., and Shaw, D.M. (1963). Mineral metabolism in melancholia. *BMJ*, 2, 1439–1444.

Coppen, A., Shaw, D.M., Malleson, A., and Costain, R. (1966). Mineral metabolism in mania. *BMJ*, 5479, 71–75.

Coppen, A., Prange, A.J. Jr., Hill, C., Whybrow, P.C., and Noguera, R. (1972). Abnormalities of indoleamines in affective disorders. *Arch Gen Psychiatry*, 26, 474–478.

Coppen, A., Swade, C., and Wood, K. (1980). Lithium restores abnormal platelet 5-HT transport in patients with affective disorders. *Br J Psychiatry*, 136, 235–238.

Cordeiro, M.L., Umbach, J.A., and Gundersen, C.B. (2000). Lithium ions up-regulate mRNAs encoding dense-core vesicle proteins in nerve growth factor-differentiated PC12 cells. *J Neurochem*, 75, 2622–2625.

Corona, G.L., Cucchi, M.L., Santagostino, G., Frattini, P., Zerbi, F., Fenoglio, L., and Savoldi, F. (1982). Blood noradrenaline and 5-HT levels in depressed women during amitriptyline or lithium treatment. *Psychopharmacology (Berl)*, 77, 236–241.

Corrigan, M.H., Denahan, A.Q., Wright, C.E., Ragual, R.J., and Evans, D.L. (2000). Comparison of pramipexole, fluoxetine, and placebo in patients with major depression. *Depress Anxiety*, 11, 58–65.

Corvol, J.C., Studler, J.M., Schonn, J.S., Girault, J.A., and Herve, D. (2001). Gα(olf) is necessary for coupling D1 and A2a receptors to adenylyl cyclase in the striatum. *J Neurochem*, 76, 1585–1588.

Costa, E., Davis, J., Grayson, D.R., Guidotti, A., Pappas, G.D., and Pesold, C. (2001). Dendritic spine hypoplasticity and down-regulation of reelin and GABAergic tone in schizophrenia vulnerability. *Neurobiol Dis*, 8, 723–742.

Costa, E., Chen, Y., Davis, J., Dong, E., Noh, J.S., Tremolizzo, L., Veldic, M., Grayson, D.R., and Guidotti, A. (2002). REELIN and schizophrenia: A disease at the interface of the genome and the epigenome. *Mol Intervent*, 2, 47–57.

Cotter, D., Mackay, D., Landau, S., Kerwin, R., and Everall, I. (2001). Reduced glial cell density and neuronal size in the anterior cingulate cortex in major depressive disorder. *Arch Gen Psychiatry*, 58, 545–553.

Cotter, D., Landau, S., Beasley, C., Stevenson, R., Chana, G., MacMillan, L., and Everall, I. (2002a). The density and spatial distribution of GABAergic neurons, labelled using calcium binding proteins, in the anterior cingulate cortex in major depressive disorder, bipolar disorder, and schizophrenia. *Biol Psychiatry*, 51, 377–386.

Cotter, D., Mackay, D., Chana, G., Beasley, C., Landau, S., and Everall, I.P. (2002b). Reduced neuronal size and glial cell density in area 9 of the dorsolateral prefrontal cortex in subjects with major depressive disorder. *Cereb Cortex*, 12, 386–394.

Couldwell, W.T., Weiss, M.H., DeGiorgio, C.M., Weiner, L.P., Hinton, D.R., Ehresmann, G.R., Conti, P.S., and Apuzzo, M.L. (1993). Clinical and radiographic response in a minority of patients with recurrent malignant gliomas treated with high-dose tamoxifen. *Neurosurgery*, 32(3), 485–489; discussion 489–490.

Couldwell, W.T., Hinton, D.R., Surnock, A.A., DeGiorgio, C.M., Weiner, L.P., Apuzzo, M.L., Masri, L., Law, R.E., and Weiss, M.H. (1996). Treatment of recurrent malignant gliomas with chronic oral high-dose tamoxifen. *Clin Cancer Res*, 2(4), 619–622.

Coull, M.A., Lowther, S., Katona, C.L., and Horton, R.W. (2000). Altered brain protein kinase C in depression: A post-mortem study. *Eur Neuropsychopharmacol*, 10, 283–288.

Cowan, W.M., Kopnisky, K.L., and Hyman, S.E. (2002). The human genome project and its impact on psychiatry. *Annu Rev Neurosci*, 25, 1–50.

Cowdry, R.W., Wehr, T.A., Zis, A.P., and Goodwin, F.K. (1983). Thyroid abnormalities associated with rapid-cycling bipolar illness. *Arch Gen Psychiatry*, 40, 414–420.

Cowell, H.E., and Garrod, D.R. (1999). Activation of protein kinase C modulates cell–cell and cell–substratum adhesion of a human colorectal carcinoma cell line and restores 'normal' epithelial morphology. *Int J Cancer*, 80(3), 455–464.

Cowen, P.J. (2000). Psychopharmacology of 5-HT(1A) receptors. *Nucl Med Biol*, 27, 437–439.

Cowen, P.J., Charig, E.M., Fraser, S., and Elliott, J.M. (1987). Platelet 5-HT receptor binding during depressive illness and tricyclic antidepressant treatment. *J Affect Disord*, 13, 45–50.

Cowen, P.J., Parry-Billings, M., and Newsholme, E.A. (1989). Decreased plasma tryptophan levels in major depression. *J Affect Disord*, 16, 27–31.

Coyle, J.T., and Manji, H.K. (2002). Getting balance: Drugs for bipolar disorder share target. *Nat Med*, 8, 557–558.

Coyle, J.T., and Schwarcz, R. (2000). Mind glue: Implications of glial cell biology for psychiatry. *Arch Gen Psychiatry*, 57, 90–93.

Coyle, N., Jones, I., Robertson, E., Lendon, C., and Craddock, N. (2000). Variation at the serotonin transporter gene influences susceptibility to bipolar affective puerperal psychosis. *Lancet*, 356, 1490–1491.

Craddock, N., O'Donovan, M.C., and Owen, M.J. (2005). The genetics of schizophrenia and bipolar disorder: Dissecting psychosis. *J Med Genet*, 42(3), 193–204.

Cremona, O., Di Paolo, G., Wenk, M.R., Luthi, A., Kim, W.T., Takei, K., Daniell, L., Nemoto, Y., Shears, S.B., Flavell, R.A., McCormick, D.A., and De Camilli, P. (1999). Essential role of phosphoinositide metabolism in synaptic vesicle recycling. *Cell*, 99, 179–188.

Cross, D.A., Culbert, A.A., Chalmers, K.A., Facci, L., Skaper, S.D., and Reith, A.D. (2001). Selective small-molecule inhibitors of glycogen synthase kinase-3 activity protect primary neurones from death. *J Neurochem*, 77, 94–102.

Crow, T.J., Cross, A.J., Cooper, S.J., Deakin, J.F., Ferrier, I.N., Johnson, J.A., Joseph, M.H., Owen, F., Poulter, M., and Lofthouse, R. (1984). Neurotransmitter receptors and monoamine metabolites in the brains of patients with Alzheimer-type dementia and depression, and suicides. *Neuropharmacology*, 23, 1561–1569.

Crowder, R.J., and Freeman, R.S. (2000). Glycogen synthase kinase-3 beta activity is critical for neuronal death caused by inhibiting phosphatidylinositol 3-kinase or Akt but not for death caused by nerve growth factor withdrawal. *J Biol Chem*, 275, 34266–34271.

Crunelli, V., Bernasconi, S., and Samanin, R. (1979). Evidence against serotonin involvement in the tonic component of electrically induced convulsions and in carbamazepine anticonvulsant activity. *Psychopharmacology (Berl)*, 66(1), 79.

Cusin, C., Serretti, A., Lattuada, E., Lilli, R., Lorenzi, C., Mandelli, L., Pisati, E., and Smeraldi, E. (2001). Influence of 5-HTTLPR and TPH variants on illness time course in mood disorders. *J Psychiatr Res*, 35, 217–223.

Cutler, N.R., and Post, R.M. (1982). State-related cyclical dyskinesias in manic-depressive illness. *J Clin Psychopharmacol*, 2, 350–354.

Czeh, B., Michaelis, T., Watanabe, T., Frahm, J., de Biurrun, G., van Kampen, M., Bartolomucci, A., and Fuchs, E. (2001). Stress-induced changes in cerebral metabolites, hippocampal volume, and cell proliferation are prevented by antidepressant treatment with tianeptine. *Proc Natl Acad Sci USA*, 98, 12796–12801.

Dafflon, M., Decosterd, L.A., Biollaz, J., Preisig, M., Dufour, H., and Buclin, T. (1999). Trace lithium in mood disorders. *J Affect Disord*, 54(1-2), 199–203.

Dagher, G., Gay, C., Brossard, M., Feray, J.C., Olie, J.P., Garay, R.P., Loo, H., and Meyer, P. (1984). Lithium, sodium and potassium transport in erythrocytes of manic-depressive patients. *Acta Psychiatr Scand*, 69(1), 24–36.

Daigen, A., Akiyama, K., Itoh, T., Kohira, I., Sora, I., Morimoto, K., and Otsuki, S. (1991). Long-lasting enhancement of the membrane-associated protein kinase C activity in the hippocampal kindled rat. *Jpn J Psychiatry Neurol*, 45, 297–301.

Dailey, J.W., Cheong, J.H., Ko, K.H., Adams-Curtis, L.E., and Jobe, P.C. (1995). Anticonvulsant properties of D-20443 in genetically epilepsy-prone rats: prediction of clinical response. *Neurosci Lett*, 195, 77–80.

D'Aquila, P.S., Collu, M., Devoto, P., and Serra, G. (2000). Chronic lithium chloride fails to prevent imipramine-induced sensitization to the dopamine D(2)-like receptor agonist quinpirole. *Eur J Pharmacol*, 395, 157–160.

D'Aquila, P.S., Peana, A.T., Tanda, O., and Serra, G. (2001). Carbamazepine prevents imipramine-induced behavioural sensitization to the dopamine D(2)-like receptor agonist quinpirole. *Eur J Pharmacol*, 416, 107–111.

Davanzo, P., Thomas, M.A., Yue, K., Oshiro, T., Belin, T., Strober, M., and McCracken, J. (2001). Decreased anterior cingulate myo-inositol/creatine spectroscopy resonance with lithium treatment in children with bipolar disorder. *Neuropsychopharmacology*, 24, 359–369.

David, M.M., Owen, J.A., Abraham, G., Delva, N.J., Southmayd, S.E., Wooltorton, E., and Lawson, J.S. (2000). Thyroid function and response to 48-hour sleep deprivation in treatment-resistant depressed patients. *Biol Psychiatry*, 48(4), 323–326.

Davies, J.A. (1995). Mechanisms of action of antiepileptic drugs. *Seizure*, 4, 267–271.

Davis, G.C., Bunney, W.E., Buchsbaum, M., DeFraties, E.G., Duncan, W., Gillin, J.C., Van Kammen, D.P., Kleinman, J., Murphy, D.L., Post, R.M., Reus, V., and Wyatt, R.J. (1979). Use of narcotic antagonists to study the role of endorphins in normal and psychiatric patients. In E. Usdin, W.E. Bunney, and N.S. Kline (Eds.), *Endorphins in Mental Health Research* (pp. 393–406). New York: Oxford University Press.

Davis, G.C., Extein, I., Reus, V.I., Hamilton, W., Post, R.M., Goodwin, F.K., and Bunney, W.E. Jr. (1980). Failure of naloxone to reduce manic symptoms. *Am J Psychiatry*, 137, 1583–1585.

Davis, J.M., and Bresnahan, D.B. (1987). Psychopharmacology in clinical psychiatry. In R.E. Hales and A.J. Frances (Eds), *American Psychiatric Association Annual Review* (Vol. 6) (pp. 159–187). Washington, DC: American Psychiatric Press.

Davis, J.M., Koslow, S.H., Gibbons, R.D., Maas, J.W., Bowden, C.L., Casper, R., Hanin, I., Javaid, J.I., Chang, S.S., and Stokes, P.E. (1988). Cerebrospinal fluid and urinary biogenic amines in depressed patients and healthy controls. *Arch Gen Psychiatry*, 45, 705–717.

Davis, K.L., Berger, P.A., Hollister, L.E., and Defraites, E. (1978). Physostigmine in mania. *Arch Gen Psychiatry*, 35, 119–122.

Deakin, J.F., Pennell, I., Upadhyaya, A.J., and Lofthouse, R. (1990). A neuroendocrine study of 5-HT function in depression: Evidence for biological mechanisms of endogenous and psychosocial causation. *Psychopharmacology (Berl)*, 101, 85–92.

Dean, B., Pavey, G., McLeod, M., Opeskin, K., Keks, N., and Copolov, D. (2001). A change in the density of [(3)H]flumazenil, but not [(3)H]muscimol binding, in Brodmann's area 9 from subjects with bipolar disorder. *J Affect Disord*, 66, 147–158.

Dean, B., Scarr, E., and McLeod, M. (2005). Changes in hippocampal GABAA receptor subunit composition in bipolar 1 disorder. *Brain Res Mol Brain Res*, 138(2), 145–155.

Dean, C., Williams, R.J., and Brockington, I.F. (1989). Is puerperal psychosis the same as bipolar manic-depressive disorder? A family study. *Psychol Med*, 19(3), 637–647.

Deans, Z.C., Dawson, S.J., Kilimann, M.W., Wallace, D., Wilson, M.C., and Latchman, D.S. (1997). Differential regulation of genes encoding synaptic proteins by the Oct-2 transcription factor. *Brain Res Mol Brain Res*, 51, 1–7.

DeBattista, C., Posener, J.A., Kalehzan, B.M., and Schatzberg, A.F. (2000). Acute antidepressant effects of intravenous hydrocortisone and CRH in depressed patients: A double-blind, placebo-controlled study. *Am J Psychiatry*, 157, 1334–1337.

DeBattista, C., Solvason, H.B., Poirier, J., Kendrick, E., and Schatzberg, A.F. (2003). A prospective trial of bupropion sr augmentation of partial and non-responders to serotonergic antidepressants. *J Clin Psychopharmacol*, 23(1), 27–30.

Degkwitz, R., Koufen, H., Consbruch, U., Becker, W., and Knauf, H. (1979). Lithium balance in mania. *Int Pharmacopsychiatry*, 14, 199–212.

Delgado, P.L., Charney, D.S., Price, L.H., Aghajanian, G.K., Landis, H., and Heninger, G.R. (1990). Serotonin function and the mechanism of antidepressant action. Reversal of antidepressant-induced remission by rapid depletion of plasma tryptophan. *Arch Gen Psychiatry*, 47, 411–418.

Delgado, P.L., Price, L.H., Miller, H.L., Salomon, R.M., Licinio, J., Krystal, J.H., Heninger, G.R., and Charney, D.S. (1991). Rapid serotonin depletion as a provocative challenge test for patients with major depression: Relevance to antidepressant action and the neurobiology of depression. *Psychopharmacol Bull*, 27, 321–330.

Delgado, P.L., Miller, H.L., Salomon, R.M., Licinio, J., Krystal, J.H., Moreno, F.A., Heninger, G.R., and Charney, D.S. (1999). Tryptophan-depletion challenge in depressed patients treated with desipramine or fluoxetine: Implications for the role of serotonin in the mechanism of antidepressant action. *Biol Psychiatry*, 46, 212–220.

Del Vecchio, M., Farzati, B., Maj, M., Minucci, P., Guida, L., and Kemali, D. (1981). Cell membrane predictors of response to lithium prophylaxis of affective disorders. *Neuropsychobiology*, 7(5), 243–247.

Demeester-Mirkine, N., and Dumont, J.E. (1980). The hypothalamo-pituitary thyroid axis. In M. deVisscher (Ed.), *The Thyroid Gland* (pp. 145–152). New York: Raven Press.

DeMet, E.M., and Sokolski, K.N. (1999). Sodium valproate increases pupillary responsiveness to a cholinergic agonist in responders with mania. *Biol Psychiatry*, 46, 432–436.

Demitrack, M.A., and Gold, P.W. (1988). Oxytocin: Neurobiologic considerations and their implications for affective illness. *Prog Neuropsychopharmacol Biol Psychiatry*, 12(Suppl.), S23–S51.

de Montigny, C. (1981). Enhancement of the 5-HT neurotransmission by antidepressant treatments. *J Physiol (Paris)*, 77(2-3), 455–461.

de Montigny, C., Grunberg, F., Mayer, A., and Deschenes, J.P. (1981). Lithium induces rapid relief of depression in tricyclic antidepressant drug non-responders. *Br J Psychiatry*, 138, 252–256.

de Montigny, C., Cournoyer, G., Morissette, R., Langlois, R., and Caille, G. (1983). Lithium carbonate addition in tricyclic antidepressant-resistant unipolar depression. Correlations with the neurobiologic actions of tricyclic antidepressant drugs and lithium ion on the serotonin system. *Arch Gen Psychiatry*, 40(12), 1327–1334.

DeMontis, M.G., Fadda, P., Devoto, P., Martellotta, M.C., and Fratta, W. (1990). Sleep deprivation increases dopamine D1 receptor antagonist [3H]SCH 23390 binding and dopamine-stimulated adenylate cyclase in the rat limbic system. *Neurosci Lett*, 117, 224–227.

De Paermentier, F., Cheetham, S.C., Crompton, M.R., Katona, C.L., and Horton, R.W. (1990). Brain beta-adrenoreceptor binding sites in antidepressant-free depressed suicide victims. *Brain Res*, 525, 71–77.

De Paermentier, F., Cheetham, S.C., Crompton, M.R., Katona, C.L., and Horton, R.W. (1991). Brain beta-adrenoreceptor binding sites in depressed suicide victims: Effects of antidepressant treatment. *Psychopharmacology*, 105, 283–288.

De Paermentier, F., Lowther, S., Crompton, M.R., Katona, C.L., and Horton, R.W. (1997a). Beta-adrenoceptors in human pineal glands are unaltered in depressed suicides. *J Psychopharmacol*, 11, 295–299.

De Paermentier, F., Mauger, J.M., Lowther, S., Crompton, M.R., Katona, C.L., and Horton, R.W. (1997b). Brain alpha-adrenoceptors in depressed suicides. *Brain Res*, 757, 60–68.

Depue, R.A., Kleiman, R.M., Davis, P., Hutchinson, M., and Krauss, S.P. (1985). The behavioral high-risk paradigm and bipolar affective disorder: VIII. Serum free cortisol in nonpatient cyclothymic subjects selected by the General Behavior Inventory. *Am J Psychiatry*, 142, 175–181.

Deshauer, D., Grof, E., Alda, M., and Grof, P. (1999). Patterns of DST positivity in remitted affective disorders. *Biol Psychiatry*, 45, 1023–1029.

Deuschle, M., Schweiger, U., Gotthardt, U., Weber, B., Korner, A., Schmider, J., Standhardt, H., Lammers, C.H., Krumm, B., and Heuser, I. (1998). The combined dexamethasone/corticotropin-releasing hormone stimulation test is more closely associated with features of diurnal activity of the hypothalamo-pituitary-adrenocortical system than the dexamethasone suppression test. *Biol Psychiatry*, 43, 762–766.

Devanand, D.P., Lo, I., Sackeim, H.A., Halbreich, U., Ross, F., and Cooper, T. (1987). *Acute and subacute effects of electroconvulsive therapy on plasma oxytocin and vasopressin in depressed patients*. 42nd Annual meeting of the Society of Biological Psychiatry.

de Villiers, A.S., Russell, V.A., Carstens, M.E., Searson, J.A., van Zyl, A.M., Lombard, C.J., and Taljaard, J.J. (1989). Noradrenergic function and hypothalamic–pituitary–adrenal axis activity in adolescents with major depressive disorder. *Psychiatry Res*, 27(2), 101–109.

De Wied, D., Bohus, B., and Van Wimersma, Tj.B. (1975). Memory deficit in rats with hereditary diabetes insipidus. *Brain Research*, 85(1), 152–156.

D'Haenen, H.A., and Bossuyt, A. (1994). Dopamine D2 receptors in depression measured with single photon emission computed tomography. *Biol Psychiatry*, 35(2), 128–132.

D'Haenen, H., Bossuyt, A., Mertens, J., Bossuyt-Piron, C., Gijsemans, M., and Kaufman, L. (1992). SPECT imaging of serotonin2 receptors in depression. *Psychiatry Res*, 45, 227–237.

Diacicov, S., and Tudorache, B. (1990). Clonidine treatment in manic episodes. *Rev Med Int Neurol Psihiatr Neurochir Dermatovenerol Neurol Psihiatr Neurochir*, 35, 29–32.

Dick, D.A.T., Naylor, G.J., and Dick, E.G. (1978). Effects of Lithium on sodium transport across membranes. In F.N. Johnson, S. Johnson (Eds.), *Lithium in Medical Practice* (pp. 173–182). Baltimore: University Park Press.

Dillon, K.A., Gross-Isseroff, R., Israeli, M., and Biegon, A. (1991). Autoradiographic analysis of serotonin 5-HT1A receptor binding in the human brain postmortem: Effects of age and alcohol. *Brain Res*, 554, 56–64.

Dilsaver, S.C., and Coffman, J.A. (1989). Cholinergic hypothesis of depression: A reappraisal. *J Clin Psychopharmacol*, 9, 173–179.

Dilsaver, S.C., and Hariharan, M. (1988). Amitriptyline-induced supersensitivity of a central muscarinic mechanism: Lithium blocks amitriptyline-induced supersensitivity. *Psychiatry Res*, 25, 181–186.

Dilsaver, S.C., and Hariharan, M. (1989). Chronic treatment with lithium produces supersensitivity to nicotine. *Biol Psychiatry*, 25, 795–799.

Dilsaver, S.C., Peck, J.A., Traumata, D., and Swan, A.C. (1993). Treatment with carbamazepine may enhance alpha 2-noradrenergic autoreceptor sensitivity. *Biol Psychiatry*, 34, 551–557.

Dinan, T.G., Yatham, L.N., O'Keane, V., and Barry, S. (1991). Blunting of noradrenergic-stimulated growth hormone release in mania. *Am J Psychiatry*, 148, 936–938.

Dinan, T.G., O'Keane, V., and Thakore, J. (1994). Pyridostigmine induced growth hormone release in mania: focus on the cholinergic/somatostatin system. *Clin Endocrinol (Oxf)*, 40, 93–96.

Divish, M.M., Sheftel, G., Boyle, A., Kalasapudi, V.D., Papolos, D.F., and Lachman, H.M. (1991). Differential effect of lithium on fos protooncogene expression mediated by receptor and postreceptor activators of protein kinase C and cyclic adenosine monophosphate: Model for its antimanic action. *J Neurosci Res*, 28, 40–48.

Dixon, J.F., and Hokin, L.E. (1997). The antibipolar drug valproate mimics lithium in stimulating glutamate release and inositol 1,4,5-trisphosphate accumulation in brain cortex slices but not accumulation of inositol monophosphates and bisphosphates. *Proc Natl Acad Sci USA*, 94, 4757–4760.

Dixon, J.F., and Hokin, L.E. (1998). Lithium acutely inhibits and chronically up-regulates and stabilizes glutamate uptake by presynaptic nerve endings in mouse cerebral cortex. *Proc Natl Acad Sci USA*, 95(14), 8363–8368.

D'Mello, S.R., Anelli, R., and Calissano, P. (1994). Lithium induces apoptosis in immature cerebellar granule cells but promotes survival of mature neurons. *Exp Cell Res*, 211, 332–338.

Dobner, P.R., Tischler, A.S., Lee, Y.C., Bloom, S.R., and Donahue, S.R. (1988). Lithium dramatically potentiates neurotensin/neuromedin N gene expression. *J Biol Chem*, 263, 13983–13986.

Doraiswamy, P.M., MacFall, J., Krishnan, K.R., O'Connor, C., Wan, X., Benaur, M., Lewandowski, M., and Fortner, M. (1999). Magnetic resonance assessment of cerebral perfusion in depressed cardiac patients: Preliminary findings. *Am J Psychiatry*, 156, 1641–1643.

Doran, A.R., Rubinow, D.R., Roy, A., and Pickar, D. (1986). CSF somatostatin and abnormal response to dexamethasone administration in schizophrenic and depressed patients. *Arch Gen Psychiatry*, 43, 365–369.

Dowlatshahi, D., MacQueen, G.M., Wang, J.F., and Young, L.T. (1998). Increased temporal cortex CREB concentrations and antidepressant treatment in major depression. *Lancet*, 352, 1754–1755.

Drevets, W.C. (2000). Neuroimaging studies of mood disorders. *Biol Psychiatry*, 48, 813–829.

Drevets, W.C. (2001). Neuroimaging and neuropathological studies of depression: Implications for the cognitive-emotional features of mood disorders. *Curr Opin Neurobiol*, 11, 240–249.

Drevets, W.C., Frank, E., Price, J.C., Kupfer, D.J., Holt, D., Greer, P.J., Huang, Y., Gautier, C., and Mathis, C. (1999). PET imaging of serotonin 1A receptor binding in depression. *Biol Psychiatry*, 46, 1375–1387.

Drevets, W.C., Frank, E., Price, J.C., Kupfer, D.J., Greer, P.J., and Mathis, C. (2000). Serotonin type-1A receptor imaging in depression. *Nucl Med Biol*, 27, 499–507.

Drevets, W.C., Price, J.L., Bardgett, M.E., Reich, T., Todd, R.D., and Raichle, M.E. (2002). Glucose metabolism in the amygdala in depression: Relationship to diagnostic subtype and plasma cortisol levels. *Pharmacol Biochem Behav*, 71, 431–447.

D'Sa, C., and Duman, R.S. (2002). Antidepressants and neuroplasticity. *Bipolar Disord*, 4, 183–194.

Du, J., Gray, N., Falke, C., Yuan, P., Szabo, S., and Manji, H. (2003). Structurally dissimilar antimanic agents modulate synaptic plasticity by regulating AMPA glutamate receptor subunit GluR1 synaptic expression. *Ann NY Acad Sci*, 1003, 378–380.

Dubovsky, S.L., Christiano, J., Daniell, L.C., Franks, R.D., Murphy, J., Adler, L., Baker, N., and Harris, R.A. (1989). Increased platelet intracellular calcium concentration in patients with bipolar affective disorders. *Arch Gen Psychiatry*, 46, 632–638.

Dubovsky, S.L., Lee, C., Christiano, J., and Murphy, J. (1991). Elevated platelet intracellular calcium concentration in bipolar depression. *Biol Psychiatry*, 29, 441–450.

Dubovsky, S.L., Murphy, J., Christiano, J., and Lee, C. (1992a). The calcium second messenger system in bipolar disorders: Data supporting new research directions. *J Neuropsychiatry Clin Neurosci*, 4, 3–14.

Dubovsky, S.L., Murphy, J., Thomas, M., and Rademacher, J. (1992b). Abnormal intracellular calcium ion concentration in platelets and lymphocytes of bipolar patients. *Am J Psychiatry*, 149, 118–120.

Dubovsky, S.L., Thomas, J., Hijazi, A., and Murphy, J. (1994). Intracellular calcium signaling in peripheral cells of patients with bipolar affective disorder. *Eur Arch Psychiatry Clin Neurosci*, 243, 229–234.

Ducottet, C., Griebel, G., and Belzung, C. (2003). Effects of the selective nonpeptide corticotropin-releasing factor receptor 1 antagonist antalarmin in the chronic mild stress model of depression in mice. *Prog Neuropsychopharmacol Biol Psychiatry*, 27(4), 625–631.

Duman, RS. (2004). Role of neurotrophic factors in the etiology and treatment of mood disorders. *Neuromol Med*, 5(1), 11–25.

Duman, R.S., Heninger, G.R., and Nestler, E.J. (1997). A molecular and cellular theory of depression. *Arch Gen Psychiatry*, 54, 597–606.

Duman, R.S., Malberg, J., and Thome, J. (1999). Neural plasticity to stress and antidepressant treatment. *Biol Psychiatry*, 46, 1181–1191.

Duman, R.S., Malberg, J., Nakagawa, S., and D'Sa, C. (2000). Neuronal plasticity and survival in mood disorders. *Biol Psychiatry*, 48, 732–739.

Dunner, D.L., Levitt, M., Kumbaraci, T., and Fieve, R.R. (1977). Erythrocyte catechol-O-methyltransferase activity in primary affective disorder. *Biol Psychiatry*, 12, 237–244.

Duval, F., Macher, J.P., and Mokrani, M.C. (1990). Difference between evening and morning thyrotropin responses to protirelin in major depressive episode. *Arch Gen Psychiatry*, 47, 443–448.

Dwivedi, Y., and Pandey, G.N. (1999). Administration of dexamethasone up-regulates protein kinase C activity and the expression of gamma and epsilon protein kinase C isozymes in the rat brain. *J Neurochem*, 72, 380–387.

Eastwood, S.L., and Harrison, P.J. (2001). Synaptic pathology in the anterior cingulate cortex in schizophrenia and mood disorders. A review and a Western blot study of synaptophysin, GAP-43 and the complexins. *Brain Res Bull*, 55, 569–78.

Ebert, D., and Ebmeier, K.P. (1996). The role of the cingulate gyrus in depression: From functional anatomy to neurochemistry. *Biol Psychiatry*, 39, 1044–1050.

Ebstein, R.P., Lerer, B., Shlaufman, M., and Belmaker, R.H. (1983). The effect of repeated electroconvulsive shock treatment and chronic lithium feeding on the release of norepinephrine from rat cortical vesicular preparations. *Cell Mol Neurobiol*, 3, 191–201.

Ebstein, R.P., Moscovich, D., Zeevi, S., Amiri, Z., and Lerer, B. (1987). Effect of lithium in vitro and after chronic treatment on human platelet adenylate cyclase activity: Postreceptor modification of second-messenger signal amplification. *Psychiatry Res*, 21, 221–228.

Ebstein, R.P., Lerer, B., Bennett, E.R., Shapira, B., Kindler, S., Shemesh, Z., and Gerstenhaber, N. (1988). Lithium modulation of second messenger signal amplification in man: Inhibition of phosphatidylinositol-specific phospholipase C and adenylate cyclase activity. *Psychiatry Res*, 24, 45–52.

Eckermann, K., Beasley, A., Yang, P., Gaytan, O., Swann, A., and Dafny, N. (2001). Methylphenidate sensitization is modulated by valproate. *Life Sci*, 69, 47–57.

Eden Evins, A., Demopulos, C., Nierenberg, A., Culhane, M.A., Eisner, L., and Sachs, G. (2006). A double-blind, placebo-controlled trial of adjunctive donepezil in treatment-resistant mania. *Bipolar Disord*, 8, 75–80.

Egan, M.F., Goldberg, T.E., Kolachana, B.S., Callicott, J.H., Mazzanti, C.M., Straub, R.E., Goldman, D., and Weinberger, D.R. (2001). Effect of COMT Val108/158 Met genotype on frontal lobe function and risk for schizophrenia. *Proc Natl Acad Sci USA*, 98, 6917–6922.

Egan, M.F., Kojima, M., Callicott, J.H., Goldberg, T.E., Kolachana, B.S., Bertolino, A., Zaitsev, E., Gold, B., Goldman, D., Dean, M., Lu, B., and Weinberger, D.R. (2003). The BDNF val66met polymorphism affects activity-dependent secretion of BDNF and human memory and hippocampal function. *Cell*, 112(2), 257–269.

Egeland, J.A., Kidd, J.R., Frazer, A., Kidd, K.K., and Neuhauser, V.I. (1984). Amish study: V. Lithium-sodium countertransport and catechol O-methyltransferase in pedigrees of bipolar probands. *Am J Psychiatry*, 141, 1049–1054.

Ehrlich, B.E., and Diamond, J.M. (1979). Lithium fluxes in human erythrocytes. *Am J Physiol*, 237, C102–C110.

Ehrlich, B.E., and Diamond, J.M. (1980). Lithium, membranes, and manic-depressive illness. *J Membr Biol*, 52, 187–200.

Ehrlich, B.E., Diamond, J.M., and Gosenfeld, L. (1981). Lithium-induced changes in sodium-lithium countertransport. *Biochem Pharmacol*, 30, 2539–2543.

Ehrlich, B.E., Diamond, J.M., Fry, V., and Meier, K. (1983). Lithium's inhibition of erythrocyte cation countertransport involves a slow process in the erythrocyte. *J Membr Biol*, 75, 233–240.

Eilam, D., and Szechtman, H. (1989). Biphasic effect of D2 agonist quinpirole on locomotion and movements. *Eur J Pharmacol*, 161, 151–157.

Eilam, D., and Szechtman, H. (1990). Dosing regimen differentiates sensitization of locomotion and mouthing to D2 agonist quinpirole. *Pharmacol Biochem Behav*, 36, 989–991.

Einat, H., Einat, D., Allan, M., Talangbayan, H., Tsafnat, T., and Szechtman, H. (1996). Associational and nonassociational mechanisms in locomotor sensitization to the dopamine agonist quinpirole. *Psychopharmacology (Berl)*, 127, 95–101.

Einat, H., Kofman, O., and Belmaker, R.H. (2000). Animal models of bipolar disorder: From a single episode to progressive cycling models. In I. Weiner (Ed.), *Contemporary Issues in Modeling Psychopharmacology* (pp. 165–180). Boston: Kluwer Academic Publishers.

Einat, H., Belmaker, R.H., Zangen, A., Overstreet, D.H., and Yadid, G. (2002a). Chronic inositol treatment reduces depression-like immobility of Flinders Sensitive Line rats in the forced swim test. *Depress Anxiety*, 15, 148–151.

Einat, H., Chen, G., and Manji, H.K. (2002b). Does the ERK map kinase signaling cascade play a role in the pathophysiology and treatment of bipolar disorder? *Biol Psychiatry*, 51, 376s.

Einat, H., Belmaker, R.H., and Manji, H.K. (2003a). New aproaches to modeling bipolar disorder. *Psychopharmacol Bull*, 37, 47–63.

Einat, H., Yuan, P., Gould, T.D., Li, J., Du, J., Zhang, L., Manji, H.K., and Chen, G. (2003b). The role of the extracellular signal-regulated kinase signaling pathway in mood modulation. *J Neurosci*, 23, 7311–7316.

Elizur, A., Shopsin, B., Gershon, S., and Ehlenberger, A. (1972). Intra-extracellular lithium ratios and clinical course in affective states. *Clin Pharmacol Ther*, 13, 947–953.

Ellinwood, E.H. Jr., Sudilovsky, A., and Nelson, L. (1972). Behavioral analysis of chronic amphetamine intoxication. *Biol Psychiatry*, 4, 215–230.

Ellis, J., and Lenox, R.H. (1990). Chronic lithium treatment prevents atropine-induced supersensitivity of the muscarinic phosphoinositide response in rat hippocampus. *Biol Psychiatry*, 28, 609–619.

Ellis, P.M., and Salmond, C. (1994). Is platelet imipramine binding reduced in depression? A meta-analysis. *Biol Psychiatry*, 36:292–299.

El-Mallakh, R.S. (1983). The Na,K-ATPase hypothesis for manic-depression. II. The mechanism of action of lithium. *Med Hypotheses*, 12, 269–282.

El-Mallakh, R.S., and Jaziri, W.A. (1990). Calcium channel blockers in affective illness: Role of sodium-calcium exchange. *J Clin Psychopharmacol*, 10, 203–206.

Elphick, M., Yang, J.D., and Cowen, P.J. (1990). Effects of carbamazepine on dopamine- and serotonin-mediated neuroendocrine responses. *Arch Gen Psychiatry*, 47, 135–140.

Emamghoreishi, M., Schlichter, L., Li, P.P., Parikh, S., Sen, J., Kamble, A., and Warsh, J.J. (1997). High intracellular calcium concentrations in transformed lymphoblasts from subjects with bipolar I disorder. *Am J Psychiatry*, 154, 976–982.

Emamghoreishi, M., Li, P.P., Schlichter, L., Parikh, S.V., Cooke, R., and Warsh, J.J. (2000). Associated disturbances in calcium homeostasis and G protein–mediated cAMP signaling in bipolar I disorder. *Biol Psychiatry*, 48(7), 665–673.

Emrich, H.M., Cording, C., Piree, S., Kölling, A., Möller, H.J., VonZerssen, D., and Herz, A. (1979). Actions of naloxone in different types of psychosis. In E. Usdin, W.E. Bunney, and N.S. Kline (Eds.), *Endorphins in Mental Health Research* (pp. 452–460). New York: Oxford University Press.

Emrich, H.M., Aldenhoff, J.B., and Lux, H.D. (1982). *Basic Mechanisms in the Action of Lithium*. Amsterdam: Excerpta Medica.

Engel, J., and Berggren, U. (1980). Effects of lithium on behaviour and central monoamines. *Acta Psychiatr Scand Suppl*, 280, 133–143.

Erfurth, A., Michael, N., Stadtland, C., and Arolt, V. (2002). Bupropion as add-on strategy in difficult-to-treat bipolar depressive patients. *Neuropsychobiology*, 45(Suppl. 1), 33–36.

Eriksson, P.S., Perfilieva, E., Bjork-Eriksson, T., Alborn, A.M., Nordborg, C., Peterson, D.A., and Gage, F.H. (1998). Neurogenesis in the adult human hippocampus. *Nat Med*, 4(11), 1313–1317.

Eroglu, L., Hizal, A., and Koyuncuoglu, H. (1981). The effect of long-term concurrent administration of chlorpromazine and lithium on the striatal and frontal cortical dopamine metabolism in rats. *Psychopharmacology (Berl)*, 73, 84–86.

Esler, M. (1982). Assessment of sympathetic nervous function in humans from noradrenaline plasma kinetics. *Clin Sci (Lond)*, 62, 247–254.

Esler, M., Turbott, J., Schwarz, R., Leonard, P., Bobik, A., Skews, H., and Jackman, G. (1982). The peripheral kinetics of norepinephrine in depressive illness. *Arch Gen Psychiatry*, 39(3), 295–300.

Evans, D.L., and Nemeroff, C.B. (1983). The dexamethasone suppression test in mixed bipolar disorder. *Am J Psychiatry*, 140, 615–617.

Evans, M.S., Zorumski, C.F., and Clifford, D.B. (1990). Lithium enhances neuronal muscarinic excitation by presynaptic facilitation. *Neuroscience*, 38, 457–468.

Everitt, B.J., Hokfelt, T., Terenius, L., Tatemoto, K., Mutt, V., and Goldstein, M. (1984). Differential co-existence of neuropeptide Y (NPY)-like immunoreactivity with catecholamines in the central nervous system of the rat. *Neuroscience*, 11(2), 443–462.

Extein, I.L. (2000). High doses of levothyroxine for refractory rapid cycling. *Am J Psychiatry*, 157, 1704–1705.

Extein, I., Goodwin, F.K., Lewy, A.J., Schoenfeld, R.I., and Fakhur, L.R. (1979a). Behavioral and biochemical effects of FK 33-824, a parenterally and orally active enkephalin analog. In E. Usdin, W.E. Bunney, and N.S. Kline (Eds.), *Endorphins in Mental Health Research* (pp. 279–292). New York: Oxford University Press.

Extein, I., Lo, C., Goodwin, F.K., and Schoenfeld, R.I. (1979b). Dopamine-mediated behavior produced by the enkephalin analogue FK 33-824. *Psychiatry Res*, 1, 333–339.

Fadda, P., Tortorella, A., and Fratta, W. (1991). Sleep deprivation decreases mu and delta opioid receptor binding in the rat limbic system. *Neurosci Lett*, 129, 315–317.

Fadda, P., Martellotta, M.C., De Montis, M.G., Gessa, G.L., and Fratta, W. (1992). Dopamine D1 and opioid receptor binding changes in the limbic system of sleep deprived rats. *Neurochem Int*, 20, 153S–156S.

Fadic, R., and Johns, D.R. (1996). Clinical spectrum of mitochondrial diseases. *Semin Neurol*, 16(1), 11–20.

Fahn, S. (1978). Post-anoxic action myoclonus: Improvement with valproic acid. *N Engl J Med*, 299, 313–314.

Fahndrich, E., Coper, H., Christ, W., Helmchen, H., Muller-Oerlinghausen, B., and Pietzcker, A. (1980). Erythrocyte COMT-activity in patients with affective disorders. *Acta Psychiatr Scand*, 61, 427–437.

Farley, I.J., Price, K.S., McCullough, E., Deck, J.H., Hordynski, W., and Hornykiewicz, O. (1978). Norepinephrine in chronic paranoid schizophrenia: Above-normal levels in limbic forebrain. *Science*, 200, 456–458.

Fatemi, S.H. (2002). The role of Reelin in pathology of autism. *Mol Psychiatry*, 7, 919–920.

Fatemi, S.H., Earle, J.A., and McMenomy, T. (2000a). Hippocampal CA4 Reelin-positive neurons. *Mol Psychiatry*, 5, 571.

Fatemi, S.H., Earle, J.A., and McMenomy, T. (2000b). Reduction in Reelin immunoreactivity in hippocampus of subjects with schizophrenia, bipolar disorder and major depression. *Mol Psychiatry*, 5, 571, 654–663.

Fatemi, S.H., Earle, J.A., Stary, J.M., Lee, S., and Sedgewick, J. (2001a). Altered levels of the synaptosomal associated protein SNAP-25 in hippocampus of subjects with mood disorders and schizophrenia. *Neuroreport*, 12, 3257–3262.

Fatemi, S.H., Kroll, J.L., and Stary, J.M. (2001b). Altered levels of Reelin and its isoforms in schizophrenia and mood disorders. *Neuroreport*, 12, 3209–3215.

Fatemi, S.H., Stary, J.M., and Egan, E.A. (2002). Reduced blood levels of reelin as a vulnerability factor in pathophysiology of autistic disorder. *Cell Mol Neurobiol*, 22, 139–152.

Feinberg, M., and Carroll, B.J. (1984). Biological 'markers' for endogenous depression. Effect of age, severity of illness, weight loss, and polarity. *Arch Gen Psychiatry*, 41, 1080–1085.

Fernstrom, J.D. (1983). Role of precursor availability in control of monoamine biosynthesis in brain. *Physiol Rev*, 63, 484–546.

Fernstrom, J.D., and Wurtman, R.J. (1997). Brain serotonin content: Physiological regulation by plasma neutral amino acids. *Obes Res*, 5(4), 377–380.

Ferrari, E., Bossolo, P.A., Vailati, A., Martinelli, I., Rea, A., and Nosari, I. (1977). Effects of a vagolytic substance on the circadian rhythm of the ACTH-secreting system in man. *Ann Endocrinol (Paris)*, 38, 203–213.

Ferrendelli, J.A., and Kinscherf, D.A. (1979). Inhibitory effects of anticonvulsant drugs on cyclic nucleotide accumulation in brain. *Ann Neurol*, 5, 533–538.

Ferris, C.F., Lu, S.F., Messenger, T., Guillon, C.D., Heindel, N., Miller, M., Koppel, G., Robert Bruns, F., and Simon, N.G. (2006). Orally active vasopressin V1a receptor antagonist, SRX251, selectively blocks aggressive behavior. *Pharmacol Biochem Behav*, 83(2), 169–174.

Fields, A., Li, P.P., Kish, S.J., and Warsh, J.J. (1999). Increased cyclic AMP-dependent protein kinase activity in postmortem brain from patients with bipolar affective disorder. *J Neurochem*, 73, 1704–1710.

File, S.E. (1997). Anxiolytic action of a neurokinin1 receptor antagonist in the social interaction test. *Pharmacol Biochem Behav*, 58(3), 747–752.

Filser, J.G., Spira, J., Fischer, M., Gattaz, W.F., and Muller, W.E. (1988). The evaluation of 4-hydroxy-3-methoxyphenylglycol sulfate as a possible marker of central norepinephrine turnover. Studies in healthy volunteers and depressed patients. *J Psychiatr Res*, 22, 171–181.

Fink, M., Papakostas, Y., Lee, J., Meehan, T., and Johnson, L. (1981). Clinical trials with des-tyr-gamma-endorphin (GK-78). In C. Perris, G. Struwe, and B. Jansson (Eds.), *Biological Psychiatry 1981* (pp. 398–401). Amsterdam: Elsevier.

Fischer, W., and Muller, M. (1988). Pharmacological modulation of central monoaminergic systems and influence on the anticonvulsant effectiveness of standard antiepileptics in maximal electroshock seizure. *Biomed Biochim Acta*, 47, 631–645.

Fisher, S.K., Heacock, A.M., and Agranoff, B.W. (1992). Inositol lipids and signal transduction in the nervous system: An update. *J Neurochem*, 58, 18–38.

Fishman, S.M., Catarau, E.M., Sachs, G., Stojanovic, M., and Borsook, D. (1996). Corticosteroid-induced mania after single regional application at the celiac plexus. *Anesthesiology*, 85(5), 1194–1196.

Foley, K.M., Kourides, I.A., Inturrisi, C.E., Kaiko, R.F., Zaroulis, C.G., Posner, J.B., Houde, R.W., and Li, C.H. (1979). Beta-endorphin: Analgesic and hormonal effects in humans. *Proc Natl Acad Sci USA*, 76, 5377–5381.

Forstner, U., Bohus, M., Gebicke-Harter, P.J., Baumer, B., Berger, M., and van Calker, D. (1994). Decreased agonist-stimulated Ca2+ response in neutrophils from patients under chronic lithium therapy. *Eur Arch Psychiatry Clin Neurosci*, 243(5), 240–243.

France, R.D., Urban, B., Krishnan, K.R., Bissett, G., Banki, C.M., Nemeroff, C., and Speilman, F.J. (1988). CSF corticotropin-releasing factor-like immunoactivity in chronic pain patients with and without major depression. *Biol Psychiatry*, 23, 86–88.

Frances, H., Maurin, Y., Lecrubier, Y., Puech, A.J., and Simon, P. (1981). Effect of chronic lithium treatment on isolation-induced behavioral and biochemical effects in mice. *Eur J Pharmacol*, 72, 337–341.

Francis, D., Diorio, J., Liu, D., and Meaney, M.J. (1999). Nongenomic transmission across generations of maternal behavior and stress responses in the rat. *Science*, 286, 1155–1158.

Fratta, W., Collu, M., Martellotta, M.C., Pichiri, M., Muntoni, F., and Gessa, G.L. (1987). Stress-induced insomnia: Opioid-dopamine interactions. *Eur J Pharmacol*, 142, 437–440.

Frazer, A., Mendels, J., Brunswick, D., London, J., Pring, M., Ramsey, T.A., and Rybakowski, J. (1978). Erythrocyte concentrations of the lithium ion: Clinical correlates and mechanisms of action. *Am J Psychiatry*, 135, 1065–1069.

Frazer, A., Ramsey, T.A., Swann, A., Bowden, C., Brunswick, D., Garver, D., and Secunda, S. (1983). Plasma and erythrocyte electrolytes in affective disorders. *J Affect Disord*, 5, 103–113.

Freedman, R.R., Embury, J., Migaly, P., Keegan, D., Pandey, G.N., Javaid, J.I., and Davis, J.M. (1990). Stress-induced desensitization of alpha 2-adrenergic receptors in human platelets. *Psychosom Med*, 52, 624–630.

Friedman, E., and Gershon, S. (1973). Effect of lithium on brain dopamine. *Nature*, 243, 520–521.

Friedman, E., and Wang, H.Y. (1988). Effect of chronic lithium treatment on 5-hydroxytryptamine autoreceptors and release of 5-[3H]hydroxytryptamine from rat brain cortical, hippocampal, and hypothalamic slices. *J Neurochem*, 50, 195–201.

Friedman, E., and Wang, H.Y. (1996). Receptor-mediated activation of G proteins is increased in postmortem brains of bipolar affective disorder subjects. *J Neurochem*, 67, 1145–1152.

Friedman, E., Dallob, A., and Levine, G. (1979). The effect of long-term lithium treatment on reserpine-induced supersensitivity in dopaminergic and serotonergic transmission. *Life Sci*, 25, 1263–1266.

Friedman, E., Hoau Yan, W., Levinson, D., Connell, T.A., and Singh, H. (1993). Altered platelet protein kinase C activity in bipolar affective disorder, manic episode. *Biol Psychiatry*, 33, 520–525.

Frye, M.A., Denicoff, K.D., Bryan, A.L., Smith-Jackson, E.E., Ali, S.O., Luckenbaugh, D., Leverich, G.S., and Post, R.M. (1999a). Association between lower serum free T4 and greater mood instability and depression in lithium-maintained bipolar patients. *Am J Psychiatry*, 156, 1909–1914.

Frye, M.A., Dunn, R.T., Gary, K.A., Kimbrell, T.A., Callahan, A.M., Luckenbaugh, D.A., Cora-Locatelli, G., Vanderham, E., Winokur, A., and Post, R.M. (1999b). Lack of correlation between cerebrospinal fluid thyrotropin-releasing hormone (TRH) and TRH-stimulated thyroid-stimulating hormone in patients with depression. *Biol Psychiatry*, 45, 1049–1052.

Furlong, R.A., Ho, L., Walsh, C., Rubinsztein, J.S., Jain, S., Paykel, E.S., Easton, D.F., and Rubinsztein, D.C. (1998). Analysis and meta-analysis of two serotonin transporter gene polymorphisms in bipolar and unipolar affective disorders. *Am J Med Genet*, 81, 58–63.

Fyro, B., Petterson, U., and Sedvall, G. (1975). The effect of lithium treatment on manic symptoms and levels of monoamine metabolites in cerebrospinal fluid of manic depressive patients. *Psychopharmacologia*, 44, 99–103.

Gabriel, S.M., Knott, P.J., and Haroutunian, V. (1995). Alterations in cerebral cortical galanin concentrations following neurotransmitter-specific subcortical lesions in the rat. *J Neurosci*, 15(8), 5526–5534.

Gaillard, W.D., Zeffiro, T., Fazilat, S., DeCarli, C., and Theodore, W.H. (1996). Effect of valproate on cerebral metabolism and blood flow: An 18F-2-deoxyglucose and 15O water positron emission tomography study. *Epilepsia*, 37, 515–521.

Gallager, D.W., Pert, A., and Bunney, W.E. Jr. (1978). Haloperidol-induced presynaptic dopamine supersensitivity is blocked by chronic lithium. *Nature*, 273, 309–312.

Galva, M.D., Bondiolotti, G.P., Olasmaa, M., and Picotti, G.B. (1995). Effect of aging on lazabemide binding, monoamine oxidase activity and monoamine metabolites in human frontal cortex. *J Neural Transm Gen Sect*, 101, 83–94.

Gann, H., Riemann, D., Hohagen, F., Strauss, L.G., Dressing, H., Muller, W.E., and Berger, M. (1993). 48-hour rapid cycling: Results of psychopathometric, polysomnographic, PET imaging and neuroendocrine longitudinal investigations in a single case. *J Affect Disord*, 28, 133–140.

Garcia-Sevilla, J.A., and Fuster, M.J. (1986). Labelling of human platelet alpha 2-adrenoceptors with the full agonist [3H] (-)adrenaline. *Eur J Pharmacol*, 124, 31–41.

Garcia-Sevilla, J.A., Ugedo, L., Ulibarri, I., and Gutierrez, M. (1986a). Heroin increases the density and sensitivity of platelet alpha 2-adrenoceptors in human addicts. *Psychopharmacology (Berl)*, 88(4), 489–492.

Garcia-Sevilla, J.A., Guimon, J., Garcia-Vallejo, P., and Fuster, M.J. (1986b). Biochemical and functional evidence of supersensitive platelet alpha 2-adrenoceptors in major affective disorder. Effect of long-term lithium carbonate treatment. *Arch Gen Psychiatry*, 43(1), 51–57.

Garcia-Sevilla, J.A., Padro, D., Giralt, M.T., Guimon, J., and Areso, P. (1990). Alpha 2-adrenoceptor-mediated inhibition of platelet adenylate cyclase and induction of aggregation in major depression. Effect of long-term cyclic antidepressant drug treatment. *Arch Gen Psychiatry*, 47, 125–132.

Garcia-Sevilla, J.A., Escriba, P.V., Busquets, X., Walzer, C., and Guimon, J. (1996). Platelet imidazoline receptors and regulatory G proteins in patients with major depression. *Neuroreport*, 8, 169–172.

Garcia-Sevilla, J.A., Escriba, P.V., Ozaita, A., La Harpe, R., Walzer, C., Eytan, A., and Guimon, J. (1999). Up-regulation of immunolabeled alpha2A-adrenoceptors, Gi coupling proteins, and regulatory receptor kinases in the prefrontal cortex of depressed suicides. *J Neurochem*, 72, 282–291.

Garlow, S., Mussellman, D., and Nemeroff, C. (1999). The neurochemistry of mood disorders. In B.S. Bunney (Ed.), *Neurobiology of Mental Illness* (pp. 348–364). New York: Oxford University Press.

Gass, P., Kretz, O., Wolfer, D.P., Berger, S., Tronche, F., Reichardt, H.M., Kellendonk, C., Lipp, H.P., Schmid, W., and Schutz, G. (2000). Genetic disruption of mineralocorticoid receptor leads to impaired neurogenesis and granule cell degeneration in the hippocampus of adult mice. *EMBO Rep*, 1, 447–451.

Geracioti, T.D. Jr., Loosen, P.T., Ekhator, N.N., Schmidt, D., Chambliss, B., Baker, D.G., Kasckow, J.W., Richtand, N.M., Keck, P.E. Jr., and Ebert, M.H. (1997). Uncoupling of serotonergic and noradrenergic systems in depression: Preliminary evidence from continuous cerebrospinal fluid sampling. *Depress Anxiety*, 6, 89–94.

Gerner, R.H., and Hare, T.A. (1981). CSF GABA in normal subjects and patients with depression, schizophrenia, mania, and anorexia nervosa. *Am J Psychiatry*, 138, 1098–1101.

Gerner, R.H., and Wilkins, J.N. (1983). CSF cortisol in patients with depression, mania, or anorexia nervosa and in normal subjects. *Am J Psychiatry*, 140, 92–94.

Gerner, R.H., and Yamada, T. (1982). Altered neuropeptide concentrations in cerebrospinal fluid of psychiatric patients. *Brain Res*, 238(1), 298–302.

Gerner, R.H., Post, R.M., and Bunney, W.E. Jr. (1976). A dopaminergic mechanism in mania. *Am J Psychiatry*, 133, 1177–1180.

Gerner, R.H., Post, R.M., Gillin, J.C., and Bunney, W.E. Jr. (1979). Biological and behavioral effects of one night's sleep deprivation in depressed patients and normals. *J Psychiatr Res*, 15, 21–40.

Gerner, R.H., Catlin, D.H., Gorelick, D.A., Hui, K.K., and Li, C.H. (1980). Beta-endorphin: Intravenous infusion causes behavioral change in psychiatric inpatients. *Arch Gen Psychiatry*, 37, 642–647.

Gerner, R.H., Fairbanks, L., Anderson, G.M., Young, J.G., Scheinin, M., Linnoila, M., Hare, T.A., Shaywitz, B.A., and Cohen, D.J. (1984). CSF neurochemistry in depressed, manic, and schizophrenic patients compared with that of normal controls. *Am J Psychiatry*, 141, 1533–1540.

Gershon, E.S., and Jonas, W.Z. (1975). Erythrocyte soluble catechol-O-methyl transferase activity in primary affective disorder. A clinical and genetic study. *Arch Gen Psychiatry*, 32, 1351–1356.

Gesing, A., Bilang-Bleuel, A., Droste, S.K., Linthorst, A.C., Holsboer, F., and Reul, J.M. (2001). Psychological stress increases hippocampal mineralocorticoid receptor levels: Involvement of corticotropin-releasing hormone. *J Neurosci*, 21, 4822–4829.

Gessa, G.L., Pani, L., Serra, G., and Fratta, W. (1995). Animal models of mania. *Adv Biochem Psychopharmacol*, 49, 43–66.

Giambalvo, C.T. (1992a). Protein kinase C and dopamine transport: 1. Effects of amphetamine in vivo. *Neuropharmacology*, 31, 1201–1210.

Giambalvo, C.T. (1992b). Protein kinase C and dopamine transport: 2. Effects of amphetamine in vitro. *Neuropharmacology*, 31, 1211–1222.

Gibbons, J.L. (1964). Cortisol secretion rate in depressive illness. *Arch Gen Psychiatry*, 10, 572–575.

Gillin, J.C., Wyatt, R.J., Fram, D., and Snyder, F. (1978). The relationship between changes in REM sleep and clinical improvement in depressed patients treated with amitriptyline. *Psychopharmacology (Berl)*, 59, 267–272.

Gjerris, A., Fahrenkrug, J., Bojhold, S., and Rafaelsen, O.J. (1981). Vasoactive intestinal polypeptide in cerebrospinal fluid in psychiatric disorders. In C. Perris, G. Struwe, and B. Jansson (Eds.), *Biological Psychiatry 1981* (pp. 359–362). Amsterdam: Elsevier.

Gjerris, A., Rafaelsen, O.J., Vendsborg, P., Fahrenkrug, J., and Rehfeld, J.F. (1984). Vasoactive intestinal polypeptide decreased in cerebrospinal fluid (CSF) in atypical depression. Vasoactive intestinal polypeptide, cholecystokinin and gastrin in CSF in psychiatric disorders. *J Affect Disord*, 7, 325–337.

Gjerris, A., Hammer, M., Vendsborg, P., Christensen, N.J., and Rafaelsen, O.J. (1985). Cerebrospinal fluid vasopressin—changes in depression. *Br J Psychiatry*, 147, 696–701.

Gjessing, R. (1938). Disturbance of somatic functions in catatonia with periodic course, and their compensation. *J Ment Sci*, 84, 608–621.

Glen, A.I., and Reading, H.W. (1973). Regulatory action of lithium in manic-depressive illness. *Lancet*, 2, 1239–1241.

Glen, A.I., Ongley, G.C., and Robinson, K. (1968). Diminished membrane transport in manic-depressive psychosis and recurrent depression. *Lancet*, 2, 241–243.

Glitz, D.A., Manji, H.K., and Moore, G.J. (2002). Mood disorders: Treatment-induced changes in brain neurochemistry and structure. *Semin Clin Neuropsychiatry*, 7, 269–280.

Glue, P.W., Cowen, P.J., Nutt, D.J., Kolakowska, T., and Grahame-Smith, D.G. (1986). The effect of lithium on 5-HT-mediated neuroendocrine responses and platelet 5-HT receptors. *Psychopharmacology (Berl)*, 90, 398–402.

Gnegy, M.E., Hong, P., and Ferrell, S.T. (1993). Phosphorylation of neuromodulin in rat striatum after acute and repeated, intermittent amphetamine. *Brain Res Mol Brain Res*, 20, 289–298.

Godfrey, P.P., McClue, S.J., White, A.M., Wood, A.J., and Grahame-Smith, D.G. (1989). Subacute and chronic in vivo lithium treatment inhibits agonist- and sodium fluoride-stimulated inositol phosphate production in rat cortex. *J Neurochem*, 52, 498–506.

Godwin, C.D., Greenberg, L.B., and Shukla, S. (1984). Consistent dexamethasone suppression test results with mania and depression in bipolar illness. *Am J Psychiatry*, 141, 1263–1265.

Gold, M.S., Pottash, A.L., and Extein, I. (1981). Hypothyroidism and depression. Evidence from complete thyroid function evaluation. *JAMA*, 245, 1919–1922.

Gold, M.S., Pottash, A.L., and Extein, I. (1982). "Symptomless" autoimmune thyroiditis in depression. *Psychiatry Res*, 6, 261–269.

Gold, P.W., and Chrousos, G.P. (1985). Clinical studies with corticotropin releasing factor: Implications for the diagnosis and pathophysiology of depression, Cushing's disease, and adrenal insufficiency. *Psychoneuroendocrinology*, 10, 401–419.

Gold, P.W., and Chrousos, G.P. (2002). Organization of the stress system and its dysregulation in melancholic and atypical depression: High vs. low CRH/NE states. *Mol Psychiatry*, 7, 254–275.

Gold, P.W., Goodwin, F.K., and Reus, V.I. (1978). Vasopressin in affective illness. *Lancet*, 1, 1233–1236.

Gold, P.W., Weingartner, H., Ballenger, J.C., Goodwin, F.K., and Post, R.M. (1979). Effects of 1-desamo-8-D-arginine vasopressin on behaviour and cognition in primary affective disorder. *Lancet*, 2, 992–994.

Gold, P.W., Goodwin, F.K., Post, R.M., and Robertson, G.L. (1981). Vasopressin function in depression and mania [proceedings]. *Psychopharmacol Bull*, 17, 7–9.

Gold, P.W., Ballenger, J.C., Robertson, G.L., Wingartner, H., Rubinow, D.R., Hoban, M.C., Goodwin, F.K., and Post, R.M. (1984a). Vasopressin in affective illness: Direct measurement, clinical trials, and response to hypertonic saline. In R.M. Post and J.C. Ballenger (Eds.), *Neurobiology of Mood Disorders* (pp. 323–339). Baltimore: Williams and Wilkins.

Gold, P.W., Chrousos, G., Kellner, C., Post, R., Roy, A., Augerinos, P., Schulte, H., Oldfield, E., and Loriaux, D.L. (1984b). Psychiatric implications of basic and clinical studies with corticotropin-releasing factor. *Am J Psychiatry*, 141, 619–627.

Gold, P.W., Calabrese, J.R., Kling, M.A., Avgerinos, P., Khan, I., Gallucci, W.T., Tomai, T.P., and Chrousos, G.P. (1986). Abnormal ACTH and cortisol responses to ovine corticotropin releasing factor in patients with primary affective disorder. *Prog Neuropsychopharmacol Biol Psychiatry*, 10, 57–65.

Gold, P.W., Goodwin, F.K., and Chrousos, G.P. (1988). Clinical and biochemical manifestations of depression. Relation to the neurobiology of stress (2). *N Engl J Med*, 319, 413–420.

Goldberg, J.F., Burdick, K.E., and Endick, C.J. (2004). Preliminary randomized, double-blind, placebo-controlled trial of pramipexole added to mood stabilizers for treatment-resistant bipolar depression. *Am J Psychiatry*, 161(3), 564–566.

Goldstein, D.S., Brush, J.E. Jr., Eisenhofer, G., Stull, R., and Esler, M. (1988). In vivo measurement of neuronal uptake of norepinephrine in the human heart. *Circulation*, 78, 41–48.

Goldstein, E.T., and Preskorn, S.H. (1989). Mania triggered by a steroid nasal spray in a patient with stable bipolar disorder. *Am J Psychiatry*, 146, 1076–1077.

Goldstein, J., Van Cauter, E., Linkowski, P., Vanhaelst, L., and Mendlewicz, J. (1980). Thyrotropin nyctohemeral pattern in primary depression: Differences between unipolar and bipolar women. *Life Sci*, 27, 1695–1703.

Goldstein, M., Fuxe, K., Meller, E., Seyfried, C.A., Agnati, L., and Mascagni, F.M. (1987). The characterization of the dopaminergic profile of EMD 23,448, and indolyl-3-butylamine: Selective actions on presynaptic and supersensitive postsynaptic DA receptor populations. *J Neural Transm*, 70, 193–215.

Gomez-Piñilla, F., So, V., and Kesslak, J.P. (2001). Spatial learning induces neurotrophin receptor and synapsin I in the hippocampus. *Brain Res*, 904, 13–19.

Gonzalez-Pinto, A., Imaz, H., De Heredia, J.L., Gutierrez, M., and Mico, J.A. (2001). Mania and tramadol-fluoxetine combination. *Am J Psychiatry*, 158(6), 964–965.

Goodnick, P.J. (1990). Bupropion in chronic fatigue syndrome. *Am J Psychiatry*, 147(8), 1091.

Goodnick, P., and Gershon, S. (1984). Chemotherapy of cognitive disorders in geriatric subjects. *J Clin Psychiatry*, 45, 196–209.

Goodnick, P.J., and Meltzer, H.Y. (1984). Neurochemical changes during discontinuation of lithium prophylaxis. I. Increases in clonidine-induced hypotension. *Biol Psychiatry*, 19, 883–889.

Goodwin, F.K., and Ghaemi, S.N. (1998). Understanding manic-depressive illness. *Arch Gen Psychiatry*, 55(1), 23–25.

Goodwin, F.K., and Jamison, K.R. (1990). *Manic-Depressive Illness*. New York: Oxford University Press.

Goodwin, F., and Sack, R.L. (1973). Affective disorders: The catecholamine hypothesis revisited. In E. Usdin and S. Snyder (Eds.), *Frontiers in Catecholamine Research* (pp. 1157–1164). New York: Pergamon Press.

Goodwin, F.K., and Sack, R.L. (1974). Central dopamine function in affective illness: Evidence from precursors, enzyme inhibitors, and studies of central dopamine turnover. *Adv Biochem Psychopharmacol*, 12(0), 261–279.

Goodwin, F.K., Murphy, D.L., Brodie, H.K., and Bunney, W.E. Jr. (1970). L-DOPA, catecholamines, and behavior: A clinical and biochemical study in depressed patients. *Biol Psychiatry*, 2, 341–366.

Goodwin, F.K., Post, R.M., Dunner, D.L., and Gordon, E.K. (1973). Cerebrospinal fluid amine metabolites in affective illness: The probenecid technique. *Am J Psychiatry*, 130, 73–79.

Goodwin, F.K., Muscettola, G., Gold, P.W., and Wehr, T.A. (1978). Biochemical and pharmacological differentiation of affective disorders: An overview. In H.S. Akiskal and W.L. Webb (Eds.), *Psychiatric Diagnoses: Exploration of Biological Predictors* (pp. 313–336). New York: SP Medical and Scientific Books.

Goodwin, F.K., Prange, A.J. Jr., Post, R.M., Muscettola, G., and Lipton, M.A. (1982). Potentiation of antidepressant effects by L-triiodothyronine in tricyclic nonresponders. *Am J Psychiatry*, 139, 34–38.

Goodwin, G.M., De Souza, R.J., Wood, A.J., and Green, A.R. (1986a). The enhancement by lithium of the 5-HT$_{1A}$ mediated serotonin syndrome produced by 8-OH-DPAT in the rat: Evidence for a post-synaptic mechanism. *Psychopharmacology (Berl)*, 90, 488–493.

Goodwin, G.M., DeSouza, R.J., Wood, A.J., and Green, A.R. (1986b). Lithium decreases 5-HT$_{1A}$ and 5-HT$_2$ receptor and alpha 2-adrenoceptor mediated function in mice. *Psychopharmacology (Berl)*, 90, 482–487.

Gorkin, R.A., and Richelson, E. (1981). Lithium transport by mouse neuroblastoma cells. *Neuropharmacology*, 20, 791–801.

Gottesfeld, Z., Ebstein, B.S., and Samuel, D. (1971). Effect of lithium on concentrations of glutamate and GABA levels in amygdala and hypothalamus of rat. *Nat New Biol*, 234, 124–125.

Gottesman, I.I., and Gould, T.D. (2003). The endophenotype concept in psychiatry: Etymology and strategic intentions. *Am J Psychiatry*, 160(4), 636–645.

Gottesman, I.I., and Shields, J. (1973). Genetic theorizing and schizophrenia. *Br J Psychiatry*, 122(566), 15–30.

Gould, E., Tanapat, P., Rydel, T., and Hastings, N. (2000). Regulation of hippocampal neurogenesis in adulthood. *Biol Psychiatry*, 48, 715–720.

Gould, G.G., Mehta, A.K., Frazer, A., and Ticku, M.K. (2003). Quantitative autoradiographic analysis of the new radioligand [^{3}H](2E)-(5-hydroxy-5,7,8,9-tetrahydro-6H-benzo[a][7]annulen-6-ylidene) ethanoic acid ([^{3}H]NCS-382) at gamma-hydroxybutyric acid (GHB) binding sites in rat brain. *Brain Res*, 979, 51–56.

Gould, T.D., and Manji, H.K. (2002a). Signaling networks in the pathophysiology and treatment of mood disorders. *J Psychosom Res*, 53, 687–697.

Gould, T.D., and Manji, H.K. (2002b). The Wnt signaling pathway in bipolar disorder. *Neuroscientist*, 8(5), 497–511.

Gould, T.D., and Manji, H.K. (2004). The molecular medicine revolution and psychiatry: Bridging the gap between basic neuroscience research and clinical psychiatry. *J Clin Psychiatry*, 65, 598–604.

Gould, T.D., and Manji, H.K. (2005). Glycogen synthase kinase-3: A putative molecular target for lithium mimetic drugs. *Neuropsychopharmacology*, 30(7), 1223–1237.

Gould, T.D., Gray, N.A., and Manji, H.K. (2003). The cellular neurobiology of severe mood and anxiety disorders: Implications for the development of novel therapeutics. In D.S. Charney (Ed.), *Molecular Neurobiology for the Clinician* (pp. 123–227). Washington, DC: American Psychiatric Press.

Gould, T.D., Chen, G., and Manji, H.K. (2004a). In vivo evidence in the brain for lithium inhibition of glycogen synthase kinase-3. *Neuropsychopharmacology*, 29, 32–38.

Gould, T.D., Einat, E., Bhat, R., and Manji, H.K. (2004b). AR-A014418, a selective GSK-3 inhibitor, produces antidepressant-like effects in the forced swim test. *Int J Neuropsychopharmacol*, 7, 1–4.

Gould, T.D., Quiroz, J., Singh, J., Zarate, C., and Manji, H.K. (2004c). Emerging experimental therapeutics for bipolar disorder: Novel insights from the molecular and cellular mechanisms of action of mood stabilizers. *Mol Psychiatry*, 9, 734–755.

Graham, P.M., Booth, J., Boranga, G., Galhenage, S., Myers, C.M., Teoh, C.L., and Cox, L.S. (1982). The dexamethasone suppression test in mania. *J Affect Disord*, 4, 201–211.

Graham, Y.P., Heim, C., Goodman, S.H., Miller, A.H., and Nemeroff, C.B. (1999). The effects of neonatal stress on brain development: Implications for psychopathology. *Dev Psychopathol*, 11, 545–565.

Grahame-Smith, D.G., and Green, A.R. (1974). The role of brain 5-hydroxytryptamine in the hyperactivity produced in rats by lithium and monoamine oxidase inhibition. *Br J Pharmacol*, 52, 19–26.

Gram, L., Larsson, O.M., Johnsen, A.H., and Schousboe, A. (1988). Effects of valproate, vigabatrin and aminooxyacetic acid on release of endogenous and exogenous GABA from cultured neurons. *Epilepsy Res*, 2, 87–95.

Gray, N.A., Zhou, R., Du, J., Moore, G.J., and Manji, H.K. (2003). The use of mood stabilizers as plasticity enhancers in the treatment of neuropsychiatric disorders. *J Clin Psychiatry*, 64(Suppl. 5), 3–17.

Gray, T.S., and Morley, J.E. (1986). Neuropeptide Y: Anatomical distribution and possible function in mammalian nervous system. *Life Sci*, 38(5), 389–401.

Greden, J.F. (1982). Biological markers of melancholia and reclassification of depressive disorders. *Encephale*, 8, 193–202.

Greden, J.F., Price, H.L., Genero, N., Feinberg, M., and Levine, S. (1984). Facial emg activity levels predict treatment outcome in depression. *Psychiatry Res*, 13(4), 345–352.

Greengard, P., Valtorta, F., Czernik, A.J., and Benfenati, F. (1993). Synaptic vesicle phosphoproteins and regulation of synaptic function. *Science*, 259, 780–785.

Greenspan, K., Schildkraut, J.J., Gordon, E.K., Baer, L., Aronoff, M.S., and Durell, J. (1970). Catecholamine metabolism in affective disorders. 3. MHPG and other catecholamine metabolites in patients treated with lithium carbonate. *J Psychiatr Res*, 7, 171–183.

Greenwood, T.A., Alexander, M., Keck, P.E., McElroy, S., Sadovnick, A.D., Remick, R.A., and Kelsoe, J.R. (2001). Evidence for linkage disequilibrium between the dopamine transporter and bipolar disorder. *Am J Med Genet*, 105, 145–151.

Greil, W., Eisenried, F., Becker, B.F., and Duhm, J. (1977). Interindividual differences in the Na+-dependent Li+ counter-transport system and in the Li+ distribution ratio across the red cell membrane among Li+-treated patients. *Psychopharmacology (Berl)*, 53, 19–26.

Griebel, G., Simiand, J., Steinberg, R., Jung, M., Gully, D., Roger, P., Geslin, M., Scatton, B., Maffrand, J.P., and Soubrie, P. (2002). 4-(2-chloro-4-methoxy-5-methylphenyl)-n-[(1s)-2-cyclopropyl-1-(3-fluoro-4-methylphenyl)ethyl]5-methyl-n-(2-propynyl)-1,3-thiazol-2-amine hydrochloride (ssr125543a), a potent and selective corticotrophin-releasing factor(1) receptor antagonist. II. Characterization in rodent models of stress-related disorders. *J Pharmacol Exp Ther*, 301(1), 333–345.

Griffiths, E.C. (1985). Thyrotrophin releasing hormone: Endocrine and central effects. *Psychoneuroendocrinology*, 10, 225–235.

Grignon, S., Levy, N., Couraud, F., and Bruguerolle, B. (1996). Tyrosine kinase inhibitors and cycloheximide inhibit Li+ protection of cerebellar granule neurons switched to non-depolarizing medium. *Eur J Pharmacol*, 315, 111–114.

Grillo, C., Piroli, G., Gonzalez, S.L., Angulo, J., McEwen, B.S., and De Nicola, A.F. (1994). Glucocorticoid regulation of mRNA encoding (Na+K) ATPase alpha 3 and beta 1 subunits in rat brain measured by in situ hybridization. *Brain Res*, 657, 83–91.

Grimes, C.A., and Jope, R.S. (1999). Cholinergic stimulation of early growth response-1 DNA binding activity requires protein kinase C and mitogen-activated protein kinase kinase activation and is inhibited by sodium valproate in SH-SY5Y cells. *J Neurochem*, 73, 1384–1392.

Grof, E., Brown, G.M., Grof, P., and Van Loon, G.R. (1986). Effects of lithium administration on plasma catecholamines. *Psychiatry Res*, 19, 87–92.

Gross-Isseroff, R., Israeli, M., and Biegon, A. (1989). Autoradiographic analysis of tritiated imipramine binding in the human brain post mortem: Effects of suicide. *Arch Gen Psychiatry*, 46, 237–241.

Gross-Isseroff, G., Salama, D., Israeli, M., and Biegon, A. (1990a). Autoradiographic analysis of [3H]ketanserin binding in the human brain postmortem: Effect of suicide. *Brain Res*, 507, 208–215.

Gross-Isseroff, R., Dillon, K.A., Fieldust, S.J., and Biegon, A. (1990b). Autoradiographic analysis of α1-noradrenergic receptors in the human brain postmortem. Effect of suicide. *Arch Gen Psychiatry*, 47: 1049–1053.

Gross-Isseroff, R., Dillon, K.A., Israeli, M., and Biegon, A. (1990c). Regionally selective increases in mu opioid receptor density in the brains of suicide victims. *Brain Res*, 530, 312–316.

Grossman, F., and Potter, W.Z. (1999). Catecholamines in depression: A cumulative study of urinary norepinephrine and its major metabolites in unipolar and bipolar depressed patients versus healthy volunteers at the NIMH. *Psychiatry Res*, 87, 21–27.

Grote, S.S., Moses, S.G., Robins, E., Hudgens, R.W., and Croninger, A.B. (1974). A study of selected catecholamine metabolizing enzymes: A comparison of depressive suicides and alcoholic suicides with controls. *J Neurochem*, 23, 791–802.

Grunhage, F., Schulze, T.G., Muller, D.J., Lanczik, M., Franzek, E., Albus, M., Borrmann-Hassenbach, M., Knapp, M., Cichon, S., Maier, W., Rietschel, M., Propping, P., and Nothen, M.M. (2000). Systematic screening for DNA sequence variation in the coding region of the human dopamine transporter gene (DAT1). *Mol Psychiatry*, 5, 275–282.

Guerri, C., Ribelles, M., and Grisolia, S. (1981). Effects of lithium, and lithium and alcohol administration on (Na + K)-ATPase. *Biochem Pharmacol*, 30, 25–30.

Guidotti, A., Auta, J., Davis, J.M., Di-Giorgi-Gerevini, V., Dwivedi, Y., Grayson, D.R., Impagnatiello, F., Pandey, G.,

Pesold, C., Sharma, R., Uzunov, D., and Costa, E. (2000). Decrease in reelin and glutamic acid decarboxylase67 (GAD67) expression in schizophrenia and bipolar disorder. A post-mortem brain study. *Arch Gen Psychiatry*, 57, 1061–1069.

Gurevich, E.V., and Joyce, J.N. (1996). Comparison of [3H]paroxetine and [3H]cyanoimipramine for quantitative measurement of serotonin transporter sites in human brain. *Neuropsychopharmacology*, 14, 309–323.

Gutierrez, B., Fananas, L., Arranz, M.J., Valles, V., Guillamat, R., van Os, J., and Collier, D. (1996). Allelic association analysis of the 5-HT2C receptor gene in bipolar affective disorder. *Neurosci Lett*, 212, 65–67.

Habib, K.E., Weld, K.P., Rice, K.C., Pushkas, J., Champoux, M., Listwak, S., Webster, E.L., Atkinson, A.J., Schulkin, J., Contoreggi, C., Chrousos, G.P., McCann, S.M., Suomi, S.J., Higley, J.D., and Gold, P.W. (2000). Oral administration of a corticotropin-releasing hormone receptor antagonist significantly attenuates behavioral, neuroendocrine, and autonomic responses to stress in primates. *Proc Natl Acad Sci USA*, 97(11), 6079–6084.

Haggerty, J.J. Jr., Silva, S.G., Marquardt, M., Mason, G.A., Chang, H.Y., Evans, D.L., Golden, R.N., and Pedersen, C. (1997). Prevalence of antithyroid antibodies in mood disorders. *Depress Anxiety*, 5, 91–96.

Hahn, C.G., and Friedman, E. (1999). Abnormalities in protein kinase C signaling and the pathophysiology of bipolar disorder. *Bipolar Disord*, 1, 81–86.

Halaris, A.E. (1978). Plasma 3-methoxy-4-hydroxyphenylglycol in manic psychosis. *Am J Psychiatry*, 135, 493–494.

Hall, A.C., Brennan, A., Goold, R.G., Cleverley, K., Lucas, F.R., Gordon-Weeks, P.R., and Salinas, P.C. (2002). Valproate regulates GSK-3-mediated axonal remodeling and synapsin I clustering in developing neurons. *Mol Cell Neurosci*, 20, 257–270.

Hallcher, L.M., and Sherman, W.R. (1980). The effects of lithium ion and other agents on the activity of myo-inositol-1-phosphatase from bovine brain. *J Biol Chem*, 255, 10896–10901.

Halper, J.P., Brown, R.P., Sweeney, J.A., Kocsis, J.H., Peters, A., and Mann, J.J. (1988). Blunted beta-adrenergic responsivity of peripheral blood mononuclear cells in endogenous depression. Isoproterenol dose-response studies. *Arch Gen Psychiatry*, 45, 241–244.

Hamilton, S.R., Liu, B., Parsons, R.E., Papadopoulos, N., Jen, J., Powell, S.M., Krush, A.J., Berk, T., Cohen, Z., and Tetu B. (1995). The molecular basis of Turcot's syndrome. *N Engl J Med*, 332, 839–847.

Hao, Y.L., Creson, T., Zhang, L., Li, P., Yuan, P.X., Gould, T.D., Manji, H.K., and Chen, G. (2004). Mood-stabilizer valproate promotes ERK pathway dependent cortical neuronal growth and neurogenesis. *J Neurosci*, 24, 6590–6599.

Harder, R., and Bonisch, H. (1985). Effects of monovalent ions on the transport of noradrenaline across the plasma membrane of neuronal cells (PC-12 cells). *J Neurochem*, 45, 1154–1162.

Harrison-Read, P.E. (1979). Evidence from behavioural reactions to fenfluramine, 5-hydroxytryptophan, and 5-methoxy-N,N-dimethyltryptamine for differential effects of short-term and long-term lithium on indoleaminergic mechanisms in rats [proceedings]. *Br J Pharmacol*, 66, 144P–145P.

Harro, J., Tonissaar, M., and Eller, M. (2001). The effects of CRA 1000, a non-peptide antagonist of corticotropin-releasing factor receptor type 1, on adaptive behaviour in the rat. *Neuropeptides*, 35(2), 100–109.

Hashimoto, H., Onishi, H., Koide, S., Kai, T., and Yamagami, S. (1996). Plasma neuropeptide Y in patients with major depressive disorder. *Neurosci Lett*, 216(1), 57–60.

Hashimoto, R., Hough, C., Nakazawa, T., Yamamoto, T., and Chuang, D.M. (2002). Lithium protection against glutamate excitotoxicity in rat cerebral cortical neurons: Involvement of NMDA receptor inhibition possibly by decreasing NR2B tyrosine phosphorylation. *J Neurochem*, 80(4), 589–597.

Haskett, R.F. (1985). Diagnostic categorization of psychiatric disturbance in Cushing's syndrome. *Am J Psychiatry*, 142, 911–916.

Hasler, G., Drevets, W.C., Gould, T.D., Gottesman, I.I., and Manji, H.K. (2006). Toward constructing an endophenotype strategy for bipolar disorders. *Biol Psychiatry*, 60(2), 93–105.

Hassel, B., Iversen, E.G., Gjerstad, L., and Tauboll, E. (2001). Up-regulation of hippocampal glutamate transport during chronic treatment with sodium valproate. *J Neurochem*, 77, 1285–1292.

Hatterer, J.A., Kocsis, J.H, and Stokes, P.E. (1988). Thyroid function in patients maintained on lithium. *Psychiatry Res*, 26, 249–257.

Hayashi, T., Umemori, H., Mishina, M., and Yamamoto, T. (1999). The AMPA receptor interacts with and signals through the protein tyrosine kinase Lyn. *Nature*, 397, 72–76.

Haydon, P.G. (2001). GLIA: Listening and talking to the synapse. *Nat Rev Neurosci*, 2, 185–193.

Healy, D., Carney, P.A., and Leonard, B.E. (1983). Monoamine-related markers of depression: Changes following treatment. *J Psychiatr Res*, 17, 251–260.

Healy, D., Carney, P.A., O'Halloran, A., and Leonard, B.E. (1985). Peripheral adrenoceptors and serotonin receptors in depression. Changes associated with response to treatment with trazodone or amitriptyline. *J Affect Disord*, 9, 285–296.

Heckers, S., Stone, D., Walsh, J., Shick, J., Koul, P., and Benes, F.M. (2002). Differential hippocampal expression of glutamic acid decarboxylase 65 and 67 messenger RNA in bipolar disorder and schizophrenia. *Arch Gen Psychiatry*, 59, 521–529.

Hedge, G.A., and de Wied, D. (1971). Corticotropin and vasopressin secretion after hypothalamic implantation of atropine. *Endocrinology*, 88, 1257–1259.

Hedge, G.A., and Smelik, P.G. (1968). Corticotropin release: Inhibition by intrahypothalamic implantation of atropine. *Science*, 159, 891–892.

Hedlund, B., Abens, J., and Bartfai, T. (1983). Vasoactive intestinal polypeptide and muscarinic receptors: Supersensitivity induced by long-term atropine treatment. *Science*, 220, 519–521.

Heilig, M., and Widerlöv, E. (1990). Neuropeptide Y: An overview of central distribution, functional aspects, and possible involvement in neuropsychiatric illnesses. *Acta Psychiatr Scand*, 82(2), 95–114.

Heilig, M., Wahlestedt, C., Ekman, R., and Widerlöv, E. (1988a). Antidepressant drugs increase the concentration of neuropeptide Y (NPY)-like immunoreactivity in the rat brain. *Eur J Pharmacol*, 147, 465–467.

Heilig, M., Wahlestedt, C., and Widerlöv, E. (1988b). Neuropeptide Y (NPY)-induced suppression of activity in the rat: Evidence for NPY receptor heterogeneity and for interaction with alpha-adrenoceptors. *Eur J Pharmacol*, 157, 205–213.

Hein, M.D., and Jackson, I.M. (1990). Review: Thyroid function in psychiatric illness. *Gen Hosp Psychiatry*, 12, 232–244.

Hendrick, V., Altshuler, L., and Whybrow, P. (1998). Psychoneuroendocrinology of mood disorders. The hypothalamic–pituitary–thyroid axis. *Psychiatr Clin North Am*, 21, 277–292.

Heninger, G.R., Charney, D.S., and Sternberg, D.E. (1983). Lithium carbonate augmentation of antidepressant treatment. An effective prescription for treatment-refractory depression. *Arch Gen Psychiatry*, 40, 1335–1342.

Heninger, G.R., Charney, D.S., and Price, L.H. (1988). Alpha 2-Adrenergic receptor sensitivity in depression. The plasma MHPG, behavioral, and cardiovascular responses to yohimbine. *Arch Gen Psychiatry*, 45, 718–726.

Henn, F.A., and McKinney, W.T. (1987). Animal models in psychiatry. In H.Y. Meltzer (Ed.), *Psychopharmacology: The Third Generation of Progress* (pp. 687–695). New York: Raven Press.

Hermoni, M., Lerer, B., Ebstein, R.P., and Belmaker, R.H. (1980). Chronic lithium prevents reserpine-induced supersensitivity of adeylate cyclase. *J Pharm Pharmacol*, 32, 510–511.

Hermoni, M., Barzilai, A., and Rahimimoff, H. (1987). Modulation of the Na+-Ca2+ antiport by its ionic environment: The effect of lithium. *Isr J Med Sci*, 23, 44–48.

Hertz, M. (1964). On rhythmic phenomenon in thyroidectomized patients. *Acta Psychiatr Scand*, 40, 449–456.

Herve, D., Levi-Strauss, M., Marey-Semper, I., Verney, C., Tassin, J.P., Glowinski, J., and Girault, J.A. (1993). G(olf) and Gs in rat basal ganglia: possible involvement of G(olf) in the coupling of dopamine D1 receptor with adenylyl cyclase. *J Neurosci*, 13, 2237–2248.

Herzog, E.D., Aton, S.J., Numano, R., Sakaki, Y., and Tei, H. (2004). Temporal precision in the mammalian circadian system: A reliable clock from less reliable neurons. *J Biol Rhythms*, 19(1), 35–46.

Hesketh, J., and Glen, I. (1978). Lithium transport from cerebrospinal fluid. *Biochem Pharmacol*, 27(5), 813–814.

Hesketh, J.C., Glen, A.I.M., and Reading, H.W. (1977). Membrane ATPase activities in depressive illness. *J Neurochem*, 28, 1401–1402.

Hetman, M., Cavanaugh, J.E., Kimelman, D., and Xia, Z. (2000). Role of glycogen synthase kinase-3beta in neuronal apoptosis induced by trophic withdrawal. *J Neurosci*, 20, 2567–2574.

Heuser, I., Yassouridis, A., and Holsboer, F. (1994). The combined dexamethasone/CRH test: A refined laboratory test for psychiatric disorders. *J Psychiatr Res*, 28, 341–356.

Hicks, R.A., Moore, J.D., Hayes, C., Phillips, N., and Hawkins, J. (1979). REM sleep deprivation increases aggressiveness in male rats. *Physiol Behav*, 22, 1097–1100.

Hilfiker, S., Pieribone, V.A., Czernik, A.J., Kao, H.T., Augustine, G.J., and Greengard, P. (1999a). Synapsins as regulators of neurotransmitter release. *Philos Trans R Soc Lond B Biol Sci*, 354, 269–279.

Hilfiker, S., Pieribone, V.A., Nordstedt, C., Greengard, P., and Czernik, A.J. (1999b). Regulation of synaptotagmin I phosphorylation by multiple protein kinases. *J Neurochem*, 73, 921–932.

Himmelhoch, J.M., Thase, M.E., Mallinger, A.G., and Houck, P. (1991). Tranylcypromine versus imipramine in anergic bipolar depression. *Am J Psychiatry*, 148, 910–916.

Hirvonen, M.R., Paljarvi, L., Naukkarinen, A., Komulainen, H., and Savolainen, K.M. (1990). Potentiation of malaoxon-induced convulsions by lithium: early neuronal injury, phosphoinositide signaling, and calcium. *Toxicol Appl Pharmacol*, 104, 276–289.

Hitzemann, R. (2000). Animal models of psychiatric disorders and their relevance to alcoholism. *Alcohol Res Health*, 24, 149–158.

Hitzemann, R., Mark, C., Hirschowitz, J., and Garver, D. (1989). RBC lithium transport in the psychoses. *Biol Psychiatry*, 25, 296–304.

Ho, A.K., and Tsai, C.S. (1975). Lithium and ethanol preference. *J Pharm Pharmacol*, 27, 58–59.

Ho, A.K., Loh, H.H., Craves, F., Hitzemann, R.J., and Gershon, S. (1970). The effect of prolonged lithium treatment on the synthesis rate and turnover of monoamines in brain regions of rats. *Eur J Pharmacol*, 10, 72–78.

Hoehe, M., Valido, G., and Matussek, N. (1988). Growth hormone, noradrenaline, blood pressure and cortisol responses to clonidine in healthy male volunteers: Dose–response relations and reproducibility. *Psychoneuroendocrinology*, 13, 409–418.

Hoesche, C., Bartsch, P., and Kilimann, M.W. (1995). The CRE consensus sequence in the synapsin I gene promoter region confers constitutive activation but no regulation by cAMP in neuroblastoma cells. *Biochim Biophys Acta*, 1261, 249–256.

Hofmann, P., Gangadhar, B.N., Probst, C., Koinig, G., and Hatzinger, R. (1994). TSH response to TRH and ECT. *J Affect Disord*, 32, 127–131.

Hokfelt, T., Lundberg, J.M., Tatemoto, K., Mutt, V., Terenius, L., Polak, J., Bloom, S., Sasek, C., Elde, R., and Goldstein, M. (1983). Neuropeptide y (NPY)- and FMRFamide neuropeptide-like immunoreactivities in catecholamine neurons of the rat medulla oblongata. *Acta Physiol Scand*, 117(2), 315–318.

Hokin-Neaverson, M., and Jefferson, J.W. (1989a). Erythrocyte sodium pump activity in bipolar affective disorder and other psychiatric disorders. *Neuropsychobiology*, 22, 1–7.

Hokin-Neaverson, M., and Jefferson, J.W. (1989b). Deficient erythrocyte Na,K-ATPase activity in different affective states in bipolar affective disorder and normalization by lithium therapy. *Neuropsychobiology*, 22, 18–22.

Hokin-Neaverson, M., Spiegel, D.A., and Lewis, W.C. (1974). Deficiency of erythrocyte sodium pump activity in bipolar manic-depressive psychosis. *Life Sci*, 15, 1739–1748.

Hokin-Neaverson, M., Burckhardt, W.A., and Jefferson, J.W. (1976). Increased erythrocyte Na+ pump and NaK-ATPase activity during lithium therapy. *Res Commun Chem Pathol Pharmacol*, 14, 117–126.

Holemans, S., De Paermentier, F., Horton, R.W., Crompton, M.R., Katona, C.L., and Maloteaux, J.M. (1993). NMDA glutamatergic receptors, labelled with [3H]MK-801, in brain samples from drug-free depressed suicides. *Brain Res*, 616, 138–143.

Holian, O., and Nelson, R. (1992). Action of long-chain fatty acids on protein kinase C activity: Comparison of omega-6 and omega-3 fatty acids. *Anticancer Res*, 12, 975–980.

Holmes, A., Kinney, J.W., Wrenn, C.C., Li, Q., Yang, R.J., Ma, L., Vishwanath, J., Saavedra, M.C., Innerfield, C.E., Jacoby, A.S., Shine, J., Iismaa, T.P., and Crawley, J.N. (2003). Galanin GAL-R1 receptor null mutant mice display increased anxiety-like behavior specific to the elevated plus-maze. *Neuropsychopharmacology*, 28(6), 1031–1044.

Holsboer, F. (2000). The stress hormone system is back on the map. *Curr Psychiatry Rep*, 2(6), 454–456.

Holsboer, F. (2001). Stress, hypercortisolism and corticosteroid receptors in depression: Implications for therapy. *J Affect Disord*, 62(1-2), 77–91.

Holsboer, F., Gerken, A., Stalla, G.K., and Muller, O.A. (1985). ACTH, cortisol, and corticosterone output after ovine corticotrophin-releasing factor challenge during depression and after recovery. *Biol Psychiatry*, 20(3), 276–286.

Holsboer, F., Lauer, C. J., Schreiber, W., and Krieg, J.C. (1995). Altered hypothalamic–pituitary–adrenocortical regulation in

healthy subjects at high familial risk for affective disorders. *Neuroendocrinology*, 62(4), 340–347.

Holzbauer, M., and Youdim, M.B. (1973). The oestrous cycle and monoamine oxidase activity. *Br J Pharmacol*, 48(4), 600–608.

Honchar, M.P., Olney, J.W., and Sherman, W.R. (1983). Systemic cholinergic agents induce seizures and brain damage in lithium-treated rats. *Science*, 220, 323–325.

Honer, C., Nam, K., Fink, C., Marshall, P., Ksander, G., Chatelain, R.E., Cornell, W., Steele, R., Schweitzer, R., and Schumacher, C. (2003). Glucocorticoid receptor antagonism by cyproterone acetate and ru486. *Mol Pharmacol*, 63(5), 1012–1020.

Honer, W.G., Falkai, P., Bayer, T.A., Xie, J., Hu, L., Li, H.Y., Arango, V., Mann, J.J., Dwork, A.J., and Trimble, W.S. (2002). Abnormalities of SNARE mechanism proteins in anterior frontal cortex in severe mental illness. *Cereb Cortex*, 12, 349–356.

Hong, J.S., Tilson, H.A., and Yoshikawa, K. (1983). Effects of lithium and haloperidol administration on the rat brain levels of substance P. *J Pharmacol Exp Ther*, 224, 590–593.

Hong, S.E., Shugart, Y.Y., Huang, D.T., Shahwan, S.A., Grant, P.E., Hourihane, J.O., Martin, N.D., and Walsh, C.A. (2000). Autosomal recessive lissencephaly with cerebellar hypoplasia is associated with human *RELN* mutations. *Nat Genet*, 26, 93–96.

Horgan, K., Cooke, E., Hallett, M.B., and Mansel, R.E. (1986). Inhibition of protein kinase C mediated signal transduction by tamoxifen. Importance for antitumour activity. *Biochem Pharmacol*, 35(24), 4463–4465.

Hotsenpiller, G., Giorgetti, M., and Wolf, M.E. (2001). Alterations in behaviour and glutamate transmission following presentation of stimuli previously associated with cocaine exposure. *Eur J Neurosci*, 14(11), 1843–1855.

Hotta, I., and Yamawaki, S. (1988). Possible involvement of presynaptic 5-HT autoreceptors in effect of lithium on 5-HT release in hippocampus of rat. *Neuropharmacology*, 27, 987–992.

Hough, C.J., Irwin, R.P., Gao, X.M., Rogawski, M.A., and Chuang, D.M. (1996). Carbamazepine inhibition of *N*-methyl-D-aspartate-evoked calcium influx in rat cerebellar granule cells. *J Pharmacol Exp Ther*, 276, 143–149.

Hough, C., Lu, S.J., Davis, C.L., Chuang, D.M., and Post, R.M. (1999). Elevated basal and thapsigargin-stimulated intracellular calcium of platelets and lymphocytes from bipolar affective disorder patients measured by a fluorometric microassay. *Biol Psychiatry*, 46, 247–255.

Hovatta, I., Tennant, R.S., Helton, R., Marr, R.A., Singer, O., Redwine, J.M., Ellison, J.A., Schadt, E.E., Verma, I.M., Lockhart, D.J., and Barlow, C. (2005). Glyoxalase 1 and glutathione reductase 1 regulate anxiety in mice. *Nature*, 438(7068), 662–666.

Hrdina, P.D., Demeter, E., Vu, T.B., Sotonyi, P., and Palkovits, M. (1993). 5-HT uptake sites and 5-HT2 receptors in brain of antidepressant-free suicide victims/depressives: Increase in 5-HT2 sites in cortex and amygdala. *Brain Res*, 614, 37–44.

Hrdina, P.D., Bakish, D., Chudzik, J., Ravindran, A., and Lapierre, Y.D. (1995). Serotonergic markers in platelets of patients with major depression: Upregulation of 5-HT$_2$ receptors. *J Psychiatry Neurosci*, 20, 11–19.

Hrdina, P.D., Faludi, G., Li, Q., Bendotti, C., Tekes, K., Sotonyi, P., and Palkovits, M. (1998). Growth-associated protein (GAP-43), its mRNA, and protein kinase C (PKC) isoenzymes in brain regions of depressed suicides. *Mol Psychiatry*, 3, 411–418.

Huang, L.T., Liou, C.W., Yang, S.N., Lai, M.C., Hung, P.L., Wang, T.J., Cheng, S.C., and Wu, C.L. (2002). Aminophylline aggravates long-term morphological and cognitive damages in status epilepticus in immature rats. *Neurosci Lett*, 321(3), 137–140.

Huang, X., Wu, D.Y., Chen, G., Manji, H., and Chen, D.F. (2003). Support of retinal ganglion cell survival and axon regeneration by lithium through a Bcl-2-dependent mechanism. *Invest Ophthalmol Vis Sci*, 44, 347–354.

Hucks, D., Lowther, S., Crompton, M.R., Katona, C.L., and Horton, R.W. (1997). Corticotropin-releasing factor binding sites in cortex of depressed suicides. *Psychopharmacology (Berl)*, 134, 174–178.

Huey, L.Y., Janowsky, D.S., Judd, L.L., Abrams, A., Parker, D., and Clopton, P. (1981). Effects of lithium carbonate on methylphenidate-induced mood, behavior, and cognitive processes. *Psychopharmacology (Berl)*, 73, 161–164.

Hughes, J.H., Dunne, F., and Young, A.H. (2000). Effects of acute tryptophan depletion on mood and suicidal ideation in bipolar patients symptomatically stable on lithium. *Br J Psychiatry*, 177, 447–451.

Hunter, R., Christie, J.E., Whalley, L.J., Bennie, J., Carroll, S., Dick, H., Goodwin, G.M., Wilson, H., and Fink, G. (1989). Luteinizing hormone responses to luteinizing hormone releasing hormone (LHRH) in acute mania and the effects of lithium on LHRH and thyrotrophin releasing hormone tests in volunteers. *Psychol Med*, 19(1), 69–77.

Hurd, Y.L. (2002). Subjects with major depression or bipolar disorder show reduction of prodynorphin mRNA expression in discrete nuclei of the amygdaloid complex. *Mol Psychiatry*, 7, 75–81.

Hurd, Y.L., Herman, M.M., Hyde, T.M., Bigelow, L.B., Weinberger, D.R., and Kleinman, J.E. (1997). Prodynorphin mRNA expression is increased in the patch versus matrix compartment of the caudate nucleus in suicide subjects. *Mol Psychiatry*, 2, 495–500.

Hurley, S.C. (2002). Lamotrigine update and its use in mood disorders. *Ann Pharmacother*, 36, 860–873.

Husum, H., Vasquez, P.A., and Mathe, A.A. (2001). Changed concentrations of tachykinins and neuropeptide Y in brain of a rat model of depression: Lithium treatment normalizes tachykinins. *Neuropsychopharmacology*, 24, 183–191.

Ichikawa, J., and Meltzer, H.Y. (1999). Valproate and carbamazepine increase prefrontal dopamine release by 5-HT$_{1A}$ receptor activation. *Eur J Pharmacol*, 380, R1–R3.

Ichikawa, J., Dai, J., and Meltzer, H.Y. (2001). DOI, a 5-HT2A/2C receptor agonist, attenuates clozapine-induced cortical dopamine release. *Brain Res*, 907(1-2), 151–155.

Ichimiya, T., Suhara, T., Sudo, Y., Okubo, Y., Nakayama, K., Nankai, M., Inoue, M., Yasuno, F., Takano, A., Maeda, J., and Shibuya, H. (2002). Serotonin transporter binding in patients with mood disorders: A PET study with [11C](+)McN5652. *Biol Psychiatry*, 51(9), 715–722.

Ikeda, Y., Ijima, M., and Nomura, S. (1982). Serum dopamine-beta-hydroxylase in manic-depressive psychosis. *Br J Psychiatry*, 140, 209–210.

Ikonomov, O.C., and Manji, H.K. (1999). Molecular mechanisms underlying mood stabilization in manic-depressive illness: The phenotype challenge. *Am J Psychiatry*, 156(10), 1506–1514.

Impagnatiello, F., Guidotti, A.R., Pesold, C., Dwivedi, Y., Caruncho, H., Pisu, M.G., Uzunov, D.P., Smalheiser, N.R., Davis, J.M., Pandey, G.N., Pappas, G.D., Tueting, P., Sharma, R.P., and Costa, E. (1998). A decrease of reelin expression as a putative vulnerability factor in schizophrenia. *Proc Natl Acad Sci USA*, 95, 15718–15723.

Ingbar, S.H., and Braverman, L.E. (Eds.). (1986). *Werner's, the Thyroid: A Fundamental and Clinical Text* (5th Edition). New York: Lippincott.

Inoue, T., Tsuchiya, K., and Koyama, T. (1996). Serotonergic activation reduces defensive freezing in the conditioned fear paradigm. *Pharmacol Biochem Behav*, 53, 825–831.

Inouye, M., Yamamura, H., and Nakano, A. (1995). Lithium delays the radiation-induced apoptotic process in external granule cells of mouse cerebellum. *J Radiat Res (Tokyo)*, 36, 203–208.

Insel, T.R., Kalin, N.H., Guttmacher, L.B., Cohen, R.M., and Murphy, D.L. (1982). The dexamethasone suppression test in patients with primary obsessive-compulsive disorder. *Psychiatry Res*, 6, 153–160.

Insel, T.R., Hamilton, J.A., Guttmacher, L.B., and Murphy, D.L. (1983). D-amphetamine in obsessive-compulsive disorder. *Psychopharmacology (Berl)*, 80(3), 231–235.

Irwin, M., Brown, M., Patterson, T., Hauger, R., Mascovich, A., and Grant, I. (1991). Neuropeptide Y and natural killer cell activity: Findings in depression and Alzheimer caregiver stress. *FAESB J*, 5, 3100–3107.

Iwata, S., Hewlett, G.H., and Gnegy, M.E. (1997a). Amphetamine increases the phosphorylation of neuromodulin and synapsin I in rat striatal synaptosomes. *Synapse*, 26, 281–291.

Iwata, S.I., Hewlett, G.H., Ferrell, S.T., Kantor, L., and Gnegy, M.E. (1997b). Enhanced dopamine release and phosphorylation of synapsin I and neuromodulin in striatal synaptosomes after repeated amphetamine. *J Pharmacol Exp Ther*, 283, 1445–1452.

Jacobs, B.L., Praag, H., and Gage, F.H. (2000). Adult brain neurogenesis and psychiatry: A novel theory of depression. *Mol Psychiatry*, 5, 262–269.

Jacobs, D., and Silverstone, T. (1986). Dextroamphetamine-induced arousal in human subjects as a model for mania. *Psychol Med*, 16, 323–329.

Jahn, H., Schick, M., Kiefer, F., Kellner, M., Yassouridis, A., and Wiedemann, K. (2004). Metyrapone as additive treatment in major depression: A double-blind and placebo-controlled trial. *Arch Gen Psychiatry*, 61(12), 1235–1244.

Janowsky, D.S., and Overstreet, D.H. (1995). The role of acetylcholine mechanisms in mood disorders. In D.J. Kupfer (Ed.), *Psychopharmacology: The Fourth Generation of Progress* (pp. 945–956). New York: Raven Press.

Janowsky, D.S., and Risch, S.C. (1984). Choinomimetic and anticholinergic drugs used to investigate an acetylcholine hypothesis of affective disorders and stress. *Drug Dev Res*, 125–142.

Janowsky, D.S., el-Yousef, K., Davis, J.M., and Sekerke, H.J. (1973). Parasympathetic suppression of manic symptoms by physostigmine. *Arch Gen Psychiatry*, 28(4), 542–547.

Janowsky, D., Judd, L., Huey, L., Roitman, N., Parker, D., and Segal, D. (1978). Naloxone effects on manic symptoms and growth-hormone levels. *Lancet*, 2, 320.

Janowsky, D., Judd, L., Huey, L., Roitman, N., and Parker, D. (1979). Naloxone effects on serum growth hormone and prolactin in man. *Psychopharmacology (Berl)*, 65, 95–97.

Janowsky, D.S., Overstreet, D.H., and Nurnberger, J.I. Jr. (1994). Is cholinergic sensitivity a genetic marker for the affective disorders? *Am J Med Genet*, 54, 335–344.

Jensen, J.B., and Mork, A. (1997). Altered protein phosphorylation in the rat brain following chronic lithium and carbamazepine treatments. *Eur Neuropsychopharmacol*, 7, 173–179.

Jensen, J.B., Mikkelsen, J.D., and Mork, A. (2000). Increased adenylyl cyclase type 1 mRNA, but not adenylyl cyclase type 2 in the rat hippocampus following antidepressant treatment. *Eur Neuropsychopharmacol*, 10, 105–111.

Jimenez-Vasquez, P.A., Overstreet, D.H., and Mathe, A.A. (2000). Neuropeptide Y in male and female brains of Flinders Sensitive Line, a rat model of depression. Effects of electroconvulsive stimuli. *J Psychiatr Res*, 34, 405–412.

Jimerson, D.C., Post, R.M., Carman, J.S., van Kammen, D.P., Wood, J.H., Goodwin, F.K., and Bunney, W.E. Jr. (1979). CSF calcium: Clinical correlates in affective illness and schizophrenia. *Biol Psychiatry*, 14, 37–51.

Jimerson, D.C., Nurnberger, J.I. Jr., Post, R.M., Gershon, E.S., and Kopin, I.J. (1981). Plasma MHPG in rapid cyclers and healthy twins. *Arch Gen Psychiatry*, 38, 1287–1290.

Jimerson, D.C., van Kammen, D.P., Post, R.M., Docherty, J.P., and Bunney, W.E. Jr. (1982). Diazepam in schizophrenia: A preliminary double-blind trial. *Am J Psychiatry*, 139(4), 489–491.

Jimerson, D.C., Insel, T.R., Reus, V.I., and Kopin, I.J. (1983). Increased plasma MHPG in dexamethasone-resistant depressed patients. *Arch Gen Psychiatry*, 40(2), 173–176.

Joffe, H., and Cohen, L.S. (1998). Estrogen, serotonin, and mood disturbance: Where is the therapeutic bridge? *Biol Psychiatry*, 44, 798–811.

Joffe, R.T., Roy-Byrne, P.P., Udhe, T.W., and Post, R.M. (1984). Thyroid function and affective illness: A reappraisal. *Biol Psychiatry*, 19(12), 1685–1691.

Joffe, R.T., Post, R.M., and Uhde, T.W. (1986). Effects of carbamazepine on serum electrolytes in affectively ill patients. *Psychol Med*, 16, 331–335.

Joffe, R.T., Kutcher, S., and MacDonald, C. (1988). Thyroid function and bipolar affective disorder. *Psychiatry Res*, 25, 117–121.

Joffe, R.T., Young, L.T., Cooke, R.G., and Robb, J. (1994). The thyroid and mixed affective states. *Acta Psychiatr Scand*, 90, 131–132.

Johannessen, C.U. (2000). Mechanisms of action of valproate: A commentary. *Neurochem Int*, 37, 103–110.

Johannessen, C.U., Petersen, D., Fonnum, F., and Hassel, B. (2001). The acute effect of valproate on cerebral energy metabolism in mice. *Epilepsy Res*, 47, 247–256.

Johnson, F.N. (1980). *Handbook of Lithium Therapy*. Baltimore: University Park Press.

Johnson, L., El-Khoury, A., Aberg-Wistedt, A., Stain-Malmgren, R., and Mathe, A.A. (2001). Tryptophan depletion in lithium-stabilized patients with affective disorder. *Int J Neuropsychopharmacol*, 4, 329–336.

Johnston-Wilson, N.L., Sims, C.D., Hofmann, J.P., Anderson, L., Shore, A.D., Torrey, E.F., and Yolken, R.H. (2000). Disease-specific alterations in frontal cortex brain proteins in schizophrenia, bipolar disorder, and major depressive disorder. The Stanley Neuropathology Consortium. *Mol Psychiatry*, 5, 142–149.

Jones, F.D., Maas, J.W., Dekirmenjian, H., and Fawcett, J.A. (1973). Urinary catecholamine metabolites during behavioral changes in a patient with manic-depressive cycles. *Science*, 179, 300–302.

Jope, R.S. (1979). High affinity choline transport and acetylCoA production in brain and their roles in the regulation of acetylcholine synthesis. *Brain Res*, 180, 313–344.

Jope, R.S. (1993). Lithium selectively potentiates cholinergic activity in rat brain. *Prog Brain Res*, 98, 317–322.

Jope, R.S. (1999). A bimodal model of the mechanism of action of lithium. *Mol Psychiatry*, 4, 21–25.

Jope, R.S., and Song, L. (1997). AP-1 and NF-kappaB stimulated by carbachol in human neuroblastoma SH-SY5Y cells are differentially sensitive to inhibition by lithium. *Brain Res Mol Brain Res*, 50, 171–180.

Jope, R.S., and Williams, M.B. (1994). Lithium and brain signal transduction systems. *Biochem Pharmacol*, 47, 429–441.

Jope, R.S., Jenden, D.J., Ehrlich, B.E., and Diamond, J.M. (1978). Choline accumulates in erythrocytes during lithium therapy. *N Engl J Med*, 299, 833–834.

Jope, R.S., Jenden, D.J., Ehrlich, B.E., Diamond, J.M., and Gosenfeld, L.F. (1980). Erythrocyte choline concentrations are elevated in manic patients. *Proc Natl Acad Sci USA*, 77, 6144–6146.

Jope, R.S., Morrisett, R.A., and Snead, O.C. (1986). Characterization of lithium potentiation of pilocarpine-induced status epilepticus in rats. *Exp Neurol*, 91, 471–480.

Jope, R.S., Song, L., Li, P.P., Young, L.T., Kish, S.J., Pacheco, M.A., and Warsh, J.J. (1996). The phosphoinositide signal transduction system is impaired in bipolar affective disorder brain. *J Neurochem*, 66, 2402–2409.

Jordan, V.C. (1994). Molecular mechanisms of antiestrogen action in breast cancer. *Breast Cancer Res Treat*, 31(1), 41–52.

Jordan, V.C. (2003). Targeting antihormone resistance in breast cancer: A simple solution. *Ann Oncol*, 14(7), 969–970.

Josephson, A.M., and Mackenzie, T.B. (1979). Appearance of manic psychosis following rapid normalization of thyroid status. *Am J Psychiatry*, 136, 846–847.

Josephson, A.M., and Mackenzie, T.B. (1980). Thyroid-induced mania in hypothyroid patients. *Br J Psychiatry*, 137, 222–228.

Joyce, J.N., Lexow, N., Kim, S.J., Artymyshyn, R., Senzon, S., Lawrence, D., Cassanova, M.F., Kleinman, J.E., Bird, E.D., and Winokur, A. (1992). Distribution of beta-adrenergic receptor subtypes in human post-mortem brain: Alterations in limbic regions of schizophrenics. *Synapse*, 10, 228–246.

Joyce, J.N., Shane, A., Lexow, N., Winokur, A., Casanova, M.F., and Kleinman, J.E. (1993). Serotonin uptake sites and serotonin receptors are altered in the limbic system of schizophrenics. *Neuropsychopharmacology*, 8, 315–336.

Joyce, P.R. (1991). The prognostic significance of thyroid function in mania. *J Psychiatr Res*, 25(1-2), 1–6.

Joyce, P.R., and Paykel, E.S. (1989). Predictors of drug response in depression. *Arch Gen Psychiatry*, 46, 89–99.

Joyce, P.R., Fergusson, D.M., Woollard, G., Abbott, R.M., Horwood, L.J., and Upton, J. (1995). Urinary catecholamines and plasma hormones predict mood state in rapid cycling bipolar affective disorder. *J Affect Disord*, 33, 233–243.

Juckel, G., Hegerl, U., Mavrogiorgou, P., Gallinat, J., Mager, T., Tigges, P., Dresel, S., Schroter, A., Stotz, G., Meller, I., Greil, W., and Moller, H.J. (2000). Clinical and biological findings in a case with 48-hour bipolar ultrarapid cycling before and during valproate treatment. *J Clin Psychiatry*, 61, 585–593.

Judd, L.L., Janowsky, D.S., Segal, D.S., and Huey, L.Y. (1980). Naloxone-induced behavioral and physiological effects in normal and manic subjects. *Arch Gen Psychiatry*, 37, 583–586.

Kafka, M.S., and Paul, S.M. (1986). Platelet alpha 2-adrenergic receptors in depression. *Arch Gen Psychiatry*, 43, 91–95.

Kafka, M.S., Wirz-Justice, A., Naber, D., Marangos, P.J., O'Donohue, T.L., and Wehr, T.A. (1982). Effect of lithium on circadian neurotransmitter receptor rhythms. *Neuropsychobiology*, 8, 41–50.

Kakiuchi, C., Iwamoto, K., Ishiwata, M., Bundo, M., Kasahara, T., Kusumi, I., Tsujita, T., Okazaki, Y., Nanko, S., Kunugi, H., Sasaki, T., and Kato, T. (2003). Impaired feedback regulation of XBP1 as a genetic risk factor for bipolar disorder. *Nat Genet*, 35, 171–175.

Kakiuchi, C., Ishiwata, M., Kametani, M., Nelson, C., Iwamoto, K., and Kato, T. (2005). Quantitative analysis of mitochondrial DNA deletions in the brains of patients with bipolar disorder and schizophrenia. *Int J Neuropsychopharmacol*, 8(4), 515–522.

Kalin, N.H., Gibbs, D.M., Barksdale, C.M., Shelton, S.E., and Carnes, M. (1985). Behavioral stress decreases plasma oxytocin concentrations in primates. *Life Sci*, 36, 1275–1280.

Kao, H.T., Song, H.J., Porton, B., Ming, G.L., Hoh, J., Abraham, M., Czernik, A.J., Pieribone, V.A., Poo, M.M., and Greengard, P. (2002). A protein kinase A–dependent molecular switch in synapsins regulates neurite outgrowth. *Nat Neurosci*, 5, 431–437.

Karege, F., Bovier, P., Gaillard, J.M., and Tissot, R. (1987). The decrease of erythrocyte catechol-O-methyltransferase activity in depressed patients and its diagnostic significance. *Acta Psychiatr Scand*, 76, 303–308.

Karege, F., Bovier, P., Widmer, J., Gaillard, J.M., and Tissot, R. (1992). Platelet membrane alpha 2-adrenergic receptors in depression. *Psychiatry Res*, 43(3), 243–252.

Karege, F., Golaz, J., Schwald, M., and Malafosse, A. (1999). Lithium and haloperidol treatments differently affect the mononuclear leukocyte Gαs protein levels in bipolar affective disorder. *Neuropsychobiology*, 39(4), 181–186.

Karson, C.N., Mrak, R.E., Schluterman, K.O., Sturner, W.Q., Sheng, J.G., and Griffin, W.S. (1999). Alterations in synaptic proteins and their encoding mRNAs in prefrontal cortex in schizophrenia: A possible neurochemical basis for 'hypofrontality.' *Mol Psychiatry*, 4, 39–45.

Kasper, S., Sack, D.A., Wehr, T.A., Kick, H., Voll, G., and Vieira, A. (1988). Nocturnal TSH and prolactin secretion during sleep deprivation and prediction of antidepressant response in patients with major depression. *Biol Psychiatry*, 24, 631–641.

Kastin, A.J., Ehrensing, R.H., Schalch, D.S., and Anderson, M.S. (1972). Improvement in mental depression with decreased thyrotropin response after administration of thyrotropin-releasing hormone. *Lancet*, 2, 740–742.

Kato, T. (2001). The other, forgotten genome: Mitochondrial DNA and mental disorders. *Mol Psychiatry*, 6(6), 625–633.

Kato, T., and Kato, N. (2000). Mitochondrial dysfunction in bipolar disorder. *Bipolar Disord*, 2(3 Pt. 1), 180–190.

Kato, T., Hamakawa, H., Shioiri, T., Murashita, J., Takahashi, Y., Takahashi, S., and Inubushi, T. (1996). Choline-containing compounds detected by proton magnetic resonance spectroscopy in the basal ganglia in bipolar disorder. *J Psychiatry Neurosci*, 21, 248–254.

Kato, T., Ishiwata, M., Mori, K., Washizuka, S., Tajima, O., Akiyama, T., and Kato, N. (2003). Mechanisms of altered CA2+ signalling in transformed lymphoblastoid cells from patients with bipolar disorder. *Int J Neuropsychopharmacol*, 6(4), 379–389.

Katona, C.L., Theodorou, A.E., and Horton, R.W. (1987). Alpha 2-adrenoceptors in depression. *Psychiatr Dev*, 5, 129–49.

Katz, M.M., Maas, J.W., Frazer, A., Koslow, S.H., Bowden, C.L., Berman, N., Swann, A.C., and Stokes, P.E. (1994). Drug-induced actions on brain neurotransmitter systems and changes in the behaviors and emotions of depressed patients. *Neuropsychopharmacology*, 11(2), 89–100.

Katzenellenbogen, J.A., O'Malley, B.W., and Katzenellenbogen, B.S. (1996). Tripartite steroid hormone receptor pharmacology: Interaction with multiple effector sites as a basis for the cell- and promoter-specific action of these hormones. *Mol Endocrinol*, 10, 119–131.

Katzman, R., and Pappius, H.M. (1973). *Brain Electrolytes and Fluid Metabolism.* Baltimore: Williams & Wilkins.

Kaufmann, C.A., Gillin, J.C., Hill, B., O'Laughlin, T., Phillips, I., Kleinman, J.E., and Wyatt, R.J. (1984). Muscarinic binding in suicides. *Psychiatry Res*, 12, 47–55.

Kay, G., Sargeant, M., McGuffin, P., Whatley, S., Marchbanks, R., Baldwin, D., Montgomery, S., and Elliott, J.M. (1993). The lymphoblast beta-adrenergic receptor in bipolar depressed patients: Characterization and down-regulation. *J Affect Disord*, 27, 163–172.

Kay, G., Sargeant, M., McGuffin, P., Whatley, S., Marchbanks, R., Bullock, T., Montgomery, S., and Elliott, J.M. (1994). The lymphoblast beta-adrenergic receptor in bipolar depressed patients: Effect of chronic incubation with lithium chloride. *J Affect Disord*, 30, 185–192.

Keck, M.E., Welt, T., Muller, M.B., Uhr, M., Ohl, F., Wigger, A., Toschi, N., Holsboer, F., and Landgraf, R. (2003). Reduction of hypothalamic vasopressinergic hyperdrive contributes to clinically relevant behavioral and neuroendocrine effects of chronic paroxetine treatment in a psychopathological rat model. *Neuropsychopharmacology*, 28(2), 235–243.

Kelly, W.F., Kelly, M.J., and Faragher, B. (1996). A prospective study of psychiatric and psychological aspects of cushing's syndrome. *Clin Endocrinol (Oxf)*, 45(6), 715–720.

Kempermann, G. (2002). Why new neurons? Possible functions for adult hippocampal neurogenesis. *J Neurosci*, 22, 635–638.

Kempermann, G., and Gage, F.H. (1999). Experience-dependent regulation of adult hippocampal neurogenesis: Effects of long-term stimulation and stimulus withdrawal. *Hippocampus*, 9, 321–332.

Kempermann, G., Kuhn, H.G., and Gage, F.H. (1997). More hippocampal neurons in adult mice living in an enriched environment. *Nature*, 386, 493–495.

Kendall, D.A., and Nahorski, S.R. (1987). Acute and chronic lithium treatments influence agonist and depolarization-stimulated inositol phospholipid hydrolysis in rat cerebral cortex. *J Pharmacol Exp Ther*, 241, 1023–1027.

Kendall, D.A., Stancel, G.M., and Enna, S.J. (1982). The influence of sex hormones on antidepressant-induced alterations in neurotransmitter receptor binding. *J Neurosci*, 2, 354–360.

Kennedy, S.H., Tighe, S., McVey, G., and Brown, G.M. (1989). Melatonin and cortisol "switches" during mania, depression, and euthymia in a drug-free bipolar patient. *J Nerv Ment Dis*, 177, 300–303.

Kessler, R.C., McGonagle, K.A., Swartz, M., Blazer, D.G., and Nelson, C.B. (1993). Sex and depression in the National Comorbidity Survey. I: Lifetime prevalence, chronicity and recurrence. *J Affect Disord*, 29, 85–96.

Keynes, R.D., and Swan, R.C. (1959). The permeability of frog muscle fibres to lithium ions. *J Physiol*, 147, 626–638.

Khaitan, L., Calabrese, J.R., and Stockmeier, C.A. (1994). Effects of chronic treatment with valproate on serotonin-1A receptor binding and function. *Psychopharmacology (Berl)*, 113, 539–542.

Kilbey, M.M., and Ellinwood, E.H. Jr. (1977). Reverse tolerance to stimulant-induced abnormal behavior. *Life Sci*, 20, 1063–1075.

Kilts, C.D. (2001). Imaging the roles of the amygdala in drug addiction. *Psychopharmacol Bull*, 35(1), 84–94.

Kim, C.H., Chung, H.J., Lee, H.K., and Huganir, R.L. (2001). Interaction of the AMPA receptor subunit GluR2/3 with PDZ domains regulates hippocampal long-term depression. *Proc Natl Acad Sci USA*, 98, 11725–11730.

Kim, J.S., Chang, M.Y., Yu, I.T., Kim, J.H., Lee, S.H., Lee, Y.S., and Son, H. (2004). Lithium selectively increases neuronal differentiation of hippocampal neural progenitor cells both in vitro and in vivo. *J Neurochem*, 89(2), 324–336.

Kim, M.H., and Neubig, R.R. (1987). Membrane reconstitution of high-affinity alpha 2 adrenergic agonist binding with guanine nucleotide regulatory proteins. *Biochemistry*, 26, 3664–3672.

Kim, Y.B., Dunner, D.L., Meltzer, H.L., and Fieve, R.R. (1978). Lithium erythrocyte: Plasma ratio in primary affective disorder. *Compr Psychiatry*, 19(2), 129–134.

Kiriike, N., Izumiya, Y., Nishiwaki, S., Maeda, Y., Nagata, T., and Kawakita, Y. (1988). TRH test and DST in schizoaffective mania, mania, and schizophrenia. *Biol Psychiatry*, 24, 415–422.

Kirkegaard, C., Faber, J., Hummer, L., and Rogowski, P. (1979). Increased levels of TRH in cerebrospinal fluid from patients with endogenous depression. *Psychoneuroendocrinology*, 4, 227–235.

Kirov, G., Murphy, K.C., Arranz, M.J., Jones, I., McCandles, F., Kunugi, H., Murray, R.M., McGuffin, P., Collier, D.A., Owen, M.J., and Craddock, N. (1998). Low activity allele of catechol-O-methyltransferase gene associated with rapid cycling bipolar disorder. *Mol Psychiatry*, 3(4), 342–345.

Kirov, G., Rees, M., Jones, I., MacCandless, F., Owen, M.J., and Craddock, N. (1999). Bipolar disorder and the serotonin transporter gene: A family-based association study. *Psychol Med*, 29, 1249–1254.

Kjellman, B.F., Beck-Friis, J., Ljunggren, J.G., and Wetterberg, L. (1984). Twenty-four-hour serum levels of TSH in affective disorders. *Acta Psychiatr Scand*, 69(6), 491–502.

Kjellman, B.F., Beck-Friis, J., Ljunggren, J.G., Ross, S.B., Unden, F., and Wetterberg, L. (1986). Serum dopamine-beta-hydroxylase activity in patients with major depressive disorders. *Acta Psychiatr Scand*, 73, 266–270.

Klaiber, E.L., Kobayashi, Y., Broverman, D.M., and Hall, F. (1971). Plasma monoamine oxidase activity in regularly menstruating women and in amenorrheic women receiving cyclic treatment with estrogens and a progestin. *J Clin Endocrinol Metab*, 33, 630–638.

Klawans, H.L., Weiner, W.J., and Nausieda, P.A. (1977). The effect of lithium on an animal model of tardive dyskinesia. *Prog Neuropsychopharmacol*, 1, 53–60.

Klein, P.S., and Melton, D.A. (1996). A molecular mechanism for the effect of lithium on development. *Proc Natl Acad Sci USA*, 93, 8455–8459.

Klein, E., Lerer, B., Newman, M., Belmaker, R.H., and Bhargava, H.N. (1984). Effect of cyclo(Leu-Gly) on reserpine-induced hypomotility and increases in cortical beta-adrenergic receptors. *Psychopharmacology (Berl)*, 83, 76–78.

Klemfuss, H. (1992). Diminishing toxic effects of lithium administration. *Am J Psychiatry*, 149(6), 846.

Kline, N.S., and Lehmann, H.E. (1979). β-Endorphin therapy in psychiatric patients. In E. Usdin, W.E. Bunney, and N.S. Kline (Eds.), *Endorphins in Mental Health Research* (pp. 500–517). New York: Oxford University Press.

Kling, M.A., Rubinow, D.R., Doran, A.R., Roy, A., Davis, C.L., Calabrese, J.R., Nieman, L.K., Post, R.M., Chrousos, G.P., and Gold, P.W. (1993). Cerebrospinal fluid immunoreactive somatostatin concentrations in patients with Cushing's disease and major depression: Relationship to indices of corticotrophin-releasing hormone and cortisol secretion. *Neuroendocrinology*, 57(1), 79–88.

Klysner, R., Geisler, A., and Rosenberg, R. (1987). Enhanced histamine- and beta-adrenoceptor-mediated cyclic AMP formation in leukocytes from patients with endogenous depression. *J Affect Disord*, 13, 227–232.

Knapp, S., and Mandell, A.J. (1973). Short- and long-term lithium administration: Effects on the brain's serotonergic biosynthetic systems. *Science*, 180, 645–670.

Koenig, R.J., Leonard, J.L., Senator, D., Rappaport, N., Watson, A.Y., and Larsen, P.R. (1984). Regulation of thyroxine 5'-deiodinase activity by 3,5,3'-triiodothyronine in cultured rat anterior pituitary cells. *Endocrinology*, 115, 324–329.

Kofman, O., and Belmaker, R.H. (1990). Intracerebroventricular myo-inositol antagonizes lithium-induced suppression of rearing behaviour in rats. *Brain Res*, 534, 345–347.

Kofman, O., and Belmaker, R.H. (1991). Animal models of mania and bipolar affective disorders. In P. Soubrie. (Ed.), *Anxiety, Depression and Mania.* New York: Karger.

Kofman, O., and Belmaker, R.H. (1993). Ziskind-Somerfeld Research Award 1993. Biochemical, behavioral, and clinical studies of the role of inositol in lithium treatment and depression. *Biol Psychiatry*, 34, 839–852.

Kofman, O., Belmaker, R.H., Grisaru, N., Alpert, C., Fuchs, I., Katz, V., and Rigler, O. (1991). Myo-inositol attenuates two specific behavioral effects of acute lithium in rats. *Psychopharmacol Bull*, 27, 185–190.

Kofman, O., Bersudsky, Y., Vinnitsky, I., Alpert, C., and Belmaker, R.H. (1993). The effect of peripheral inositol injection on rat motor activity models of depression. *Isr J Med Sci*, 29, 580–586.

Kofman, O., Li, P.P., and Warsh, J.J. (1998). Lithium, but not carbamazepine, potentiates hyperactivity induced by intra-accumbens cholera toxin. *Pharmacol Biochem Behav*, 59, 191–200.

Konradi, C., Eaton, M., MacDonald, M.L., Walsh, J., Benes, F.M., and Heckers, S. (2004). Molecular evidence for mitochondrial dysfunction in bipolar disorder. *Arch Gen Psychiatry*, 61(3), 300–308.

Kontaxakis, V., Markianos, M., Markidis, M., and Stefanis, C. (1989). Clonidine in the treatment of mixed bipolar disorder. *Acta Psychiatr Scand*, 79, 108.

Kopin, I.J. (1985). Catecholamine metabolism: Basic aspects and clinical significance. *Pharmacol Rev*, 37, 333–364.

Korpi, E.R., Kleinman, J.E., Goodman, S.I., Phillips, I., DeLisi, L.E., Linnoila, M., and Wyatt, R.J. (1986). Serotonin and 5-hydroxyindoleacetic acid in brains of suicide victims: Comparison in chronic schizophrenic patients with suicide as cause of death. *Arch Gen Psychiatry*, 43, 594–600.

Korpi, E.R., Kleinman, J.E., and Wyatt, R.J. (1988). GABA concentrations in forebrain areas of suicide victims. *Biol Psychiatry*, 23, 109–114.

Korte, M., Griesbeck, O., Gravel, C., Carroll, P., Staiger, V., Thoenen, H., and Bonhoeffer, T. (1996). Virus-mediated gene transfer into hippocampal CA1 region restores long-term potentiation in brain-derived neurotrophic factor mutant mice. *Proc Natl Acad Sci USA*, 93, 12547–12552.

Koslow, S.H., Maas, J.W., Bowden, C.L., Davis, J.M., Hanin, I., and Javaid, J. (1983). CSF and urinary biogenic amines and metabolites in depression and mania. A controlled, univariate analysis. *Arch Gen Psychiatry*, 40, 999–1010.

Kostic, V., Jackson-Lewis, V., de Bilbao, F., Dubois-Dauphin, M., and Przedborski, S. (1997). Bcl-2: Prolonging life in a transgenic mouse model of familial amyotrophic lateral sclerosis. *Science*, 277(5325), 559–562.

Kraemer, G.W., Ebert, M.H., Lake, C.R., and McKinney, W.T. (1984). Cerebrospinal fluid measures of neurotransmitter changes associated with pharmacological alteration of the despair response to social separation in rhesus monkeys. *Psychiatry Res*, 11, 303–315.

Kramer, M.S., Cutler, N., Feighner, J., Shrivastava, R., Carman, J., Sramek, J.J., Reines, S.A., Liu, G., Snavely, D., Wyatt-Knowles, E., Hale, J.J., Mills, S.G., MacCoss, M., Swain, C.J., Harrison, T., Hill, R.G., Hefti, F., Scolnick, E.M., Cascieri, M.A., Chicchi, G.G., Sadowski, S., Williams, A.R., Hewson, L., Smith, D., Carlson, E.J., Hargreaves, R.J., and Rupniak, N.M. (1998). Distinct mechanism for antidepressant activity by blockade of central substance P receptors. *Science*, 281, 1640–1645.

Krell, R.D., and Goldberg, A.M. (1973). Effect of acute and chronic administration of lithium on steady-state levels of mouse brain choline and acetylcholine. *Biochem Pharmacol*, 22, 3289–3291.

Krieger, D.T., Silverberg, A.I., Rizzo, F., and Krieger, H.P. (1968). Abolition of circadian periodicity of plasma 17-OHCS levels in the cat. *Am J Physiol*, 215, 959–967.

Krishnan, R.R., Maltbie, A.A., and Davidson, J.R. (1983). Abnormal cortisol suppression in bipolar patients with simultaneous manic and depressive symptoms. *Am J Psychiatry*, 140, 203–205.

Krystal, A., Krishnan, K.R., Raitiere, M., Poland, R., Ritchie, J.C., Dunnick, N.R., Hanada, K., and Nemeroff, C.B. (1990). Differential diagnosis and pathophysiology of Cushing's syndrome and primary affective disorder. *J Neuropsychiatry Clin Neurosci*, 2(1), 34–43.

Krystal, J.H., Sanacora, G., Blumberg, H., Anand, A., Charney, D.S., Marek, G., Epperson, C.N., Goddard, A., and Mason, G.F. (2002). Glutamate and GABA systems as targets for novel antidepressant and mood-stabilizing treatments. *Mol Psychiatry*, 7(Suppl. 1), S71–S80.

Kucinski, B.J., Antelman, S.M., Caggiula, A.R., Fowler, H., Gershon, S., and Edwards, D.J. (1999). Cocaine-induced oscillation is conditionable. *Pharmacol Biochem Behav*, 63, 449–455.

Kuhn, H.G., Biebl, M., Wilhelm, D., Li, M., Friedlander, R.M., and Winkler, J. (2005). Increased generation of granule cells in adult Bcl-2-overexpressing mice: A role for cell death during continued hippocampal neurogenesis. *Eur J Neurosci*, 22(8), 1907–1915.

Kuhs, H., Farber, D., and Tolle, R. (1996). Serum prolactin, growth hormone, total corticoids, thyroid hormones and thyrotropine during serial therapeutic sleep deprivation. *Biol Psychiatry*, 39(10), 857–864.

Künig, G., Niedermeyer, B., Deckert, J., Gsell, W., Ransmayr, G., and Riederer, P. (1998). Inhibition of [3H]alpha-amino-3-hydroxy-5-methyl-4-isoxazole-propionic acid [AMPA] binding by the anticonvulsant valproate in clinically relevant concentrations: An autoradiographic investigation in human hippocampus. *Epilepsy Res*, 31, 153–157.

Kunugi, H., Hattori, M., Kato, T., Tatsumi, M., Sakai, T., Sasaki, T., Hirose, T., and Nanko, S. (1997). Serotonin transporter gene polymorphisms: Ethnic difference and possible association with bipolar affective disorder. *Mol Psychiatry*, 2, 457–462.

Kunzel, H.E., Zobel, A.W., Nickel, T., Ackl, N., Uhr, M., Sonntag, A., Ising, M., and Holsboer, F. (2003). Treatment of depression with the CRH-1-receptor antagonist R121919: Endocrine changes and side effects. *J Psychiatr Res*, 37(6), 525–533.

Kuriyama, K., and Kakita, K. (1980). Cholera toxin induced epileptogenic focus: An animal model for studying roles of cyclic AMP in the establishment of epilepsy. *Prog Clin Biol Res*, 39, 141–155.

Kuruvilla, A., and Uretsky, N.J. (1981). Effect of sodium valproate on motor function regulated by the activation of GABA receptors. *Psychopharmacology (Berl)*, 72(2), 167–172.

Kusalic, M. (1992). Grade II and grade III hypothyroidism in rapid-cycling bipolar patients. *Neuropsychobiology*, 25, 177–181.

Kusalic, M., and Engelsmann, F. (1996). Effect of lithium maintenance treatment on hypothalamic pituitary gonadal axis in bipolar men. *J Psychiatry Neurosci*, 21, 181–186.

Kusumi, I., Koyama, T., and Yamashita, I. (1991). Effects of various factors on serotonin-induced Ca2+ response in human platelets. *Life Sci*, 48, 999–1010.

Kusumi, I., Koyama, T., and Yamashita, I. (1994a). Serotonin-induced platelet intracellular calcium mobilization in depressed patients. *Psychopharmacology (Berl)*, 113, 322–327.

Kusumi, I., Koyama, T., and Yamashita, I. (1994b). Effect of mood stabilizing agents on agonist-induced calcium mobilization in human platelets. *J Psychiatr Neurosci*, 19, 222–225.

Kusumi, I., Suzuki, K., Sasaki, Y., Kameda, K., and Koyama, T. (2000). Treatment response in depressed patients with enhanced Ca mobilization stimulated by serotonin. *Neuropsychopharmacology*, 23, 690–696.

Laakso, M.L., and Oja, S.S. (1979). Transport of tryptophan and tyrosine in rat brain slices in the presence of lithium. *Neurochem Res*, 4, 411–423.

Lachman, H.M., Morrow, B., Shprintzen, R., Veit, S., Parsia, S.S., Faedda, G., Goldberg, R., Kucherlapati, R., and Papolos, D.F. (1996). Association of codon 108/158 catechol-O-methyltransferase gene polymorphism with the psychiatric manifestations of velo-cardio-facial syndrome. *Am J Med Genet*, 67, 468.

Ladd, C.O., Huot, R.L., Thrivikraman, K.V., Nemeroff, C.B., Meaney, M.J., and Plotsky, P.M. (2000). Long-term behavioral and neuroendocrine adaptations to adverse early experience. *Prog Brain Res*, 122, 81–103.

Laeng, P., Pitts, R.L., Lemire, A.L., Drabik, C.E., Weiner, A., Tang, H., Thyagarajan, R., Mallon, B.S., and Altar, C.A. (2004). The mood stabilizer valproic acid stimulates GABA neurogenesis from rat forebrain stem cells. *J Neurochem*, 91(1), 238–251.

Laruelle, M., Abi-Dargham, A., Casanova, M.F., Toti, R., Weinberger, D.R., and Kleinman, J.E. (1993). Selective abnormalities of prefrontal serotonergic receptors in schizophrenia. A postmortem study. *Arch Gen Psychiatry*, 50, 810–818.

Lattanzi, L., Dell'Osso, L., Cassano, P., Pini, S., Rucci, P., Houck, P.R., Gemignani, A., Battistini, G., Bassi, A., Abelli, M., and Cassano, G.B. (2002). Pramipexole in treatment-resistant depression: A 16-week naturalistic study. *Bipolar Disord*, 4, 307–314.

Lauterborn, J.C., Lynch, G., Vanderklish, P., Arai, A., and Gall, C.M. (2000). Positive modulation of AMPA receptors increases neurotrophin expression by hippocampal and cortical neurons. *J Neurosci*, 20, 8–21.

Lawrence, K.M., De Paermentier, F., Cheetham, S.C., Crompton, M.R., Katona, C.L., and Horton, R.W. (1990). Brain 5-HT uptake sites, labelled with [3H]paroxetine, in antidepressant-free depressed suicides. *Brain Res*, 526, 17–22.

Lawrence, K.M., De Paermentier, F., Lowther, S., Crompton, M.R., Katona, C.L., and Horton, R.W. (1997). Brain 5-hydroxytryptamine uptake sites labeled with [3H]paroxetine in antidepressant drug-treated depressed suicide victims and controls. *J Psychiatry Neurosci*, 22, 185–191.

Lawrence, K.M., Kanagasundaram, M., Lowther, S., Katona, C.L., Crompton, M.R., and Horton, R.W. (1998). [3H]imipramine binding in brain samples from depressed suicides and controls: 5-HT uptake sites compared with sites defined by desmethylimipramine. *J Affect Disord*, 47, 105–112.

Lawrence, M.S., Ho, D.Y., Sun, G.H., Steinberg, G.K., and Sapolsky, R.M. (1996). Overexpression of bcl-2 with herpes simplex virus vectors protects cns neurons against neurological insults in vitro and in vivo. *J Neurosci*, 16(2), 486–496.

Lazarus, J.H., and Muston, H.L. (1978). The effect of lithium on the iodide concentrating mechanism in mouse salivary gland. *Acta Pharmacol Toxicol (Copenh)*, 43, 55–58.

Leach, M.J., Marden, C.M., and Miller, A.A. (1986). Pharmacological studies on lamotrigine, a novel potential antiepileptic drug: II. Neurochemical studies on the mechanism of action. *Epilepsia*, 27, 490–497.

Leake, A., Fairbairn, A.F., McKeith, I.G., and Ferrier, I.N. (1991). Studies on the serotonin uptake binding site in major depressive disorder and control post-mortem brain: Neurochemical and clinical correlates. *Psychiatry Res*, 39, 155–165.

Leboyer, M., Quintin, P., Manivet, P., Varoquaux, O., Allilaire, J.F., and Launay, J.M. (1999). Decreased serotonin transporter binding in unaffected relatives of manic depressive patients. *Biol Psychiatry*, 46, 1703–1706.

Lechin, F., van der Dijs, B., Jakubowicz, D., Camero, R.E., Villa, S., Arocha, L., and Lechin, A.E. (1985). Effects of clonidine on blood pressure, noradrenaline, cortisol, growth hormone, and prolactin plasma levels in high and low intestinal tone depressed patients. *Neuroendocrinology*, 41, 156–162.

Lecuona, E., Luquin, S., Avila, J., Garcia-Segura, L.M., and Martin-Vasallo, P. (1996). Expression of the beta 1 and beta 2(AMOG) subunits of the Na,K-ATPase in neural tissues: Cellular and developmental distribution patterns. *Brain Res Bull*, 40, 167–174.

Lee, P.L. (1974). Single-column system for accelerated amino acid analysis of physiological fluids using five lithium buffers. *Biochem Med*, 10, 107–121.

Legutko, B., Li, X., and Skolnick, P. (2001). Regulation of BDNF expression in primary neuron culture by LY392098, a novel AMPA receptor potentiator. *Neuropharmacology*, 40, 1019–1027.

Leibenluft, E. (1996). Women with bipolar illness: Clinical and research issues. *Am J Psychiatry*, 153, 163–173.

Leibenluft, E., Ashman, S.B., Feldman-Naim, S., and Yonkers, K.A. (1999). Lack of relationship between menstrual cycle phase and mood in a sample of women with rapid cycling bipolar disorder. *Biol Psychiatry*, 46, 577–580.

Leiderman, D.B., Balish, M., Bromfield, E.B., and Theodore, W.H. (1991). Effect of valproate on human cerebral glucose metabolism. *Epilepsia*, 32, 417–422.

Lenox, R.H., and Hahn, C.G. (2000). Overview of the mechanism of action of lithium in the brain: Fifty-year update. *J Clin Psychiatry*, 61, 5–15.

Lenox, R.H., and Manji, H.K. (1995). Lithium. In A.F. Schatzberg, C.B. Nemeroff (Eds.), *The American Psychiatric Press Textbook of Psychopharmacology* (pp. 303–349). Washington, DC: American Psychiatric Press.

Lenox, R.H., and Manji, H. (1998). Drugs for treatment of bipolar disorder: Lithium. In C.B. Nemeroff (Ed.), *Textbook of psychopharmacology* (2nd Edition) (pp. 379–429). Washington, DC: American Psychiatry Press.

Lenox, R.H., Watson, D.G., Patel, J., and Ellis, J. (1992). Chronic lithium administration alters a prominent PKC substrate in rat hippocampus. *Brain Res*, 570, 333–340.

Lenox, R.H., Gould, T.D., and Manji, H.K. (2002). Endophenotypes in bipolar disorder. *Am J Med Genet*, 114, 391–406.

Lerer, B., and Stanley, M. (1985). Does lithium stabilize muscarinic receptors? *Biol Psychiatry*, 20, 1247–1250.

Lerer, B., Globus, M., Brik, E., Hamburger, R., and Belmaker, R.H. (1984). Effect of treatment and withdrawal from chronic lithium in rats on stimulant-induced responses. *Neuropsychobiology*, 11, 28–32.

Lerer, B., Macciardi, F., Segman, R.H., Adolfsson, R., Blackwood, D., Blairy, S., Del Favero, J., Dikeos, D.G., Kaneva, R., Lilli, R., Massat, I., Milanova, V., Muir, W., Noethen, M., Oruc, L., Petrova, T., Papadimitriou, G.N., Rietschel, M., Serretti, A., Souery, D., Van Gestel, S., Van Broeckhoven, C., and Mendlewicz, J. (2001). Variability of 5-HT2C receptor cys23ser polymorphism among European populations and vulnerability to affective disorder. *Mol Psychiatry*, 6, 579–585.

Leverich, G.S., Altshuler, L.L., Frye, M.A., Suppes, T., Keck, P.E. Jr., McElroy, S.L., Denicoff, K.D., Obrocea, G., Nolen, W.A., Kupka, R., Walden, J., Grunze, H., Perez, S., Luckenbaugh, D.A., and Post, R.M. (2003). Factors associated with suicide attempts in 648 patients with bipolar disorder in the Stanley Foundation Bipolar Network. *J Clin Psychiatry*, 64(5), 506–515.

Leviel, V., and Naquet, R. (1977). A study of the action of valproic acid on the kindling effect. *Epilepsia*, 18, 229–234.

Levine, J., Panchalingam, K., Rapoport, A., Gershon, S., McClure, R.J., and Pettegrew, J.W. (2000). Increased cerebrospinal fluid glutamine levels in depressed patients. *Biol Psychiatry*, 47, 586.

Levitt, M., Dunner, D.L., Mendlewicz, J., Frewin, D.B., Lawlor, W., Fleiss, J.L., Stallone, F., and Fieve, R.R. (1976). Plasma dopamine beta hydroxylase activity in affective disorders. *Psychopharmacologia*, 46, 205–210.

Levy, A., Zohar, J., and Belmaker, R.H. (1982). The effect of chronic lithium pretreatment on rat brain muscarinic receptor regulation. *Neuropharmacology*, 21(11), 1199–1201.

Lewin, E., and Bleck, V. (1977). Cyclic AMP accumulation in cerebral cortical slices: Effect of carbamazepine, phenobarbital, and phenytoin. *Epilepsia*, 18, 237–242.

Lewis, D.A., and Smith, R.E. (1983). Steroid-induced psychiatric syndromes. A report of 14 cases and a review of the literature. *J Affect Disord*, 5(4), 319–332.

Lewis, L.D., and Cochrane, G.M. (1983). Psychosis in a child inhaling budesonide. *Lancet*, 2(8350), 634.

Leyton, M., Young, S.N., and Benkelfat, C. (1997). Relapse of depression after rapid depletion of tryptophan. *Lancet*, 349, 1840–1841.

Li, R., and El-Mallakh, R.S. (2000). A novel evidence of different mechanisms of lithium and valproate neuroprotective action on human sy5y neuroblastoma cells: Caspase-3 dependency. *Neurosci Lett*, 294(3), 147–150.

Li, R., Shen, Y., and El-Mallahk, R.S. (1994). Lithium protects against ouabain-induced cell death. *Lithium*, 5, 211–216.

Li, T., Vallada, H., Curtis, D., Arranz, M., Xu, K., Cai, G., Deng, H., Liu, J., Murray, R., Liu, X., and Collier, D.A. (1997). Catechol-O-methyltransferase Val158Met polymorphism: Frequency analysis in Han Chinese subjects and allelic association of the low activity allele with bipolar affective disorder. *Pharmacogenetics*, 7, 349–353.

Li, T., Liu, X., Sham, P.C., Aitchison, K.J., Cai, G., Arranz, M.J., Deng, H., Liu, J., Kirov, G., Murray, R.M., and Collier, D.A. (1999). Association analysis between dopamine receptor genes and bipolar affective disorder. *Psychiatry Res*, 86(3), 193–201.

Li, X., Tizzano, J.P., Griffey, K., Clay, M., Lindstrom, T., and Skolnick, P. (2001). Antidepressant-like actions of an AMPA receptor potentiator (LY392098). *Neuropharmacology*, 40, 1028–1033.

Li, X., Bijur, G.N., and Jope, R.S. (2002). Glycogen synthase kinase-3beta, mood stabilizers, and neuroprotection. *Bipolar Disord*, 4(2), 137–144.

Li, Y.W., Hill, G., Wong, H., Kelly, N., Ward, K., Pierdomenico, M., Ren, S., Gilligan, P., Grossman, S., Trainor, G., Taub, R., McElroy, J., and Zazcek, R. (2003). Receptor occupancy of nonpeptide corticotropin-releasing factor 1 antagonist DMP696: Correlation with drug exposure and anxiolytic efficacy. *J Pharmacol Exp Ther*, 305(1), 86–96.

Lieberman, K.W., and Stokes, P. (1980). Lithium distribution ratios in psychiatrically normal subjects. *Pharmacol Biochem Behav*, 13(2), 205–208.

Lieblich, I., and Yirmiya, R. (1987). Naltrexone reverses a long-term depressive effect of a toxic lithium injection on saccharin preference. *Physiol Behav*, 39, 547–550.

Lingsch, C., and Martin, K. (1976). An irreversible effect of lithium administration to patients. *Br J Pharmacol*, 57, 323–327.

Linkowski, P., Kerkhofs, M., Van Onderbergen, A., Hubain, P., Copinschi, G., L'Hermite-Baleriaux, M., Leclercq, R., Brasseur, M., Mendlewicz, J., and Van Cauter, E. (1994). The 24-hour profiles of cortisol, prolactin, and growth hormone secretion in mania. *Arch Gen Psychiatry*, 51(8), 616–624.

Linnoila, M., Karoum, F., and Potter, W.Z. (1983a). Effects of antidepressant treatments on dopamine turnover in depressed patients. *Arch Gen Psychiatry*, 40, 1015–1017.

Linnoila, M., Karoum, F., Rosenthal, N., and Potter, W.Z. (1983b). Electroconvulsive treatment and lithium carbonate. Their effects on norepinephrine metabolism in patients with primary, major depressions. *Arch Gen Psychiatry*, 40, 677–680.

Linnoila, M., Miller, T.L., Bartko, J., and Potter, W.Z. (1984). Five antidepressant treatments in depressed patients. Effects on urinary serotonin and 5-hydroxyindoleacetic acid output. *Arch Gen Psychiatry*, 41, 688–692.

Linnoila, M., Guthrie, S., Lane, E.A., Karoum, F., Rudorfer, M., and Potter, W.Z. (1986). Clinical studies on norepinephrine metabolism: how to interpret the numbers. *Psychiatry Res*, 17, 229–239.

Little, K., Clark, T.B., Ranc, J., and Duncan, G.E. (1993). Beta-adrenergic receptor binding in frontal cortex from suicide victims. *Biol Psychiatry*, 34, 596–605.

Little, K.Y., McLauglin, D.P., Ranc, J., Gilmore, J., Lopez, J.F., Watson, S.J., Carroll, F.I., and Butts, J.D. (1997). Serotonin transporter binding sites and mRNA levels in depressed persons committing suicide. *Biol Psychiatry*, 41, 1156–1164.

Lloyd, K.G., Farley, I.J., Deck, J.H., and Hornykiewicz, O. (1974). Serotonin and 5-hydroxyindoleacetic acid in discrete areas of the brainstem of suicide victims and control patients. *Adv Biochem Psychopharmacol*, 11, 387–397.

Lloyd, K.G., Morselli, P.L., and Bartholini, G. (1987). GABA and affective disorders. *Med Biol*, 65, 159–165.

Lloyd, R.L., Pekary, A.E., Sattin, A., and Amundson, T. (2001). Antidepressant effects of thyrotropin-releasing hormone analogues using a rodent model of depression. *Pharmacol Biochem Behav*, 70, 15–22.

Looney, S.W., and el-Mallakh, R.S. (1997). Meta-analysis of erythrocyte Na,K-ATPase activity in bipolar illness. *Depress Anxiety*, 5(2), 53–65.

Loosen, P.T., Marciniak, R., and Thadani, K. (1987). TRH-induced TSH response in healthy volunteers: Relationship to psychiatric history. *Am J Psychiatry*, 144(4), 455–459.

López, J.F., Palkovits, M., Arato, M., Mansour, A., Akil, H., and Watson, S.J. (1992). Localization and quantification of pro-opiomelanocortin mRNA and glucocorticoid receptor mRNA in pituitaries of suicide victims. *Neuroendocrinology*, 56, 491–501.

López, J.F., Chalmers, D.T., Little, K.Y., and Watson, S.J. (1998). A.E. Bennett Research Award. Regulation of serotonin1A, glucocorticoid, and mineralocorticoid receptor in rat and human hippocampus: Implications for the neurobiology of depression. *Biol Psychiatry*, 43, 547–573.

Loscher, W. (1993). Effects of the antiepileptic drug valproate on metabolism and function of inhibitory and excitatory amino acids in the brain. *Neurochem Res*, 18, 485–502.

Loscher, W. (1999). Valproate: A reappraisal of its pharmacodynamic properties and mechanisms of action. *Prog Neurobiol*, 58, 31–59.

Loscher, W., and Honack, D. (1996). Valproate and its major metabolite E-2-en-valproate induce different effects on behaviour and brain monoamine metabolism in rats. *Eur J Pharmacol*, 299, 61–67.

Loscher, W., and Schmidt, D. (1980). Increase of human plasma GABA by sodium valproate. *Epilepsia*, 21, 611–615.

Loscher, W., and Siemes, H. (1984). Valproic acid increases gamma-aminobutyric acid in CSF of epileptic children. *Lancet*, 2, 225.

LoTurco, J.J. (2000). Neural circuits in the 21st century: Synaptic networks of neurons and glia. *Proc Natl Acad Sci USA*, 97, 8196–8197.

Louis, W.J., Doyle, A.E., and Anavekar, S.N. (1975). Plasma noradrenaline concentration and blood pressure in essential hypertension, phaeochromocytoma and depression. *Clin Sci Mol Med Suppl*, 2, 239s–242s.

Lowther, S., Crompton, M.R., Katona, C.L., and Horton, R.W. (1996). GTP gamma S and forskolin-stimulated adenylyl cyclase activity in post-mortem brain from depressed suicides and controls. *Mol Psychiatry*, 1, 470–477.

Lowther, S., De Paermentier, F., Cheetham, S.C., Crompton, M.R., Katona, C.L., and Horton, R.W. (1997a). 5-HT1A receptor binding sites in post-mortem brain samples from depressed suicides and controls. *J Affect Disord*, 42, 199–207.

Lowther, S., Katona, C.L., Crompton, M.R., and Horton, R.W. (1997b). 5-HT1D and 5-HT1E/1F binding sites in depressed suicides: Increased 5-HT1D binding in globus pallidus but not cortex. *Molec Psychiatry*, 2, 314–321.

Lowther, S., Katona, C.L., Crompton, M.R., and Horton, R.W. (1997c). Brain [3H]cAMP binding sites are unaltered in depressed suicides, but decreased by antidepressants. *Brain Res*, 758, 223–228.

Lu, R., Song, L., and Jope, R.S. (1999). Lithium attenuates p53 levels in human neuroblastoma SH-SY5Y cells. *Neuroreport*, 10, 1123–1125.

Lucas, F.R., and Salinas, P.C. (1997). WNT-7a induces axonal remodeling and increases synapsin I levels in cerebellar neurons. *Dev Biol*, 192, 31–44.

Lucca, A., Lucini, V., Piatti, E., Ronchi, P., and Smeraldi, E. (1992). Plasma tryptophan levels and plasma tryptophan/neutral amino acids ratio in patients with mood disorder, patients with obsessive-compulsive disorder, and normal subjects. *Psychiatry Res*, 44, 85–91.

Lucki, I. (1997). The forced swimming test as a model for core and component behavioral effects of antidepressant drugs. *Behav Pharmacol*, 8(6-7), 523–532.

Ludvig, N., and Moshe, S.L. (1989). Different behavioral and electrographic effects of acoustic stimulation and dibutyryl cyclic AMP injection into the inferior colliculus in normal and in genetically epilepsy-prone rats. *Epilepsy Res*, 3185–3190.

Lyon, M. (1991). Animal models of mania and schizophrenia. In P. Willner (Ed.), *Behavioral Models in Psychopharmacology: Theoretical, Industrial and Clinical Perspectives* (pp. 253–310). Cambridge, MA: Cambridge University Press.

Lyons, D.M. (2002). Stress, depression, and inherited variation in primate hippocampal and prefrontal brain development. *Psychopharmacol Bull*, 36, 27–43.

Lyons, D.M., Yang, C., Sawyer-Glover, A.M., Moseley, M.E., and Schatzberg, A.F. (2001). Early life stress and inherited variation in monkey hippocampal volumes. *Arch Gen Psychiatry*, 58, 1145–1151.

Lyttkens, L., Soderberg, U., and Wetterberg, L. (1976). Relation between erythrocyte and plasma lithium concentrations as an index in psychiatric disease. *Ups J Med Sci*, 81(2), 123.

Maas, J.W. (1972). Adrenocortical steroid-hormones, electrolytes, and disposition of catecholamines with particular reference to depressive states. *J Psychiatr Res*, 9, 227–241.

Maas, J.W., Koslow, S.H., Katz, M.M., Bowden, C.L., Gibbons, R.L., Stokes, P.E., Robins, E., and Davis, J.M. (1984). Pretreatment neurotransmitter metabolite levels and response to tricyclic antidepressant drugs. *Am J Psychiatry*, 141, 1159–1171.

Maas, J.W., Koslow, S.H., Davis, J., Katz, M., Frazer, A., Bowden, C.L., Berman, N., Gibbons, R., Stokes, P., and Landis, D.H. (1987). Catecholamine metabolism and disposition in healthy and depressed subjects. *Arch Gen Psychiatry*, 44(4), 337–344.

Machado-Vieira, R., Kapczinski, F., and Soares, J.C. (2004). Perspectives for the development of animal models of bipolar disorder. *Prog Neuropsychopharmacol Biol Psychiatry*, 28(2), 209–224.

MacMillan, V., Leake, J., Chung, T., and Bovell, M. (1987). The effect of valproic acid on the 5-hydroxyindoleacetic, homovanillic and lactic acid levels of cerebrospinal fluid. *Brain Res*, 420, 268–276.

MacQueen, G.M., Campbell, S., McEwen, B.S., Macdonald, K., Amano, S., Joffe, R.T., Nahmias, C., and Young, L.T. (2003). Course of illness, hippocampal function, and hippocampal volume in major depression. *Proc Natl Acad Sci USA*, 100(3), 1387–1392.

Maes, M.H., De Ruyter, M., and Suy, E. (1987). Prediction of subtype and severity of depression by means of dexamethasone suppression test, l-tryptophan: Competing amino acid ratio, and mhpg flow. *Biol Psychiatry*, 22(2), 177–188.

Maes, M., Vandewoude, M., Schotte, C., Martin, M., D'Hondt, P., Scharpe, S., and Blockx, P. (1990). The decreased availability of L-tryptophan in depressed females: Clinical and biological correlates. *Prog Neuropsychopharmacol Biol Psychiatry*, 14, 903–919.

Maes, M., Meltzer, H., D'Hondt, P., Cosyns, P., and Blockx, P. (1995). Effects on serotonin precursors on the negative feedback effects of glucocorticoids on hypothalamic–pituitary–adrenal axis function in depression. *Psychoneuroendocrinology*, 20, 149–167.

Maes, M., Calabrese, J., Jayathilake, K., and Meltzer, H.Y. (1997). Effects of subchronic treatment with valproate on l-5-HTP-induced cortisol responses in mania: Evidence for increased central serotonergic neurotransmission. *Psychiatry Res*, 71(2), 67–76.

Maes, M., Verkerk, R., Vandoolaeghe, E., Lin, A., and Scharpe, S. (1998). Serum levels of excitatory amino acids, serine, glycine, histidine, threonine, taurine, alanine and arginine in treatment-resistant depression: Modulation by treatment with antidepressants and prediction of clinical responsivity. *Acta Psychiatr Scand*, 97, 302–308.

Maggi, A., and Enna, S.J. (1980). Regional alterations in rat brain neurotransmitter systems following chronic lithium treatment. *J Neurochem*, 34, 888–892.

Maggirwar, S.B., Sarmiere, P.D., Dewhurst, S., and Freeman, R.S. (1998). Nerve growth factor–dependent activation of NF-kappaB contributes to survival of sympathetic neurons. *J Neurosci*, 18, 10356–10365.

Magistretti, P.J., and Pellerin, L. (1996). Cellular mechanisms of brain energy metabolism. Relevance to functional brain imaging and to neurodegenerative disorders. *Ann NY Acad Sci*, 777, 380–387.

Magliozzi, J.R., Gietzen, D., Maddock, R.J., Haack, D., Doran, A.R., Goodman, T., and Weiler, P.G. (1989). Lymphocyte beta-adrenoreceptor density in patients with unipolar depression and normal controls. *Biol Psychiatry*, 26(1), 15–25.

Mahan, L.C., Burch, R.M., Monsma, F.J. Jr., and Sibley, D.R. (1990). Expression of striatal D1 dopamine receptors coupled to inositol phosphate production and Ca2+ mobilization in *Xenopus* oocytes. *Proc Natl Acad Sci USA*, 87, 2196–2200.

Mahmood, T., and Silverstone, T. (2001). Serotonin and bipolar disorder. *J Affect Disord*, 66, 1–11.

Mahmood, T., Silverstone, T., Connor, R., and Herbison, P. (2002). Sumatriptan challenge in bipolar patients with and without migraine: A neuroendocrine study of 5-HT1D receptor function. *Int Clin Psychopharmacol*, 17, 33–36.

Maisel, A.S., Harris, T., Rearden, C.A., and Michel, M.C. (1990). Beta-adrenergic receptors in lymphocyte subsets after exercise. Alterations in normal individuals and patients with congestive heart failure. *Circulation*, 82, 2003–2010.

Maitre, L., Baltzer, V., Mondadori, C., Olpe, H.R., Baumann, P.A., and Waldmeier, P.C. (1984). Psychopharmacological and behavioral effects of anti-epileptic drugs in animals. In A.A. Muller (Ed.), *Anticonvulsants in Affective Disorders* (pp. 3–13). Amsterdam: Elsevier.

Maizels, E.T., Miller, J.B., Cutler, R.E. Jr., Jackiw, V., Carney, E.M., Mizuno, K., Ohno, S., and Hunzicker-Dunn, M. (1992). Estrogen modulates Ca(2+)-independent lipid-stimulated kinase in the rabbit corpus luteum of pseudopregnancy. Identification of luteal estrogen-modulated lipid-stimulated kinase as protein kinase C delta. *J Biol Chem*, 267, 17061–17068.

Maj, J., and Wedzony, K. (1985). Repeated treatment with imipramine or amitriptyline increases the locomotor response of rats to (+)-amphetamine given into the nucleus accumbens. *J Pharm Pharmacol*, 37, 362–364.

Maj, M., Ariano, M.G., Arena, F., and Kemali, D. (1984). Plasma cortisol, catecholamine and cyclic AMP levels, response to dexamethasone suppression test and platelet MAO activity in manic-depressive patients. A longitudinal study. *Neuropsychobiology*, 11, 168–173.

Maj, J., Chojnacka-Wojcik, E., Lewandowska, A., Tatarczynska, E., and Wiczynska, B. (1985). The central action of carbamazepine as a potential antidepressant drug. *Pol J Pharmacol Pharm*, 37(1), 47–56.

Malik, N., Canfield, V.A., Beckers, M.C., Gros, P., and Levenson, R. (1996). Identification of the mammalian Na,K-ATPase 3 subunit. *J Biol Chem*, 271, 22754–22758.

Malison, R.T., Anand, A., Pelton, G.H., Kirwin, P., Carpenter, L., McDougle, C.J., Heninger, G.R., and Price, L.H. (1999). Limited efficacy of ketoconazole in treatment-refractory major depression. *J Clin Psychopharmacol*, 19(5), 466–470.

Mallinger, A.G., Mallinger, J., Himmelhoch, J.M., Neil, J.F., and Hanin, I. (1980). Transmembrane distribution of lithium and sodium in erythrocytes of depressed patients. *Psychopharmacology (Berl)*, 68(3), 249.

Mallinger, A.G., Mallinger, J., Himmelhoch, J.M., Rossi, A., and Hanin, I. (1983). Essential hypertension and membrane lithium transport in depressed patients. *Psychiatry Res*, 10, 11–16.

Mallinger, A.G., Hanin, I., Himmelhoch, J.M., Thase, M.E., and Knopf, S. (1987). Stimulation of cell membrane sodium transport activity by lithium: Possible relationship to therapeutic action. *Psychiatry Res*, 22, 49–59.

Mallinger, A.G., Frank, E., Thase, M.E., Dippold, C.S., and Kupfer, D.J. (1997). Low rate of membrane lithium transport during treatment correlates with outcome of maintenance pharmacotherapy in bipolar disorder. *Neuropsychopharmacology*, 16(5), 325–332.

Malone, K.M., Thase, M.E., Mieczkowski, T., Myers, J.E., Stull, S.D., Cooper, T.B., and Mann, J.J. (1993). Fenfluramine challenge test as a predictor of outcome in major depression. *Psychopharmacol Bull*, 29, 155–161.

Manev, H., Uz, T., Smalheiser, N.R., and Manev, R. (2001). Antidepressants alter cell proliferation in the adult brain in vivo and in neural cultures in vitro. *Eur J Pharmacol*, 411, 67–70.

Manji, H.K. (1992). G proteins: Implications for psychiatry. *Am J Psychiatry*, 149, 746–760.

Manji, H.K., and Chen, G. (2000). Post-receptor signaling pathways in the pathophysiology and treatment of mood disorders. *Curr Psychiatry Rep*, 2, 479–489.

Manji, H., and Duman, R. (2001). Impairments of neuroplasticity and cellular resilience in severe mood disorder: Implications for the development of novel therapeutics. *Psychopharmacol Bull*, 35, 5–49.

Manji, H.K., and Lenox, R.H. (1994). Long-term action of lithium: A role for transcriptional and posttranscriptional factors regulated by protein kinase C. *Synapse*, 16, 11–28.

Manji, H.K., and Lenox, R.H. (1998). Lithium: A molecular transducer of mood-stabilization in the treatment of bipolar disorder. *Neuropsychopharmacology*, 19, 161–166.

Manji, H.K., and Lenox, R.H. (1999). Ziskind-Somerfeld Research Award. Protein kinase C signaling in the brain: Molecular transduction of mood stabilization in the treatment of manic-depressive illness. *Biol Psychiatry*, 46, 1328–1351.

Manji, H.K., and Lenox, R.H. (2000a). The nature of bipolar disorder. *J Clin Psychiatry*, 61(Suppl. 13), 42–57.

Manji, H.K., and Lenox, R.H. (2000b). Signaling: Cellular insights into the pathophysiology of bipolar disorder. *Biol Psychiatry*, 48, 518–530.

Manji, H.K., and Potter, W. (1997). Monoaminergic mechanisms in bipolar disorder. In R.T. Joffe (Ed.), *Bipolar Disorder: Biological Models and Their Clinical Application* (pp. 235–254). New York: Marcel Dekker.

Manji, H.K., Chen, G.A., Bitran, J.A., and Potter, W.Z. (1991a). Down-regulation of beta receptors by desipramine in vitro involves PKC/phospholipase A2. *Psychopharmacol Bull*, 27, 247–253.

Manji, H.K., Hsiao, J.K., Risby, E.D., Oliver, J., Rudorfer, M.V., and Potter, W.Z. (1991b). The mechanisms of action of lithium. I. Effects on serotoninergic and noradrenergic systems in normal subjects. *Arch Gen Psychiatry*, 48, 505–512.

Manji, H.K., Etcheberrigaray, R., Chen, G., and Olds, J.L. (1993). Lithium decreases membrane-associated protein kinase C in hippocampus: selectivity for the alpha isozyme. *J Neurochem*, 61, 2303–2310.

Manji, H.K., Chen, G., Shimon, H., Hsiao, J.K., Potter, W.Z., and Belmaker, R.H. (1995a). Guanine nucleotide-binding proteins in bipolar affective disorder. Effects of long-term lithium treatment. *Arch Gen Psychiatry*, 52, 135–144.

Manji, H.K., Potter, W.Z., and Lenox, R.H. (1995b). Signal transduction pathways. Molecular targets for lithium's actions. *Arch Gen Psychiatry*, 52, 531–543.

Manji, H.K., Bersudsky, Y., Chen, G., Belmaker, R.H., and Potter, W.Z. (1996). Modulation of protein kinase C isozymes and substrates by lithium: The role of myo-inositol. *Neuropsychopharmacology*, 15, 370–381.

Manji, H.K., Chen, G., Potter, W., and Kosten, T.R. (1997a). Guanine nucleotide binding proteins in opioid-dependent patients. *Biol Psychiatry*, 41(2), 130–134.

Manji, H.K., Moore, G.J., and Bebchuk, J.M. (1997b). Modulation of brain phosphoinositide signaling by lithium: Relationship to therapeutic response. *Biol Psychiatry*, 42, 290S.

Manji, H.K., McNamara, R., Chen, G., and Lenox, R.H. (1999a). Signalling pathways in the brain: Cellular transduction of mood stabilisation in the treatment of manic-depressive illness. *Aust N Z J Psychiatry*, 33(Suppl.), S65–S83.

Manji, H.K., Moore, G.J., and Chen, G. (1999b). Lithium at 50: Have the neuroprotective effects of this unique cation been overlooked? *Biol Psychiatry*, 46, 929–940.

Manji, H.K., Moore, G.J., and Chen, G. (2000a). Clinical and preclinical evidence for the neurotrophic effects of mood stabilizers: Implications for the pathophysiology and treatment of manic-depressive illness. *Biol Psychiatry*, 48(8), 740–754.

Manji, H.K., Moore, G.J., and Chen, G. (2000b). Lithium upregulates the cytoprotective protein Bcl-2 in the CNS in vivo: A role for neurotrophic and neuroprotective effects in manic-depressive illness. *J Clin Psychiatry*, 61(Suppl. 9), 82–96.

Manji, H.K., Drevets, W.C., and Charney, D.S. (2001a). The cellular neurobiology of depression. *Nat Med*, 7, 541–547.

Manji, H.K., Moore, G.J., and Chen, G. (2001b). Bipolar disorder: Leads from the molecular and cellular mechanisms of action of mood stabilizers. *Br J Psychiatry Suppl*, 41, s107–s119.

Manji, H.K., Gottesman, I.I., and Gould, T.D. (2003a). Signal transduction and genes-to-behaviors pathways in psychiatric diseases. *Sci STKE*, 207, pe49.

Manji, H.K., Quiroz, J.A., Sporn, J., Payne, J.L., Denicoff, K.A., Gray, N., Zarate, C.A. Jr., and Charney, D.S. (2003b). Enhancing neuronal plasticity and cellular resilience to develop novel, improved therapeutics for difficult-to-treat depression. *Biol Psychiatry*, 53, 707–742.

Mann, J.J., and Stanley, M. (1984). Postmortem monoamine oxidase enzyme kinetics in the frontal cortex of suicide victims and controls. *Acta Psychiatr Scand*, 69, 135–139.

Mann, J.J., Brown, R.P., Halper, J.P., Sweeney, J.A., Kocsis, J.H., Stokes, P.E., and Bilezikian, J.P. (1985). Reduced sensitivity of lymphocyte beta-adrenergic receptors in patients with endogenous depression and psychomotor agitation. *N Engl J Med*, 313, 715–720.

Mann, J.J., Stanley, M., McBride, P.A., and McEwen, B.S. (1986). Increased serotonin2 and beta-adrenergic receptor binding in the frontal cortices of suicide victims. *Arch Gen Psychiatry*, 43(10), 954–959.

Mann, J.J., McBride, P.A., Brown, R.P., Linnoila, M., Leon, A.C., DeMeo, M., Mieczkowski, T., Myers, J.E., and Stanley, M. (1992). Relationship between central and peripheral serotonin indexes in depressed and suicidal psychiatric inpatients. *Arch Gen Psychiatry*, 49, 442–446.

Mann, J.J., Henteleff, R.A., Lagattuta, T.F., Perper, J.A., Li, S., and Arango, V. (1996a). Lower 3H-paroxetine binding in cerebral cortex of suicide victims is partly due to fewer high affinity, non-transporter sites. *J Neural Transm*, 103, 1337–1350.

Mann, J.J., Arango, V., Henteleff, R.A., Lagattuta, T.F., and Wong, D.T. (1996b). Serotonin 5-HT3 receptor binding kinetics in the cortex of suicide victims are normal. *J Neural Transm*, 103, 165–171.

Mannel, M., Muller-Oerlinghausen, B., Czernik, A., and Sauer, H. (1997). 5-HT brain function in affective disorder: d,l-fenfluramine-induced hormone release and clinical outcome in long-term lithium/carbamazepine prophylaxis. *J Affect Disord*, 46, 101–113.

Mansbach, R.S., Brooks, E.N., and Chen, Y.L. (1997). Antidepressant-like effects of CP-154,526, a selective CRF1 receptor antagonist. *Eur J Pharmacol*, 323, 21–26.

Marangell, L.B., George, M.S., Callahan, A.M., Ketter, T.A., Pazzaglia, P.J., L'Herrou, T.A., Leverich, G.S., and Post, R.M. (1997). Effects of intrathecal thyrotropin-releasing hormone (protirelin) in refractory depressed patients. *Arch Gen Psychiatry*, 54, 214–222.

Marazziti, D., Lenzi, A., Galli, L., San Martino, S., and Cassano, G.B. (1991). Decreased platelet serotonin uptake in bipolar I patients. *Int Clin Psychopharmacol*, 6, 25–30.

Mark, R.J., Ashford, J.W., Goodman, Y., and Mattson, M.P. (1995). Anticonvulsants attenuate amyloid beta-peptide neurotoxicity, Ca2+ deregulation, and cytoskeletal pathology. *Neurobiol Aging*, 16, 187–198.

Martinek, S., Inonog, S., Manoukian, A.S., and Young, M.W. (2001). A role for the segment polarity gene *shaggy/GSK-3* in the *Drosophila* circadian clock. *Cell*, 105, 769–779.

Masana, M.I., Bitran, J.A., Hsiao, J.K., and Potter, W.Z. (1992). In vivo evidence that lithium inactivates Gi modulation of adenylate cyclase in brain. *J Neurochem*, 59, 200–205.

Masand, P.S., Pickett, P., and Murray, G.B. (1995). Hypomania precipitated by psychostimulant use in depressed medically ill patients. *Psychosomatics*, 36(2), 145–147.

Mason, J.W., Giller, E.L., and Kosten, T.R. (1988). Serum testosterone differences between patients with schizophrenia and those with affective disorder. *Biol Psychiatry*, 23, 357–366.

Massat, I., Souery, D., Del-Favero, J., Oruc, L., Noethen, M.M., Blackwood, D., Thomson, M., Muir, W., Papadimitriou, G.N., Dikeos, D.G., Kaneva, R., Serretti, A., Lilli, R., Smeraldi, E., Jakovljevic, M., Folnegovic, V., Rietschel, M., Milanova, V., Valente, F., Van Broeckhoven, C., and Mendlewicz, J. (2002). Excess of allele1 for alpha3 subunit GABA receptor gene (GABRA3) in bipolar patients: A multicentric association study. *Mol Psychiatry*, 7, 201.

Mastronardi, L., Puzzilli, F., and Ruggeri, A. (1998). Tamoxifen as a potential treatment of glioma. *Anticancer Drugs*, 9(7), 581–586.

Mathe, A.A., Jousisto-Hanson, J., Stenfors, C., and Theodorsson, E. (1990). Effect of lithium on tachykinins, calcitonin gene-related peptide, and neuropeptide Y in rat brain. *J Neurosci Res*, 26, 233–237.

Mathe, A.A., Agren, H., Lindstrom, L., and Theodorsson, E. (1994). Increased concentration of calcitonin gene-related peptide in cerebrospinal fluid of depressed patients. A possible trait marker of major depressive disorder. *Neurosci Lett*, 182(2), 138–142.

Mathews, R., Li, P.P., Young, L.T., Kish, S.J., and Warsh, J.J. (1997). Increased G alpha q/11 immunoreactivity in postmortem occipital cortex from patients with bipolar affective disorder. *Biol Psychiatry*, 41, 649–656.

Mathis, P., Schmitt, L., Benatia, M., Granier, F., Ghisolfi, J., and Moron, P. (1988). Plasma amino acid disturbances and depression. *Encephale*, 14, 77–82.

Matsubara, S., Arora, R.C., and Meltzer, H.Y. (1991). Serotonergic measures in suicide brain: 5-HT$_{1A}$ binding sites in frontal cortex of suicide victims. *J Neural Transm Gen Sect*, 85, 181–194.

Mattson, M.P., LaFerla, F.M., Chan, S.L., Leissring, M.A., Shepel, P.N., and Geiger, J.D. (2000). Calcium signaling in the ER: Its role in neuronal plasticity and neurodegenerative disorders. *Trends Neurosci*, 23(5), 222–229.

Matussek, N., Ackenheil, M., Hippius, H., Muller, F., Schroder, H.T., Schultes, H., and Wasilewski, B. (1980). Effect of clonidine on growth hormone release in psychiatric patients and controls. *Psychiatry Res*, 2, 25–36.

Mauri, M.C., Ferrara, A., Boscati, L., Bravin, S., Zamberlan, F., Alecci, M., and Invernizzi, G. (1998). Plasma and platelet amino acid concentrations in patients affected by major depression and under fluvoxamine treatment. *Neuropsychobiology*, 37, 124–129.

McBride, P.A., Brown, R.P., DeMeo, M., Keilp, J., Mieczkowski, T., and Mann, J.J. (1994). The relationship of platelet 5-HT$_2$ receptor indices to major depressive disorder, personality traits, and suicidal behavior. *Biol Psychiatry*, 35, 295–308.

McCance, S.L., Cohen, P.R., and Cowen, P.J. (1989). Lithium increases 5-HT-mediated prolactin release. *Psychopharmacology (Berl)*, 99, 276–281.

McCullumsmith, R.E., and Meador-Woodruff, J.H. (2002). Striatal excitatory amino acid transporter transcript expression in schizophrenia, bipolar disorder, and major depressive disorder. *Neuropsychopharmacology*, 26, 368–375.

McDonald, W.M., Tupler, L.A., Marsteller, F.A., Figiel, G.S., DiSouza, S., Nemeroff, C.B., and Krishnan, K.R. (1999). Hyperintense lesions on magnetic resonance images in bipolar disorder. *Biol Psychiatry*, 45, 965–971.

McEwen, B.S. (1999a). Stress and the aging hippocampus. *Front Neuroendocrinol*, 20(1), 49–70.

McEwen, B.S. (1999b). Stress and hippocampal plasticity. *Annu Rev Neurosci*, 22, 105–122.

McEwen, B.S. (2000). The neurobiology of stress: From serendipity to clinical relevance. *Brain Res*, 886, 172–189.

McEwen, B.S. (2003). Interacting mediators of allostasis and allostatic load: Towards an understanding of resilience in aging. *Metabolism*, 52(10 Suppl. 2), 10–16.

McEwen, B.S., and Magarinos, A.M. (2001). Stress and hippocampal plasticity: Implications for the pathophysiology of affective disorders. *Hum Psychopharmacol*, 16, S7–S19.

McGrath, P.J., Stewart, J.W., Harrison, W., and Quitkin, F.M. (1987). Treatment of tricyclic refractory depression with a monoamine oxidase inhibitor antidepressant. *Psychopharmacol Bull*, 23, 169–172.

McGrath, P.J., Stewart, J.W., Nunes, E.V., Ocepek-Welikson, K., Rabkin, J.G., Quitkin, F.M., and Klein, D.F. (1993). A double-blind crossover trial of imipramine and phenelzine for outpatients with treatment-refractory depression. *Am J Psychiatry*, 150, 118–123.

McGrath, P.J., Quitkin, F.M., and Klein, D.F. (1995). Bromocriptine treatment of relapses seen during selective serotonin reuptake inhibitor treatment of depression. *J Clin Psychopharmacol*, 15, 289–291.

McKinney, W.T. (1986). Electroconvulsive therapy and animal models of depression. *Ann NY Acad Sci*, 462, 65–69.

McKinney, W.T. (1988). *Models of Mental Disorders: A New Comparative Psychiatry*. New York: Plenum Medical Book Co.

McKinney, W.T. (2001). Overview of the past contributions of animal models and their changing place in psychiatry. *Semin Clin Neuropsychiatry*, 6, 68–78.

McKinney, W.T., Jr., Young, L.D., Suomi, S.J., and Davis, J.M. (1973). Chlorpromazine treatment of disturbed monkeys. *Arch Gen Psychiatry*, 29, 490–494.

McMahon, F.J., Buervenich, S., Charney, D., Lipsky, R., Rush, A.J., Wilson, A.F., Sorant, A.J., Papanicolaou, G.J., Laje, G., Fava, M., Trivedi, M.H., Wisniewski, S.R., and Manji, H. (2006). Variation in the gene encoding the serotonin 2a receptor is associated with outcome of antidepressant treatment. *Am J Hum Genet*, 78(5), 804–814.

McManamy, J. (2006). *Living Well with Depression and Bipolar Disorder: What Your Doctor Doesn't Tell You*. New York: Collins.

McNamara, R.K., Hyde, T.M., Kleinman, J.E., and Lenox, R.H. (1999). Expression of the myristoylated alanine-rich C kinase substrate (MARCKS) and MARCKS-related protein (MRP) in the prefrontal cortex and hippocampus of suicide victims. *J Clin Psychiatry*, 60(Suppl. 2), 21–26.

McTavish, S.F., McPherson, M.H., Harmer, C.J., Clark, L., Sharp, T., Goodwin, G.M., and Cowen, P.J. (2001). Antidopaminergic effects of dietary tyrosine depletion in healthy subjects and patients with manic illness. *Br J Psychiatry*, 179, 356–360.

Meador-Woodruff, J.H., Hogg, A.J. Jr., and Smith, R.E. (2001). Striatal ionotropic glutamate receptor expression in schizophrenia,

bipolar disorder, and major depressive disorder. *Brain Res Bull*, 55, 631–640.

Meagher, J.B., O'Halloran, A., Carney, P.A., and Leonard, B.E. (1990). Changes in platelet 5-hydroxytryptamine uptake in mania. *J Affect Disord*, 19, 191–196.

Meana, J.J., and Garcia-Sevilla, J.A. (1987). Increased alpha 2-adrenoceptor density in the frontal cortex of depressed suicide victims. *J Neural Transm*, 70, 377–381.

Meana, J.J., Barturen, F., and García-Sevilla, J.A. (1992). α2-Adrenoceptors in the brain of suicide victims: Increased receptor density associated with major depression. *Biol Psychiatry*, 31, 471–490.

Meaney, M.J., Diorio, J., Francis, D., LaRocque, S., O'Donnell, D., Smythe, J.W., Sharma, S., and Tannenbaum, B. (1994). Environmental regulation of the development of glucocorticoid receptor systems in the rat forebrain. The role of serotonin. *Ann NY Acad Sci*, 746, 260–273; discussion 274, 289–293.

Medini, L., Colli, S., Mosconi, C., Tremoli, E., and Galli, C. (1990). Diets rich in n-9, n-6 and n-3 fatty acids differentially affect the generation of inositol phosphates and of thromboxane by stimulated platelets, in the rabbit. *Biochem Pharmacol*, 39, 129–133.

Mellerup, E.T., and Rafaelsen, O.J. (1981). Depression and cerebrospinal fluid citrate. *Acta Psychiatr Scand*, 63, 57–60.

Meltzer, H.Y., and Lowy, M.T. (1987). The serotonin hypothesis of depression. In H.Y. Meltzer (Ed.), *Psychopharmacology: The Third Generation of Progress* (pp. 513–526). New York: Raven Press.

Meltzer, H.Y., Arora, R.C., Baber, R., and Tricou, B.J. (1981). Serotonin uptake in blood platelets of psychiatric patients. *Arch Gen Psychiatry*, 38, 1322–1326.

Meltzer, H.Y., Tueting, P., and Jackman, H. (1982). The effect of lithium on platelet monoamine oxidase activity in bipolar and schizoaffective disorders. *Br J Psychiatry*, 140, 192–198.

Meltzer, H.Y., Arora, R.C., and Goodnick, P. (1983). Effect of lithium carbonate on serotonin uptake in blood platelets of patients with affective disorders. *J Affect Disord*, 5, 215–21.

Meltzer, H.Y., Umberkoman-Wiita, B., Robertson, A., Tricou, B.J., Lowy, M., and Perline, R. (1984). Effect of 5-hydroxytryptophan on serum cortisol levels in major affective disorders. I. Enhanced response in depression and mania. *Arch Gen Psychiatry*, 41, 366–374.

Mendels, J., and Frazer, A. (1973). Intracellular lithium concentration and clinical response: Towards a membrane theory of depression. *J Psychiatr Res*, 10, 9–18.

Mendlewicz, J., Verbanck, P., Linkowski, P., and Wilmotte, J. (1978). Lithium accumulation in erythrocytes of manic-depressive patients: An in vivo twin study. *Br J Psychiatry*, 133, 436–444.

Merry, D.E., and Korsmeyer, S.J. (1997). Bcl-2 gene family in the nervous system. *Annu Rev Neurosci*, 20, 245–267.

Meurs, E., Rougeot, C., Svab, J., Laurent, A.G., Hovanessian, A.G., Robert, N., Gruest, J., Montagnier, L., and Dray, F. (1982). Use of an anti-human leukocyte interferon monoclonal antibody for the purification and radioimmunoassay of human alpha interferon. *Infect Immun*, 37(3), 919–926.

Meyer, J.H., Kapur, S., Houle, S., DaSilva, J., Owczarek, B., Brown, G.M., Wilson, A.A., and Kennedy, S.H. (1999). Prefrontal cortex 5-HT$_2$ receptors in depression: An [18F]setoperone PET imaging study. *Am J Psychiatry*, 156, 1029–1034.

Meyerson, L.R., Wennogle, L.P., Abel, M.S., Coupet, J., Lippa, A.S., Rauh, C.E., and Beer, B. (1982). Human brain receptor alterations in suicide victims. *Pharmacol Biochem Behav*, 17, 159–163.

Michael-Titus, A.T., Bains, S., Jeetle, J., and Whelpton, R. (2000). Imipramine and phenelzine decrease glutamate overflow in the prefrontal cortex: A possible mechanism of neuroprotection in major depression? *Neuroscience*, 100(4), 681.

Michel, A.D., Loury, D.N., and Whiting, R.L. (1990). Assessment of imiloxan as a selective alpha 2B-adrenoceptor antagonist. *Br J Pharmacol*, 99, 560–564.

Miguel-Hidalgo, J., and Rajkowska, G. (2002). Reduction of glia in the prefrontal cortex: A hypothesis of its role in the pathophysiology of major depressive disorder. *Biol Psychiatry*, 51, 98S.

Miguel-Hidalgo, J.J., Baucom, C., Dilley, G., Overholser, J.C., Meltzer, H.Y., Stockmeier, C.A., and Rajkowska, G. (2000). Glial fibrillary acidic protein immunoreactivity in the prefrontal cortex distinguishes younger from older adults in major depressive disorder. *Biol Psychiatry*, 48(8), 861–873.

Miki, M., Hamamura, T., Ujike, H., Lee, Y., Habara, T., Kodama, M., Ohashi, K., Tanabe, Y., and Kuroda, S. (2001). Effects of subchronic lithium chloride treatment on G-protein subunits (G_{olf}, $G\gamma7$) and adenylyl cyclase expressed specifically in the rat striatum. *Eur J Pharmacol*, 428, 303–309.

Miller, H.L., Delgado, P.L., Salomon, R.M., Berman, R., Krystal, J.H., Heninger, G.R., and Charney, D.S. (1996). Clinical and biochemical effects of catecholamine depletion on antidepressant-induced remission of depression. *Arch Gen Psychiatry*, 53(2), 117–128.

Milligan, G., and Wakelam, M. (1992). *G Proteins: Signal Transduction and Disease*. San Diego: Academic Press.

Minabe, Y., Tanii, Y., Tsunoda, M., and Kurachi, M. (1987). Acute effect of TRH, flunarizine, lithium and zotepine on amygdaloid kindled seizures induced with low-frequency stimulation. *Jpn J Psychiatry Neurol*, 41, 685–691.

Minabe, Y., Emori, K., and Kurachi, M. (1988). Effects of chronic lithium treatment on limbic seizure generation in the cat. *Psychopharmacology (Berl)*, 96, 391–394.

Minden, S.L., Orav, J., and Schildkraut, J.J. (1988). Hypomanic reactions to ACTH and prednisone treatment for multiple sclerosis. *Neurology*, 38(10), 1631–1634.

Mineka, S., and Suomi, S.J. (1978). Social separation in monkeys. *Psychol Bull*, 85, 1376–1400.

Miner, J.N., Tyree, C., Hu, J., Berger, E., Marschke, K., Nakane, M., Coghlan, M.J., Clemm, D., Lane, B., and Rosen, J. (2003). A nonsteroidal glucocorticoid receptor antagonist. *Mol Endocrinol*, 17(1), 117–127.

Minneman, K.P., Dibner, M.D., Wolfe, B.B., and Molinoff, P.B. (1979). Beta1- and beta2-adrenergic receptors in rat cerebral cortex are independently regulated. *Science*, 204, 866–868.

Mirnikjoo, B., Brown, S.E., Kim, H.F., Marangell, L.B., Sweatt, J.D., and Weeber, E.J. (2001). Protein kinase inhibition by omega-3 fatty acids. *J Biol Chem*, 276, 10888–10896.

Mitchell, P.B., and Smythe, G. (1990). Hormonal responses to fenfluramine in depressed and control subjects. *J Affect Disord*, 19, 43–51.

Mitchell, P.B., Manji, H.K., Chen, G., Jolkovsky, L., Smith-Jackson, E., Denicoff, K., Schmidt, M., and Potter, W.Z. (1997). High levels of Gs alpha in platelets of euthymic patients with bipolar affective disorder. *Am J Psychiatry*, 154, 218–223.

Mizuno, K., Okada, M., Murakami, T., Kamata, A., Zhu, G., Kawata, Y., Wada, K., and Kaneko, S. (2000). Effects of carbamazepine on acetylcholine release and metabolism. *Epilepsy Res*, 40, 187–195.

Mizuta, T., and Segawa, T. (1989). Chronic effects of imipramine and lithium on 5-HT receptor subtypes in rat frontal cortex, hippocampus and choroid plexus: Quantitative receptor autoradiographic analysis. *Jpn J Pharmacol*, 50, 315–326.

Modell, S., Lauer, C.J., Schreiber, W., Huber, J., Krieg, J.C., and Holsboer, F. (1998). Hormonal response pattern in the combined DEX-CRH test is stable over time in subjects at high familial risk for affective disorders. *Neuropsychopharmacology*, 18, 253–262.

Modestin, J., Hunger, J., and Schwartz, R.B. (1973a). Depressive effects of physostigmine. *Arch Psychiatr Nervenkr*, 218, 67–77.

Modestin, J., Schwartz, R.B., and Hunger, J. (1973b). Investigation about an influence of physostigmine on schizophrenic symptoms. *Pharmakopsychiatr Neuropsychopharmakol*, 6, 300–304.

Moises, H.C., Smith, C.B., Spengler, R.N., and Hollingsworth, P.J. (1986). Presynaptic alpha 2 adrenoreceptor function in dependent rats before and after morphine withdrawal. *NIDA Res Monogr*, 75, 579–582.

Molchan, S.E., Lawlor, B.A., Hill, J.L., Mellow, A.M., Davis, C.L., Martinez, R., and Sunderland, T. (1991). The TRH stimulation test in Alzheimer's disease and major depression: Relationship to clinical and CSF measures. *Biol Psychiatry*, 30, 567–576.

Moller, S.E., de Beurs, P., Timmerman, L., Tan, B.K., Leijnse-Ybema, H.J., Stuart, M.H., and Petersen, H.E. (1986). Plasma tryptophan and tyrosine ratios to competing amino acids in relation to antidepressant response to citalopram and maprotiline. A preliminary study. *Psychopharmacology (Berl)*, 88, 96–100.

Mooney, J.J., Samson, J.A., McHale, N.L., Colodzin, R., Alpert, J., Koutsos, M., and Schildkraut, J.J. (1998). Signal transduction by platelet adenylate cyclase: Alterations in depressed patients may reflect impairment in the coordinated integration of cellular signals (coincidence detection). *Biol Psychiatry*, 43, 574–583.

Moore, C.M., Breeze, J.L., Kukes, T.J., Rose, S.L., Dager, S.R., Cohen, B.M., and Renshaw, P.F. (1999a). Effects of myo-inositol ingestion on human brain myo-inositol levels: A proton magnetic resonance spectroscopic imaging study. *Biol Psychiatry*, 45, 1197–1202.

Moore, C.M., Frederick, B.B., and Renshaw, P.F. (1999b). Brain biochemistry using magnetic resonance spectroscopy: Relevance to psychiatric illness in the elderly. *J Geriatr Psychiatry Neurol*, 12, 107–117.

Moore, C.M., Biederman, J., Wozniak, J., Mick, E., Aleardi, M., Wardrop, M., Dougherty, M., Harpold, T., Hammerness, P., Randall, E., and Renshaw, P.F. (2006). Differences in brain chemistry in children and adolescents with attention deficit hyperactivity disorder with and without comorbid bipolar disorder: A proton magnetic resonance spectroscopy study. *Am J Psychiatry*, 163(2), 316–318.

Moore, G.J., and Galloway, M.P. (2002). Magnetic resonance spectroscopy: Neurochemistry and treatment effects in affective disorders. *Psychopharmacol Bull*, 36, 5–23.

Moore, G.J., Bebchuk, J.M., Parrish, J.K., Faulk, M.W., Arfken, C.L., Strahl-Bevacqua, J., and Manji, H.K. (1999). Temporal dissociation between lithium-induced changes in frontal lobe myo-inositol and clinical response in manic-depressive illness. *Am J Psychiatry*, 156, 1902–1908.

Moore, G.J., Bebchuk, J.M., Hasanat, K., Chen, G., Seraji-Bozorgzad, N., Wilds, I.B., Faulk, M.W., Koch, S., Glitz, D.A.,

Jolkovsky, L., and Manji, H.K. (2000). Lithium increases N-acetyl-aspartate in the human brain: In vivo evidence in support of Bcl-2's neurotrophic effects? *Biol Psychiatry*, 48, 1–8.

Moore, P., Gillin, C., Bhatti, T., DeModena, A., Seifritz, E., Clark, C., Stahl, S., Rapaport, M., and Kelsoe, J. (1998). Rapid tryptophan depletion, sleep electroencephalogram, and mood in men with remitted depression on serotonin reuptake inhibitors. *Arch Gen Psychiatry*, 55, 534–539.

Moore, P.B., Shepherd, D.J., Eccleston, D., Macmillan, I.C., Goswami, U., McAllister, V.L., and Ferrier, I.N. (2001). Cerebral white matter lesions in bipolar affective disorder: Relationship to outcome. *Br J Psychiatry*, 178, 172–176.

Mora, A., Gonzalez-Polo, R.A., Fuentes, J.M., Soler, G., and Centeno, F. (1999). Different mechanisms of protection against apoptosis by valproate and Li+. *Eur J Biochem*, 266, 886–891.

Mora, A., Sabio, G., Gonzalez-Polo, R.A., Cuenda, A., Alessi, D.R., Alonso, J.C., Fuentes, J.M., Soler, G., and Centeno, F. (2001). Lithium inhibits caspase 3 activation and dephosphorylation of PKB and GSK3 induced by K+ deprivation in cerebellar granule cells. *J Neurochem*, 78, 199–206.

Morden, B., Mullins, R., Levine, S., Cohen, H., and Dement, W. (1968). Effect of REM deprivation on the mating behavior of male rats. *Psychophysiology*, 5, 241.

Mori, S., Tardito, D., Dorigo, A., Zanardi, R., Smeraldi, E., Racagni, G., and Perez, J. (1998). Effects of lithium on cAMP-dependent protein kinase in rat brain. *Neuropsychopharmacology*, 19, 233–240.

Mork, A., and Geisler, A. (1989). The effects of lithium in vitro and ex vivo on adenylate cyclase in brain are exerted by distinct mechanisms. *Neuropharmacology*, 28, 307–311.

Mork, A., Klysner, R., and Geisler, A. (1990). Effects of treatment with a lithium-imipramine combination on components of adenylate cyclase in the cerebral cortex of the rat. *Neuropharmacology*, 29, 261–267.

Mork, A., Geisler, A., and Hollund, P. (1992). Effects of lithium on second messenger systems in the brain. *Pharmacol Toxicol*, 71(Suppl. 1), 4–17.

Morris, P.J., Lakin, N.D., Dawson, S.J., Ryabinin, A.E., Kilimann, M.W., Wilson, M.C., and Latchman, D.S. (1996). Differential regulation of genes encoding synaptic proteins by members of the Brn-3 subfamily of POU transcription factors. *Brain Res Mol Brain Res*, 43, 279–285.

Moscovich, D.G., Belmaker, R.H., Agam, G., and Livne, A. (1990). Inositol-1-phosphatase in red blood cells of manic-depressive patients before and during treatment with lithium. *Biol Psychiatry*, 27(5), 552–555.

Moses, S.G., and Robins, E. (1975). Regional distribution of norepinephrine and dopamine in brains of depressive suicides and alcoholic suicides. *Psychopharmacol Commun*, 1, 327–337.

Mota de Freitas, D., Silberberg, J., Espanol, M.T., Dorus, E., Abraha, A., Dorus, W., Elenz, E., and Whang, W. (1990). Measurement of lithium transport in RBC from psychiatric patients receiving lithium carbonate and normal individuals by 7Li NMR spectroscopy. *Biol Psychiatry*, 28, 415–424.

Motohashi, N., Ikawa, K., and Kariya, T. (1989). GABAB receptors are up-regulated by chronic treatment with lithium or carbamazepine. GABA hypothesis of affective disorders? *Eur J Pharmacol*, 166, 95–99.

Moudy, A.M., Handran, S.D., Goldberg, M.P., Ruffin, N., Karl, I., Kranz-Eble, P., DeVivo, D.C., and Rothman, S.M. (1995). Abnormal calcium homeostasis and mitochondrial polarization in a human encephalomyopathy. *Proc Natl Acad Sci USA*, 92(3), 729–733.

Mucha, R.F., Millan, M.J., and Herz, A. (1985). Aversive properties of naloxone in non-dependent (naive) rats may involve blockade of central beta-endorphin. *Psychopharmacology (Berl)*, 86, 281–285.

Muhlbauer, H.D. (1984). The influence of fenfluramine stimulation on prolactin plasma levels in lithium long-term-treated manic-depressive patients and healthy subjects. *Pharmacopsychiatry*, 17(6), 191–193.

Muhlbauer, H.D., and Muller-Oerlinghausen, B. (1985). Fenfluramine stimulation of serum cortisol in patients with major affective disorders and healthy controls: Further evidence for a central serotonergic action of lithium in man. *J Neural Transm*, 61, 81–94.

Muller, W., Brunner, H., and Misgeld, U. (1989). Lithium discriminates between muscarinic receptor subtypes on guinea pig hippocampal neurons in vitro. *Neurosci Lett*, 100, 135.

Mullins, L.J., and Brinley, F.J. Jr. (1967). Some factors influencing sodium extrusion by internally dialyzed squid axons. *J Gen Physiol*, 50, 2333–2355.

Mundo, E., Walker, M., Cate, T., Macciardi, F., and Kennedy, J.L. (2001). The role of serotonin transporter protein gene in antidepressant-induced mania in bipolar disorder: Preliminary findings. *Arch Gen Psychiatry*, 58, 539–544.

Munzer, J.S., Daly, S.E., Jewell-Motz, E.A., Lingrel, J.B., and Blostein, R. (1994). Tissue- and isoform-specific kinetic behavior of the Na,K-ATPase. *J Biol Chem*, 269, 16668–16676.

Murakami, T., Okada, M., Kawata, Y., Zhu, G., Kamata, A., and Kaneko, S. (2001). Determination of effects of antiepileptic drugs on SNAREs-mediated hippocampal monoamine release using in vivo microdialysis. *Br J Pharmacol*, 134, 507–520.

Murashita, J., Kato, T., Shioiri, T., Inubushi, T., and Kato, N. (2000). Altered brain energy metabolism in lithium-resistant bipolar disorder detected by photic stimulated 31P-MR spectroscopy. *Psychol Med*, 30(1), 107–115.

Murphy, B.E., Filipini, D., and Ghadirian, A.M. (1993). Possible use of glucocorticoid receptor antagonists in the treatment of major depression: Preliminary results using RU486. *J Psychiatry Neurosci*, 18(5), 209–213.

Murphy, D.L., Brodie, H.K., Goodwin, F.K., and Bunney, W.E. Jr. (1971). Regular induction of hypomania by L-dopa in "bipolar" manic-depressive patients. *Nature*, 229, 135–136.

Murphy, D.L., Donnelly, C., and Moskowitz, J. (1974). Catecholamine receptor function in depressed patients. *Am J Psychiatry*, 131, 1389–1391.

Murphy, D.L., Lipper, S., Campbell, I.C., Major, M.F., Slater, S., and Buchsbaum, M.S. (1979). Comparative studies of MAO-A and MAO-B inhibitors in man. In T.P. Singer, R.W. Von Korff, and D.L. Murphy (Eds.), *Monamine Oxidase: Structure Function and Altered Functions* (pp. 457–475). New York: Academic Press.

Murphy, D.L., Coursey, R.D., Haenel, T., Aloi, J., and Buchsbaum, M.S. (1982a). Platelet monoamine oxidase as a biological marker in the affective disorders and alcoholism. In E.H. Usdin (Ed.), *Biological Markers in Psychiatry and Neurology* (pp. 123–134). Oxford: Pergamon Press.

Murphy, D.L., Pickar, D., and Alterman, I.S. (1982b). Methods for the quantitative assessment of depressive and manic behavior. In E.I. Burdock, A. Sudilovsky, and S. Gershon (Eds.), *The Behavior of Psychiatric Patients: Quantitative Techniques for Evaluation* (pp. 355–392). New York: Marcel Dekker.

Murray, M., and Greenberg, M.L. (2000). Expression of yeast INM1 encoding inositol monophosphatase is regulated by inositol, carbon source and growth stage and is decreased by lithium and valproate. *Mol Microbiol*, 36, 651–661.

Muscettola, G., Potter, W.Z., Pickar, D., and Goodwin, F.K. (1984). Urinary 3-methoxy-4-hydroxyphenylglycol and major affective disorders. A replication and new findings. *Arch Gen Psychiatry*, 41, 337–342.

Musselman, D.L., and Nemeroff, C.B. (1996). Depression and endocrine disorders: Focus on the thyroid and adrenal system. *Br J Psychiatry Suppl*, 123–128.

Musselman, D.L., Evans, D.L., and Nemeroff, C.B. (1998). The relationship of depression to cardiovascular disease: epidemiology, biology, and treatment. *Arch Gen Psychiatry*, 55, 580–592.

Mynett-Johnson, L.A., Murphy, V.E., Claffey, E., Shields, D.C., and McKeon, P. (1998). Preliminary evidence of an association between bipolar disorder in females and the catechol-O-methyltransferase gene. *Psychiatr Genet*, 8, 221–225.

Mynett-Johnson, L., Kealey, C., Claffey, E., Curtis, D., Bouchier-Hayes, L., Powell, C., and McKeon, P. (2000). Multimarker haplotypes within the serotonin transporter gene suggest evidence of an association with bipolar disorder. *Am J Med Genet*, 96(6), 845–849.

Naber, D., Sand, P., and Heigl, B. (1996). Psychopathological and neuropsychological effects of 8-days' corticosteroid treatment. A prospective study. *Psychoneuroendocrinology*, 21(1), 25–31.

Nahorski, S.R., Ragan, C.I., and Challiss, R.A. (1991). Lithium and the phosphoinositide cycle: An example of uncompetitive inhibition and its pharmacological consequences. *Trends Pharmacol Sci*, 12, 297–303.

Nahorski, S.R., Jenkinson, S., and Challiss, R.A. (1992). Disruption of phosphoinositide signalling by lithium. *Biochem Soc Trans*, 20, 430–434.

Nakamura, S. (1990). Antidepressants induce regeneration of catecholaminergic axon terminals in the rat cerebral cortex. *Neurosci Lett*, 111, 64–68.

Nalepa, I. (1993). The effects of chlorpromazine and haloperidol on second messenger systems related to adrenergic receptors. *Pol J Pharmacol*, 45, 399–412.

Nalepa, I. (1994). The effect of psychotropic drugs on the interaction of protein kinase C with second messenger systems in the rat cerebral cortex. *Pol J Pharmacol*, 46, 1–14.

Narita, M., Aoki, T., Ozaki, S., Yajima, Y., and Suzuki, T. (2001). Involvement of protein kinase Cγ isoform in morphine-induced reinforcing effects. *Neuroscience*, 103(2), 309–314.

Nau, H., and Loscher, W. (1982). Valproate: Brain and plasma levels of the drug and its metabolites, anticonvulsant effects and gamma-aminobutyric acid (GABA) metabolism in the mouse. *J Pharmacol Exp Ther*, 220, 654–659.

Naylor, G.J., and Smith, A.H. (1981). Vanadium: A possible aetiological factor in manic depressive illness. *Psychol Med*, 11, 249–256.

Naylor, G.J., McNamee, H.B., and Moody, J.P. (1970). The plasma control of erythrocyte sodium and potassium metabolism in depressive illness. *J Psychosom Res*, 14, 179–186.

Naylor, G.J., McNamee, H.B., and Moody, J.P. (1971). Changes in erythrocyte sodium and potassium on recovery from a depressive illness. *Br J Psychiatry*, 118, 219–223.

Naylor, G.J., Dick, D.A., Dick, E.G., and Moody, J.P. (1974a). Lithium therapy and erythrocyte membrane cation carrier. *Psychopharmacologia*, 37, 81–86.

Naylor, G.J., Donald, J.M., Le Poidevin, D., and Reid, A.H. (1974b). A double-blind trial of long-term lithium therapy in mental defectives. *Br J Psychiatry*, 124, 52–57.

Naylor, G.J., Reid, A.H., Dick, D.A.T., and Dick, E.G. (1976). A biochemical study of short-cycle manic-depressive psychosis in mental defectives. *Br J Psychiatry*, 128, 1690–1180.

Naylor, G.J., Smith, A.H., Dick, E.G., Dick, D.A., McHarg, A.M., and Chambers, C.A. (1980). Erythrocyte membrane cation carrier in manic-depressive psychosis. *Psychol Med*, 10, 521–525.

Nemanov, L., Ebstein, R.P., Belmaker, R.H., Osher, Y., and Agam, G. (1999). Effect of bipolar disorder on lymphocyte inositol monophosphatase mRNA levels. *Int J Neuropsychopharmcol*, 2, 25–29.

Nemeroff, C.B., Kalivas, P.W., Golden, R.N., and Prange, A.J. Jr. (1984a). Behavioral effects of hypothalamic hypophysiotropic hormones, neurotensin, substance P and other neuropeptides. *Pharmacol Ther*, 24, 1–56.

Nemeroff, C.B., Widerlöv, E., Bissette, G., Walleus, H., Karlsson, I., Eklund, K., Kilts, C.D., Loosen, P.T., and Vale, W. (1984b). Elevated concentrations of CSF corticotropin-releasing factor-like immunoreactivity in depressed patients. *Science*, 226, 1342–1344.

Nemeroff, C.B., Simon, J.S., Haggerty, J.J. Jr., and Evans, D.L. (1985). Antithyroid antibodies in depressed patients. *Am J Psychiatry*, 142, 840–843.

Nemeroff, C.B., Owens, M.J., Bissette, G., Andorn, A.C., and Stanley, M. (1988). Reduced corticotropin releasing factor binding sites in the frontal cortex of suicide victims. *Arch Gen Psychiatry*, 45, 577–579.

Nemeroff, C.B., Bissette, G., Akil, H., and Fink, M. (1991). Neuropeptide concentrations in the cerebrospinal fluid of depressed patients treated with electroconvulsive therapy. Corticotrophin-releasing factor, beta-endorphin and somatostatin. *Br J Psychiatry*, 158, 59–63.

Nemeroff, C.B., Evans, D.L., Gyulai, L., Sachs, G.S., Bowden, C.L., Gergel, I.P., Oakes, R., and Pitts, C.D. (2001). Double-blind, placebo-controlled comparison of imipramine and paroxetine in the treatment of bipolar depression. *Am J Psychiatry*, 158, 906–912.

Nestler, E.J., Terwilliger, R.Z., and Duman, R.S. (1989). Chronic antidepressant administration alters the subcellular distribution of cyclic AMP–dependent protein kinase in rat frontal cortex. *J Neurochem*, 53, 1644–1647.

Nestler, E.J., Terwilliger, R.Z., and Duman, R.S. (1995). Regulation of endogenous ADP-ribosylation by acute and chronic lithium in rat brain. *J Neurochem*, 64, 2319–2324.

Nestler, E.J., Barrot, M., DiLeone, R.J., Eisch, A.J., Gold, S.J., and Monteggia, L.M. (2002a). Neurobiology of depression. *Neuron*, 34, 13–25.

Nestler, E.J., Gould, E., Manji, H., Buncan, M., Duman, R.S., Greshenfeld, H.K., Hen, R., Koester, S., Lederhendler, I., Meaney, M., Robbins, T., Winsky, L., and Zalcman, S. (2002b). Preclinical models: status of basic research in depression. *Biol Psychiatry*, 52, 503–528.

Neubig, R.R., Gantzos, R.D., and Thomsen, W.J. (1988). Mechanism of agonist and antagonist binding to alpha 2 adrenergic receptors: Evidence for a precoupled receptor-guanine nucleotide protein complex. *Biochemistry*, 27, 2374–2384.

Neumeister, A. (2003). Tryptophan depletion, serotonin, and depression: Where do we stand? *Psychopharmacol Bull*, 37, 99–115.

Neumeister, A., Praschak-Rieder, N., Hesselmann, B., Vitouch, O., Rauh, M., Barocka, A., and Kasper, S. (1997). Rapid tryptophan depletion in drug-free depressed patients with seasonal affective disorder. *Am J Psychiatry*, 154(8), 1153–1155.

Neumeister, A., Praschak-Rieder, N., Hesselmann, B., Vitouch, O., Rauh, M., Barocka, A., Tauscher, J., and Kasper, S. (1998). Effects of tryptophan depletion in drug-free depressed patients who responded to total sleep deprivation. *Arch Gen Psychiatry*, 55, 167–172.

Neumeister, A., Young, T., and Stastny, J. (2004). Implications of genetic research on the role of the serotonin in depression: Emphasis on the serotonin type 1a receptor and the serotonin transporter. *Psychopharmacology (Berl)*, 174(4), 512–524.

Newman, M.E., and Belmaker, R.H. (1987). Effects of lithium in vitro and ex vivo on components of the adenylate cyclase system in membranes from the cerebral cortex of the rat. *Neuropharmacology*, 26, 211–217.

Newman, M.E., Drummer, D., and Lerer, B. (1990). Single and combined effects of desimipramine and lithium on serotonergic receptor number and second messenger function in rat brain. *J Pharmacol Exp Ther*, 252, 826–831.

Newman, M.E., Shapira, B., and Lerer, B. (1998). Evaluation of central serotonergic function in affective and related disorders by the fenfluramine challenge test: A critical review. *Int J Neuropsychopharmcol*, 1, 49–69.

Nibuya, M., Morinobu, S., and Duman, R.S. (1995). Regulation of BDNF and TrkB mRNA in rat brain by chronic electroconvulsive seizure and antidepressant drug treatments. *J Neurosci*, 15, 7539–7547.

Nibuya, M., Nestler, E.J., and Duman, R.S. (1996). Chronic antidepressant administration increases the expression of cAMP response element binding protein (CREB) in rat hippocampus. *J Neurosci*, 16, 2365–2372.

Nibuya, M., Takahashi, M., Russell, D.S., and Duman, R.S. (1999). Repeated stress increases catalytic TrkB mRNA in rat hippocampus. *Neurosci Lett*, 267, 81–84.

Nicholas, L., Dawkins, K., and Golden, R.N. (1998). Psychoneuroendocrinology of depression. Prolactin. *Psychiatr Clin North Am*, 21, 341–358.

Niesler, B., Flohr, T., Nothen, M.M., Fischer, C., Rietschel, M., Franzek, E., Albus, M., Propping, P., and Rappold, G.A. (2001). Association between the 5' UTR variant C178T of the serotonin receptor gene HTR3A and bipolar affective disorder. *Pharmacogenetics*, 11, 471–475.

Nikaido, T., Akiyama, M., Moriya, T., and Shibata, S. (2001). Sensitized increase of period gene expression in the mouse caudate/putamen caused by repeated injection of methamphetamine. *Mol Pharmacol*, 59(4), 894–900.

Nilsson, C., Karlsson, G., Blennow, K., Heilig, M., and Ekman, R. (1996). Differences in the neuropeptide Y–like immunoreactivity of the plasma and platelets of human volunteers and depressed patients. *Peptides*, 17(3), 359–362.

Nilsson, M., Hansson, E., and Ronnback, L. (1990). Transport of valproate and its effects on GABA uptake in astroglial primary culture. *Neurochem Res*, 15, 763–767.

Nishizuka, Y. (1992). Intracellular signaling by hydrolysis of phospholipids and activation of protein kinase C. *Science*, 258, 607–614.

Noble, A.B., McKinney, W.T. Jr., Mohr, C., and Moran, E. (1976). Diazepam treatment of socially isolated monkeys. *Am J Psychiatry*, 133, 1165–1170.

Noga, J.T., Hyde, T.M., Herman, M.M., Spurney, C.F., Bigelow, L.B., Weinberger, D.R., and Kleinman, J.E. (1997). Glutamate receptors in the postmortem striatum of schizophrenic, suicide, and control brains. *Synapse*, 27, 168–176.

Nolen, W.A., van de Putte, J.J., Dijken, W.A., Kamp, J.S., Blansjaar, B.A., Kramer, H.J., and Haffmans, J. (1988). Treatment strategy in depression. II. MAO inhibitors in depression resistant to cyclic antidepressants: Two controlled crossover studies with tranylcypromine versus L-5-hydroxytryptophan and nomifensine. *Acta Psychiatr Scand*, 78, 676–683.

Nolen-Hoeksema, S. (1987). Sex differences in unipolar depression: Evidence and theory. *Psychol Bull*, 101, 259–282.

Nonaka, S., and Chuang, D.M. (1998). Neuroprotective effects of chronic lithium on focal cerebral ischemia in rats. *Neuroreport*, 9, 2081–2084.

Nonaka, S., Hough, C.J., and Chuang, D.M. (1998). Chronic lithium treatment robustly protects neurons in the central nervous system against excitotoxicity by inhibiting N-methyl-D-aspartate receptor-mediated calcium influx. *Proc Natl Acad Sci USA*, 95, 2642–2647.

Nowak, G., Trullas, R., Layer, R.T., Skolnick, P., and Paul, I.A. (1993). Adaptive changes in the N-methyl-D-aspartate receptor complex after chronic treatment with imipramine and 1-aminocyclopropanecarboxylic acid. *J Pharmacol Exp Ther*, 265, 1380–1386.

Nowak, G., Ordway, G.A., and Paul, I.A. (1995a). Alterations in the N-methyl-D-aspartate (NMDA) receptor complex in the frontal cortex of suicide victims. *Brain Res*, 675, 157–164.

Nowak, G., Redmond, A., McNamara, M., and Paul, I.A. (1995b). Swim stress increases the potency of glycine at the N-methyl-D-aspartate receptor complex. *J Neurochem*, 64, 925–927.

Nurnberger, J.I. Jr., Jimerson, D.C., Allen, J.R., Simmons, S., and Gershon, E. (1982). Red cell ouabain-sensitive Na+-K+-adenosine triphosphatase: Astate marker in affective disorder inversely related to plasma cortisol. *Biol Psychiatry*, 17, 981–992.

Nurnberger, J.I. Jr., Jimerson, D.C., Simmons-Alling, S., Tamminga, C., Nadi, N.S., Lawrence, D., Sitaram, N., Gillin, J.C., and Gershon, E.S. (1983). Behavioral, physiological, and neuroendocrine responses to arecoline in normal twins and "well state" bipolar patients. *Psychiatry Res*, 9, 191–200.

Nurnberger, J.I. Jr., Berrettini, W., Mendelson, W., Sack, D., and Gershon, E.S. (1989). Measuring cholinergic sensitivity: I. Arecoline effects in bipolar patients. *Biol Psychiatry*, 25, 610–617.

Nurnberger, J.I. Jr., Berrettini, W., Simmons-Alling, S., Lawrence, D., and Brittain, H. (1990). Blunted ACTH and cortisol response to afternoon tryptophan infusion in euthymic bipolar patients. *Psychiatry Res*, 31, 57–67.

Nurnberger, J.I., Adkins, S., Lahiri, D.K., Mayeda, A., Hu, K., Lewy, A., Miller, A., Bowman, E.S., Miller, M.J., Rau, L., Smiley, C., and Davis-Singh, D. (2000). Melatonin suppression by light in euthymic bipolar and unipolar patients. *Arch Gen Psychiatry*, 57(6), 572–579.

Nutt, D.J. (1989). Altered central alpha 2-adrenoceptor sensitivity in panic disorder. *Arch Gen Psychiatry*, 46, 165–169.

O'Brian, C.A., Ward, N.E., and Anderson, B.W. (1988). Role of specific interactions between protein kinase C and triphenylethylenes in inhibition of the enzyme. *J Natl Cancer Inst*, 80(20), 1628–1633.

Odagaki, Y., Koyama, T., Matsubara, S., Matsubara, R., and Yamashita, I. (1990). Effects of chronic lithium treatment on serotonin binding sites in rat brain. *J Psychiatr Res*, 24, 271–277.

Ohmori, T., Arora, R.C., and Meltzer, H.Y. (1992). Serotonergic measures in suicide brain: The concentration of 5-HIAA, HVA, and tryptophan in frontal cortex of suicide victims. *Biol Psychiatry*, 32, 57–71.

Okamoto, Y., Kagaya, A., Shinno, H., Motohashi, N., and Yamawaki, S. (1995). Serotonin-induced platelet calcium mobilization is enhanced in mania. *Life Sci*, 56, 327–332.

Okuyama, S., Chaki, S., Kawashima, N., Suzuki, Y., Ogawa, S., Nakazato, A., Kumagai, T., Okubo, T., and Tomisawa, K. (1999). Receptor binding, behavioral, and electrophysiological profiles of nonpeptide corticotropin-releasing factor subtype 1 receptor antagonists CRA1000 and CRA1001. *J Pharmacol Exp Ther*, 289(2), 926–935.

Olive, M.F., Mehmert, K.K., Messing, R.O., and Hodge, C.W. (2000). Reduced operant ethanol self-administration and in vivo mesolimbic dopamine responses to ethanol in PKCepsilon-deficient mice. *Eur J Neurosci*, 12, 4131–4140.

Ongur, D., Drevets, W.C., and Price, J.L. (1998). Glial reduction in the subgenual prefrontal cortex in mood disorders. *Proc Natl Acad Sci USA*, 95, 13290–13295.

Oomen, H.A., Schipperijn, A.J., and Drexhage, H.A. (1996). The prevalence of affective disorder and in particular of a rapid cycling of bipolar disorder in patients with abnormal thyroid function tests. *Clin Endocrinol (Oxf)*, 45, 215–223.

Oppenheim, G., Ebstein, R.P., and Belmaker, R.H. (1979). Effect of lithium on the physostigmine-induced behavioral syndrome and plasma cyclic GMP. *J Psychiatr Res*, 15, 133–138.

Ordway, G.A., Smith, K.S., and Haycock, J.W. (1994a). Elevated tyrosine hydroxylase in the locus coeruleus of suicide victims. *J Neurochem*, 62, 680–685.

Ordway, G.A., Widdowson, P.S., Smith, K.S., and Halaris, A. (1994b). Agonist binding to α2-adrenoceptors is elevated in the locus coeruleus from victims of suicide. *J Neurochem*, 63, 617–624.

Ordway, G.A., Farley, J.T., Dilley, G.E., Overholser, J.C., Meltzer, H.Y., Balraj, E.K., Stockmeier, C.A., and Klimek, V. (1999). Quantitative distribution of monoamine oxidase A in brainstem monoamine nuclei is normal in major depression. *Brain Res*, 847, 71–79.

Orlovskaya, D.D., Vostrikov, V.M., Rachmanova, V.I., and Uranova, N.A. (2000). Decreased numerical density of oligodendroglial cells in postmortem prefrontal cortex in schizophrenia, bipolar affective disorder and major depression. *Schizophr Res*, 41, 105.

Ormandy, G.C., and Jope, R.S. (1991). Pertussis toxin potentiates seizures induced by pilocarpine, kainic acid and N-methyl-D-aspartate. *Brain Res*, 553, 51–57.

Orr, K.G., Mostert, J., and Castle, D.J. (1998). Mania associated with codeine and paracetamol. *Aust N Z J Psychiatry*, 32, 586–588.

Orth, D.N., Shelton, R.C., Nicholson, W.E., Beck-Peccoz, P., Tomarken, A.J., Persani, L., and Loosen, P.T. (2001). Serum thyrotropin concentrations and bioactivity during sleep deprivation in depression. *Arch Gen Psychiatry*, 58, 77–83.

Oruc, L., Verheyen, G.R., Furac, I., Jakovljevic, M., Ivezic, S., Raeymaekers, P., and Van Broeckhoven C. (1997). Association analysis of the 5-HT2C receptor and 5-HT transporter genes in bipolar disorder. *Am J Med Genet*, 74(5), 504–506.

Oshima, A., Yamashita, S., Owashi, T., Murata, T., Tadokoro, C., Miyaoka, H., Kamijima, K., and Higuchi, T. (2000). The differential ACTH responses to combined dexamethasone/CRH administration in major depressive and dysthymic disorders. *J Psychiatr Res*, 34(4-5), 325–328.

Ostrow, D.G., Pandey, G.N., Davis, J.M., Hurt, S.W., and Tosteson, D.C. (1978). A heritable disorder of lithium transport in erythrocytes of a subpopulation of manic-depressive patients. *Am J Psychiatry*, 135, 1070–1078.

Ostrow, D.G., and Davis, J.M. (1982). Laboratory measurements in the clinical use of lithium. *Clin Neuropharmacol*, 5(3), 317–336.

Owen, F., Cross, A.J., Crow, T.J., Deakin, J.F., Ferrier, I.N., Lofthouse, R., and Poulter, M. (1983). Brain 5-HT2 receptors and suicide. *Lancet*, ii, 1256.

Owen F., Chambers, D.R., Cooper, S.J., Crow, T.J., Johnson, J.A., Lofthouse, R., and Poulter, M. (1986). Serotonergic mechanisms in brains of suicide victims. *Brain Res*, 362, 185–188.

Owens, D.F., and Kriegstein, A.R. (2002). Is there more to GABA than synaptic inhibition? *Nat Rev Neurosci*, 3(9), 715–727.

Owens, M.J., and Nemeroff, C.B. (1998). The serotonin transporter and depression. *Depress Anxiety*, 8(Suppl. 1), 5–12.

Oyama, T., Yamaya, R., Jin, T., and Kudo, T. (1982). Effect of exogenous beta-endorphin on anterior pituitary hormone secretion in man. *Acta Endocrinol (Copenh)*, 99, 9–13.

Ozaki, N., and Chuang, D.M. (1997). Lithium increases transcription factor binding to AP-1 and cyclic AMP-responsive element in cultured neurons and rat brain. *J Neurochem*, 69, 2336–2344.

Pacheco, M.A., Stockmeier, C., Meltzer, H.Y., Overholser, J.C., Dilley, G.E., and Jope, R.S. (1996). Alterations in phosphoinositide signaling and G-protein levels in depressed suicide brain. *Brain Res*, 723, 37–45.

Palmer, G.C. (1979). Interactions of antiepileptic drugs on adenylate cyclase and phosphodiesterases in rat and mouse cerebrum. *Exp Neurol*, 63, 322–335.

Palmer, A.M., Burns, M.A., Arango, V., and Mann, J.J. (1994). Similar effects of glycine, zinc and an oxidizing agent on [3H]dizocilpine binding to the N-methyl-D-aspartate receptor in neocortical tissue from suicide victims and controls. *J Neural Transm Gen Sect*, 96, 1–8.

Pandey, G.N., and Davis, J.M. (1986). Leukocyte β-adrenergic receptors: A marker for central β-adrenergic receptor function in depression. *Clin Neuropharmacol*, 14(Suppl. 9), 353–355.

Pandey, G.N., Ostrow, D.G., Haas, M., Dorus, E., Casper, R.C., Davis, J.M., and Tosteson, D.C. (1977). Abnormal lithium and sodium transport in erythrocytes of a manic patient and some members of his family. *Proc Natl Acad Sci USA*, 74(8), 3607–3611.

Pandey, G.N., Dysken, M.W., Garver, D.L., and Davis, J.M. (1979). Beta-adrenergic receptor function in affective illness. *Am J Psychiatry*, 136, 675–678.

Pandey, G.N., Sudershan, P., and Davis, J.M. (1985). Beta-adrenergic receptor function in depression and the effect of antidepressant drugs. *Acta Pharmacol Toxicol (Copenh)*, 56 (Suppl. 1), 66–79.

Pandey, G.N., Janicak, P.G., and Davis, J.M. (1987). Decreased beta-adrenergic receptors in the leukocytes of depressed patients. *Psychiatry Res*, 22, 265–273.

Pandey, G.N., Janicak, P.G., Javaid, J.I., and Davis, J.M. (1989). Increased 3H-clonidine binding in the platelets of patients with depressive and schizophrenic disorders. *Psychiatry Res*, 28, 73–88.

Pandey, G.N., Pandey, S.C., Janicak, P.G., Marks, R.C., and Davis, J.M. (1990). Platelet serotonin-2 receptor binding sites in depression and suicide. *Biol Psychiatry*, 28, 215–222.

Pandey, G.N., Pandey, S.C., Dwivedi, Y., Sharma, R.P., Janicak, P.G., and Davis, J.M. (1995). Platelet serotonin-2A receptors: A potential biological marker for suicidal behavior. *Am J Psychiatry*, 152, 850–855.

Pandey, G.N., Dwivedi, Y., Pandey, S.C., Conley, R.R., Roberts, R.C., and Tamminga, C.A. (1997a). Protein kinase C in the postmortem brain of teenage suicide victims. *Neurosci Lett*, 228, 111–114.

Pandey, G.N., Conley, R.R., Pandey, S.C., Goel, S., Roberts, R.C., Tamminga, C.A., Chute, D., and Smialek, J. (1997b). Benzodiazepine receptors in the post-mortem brain of suicide victims and schizophrenic subjects. *Psychiatry Res*, 71, 137–149.

Pap, M., and Cooper, G.M. (1998). Role of glycogen synthase kinase-3 in the phosphatidylinositol 3-kinase/Akt cell survival pathway. *J Biol Chem*, 273, 19929–19932.

Papadimitriou, G.N., Dikeos, D.G., Karadima, G., Avramopoulos, D., Daskalopoulou, E.G., Vassilopoulos, D., and Stefanis, C.N. (1998). Association between the GABA(A) receptor alpha5 subunit gene locus (GABRA5) and bipolar affective disorder. *Am J Med Genet*, 81, 73–80.

Papolos, D.F., Veit, S., Faedda, G.L., Saito, T., and Lachman, H.M. (1998). Ultra-ultra rapid cycling bipolar disorder is associated with the low activity catecholamine-O-methyltransferase allele. *Mol Psychiatry*, 3, 346–349.

Papp, M., Willner, P., and Muscat, R. (1991). An animal model of anhedonia: Attenuation of sucrose consumption and place preference conditioning by chronic unpredictable mild stress. *Psychopharmacology (Berl)*, 104, 255–259.

Pare, C.M.B., Yeung, D.P., Price, K., and Stacey, R.S. (1969). 5-Hydroxytryptamine, noradrenaline, and dopamine in brainstem, hypothalamus, and caudate nucleus of controls and of patients committing suicide by coal-gas poisoning. *Lancet*, ii, 133–135.

Parekh, P.I., Ketter, T.A., Altshuler, L., Frye, M.A., Callahan, A., Marangell, L., and Post, R.M. (1998). Relationships between thyroid hormone and antidepressant responses to total sleep deprivation in mood disorder patients. *Biol Psychiatry*, 43, 392–394.

Parry, B.L., Hauger, R., LeVeau, B., Mostofi, N., Cover, H., Clopton, P., and Gillin, J.C. (1996). Circadian rhythms of prolactin and thyroid-stimulating hormone during the menstrual cycle and early versus late sleep deprivation in premenstrual dysphoric disorder. *Psychiatry Res*, 62(2), 147–160.

Parsian, A., Chakraverty, S., and Todd, R.D. (1995). Possible association between the dopamine D3 receptor gene and bipolar affective disorder. *Am J Med Genet*, 60, 234–237.

Pascual, T., and Gonzalez, J.L. (1995). A protective effect of lithium on rat behaviour altered by ibotenic acid lesions of the basal forebrain cholinergic system. *Brain Res*, 695, 289–292.

Patel, P.D., Lopez, J.F., Lyons, D.M., Burke, S., Wallace, M., and Schatzberg, A.F. (2000). Glucocorticoid and mineralocorticoid receptor mRNA expression in squirrel monkey brain. *J Psychiatr Res*, 34, 383–392.

Patsalos, P.N., and Lascelles, P.T. (1981). Changes in regional brain levels of amino acid putative neurotransmitters after prolonged treatment with the anticonvulsant drugs diphenylhydantoin, phenobarbitone, sodium valproate, ethosuximide, and sulthiame in the rat. *J Neurochem*, 36, 688–695.

Paul, I.A., Trullas, R., Skolnick, P., and Nowak, G. (1992). Downregulation of cortical beta-adrenoceptors by chronic treatment with functional NMDA antagonists. *Psychopharmacology (Berl)*, 106, 285–287.

Paul, S.M., Rehavi, M., Skolnick, P., and Goodwin, F.K. (1984). High affinity binding of antidepressants to biogenic amine transport sites in human brain and platelet: Studies in depression. In M. Post and J.C. Ballenger (Eds.), *Neurobiology of Mood Disorders* (pp. 846–853). Baltimore: Williams & Wilkins.

Payne, J.L., Quiroz, J.A., Carlos, A., Zarate, J., and Manji, H.K. (2002). Timing is everything: Does the robust upregulation of noradrenergically regulated plasticity genes underlie the rapid antidepressant effects of sleep deprivation? *Biol Psychiatry*, 52, 921–926.

Pearlson, G.D., Wong, D.F., Tune, L.E., Ross, C.A., Chase, G.A., Links, J.M., Dannals, R.F., Wilson, A.A., Ravert, H.T., and Wagner, H.N. Jr. (1995). In vivo D2 dopamine receptor density in psychotic and nonpsychotic patients with bipolar disorder. *Arch Gen Psychiatry*, 52, 471–477.

Peckys, D., and Hurd, Y.L. (2001). Prodynorphin and kappa opioid receptor mRNA expression in the cingulate and prefrontal cortices of subjects diagnosed with schizophrenia or affective disorders. *Brain Res Bull*, 55, 619–624.

Pepe, S., Bogdanov, K., Hallaq, H., Spurgeon, H., Leaf, A., and Lakatta, E. (1994). Omega 3 polyunsaturated fatty acid modulates dihydropyridine effects on L-type Ca2+ channels, cytosolic Ca2+, and contraction in adult rat cardiac myocytes. *Proc Natl Acad Sci USA*, 91, 8832–8836.

Pepper, G.M., and Krieger, D.T. (1984). Hypothalamic–pituitary–adrenal abnormalities in affective illness. In R.M. Post and J.C. Ballenger (Eds.), *Neurobiology of the Mood Disorders*, Vol. I (pp. 245–270). Baltimore: Williams and Wilkins.

Perera, T.F., Coplan, J.D., Lisanby, S.H., et al. (2006, submitted). ECS induced neurogenesis in the adult monkey dentate gyrus. Submitted to *Proc Natl Acad Sci USA*.

Perez, J., Zanardi, R., Mori, S., Gasperini, M., Smeraldi, E., and Racagni, G. (1995). Abnormalities of cAMP dependent endogenous phosphorylation in platelets from patients with bipolar disorder. *Am J Psychiatry*, 152(8), 1204–1206.

Perez, J., Tardito, D., Mori, S., Racagni, G., Smeraldi, E., and Zanardi, R. (2000). Altered Rap1 endogenous phosphorylation and levels in platelets from patients with bipolar disorder. *J Psychiatr Res*, 34, 99–104.

Perez de Castro, I., Santos, J., Torres, P., Visedo, G., Saiz-Ruiz, J., Llinares, C., and Fernandez-Piqueras, J. (1995). A weak association between TH and DRD2 genes and bipolar affective disorder in a Spanish sample. *J Med Genet*, 32, 131–134.

Perlman, W.R., Webster, M.J., Kleinman, J.E., and Weickert, C.S. (2004). Reduced glucocorticoid and estrogen receptor alpha messenger ribonucleic acid levels in the amygdala of patients with major mental illness. *Biol Psychiatry*, 56(11), 844–852.

Perlow, M.J., Reppert, S.M., Artman, H.A., Fisher, D.A., Self, S.M., and Robinson, A.G. (1982). Oxytocin, vasopressin, and estrogen-stimulated neurophysin: Daily patterns of concentration in cerebrospinal fluid. *Science*, 216, 1416–1418.

Pernow, J., Lundberg, J.M., and Kaijser, L. (1988). Alpha-adrenoceptor influence on plasma levels of neuropeptide Y–like immunoreactivity and catecholamines during rest and sympathoadrenal activation in humans. *J Cardiovasc Pharmacol*, 12(5), 593–599.

Persico, A.M., D'Agruma, L., Maiorano, N., Totaro, A., Militerni, R., Bravaccio, C., Wassink, T.H., Schneider, C., Melmed, R., Trillo, S., Montecchi, F., Palermo, M., Pascucci, T., Puglisi-Allegra, S., Reichelt, K.L., Conciatori, M., Marino, R., Quattrocchi, C.C., Baldi, A., Zelante, L., Gasparini, P., Keller, F., and Collaborative Linkage Study of Autism. (2001). *Reelin* gene alleles and haplotypes as a factor predisposing to autistic disorder. *Mol Psychiatry*, 6, 150–159.

Persinger, M.A., Makarec, K., and Bradley, J.C. (1988). Characteristics of limbic seizures evoked by peripheral injections of lithium and pilocarpine. *Physiol Behav*, 44, 27–37.

Pert, A., Rosenblatt, J.E., Sivit, C., Pert, C.B., and Bunney, W.E. Jr. (1978). Long-term treatment with lithium prevents the development of dopamine receptor supersensitivity. *Science*, 201(4351), 171–173.

Pert, C.B., and Snyder, S.H. (1973). Properties of opiate-receptor binding in rat brain. *Proc Natl Acad Sci USA*, 70(8), 2243–2247.

Perugi, G., Toni, C., Ruffolo, G., Frare, F., and Akiskal, H. (2001). Adjunctive dopamine agonists in treatment-resistant bipolar II depression: An open case series. *Pharmacopsychiatry*, 34, 137–141.

Pesold, C., Impagnatiello, F., Pisu, M.G., Uzunov, D.P., Costa, E., Guidotti, A., and Caruncho, H.J. (1998a). Reelin is preferentially expressed in neurons synthesizing gamma-aminobutyric acid in cortex and hippocampus of adult rats. *Proc Natl Acad Sci USA*, 95, 3221–3226.

Pesold, C., Pisu, M.G., Impagnatiello, F., Uzunov, D.P., and Caruncho, H.J. (1998b). Simultaneous detection of glutamic acid decarboxylase and reelin mRNA in adult rat neurons using in situ hybridization and immunofluorescence. *Brain Res Brain Res Protoc*, 3, 155–160.

Petronis, A. (2003). Epigenetics and bipolar disorder: New opportunities and challenges. *Am J Med Genet C Semin Med Genet*, 123(1), 65–75.

Petronis, A. (2004). The origin of schizophrenia: Genetic thesis, epigenetic antithesis, and resolving synthesis. *Biol Psychiatry*, 55(10), 965–970.

Petty, F., and Schlesser, M.A. (1981). Plasma GABA in affective illness. A preliminary investigation. *J Affect Disord*, 3, 339–343.

Petty, F., and Sherman, A.D. (1981). A pharmacologically pertinent animal model of mania. *J Affect Disord*, 3, 381–387.

Petty, F., and Sherman, A.D. (1984). Plasma GABA levels in psychiatric illness. *J Affect Disord*, 6, 131–138.

Petty, F., Kramer, G.L., Dunnam, D., and Rush, A.J. (1990). Plasma GABA in mood disorders. *Psychopharmacol Bull*, 26, 157–161.

Petty, F., Kramer, G.L., Fulton, M., Moeller, F.G., and Rush, A.J. (1993). Low plasma GABA is a trait-like marker for bipolar illness. *Neuropsychopharmacology*, 9, 125–132.

Petty, F., Rush, A.J., Davis, J.M., Calabrese, J.R., Kimmel, S.E., Kramer, G.L., Small, J.G., Miller, M.J., Swann, A.E., Orsulak, P.J., Blake, M.E., and Bowden, C.L. (1996). Plasma GABA predicts acute response to divalproex in mania. *Biol Psychiatry*, 39, 278–284.

Phelan, M.C. (1989). Beclomethasone mania. *Br J Psychiatry*, 155, 871–872.

Phelps, J. (2006). *Why Am I Still Depressed? Recognizing and Managing the Ups and Downs of Bipolar II and Soft Bipolar Disorder.* New York: McGraw-Hill.

Phiel, C.J., and Klein, P.S. (2001). Molecular targets of lithium action. *Annu Rev Pharmacol Toxicol*, 41, 789–813.

Pickar, D., Sweeney, D.R., Maas, J.W., and Heninger, G.R. (1978). Primary affective disorder, clinical state change, and MHPG excretion: A longitudinal study. *Arch Gen Psychiatry*, 35, 1378–1383.

Pickar, D., Davis, G.C., Schulz, S.C., Extein, I., Wagner, R., Naber, D., Gold, P.W., van Kammen, D.P., Goodwin, F.K., Wyatt, R.J.,

Li, C.H., and Bunney, W.E. Jr. (1981). Behavioral and biological effects of acute beta-endorphin injection in schizophrenic and depressed patients. *Am J Psychiatry*, 138, 160–166.

Pickar, D., Naber, D., Post, R.M., van Kammen, D.P., Kaye, W., Rubinow, D.R., Ballenger, J.C., and Bunney, W.E. Jr. (1982a). Endorphins in the cerebrospinal fluid of psychiatric patients. *Ann NY Acad Sci*, 398, 399–412.

Pickar, D., Vartanian, F., Bunney, W.E. Jr., Maier, H.P., Gastpar, M.T., Prakash, R., Sethi, B.B., Lideman, R., Belyaev, B.S., Tsutsulkovskaja, M.V., Jungkunz, G., Nedopil, N., Verhoeven, W., and van Praag, H. (1982b). Short-term naloxone administration in schizophrenic and manic patients. A World Health Organization collaborative study. *Arch Gen Psychiatry*, 39, 313–319.

Pickar, D., Dubois, M., and Cohen, M.R. (1984). Behavioral change in a cancer patient following intrathecal beta-endorphin administration. *Am J Psychiatry*, 141, 103–104.

Pilc, A., Branski, P., Palucha, A., and Aronowski, J. (1999). The effect of prolonged imipramine and electroconvulsive shock treatment on calcium/calmodulin-dependent protein kinase II in the hippocampus of rat brain. *Neuropharmacology*, 38, 597–603.

Piletz, J.E., Schubert, D.S., and Halaris, A. (1986). Evaluation of studies on platelet alpha 2 adrenoreceptors in depressive illness. *Life Sci*, 39, 1589–1616.

Piletz, J.E., Halaris, A., Saran, A., and Marler, M. (1990). Elevated 3H-para-aminoclonidine binding to platelet purified plasma membranes from depressed patients. *Neuropsychopharmacology*, 3, 201–210.

Pilgrim, C., and Hutchison, J.B. (1994). Developmental regulation of sex differences in the brain: Can the role of gonadal steroids be redefined? *Neuroscience*, 60, 843–855.

Plotsky, P.M., Owens, M.J., and Nemeroff, C.B. (1995). Neuropeptide alterations in mood disorder. In R.E. Bloom, D.J. Kupfer (Eds.), *Psychopharmacology: The Fourth Generation of Progress* (pp. 971–981). New York: Raven Press.

Plyte, S.E., Hughes, K., Nikolakaki, E., Pulverer, B.J., and Woodgett, J.R. (1992). Glycogen synthase kinase-3: Functions in oncogenesis and development. *Biochim Biophys Acta*, 1114, 147–162.

Poirier, M.F., Galzin, A.M., Pimoule, C., Schoemaker, H., Le Quan Bui, K.H., Meyer, P., Gay, C., Loo, H., and Langer, S.Z. (1988). Short-term lithium administration to healthy volunteers produces long-lasting pronounced changes in platelet serotonin uptake but not imipramine binding. *Psychopharmacology (Berl)*, 94, 521–526.

Poirier-Littre, M.F., Loo, H., Dennis, T., and Scatton, B. (1993). Lithium treatment increases norepinephrine turnover in the plasma of healthy subjects. *Arch Gen Psychiatry*, 50, 72–73.

Poitou, P., and Bohuon, C. (1975). Catecholamine metabolism in the rat brain after short- and long-term lithium administration. *J Neurochem*, 25, 535–537.

Pollack, I.F., DaRosso, R.C., Robertson, P.L., Jakacki, R.L., Mirro, J.R. Jr., Blatt, J., Nicholson, S., Packer, R.J., Allen, J.C., Cisneros, A., and Jordan, V.C. (1997). A phase I study of high-dose tamoxifen for the treatment of refractory malignant gliomas of childhood. *Clin Cancer Res*, 3(7), 1109–1115.

Poncelet, M., Dangoumau, L., Soubrie, P., and Simon, P. (1987). Effects of neuroleptic drugs, clonidine and lithium on the expression of conditioned behavioral excitation in rats. *Psychopharmacology (Berl)*, 92, 393–397.

Pontzer, N.J., and Crews, F.T. (1990). Desensitization of muscarinic stimulated hippocampal cell firing is related to phosphoinositide hydrolysis and inhibited by lithium. *J Pharmacol Exp Ther*, 253, 921–929.

Pope, H.G. Jr., and Katz, D.L. (1988). Affective and psychotic symptoms associated with anabolic steroid use. *Am J Psychiatry*, 145, 487–490.

Pope, H.G., Kourie, E.M., and Hudson, J.I. (2000). Effects of supraphysiologic doses of testosterone on mood and aggression in normal men. *Arch Gen Psychiatry*, 57, 133–140.

Popoli, M., Vocaturo, C., Perez, J., Smeraldi, E., and Racagni, G. (1995). Presynaptic Ca2+/calmodulin-dependent protein kinase II: Autophosphorylation and activity increase in the hippocampus after long-term blockade of serotonin reuptake. *Mol Pharmacol*, 48, 623–629.

Popoli, M., Brunello, N., Perez, J., and Racagni, G. (2000). Second messenger–regulated protein kinases in the brain: Their functional role and the action of antidepressant drugs. *J Neurochem*, 74, 21–33.

Porsolt, R.D. (2000). Animal models of depression: Utility for transgenic research. *Rev Neurosci*, 11, 53–58.

Post, R.M., and Ballenger, J.C. (1981). *Kindling Models for the Progressive Development of Psychopathology. Handbook of Biological Psychiatry.* New York: Dekker.

Post, R., and Kopanda, R.T. (1976). Cocaine, kindling, and psychosis. *Am J Psychiatry*, 133, 627–634.

Post, R.M., and Weiss, S.R. (1989). Sensitization, kindling, and anticonvulsants in mania. *J Clin Psychiatry*, 50, 23–30; discussion 45–47.

Post, R.M., and Weiss, S.R. (1992). Ziskind-Somerfeld Research Award 1992. Endogenous biochemical abnormalities in affective illness: Therapeutic versus pathogenic. *Biol Psychiatry*, 32, 469–484.

Post, R.M., and Weiss, S.R. (1996). A speculative model of affective illness cyclicity based on patterns of drug tolerance observed in amygdala-kindled seizures. *Mol Neurobiol*, 13, 33–60.

Post, R.M., and Weiss, S.R. (1997). Emergent properties of neural systems: How focal molecular neurobiological alterations can affect behavior. *Dev Psychopathol*, 9, 907–929.

Post, R.M., Kotin, J., and Goodwin, F.K. (1976). Effect of sleep deprivation on mood and central amine metabolism in depressed patients. *Arch Gen Psychiatry*, 33, 627–632.

Post, R.M., Cramer, H., and Goodwin, F.K. (1977). Cyclic AMP in cerebrospinal fluid of manic and depressive patients. *Psychol Med*, 7, 599–605.

Post, R.M., Gerner, R.H., Carman, J.S., Gillin, J.C., Jimerson, D.C., Goodwin, F.K., and Bunney, W.E. Jr. (1978). Effects of a dopamine agonist piribedil in depressed patients: Relationship of pretreatment homovanillic acid to antidepressant response. *Arch Gen Psychiatry*, 35, 609–615.

Post, R.M., Ballenger, J.C., Hare, T.A., and Bunney, W.E. Jr. (1980a). Lack of effect of carbamazepine on gamma-aminobutyric acid in cerebrospinal fluid. *Neurology* 30, 1008–1011.

Post, R.M., Jimerson, D.C., Bunney, W.E., Jr., and Goodwin, F.K. (1980b). Dopamine and mania: Behavioral and biochemical effects of the dopamine receptor blocker pimozide. *Psychopharmacology (Berl)*, 67, 297–305.

Post, R.M., Lockfeld, A., Squillace, K.M., and Contel, N.R. (1981). Drug–environment interaction: Context dependency of cocaine-induced behavioral sensitization. *Life Sci*, 28(7), 755–760.

Post, R.M., Contel, N.R., and Gold, P. (1982a). Impaired behavioral sensitization to cocaine in vasopressin-deficient rats. *Life Sci*, 31(24), 2745–2750.

Post, R.M., Ballenger, J.C., Uhde, T.W., Smith, C., Rubinow, D.R., and Bunney, W.E. (1982b). Effect of carbamazepine on cyclic nucleotides in CSF of patients with affective illness. *Biol Psychiatry*, 17, 1037–1045.

Post, R.M., Jimerson, D.C., Ballenger, J.C., Lake, C.R., Uhde, T.W., and Goodwin, F.K. (1984a). Cerebrospinal fluid norepinephrine and its metabolites in manic-depressive illness. In R.M. Post and J.C. Ballenger (Eds.), *Neurobiology of Mood Disorders* (pp. 539–553). Baltimore: Williams & Wilkins.

Post, R.M., Putnam, F., Contel, N.R., and Goldman, B. (1984b). Electroconvulsive seizures inhibit amygdala kindling: Implications for mechanisms of action in affective illness. *Epilepsia*, 25, 234–239.

Post, R.M., Rubinow, D.R., and Ballenger, J.C. (1984c). Conditioning, sensitization, and kindling: Implications for the course of affective illness. In R.M. Post and J.C. Ballenger (Eds.), *The Neurobiology of Mood Disorders* (pp. 432–466). Baltimore: Williams & Wilkins.

Post, R.M., Uhde, T.W., and Ballenger, J.C. (1984d). The efficacy of carbamazepine in affective illness. *Adv Biochem Psychopharmacol*, 39, 421–437.

Post, R.M., Weiss, S.R., and Pert, A. (1984e). Differential effects of carbamazepine and lithium on sensitization and kindling. *Prog Neuropsychopharmacol Biol Psychiatry*, 8, 425–434.

Post, R.M., Rubinow, D.R., Uhde, T.W., Ballenger, J.C., Lake, C.R., Linnoila, M., Jimerson, D.C., and Reus, V. (1985). Effects of carbamazepine on noradrenergic mechanisms in affectively ill patients. *Psychopharmacology (Berl)*, 87, 59–63.

Post, R.M., Uhde, T.W., Rubinow, D.R., and Huggins, T. (1987). Differential time course of antidepressant effects after sleep deprivation, ECT, and carbamazepine: Clinical and theoretical implications. *Psychiatry Res*, 22, 11–19.

Post, R.M., Rubinow, D.R., Uhde, T.W., Roy-Byrne, P.P., Linnoila, M., Rosoff, A., and Cowdry, R. (1989). Dysphoric mania. Clinical and biological correlates. *Arch Gen Psychiatry*, 46(4), 353–358.

Post, R.M., Ketter, T.A., Joffe, R.T., and Kramlinger, K.L. (1991). Lack of beneficial effects of l-baclofen in affective disorder. *Int Clin Psychopharmacol*, 6(4), 197–207.

Post, R.M., Weiss, S.R., Smith, M., Rosen, J., and Frye, M. (1995). Stress, conditioning, and the temporal aspects of affective disorders. *Ann N Y Acad Sci*, 771, 677–696.

Post, R.M., Kramlinger, K.G., Joffe, R.T., Roy-Byrne, P.P., Rosoff, A., Frye, M.A., and Huggins, T. (1997). Rapid cycling bipolar affective disorder: Lack of relation to hypothyroidism. *Psychiatry Res*, 72(1), 1–7.

Post, R.M., Weiss, S.R., Li, H., Smith, M.A., Zhang, L.X., Xing, G., Osuch, E.A., and McCann, U.D. (1998). Neural plasticity and emotional memory. *Dev Psychopathol*, 10, 829–855.

Potter, W.Z., and Linnoila, M. (1989). Biochemical classifications of diagnostic subgroups and D-type scores. *Arch Gen Psychiatry*, 46(3), 269–271.

Potter, W.Z., and Manji, H.K. (1994). Catecholamines in depression: An update. *Clin Chem*, 40(2), 279–287.

Potter, W.Z., Rudorfer, M.V., and Goodwin, F.K. (1987). Biological findings in bipolar disorders. In D. Francis (Ed.), *American Psychiatric Association Annual Review* (Vol. 6) (pp. 32–60). Washington, DC: American Psychiatric Press.

Prange, A.J., Jr., Lara, P.P., Wilson, I.C., Alltop, L.B., and Breese, G.R. (1972). Effects of thyrotropin-releasing hormone in depression. *Lancet*, 2, 999–1002.

Prange, A.J.W., Lara, P.P., and Alltop, P.P. (1974). Effects of thyrotropin-releasing hormones in depression. In A.J. Prange (Ed.), *The Thyroid Axis, Drugs and Behavior* (pp. 135–145). New York: Raven Press.

Preisig, M., Bellivier, F., Fenton, B.T., Baud, P., Berney, A., Courtet, P., Hardy, P., Golaz, J., Leboyer, M., Mallet, J., Matthey, M.L., Mouthon, D., Neidhart, E., Nosten-Bertrand, M., Stadelmann-Dubuis, E., Guimon, J., Ferrero, F., Buresi, C., and Malafosse, A. (2000). Association between bipolar disorder and monoamine oxidase A gene polymorphisms: Results of a multicenter study. *Am J Psychiatry*, 157, 948–955.

Price, L.H., Charney, D.S., Rubin, A.L., and Heninger, G.R. (1986). Alpha 2-adrenergic receptor function in depression. The cortisol response to yohimbine. *Arch Gen Psychiatry*, 43, 849–858.

Price, L.H., Charney, D.S., Delgado, P.L., and Heninger, G.R. (1989). Lithium treatment and serotoninergic function. Neuroendocrine and behavioral responses to intravenous tryptophan in affective disorder. *Arch Gen Psychiatry*, 46, 13–19.

Price, L.H., Charney, D.S., Delgado, P.L., and Heninger, G.R. (1990). Lithium and serotonin function: Implications for the serotonin hypothesis of depression. *Psychopharmacology (Berl)*, 100, 3–12.

Price, L.H., Charney, D.S., Delgado, P.L., and Heninger, G.R. (1991). Serotonin function and depression: Neuroendocrine and mood responses to intravenous L-tryptophan in depressed patients and healthy comparison subjects. *Am J Psychiatry*, 148, 1518–1525.

Price, W.A., and DeMarzio, L. (1986). Premenstrual tension syndrome in rapid-cycling bipolar affective disorder. *J Clin Psychiatry*, 47, 415–417.

Purba, J.S., Hoogendijk, W.J., Hofman, M.A., and Swaab, D.F. (1996). Increased number of vasopressin- and oxytocin-expressing neurons in the paraventricular nucleus of the hypothalamus in depression. *Arch Gen Psychiatry*, 53, 137–143.

Purdy, R.E., Julien, R.M., Fairhurst, A.S., and Terry, M.D. (1977). Effect of carbamazepine on the in vitro uptake and release of norepinephrine in adrenergic nerves of rabbit aorta and in whole brain synaptosomes. *Epilepsia*, 18, 251–257.

Puzynski, S., Rode, A., and Zaluska, M. (1983). Studies on biogenic amine metabolizing enzymes (DBH, COMT, MAO) and pathogenesis of affective illness. I. Plasma dopamine-β-hydroxylase activity in endogenous depression. *Acta Psychiatr Scand*, 67, 89–95.

Quattrone, A., and Samanin, R. (1977). Decreased anticonvulsant activity of carbamazepine in 6-hydroxydopamine-treated rats. *Eur J Pharmacol*, 41, 336.

Quattrone, A., Crunelli, V., and Samanin, R. (1978). Seizure susceptibility and anticonvulsant activity of carbamazepine, diphenylhydantoin and phenobarbital in rats with selective depletions of brain monoamines. *Neuropharmacology*, 17, 643–647.

Quattrone, A., Annunziato, L., Aguglia, U., and Preziosi, P. (1981). Carbamazepine, phenytoin and phenobarbital do not influence brain catecholamine uptake, in vivo, in male rats. *Arch Int Pharmacodyn Ther*, 252, 180–185.

Quigley, H.A., Nickells, R.W., Kerrigan, L.A., Pease, M.E., Thibault, D.J., and Zack, D.J. (1995). Retinal ganglion cell death in experimental glaucoma and after axotomy occurs by apoptosis. *Invest Ophthalmol Vis Sci*, 36, 774–786.

Quintin, P., Benkelfat, C., Launay, J.M., Arnulf, I., Pointereau-Bellenger, A., Barbault, S., Alvarez, J.C., Varoquaux, O., Perez-Diaz, F., Jouvent, R., and Leboyer, M. (2001). Clinical and neurochemical effect of acute tryptophan depletion in unaffected relatives of patients with bipolar affective disorder. *Biol Psychiatry*, 50, 184–190.

Quiroz, J., Singh, J., Gould, T.D., Denicoff, K., Zarate, C., and Manji, H.K. (2004). Emerging experimental therapeutics for bipolar disorder: Clues from the molecular neurobiology of the disorder. *Mol Psychiatry*, 9, 756–776.

Raadsheer, F.C., Hoogendijk, W.J., Stam, F.C., Tilders, F.J., and Swaab, D.F. (1994). Increased numbers of corticotropin-releasing hormone expressing neurons in the hypothalamic paraventricular nucleus of depressed patients. *Neuroendocrinology*, 60(4), 436–444.

Racine, R. (1978). Kindling: The first decade. *Neurosurgery*, 3, 234–252.

Raeburn, P. (2004). *Acquainted with the Night: A Parent's Quest to Understand Depression and Bipolar Disorder in His Children.* New York: Broadway.

Rahman, S., Li, P.P., Young, L.T., Kofman, O., Kish, S.J., and Warsh, J.J. (1997). Reduced [3H]cyclic AMP binding in postmortem brain from subjects with bipolar affective disorder. *J Neurochem*, 68, 297–304.

Rajkowska, G. (1997). Morphometric methods for studying the prefrontal cortex in suicide victims and psychiatric patients. *Ann NY Acad Sci*, 836, 253–268.

Rajkowska, G. (2000). Postmortem studies in mood disorders indicate altered numbers of neurons and glial cells. *Biol Psychiatry*, 48, 766–777.

Rajkowska, G. (2002a). Cell pathology in bipolar disorder. *Bipolar Disord*, 4, 105–116.

Rajkowska, G. (2002b). Cell pathology in mood disorders. *Semin Clin Neuropsychiatry*, 7, 281–292.

Rajkowska, G., Miguel-Hidalgo, J.J., Wei, J., Dilley, G., Pittman, S.D., Meltzer, H.Y., Overholser, J.C., Roth, B.L., and Stockmeier, C.A. (1999). Morphometric evidence for neuronal and glial prefrontal cell pathology in major depression. *Biol Psychiatry*, 45, 1085–1098.

Rajkowska, G., Halaris, A., and Selemon, L.D. (2001). Reductions in neuronal and glial density characterize the dorsolateral prefrontal cortex in bipolar disorder. *Biol Psychiatry*, 49(9), 741–752.

Rajkowska, G., Stockmeier, C.A., Mahajan, G.J., and Konick, L.C. (2004). Cellular changes in the postmortem hippocampus in major depression. *Biol Psychiatry*, 56(9), 640–650.

Ram, A., Guedj, F., Cravchik, A., Weinstein, L., Cao, Q., Badner, J.A., Goldin, L.R., Grisaru, N., Manji, H.K., Belmaker, R.H., Gershon, E.S., and Gejman, P.V. (1997). No abnormality in the gene for the G protein stimulatory alpha subunit in patients with bipolar disorder. *Arch Gen Psychiatry*, 54, 44–48.

Ramsey, T.A., Frazer, A., Mendels, J., and Dyson, W.L. (1979). The erythrocyte lithium-plasma lithium ratio in patients with primary affective disorder. *Arch Gen Psychiatry*, 36, 457–461.

Rana, R.S., and Hokin, L.E. (1990). Role of phosphoinositides in transmembrane signaling. *Physiol Rev*, 70, 115–164.

Rasenick, M.M., Chen, J., and Ozawa, H. (2000). Effects of antidepressant treatments on the G protein–adenylyl cyclase axis as the possible basis of therapeutic action. In R.H. Belmaker

(Ed.), *Bipolar Medications: Mechanisms of Action* (1st Edition) (pp. 87–108). Washington, DC: American Psychiatric Press.

Rasmusson, A.M., Southwick, S.M., Hauger, R.L., and Charney, D.S. (1998). Plasma neuropeptide Y (NPY) increases in humans in response to the alpha 2 antagonist yohimbine. *Neuropsychopharmacology*, 19(1), 95–98.

Rausch, J.L., Janowsky, D.S., Risch, S.C., and Huey, L.Y. (1986). A kinetic analysis and replication of decreased platelet serotonin uptake in depressed patients. *Psychiatry Res*, 19, 105–112.

Rebas, E., Lachowicz, A., and Lachowicz, L. (1995). Estradiol and pregnenolone sulfate could modulate PMA-stimulated and Ca2+/calmodulin-dependent synaptosomal membrane protein phosphorylation from rat brain in vivo. *Biochem Biophys Res Commun*, 207, 606–612.

Reddy, P.L., Khanna, S., Subhash, M.N., Channabasavanna, S.M., and Rao, B.S. (1989). Erythrocyte membrane Na-K ATPase activity in affective disorder. *Biol Psychiatry*, 26, 533–537.

Reddy, P.L., Khanna, S., Subhash, M.N., Channabasavanna, S.M., and Rao, B.S. (1992). Erythrocyte membrane sodium-potassium adenosine triphosphatase activity in affective disorders. *J Neural Transm [Gen Sect]*, 89, 209–218.

Redei, E., Organ, M., and Hart, S. (1999). Antidepressant-like properties of prepro-TRH 178–199: Acute effects in the forced swim test. *Neuroreport*, 10, 3273–3276.

Redmond, D.E. Jr., Katz, M.M., Maas, J.W., Swann, A., Casper, R., and Davis, J.M. (1986). Cerebrospinal fluid amine metabolites. Relationships with behavioral measurements in depressed, manic, and healthy control subjects. *Arch Gen Psychiatry*, 43, 938–947.

Rees, M., Norton, N., Jones, I., McCandless, F., Scourfield, J., Holmans, P., Moorhead, S., Feldman, E., Sadler, S., Cole, T., Redman, K., Farmer, A., McGuffin, P., Owen, M.J., and Craddock, N. (1997). Association studies of bipolar disorder at the human serotonin transporter gene (hSERT; 5HTT). *Mol Psychiatry*, 2, 398–402.

Reiach, J.S., Li, P.P., Warsh, J.J., Kish, S.J., and Young, L.T. (1999). Reduced adenylyl cyclase immunolabeling and activity in postmortem temporal cortex of depressed suicide victims. *J Affect Disord*, 56(23), 141–151.

Reich, T., and Winokur, G. (1970). Postpartum psychoses in patients with manic depressive disease. *J Nerv Ment Dis*, 151, 60–68.

Reisine, T.D. (1984). Cellular mechanisms regulating adrenocorticotropin release. *J Recept Res*, 4, 291–300.

Ren, M., Senatorov, V.V., Chen, R.W., and Chuang, D.M. (2003). Postinsult treatment with lithium reduces brain damage and facilitates neurological recovery in a rat ischemia/reperfusion model. *Proc Natl Acad Sci USA*, 100(10), 6210–6215.

Ren, M., Leng, Y., Jeong, M., Leeds, P.R., and Chuang, D.M. (2004). Valproic acid reduces brain damage induced by transient focal cerebral ischemia in rats: Potential roles of histone deacetylase inhibition and heat shock protein induction. *J Neurochem*, 89(6), 1358–1367.

Renshaw, P.F., and Cohen, B.M. (1993). Functional brain imaging in the elderly. *J Nucl Med*, 34, 1101–1102.

Reppert, S.M., and Weaver, D.R. (2001). Molecular analysis of mammalian circadian rhythms. *Annu Rev Physiol*, 63, 647–676.

Reul, J.M., and Holsboer, F. (2002). Corticotropin-releasing factor receptors 1 and 2 in anxiety and depression. *Curr Opin Pharmacol*, 2, 23–33.

Reus, V.I., Joseph, M., and Dallman, M. (1983). Regulation of ACTH and cortisol in depression. *Peptides*, 4, 785–788.

Reynolds, G.P., Beasley, C.L., and Zhang, Z.J. (2002). Understanding the neurotransmitter pathology of schizophrenia: Selective deficits of subtypes of cortical GABAergic neurons. *J Neural Transm*, 109, 881–889.

Reynolds, J.N., and Wickens, J.R. (2000). Substantia nigra dopamine regulates synaptic plasticity and membrane potential fluctuations in the rat neostriatum, in vivo. *Neuroscience*, 99(2), 199–203.

Richelson, E. (1977). Lithium ion entry through the sodium channel of cultured mouse neuroblastoma cells: A biochemical study. *Science*, 196, 1001–1002.

Richelson, E., Snyder, K., Carlson, J., Johnson, M., Turner, S., Lumry, A., Boerwinkle, E., and Sing, C.F. (1986). Lithium ion transport by erythrocytes of randomly selected blood donors and manic-depressive patients: Lack of association with affective illness. *Am J Psychiatry*, 143, 457–462.

Riddell, F.G., Patel, A., and Hughes, M.S. (1990). Lithium uptake rate and lithium: Lithium exchange rate in human erythrocytes at a nearly pharmacologically normal level monitored by 7Li NMR. *J Inorg Biochem*, 39(3), 187–192.

Rihmer, Z., Bagdy, G., and Arato, M. (1983). Serum dopamine-beta-hydroxylase activity and family history of patients with bipolar manic-depressive illness. *Acta Psychiatr Scand*, 68, 140–141.

Rimon, R., Terenius, L., Averbuch, I., and Belmaker, R.H. (1983). High-dose haloperidol increases CSF opioid activity in patients with chronic schizophrenia. *Pharmacopsychiatria*, 16, 9–12.

Rimon, R., Le Greves, P., Nyberg, F., Heikkila, L., Salmela, L., and Terenius, L. (1984). Elevation of substance P–like peptides in the CSF of psychiatric patients. *Biol Psychiatry*, 19(4), 509–516.

Risby, E.D., Hsiao, J.K., Manji, H.K., Bitran, J., Moses, F., Zhou, D.F., and Potter, W.Z. (1991). The mechanisms of action of lithium. II. Effects on adenylate cyclase activity and beta-adrenergic receptor binding in normal subjects. *Arch Gen Psychiatry*, 48, 513–524.

Risch, S.C., Cohen, R.M., Janowsky, D.S., Kalin, N.H., and Murphy, D.L. (1980). Mood and behavioral effects of physostigmine on humans are accompanied by elevations in plasma beta-endorphin and cortisol. *Science*, 209, 1545–1546.

Risch, S.C., Cohen, R.M., Janowsky, D.S., Kalin, N.H., Sitaram, N., Gillin, J.C., and Murphy, D.L. (1981). Physostigmine induction of depressive symptomatology in normal human subjects. *Psychiatry Res*, 4, 89–94.

Risch, S.C., Janowsky, D.S., and Gillin, J.C. (1983). Muscarinic supersensitivity of anterior pituitary ACTH and β-endorphin release in major depressive illness. *Peptides*, 4, 789–792.

Ritchie, E.A. (1956). Toxic psychosis under cortisone and corticotrophin. *J Ment Sci*, 102(429), 830–837.

Ritchie, J.M., and Straub, R.W. (1980). Observations on the mechanism for the active extrusion of lithium in mammalian non-myelinated nerve fibres. *J Physiol*, 304, 123–134.

Rizzo, N.D., Fox, H.M., Laidlaw, J.C., and Thorn, G.W. (1954). Concurrent observations of behavior changes and of adrenocortical variations in a cyclothymic patient during a period of 12 months. *Ann Intern Med*, 41, 798–815.

Robbins, T.W., and Sahakian, B.J. (1980). Animal models of mania. In R.H. Belmaker (Ed.), *Mania, an Evolving Concept* (pp. 143–216). Jamaica: MTP Press/Spectrum Publications.

Robinson, P.J. (1991). The role of protein kinase C and its neuronal substrates dephosphin, B-50, and MARCKS in neurotransmitter release. *Mol Neurobiol*, 5(2-4), 87–130.

Robinson, T.E., and Becker, J.B. (1986). Enduring changes in brain and behavior produced by chronic amphetamine administration: A review and evaluation of animal models of amphetamine psychosis. *Brain Res*, 396, 157–198.

Rochet, T., Tonon, M.C., Kopp, N., Vaudry, H., and Miachon, S. (1998). Evaluation of endozepine-like immuoreactivity in the frontal cortex of suicide victims. *Neuroreport*, 9, 53–56.

Ronai, A.Z., and Vizi, S.E. (1975). The effect of lithium treatment on the acetylcholine content of rat brain. *Biochem Pharmacol*, 24, 1819–1820.

Rose, A.M., Mellett, B.J., Valdes, R. Jr., Kleinman, J.E., Herman, M.M., Li, R., and el-Mallakh, R.S. (1998). Alpha 2 isoform of the Na,K-adenosine triphosphatase is reduced in temporal cortex of bipolar individuals. *Biol Psychiatry*, 44, 892–897.

Rosel, P., Arranz, B., Vallejo, J., Oros, M., Menchon, J.M., Alvarez, P., and Navarro, M.A. (1997). High affinity [3H]imipramine and [3H]paroxetine binding sites in suicide brains. *J Neural Transm*, 104, 921–929.

Rosel, P., Arranz, B., Vallejo, J., Oros, M., Crespo, J.M., Menchon, J.M., and Navarro, M.A. (1998). Variations in [3H]imipramine and 5-HT2A but not [3H]paroxetine binding sites in suicide brains. *Psychiatry Res Neuroimaging Sect*, 82, 161–170.

Rosenblatt, J.E., Pert, C.B., Tallman, J.F., Pert, A., and Bunney, W.E. Jr. (1979). The effect of imipramine and lithium on alpha- and beta-receptor binding in rat brain. *Brain Res*, 160, 186–191.

Rosenblatt, J.E., Pert, A., Layton, B., and Bunney, W.E. Jr. (1980). Chronic lithium reduces [3H]spiroperidol binding in rat striatum. *Eur J Pharmacol*, 67, 321–322.

Rothman, S.M. (1999). Mutations of the mitochondrial genome: Clinical overview and possible pathophysiology of cell damage. *Biochem Soc Symp*, 66, 111–122.

Rothschild, A.J., Schatzberg, A.F., Rosenbaum, A.H., Stahl, J.B., and Cole, J.O. (1982). The dexamethasone suppression test as a discriminator among subtypes of psychotic patients. *Br J Psychiatry*, 141, 471–474.

Rotondo, A., Mazzanti, C., Dell'Osso, L., Rucci, P., Sullivan, P., Bouanani, S., Gonnelli, C., Goldman, D., and Cassano, G.B. (2002). Catechol O-methyltransferase, serotonin transporter, and tryptophan hydroxylase gene polymorphisms in bipolar disorder patients with and without comorbid panic disorder. *Am J Psychiatry*, 159(1), 23–29.

Rousseva, A., Henry, C., van den Bulke, D., Fournier, G., Laplanche, J.L., Leboyer, M., Bellivier, F., Aubry, J.M., Baud, P., Boucherie, M., Buresi, C., Ferrero, F., and Malafosse, A. (2003). Antidepressant-induced mania, rapid cycling and the serotonin transporter gene polymorphism. *Pharmacogenomics J*, 3(2), 101–104.

Rowntree, D.W., Neven, S., and Wilson, A. (1950). The effect of diisopropylflurophosphonate in schizophrenia and manic depressive psychosis. *J Neurol Neuroserg Psychiatry*, 47–62.

Roy, A., Pickar, D., Linnoila, M., and Potter, W.Z. (1985). Plasma norepinephrine level in affective disorders. Relationship to melancholia. *Arch Gen Psychiatry*, 42, 1181–1185.

Roy, A., Jimerson, D.C., and Pickar, D. (1986). Plasma MHPG in depressive disorders and relationship to the dexamethasone suppression test. *Am J Psychiatry*, 143, 846–851.

Roy, A., Everett, D., Pickar, D., Paul, S.M. (1987a). Platelet tritiated imipramine binding and serotonin uptake in depressed patients and controls. *Arch Gen Psychiatry*, 44, 320–327.

Roy, A., Guthrie, S., Pickar, D., and Linnoila, M. (1987b). Plasma norepinephrine responses to cold challenge in depressed patients and normal controls. *Psychiatry Res*, 21, 161–168.

Roy, A., Pickar, D., Paul, S., Doran, A., Chrousos, G.P., and Gold, P.W. (1987c). CSF corticotrophin-releasing hormone in depressed patients and normal control subjects. *Am J Psychiatry*, 144, 641–645.

Roy, A., Guthrie, S., Karoum, F., Pickar, D., and Linnoila, M. (1988). High intercorrelations among urinary outputs of norepinephrine and its major metabolites. A replication in depressed patients and controls. *Arch Gen Psychiatry*, 45(2), 158–161.

Roy, A., Wolkowitz, O.M., Bissette, G., and Nemeroff, C.B. (1994). Differences in CSF concentrations of thyrotropin-releasing hormone in depressed patients and normal subjects: Negative findings. *Am J Psychiatry*, 151, 600–602.

Rubin, A.L., Price, L.H., Charney, D.S., and Heninger, G.R. (1985). Noradrenergic function and the cortisol response to dexamethasone in depression. *Psychiatry Res*, 15, 5–15.

Rubin, R.T., O'Toole, S.M., Rhodes, M.E., Sekula, L.K., and Czambel, R.K. (1999). Hypothalamo–pituitary–adrenal cortical responses to low-dose physostigmine and arginine vasopressin administration: Sex differences between major depressives and matched control subjects. *Psychiatry Res*, 89, 1–20.

Rubinow, D.R. (1986). Cerebrospinal fluid somatostatin and psychiatric illness. *Biol Psychiatry*, 21, 341–365.

Rubinow, D.R., Gold, P.W., Post, R.M., Ballenger, J.C., Cowdry, R., Bollinger, J., and Reichlin, S. (1983). CSF somatostatin in affective illness. *Arch Gen Psychiatry*, 40, 409–412.

Rubinow, D.R., Post, R.M., Savard, R., and Gold, P.W. (1984). Cortisol hypersecretion and cognitive impairment in depression. *Arch Gen Psychiatry*, 41, 279–283.

Rudorfer, M.V., Golden, R.N., and Potter, W.Z. (1984). Second-generation antidepressants. *Psychiatr Clin North Am*, 7, 519–534.

Rudorfer, M.V., Ross, R.J., Linnoila, M., Sherer, M.A., and Potter, W.Z. (1985). Exaggerated orthostatic responsivity of plasma norepinephrine in depression. *Arch Gen Psychiatry*, 42, 1186–1192.

Rudorfer, M.V., Sherer, M.A., Lane, E.A., Golden, R.N., Linnoila, M., and Potter, W.Z. (1991). Acute noradrenergic effects of desipramine in depression. *J Clin Psychopharmacol*, 11, 22–27.

Rush, A.J., Giles, D.E., Schlesser, M.A., Orsulak, P.J., Parker, C.R. Jr., Weissenburger, J.E., Crowley, G.T., Khatami, M., and Vasavada, N. (1996). The dexamethasone suppression test in patients with mood disorders. *J Clin Psychiatry*, 57(10), 470–484.

Rush, A.J., Giles, D.E., Schlesser, M.A., Orsulak, P.J., Weissenburger, J.E., Fulton, C.L., Fairchild, C.J., and Roffwarg, H.P. (1997). Dexamethasone response, thyrotropin-releasing hormone stimulation, rapid eye movement latency, and subtypes of depression. *Biol Psychiatry*, 41, 915–928.

Russell, R.W., Pechnick, R., and Jope, R.S. (1981). Effects of lithium on behavioral reactivity: Relation to increases in brain cholinergic activity. *Psychopharmacology (Berl)*, 73, 120–125.

Ryabinin, A.E., Sato, T.N., Morris, P.J., Latchman, D.S., and Wilson, M.C. (1995). Immediate upstream promoter regions required for neurospecific expression of SNAP-25. *J Mol Neurosci*, 6, 201–210.

Ryan, W.G., Richards, J.M., and Lee, J.Y. (1989). Characteristics of the in vivo RBC: Plasma lithium ratio in a clinical setting. *Biol Psychiatry*, 26(5), 537–540.

Rybakowski, J.K., and Twardowska, K. (1999). The dexamethasone/corticotropin-releasing hormone test in depression in bipolar and unipolar affective illness. *J Psychiatr Res*, 33, 363–370.

Rybakowski, J., Chlopocka, M., Kapelski, Z., Hernacka, B., Szajnerman, Z., and Kasprzak, K. (1974). Red blood cell lithium index in patients with affective disorders in the course of lithium prophylaxis. *Int Pharmacopsychiatry*, 9(3), 166–171.

Rybakowski, J., Frazer, A., Mendels, J., and Ramsey, T.A. (1978). Erythrocyte accumulation of the lithium ion in control subjects and patients with primary affective disorder. *Commun Psychopharmacol*, 2(2), 99–104.

Rybakowski, J., Potok, E., and Strzyzewski, W. (1981). Erythrocyte membrane adenosine triphosphatase activities in patients with endogenous depression and healthy subject. *Eur J Clin Invest*, 11, 61–64.

Rybakowski, J.K., Borkowska, A., Czerski, P.M., Skibinska, M., and Hauser, J. (2003). Polymorphism of the brain-derived neurotrophic factor gene and performance on a cognitive prefrontal test in bipolar patients. *Bipolar Disord*, 5(6), 468–472.

Ryves, W.J., and Harwood, A.J. (2001). Lithium inhibits glycogen synthase kinase-3 by competition for magnesium. *Biochem Biophys Res Commun*, 80, 720–725.

Sachar, E.J., Hellman, L., Roffwarg, H.P., Halpern, F.S., Fukushima, D.K., and Gallagher, T.F. (1973). Disrupted 24-hour patterns of cortisol secretion in psychotic depression. *Arch Gen Psychiatry*, 28, 19–24.

Sack, D.A., Duncan, W., Rosenthal, N.E., Mendelson, W.E., and Wehr, T.A. (1988). The timing and duration of sleep in partial sleep deprivation therapy of depression. *Acta Psychiatr Scand*, 77, 219–224.

Sahin-Erdemli, I., Medford, R.M., and Songu-Mize, E. (1995). Regulation of Na+,K(+)-ATPase alpha-subunit isoforms in rat tissues during hypertension. *Eur J Pharmacol*, 292, 163–171.

Saito, T., Parsia, S., Papolos, D.F., and Lachman, H.M. (2000). Analysis of the pseudoautosomal X-linked gene *SYBL1* in bipolar affective disorder: Description of a new candidate allele for psychiatric disorders. *Am J Med Genet*, 96, 317–323.

Saito, T., Guan, F., Papolos, D.F., Lau, S., Klein, M., Fann, C.S., and Lachman, H.M. (2001a). Mutation analysis of *SYNJ1*: A possible candidate gene for chromosome 21q22-linked bipolar disorder. *Mol Psychiatry*, 6, 387–395.

Saito, T., Guan, F., Papolos, D.F., Rajouria, N., Fann, C.S., and Lachman, H.M. (2001b). Polymorphism in SNAP29 gene promoter region associated with schizophrenia. *Mol Psychiatry*, 6, 193–201.

Sanacora, G., Mason, G.F., Rothman, D.L., Behar, K.L., Hyder, F., Petroff, O.A., Berman, R.M., Charney, D.S., and Krystal, J.H. (1999). Reduced cortical gamma-aminobutyric acid levels in depressed patients determined by proton magnetic resonance spectroscopy. *Arch Gen Psychiatry*, 56, 1043–1047.

Sanacora, G., Gueorguieva, R., Epperson, C.N., Wu, Y.T., Appel, M., Rothman, D.L., Krystal, J.H., and Mason, G.F. (2004). Subtype-specific alterations of gamma-aminobutyric acid and glutamate in patients with major depression. *Arch Gen Psychiatry*, 61(7), 705–713.

Sanchez, M.M., Young, L.J., Plotsky, P.M., and Insel, T.R. (2000). Distribution of corticosteroid receptors in the rhesus brain: Relative absence of glucocorticoid receptors in the hippocampal formation. *J Neurosci*, 20, 4657–4668.

Sanchez, R.S., Murthy, G.G., Mehta, J., Shreeve, W.W., and Singh, F.R. (1976). Pituitary–testicular axis in patients on lithium therapy. *Fertil Steril*, 27, 667–669.

Sands, S.A., Guerra, V., and Morilak, D.A. (2000). Changes in tyrosine hydroxylase mRNA expression in the rat locus coeruleus following acute or chronic treatment with valproic acid. *Neuropsychopharmacology*, 22(1), 27–35.

Santarelli, L., Saxe, M., and Gross, C. (2003). Requirement of hippocampal neurogenesis for the behavioral effects of antidepressants. *Science*, 301(5634), 805–809.

Sapolsky, R.M. (1996). Stress, glucocorticoids, and damage to the nervous system: The current state of confusion. *Stress*, 1, 1–19.

Sapolsky, R.M. (2000a). The possibility of neurotoxicity in the hippocampus in major depression: A primer on neuron death. *Biol Psychiatry*, 48, 755–765.

Sapolsky, R.M. (2000b). Glucocorticoids and hippocampal atrophy in neuropsychiatric disorders. *Arch Gen Psychiatry*, 57, 925–935.

Sapolsky, R.M., Romero, L.M., and Munck, A.U. (2000). How do glucocorticoids influence stress responses? Integrating permissive, suppressive, stimulatory, and preparative actions. *Endocr Rev*, 21, 55–89.

Sarai, M., Taniguchi, N., Kagomoto, T., Kameda, H., Uema, T., and Hishikawa, Y. (1982). Major depressive episode and low dose dexamethasone suppression test. *Folia Psychiatr Neurol Jpn*, 36(2), 109–114.

Sargent, P.A., Kjaer, K.H., Bench, C.J., Rabiner, E.A., Messa, C., Meyer, J., Gunn, R.N., Grasby, P.M., and Cowen, P.J. (2000). Brain serotonin1A receptor binding measured by positron emission tomography with [11C]WAY-100635: Effects of depression and antidepressant treatment. *Arch Gen Psychiatry*, 57, 174–180.

Sarkadi, B., Alifimoff, J.K., Gunn, R.B., and Tosteson, D.C. (1978). Kinetics and stoichiometry of Na-dependent Li transport in human red blood cells. *J Gen Physiol*, 72, 249–265.

Sastre, M., and García-Sevilla, J.A. (1997). Densities of I2-imidazoline receptors, α2-adrenoceptors and monoamine oxidase B in brains of suicide victims. *Neurochem Int*, 30, 63–72.

Sastre, M., Escriba, P.V., Reis, D.J., and Garcia-Sevilla, J.A. (1995). Decreased number and immunoreactivity of I2-imidazoline receptors in the frontal cortex of suicide victims. *Ann NY Acad Sci*, 763, 520–522.

Sattin, A. (1999). The role of TRH and related peptides in the mechanism of action of ECT. *J ECT*, 15, 76–92.

Saunders, J., and Williams, J. (2003). Antagonists of the corticotropin releasing factor receptor. *Prog Med Chem*, 41, 195–247.

Sawaya, M.C., Horton, R.W., and Meldrum, B.S. (1975). Effects of anticonvulsant drugs on the cerebral enzymes metabolizing GABA. *Epilepsia*, 16, 649–655.

Scappa, S., Teverbaugh, P., and Ananth, J. (1993). Episodic tardive dyskinesia and parkinsonism in bipolar disorder patients. *Can J Psychiatry*, 38, 633–634.

Schaefer, E., Leimer, I., Haeselbarth, V., and Meier, D. (1996). Tolerability of pramipexole in patients hospitalized for major depressive disorder: An open-label study to assess the maximum tolerated dose of pramipexole with repeated dosing. Clinical Report No. U96-0084, February 5, 1996.

Schatzberg, A.F., and Schildkraut, J.J. (1995). Recent studies on norepinephrine systems in mood disorders. In D.J. Kupfer (Ed.), *Psychopharmacology: The Fourth Generation of Progress* (pp. 957–969). New York: Raven Press.

Schatzberg, A.F., Orsulak, P.J., Rosenbaum, A.H., Maruta, T., Kruger, E.R., Cole, J.O., and Schildkraut, J.J. (1982). Toward a biochemical classification of depressive disorders: V. Heterogeneity of unipolar depressions. *Am J Psychiatry*, 139, 471–475.

Schatzberg, A.F., Samson, J.A., Bloomingdale, K.L., Orsulak, P.J., Gerson, B., Kizuka, P.P., Cole, J.O., and Schildkraut, J.J. (1989). Toward a biochemical classification of depressive disorders. X. Urinary catecholamines, their metabolites, and D-type scores in subgroups of depressive disorders. *Arch Gen Psychiatry*, 46, 260–268.

Schildkraut, J.J. (1965). The catecholamine hypothesis of affective disorders: A review of supporting evidence. *Am J Psychiatry*, 122, 509–522.

Schildkraut, J.J. (1973). Norepinephrine metabolites as biochemical criteria for classifying depressive disorders and predicting responses to treatment: Preliminary findings. *Am J Psychiatry*, 130, 695–699.

Schildkraut, J.J. (1974). The effects of lithium on norepinephrine turnover and metabolism: Basic and clinical studies. *J Nerv Ment Dis*, 158, 348–360.

Schildkraut, J.J., Schanberg, S.M., and Kopin, I.J. (1966). The effects of lithium ion on H3-norepinephrine metabolism in brain. *Life Sci*, 5, 1479–1483.

Schildkraut, J.J., Logue, M.A., and Dodge, G.A. (1969). The effects of lithium salts on the turnover and metabolism of norepinephrine in rat brain. *Psychopharmacologia*, 14, 135–141.

Schildkraut, J.J., Keeler, B.A., Grab, E.L., Kantrowich, J., and Hartmann, E. (1973). M.H.P.G. excretion and clinical classification in depressive disorders. *Lancet*, 1, 1251–1252.

Schmider, J., Lammers, C.H., Gotthardt, U., Dettling, M., Holsboer, F., and Heuser, I.J. (1995). Combined dexamethasone/corticotropin-releasing hormone test in acute and remitted manic patients, in acute depression, and in normal controls: I. *Biol Psychiatry*, 38, 797–802.

Schmidt, P.J., Daly, R.C., Bloch, M., Smith, M.J., Danaceau, M.A., St Clair, L.S., Murphy, J.H., Haq, N., and Rubinow, D.R. (2005). Dehydroepiandrosterone monotherapy in midlife-onset major and minor depression. *Arch Gen Psychiatry*, 62(2), 154–162.

Schoch, S., Deak, F., Konigstorfer, A., Mozhayeva, M., Sara, Y., Sudhof, T.C., and Kavalali, E.T. (2001). SNARE function analyzed in synaptobrevin/VAMP knockout mice. *Science*, 294(5544), 1117–1122.

Schreiber, G., Avissar, S., Danon, A., and Belmaker, R.H. (1991). Hyperfunctional G proteins in mononuclear leukocytes of patients with mania. *Biol Psychiatry*, 29(3), 273–280.

Schreiber, S., and Lerer, B. (1997). "Failure to thrive" in elderly depressed patients: A new concept or a different name for an old problem? *Isr J Psychiatry Relat Sci*, 34(2), 108–114.

Schultz, J.E., Siggins, G.R., Schocker, F.W., Turck, M., and Bloom, F.E. (1981). Effects of prolonged treatment with lithium and tricyclic antidepressants on discharge frequency, norepinephrine responses and beta receptor binding in rat cerebellum: Electrophysiological and biochemical comparison. *J Pharmacol Exp Ther*, 216, 28–38.

Scott, M., and Reading, H.W. (1978). A comparison of platelet membrane and erythrocyte membrane adenosine triphosphatase-specific activities in affective disorders. *Biochem Soc Trans*, 6, 642–644.

Scott, M., Reading, H.W., and Loudon, J.B. (1979). Studies on human blood platelets in affective disorder. *Psychopharmacology (Berl)*, 60, 131–135.

Segal, D.S., Callaghan, M., and Mandell, A.J. (1975). Alterations in behaviour and catecholamine biosynthesis induced by lithium. *Nature*, 254, 58–59.

Seligman, M.E., and Maier, S.F. (1967). Failure to escape traumatic shock. *J Exp Psychol*, 74, 1–9.

Senatorov, V.V., Ren, M., Kanai, H., Wei, H., and Chunag, D.M. (2004). Short-term lithium treatment promotes neuronal survival and proliferation in rat striatum infused with quinolinic acid, and excitotoxic model of Huntington's disease. *Mol Psychiatry*, 9, 371–385.

Sengupta, N., Datta, S.C., Sengupta, D., and Bal, S. (1980). Platelet and erythrocyte-membrane adenosine triphosphatase activity in depressive and manic-depressive illness. *Psychiatry Res*, 3, 337–344.

Serretti, A., Macciardi, F., Verga, M., Cusin, C., Pedrini, S., and Smeraldi, E. (1998). Tyrosine hydroxylase gene associated with depressive symptomatology in mood disorder. *Am J Med Genet*, 81, 127–130.

Serretti, A., Lattuada, E., Lorenzi, C., Lilli, R., and Smeraldi, E. (2000). Dopamine receptor D2 Ser/Cys 311 variant is associated with delusion and disorganization symptomatology in major psychoses. *Mol Psychiatry*, 5, 270–274.

Serretti, A., Lilli, R., Lorenzi, C., Lattuada, E., Cusin, C., and Smeraldi, E. (2001). Tryptophan hydroxylase gene and major psychoses. *Psychiatry Res*, 103, 79–86.

Seymour, P.A., Schmidt, A.W., and Schulz, D.W. (2003). The pharmacology of CP-154,526, a non-peptide antagonist of the CRH1 receptor: A review. *CNS Drug Rev*, 9(1), 57–96.

Shah, P.J., Ogilvie, A.D., Goodwin, G.M., and Ebmeier, K.P. (1997). Clinical and psychometric correlates of dopamine D2 binding in depression. *Psychol Med*, 27, 1247–1256.

Shaldubina, A., Einat, H., Szechtman, H., Shimon, H., and Belmaker, R.H. (2002). Preliminary evaluation of oral anticonvulsant treatment in the quinpirole model of bipolar disorder. *J Neural Transm*, 109, 433–440.

Shapira, B., Cohen, J., Newman, M.E., and Lerer, B. (1993). Prolactin response to fenfluramine and placebo challenge following maintenance pharmacotherapy withdrawal in remitted depressed patients. *Biol Psychiatry*, 33, 531–535.

Sharfstein, S.S., Sack, D.S., and Fauci, A.S. (1982). Relationship between alternate-day corticosteroid therapy and behavioral abnormalities. *JAMA*, 248(22), 2987–2989.

Sharma, R., Venkatasubramanian, P.N., Barany, M., and Davis, J.M. (1992). Proton magnetic resonance spectroscopy of the brain in schizophrenic and affective patients. *Schizophr Res*, 8, 43–49.

Shaughnessy, R., Greene, S.C., Pandey, G.N., and Dorus, E. (1985). Red-cell lithium transport and affective disorders in a multigeneration pedigree: Evidence for genetic transmission of affective disorders. *Biol Psychiatry*, 20, 451–454.

Shaw, D.M., Camps, F.E., and Eccleston, E.G. (1967). 5-Hydroxytryptamine in the hind-brain of depressive suicides. *Br J Psychiatry*, 113, 1407–1411.

Sheffield, A. (1999). *How You Can Survive When They're Depressed: Living and Coping with Depression Fallout*. New York: HarperCollins.

Sheline, Y.I., Black, K.J., Bardgett, M.E., and Csernansky, J.G. (1995). Platelet binding characteristics distinguish placebo responders from nonresponders in depression. *Neuropsy-chopharmacology*, 12, 315–322.

Sheline, Y.I., Wang, P.W., Gado, M.H., Csernansky, J.G., and Vannier, M.W. (1996). Hippocampal atrophy in recurrent major depression. *Proc Natl Acad Sci USA*, 93(9), 3908–3913.

Sheline, Y.I., Gado, M.H., and Kraemer, H.C. (2003). Untreated depression and hippocampal volume loss. *Am J Psychiatry*, 160(8), 1516–1518.

Sherif, F., Marcusson, J., and Oreland, L. (1991). Brain gamma-aminobutyrate transaminase and monoamine oxidase activities in suicide victims. *Eur Arch Psychiatry Clin Neurosci*, 241, 139–144.

Sherman, W.R., Munsell, L.Y., Gish, B.G., and Honchar, M.P. (1985). Effects of systemically administered lithium on phosphoinositide metabolism in rat brain, kidney, and testis. *J Neurochem*, 44(3), 798–807.

Sherman, W.R., Gish, B.G., Honchar, M.P., and Munsell, L.Y. (1986). Effects of lithium on phosphoinositide metabolism in vivo. *Fed Proc*, 45(11), 2639–2646.

Shiah, I.S., and Yatham, L.N. (2000). Serotonin in mania and in the mechanism of action of mood stabilizers: A review of clinical studies. *Bipolar Disord*, 2, 77–92.

Shiah, I.S., Yatham, L.N., Lam, R.W., and Zis, A.P. (1997). Effects of divalproex sodium on 5-HT$_{1A}$ receptor function in healthy human males: Hypothermic, hormonal, and behavioral responses to ipsapirone. *Neuropsychopharmacology*, 17, 382–390.

Shibata, K., Morita, K., Kitayama, S., Okamoto, H., and Dohi, T. (1996). Ca2+ entry induced by calcium influx factor and its regulation by protein kinase C in rabbit neutrophils. *Biochem Pharmacol*, 52, 167–171.

Shimon, H., Agam, G., Belmaker, R.H., Hyde, T.M., and Kleinman, J.E. (1997). Reduced frontal cortex inositol levels in postmortem brain of suicide victims and patients with bipolar disorder. *Am J Psychiatry*, 154, 1148–1150.

Shippenberg, T.S., and Herz, A. (1991). Influence of chronic lithium treatment upon the motivational effects of opioids: Alteration in the effects of mu- but not kappa-opioid receptor ligands. *J Pharmacol Exp Ther*, 256, 1101–1106.

Shippenberg, T.S., Millan, M.J., Mucha, R.F., and Herz, A. (1988). Involvement of beta-endorphin and mu-opioid receptors in mediating the aversive effect of lithium in the rat. *Eur J Pharmacol*, 154, 135–144.

Shukla, G.S. (1985). Combined lithium and valproate treatment and subsequent withdrawal: Serotonergic mechanism of their interaction in discrete brain regions. *Prog Neuropsychopharmacol Biol Psychiatry*, 9, 153–156.

Siegel, J.M., and Rogawski, M.A. (1988). A function for REM sleep: Regulation of noradrenergic receptor sensitivity. *Brain Res*, 472(3), 213–233.

Siever, L.J. (1987). Role of noradrenergic mechanisms in the etiology of the affective disorders. In H.Y. Meltzer (Ed.), *Psychopharmacology: The Third Generation of Progress* (pp. 493–504). New York: Raven Press.

Siever, L.J., and Uhde, T.W (1984). New studies and perspectives on the noradrenergic receptor system in depression: Effects of the alpha 2-adrenergic agonist clonidine. *Biol Psychiatry*, 19, 131–156.

Siever, L.J., Uhde, T.W., Silberman, E.K., Jimerson, D.C., Aloi, J.A., Post, R.M., and Murphy, D.L. (1982). Growth hormone response to clonidine as a probe of noradrenergic receptor responsiveness in affective disorder patients and controls. *Psychiatry Res*, 6, 171–183.

Siever, L.J., Insel, T.R., Jimerson, D.C., Lake, C.R., Uhde, T.W., Aloi, J., and Murphy, D.L. (1983). Growth hormone response to clonidine in obsessive-compulsive patients. *Br J Psychiatry*, 142, 184–187.

Siever, L.J., Uhde, T.W., Jimerson, D.C., Lake, C.R., Silberman, E.R., Post, R.M., and Murphy, D.L. (1984). Differential inhibitory noradrenergic responses to clonidine in 25 depressed patients and 25 normal control subjects. *Am J Psychiatry*, 141, 733–741.

Silverstone, T. (1978). Dopamine, mood and manic-depressive psychosis. In S. Garattini (Ed.), *Depressive Disorders* (pp. 419–430). Stuttgart: FK Schattauer Verlag.

Silverstone, T. (1984). Response to bromocriptine distinguishes bipolar from unipolar depression. *Lancet*, 1, 903–904.

Simmons, N.E., Alden, T.D., Thorner, M.O., and Laws, E.R. Jr. (2001). Serum cortisol response to transsphenoidal surgery for cushing disease. *J Neurosurg*, 95(1), 1–8.

Simon, J.R., and Kuhar, M.J. (1976). High-affinity choline uptake: Ionic and energy requirements. *J Neurochem*, 27, 93–99.

Simpkins, J.W., Green, P.S., Gridley, K.E., Singh, M., de Fiebre, N.C., and Rajakumar, G. (1997). Role of estrogen replacement therapy in memory enhancement and the prevention of neuronal loss associated with Alzheimer's disease. *Am J Med*, 103, 19S–25S.

Simpson, H.B., Nee, J.C., and Endicott, J. (1997). First-episode major depression. Few sex differences in course. *Arch Gen Psychiatry*, 54, 633–639.

Singh, M., Meyer, E.M., and Simpkins, J.W. (1995). The effect of ovariectomy and estradiol replacement on brain-derived neurotrophic factor messenger ribonucleic acid expression in cortical and hippocampal brain regions of female Sprague-Dawley rats. *Endocrinology*, 136, 2320–2324.

Sirois, F. (2003). Steroid psychosis: A review. *Gen Hosp Psychiatry*, 25(1), 27–33.

Si-Tahar, M., Renesto, P., Falet, H., Rendu, F., and Chignard, M. (1996). The phospholipase C/protein kinase C pathway is involved in cathepsin G-induced human platelet activation: Comparison with thrombin. *Biochem J*, 313(Pt. 2), 401–408.

Sitaram, N., Wyatt, R.J., Dawson, S., and Gillin, J.C. (1976). REM sleep induction by physostigmine infusion during sleep. *Science*, 191, 1281–1283.

Sitaram, N., Moore, A.M., and Gillin, J.C. (1978a). Experimental acceleration and slowing of REM sleep ultradian rhythm by cholinergic agonist and antagonist. *Nature*, 274, 490–492.

Sitaram, N., Moore, A.M., and Gillin, J.C. (1978b). Induction and resetting of REM sleep rhythm in normal man by arecholine: Blockade by scopolamine. *Sleep*, 1, 83–90.

Sitaram, N., Weingartner, H., and Gillin, J.C. (1978c). Human serial learning: Enhancement with arecholine and choline impairment with scopolamine. *Science*, 201, 274–276.

Sitaram, N., Moore, A.M., and Gillin, J.C. (1979). Scopolamine-induced muscarinic supersensitivity in normal man: Changes in sleep. *Psychiatry Res*, 1, 9–16.

Sitaram, N., Nurnberger, J.I. Jr., Gershon, E.S., and Gillin, J.C. (1980). Faster cholinergic REM sleep induction in euthymic patients with primary affective illness. *Science*, 208, 200–202.

Sitaram, N., Nurnberger, J.I. Jr., Gershon, E.S., and Gillin, J.C. (1982). Cholinergic regulation of mood and REM sleep: Potential model and marker of vulnerability to affective disorder. *Am J Psychiatry*, 139, 571–576.

Sitaram, N., Dube, S., Keshavan, M., Davies, A., and Reynal, P. (1987). The association of supersensitive cholinergic REM-induction and affective illness within pedigrees. *J Psychiatr Res*, 21, 487–497.

Sivam, S.P., Breese, G.R., Napier, T.C., Mueller, R.A., and Hong, J.S. (1986). Dopaminergic regulation of proenkephalin-A gene expression in the basal ganglia. *NIDA Res Monogr*, 75, 389–392.

Sivam, S.P., Takeuchi, K., Li, S., Douglass, J., Civelli, O., Calvetta, L., Herbert, E., McGinty, J.F., and Hong, J.S. (1988). Lithium increases dynorphin A(1-8) and prodynorphin mRNA levels in the basal ganglia of rats. *Brain Res*, 427, 155–163.

Sivam, S.P., Krause, J.E., Takeuchi, K., Li, S., McGinty, J.F., and Hong, J.S. (1989). Lithium increases rat striatal beta- and gamma-preprotachykinin messenger RNAs. *J Pharmacol Exp Ther*, 248(3), 1297–1301.

Skolnick, P. (1999). Antidepressants for the new millennium. *Eur J Pharmacol*, 375, 31–40.

Skolnick, P., Legutko, B., Li, X., and Bymaster, F.P. (2001). Current perspectives on the development of non-biogenic amine-based antidepressants. *Pharmacol Res*, 43, 411–423.

Slater, S.J., Kelly, M.B., Taddeo, F.J., Ho, C., Rubin, E., and Stubbs, C.D. (1994). The modulation of protein kinase C activity by membrane lipid bilayer structure. *J Biol Chem*, 269, 4866–4871.

Smeraldi, E., Benedetti, F., Barbini, B., Campori, E., and Colombo, C. (1999). Sustained antidepressant effect of sleep deprivation combined with pindolol in bipolar depression. A placebo-controlled trial. *Neuropsychopharmacology*, 20, 380–385.

Smith, A.D., and Winkler, H. (1972). Fundamental mechanisms in the release of Catecholamines. In H. Blaschko and E. Muscholl (Eds.), *Handbook of Experimental Pharmacology, Vol. 33 Catecholamines* (pp. 538–617). Berlin: Springer-Verlag.

Smith, D.F. (1988). Lithium attenuates clonidine-induced hypoactivity: Further studies in inbred mouse strains. *Psychopharmacology (Berl)*, 94, 428–430.

Smith, M.A., Makino, S., Kvetnansky, R., and Post, R.M. (1995). Stress and glucocorticoids affect the expression of brain-derived neurotrophic factor and neurotrophin-3 mRNAs in the hippocampus. *J Neurosci*, 15, 1768–1777.

Smith, R.C., Chua, J.W., Lipetsker, B., and Bhattacharyya, A. (1996). Efficacy of risperidone in reducing positive and negative symptoms in medication-refractory schizophrenia: An open prospective study. *J Clin Psychiatry*, 57, 460–466.

Smith, R.E., and Helms, P.M. (1982). Adverse effects of lithium therapy in the acutely ill elderly patient. *J Clin Psychiatry*, 43(3), 94–99.

Soares, J.C., and Mallinger, A.G. (1997). Intracellular phosphatidylinositol pathway abnormalities in bipolar disorder patients. *Psychopharmacol Bull*, 33(4), 685–691.

Soares, J.C., Dippold, C.S., and Mallinger, A.G. (1997). Platelet membrane phosphatidylinositol-4,5-bisphosphate alterations in bipolar disorder—evidence from a single case study. *Psychiatry Res*, 69(2-3), 197–202.

Soares, J.C., Mallinger, A.G., Dippold, C.S., Frank, E., and Kupfer, D.J. (1999). Platelet membrane phospholipids in euthymic bipolar disorder patients: Are they affected by lithium treatment? *Biol Psychiatry*, 45(4), 453–457.

Soares, J.C., Mallinger, A.G., Dippold, C.S., Forster Wells, K., Frank, E., and Kupfer, D.J. (2000a). Effects of lithium on platelet membrane phosphoinositides in bipolar disorder patients: A pilot study. *Psychopharmacology (Berl)*, 149(1), 12–16.

Soares, J.C., Chen, G., Dippold, C.S., Wells, K.F., Frank, E., Kupfer, D.J., Manji, H.K., and Mallinger, A.G. (2000b). Concurrent measures of protein kinase C and phosphoinositides in lithium-treated bipolar patients and healthy individuals: A preliminary study. *Psychiatry Res.* 95(2), 109–118.

Soares, J.C., Dippold, C.S., Wells, K.F., Frank, E., Kupfer, D.J., and Mallinger, A.G. (2001). Increased platelet membrane phosphatidylinositol-4,5-bisphosphate in drug-free depressed bipolar patients. *Neurosci Lett*, 299, 150–152.

Sobczak, S., Riedel, W.J., Booij, I., Aan Het Rot, M., Deutz, N.E., and Honig, A. (2002). Cognition following acute tryptophan depletion: Difference between first-degree relatives of bipolar disorder patients and matched healthy control volunteers. *Psychol Med*, 32, 503–515.

Sofuoglu, S., Dogan, P., Kose, K., Esel, E., Basturk, M., Oguz, H., and Gonul, A.S. (1995). Changes in platelet monoamine oxidase and plasma dopamine-beta-hydroxylase activities in lithium-treated bipolar patients. *Psychiatry Res*, 59, 165–170.

Sohrabji, F., Miranda, R.C., and Toran-Allerand, C.D. (1994). Estrogen differentially regulates estrogen and nerve growth factor receptor mrnas in adult sensory neurons. *J Neurosci*, 14(2), 459–471.

Sokolski, K.N., and DeMet, E.M. (1999). Pupillary cholinergic sensitivity to pilocarpine increases in manic lithium responders. *Biol Psychiatry*, 45, 1580–1584.

Sokolski, K.N., and DeMet, E.M. (2000). Cholinergic sensitivity predicts severity of mania. *Psychiatry Res*, 95(3), 195–200.

Sonawalla, S.B., Renshaw, P.F., Moore, C.M., Alpert, J.E., Nierenberg, A.A., Rosenbaum, J.F., and Fava, M. (1999). Compounds containing cytosolic choline in the basal ganglia: A potential biological marker of true drug response to fluoxetine. *Am J Psychiatry*, 156, 1638–1640.

Song, L., and Jope, R.S. (1992). Chronic lithium treatment impairs phosphatidylinositol hydrolysis in membranes from rat brain regions. *J Neurochem*, 58, 2200–2206.

Sonino, N., and Fava, G.A. (2001). Psychiatric disorders associated with Cushing's syndrome. Epidemiology, pathophysiology and treatment. *CNS Drugs*, 15(5), 361–373.

Sorensen, P.S., Gjerris, A., and Hammer, M. (1985). Cerebrospinal fluid vasopressin in neurological and psychiatric disorders. *J Neurol Neurosurg Psychiatry*, 48, 50–57.

Soucek, K., Zvolsky, P., Krulik, R., Filip, V., Vinarova, E., and Dostal, T. (1974). The levels of lithium in serum and in red blood cells and its ratios in manic-depressive patients. *Act Nerv Super (Praha)*, 16(3), 193–194.

Souetre, E., Salvati, E., Pringuey, D., Krebs, B., Plasse, Y., and Darcourt, G. (1986). The circadian rhythm of plasma thyrotropin in depression and recovery. *Chronobiol Int*, 3, 197–205.

Souetre, E., Salvati, E., Wehr, T.A., Sack, D.A., Krebs, B., and Darcourt, G. (1988). Twenty-four-hour profiles of body temperature and plasma TSH in bipolar patients during depression and during remission and in normal control subjects. *Am J Psychiatry*, 145, 1133–1137.

Souza, F.G., Mander, A.J., Foggo, M., Dick, H., Shearing, C.H., and Goodwin, G.M. (1991). The effects of lithium discontinuation and the non-effect of oral inositol upon thyroid hormones and cortisol in patients with bipolar affective disorder. *J Affect Disord*, 22, 165–170.

Sparapani, M., Virgili, M., Ortali, F., and Contestabile, A. (1997). Effects of chronic lithium treatment on ornithine decarboxylase induction and excitotoxic neuropathology in the rat. *Brain Res*, 765, 164–168.

Sperling, R.I., Benincaso, A.I., Knoell, C.T., Larkin, J.K., Austen, K.F., and Robinson, D.R. (1993). Dietary omega-3 polyunsaturated fatty acids inhibit phosphoinositide formation and chemotaxis in neutrophils. *J Clin Invest*, 91, 651–660.

Spiegel, A. (1998). *G Proteins, Receptors, and Disease*. Totowa, NJ: Humana Press.

Spitz, R.A. (1946). Anaclitic depression: An inquiry into the genesis of psychiatric conditions in early childhood: II. *Psychoanal Study Child*, 2, 313–347.

Spleiss, O., van Calker, D., Scharer, L., Adamovic, K., Berger, M., and Gebicke-Haerter, P.J. (1998). Abnormal G protein alpha(s)–and alpha(i2)–subunit mRNA expression in bipolar affective disorder. *Mol Psychiatry*, 3, 512–520.

Sporn, J., and Sachs, G. (1997). The anticonvulsant lamotrigine in treatment-resistant manic-depressive illness. *J Clin Psychopharmacol*, 17, 185–189.

Sporn, J., Ghaemi, S.N., Sambur, M.R., Rankin, M.A., Recht, J., Sachs, G.S., Rosenbaum, J.F., and Fava, M. (2000). Pramipexole augmentation in the treatment of unipolar and bipolar depression: A retrospective chart review. *Ann Clin Psychiatry*, 12, 137–140.

Stambolic, V., Ruel, L., and Woodgett, J.R. (1996). Lithium inhibits glycogen synthase kinase-3 activity and mimics wingless signalling in intact cells. *Curr Biol.*, 6(12):1664–1668. Erratum in *Curr Biol* 1997 7(3), 196.

Stancer, H.C., and Persad, E. (1982). Treatment of intractable rapid-cycling manic-depressive disorder with levothyroxine. Clinical observations. *Arch Gen Psychiatry*, 39, 311–312.

Staner, L., Hilger, C., Hentges, F., Monreal, J., Hoffmann, A., Couturier, M., Le Bon, O., Stefos, G., Souery, D., and Mendlewicz, J. (1998). Association between novelty-seeking and the dopamine D3 receptor gene in bipolar patients: A preliminary report. *Am J Med Genet*, 81, 192–194.

Stanley, M., and Mann, J.J. (1983). Increased serotonin-2 binding sites in frontal cortex of suicide victims. *Lancet*, I, 214–216.

Stanley, M., Virgilio, J., and Gershon, S. (1982). Tritiated imipramine binding sites are decreased in the frontal cortex of suicides. *Science*, 216, 1337–1339.

Stanley, M., Mann, J.J., and Gershon, S. (1983). Alterations in pre- and postsynaptic serotonergic neurons in suicide victims. *Psychopharmacol Bull*, 19, 684–687.

Starkman, M.N., Giordani, B., Gebarski, S.S., Berent, S., Schork, M.A., and Schteingart, D.E. (1999). Decrease in cortisol reverses human hippocampal atrophy following treatment of Cushing's disease. *Biol Psychiatry*, 46(12), 1595–1602.

Staunton, D.A., Magistretti, P.J., Shoemaker, W.J., and Bloom, F.E. (1982a). Effects of chronic lithium treatment on dopamine receptors in the rat corpus striatum. I. Locomotor activity and behavioral supersensitivity. *Brain Res*, 232, 391–400.

Staunton, D.A., Magistretti, P.J., Shoemaker, W.J., Deyo, S.N., and Bloom, F.E. (1982b). Effects of chronic lithium treatment on dopamine receptors in the rat corpus striatum. II. No effect on denervation or neuroleptic-induced supersensitivity. *Brain Res*, 232, 401–412.

Steffens, D.C., and Krishnan, K.R. (1998). Structural neuroimaging and mood disorders: Recent findings, implications for classification, and future directions. *Biol Psychiatry*, 43, 705–712.

Steffens, D.C, Helms, M.J., Krishnan, K.R., and Burke, G.L. (1999). Cerebrovascular disease and depression symptoms in the cardiovascular health study. *Stroke*, 30, 2159–2166.

Stein, M.B., Chen, G., Potter, W.Z., and Manji, H.K. (1996). G-protein level quantification in platelets and leukocytes from patients with panic disorder. *Neuropsychopharmacology*, 15, 180–186.

Steketee, J.D. (1993). Injection of the protein kinase inhibitor H7 into the A10 dopamine region blocks the acute responses to cocaine: Behavioral and in vivo microdialysis studies. *Neuropharmacology*, 32, 1289–1297.

Steketee, J.D. (1994). Intra-A10 injection of H7 blocks the development of sensitization to cocaine. *Neuroreport*, 6, 69–72.

Steketee, J.D., and Kalivas, P.W. (1991). Sensitization to psychostimulants and stress after injection of pertussis toxin into the A10 dopamine region. *J Pharmacol Exp Ther*, 259, 916–924.

Steketee, J.D., Striplin, C.D., Murray, T.F., and Kalivas, P.W. (1991). Possible role for G-proteins in behavioral sensitization to cocaine. *Brain Res*, 545, 287–291.

Stenfors, C., Theodorsson, E., and Mathe, A.A. (1989). Effect of repeated electroconvulsive treatment on regional concentrations of tachykinins, neurotensin, vasoactive intestinal polypeptide, neuropeptide Y, and galanin in rat brain. *J Neurosci Res*, 24, 445–450.

Stengaard-Pedersen, K., and Schou, M. (1982). In vitro and in vivo inhibition by lithium of enkephalin binding to opiate receptors in rat brain. *Neuropharmacology*, 21, 817–823.

Steppuhn, K.G., and Turski, L. (1993). Modulation of the seizure threshold for excitatory amino acids in mice by antiepileptic drugs and chemoconvulsants. *J Pharmacol Exp Ther*, 265, 1063–1070.

Stewart, J., and Badiani, A. (1993). Tolerance and sensitization to the behavioral effects of drugs. *Behav Pharmacol*, 4(4), 289–312.

Stockmeier, C.A. (1997). Neurobiology of serotonin in depression and suicide. *Ann NY Acad Sci*, 836, 220–232.

Stockmeier, C.A. (2003). Involvement of serotonin in depression: Evidence from postmortem and imaging studies of serotonin receptors and the serotonin transporter. *J Psychiatr Res*, 37, 357–373.

Stockmeier, C.A., and Meltzer, H.Y. (1991). Beta-adrenergic receptor binding in frontal cortex of suicide victims. *Biol Psychiatry*, 29, 183–191.

Stockmeier, C.A., Dilley, G.E., Shapiro, L.A., Overholser, J.C., Thompson, P.A., and Meltzer, H.Y. (1996). Serotonin receptors in suicide victims with major depression. *Neuropsychopharmacology*, 16, 162–173.

Stockmeier, C.A., Dilley, G.E., Shapiro, L.A., Overholser, J.C., Thompson, P.A., and Meltzer, H.Y. (1997). Serotonin receptors in suicide victims with major depression. *Neuropsychopharmacology*, 16, 162–173.

Stockmeier, C.A., Shapiro, L.A., Dilley, G.E., Kolli, T.N., Friedman, L., and Rajkowska, G. (1998). Increase in serotonin-1A autoreceptors in the midbrain of suicide victims with major depression-postmortem evidence for decreased serotonin activity. *J Neurosci*, 18, 7394–7401.

Stockmeier, C.A., Mahajan, G.J., Konick, L.C., Overholser, J.C., Jurjus, G.J., Meltzer, H.Y., Uylings, H.B., Friedman, L., and Rajkowska, G. (2004). Cellular changes in the postmortem hippocampus in major depression. *Biol Psychiatry*, 56(9), 640–650.

Stokes, P.E., Pick, G.R., Stoll, P.M., and Nunn, W.D. (1975). Pituitary–adrenal function in depressed patients: Resistance to dexamethasone suppression. *J Psychiatr Res*, 12, 271–281.

Stokes, P.E., Frazer, A., and Casper, R. (1981). Unexpected neuroendocrine-transmitter relationships [proceedings]. *Psychopharmacol Bull*, 17, 72–75.

Stokes, P.E., Stoll, P.M., Koslow, S.H., Maas, J.W., Davis, J.M., Swann, A.C., and Robins, E. (1984). Pretreatment DST and hypothalamic–pituitary–adrenocortical function in depressed patients and comparison groups. A multicenter study. *Arch Gen Psychiatry*, 41, 257–267.

Stoll, A.L., Cohen, B.M., Snyder, M.B., and Hanin, I. (1991). Erythrocyte choline concentration in bipolar disorder: A predictor of clinical course and medication response. *Biol Psychiatry*, 29, 1171–1180.

Stoll, A.L., Renshaw, P.F., Sachs, G.S., Guimaraes, A.R., Miller, C., Cohen, B.M., Lafer, B., and Gonzalez, R.G. (1992). The human brain resonance of choline-containing compounds is similar in patients receiving lithium treatment and controls: An in vivo proton magnetic resonance spectroscopy study. *Biol Psychiatry*, 32, 944–949.

Stoll, A.L., Sachs, G.S., Cohen, B.M., Lafer, B., Christensen, J.D., and Renshaw, P.F. (1996). Choline in the treatment of rapid-cycling bipolar disorder: Clinical and neurochemical findings in lithium-treated patients. *Biol Psychiatry*, 40(5), 382–388.

Stork, C., and Renshaw, P.F. (2005). Mitochondrial dysfunction in bipolar disorder: Evidence from magnetic resonance spectroscopy research. *Mol Psychiatry*, 10(10), 900–919.

Strakowski, S.M., Wilson, D.R., Tohen, M., Woods, B.T., Douglass, A.W., and Stoll, A.L. (1993). Structural brain abnormalities in first-episode mania. *Biol Psychiatry*, 33, 602–609.

Strakowski, S.M., Adler, C.M., and DelBello, M.P. (2002). Volumetric MRI studies of mood disorders: Do they distinguish unipolar and bipolar disorder? *Bipolar Disord*, 4, 80–88.

Strandman, E., Wetterberg, L., Perris, C., and Ross, S.B. (1978). Serum dopamine-beta-hydroxylase in affective disorders. *Neuropsychobiology*, 4, 248–255.

Stratakis, C.A., Sarlis, N.J., Berrettini, W.H., Badner, J.A., Chrousos, G.P., Gershon, E.S., and Detera-Wadleigh, S.D. (1997). Lack of linkage between the corticotropin-releasing hormone (CRH) gene and bipolar affective disorder. *Mol Psychiatry*, 2, 483–485.

Strzyzewski, W., Rybakowski, J., Potok, E., and Zelechowska-Ruda, E. (1984). Erythrocyte cation transport in endogenous depression: Clinical and psychophysiological correlates. *Acta Psychiatr Scand*, 70, 248–253.

Styra, R., Joffe, R., and Singer, W. (1991). Hyperthyroxinemia in major affective disorders. *Acta Psychiatr Scand*, 83, 61–63.

Styron, W. (1990). *Darkness Visible: A Memoir of Madness*. New York: Random House.

Suhara, T., Nakayama, K., Inoue, O., Fukuda, H., Shimizu, M., Mori, A., and Tateno, Y. (1992). D1 dopamine receptor binding in mood disorders measured by positron emission tomography. *Psychopharmacology (Berl)*, 106, 14–18.

Sulser, F. (1978). Functional aspects of the norepinephrine receptor coupled adenylate cyclase system in the limbic forebrain and its modification by drugs which precipitate or alleviate depression: molecular approaches to an understanding of affective disorders. *Pharmakopsychiatr Neuropsychopharmakol*, 11, 43–52.

Sunahara, G.I., and Chiesa, A. (1992). Phorone (diisopropylidene acetone), a glutathione depletor, decreases rat glucocorticoid receptor binding in vivo. *Carcinogenesis*, 13(7), 1083–1089.

Sunahara, R.K., Guan, H.C., O'Dowd, B.F., Seeman, P., Laurier, L.G., Ng, G., George, S.R., Torchia, J., Van Tol, H.H., and Niznik, H.B. (1991). Cloning of the gene for a human dopamine D5 receptor with higher affinity for dopamine than D1. *Nature*, 350, 614–619.

Suomi, S.J. (1982). The development of social competence by rhesus monkeys. *Ann Ist Super Sanita*, 18, 193–202.

Suomi, S.J., Seaman, S.F., Lewis, J.K., DeLizio, R.D., and McKinney, W.T. Jr. (1978). Effects of imipramine treatment of separation-induced social disorders in rhesus monkeys. *Arch Gen Psychiatry*, 35, 321–325.

Suzuki, K., Kusumi, I., Sasaki, Y., and Koyama, T. (2001). Serotonin-induced platelet intracellular calcium mobilization in various psychiatric disorders: Is it specific to bipolar disorder? *J Affect Disord*, 64, 291–296.

Swann, A.C. (1984). Caloric intake and Na+-K+-ATPase: Differential regulation by alpha 1- and beta-noradrenergic receptors. *Am J Physiol*, 247(3 Pt. 2), R449–R455.

Swann, A.C. (1988). Norepinephrine and (Na+, K+)-ATPase: Evidence for stabilization by lithium or imipramine. *Neuropharmacology*, 27, 261–267.

Swann, A.C., Maas, J.W., Hattox, S.E., and Landis, H. (1980). Catecholamine metabolites in human plasma as indices of brain function: Effects of debrisoquin. *Life Sci*, 27, 1857–1862.

Swann, A.C., Secunda, S.K., Katz, M.M., Koslow, S.H., Maas, J.W., Chang, S., and Robins, E. (1986). Lithium treatment of mania: Clinical characteristics, specificity of symptom change, and outcome. *Psychiatry Res*, 18(2), 127–141.

Swann, A.C., Koslow, S.H., Katz, M.M., Maas, J.W., Javaid, J., Secunda, S.K., and Robins, E. (1987). Lithium carbonate treatment of mania. Cerebrospinal fluid and urinary monoamine metabolites and treatment outcome. *Arch Gen Psychiatry*, 44, 345–354.

Swann, A.C., Secunda, S.K., Stokes, P.E., Croughan, J., Davis, J.M., Koslow, S.H., and Maas, J.W. (1990). Stress, depression, and mania: Relationship between perceived role of stressful events and clinical and biochemical characteristics. *Acta Psychiatr Scand*, 81, 389–397.

Swann, A.C., Secunda, S.K., Koslow, S.H., Katz, M.M., Bowden, C.L., Maas, J.W., Davis, J.M., and Robins, E. (1991). Mania: Sympathoadrenal function and clinical state. *Psychiatry Res*, 37, 195–205.

Swann, A.C., Stokes, P.E., Casper, R., Secunda, S.K., Bowden, C.L., Berman, N., Katz, M.M., and Robins, E. (1992). Hypothalamic–pituitary–adrenocortical function in mixed and pure mania. *Acta Psychiatr Scand*, 85, 270–274.

Swann, A.C., Stokes, P.E., Secunda, S.K., Maas, J.W., Bowden, C.L., Berman, N., and Koslow, S.H. (1994). Depressive mania versus agitated depression: Biogenic amine and hypothalamic–pituitary–adrenocortical function. *Biol Psychiatry*, 35, 803–813.

Swann, A.C., Petty, F., Bowden, C.L., Dilsaver, S.C., Calabrese, J.R., and Morris, D.D. (1999). Mania: Gender, transmitter function, and response to treatment. *Psychiatry Res*, 88, 55–61.

Szabo, S., Gould, T.D., and Manji, H.K. (2003). Neurotransmitters, receptors, signal transduction pathways and second messengers. In C.B. Nemeroff and A.F. Schatzberg (Eds.), *American Psychiatric Textbook of Psychopharmacology* (pp. 3–52). Arlington, VA: American Psychiatric Publishing.

Szentistvanyi, I., and Janka, Z. (1979). Correlation between the lithium ratio and Na-dependent Li transport of red blood cells during lithium prophylaxis. *Biol Psychiatry*, 14, 973–977.

Szuba, M. P., Baxter, L.R. Jr., Fairbanks, L.A., Guze, B.H., and Schwartz, J.M. (1991). Effects of partial sleep deprivation on the diurnal variation of mood and motor activity in major depression. *Biol Psychiatry*, 30(8), 817–829.

Szuba, M.P., Baxter, L.R. Jr., Altshuler, L.L., Allen, E.M., Guze, B.H., Schwartz, J.M., and Liston, E.H. (1994). Lithium sustains the acute antidepressant effects of sleep deprivation: Preliminary findings from a controlled study. *Psychiatry Res*, 51, 283–295.

Szuba, M.P., Amsterdam, J.D., Fernando, A.T. III, Gary, K.A., Whybrow, P.C., and Winokur, A. (2005). Rapid antidepressant response after nocturnal TRH administration in patients with bipolar type I and bipolar type II major depression. *J Clin Psychopharmacol*, 25(4), 325–330.

Takashima, A., Yamaguchi, H., Noguchi, K., Michel, G., Ishiguro, K., Sato, K., Hoshino, T., Hoshi, M., and Imahori, K. (1995). Amyloid beta peptide induces cytoplasmic accumulation of amyloid protein precursor via tau protein kinase I/glycogen synthase kinase-3 beta in rat hippocampal neurons. *Neurosci Lett*, 198, 83–86.

Tan, C.H., Javors, M.A., Seleshi, E., Lowrimore, P.A., and Bowden, C.L. (1990). Effects of lithium on platelet ionic intracellular calcium concentration in patients with bipolar (manic-depressive) disorder and healthy controls. *Life Sci*, 46(16), 1175–1180.

Tan, C.H., Lee, H.S., Kua, E.H., and Peh, L.H. (1995). Resting and thrombin-stimulated cytosolic calcium in platelets of patients with alcoholic withdrawal, bipolar manic disorder and chronic schizophrenia. *Life Sci*, 56(21), 1817–1823.

Tandon, R., Channabasavanna, S.M., and Greden, J.F. (1988). CSF biochemical correlates of mixed affective states. *Acta Psychiatr Scand*, 78, 289–297.

Tanimoto, K., Maeda, K., and Terada, T. (1983). Inhibitory effect of lithium on neuroleptic and serotonin receptors in rat brain. *Brain Res*, 265, 148–151.

Tartaglia, N., Du, J., Tyler, W.J., Neale, E., Pozzo-Miller, L., and Lu, B. (2001). Protein synthesis-dependent and -independent regulation of hippocampal synapses by brain-derived neurotrophic factor. *J Biol Chem*, 276, 37585–37593.

Taylor, M.P., Reynolds, C.F. III, Frank, E., Cornes, C., Miller, M.D., Stack, J.A., Begley, A.E., Mazumdar, S., Dew, M.A., and Kupfer, D.J. (1999). Which elderly depressed patients remain well on maintenance interpersonal psychotherapy alone?: Report from the pittsburgh study of maintenance therapies in late-life depression. *Depress Anxiety*, 10(2), 55–60.

Terenius, L., and Wahlstrom, A. (1976). A method for site selectivity analysis applied to opiate receptors. *Eur J Pharmacol*, 40, 241–248.

Terenius, L., Wahlström, A., Lindström, L., and Widerlöv, E. (1976). Increased CSF levels of endorphins in chronic psychosis. *Neurosci Lett*, 3, 157–162.

Terenius, L., Wahlstrom, A., and Agren, H. (1977). Naloxone (Narcan) treatment in depression: Clinical observations and effects on CSF endorphins and monoamine metabolites. *Psychopharmacology (Berl)*, 54, 31–33.

Terry, J.B., Padzernik, T.L., and Nelson, S.R. (1990). Effect of LiCl pretreatment on cholinomimetic-induced seizures and seizure-induced brain edema in rats. *Neurosci Lett*, 114, 123–127.

Thakar, J.H., Lapierre, Y.D., and Waters, B.G. (1985). Erythrocyte membrane sodium-potassium and magnesium ATPase in primary affective disorder. *Biol Psychiatry*, 20, 734–740.

Thakore, J.H., O'Keane, V., and Dinan, T.G. (1996). d-fenfluramine-induced prolactin responses in mania: Evidence for serotonergic subsensitivity. *Am J Psychiatry*, 153, 1460–1463.

Thase, M.E., Mallinger, A.G., McKnight, D., and Himmelhoch, J.M. (1992). Treatment of imipramine-resistant recurrent depression: IV. A double-blind crossover study of tranylcypromine for anergic bipolar depression. *Am J Psychiatry*, 149, 195–198.

Thome, J., Sakai, N., Shin, K., Steffen, C., Zhang, Y.J., Impey, S., Storm, D., and Duman, R.S. (2000). cAMP response element–mediated gene transcription is upregulated by chronic antidepressant treatment. *J Neurosci*, 20, 4030–4036.

Thome, J., Pesold, B., Baader, M., Hu, M., Gewirtz, J.C., Duman, R.S., and Henn, F.A. (2001). Stress differentially regulates synaptophysin and synaptotagmin expression in hippocampus. *Biol Psychiatry*, 50, 809–812.

Thompson, P.M., Rosenberger, C., and Qualls, C. (1999). CSF SNAP-25 in schizophrenia and bipolar illness. A pilot study. *Neuropsychopharmacology*, 21, 717–722.

Tkachev, D., Mimmack, M.L., Ryan, M.M., Wayland, M., Freeman, T., Jones, P.B., Starkey, M., Webster, M.J., Yolken, R.H., and Bahn, S. (2003). Oligodendrocyte dysfunction in schizophrenia and bipolar disorder. *Lancet*, 362, 798–805.

Tollefson, G.D., Senogles, S.E., and Frey, W.H. II. (1982). Ionic regulation of antagonist binding to the human muscarinic cholinergic receptor of caudate nucleus. *J Psychiatr Res*, 17, 275–283.

Torok, T.L. (1989). Neurochemical transmission and the sodium-pump. *Prog Neurobiol*, 32(1), 11–76.

Traskman, L., Asberg, M., Bertilsson, L., and Sjostrand, L. (1981). Monoamine metabolites in CSF and suicidal behavior. *Arch Gen Psychiatry*, 38, 631–636.

Treiser, S., and Kellar, K.J. (1979). Lithium effects on adrenergic receptor supersensitivity in rat brain. *Eur J Pharmacol*, 58, 85–86.

Treiser, S., and Kellar, K.J. (1980). Lithium: Effects on serotonin receptors in rat brain. *Eur J Pharmacol*, 64, 183–185.

Treiser, S.L., Cascio, C.S., O'Donohue, T.L., Thoa, N.B., Jacobowitz, D.M., and Kellar, K.J. (1981). Lithium increases serotonin release and decreases serotonin receptors in the hippocampus. *Science*, 213, 1529–1531.

Tremolizzo, L., Doueiri, M.S., Dong, E., Grayson, D.R., Davis, J., Pinna, G., Tueting, P., Rodriguez-Menendez, V., Costa, E., and Guidotti, A. (2005). Valproate corrects the schizophrenia-like epigenetic behavioral modifications induced by methionine in mice. *Biol Psychiatry*, 57(5), 500–509.

Tricklebank, M.D., Singh, L., Jackson, A., and Oles, R.J. (1991). Evidence that a proconvulsant action of lithium is mediated by inhibition of myo-inositol phosphatase in mouse brain. *Brain Res*, 558, 145–148.

Trottier, E., Belzil, A., Stoltz, C., and Anderson, A. (1995). Localization of a phenobarbital-responsive element (PBRE) in the 5'-flanking region of the rat CYP2B2 gene. *Gene*, 158(2), 263–268.

Tsai, G., and Coyle, J.T. (1995). N-acetylaspartate in neuropsychiatric disorders. *Prog Neurobiol*, 46, 531–540.

Tsankova, N.M., Berton, O., Renthal, W., Kumar, A., Neve, R.L., and Nestler, E.J. (2006). Sustained hippocampal chromatin regulation in a mouse model of depression and antidepressant action. *Nat Neurosci*, 9(4), 519–525.

Tudorache, B., and Diacicov, S. (1991). The effect of clonidine in the treatment of acute mania. *Rom J Neurol Psychiatry*, 29, 209–213.

Turktas, L., Gucuyener, K., and Ozden, A. (1997). Medication-induced psychotic reaction. *J Am Acad Child Adolesc Psychiatry*, 36(8), 1017–1018.

Turner, K.M., Burgoyne, R.D., and Morgan, A. (1999). Protein phosphorylation and the regulation of synaptic membrane traffic. *Trends Neurosci*, 22, 459–464.

Turski, L. (1990). The *N*-methyl-D-aspartate receptor complex. Various sites of regulation and clinical consequences. *Arzneimittelforschung*, 40, 511–514.

Tzschentke, T.M., and Schmidt, W.J. (1997). Interactions of MK-801 and GYKI 52466 with morphine and amphetamine in place preference conditioning and behavioural sensitization. *Behav Brain Res*, 84, 99–107.

Ueda, Y., and Willmore, L.J. (2000). Molecular regulation of glutamate and GABA transporter proteins by valproic acid in rat hippocampus during epileptogenesis. *Exp Brain Res*, 133, 334–339.

Uhde, T.W., Vittone, B.J., Siever, L.J., Kaye, W.H., and Post, R.M. (1986). Blunted growth hormone response to clonidine in panic disorder patients. *Biol Psychiatry*, 21, 1081–1085.

Ullian, E.M., Sapperstein, S.K., Christopherson, K.S., and Barres, B.A. (2001). Control of synapse number by glia. *Science*, 291, 657–661.

Uney, J.B., Marchbanks, R.M., and Marsh, A. (1985). The effect of lithium on choline transport in human erythrocytes. *J Neurol Neurosurg Psychiatry*, 48, 229–233.

Ur, E., Turner, T.H., Goodwin, T.J., Grossman, A., and Besser, G.M. (1992). Mania in association with hydrocortisone replacement for Addison's disease. *Postgrad Med J*, 68, 41–43.

Uranova, N., Orlovskaya, D., Vikhreva, O., Zimina, I., Kolomeets, N., Vostrikov, V., and Rachmanova, V. (2001). Electron microscopy of oligodendroglia in severe mental illness. *Brain Res Bull*, 55, 597–610.

Ushijama, I., Yamada, K., and Furukawa, T. (1986). Behavioral effects of lithium on presynaptic sites of catecholaminergic neurons in the mouse. *Arch Int Pharmachodyn*, 282, 58–67.

Vacheron-Trystram, M.N., Cheref, S., and Gauillard, J. (2002). A case report of mania precipitated by use of DHEA. *Encephale*, 28(6 Pt. 1), 563–566.

Vaden, D.L., Ding, D., Peterson, B., and Greenberg, M.L. (2001). Lithium and valproate decrease inositol mass and increase expression of the yeast *INO1* and *INO2* genes for inositol biosynthesis. *J Biol Chem*, 276, 15466–15471.

Valberde, O., Tzavara, E., Hanoune, J., Roques, B.P., and Maldonado, R. (1996). Protein kinases in the rat nucleus accumbens are involved in the aversive component of opiate withdrawal. *Eur J Neurosci*, 8, 2671–2678.

Vallar, L., Muca, C., Magni, M., Albert, P., Bunzow, J., Meldolesi, J., and Civelli, O. (1990). Differential coupling of dopaminergic D2 receptors expressed in different cell types. Stimulation of phosphatidylinositol 4,5-bisphosphate hydrolysis in LtK-fibroblasts, hyperpolarization, and cytosolic-free Ca2+ concentration decrease in GH4C1 cells. *J Biol Chem*, 265, 10320–10326.

Valle, J., Ayuso-Gutierrez, J.L., and Abril, A. (1999). Evaluation of thyroid function in lithium-naive bipolar patients. *Eur Psychiatry*, 14(6), 341–345.

van Calker, D., and Belmaker, R.H. (2000). The high-affinity inositol transport system: Implications for the pathophysiology and treatment of bipolar disorder. *Bipolar Disord*, 2, 102–107.

van Calker, D., Steber, R., Klotz, K.N., and Greil, W. (1991). Carbamazepine distinguishes between adenosine receptors that mediate different second messenger responses. *Eur J Pharmacol*, 206, 285–290.

van Calker, D., Forstner, U., Bohus, M., Gebicke Harter, P., Hecht, H., Wark, H.J., and Berger, M. (1993). Increased sensitivity to agonist stimulation of the Ca2+ response in neutrophils of manic-depressive patients: Effect of lithium therapy. *Neuropsychobiology*, 27(3), 180–183.

van der Laan, J.W., de Boer, T., and Bruinvels, J. (1979). Di-n-propylacetate and GABA degradation. Preferential inhibition of succinic semialdehyde dehydrogenase and indirect inhibition of GABA-transaminase. *J Neurochem*, 32, 1769–1780.

Vanelle, J.M., Poirier, M.F., Benkelfat, C., Galinowski, A., Sechter, D., Suzini de Luca, H., and Loo, H. (1990). Diagnostic and therapeutic value of testing stimulation of thyroid-stimulating hormone by thyrotropin-releasing hormone in 100 depressed patients. *Acta Psychiatr Scand*, 81, 156–161.

Van Kammen, D.P., and Murphy, D.L. (1975). Attenuation of the euphoriant and activating effects of d- and l-amphetamine by lithium carbonate treatment. *Psychopharmacologia*, 44(3), 215–224.

Van Kammen, D.P., Docherty, J.P., Marder, S.R., Rosenblatt, J.E., and Bunney, W.E. Jr. (1985). Lithium attenuates the activation–euphoria but not the psychosis induced by d-amphetamine in schizophrenia. *Psychopharmacology (Berl)*, 87, 111–115.

Van Praag, H.M. (1982). Depression, suicide and the metabolism of serotonin in the brain. *J Affect Disord*, 4, 275–290.

Van Praag, H.M., and de Haan, S. (1979). Central serotonin metabolism and frequency of depression. *Psychiatry Res*, 1, 219–224.

Van Praag, H.M., and Korf, J. (1975). Central monoamine deficiency in depressions: Causative of secondary phenomenon? *Pharmakopsychiatr Neuropsychopharmakol*, 8, 322–326.

Van Praag, H., Christie, B.R., Sejnowski, T.J., and Gage, F.H. (1999). Running enhances neurogenesis, learning, and long-term potentiation in mice. *Proc Natl Acad Sci USA*, 96(23), 13427–13431.

Van Tits, L.J., Michel, M.C., Grosse-Wilde, H., Happel, M., Eigler, F.W., Soliman, A., and Brodde, O.E. (1990). Catecholamines increase lymphocyte beta 2-adrenergic receptors via a beta 2-adrenergic, spleen-dependent process. *Am J Physiol*, 258, E191–E202.

Vawter, M.P., Freed, W.J., and Kleinman, J.E. (2000). Neuropathology of bipolar disorder. *Biol Psychiatry*, 48(6), 486–504.

Vawter, M.P., Thatcher, L., Usen, N., Hyde, T.M., Kleinman, J.E., and Freed, W.J. (2002). Reduction of synapsin in the hippocampus of patients with bipolar disorder and schizophrenia. *Mol Psychiatry*, 7, 571–578.

Vecsei, L., and Widerlöv, E. (1988). Brain and CSF somatostatin concentrations in patients with psychiatric or neurological illness. An overview. *Acta Psychiatr Scand*, 78, 657–667.

Veith, R.C., Raskind, M.A., Barnes, R.F., Gumbrecht, G., Ritchie, J.L., and Halter, J.B. (1983). Tricyclic antidepressants and supine, standing, and exercise plasma norepinephrine levels. *Clin Pharmacol Ther*, 33, 763–769.

Veith, R.C., Halter, J.B., Murburg, M.M., et al. (1985). *Increased plasma NE appearance rate in dexamethasone resistant depression*. Fourth World Congress of Biological Psychiatry, Athens, Greece, October 13–17.

Veith, R.C., Barnes, R.F., Villacres, E., Murburg, M.M., Raskind, M.A., and Borson, S. (1988). Plasma catecholamines and norepinephrine kinetics in depression and panic disorder. In

R. Belmaker R (Ed.), *Catecholamines: Clinical Aspects* (pp. 197–202). New York: Alan R. Liss.

Veith, R.C., Lewis, N., Linares, O.A., Barnes, R.F., Raskind, M.A., Villacres, E.C., Murburg, M.M., Ashleigh, E.A., Castillo, S., and Peskind, E.R. (1994). Sympathetic nervous system activity in major depression. Basal and desipramine-induced alterations in plasma norepinephrine kinetics. *Arch Gen Psychiatry*, 51, 411–422.

Velayudhan, A., Sunitha, T.A., Balachander, S., Reddy, J.Y., and Khanna, S. (1999). A study of platelet serotonin receptor in mania. *Biol Psychiatry*, 45, 1059–1062.

Verbanck, P.M., Lotstra, F., Gilles, C., Linkowski, P., Mendlewicz, J., and Vanderhaeghen, J.J. (1984). Reduced cholecystokinin immunoreactivity in the cerebrospinal fluid of patients with psychiatric disorders. *Life Sci*, 34, 67–72.

Verimer, T., Goodale, D.B., Long, J.P., and Flynn, J.R. (1980). Lithium effects on haloperidol-induced pre- and postsynaptic dopamine receptor supersensitivity. *J Pharm Pharmacol*, 32, 665–666.

Virkkunen, M., De Jong, J., Bartko, J., and Linnoila, M. (1989). Psychobiological concomitants of history of suicide attempts among violent offenders and impulsive fire setters. *Arch Gen Psychiatry*, 46, 604–606.

Vogt, I.R., Shimron-Abarbanell, D., Neidt, H., Erdmann, J., Cichon, S., Schulze, T.G., Muller, D.J., Maier, W., Albus, M., Borrmann-Hassenbach, M., Knapp, M., Rietschel, M., Propping, P., and Nothen, M.M. (2000). Investigation of the human serotonin 6 [5-HT6] receptor gene in bipolar affective disorder and schizophrenia. *Am J Med Genet*, 96, 217–221.

Vollenweider, F.X., Maguire, R.P., Leenders, K.L., Mathys, K., and Angst, J. (1998). Effects of high amphetamine dose on mood and cerebral glucose metabolism in normal volunteers using positron emission tomography (PET). *Psychiatry Res*, 83(3), 149–162.

Volonte, C., and Rukenstein, A. (1993). Lithium chloride promotes short-term survival of PC12 cells after serum and NGF-deprivation. *Lithium*, 4, 211–219.

von Knorring, L., Oreland, L., Perris, C., and Runeberg, S. (1976). Lithium RBC/plasma ratio in subgroups of patients with affective disorders. *Neuropsychobiology*, 2(2-3), 74–80.

Vriend, J.P., and Alexiuk, N.A. (1996). Effects of valproate on amino acid and monoamine concentrations in striatum of audiogenic seizure-prone Balb/c mice. *Mol Chem Neuropathol*, 27, 307–324.

Vrontakis, M.E. (2002). Galanin: A biologically active peptide. *Curr Drug Targets CNS Neurol Disord*, 1(6), 531–541.

Wada, J.A., Osawa, T., Sato, M., Wake, A., Corcoran, M.E., and Troupin, A.S. (1976). Acute anticonvulsant effects of diphenylhydantoin, phenobarbital, and carbamazepine: A combined electroclinical and serum level study in amygdaloid kindled cats and baboons. *Epilepsia*, 17, 77–88.

Wada, K., Yamada, N., Suzuki, H., Lee, Y., and Kuroda, S. (2000). Recurrent cases of corticosteroid-induced mood disorder: Clinical characteristics and treatment. *J Clin Psychiatry*, 61(4), 261–267.

Wager-Smith, K., and Kay, S.A. (2000). Circadian rhythm genetics: From flies to mice to humans. *Nat Genet*, 26, 23–27.

Wahlestedt, C., Blendy, J.A., Kellar, K.J., Heilig, M., Widerlöv, E., and Ekman, R. (1990). Electroconvulsive shocks increase the concentration of neocortical and hippocampal neuropeptide Y (NPY)–like immunoreactivity in the rat. *Brain Res*, 507, 65–68.

Wakoh, H., and Hatotani, N. (1973). Endocrinological treatment of psychoses. In K. Lissák (Ed.), *Hormones and Brain Function* (pp. 491–498). New York: Plenum Press.

Waldman, I.D., Robinson, B.F., and Feigon, S.A. (1997). Linkage disequilibrium between the dopamine transporter gene (DAT1) and bipolar disorder: Extending the transmission disequilibrium test (TDT) to examine genetic heterogeneity. *Genet Epidemiol*, 14, 699–704.

Waldmeier, P.C., Baumann, P.A., Fehr, B., De Herdt, P., and Maitre, L. (1984). Carbamazepine decreases catecholamine turnover in the rat brain. *J Pharmacol Exp Ther*, 231, 166–172.

Wang, H.G., Rapp, U.R., and Reed, J.C. (1996). Bcl-2 targets the protein kinase Raf-1 to mitochondria. *Cell*, 87, 629–638.

Wang, H.Y., and Friedman, E. (1988). Chronic lithium: Desensitization of autoreceptors mediating serotonin release. *Psychopharmacology (Berl)*, 94, 312–314.

Wang, H.Y., and Friedman, E. (1996). Enhanced protein kinase C activity and translocation in bipolar affective disorder brains. *Biol Psychiatry*, 40, 568–575.

Wang, H.Y., and Friedman, E. (1999). Effects of lithium on receptor-mediated activation of G proteins in rat brain cortical membranes. *Neuropharmacology*, 38, 403–414.

Wang, H., and Friedman, E. (2001). Increased association of brain protein kinase C with the receptor for activated c kinase-1 (RACK1) in bipolar affective disorder. *Biol Psychiatry*, 50(5), 364–370.

Wang, H.Y., Markowitz, P., Levinson, D., Undie, A.S., and Friedman, E. (1999). Increased membrane-associated protein kinase C activity and translocation in blood platelets from bipolar affective disorder patients. *J Psychiatr Res*, 33, 171–179.

Wang, J.-F., Young, L.T., Li, P.P., and Warsh, J.J. (1997). Signal transduction abnormalities in bipolar disorder. In R.T. Joffe (Ed.), *Bipolar Disorder: Biological Models and Their Clinical Application* (pp. 41–79). New York: Dekker.

Wang, J.F., Asghari, V., Rockel, C., and Young, L.T. (1999). Cyclic AMP responsive element binding protein phosphorylation and DNA binding is decreased by chronic lithium but not valproate treatment of SH-SY5Y neuroblastoma cells. *Neuroscience*, 91, 771–776.

Wang, S.J., Huang, C.C., Hsu, K.S., Tsai, J.J., and Gean, P.W. (1996). Presynaptic inhibition of excitatory neurotransmission by lamotrigine in the rat amygdalar neurons. *Synapse*, 24, 248–255.

Warner-Schmidt, J.L., and Duman, R.S. (2006). Hippocampal neurogenesis: Opposing effects of stress and antidepressant treatment. *Hippocampus*, 16(3), 239–249.

Warsh, J., Young, L., and Li, P. (2000). Guanine nucleotide binding (G) protein disturbances. In R. Belmaker (Ed.), *Bipolar Affective Disorder in Bipolar Medications: Mechanisms of Action* (pp. 299–329). Washington, DC: American Psychiatric Press.

Watanabe, Y., Gould, E., Daniels, D.C., Cameron, H., and McEwen, B.S. (1992). Tianeptine attenuates stress-induced morphological changes in the hippocampus. *Eur J Pharmacol*, 222, 157–162.

Watson, D.G., Watterson, J.M., and Lenox, R.H. (1998). Sodium valproate down-regulates the myristoylated alanine-rich C kinase substrate (MARCKS) in immortalized hippocampal cells: A property of protein kinase C–mediated mood stabilizers. *J Pharmacol Exp Ther*, 285(1), 307–316.

Watts, B.V., and Grady, T.A. (1997). Tramadol-induced mania. *Am J Psychiatry*, 154, 1624.

Weaver, I.C., Cervoni, N., Champagne, F.A., D'Alessio, A.C., Sharma, S., Seckl, J.R., Dymov, S., Szyf, M., and Meaney, M.J. (2004). Epigenetic programming by maternal behavior. *Nat Neurosci*, 7(8), 847–854.

Webster, E.L., Lewis, D.B., Torpy, D.J., Zachman, E.K., Rice, K.C., and Chrousos, G.P. (1996). In vivo and in vitro characterization of antalarmin, a nonpeptide corticotropin-releasing hormone (CRH) receptor antagonist: Suppression of pituitary ACTH release and peripheral inflammation. *Endocrinology*, 137(12), 5747–5750.

Webster, M.J., Knable, M.B., O'Grady, J., Orthmann, J., and Weickert, C.S. (1999). Decreased glucocorticoid receptor mRNA levels in individuals with depression, bipolar disorder and schizophrenia. *Schizophr Res*, 41, 111.

Webster, M.J., Knable, M.B., O'Grady, J., Orthmann, J., and Weickert, C.S. (2002). Regional specificity of brain glucocorticoid receptor mRNA alterations in subjects with schizophrenia and mood disorders. *Mol Psychiatry*, 7(9), 924, 985–994.

Weeke, A., and Weeke, J. (1978). Disturbed circadian variation of serum thyrotropin in patients with endogenous depression. *Acta Psychiatr Scand*, 57, 281–289.

Weeke, J. (1973). Circadian variation of the serum thyrotropin level in normal subjects. *Scand J Clin Lab Invest*, 31, 337–342.

Wehr, T.A. (1977). Phase and biorhythm studies of affective illness. In W.E. Bunney Jr. (Ed.), The switch process in manic-depressive psychosis. *Ann Intern Med*, 87, 319–335.

Wehr, T.A., and Goodwin, F.K. (1987). Can antidepressants cause mania and worsen the course of affective illness? *Am J Psychiatry*, 144, 1403–1411.

Wehr, T.A., Sack, D.A., and Rosenthal, N.E. (1987). Sleep reduction as a final common pathway in the genesis of mania. *Am J Psychiatry*, 144, 201–204.

Wehr, T.A., Sack, D.A., Rosenthal, N.E., and Cowdry, R.W. (1988). Rapid cycling affective disorder: Contributing factors and treatment responses in 51 patients. *Am J Psychiatry*, 145, 179–184.

Wei, H., Qin, Z.H., Senatorov, V.V., Wei, W., Wang, Y., Qian, Y., and Chuang, D.M. (2001). Lithium suppresses excitotoxicity-induced striatal lesions in a rat model of Huntington's disease. *Neuroscience*, 106(3), 603–612.

Wei, Q., Lu, X.Y., Liu, L., Schafer, G., Shieh, K.R., Burke, S., Robinson, T.E., Watson, S.J., Seasholtz, A.F., and Akil, H. (2004). Glucocorticoid receptor overexpression in forebrain: A mouse model of increased emotional lability. *Proc Natl Acad Sci USA*, 101(32), 11851–11856.

Weinberger, D.R., Egan, M.F., Bertolino, A., Callicott, J.H., Mattay, V.S., Lipska, B.K., Berman, K.F., and Goldberg, T.E. (2001). Prefrontal neurons and the genetics of schizophrenia. *Biol Psychiatry*, 50, 825–844.

Weiner, R.D., Krystal, A.D., Coffey, C.E., and Smith, P. (1992). The electrophysiology of ECT: Relevance to mechanism of action. *Clin Neuropharmacol*, 15(Suppl. 1, Pt. A), 671A–672A.

Weingartner, H., Gold, P., Ballenger, J.C., Smallberg, S.A., Summers, R., Rubinow, D.R., Post, R.M., and Goodwin, F.K. (1981). Effects of vasopressin on human memory functions. *Science*, 211, 601–603.

Weintraub, B. (1995). *Molecular Endocrinology: Basic Concepts and Clinical Correlations*. New York: Raven Press.

Weiss, S.R., and Post, R.M. (1994). Caveats in the use of the kindling model of affective disorders. *Toxicol Ind Health*, 10, 421–447.

Weiss, E.L., Bowers, M.B. Jr., and Mazure, C.M. (1999). Testosterone-patch-induced psychotic mania. *Am J Psychiatry*, 156, 969.

Weiss, J.M., and Kilts, C.D. (1998). Animal models of depression and schizophrenia. In A.F. Schatzerg and C.B. Nemeroff (Eds.), *Textbook of Psychopharmacology* (pp. 89–131). Washington, DC: American Psychiatric Press.

Weiss, J.M., Goodman, P., Ambrose, M.J., Webster, A., and Hoffman, L.J. (1984). Neurochemical basis of behavioral depression. In E. Katkin and S. Manuck (Eds.), *Advances in Behavioral Medicine* (pp. 233–276). Greenwich, CT: JAI Press.

Weiss, J.M., Bonsall, R.W., Demetrikopoulos, M.K., Emery, M.S., and West, C.H. (1998). Galanin: A significant role in depression? *Ann NY Acad Sci*, 863, 364–382.

Weiss, S.R., Post, R.M., Costello, M., Nutt, D.J., and Tandeciarz, S. (1990). Carbamazepine retards the development of cocaine-kindled seizures but not sensitization to cocaine-induced hyperactivity. *Neuropsychopharmacology*, 3, 273–281.

Weiss, S.R., Post, R.M., Sohn, E., Berger, A., and Lewis R. (1993). Cross-tolerance between carbamazepine and valproate on amygdala-kindled seizures. *Epilepsy Res*, 16(1), 37–44.

Weiss, S.R., Li, X.L., Rosen, J.B., Li, H., Heynen, T., and Post, R.M. (1995). Quenching: Inhibition of development and expression of amygdala kindled seizures with low frequency stimulation. *Neuroreport*, 6(16), 2171–2176.

Weissman, M.M., Leaf, P.J., Tischler, G.L., Blazer, D.G., Karno, M., Bruce, M.L., and Florio, L.P. (1988). Affective disorders in five United States communities. *Psychol Med*, 18, 141–153.

Weller, E.B., and Weller, R.A. (1988). Neuroendocrine changes in affectively ill children and adolescents. *Neurol Clin*, 6, 41–54.

Wellman, C.L. (2001). Dendritic reorganization in pyramidal neurons in medial prefrontal cortex after chronic corticosterone administration. *J Neurobiol*, 49, 245–253.

Weng, G., Bhalla, U.S., and Iyengar, R. (1999). Complexity in biological signaling systems. *Science*, 284, 92–96.

Wersinger, S.R., Ginns, E.I., O'Carroll, A.M., Lolait, S.J., and Young, W.S. III. (2002). Vasopressin v1b receptor knockout reduces aggressive behavior in male mice. *Mol Psychiatry*, 7(9), 975–984.

Werstiuk, E.S., Steiner, M., and Burns, T. (1990). Studies on leukocyte beta-adrenergic receptors in depression: A critical appraisal. *Life Sci*, 47(2), 85–105. Review. Erratum in: *Life Sci*, 47(21), 1979–1980.

Weston, P.G., and Howard, M.Q. (1922). The determination of Na, K, Ca, and Mg in the blood and spinal fluid of patients suffering from manic-depressive insanity. *Arch Neurol Psychiatry*, 8, 179–183.

Whalley, L.J., Christie, J.E., Bennie, J., Dick, H., Blackburn, I.M., Blackwood, D., Sanchez Watts, G., and Fink, G. (1985). Selective increase in plasma luteinising hormone concentrations in drug free young men with mania. *BMJ (Clin Res Ed)*, 290, 99–102.

Whalley, L.J., Kutcher, S., Blackwood, D.H., Bennie, J., Dick, H., and Fink, G. (1987). Increased plasma LH in manic-depressive illness: Evidence of a state-independent abnormality. *Br J Psychiatry*, 150, 682–684.

Whittle, S.R., and Turner, A.J. (1978). Effects of the anticonvulsant sodium valproate on gamma-aminobutyrate and aldehyde metabolism in ox brain. *J Neurochem*, 31, 1453–1459.

Whitworth, P., and Kendall, D.A. (1989). Effects of lithium on inositol phospholipid hydrolysis and inhibition of dopamine

D1 receptor-mediated cyclic AMP formation by carbachol in rat brain slices. *J Neurochem*, 53, 536–541.

Whybrow, P.C. (1994). The therapeutic use of triiodothyronine and high dose thyroxine in psychiatric disorder. *Acta Med Austriaca*, 21, 47–52.

Wiborg, O., Kruger, T., and Jakobsen, S.N. (1999). Region-selective effects of long-term lithium and carbamazepine administration on cyclic AMP levels in rat brain. *Pharmacol Toxicol*, 84(2), 88–93.

Widdowson, P.S., Ordway, G.A., and Halaris, A.E. (1992). Reduced neuropeptide Y concentrations in suicide brain. *J Neurochem*, 59, 73–80.

Widerlöv, E., Bissette, G., and Nemeroff, C.B. (1988a). Monoamine metabolites, corticotropin releasing factor and somatostatin as CSF markers in depressed patients. *J Affect Disord*, 14, 99–107.

Widerlöv, E., Lindstrom, L.H., Wahlestedt, C., and Ekman, R. (1988b). Neuropeptide Y and peptide YY as possible cerebrospinal fluid markers for major depression and schizophrenia, respectively. *J Psychiatr Res*, 22, 69–79.

Widner, B., Leblhuber, F., Walli, J., Tilz, G.P., Demel, U., and Fuchs, D. (1999). Degradation of tryptophan in neurodegenerative disorders. *Adv Exp Med Biol*, 467, 133–138.

Williams, D., Lee, T.D., Dinh, N., and Young, M.K. (2000). Oligosaccharide profiling: The facile detection of mono-, di- and oligosaccharides by electrospray orthogonal time-of-flight mass spectrometry using 3-aminophenylboronic acid derivatization. *Rapid Commun Mass Spectrom*, 14(16), 1530–1537.

Williams, J.A., and Sehgal, A. (2001). Molecular components of the circadian system in *Drosophila*. *Annu Rev Physiol*, 63, 729–755.

Williams, N., Layden, B.T., Suhy, J., Metreger, T., Foley, K., Abukhdeir, A.M., Borge, G., Crayton, J., Bryant, F.B., and Mota de Freitas, D. (2003). Testing competing path models linking the biochemical variables in red blood cells from li+-treated bipolar patients. *Bipolar Disord*, 5(5), 320–329.

Willner, P. (1983). Dopamine and depression: A review of recent evidence. I. Empirical studies. *Brain Res*, 287(3), 211–224.

Willner, P. (1984). The validity of animal models of depression. *Psychopharmacology*, 83, 1–16.

Willner, P. (1991). Animal models as simulations of depression. *Trends Pharmacol Sci*, 12, 131–136.

Willner, P. (1995). Animal models of depression: Validity and applications. In G. Serra (Ed.), *Depression and Mania: From Neurobiology to Treatment* (Vol. 49) (pp. 19–42). New York: Raven Press.

Witkin, J.M. (1993). Blockade of the locomotor stimulant effects of cocaine and methamphetamine by glutamate antagonists. *Life Sci*, 53(24), PL405–410.

Wolfe, N., Katz, D.I., Albert, M.L., Almozlino, A., Durso, R., Smith, M.C., and Volicer, L. (1990). Neuropsychological profile linked to low dopamine. In Alzheimer's disease, major depression, and Parkinson's disease. *J Neurol Neurosurg Psychiatry*, 53, 915–917.

Wolkowitz, O.M., and Reus, V.I. (1999). Treatment of depression with antiglucocorticoid drugs. *Psychosom Med*, 61(5), 698–711.

Wolkowitz, O.M., Reus, V.I., Weingartner, H., Thompson, K., Breier, A., Doran, A., Rubinow, D., and Pickar, D. (1990). Cognitive effects of corticosteroids. *Am J Psychiatry*, 147(10), 1297–1303.

Wolkowitz, O.M., Reus, V.I., Roberts, E., Manfredi, F., Chan, T., Raum, W.J., Ormiston, S., Johnson, R., Canick, J., Brizendine, L., and Weingartner, H. (1997). Dehydroepiandrosterone (DHEA) treatment of depression. *Biol Psychiatry*, 41(3), 311–318.

Wolkowitz, O.M., Reus, V.I., Keebler, A., Nelson, N., Friedland, M., Brizendine, L., and Roberts, E. (1999). Double-blind treatment of major depression with dehydroepiandrosterone. *Am J Psychiatry*, 156(4), 646–649.

Wong, M.L., Kling, M.A., Munson, P.J., Listwak, S., Licinio, J., Prolo, P., Karp, B., McCutcheon, I.E., Geracioti, T.D. Jr., DeBellis, M.D., Rice, K.C., Goldstein, D.S., Veldhuis, J.D., Chrousos, G.P., Oldfield, E.H., McCann, S.M., and Gold, P.W. (2000). Pronounced and sustained central hypernoradrenergic function in major depression with melancholic features: Relation to hypercortisolism and corticotropin-releasing hormone. *Proc Natl Acad Sci USA*, 97(1), 325–330.

Wood, A.J., Elphick, M., and Grahame-Smith, D.G. (1989). Effect of lithium and of other drugs used in the treatment of manic illness on the cation-transporting properties of Na+,K+-ATPase in mouse brain synaptosomes. *J Neurochem*, 52, 1042–1049.

Wood, K., and Coppen, A. (1983). Prophylactic lithium treatment of patients with affective disorders is associated with decreased platelet [3H]dihydroergocryptine binding. *J Affect Disord*, 5, 253–258.

Woodgett, J.R. (2001). Judging a protein by more than its name: GSK–3. *Sci STKE*, 2001, RE12.

Woodside, B., Zilli, C., and Fisman, S. (1989). Biologic markers and bipolar disease in children. *Can J Psychiatry*, 34, 128–131.

Wright, A.F., Crichton, D.N., Loudon, J.B., Morten, J.E., and Steel, C.M. (1984). Beta-adrenoceptor binding defects in cell lines from families with manic-depressive disorder. *Ann Hum Genet*, 48(Pt. 3), 201–214.

Wyatt, R.J., Portnoy, B., Kupfer, D.J., Snyder, F., and Engelman, K. (1971). Resting plasma catecholamine concentrations in patients with depression and anxiety. *Arch Gen Psychiatry*, 24, 65–70.

Xing, G.Q., Russell, S., Webster, M.J., and Post, R.M. (2004). Decreased expression of mineralocorticoid receptor mRNA in the prefrontal cortex in schizophrenia and bipolar disorder. *Int J Neuropsychopharmacol*, 7(2), 143–153.

Xu, J., Culman, J., Blume, A., Brecht, S., and Gohlke, P. (2003). Chronic treatment with a low dose of lithium protects the brain against ischemic injury by reducing apoptotic death. *Stroke*, 34(5), 1287–1292.

Yamawaki, S., Kagaya, A., Okamoto, Y., Shimizu, M., Nishida, A., and Uchitomi, Y. (1996). Enhanced calcium response to serotonin in platelets from patients with affective disorders. *J Psychiatry Neurosci*, 21, 321–324.

Yan, Q.S., Mishra, P.K., Burger, R.L., Bettendorf, A.F., Jobe, P.C., and Dailey, J.W. (1992). Evidence that carbamazepine and antiepilepsirine may produce a component of their anticonvulsant effects by activating serotonergic neurons in genetically epilepsy-prone rats. *J Pharmacol Exp Ther*, 261, 652–659.

Yang, J.C., and Cortopassi, G.A. (1998). Induction of the mitochondrial permeability transition causes release of the apoptogenic factor cytochrome c. *Free Radic Biol Med*, 24(4), 624–631.

Yatham, L.N. (1996). Prolactin and cortisol responses to fenfluramine challenge in mania. *Biol Psychiatry*, 39(4), 285–288.

Yatham, L.N., Zis, A.P., Lam, R.W., Tam, E., and Shiah, I.S. (1997). Sumatriptan-induced growth hormone release in patients with major depression, mania, and normal controls. *Neuropsychopharmacology*, 17, 258–263.

Yatham, L.N., Liddle, P.F., Shiah, I.S., Scarrow, G., Lam, R.W., Adam, M.J., Zis, A.P., and Ruth, T.J. (2000). Brain serotonin2 receptors in major depression: A positron emission tomography study. *Arch Gen Psychiatry*, 57, 850–858.

Yatham, L.N., Liddle, P.F., Shiah, I.S., Lam, R.W., Ngan, E., Scarrow, G., Imperial, M., Stoessl, J., Sossi, V., and Ruth, T.J. (2002). PET study of [¹⁸F]6-fluoro-L-dopa uptake in neuroleptic- and mood-stabilizer-naive first-episode nonpsychotic mania: Effects of treatment with divalproex sodium. *Am J Psychiatry*, 159, 768–774.

Yehuda, S., Carasso, R.L., and Mostofsky, D.I. (1994). Essential fatty acid preparation (SR-3) raises the seizure threshold in rats. *Eur J Pharmacol*, 254, 193–198.

Yildiz, A., Demopulos, C.M., Moore, C.M., Renshaw, P.F., and Sachs, G.S. (2001). Effect of lithium on phosphoinositide metabolism in human brain: A proton decoupled (31)P magnetic resonance spectroscopy study. *Biol Psychiatry*, 50, 3–7.

Yoon, I.S., Li, P.P., Siu, K.P., Kennedy, J.L., Cooke, R.G., Parikh, S.V., and Warsh, J.J. (2001). Altered *IMPA2* gene expression and calcium homeostasis in bipolar disorder. *Mol Psychiatry*, 6, 678–683.

Young, A.H. (2006) Antiglucocoticoid treatments for depression. *Aust N Z J Psychiatry*, 40(5), 402–405.

Young, A.H., Gallagher, P., Watson, S., Del-Estal, D., Owen, B.M., and Ferrier, I.N. (2004). Improvements in neurocognitive function and mood following adjunctive treatment with mifepristone (RU-486) in bipolar disorder. *Neuropsychopharmacology*, 29(8), 1538–1545.

Young, C.E., Arima, K., Xie, J., Hu, L., Beach, T.G., Falkai, P., and Honer, W.G. (1998). SNAP-25 deficit and hippocampal connectivity in schizophrenia. *Cereb Cortex*, 8(3), 261–268.

Young, E.A., Watson, S.J., Kotun, H., Haskett, R.J., Grunhaus, L., Murphy-Weinberg, V., Vale, W., Rivier, J., and Akil, H. (1990). Beta-lipotropin-beta-endorphin response to low-dose ovine corticotropin releasing factor in endogenous depression. *Arch Gen Psychiatry*, 47(5), 449–457.

Young, E.A., Lopez, J.F., Murphy-Weinberg, V., Watson, S.J., and Akil, H. (2003). Mineralocorticoid receptor function in major depression. *Arch Gen Psychiatry*, 60(1), 24–28.

Young, L.T., and Woods, C.M. (1996). Mood stabilizers have differential effects on endogenous ADP ribosylation in C6 glioma cells. *Eur J Pharmacol*, 309, 215–218.

Young, L.T., Li, P.P., Kish, S.J., Siu, K.P., Kamble, A, Hornykiewicz, O., and Warsh, J.J. (1993). Cerebral cortex Gs alpha protein levels and forskolin-stimulated cyclic AMP formation are increased in bipolar affective disorder. *J Neurochem*, 61, 890–898.

Young, L.T., Li, P.P., Kamble, A., Siu, K.P., and Warsh, J.J. (1994a). Mononuclear leukocyte levels of G proteins in depressed patients with bipolar disorder or major depressive disorder. *Am J Psychiatry*, 151(4), 594–596.

Young, L.T., Li, P.P., Kish, S.J., and Warsh, J.J. (1994b). Cerebral cortex beta-adrenoceptor binding in bipolar affective disorder. *J Affect Disord*, 30, 89–92.

Young, L.T., Warsh, J.J., Kish, S.J., Shannak, K., and Hornykeiwicz, O. (1994c). Reduced brain 5-HT and elevated NE turnover and metabolites in bipolar affective disorder. *Biol Psychiatry*, 35, 121–127.

Young, L.T., Wang, J.F., Woods, C.M., and Robb, J.C. (1999). Platelet protein kinase C alpha levels in drug-free and lithium-treated subjects with bipolar disorder. *Neuropsychobiology*, 40(2), 63–66.

Young, R.C., Moline, M., and Kleyman, F. (1997). Hormone replacement therapy and late-life mania. *Am J Geriatr Psychiatry*, 5, 179–181.

Yuan, P.X., Chen, G., Huang, L.D., and Manji, H.K. (1998). Lithium stimulates gene expression through the AP-1 transcription factor pathway. *Brain Res Mol Brain Res*, 58, 225–230.

Yuan, P.X., Huang, L.D., Jiang, Y.M., Gutkind, J.S., Manji, H.K., and Chen, G. (2001). The mood stabilizer valproic acid activates mitogen-activated protein kinases and promotes neurite growth. *J Biol Chem*, 276, 31674–31683.

Yuan, P.X., Gould, T.D., Gray, N.A., Bachmann, R.F., Schloesser, R.J., Lan, M., Du, J., Moore, G.J., and Manji, H.K. (2004). Neurotrophic signaling cascades are major long-term targets for lithium: Clinical implications. *Clin Neurosci Res*, 4, 137–153.

Yuan, P.X., Zhou, R., Farzad, N., Gould, T.D., Gray, N.A., Du, J., and Manji, H.K. (2005). Enhancing resilience to stress: The role of signaling cascades. In N. Steckler, J.M. Kalin, and H.M. Reul (Eds.), *Handbook on Stress, Immunology and Behaviour*. Amsterdam: Elsevier.

Zach, J., and Ackerman, S.H. (1988). Thyroid function, metabolic regulation, and depression. *Psychosom Med*, 50(5), 454–468.

Zachrisson, O., Mathe, A.A., Stenfors, C., and Lindefors, N. (1995). Limbic effects of repeated electroconvulsive stimulation on neuropeptide Y and somatostatin mRNA expression in the rat brain. *Brain Res Mol Brain Res*, 31, 71–85.

Zachrisson, O., Mathe, A.A., and Lindefors, N. (1996). Effects of chronic lithium and electroconvulsive stimuli on cholecystokinin mRNA expression in the rat brain. *Brain Res Mol Brain Res*, 43, 347–350.

Zanardi, R., Racagni, G., Smeraldi, E., and Perez, J. (1997). Differential effects of lithium on platelet protein phosphorylation in bipolar patients and healthy subjects. *Psychopharmacology (Berl)*, 129(1), 44–47.

Zanardi, R., Serretti, A., Rossini, D., Franchini, L., Cusin, C., Lattuada, E., Dotoli, D., and Smeraldi, E. (2001). Factors affecting fluvoxamine antidepressant activity: Influence of pindolol and 5-HTTLPR in delusional and nondelusional depression. *Biol Psychiatry*, 50, 323–330.

Zarate, C.A. Jr., and Quiroz, J.A. (2003). Combination treatment in bipolar disorder: A review of controlled trials. *Bipolar Disord*, 5(3), 217–225.

Zarate, C.A., Tohen, M., and Zarate, S.B. (1997). Thyroid function tests in first-episode bipolar disorder manic and mixed types. *Biol Psychiatry*, 42(4), 302–304.

Zarate, C.A. Jr., Quiroz J.A., Payne, J.L., and Manji, H.K. (2002). Modulators of the glutamatergic system: Implications for the development of improved therapeutics in mood disorders. *Psychopharmacol Bull*, 36, 35–83.

Zarate, C.A., Du, J., Quiroz, J., Gray, N.A., Denicoff, K.D., Singh, J., Charney, D.S., and Manji, H.K. (2003). Regulation of cellular plasticity cascades in the pathophysiology and treatment of mood disorder: Role of the glutamatergic system. *Ann N Y Acad Sci*, 1003, 273–291.

Zarate, C.A. Jr., Payne, J.L., Quiroz, J., Sporn, J., Denicoff, K.K., Luckenbaugh, D., Charney, D.S., and Manji, H.K. (2004a). An open-label trial of riluzole in patients with treatment-resistant major depression. *Am J Psychiatry*, 161(1), 171–174.

Zarate, C.A., Singh, J., Payne, J.L., Quiroz, J., Denicoff, K., Luckenbaugh, D.A., Charney, D.S., and Manji, H.K. (2004b). A double-blind, randomized, placebo-controlled pilot study examining the efficacy of pramipexole in bipolar II depression. *Biol Psychiatry*, 56, 54–60.

Zarate, C.A. Jr., Payne, J.L., Singh, J., Quiroz, J.A., Luckenbaugh, D.A., Denicoff, K.D., Charney, D.S., and Manji, H.K. (2004c). Pramipexole for bipolar II depression: A placebo-controlled proof of concept study. *Biol Psychiatry*, 56(1), 54–60.

Zarate, C.A., Quiroz, J.A., Singh, J., Denicoff, K., De Jesus, G., Luckenbaugh, D., Charney, D.S., and Manji, H.K. (2005). An openlabel trial of the antiglutamatergic agent riluzole in treatmentresistant bipolar depression. *Biol Psychiatry*, 57, 430–432.

Zarate, C.A., Singh, J., Quiroz, J.A., DeJesus, G., Denicoff, K., Luckenbaugh, D.A., Manji, H.K., and Charney, D.S. (2006a). A double-blind, placebo-controlled study of memantine in the treatment of major depression. *Am J Psychiatry*, 163, 153–155.

Zarate, C.A. Jr., Singh, J., and Manji, H.K. (2006b). Cellular plasticity cascades: Targets for the development of novel therapeutics for bipolar disorder. *Biol Psychiatry*, 59(11), 1006–1020.

Zerahn, K. (1955). Studies on the active transport of lithium in the isolated frog skin. *Acta Physiol Scand*, 33, 347–358.

Zhang, L., Elmer, L.W., and Little, K.Y. (1998). Expression and regulation of the human dopamine transporter in a neuronal cell line. *Brain Res Mol Brain Res*, 59, 66–73.

Zhou, J.N., Riemersma, R.F., Unmehopa, U.A., Hoogendijk, W.J., van Heerikhuize, J.J., Hofman, M.A., and Swaab, D.F. (2001). Alterations in arginine vasopressin neurons in the suprachiasmatic nucleus in depression. *Arch Gen Psychiatry*, 58(7), 655–662.

Zhou, L., An, N., Jiang, W., Haydon, R., Cheng, H., Zhou, Q., Breyer, B., Feng, T., and He, T.C. (2002). Fluorescence-based functional assay for Wnt/beta-catenin signaling activity. *Biotechniques*, 33, 1126–1128, 1130, 1132 passim.

Zhou, R., Gray, N., Yuan, P., Li, X., Chen, J.S., Chen, G., Damschroder-Williams, P., Du, J., Zhang, L., and Manji, H.K. (2005). The anti-apoptotic, glucocorticoid receptor cochaperone protein BAG-1 is a long-term target for the actions of mood stabilizers. *J Neurosci*, 25, 4493–4502.

Zhu, G., Okada, M., Murakami, T., Kawata, Y., Kamata, A., and Kaneko, S. (2002). Interaction between carbamazepine, zonisamide and voltage-sensitive Ca2+ channel on acetylcholine release in rat frontal cortex. *Epilepsy Res*, 49, 49–60.

Zigova, T., Willing, A.E., Tedesco, E.M., Borlongan, C.V., Saporta, S., Snable, G.L., and Sanberg, P.R. (1999). Lithium chloride induces the expression of tyrosine hydroxylase in hNT neurons. *Exp Neurol*, 157, 251–258.

Zobel, A.W., Yassouridis, A., Frieboes, R.M., and Holsboer, F. (1999). Prediction of medium-term outcome by cortisol response to the combined dexamethasone-CRH test in patients with remitted depression. *Am J Psychiatry*, 156, 949–951.

Zobel, A.W., Nickel, T., Kunzel, H.E., Ackl, N., Sonntag, A., Ising, M., and Holsboer, F. (2000). Effects of the high-affinity corticotropin-releasing hormone receptor 1 antagonist R121919 in major depression: The first 20 patients treated. *J Psychiatr Res*, 34, 171–181.

Zohar, J., Bannet, J., Drummer, D., Fisch, R., Epstein, R.P., and Belmaker, R.H. (1983). The response of lymphocyte betaadrenergic receptors to chronic propranolol treatment in depressed patients, schizophrenic patients, and normal controls. *Biol Psychiatry*, 18, 553–560.

Zohar, J., Drummer, D., Edelstein, E.D., Kaiser, N., Belmaker, R.H., and Nir, I. (1985). Effect of lysine vasopressin in depressed patients on mood and 24-hour rhythm of growth hormone, cortisol, melatonin and prolactin. *Psychoneuroendocrinology*, 10, 273–279.

Zubieta, J.K., Huguelet, P., Ohl, L.E., Koeppe, R.A., Kilbourn, M.R., Carr, J.M., Giordani, B.J., and Frey, K.A. (2000). High vesicular monoamine transporter binding in asymptomatic bipolar I disorder: Sex differences and cognitive correlates. *Am J Psychiatry*, 157, 1619–1628.

Zubieta, J.K., Huguelet, P., O'Neil, R.L., and Giordani, B.J. (2001). Cognitive function in euthymic bipolar I disorder. *Psychiatry Res*, 102, 9–20.

Zucker, M., Weizman, A., Harel, D., and Rehavi, M. (2001). Changes in vesicular monoamine transporter (VMAT2) and synaptophysin in rat substantia nigra and prefrontal cortex induced by psychotropic drugs. *Neuropsychobiology*, 44, 187–191.

CHAPTER 15

Abas, M.A., Sahakian, B.J., and Levy, R. (1990). Neuropsychological deficits and CT scan changes in elderly depressives. *Psychol Med*, 20(3), 507–520.

Abercrombie, H.C., Schaefer, S.M., Larson, C.L., Oakes, T.R., Lindgren, K.A., Holden, J.E., Perlman, S.B., Turski, P.A., Krahn, D.D., Benca, R.M., and Davidson, R.J. (1998). Metabolic rate in the right amygdala predicts negative affect in depressed patients. *Neuroreport*, 9(14), 3301–3307.

Abou-Saleh, M.T., Al Suhaili, A.R., Karim, L., Prais, V., and Hamdi, E. (1999). Single photon emission tomography with 99mTc-HMPAO in Arab patients with depression. *J Affect Disord*, 55(2-3), 115–123.

Adler, C.M., Holland, S.K., Schmithorst, V., Wilke, M., Weiss, K.L., Pan, H., and Strakowski, S.M. (2004). Abnormal frontal white matter tracts in bipolar disorder: A diffusion tensor imaging study. *Bipolar Disord*, 6(3), 197–203.

Adler, C.M., Levine, A.D., DelBello, M.P., and Strakowski, S.M. (2005). Changes in gray matter volume in patients with bipolar disorder. *Biol Psychiatry*, 58(2), 151–157.

Adler, C.M., Adams, J., DelBello, M.P., Holland, S.K., Schmithorst, V., Levine, A., Jarvis, K., and Strakowski, S.M. (2006). Evidence of white matter pathology in bipolar disorder adolescents experiencing their first episode of mania: A diffusion tensor imaging study. *Am J Psychiatry*, 163(2), 322–324.

Agam, G., and Shimon, H. (2000). Human evidence of the role of inositol in bipolar disorder and antibipolar treatment. In C.L. Bowden and R.H. Belmaker (Eds.), *Bipolar Medications: Mechanisms of Action* (pp. 31–45). Washington, DC: American Psychiatric Press.

Ahearn, E.P., Steffens, D.C., Cassidy, F., Van Meter, S.A., Provenzale, J.M., Seldin, M.F., Weisler, R.H., and Krishnan, K.R. (1998). Familial leukoencephalopathy in bipolar disorder. *Am J Psychiatry*, 155(11), 1605–1607.

Alexander, G.E., Crutcher, M.D., and DeLong, M.R. (1990). Basal ganglia–thalamocortical circuits: Parallel substrates for motor, oculomotor, prefrontal and limbic functions. *Prog Brain Res*, 85, 119–146.

Alexopoulos, G.S., Young, R.C., and Shindledecker, R.D. (1992). Brain computed tomography findings in geriatric depression and primary degenerative dementia. *Biol Psychiatry*, 31(6), 591–599.

Alexopoulos, G.S., Meyers, B.S., Young, R.C., Kakuma, T., Silbersweig, D., and Charlson, M. (1997). Clinically defined vascular depression. *Am J Psychiatry*, 154(4), 562–565.

Ali, S.O., Denicoff, K.D., Altshuler, L.L., Hauser, P., Li, X., Conrad, A.J., Mirsky, A.F., Smith-Jackson, E.E., and Post, R.M. (2000). A preliminary study of the relation of neuropsychological performance to neuroanatomic structures in bipolar disorder. *Neuropsychiatry Neuropsychol Behav Neurol*, 13(1), 20–28.

al-Mousawi, A.H., Evans, N., Ebmeier, K.P., Roeda, D., Chaloner, F., and Ashcroft, G.W. (1996). Limbic dysfunction in schizophrenia and mania. A study using ^{18}F-labelled fluorodeoxyglucose and positron emission tomography. *Br J Psychiatry*, 169(4), 509–516.

Altshuler, L.L., Devinsky, O., Post, R.M., and Theodore, W. (1990). Depression, anxiety, and temporal lobe epilepsy. Laterality of focus and symptoms. *Arch Neurol*, 47(3), 284–288.

Altshuler, L.L., Conrad, A., Hauser, P., Li, X.M., Guze, B.H., Denikoff, K., Tourtellotte, W., and Post, R. (1991). Reduction of temporal lobe volume in bipolar disorder: A preliminary report of magnetic resonance imaging [letter]. *Arch Gen Psychiatry*, 48(5), 482–483.

Altshuler, L.L., Curran, J.G., Hauser, P., Mintz, J., Denicoff, K., and Post, R. (1995). T$_2$ hyperintensities in bipolar disorder: Magnetic resonance imaging comparison and literature meta-analysis. *Am J Psychiatry*, 152(8), 1139–1144.

Altshuler, L.L., Bartzokis, G., Grieder, T., Curran, J., and Mintz, J. (1998). Amygdala enlargement in bipolar disorder and hippocampal reduction in schizophrenia: An MRI study demonstrating neuroanatomic specificity [letter]. *Arch Gen Psychiatry*, 55(7), 663–664.

Altshuler, L.L., Bartzokis, G., Grieder, T., Curran, J., Jimenez, T., Leight, K., Wilkins, J., Gerner, R., and Mintz, J. (2000). An MRI study of temporal lobe structures in men with bipolar disorder or schizophrenia. *Biol Psychiatry*, 48(2), 147–162.

Amaral, J.A., Lafer, B., et al. (2002). *A H-MRS study of the anterior cingulate gyrus in euthymic bipolar patients taking lithium.* 57th Annual Convention and Scientific Program of the Society of Biological Psychiatry, Philadelphia, PA, May 16–18.

Ames, D., Dolan, R., and Mann, A. (1990). The distinction between depression and dementia in the very old. *Int J Geriatr Psychiatry*, 5, 193–198.

Amsterdam, J.D. and Mozley, P.D. (1992). Temporal lobe asymmetry with iofetamine (IMP) SPECT imaging in patients with major depression. *J Affect Disord*, 24(1), 43–53.

Amsterdam, J.D., Mozley, P.D., et al. (1995). ^{123}I-iofetamine (IMP) SPECT brain imaging in depressed patients: Normalization of temporal lobe asymmetry during clinical recovery. *Depression*, 6(3), 273–283.

Andreasen, N.C., Swayze, V.W. II, Flaum, M., Alliger, R., and Cohen, G. (1990). Ventricular abnormalities in affective disorder: Clinical and demographic correlates. *Am J Psychiatry*, 147(7), 893–900.

Andreason, P.J., Altemus, M., Zametkin, A.J., King, A.C., Lucinio, J., and Cohen, R.M. (1992). Regional cerebral glucose metabolism in bulimia nervosa. *Am J Psychiatry*, 149(11), 1506–1513.

Andreason, P.J., Zametkin, A.J., Guo, A.C., Baldwin, P., and Cohen, R.M. (1994). Gender-related differences in regional cerebral glucose metabolism in normal volunteers. *Psychiatry Res*, 51(2), 175–183.

Anzalone, S.P., Pegues, M., et al. (2002). *Reduced hippocampal volumes in familial bipolar I disorder.* 57th Annual Convention and Scientific Program of the Society of Biological Psychiatry, Philadelphia, PA, May 16–18.

Ashtari, M., Greenwald, B.S., Kramer-Ginsberg, E., Hu, J., Wu, H., Patel, M., Aupperle, P., and Pollack, S. (1999). Hippocampal/amygdala volumes in geriatric depression. *Psychol Med*, 29(3), 629–638.

Auer, D.P., Putz, B., Kraft, E., Lipinski, B., Schill, J., and Holsboer, F. (2000). Reduced glutamate in the anterior cingulate cortex in depression: An in vivo proton magnetic resonance spectroscopy study. *Biol Psychiatry*, 47(4), 305–313.

Austin, M.P., Dougall, N., Ross, M., Murray, C., O'Carroll, R.E., Moffoot, A., Ebmeier, K.P., and Goodwin, G.M. (1992). Single photon emission tomography with ^{99m}Tc-exametazime in major depression and the pattern of brain activity underlying the psychotic/neurotic continuum. *J Affect Disord*, 26(1), 31–43.

Awata, S., Ito, H., Konno, M., Ono, S., Kawashima, R., Fukuda, H., and Sato, M. (1998). Regional cerebral blood flow abnormalities in late-life depression: Relation to refractoriness and chronification. *Psychiatry Clin Neurosci*, 52(1), 97–105.

Axelson, D.A., Doraiswamy, P.M., Boyko, O.B., Rodrigo Escalona, P., McDonald, W.M., Ritchie, J.C., Patterson, L.J., Ellinwood, E.H. Jr., Nemeroff, C.B., and Krishnan, K.R. (1992). In vivo assessment of pituitary volume with magnetic resonance imaging and systematic stereology: Relationship to dexamethasone suppression test results in patients. *Psychiatry Res*, 44(1), 63–70.

Axelson, D.A., Doraiswamy, P.M., McDonald, W.M., Boyko, O.B., Tupler, L.A., Patterson, L.J., Nemeroff, C.B., Ellinwood, E.H. Jr., and Krishnan, K.R. (1993). Hypercortisolemia and hippocampal changes in depression. *Psychiatry Res*, 47(2), 163–173.

Aylward, E.H., Roberts-Twille, J.V., Barta, P.E., Kumar, A.J., Harris, G.J., Geer, M., Peyser, C.E., and Pearlson, G.D. (1994). Basal ganglia volumes and white matter hyperintensities in patients with bipolar disorder. *Am J Psychiatry*, 151(5), 687–693.

Babb, S.M., Ke, Y., Lange, N., Kaufman, M.J., Renshaw, P.F., and Cohen, B.M. (2004). Oral choline increases choline metabolites in human brain. *Psychiatry Res*, 130(1), 1–9.

Baird, A.A., Gruber, S.A., Fein, D.A., Maas, L.C., Steingard, R.J., Renshaw, P.F., Cohen, B.M., and Yurgelun-Todd, D.A. (1999). Functional magnetic resonance imaging of facial affect recognition in children and adolescents. *J Am Acad Child Adolesc Psychiatry*, 38(2), 195–199.

Baker, S.C., Frith, C.D., and Dolan, R.J. (1997). The interaction between mood and cognitive function studied with PET. *Psychol Med*, 27(3), 565–578.

Baron, J.C., Lebrun-Grandie, P., Collard, P., Crouzel, C., Mestelan, G., and Bousser, M.G. (1982). Noninvasive measurement of blood flow, oxygen consumption, and glucose utilization in the same brain regions in man by positron emission tomography: Concise communication. *J Nucl Med*, 23(5), 391–399.

Baron, J.C., Rougemont, D., Soussaline, F., Bustany, P., Crouzel, C., Bousser, M.G., and Comar, D. (1984). Local interrelationships of cerebral oxygen consumption and glucose utilization in normal subjects and in ischemic stroke patients: A positron tomography study. *J Cereb Blood Flow Metab*, 4(2), 140–149.

Bauer, M., London, E.D., Rasgon, N., Berman, S.M., Frye, M.A., Altshuler, L.L., Mandelkern, M.A., Bramen, J., Voytek, B., Woods, R., Mazziotta, J.C., and Whybrow, P.C. (2005). Supraphysiological doses of levothyroxine alter regional cerebral metabolism and improve mood in bipolar depression. *Mol Psychiatry*, 10(5), 456–469.

Baumann, B., Bornschlegl, C., Krell, D., and Bogerts, B. (1997). Changes in CSF spaces differ in endogenous and neurotic depression. A planimetric CT scan study. *J Affect Disord*, 45(3), 179–188.

Baumann, B., Danos, P., Krell, D., Diekmann, S., Leschinger, A., Stauch, R., Wurthmann, C., Bernstein, H.G., and Bogerts, B. (1999). Reduced volume of limbic system–affiliated basal ganglia in mood disorders: Preliminary data from a postmortem study. *J Neuropsychiatry Clin Neurosci*, 11(1), 71–78.

Baxter, L.R., Jr., Phelps, M.E., Mazziotta, J.C., Schwartz, J.M., Gerner, R.H., Selin, C.E., and Sumida, R.M. (1985). Cerebral metabolic rates for glucose in mood disorders. Studies with positron emission tomography and fluorodeoxyglucose F 18. *Arch Gen Psychiatry*, 42(5), 441–447.

Baxter, L.R. Jr., Phelps, M.E., Mazziotta, J.C., Guze, B.H., Schwartz, J.M., and Selin, C.E. (1987a). Local cerebral glucose metabolic rates in obsessive-compulsive disorder. A comparison with rates in unipolar depression and in normal controls. *Arch Gen Psychiatry*, 44(3), 211–218.

Baxter, L.R., Mazziotta, J.C., Phelps, M.E., Selin, C.E., Guze, B.H., and Fairbanks, L. (1987b). Cerebral glucose metabolic rates in normal human females versus normal males. *Psychiatry Res*, 21(3), 237–245.

Baxter, L.R., Jr., Schwartz, J.M., Phelps, M.E., Mazziotta, J.C., Guze, B.H., Selin, C.E., Gerner, R.H., and Sumida, R.M. (1989). Reduction of prefrontal cortex glucose metabolism common to three types of depression. *Arch Gen Psychiatry*, 46(3), 243–250.

Beats, B., Levy, R., and Forstl, H. (1991). Ventricular enlargement and caudate hyperdensity in elderly depressives. *Biol Psychiatry*, 30(5), 452–458.

Beers, C.W. ([1908] 1980). *A Mind That Found Itself*. Pittsburgh: University of Pittsburgh Press.

Bell-McGinty, S., Butters, M.A., Meltzer, C.C., Greer, P.J., Reynolds, C.F. III, and Becker, J.T. (2002). Brain morphometric abnormalities in geriatric depression: Long-term neurobiological effects of illness duration. *Am J Psychiatry*, 159(8), 1424–1427.

Bench, C.J., Friston, K.J., Brown, R.G., Scott, L.C., Frackowiak, R.S., and Dolan, R.J. (1992). The anatomy of melancholia: Focal abnormalities of cerebral blood flow in major depression. *Psychol Med*, 22(3), 607–615.

Bench, C.J., Friston, K.J., Brown, R.G., Frackowiak, R.S., and Dolan, R.J. (1993). Regional cerebral blood flow in depression measured by positron emission tomography: The relationship with clinical dimensions. *Psychol Med*, 23(3), 579–590.

Bench, C.J., Frackowiak, R.S., and Dolan, R.J. (1995). Changes in regional cerebral blood flow on recovery from depression. *Psychol Med*, 25(2), 247–261.

Benes, F.M., Kwok, E.W., Vincent, S.L., and Todtenkopf, M.S. (1998). A reduction of nonpyramidal cells in sector CA2 of schizophrenics and manic depressives. *Biol Psychiatry*, 44(2), 88–97.

Berman, K.F., Doran, A.R., Pickar, D., and Weinberger, D.R. (1993). Is the mechanism of prefrontal hypofunction in depression the same as in schizophrenia? Regional cerebral blood flow during cognitive activation. *Br J Psychiatry*, 162, 183–192.

Berridge, M.J., Downes, C.P., and Hanley, M.R. (1989). Neural and developmental actions of lithium: A unifying hypothesis. *Cell*, 59(3), 411–419.

Bertolino, A., Frye, M., Callicott, J.H., Mattay, V.S., Rakow, R., Shelton-Repella, J., Post, R., and Weinberger, D.R. (2003). Neuronal pathology in the hippocampal area of patients with bipolar disorder: A study with proton magnetic resonance spectroscopic imaging. *Biol Psychiatry*, 53(10), 906–913.

Besson, J.A., Henderson, J.G., Foreman, E.I., and Smith, F.W. (1987). An NMR study of lithium responding manic depressive patients. *Magn Reson Imaging*, 5(4), 273–277.

Beyer, J.L., Kuchibhatla, M., Payne, M.E., Moo-Young, M., Cassidy, F., Macfall, J., and Krishnan, K.R. (2004). Hippocampal volume measurement in older adults with bipolar disorder. *Am J Geriatr Psychiatry*, 12(6), 613–620.

Beyer, J.L., Taylor, W.D., MacFall, J.R., Kuchibhatia, M., Payne, M.E., Provenzale, J.M., Cassidy, F., and Krishnan, K.R. (2005). Cortical white matter microstructural abnormalities in bipolar disorder. *Neuropsychopharmacology*, 30(12), 2225–2229.

Biver, F., Goldman, S., Delvenne, V., Luxen, A., De Maertelaer, V., Hubain, P., Mendlewicz, J., and Lotstra, F. (1994). Frontal and parietal metabolic disturbances in unipolar depression. *Biol Psychiatry*, 36(6), 381–388.

Blair, R.J.R., Morris, J.S., Delvenne, V., Luxen, A., De Maertelaer, V., Hubain, P., Mendlewicz, J., and Lotstra, F. (1999). Dissociable neural responses to facial expressions of sadness and anger. *Brain*, 122(Pt. 5), 883–893.

Blumberg, H.P., Stern, E., Ricketts, S., Martinez, D., de Asis, J., White, T., Epstein, J., Isenberg, N., McBride, P.A., Kemperman, I., Emmerich, S., Dhawan, V., Eidelberg, D., Kocsis, J.H., and Silbersweig, D.A. (1999). Rostral and orbital prefrontal cortex dysfunction in the manic state of bipolar disorder. *Am J Psychiatry*, 156(12), 1986–1988.

Blumberg, H.P., Stern, E., Martinez, D., Ricketts, S., de Asis, J., White, T., Epstein, J., McBride, P.A., Eidelberg, D., Kocsis, J.H., and Silbersweig, D.A. (2000). Increased anterior cingulate and caudate activity in bipolar mania. *Biol Psychiatry*, 48(11), 1045–1052.

Blumberg, H.P., Martin, A., Kaufman, J., Leung, H.C., Skudlarski, P., Lacadie, C., Fulbright, R.K., Gore, J.C., Charney, D.S., Krystal, J.H., and Peterson, B.S. (2003a). Frontostriatal abnormalities in adolescents with bipolar disorder: Preliminary observations from functional MRI. *Am J Psychiatry*, 160(7), 1345–1347.

Blumberg, H.P., Leung, H.C., Skudlarski, P., Lacadie, C.M., Fredericks, C.A., Harris, B.C., Charney, D.S., Gore, J.C., Krystal, J.H., and Peterson, B.S. (2003b). A functional magnetic resonance imaging study of bipolar disorder: State- and trait-related dysfunction in ventral prefrontal cortices. *Arch Gen Psychiatry*, 60(6), 601–609.

Blumberg, H.P., Kaufman, J., Martin, A., Whiteman, R., Zhang, J.H., Gore, J.C., Charney, D.S., Krystal, J.H., and Peterson, B.S. (2003c). Amygdala and hippocampal volumes in adolescents and adults with bipolar disorder. *Arch Gen Psychiatry*, 60(12), 1201–1208.

Blumberg, H.P., Fredericks, C., Wang, F., Kalmar, J.H., Spencer, L., Papademetris, X., Pittman, B., Martin, A., Peterson, B.S., Fulbright, R.K., and Krystal, J.H. (2005). Preliminary evidence for persistent abnormalities in amygdale volumes in adolescents and young adults with bipolar disorder. *Bipolar Disord*, 7(6), 570–576.

Blumberg, H.P., Krystal, J.H., Bansal, R., Martin, A., Dziura, J., Durkin, K., Martin, L., Gerard, E., Charney, D.S., and Peterson, B.S. (2006). Age, rapid-cycling, and pharmacotherapy effects on ventral prefrontal cortex in bipolar disorder: A cross-sectional study. *Biol Psychiatry*, 59(7), 611–618.

Bocksberger, J.P., Young, R.C., et al. (1996). *Basal ganglia morphology in geriatric mania*. 50th Annual Meeting of the Society of Biological Psychiatry, New York, NY, May 1–5.

Bonne, O., Krausz, Y., Gorfine, M., Karger, H., Gelfin, Y., Shapira, B., Chisin, R., and Lerer, B. (1996a). Cerebral hypoperfusion in medication resistant, depressed patients assessed by Tc99m HMPAO SPECT. *J Affect Disord*, 41(3), 163–171.

Bonne, O., Krausz, Y., Shapira, B., Bocher, M., Karger, H., Gorfine, M., Chisin, R., and Lerer, B. (1996b). Increased cerebral blood flow in depressed patients responding to electroconvulsive therapy. *J Nucl Med*, 37(7), 1075–1080.

Boone, K.B., Miller, B.L., Lesser, I.M., Mehringer, C.M., Hill-Gutierrez, E., Goldberg, M.A., and Berman, N.G. (1992). Neuropsychological correlates of white-matter lesions in healthy elderly subjects. A threshold effect. *Arch Neurol*, 49(5), 549–554.

Botteron, K.N., Vannier, M.W., Geller, B., Todd, R.D., and Lee, B.C. (1995). Preliminary study of magnetic resonance imaging characteristics in 8- to 16-year-olds with mania. *J Am Acad Child Adolesc Psychiatry*, 34(6), 742–749.

Botteron, K.N., Raichle, M.E., et al. (1999). *An epidemiological twin study of prefrontal neuromorphometry in early onset depression*. 54th Annual Convention and Scientific Program of the Society of Biological Psychiatry, Washington, DC, May 13–15.

Botteron, K.N., Raichle, M.E., Drevets, W.C., Heath, A.C., and Todd, R.D. (2002). Volumetric reduction in left subgenual prefrontal cortex in early onset depression. *Biol Psychiatry*, 51(4), 342–344.

Bowley, M.P., Drevets, W.C., Ongur, D., and Price, J.L. (2002). Low glial numbers in the amygdala in major depressive disorder. *Biol Psychiatry*, 52(5), 404–412.

Brambilla, P., Harenski, K., Nicoletti, M., Mallinger, A.G., Frank, E., Kupfer, D.J., Keshavan, M.S., and Soares, J.C. (2001a). MRI study of posterior fossa structures and brain ventricles in bipolar patients. *J Psychiatr Res*, 35(6), 313–322.

Brambilla, P., Harenski, K., Nicoletti, M.A., Mallinger, A.G., Frank, E., Kupfer, D.J., Keshavan, M.S., and Soares, J.C. (2001b). Anatomical MRI study of basal ganglia in bipolar disorder patients. *Psychiatry Res*, 106(2), 65–80.

Brambilla, P., Nicoletti, M.A., Harenski, K., Sassi, R.B., Mallinger, A.G., Frank, E., Kupfer, D.J., Keshavan, M.S., and Soares, J.C. (2002). Anatomical MRI study of subgenual prefrontal cortex in bipolar and unipolar subjects. *Neuropsychopharmacology*, 27(5), 792–799.

Brambilla, P., Harenski, K., Nicoletti, M., Sassi, R.B., Mallinger, A.G., Frank, E., Kupfer, D.J., Keshavan, M.S., and Soares, J.C. (2003a). MRI investigation of temporal lobe structures in bipolar patients. *J Psychiatr Res*, 37(4), 287–295.

Brambilla, P., Nicoletti, M.A., Sassi, R.B., Mallinger, A.G., Frank, E., Kupfer, D.J., Keshavan, M.S., and Soares, J.C. (2003b). Magnetic resonance imaging study of corpus callosum abnormalities in patients with bipolar disorder. *Biol Psychiatry*, 54(11), 1294–1297.

Brambilla, P., Nicoletti, M., Sassi, R.B., Mallinger, A.G., Frank, E., Keshavan, M.S., Soares, J.C. (2004). Corpus callosum signal intensity in patients with bipolar and unipolar disorder. *J Neurol Neurosurg Psychiatry*, 75(2), 221–225.

Brambilla, P., Glahn, D.C., Balestrieri, M., and Soares, J.C. (2005). Magnetic resonance findings in bipolar disorder. *Psychiatr Clin North Am*, 28(2), 443–467.

Breiter, H.C., Etcoff, N.L., Whalen, P.J., Kennedy, W.A., Rauch, S.L., Buckner, R.L., Strauss, M.M., Hyman, S.E., and Rosen, B.R. (1996). Response and habituation of the human amygdala during visual processing of facial expression. *Neuron*, 17(5), 875–887.

Bremner, J.D., Innis, R.B., Salomon, R.M., Staib, L.H., Ng, C.K., Miller, H.L., Bronen, R.A., Krystal, J.H., Duncan, J., Rich, D., Price, L.H., Malison, R., Dey, H., Soufer, R., and Charney, D.S. (1997). Positron emission tomography measurement of cerebral metabolic correlates of tryptophan depletion–induced depressive relapse. *Arch Gen Psychiatry*, 54(4), 364–374.

Bremner, J.D., Narayan, M., Anderson, E.R., Staib, L.H., Miller, H.L., and Charney, D.S. (2000). Hippocampal volume reduction in major depression. *Am J Psychiatry*, 157(1), 115–118.

Bremner, J.D., Vythilingam, M., Vermetten, E., Nazeer, A., Adil, J., Khan, S., Staib, L.H., and Charney, D.S. (2002). Reduced volume of orbitofrontal cortex in major depression. *Biol Psychiatry*, 51(4), 273–279.

Bremner, J.D., Vythilingam, M., Ng, C.K., Vermetten, E., Nazeer, A., Oren, D.A., Berman, R.M., and Charney, D.S. (2003). Regional brain metabolic correlates of alpha-methylparatyrosine-induced depressive symptoms: Implications for the neural circuitry of depression. *JAMA*, 289(23), 3125–3134.

Bremner, J.D., Vythilingam, M., Vermetten, E., Vaccarino, V., and Charney, D.S. (2004). Deficits in hippocampal and anterior cingulate functioning during verbal declarative memory encoding in midlife major depression. *Am J Psychiatry*, 161(4), 637–645.

Broca, P. (1878). Anatomie comparée des circonvolutions cérébrales: Le grand lobe limbique et la scissure limbique dans la série des mammifères. [Anatomic considerations of cerebral convolutions: The great limbic lobe and limbic sulci in a series of mammals]. *Rev Anthropol*, 1(Ser. 2), 385–498.

Brody, A.L., Saxena, S., Mandelkern, M.A., Fairbanks, L.A., Ho, M.L., and Baxter, L.R. (2001a). Brain metabolic changes associated with symptom factor improvement in major depressive disorder. *Biol Psychiatry*, 50(3), 171–178.

Brody, A.L., Saxena, S., Stoessel, P., Gillies, L.A., Fairbanks, L.A., Alborzian, S., Phelps, M.E., Huang, S.C., Wu, H.M., Ho, M.L., Ho, M.K., Au, S.C., Maidment, K., and Baxter, L.R. Jr. (2001b). Regional brain metabolic changes in patients with major depression treated with either paroxetine or interpersonal therapy: Preliminary findings. *Arch Gen Psychiatry*, 58(7), 631–640.

Bromfield, E.B., Altshuler, L., Leiderman, D.B., Balish, M., Ketter, T.A., Devinsky, O., Post, R.M., and Theodore, W.H. (1992). Cerebral metabolism and depression in patients with complex partial seizures. *Arch Neurol*, 49(6), 617–623.

Brown, F.W., Lewine, R.J., Hudgins, P.A., and Risch, S.C. (1992). White matter hyperintensity signals in psychiatric and nonpsychiatric subjects. *Am J Psychiatry*, 149(5), 620–625.

Brühn, H., Stoppe, G., et al. (1993). *Quantitative proton MRS in vivo shows cerebral myo-inositol and cholines to be unchanged in manic-depressive patients treated with lithium* [abstract]. Proceedings of the Society of Magnetic Resonance in Medicine, New York, NY, August 14–20.

Bruno, S.D., Barker, G.J., Cercignani, M., Symms, M., and Ron, M.A. (2004). A study of bipolar disorder using magnetization transfer imaging and voxel-based morphometry. *Brain*, 127(Pt. 11), 2433–2440.

Buchsbaum, M.S., Cappelletti, J., Ball, R., Hazlett, E., King, A.C., Johnson, J., Wu, J., and DeLisi, L.E. (1984). Positron emission tomographic image measurement in schizophrenia and affective disorders. *Ann Neurol*, 15(Suppl.), S157–S165.

Buchsbaum, M.S., Wu, J., DeLisi, L.E., Holcomb, H., Kessler, R., Johnson, J., King, A.C., Hazlett, E., Langston, K., and Post, R.M. (1986). Frontal cortex and basal ganglia metabolic rates assessed by positron emission tomography with [18F]2-deoxyglucose in affective illness. *J Affect Disord*, 10(2), 137–152.

Buchsbaum, M.S., Someya, T., and Bunney, W.E. (1997a). Neuroimaging bipolar illness with positron emission tomography and magnetic resonance imaging. *Psychiatr Ann*, 27(7), 489–495.

Buchsbaum, M.S., Wu, J., Siegel, B.V., Hackett, E., Trenary, M., Abel, L., and Reynolds, C. (1997b). Effect of sertraline on regional metabolic rate in patients with affective disorder. *Biol Psychiatry*, 41(1), 15–22.

Caetano, S.C., Sassi, R., Brambilla, P., Harenski, K., Nicoletti, M., Mallinger, A.G., Frank, E., Kupfer, D.J., Keshavan, M.S., and Soares, J.C. (2001). MRI study of thalamic volumes in bipolar and unipolar patients and healthy individuals. *Psychiatry Res*, 108(3), 161–168.

Caine, E.D., and Shoulson, I. (1983). Psychiatric syndromes in Huntington's disease. *Am J Psychiatry*, 140(6), 728–733.

Campbell, S., Marriott, M., Nahmias, C., and MacQueen, G.M. (2004). Lower hippocampal volume in patients suffering from depression: A meta-analysis. *Am J Psychiatry*, 161(4), 598–607.

Caparros-Lefebvre, D., Girard-Buttaz, I., Reboul, S., Lebert, F., Cabaret, M., Verier, A., Steinling, M., Pruvo, J.P., and Petit, H. (1996). Cognitive and psychiatric impairment in herpes simplex virus encephalitis suggest involvement of the amygdalofrontal pathways. *J Neurol*, 243(3), 248–256.

Carson, A.J., MacHale, S., Allen, K., Lawrie, S.M., Dennis, M., House, A., and Sharpe, M. (2000). Depression after stroke and lesion location: A systematic review. *Lancet*, 356(9224), 122–126.

Castillo, M., Kwock, L., Courvoisie, H., and Hooper, S.R. (2000). Proton MR spectroscopy in children with bipolar affective disorder: Preliminary observations. *AJNR Am J Neuroradiol*, 21(5), 832–838.

Cecil, K.M., DelBello, M.P., Morey, R., and Strakowski, S.M. (2002). Frontal lobe differences in bipolar disorder as determined by proton MR spectroscopy. *Bipolar Disord*, 4(6), 357–365.

Cecil, K.M., DelBello, M.P., Sellars, M.C., and Strakowski, S.M. (2003). Proton magnetic resonance spectroscopy of the frontal lobe and cerebellar vermis in children with a mood disorder and a familial risk for bipolar disorders. *J Child Adolesc Psychopharmacol*, 13(4), 545–555.

Chakos, M.H., Lieberman, J.A., Bilder, R.M., Borenstein, M., Lerner, G., Bogerts, B., Wu, H., Kinon, B., and Ashtari, M. (1994). Increase in caudate nuclei volumes of first-episode schizophrenic patients taking antipsychotic drugs. *Am J Psychiatry*, 151(10), 1430–1436.

Chang, K.D., Blasey, C., Ketter, T.A., and Steiner, H. (2001). Family environment of children and adolescents with bipolar parents. *Bipolar Disord*, 3(2), 73–78.

Chang, K., Adleman, N.E., Dienes, K., Simeonova, D.I., Menon, V., and Reiss, A. (2004). Anomalous prefrontal–subcortical activation in familial pediatric bipolar disorder: A functional magnetic resonance imaging investigation. *Arch Gen Psychiatry*, 61(8), 781–792.

Charles, H.C., Lazeyras, F., Krishnan, K.R., Boyko, O.B., Patterson, L.J., Doraiswamy, P.M., and McDonald, W.M. (1994a). Proton spectroscopy of human brain: Effects of age and sex. *Prog Neuropsychopharmacol Biol Psychiatry*, 18(6), 995–1004.

Charles, H.C., Lazeyras, F., Krishnan, K.R., Boyko, O.B., Payne, M., and Moore, D. (1994b). Brain choline in depression: In vivo detection of potential pharmacodynamic effects of antidepressant therapy using hydrogen localized spectroscopy. *Prog Neuropsychopharmacol Biol Psychiatry*, 18(7), 1121–1127.

Chen, B.K., Sassi, R., Axelson, D., Hatch, J.P., Sanches, M., Nicoletti, M., Brambilla, P., Keshavan, M.S., Ryan, N.D., Birmaher, B., and Soares, J.C. (2004). Cross-sectional study of abnormal amygdala development in adolescents and young adults with bipolar disorder. *Biol Psychiatry*, 56(6), 399–405.

Choi, S.J., Lim, K.O., et al. (2002). *Differential age-related decline in white matter integrity in late-life depression*. 57th Annual Convention and Scientific Program of the Society of Biological Psychiatry, Philadelphia, PA, May 16–18.

Chugani, H.T., Phelps, M.E., and Mazziotta, J.C. (1987). Positron emission tomography study of human brain functional development. *Ann Neurol*, 22(4), 487–497.

Churchill, C.M., Priolo, C.V., Nemeroff, C.B., Krishnan, K.R.R. (1991). Occult subcortical magnetic resonance findings in elderly depressives. *Int J Geriatr Psychiatry*, 6, 213–216.

Coffey, C.E., Hinkle, P.E., Weiner, R.D., Nemeroff, C.B., Krishnan, K.R., Varia, I., and Sullivan, D.C. (1987). Electroconvulsive therapy of depression in patients with white matter hyperintensity. *Biol Psychiatry*, 22(5), 629–636.

Coffey, C.E., Figiel, G.S., Djang, W.T., Cress, M., Saunders, W.B., and Weiner, R.D. (1988a). Leukoencephalopathy in elderly depressed patients referred for ECT. *Biol Psychiatry*, 24(2), 143–161.

Coffey, C.E., Figiel, G.S., Djang, W.T., Sullivan, D.C., Herfkens, R.J., and Weiner, R.D. (1988b). Effects of ECT on brain structure: A pilot prospective magnetic resonance imaging study. *Am J Psychiatry*, 145(6), 701–706.

Coffey, C.E., Figiel, G.S., Djang, W.T., Saunders, W.B., and Weiner, R.D. (1989). White matter hyperintensity on magnetic resonance imaging: Clinical and neuroanatomic correlates in the depressed elderly. *J Neuropsychiatry Clin Neurosci*, 1(2), 135–144.

Coffey, C.E., Figiel, G.S., Djang, W.T., and Weiner, R.D. (1990). Subcortical hyperintensity on magnetic resonance imaging: A comparison of normal and depressed elderly subjects. *Am J Psychiatry*, 147(2), 187–189.

Coffey, C.E., Weiner, R.D., Djang, W.T., Figiel, G.S., Soady, S.A., Patterson, L.J., Holt, P.D., Spritzer, C.E., and Wilkinson, W.E. (1991). Brain anatomic effects of electroconvulsive therapy. A prospective magnetic resonance imaging study. *Arch Gen Psychiatry*, 48(11), 1013–1021.

Coffey, C.E., Wilkinson, W.E., Parashos, I.A., Soady, S.A., Sullivan, R.J., Patterson, L.J., Figiel, G.S., Webb, M.C., Spritzer, C.E., and Djang, W.T. (1992). Quantitative cerebral anatomy of the aging human brain: A cross-sectional study using magnetic resonance imaging. *Neurology*, 42(3 Pt. 1), 527–536.

Coffey, C.E., Wilkinson, W.E., Weiner, R.D., Parashos, I.A., Djang, W.T., Webb, M.C., Figiel, G.S., and Spritzer, C.E. (1993a). Quantitative cerebral anatomy in depression. A controlled magnetic resonance imaging study. *Arch Gen Psychiatry*, 50(1), 7–16.

Coffey, C.E., Wilkinson, W.E., Weiner, R.D., Ritchie, J.C., and Aque, M. (1993b). The dexamethasone suppression test and quantitative cerebral anatomy in depression. *Biol Psychiatry*, 33(6), 442–449.

Coffey, C.E., Lucke, J.F., Saxton, J.A., Ratcliff, G., Unitas, L.J., Billig, B., and Bryan, R.N. (1998). Sex differences in brain aging:

A quantitative magnetic resonance imaging study. *Arch Neurol*, 55(2), 169–179.

Coffman, J.A., Bornstein, R.A., Olson, S.C., Schwarzkopf, S.B., and Nasrallah, H.A. (1990). Cognitive impairment and cerebral structure by MRI in bipolar disorder. *Biol Psychiatry*, 27(11), 1188–1196.

Cohen, R.M., Semple, W.E., Gross, M., Nordahl, T.E, King, A.C., Pickar, D., and Post, R.M. (1989). Evidence for common alterations in cerebral glucose metabolism in major affective disorders and schizophrenia. *Neuropsychopharmacology*, 2(4), 241–254.

Cohen, R.M., Gross, M., Nordahl, T.E., Semple, W.E., Oren, D.A., and Rosenthal N. (1992). Preliminary data on the metabolic brain pattern of patients with winter seasonal affective disorder. *Arch Gen Psychiatry*, 49(7), 545–552.

Cohen, B.M., Renshaw, P.F., Stoll, A.L., Wurtman, R.J., Yurgelun-Todd, D., and Babb, S.M. (1995). Decreased brain choline uptake in older adults. An in vivo proton magnetic resonance spectroscopy study. *JAMA*, 274(11), 902–907.

Colla, M., Meichel, K., et al. (2002). *Hippocampal volume reduction and hypercortisolemia in major depression.* 57th Annual Convention and Scientific Program of the Society of Biological Psychiatry, Philadelphia, PA, May 16–18.

Conca, A., Fritzsche, H., Peschina, W., Konig, P., Swoboda, E., Wiederin, H., and Haas, C. (2000). Preliminary findings of simultaneous 18F-FDG and 99mTc-HMPAO SPECT in patients with depressive disorders at rest: Differential correlates with ratings of anxiety. *Psychiatry Res*, 98(1), 43–54.

Connor, S.E., Ng, V., McDonald, C., Schulze, K., Morgan, K., Dazzan, P., and Murray, R.M. (2004). A study of hippocampal shape anomaly in schizophrenia and in families multiply affected by schizophrenia or bipolar disorder. *Neuroradiology*, 46(7), 523–534.

Constant, E.L., de Volder, A.G., Ivanoiu, A., Bol, A., Labar, D., Seghers, A., Cosnard, G., Melin, J., and Daumerie, C. (2001). Cerebral blood flow and glucose metabolism in hypothyroidism: A positron emission tomography study. *J Clin Endocrinol Metab*, 86(8), 3864–3870.

Coryell, W. (2005). Rapid cycling bipolar disorder: Clinical characteristics and treatment options. *CNS Drugs*, 19(7), 557–569.

Cowell, P.E., Turetsky, B.I., Gur, R.C., Grossman, R.I., Shtasel, D.L., and Gur, R.E. (1994). Sex differences in aging of the human frontal and temporal lobes. *J Neurosci*, 14(8), 4748–4755.

Curran, S.M., Murray, C.M., Van Beck, M., Dougall, N., O'Carroll, R.E., Austin, M.P., Ebmeier, K.P., and Goodwin, G.M. (1993). A single photon emission computerised tomography study of regional brain function in elderly patients with major depression and with Alzheimer-type dementia. *Br J Psychiatry*, 163, 155–165.

Curtis, V.A., Dixon, T.A., Morris, R.G., Bullmore, E.T., Brammer, M.J., Williams, S.C., Sharma, T., Murray, R.M., and McGuire, P.K. (2001). Differential frontal activation in schizophrenia and bipolar illness during verbal fluency. *J Affect Disord*, 66(2-3), 111–121.

Dager, S.R., Friedman, S.D., Parow, A., Demopulos, C., Stoll, A.L., Lyoo, I.K., Dunner, D.L., and Renshaw, P.F. (2004). Brain metabolic alterations in medication-free patients with bipolar disorder. *Arch Gen Psychiatry*, 61(5), 450–458.

Dahabra, S., Ashton, C.H., Bahrainian, M., Britton, P.G., Ferrier, I.N., McAllister, V.A., Marsh, V.R., and Moore, P.B. (1998). Structural and functional abnormalities in elderly patients clinically recovered from early- and late-onset depression. *Biol Psychiatry*, 44(1), 34–46.

Damasio, A.R., Grabowski, T.J., et al. (1998). Neural correlates of the experience of emotion [abstract 104.1]. *Soc Neurosci Abstr*, 24, 258.

Damasio, A.R., Grabowski, T.J., et al. (1999). *The contribution of subcortical nuclei to the processing of emotion and feeling* [abstract]. 5th International Conference on Functional Mapping of the Human Brain, Düsseldorf, Germany, June 22–26.

Davanzo, P., Thomas, M.A., Yue, K., Oshiro, T., Belin, T., Strober, M., and McCracken, J. (2001). Decreased anterior cingulate myo-inositol/creatine spectroscopy resonance with lithium treatment in children with bipolar disorder. *Neuropsychopharmacology*, 24(4), 359–369.

Davanzo, P., Yue, K., Thomas, M.A., Belin, T., Mintz, J., Venkatraman, T.N., Santoro, E., Barnett, S., and McCracken, J. (2003). Proton magnetic resonance spectroscopy of bipolar disorder versus intermittent explosive disorder in children and adolescents. *Am J Psychiatry*, 160(8), 1442–1452.

Davidson, R.J., Irwin, W., Anderle, M.J., and Kalin, N.H. (2003). The neural substrates of affective processing in depressed patients treated with venlafaxine. *Am J Psychiatry*, 160(1), 64–75.

Dean, B., Scarr, E., Pavey, G., and Copolov, D. (2003). Studies on serotonergic markers in the human hippocampus: Changes in subjects with bipolar disorder. *J Affect Disord*, 75(1), 65–69.

de Asis, J.M., Stern, E., Alexopoulos, G.S., Pan, H., Van Gorp, W., Blumberg, H., Kalayam, B., Eidelberg, D., Kiosses, D., and Silbersweig, D.A. (2001). Hippocampal and anterior cingulate activation deficits in patients with geriatric depression. *Am J Psychiatry*, 158(8), 1321–1323.

DeCarli, C., Murphy, D.G., Tranh, M., Grady, C.L., Haxby, J.V., Gillette, J.A., Salerno, J.A., Gonzales-Aviles, A., Horwitz, B., and Rapoport, S.I. (1995). The effect of white matter hyperintensity volume on brain structure, cognitive performance, and cerebral metabolism of glucose in 51 healthy adults. *Neurology*, 45(11), 2077–2084.

Dechent, P., Pouwels, P.J., and Frahm J. (1999a). Neither short-term nor long-term administration of oral choline alters metabolite concentrations in human brain. *Biol Psychiatry*, 46(3), 406–411.

Dechent, P., Pouwels, P.J., Wilken, B., Hanefeld, F., and Frahm, J. (1999b). Increase of total creatine in human brain after oral supplementation of creatine-monohydrate. *Am J Physiol*, 277(3 Pt. 2), R698–R704.

de Groot, J.C., de Leeuw, F.E., Oudkerk, M., Hofman, A., Jolles, J., and Breteler, M.M. (2000). Cerebral white matter lesions and depressive symptoms in elderly adults. *Arch Gen Psychiatry*, 57(11), 1071–1076.

Deicken, R.F., Reus, V.I., Manfredi, L., and Wolkowitz, O.M. (1991). MRI deep white matter hyperintensity in a psychiatric population. *Biol Psychiatry*, 29(9), 918–922.

Deicken, R.F., Calabrese, G., Merrin, E.L., Fein, G., and Weiner, M.W. (1995a). Basal ganglia phosphorous metabolism in chronic schizophrenia. *Am J Psychiatry*, 152(1), 126–129.

Deicken, R.F., Fein, G., and Weiner, M.W. (1995b). Abnormal frontal lobe phosphorous metabolism in bipolar disorder. *Am J Psychiatry*, 152(6), 915–918.

Deicken, R.F., Eliaz, Y., Feiwell, R., and Schuff, N. (2001). Increased thalamic N-acetylaspartate in male patients with familial bipolar I disorder. *Psychiatry Res*, 106(1), 35–45.

Deicken, R.F., Pegues, M.P., Anzalone, S., Feiwell, R., and Soher, B. (2003a). Lower concentration of hippocampal N-acetylaspartate in familial bipolar I disorder. *Am J Psychiatry*, 160(5), 873–882.

Deicken, R.F., Pegues, M.P., Anzalone, S., Feiwell, R., and Soher, B. (2003b). Lower concentration of hippocampal N-acetylaspartate in familial bipolar I disorder. *Am J Psychiatry*, 160(5), 873–882.

DelBello, M.P., Strakowski, S.M., Zimmerman, M.E., Hawkins, J.M., and Sax, K.W. (1999). MRI analysis of the cerebellum in bipolar disorder: A pilot study. *Neuropsychopharmacology*, 21(1), 63–68.

DelBello, M.P., Zimmerman, M.E., Mills, N.P., Getz, G.E., and Strakowski, S.M. (2004). Magnetic resonance imaging analysis of amygdala and other subcortical brain regions in adolescents with bipolar disorder. *Bipolar Disord*, 6(1), 43–52.

de Leon, M.J., Ferris, S.H., George, A.E., Christman, D.R., Fowler, J.S., Gentes, C., Reisberg, B., Gee, B., Emmerich, M., Yonekura, Y., Brodie, J., Kricheff, I.I., and Wolf, A.P. (1983). Positron emission tomographic studies of aging and Alzheimer disease. *AJNR Am J Neuroradiol*, 4(3), 568–571.

de Leon, M.J., George, A.E., Tomanelli, J., Christman, D., Kluger, A., Miller, J., Ferris, S.H., Fowler, J., Brodie, J.D., and van Gelder, P. (1987). Positron emission tomography studies of normal aging: A replication of PET III and 18-FDG using PET VI and 11-CDG. *Neurobiol Aging*, 8(4), 319–323.

Delvenne, V., Goldman, S., Biver, F., De Maertalaer, V., Wikler, D., Damhaut, P., and Lotstra, F. (1997a). Brain hypometabolism of glucose in low-weight depressed patients and in anorectic patients: A consequence of starvation? *J Affect Disord*, 44(1), 69–77.

Delvenne, V., Goldman, S., De Maertelaer, V., Wikler, D., Damhaut, P., and Lotstra, F. (1997b). Brain glucose metabolism in anorexia nervosa and affective disorders: Influence of weight loss or depressive symptomatology. *Psychiatry Res*, 74(2), 83–92.

Demopulos, C.D., Renshaw, P.F., et al. (1996). *Rapid cycling tended to be associated with low choline in the basal ganglia.* 149th Annual Meeting of the American Psychiatric Association, New York, NY, May 4–9.

Demopulos, C.M., Renshaw, P.F., et al. (1997). *Chronic choline administration does not increase brain choline:creatine.* 150th Annual Meeting of the American Psychiatric Association, San Diego, CA, May 17–22.

Devous, M.D., Husain, M., et al. (2002). *Effects of VNS on regional cerebral blood flow in depressed subjects.* 57th Annual Convention and Scientific Program of the Society of Biological Psychiatry, Philadelphia, PA, May 16–18.

Dewan, M.J., Haldipur, C.V., Lane, E., Donnelly, M.P., Boucher, M., and Major, L.F. (1987). Normal cerebral asymmetry in bipolar patients. *Biol Psychiatry*, 22(9), 1058–1066.

Dewan, M.J., Haldipur, C.V., Boucher, M., and Major, L.F. (1988a). Is CT ventriculomegaly related to hypercortisolemia? *Acta Psychiatr Scand*, 77(2), 230–231.

Dewan, M.J., Haldipur, C.V., Boucher, M.F., Ramachandran, T., and Major, L.F. (1988b). Bipolar affective disorder. II. EEG, neuropsychological, and clinical correlates of CT abnormality. *Acta Psychiatr Scand*, 77(6), 677–682.

Dewan, M.J., Haldipur, C.V., Lane, E.E., Ispahani, A., Boucher, M.F., and Major, L.F. (1988c). Bipolar affective disorder. I. Comprehensive quantitative computed tomography. *Acta Psychiatr Scand*, 77(6), 670–676.

Dickstein, D.P., Garvey, M., Pradella, A.G., Greenstein, D.K., Sharp, W.S., Castellanos, F.X., Pine, D.S., and Leibenluft, E. (2005). Neurologic examination abnormalities in children with bipolar disorder or attention-deficit/hyperactivity disorder. *Biol Psychiatry*, 58(7), 517–524.

Dieckmann, N.F., Wang, P.W., et al. (2002). *Decreased left frontal lobe gray matter in men with bipolar I disorder.* 155th Annual Meeting of the American Psychiatric Association, Philadelphia, PA, May 18–23.

Direkze, M., Bayliss, S.G., and Cutting, J.C. (1971). Primary tumours of the frontal lobe. *Br J Clin Pract*, 25(5), 207–213.

Dolan, R.J., Calloway, S.P., and Mann, A.H. (1985). Cerebral ventricular size in depressed subjects. *Psychol Med*, 15(4), 873–878.

Dolan, R.J., Calloway, S.P., Thacker, P.F., and Mann, A.H. (1986). The cerebral cortical appearance in depressed subjects. *Psychol Med*, 16(4), 775–779.

Dolan, R.J., Bench, C.J., Brown, R.G., Scott, L.C., Friston, K.J., and Frackowiak, R.S. (1992). Regional cerebral blood flow abnormalities in depressed patients with cognitive impairment. *J Neurol Neurosurg Psychiatry*, 55(9), 768–773.

Dolan, R.J., Bench, C.J., Brown, R.G., Scott, L.C., and Frackowiak, R.S. (1994). Neuropsychological dysfunction in depression: The relationship to regional cerebral blood flow. *Psychol Med*, 24(4), 849–857.

Doris, A., Belton, E., Ebmeier, K.P., Glabus, M.F., and Marshall, I. (2004). Reduction of cingulate gray matter density in poor outcome bipolar illness. *Psychiatry Res*, 130(2), 153–159.

Drevets, W.C. (1999). Prefrontal cortical–amygdalar metabolism in major depression. *Ann NY Acad Sci*, 877, 614–637.

Drevets, W.C. (2000). Neuroimaging studies of mood disorders. *Biol Psychiatry*, 48(8), 813–829.

Drevets, W.C. (2001). Neuroimaging and neuropathological studies of depression: Implications for the cognitive-emotional features of mood disorders. *Curr Opin Neurobiol*, 11(2), 240–249.

Drevets, W.C., and Raichle, M.E. (1992). Neuroanatomical circuits in depression: Implications for treatment mechanisms. *Psychopharmacol Bull*, 28(3), 261–274.

Drevets, W.C., Videen, T.O., Price, J.L., Preskorn, S.H., Carmichael, S.T., and Raichle, M.E. (1992). A functional anatomical study of unipolar depression. *J Neurosci*, 12(9), 3628–3641.

Drevets, W.C., Price, J.L., Videen, T.O., and Todd, R.D. (1995). Metabolic abnormalities in the subgenual prefrontal cortex and ventral striatum in mood disorders. *Soc Neurosci Abstr*, 21(1), 260.

Drevets, W.C., Price, J.L., Simpson, J.R. Jr., Todd, R.D., Reich, T., Vannier, M., and Raichle, M.E. (1997). Subgenual prefrontal cortex abnormalities in mood disorders. *Nature*, 386(6627), 824–827.

Drevets, W.C., Gautier, C., Lowry, T., Bogers, W., and Greer, P. (2001). Abnormal hemodynamic responses to facially expressed emotion in major depression. *Soc Neurosci Abstr*, 31.

Drevets, W.C., Bogers, W., and Raichle, M.E. (2002a). Functional anatomical correlates of antidepressant drug treatment assessed using PET measures of regional glucose metabolism. *Eur J Neuropharmacol*, 12(6), 527–544.

Drevets, W.C., Price, J.L., Bardgett, M.E., Reich, T., Todd, R.D., and Raichle, M.E. (2002b). Glucose metabolism in the amygdala in depression: Relationship to diagnostic subtype and plasma cortisol levels. *Pharmacol Biochem Behav*, 71(3), 431–447.

Drevets, W.C., Thase, M., et al. (2002c). *Glucose metabolic correlates of depression severity and antidepressant treatment response.* 57th Annual Convention and Scientific Program of the Society of Biological Psychiatry, Philadelphia, PA, May 16–18.

Drevets, W.C., Thase, M. et al. (2002d). Antidepressant drug effects on regional glucose metabolism in major depression. *Soc Neurosci Abstr*, 32.

Drevets, W.C., Gadde, K., and Krishnan, R. (2006). Neuroimaging studies of mood disorders. In D.S. Charney and E.J. Nestler (Eds.), *The Neurobiological Foundation of Mental Illness* (Second Edition) (pp. 461–490). New York: Oxford University Press.

Dunn, R.T., Willis, M.W., Benson, B.E., Repella, J.D., Kimbrell, T.A., Ketter, T.A., Speer, A.M., Osuch, E.A., and Post, R.M. (2005). Preliminary findings of uncoupling of flow and metabolism in unipolar compared with bipolar affective illness and normal controls. *Psychiatry Res*, 140(2), 181–198.

Dupont, R.M., Jernigan, T.L., Gillin, J.C., Butters, N., Delis, D.C., and Hesselink, J.R. (1987). Subcortical signal hyperintensities in bipolar patients detected by MRI [letter]. *Psychiatry Res*, 21(4), 357–358.

Dupont, R.M., Jernigan, T.L., Butters, N., Delis, D., Hesselink, J.R., Heindel, W., and Gillin, J.C. (1990). Subcortical abnormalities detected in bipolar affective disorder using magnetic resonance imaging. Clinical and neuropsychological significance. *Arch Gen Psychiatry*, 47(1), 55–59.

Dupont, R.M., Butters, N., Schafer, K., Wilson, T., Hesselink, J., and Gillin, J.C. (1995a). Diagnostic specificity of focal white matter abnormalities in bipolar and unipolar mood disorder. *Biol Psychiatry*, 38(7), 482–486.

Dupont, R.M., Jernigan, T.L., Heindel, W., Butters, N., Shafer, K., Wilson, T., Hesselink, J., and Gillin, J.C. (1995b). Magnetic resonance imaging and mood disorders. Localization of white matter and other subcortical abnormalities. *Arch Gen Psychiatry*, 52(9), 747–755.

Ebert, D., Feistel, H., and Barocka, A. (1991). Effects of sleep deprivation on the limbic system and the frontal lobes in affective disorders: A study with Tc-99m-HMPAO SPECT. *Psychiatry Res*, 40(4), 247–251.

Ebert, D., Feistel, H., Barocka, A., Kaschka, W., and Mokrusch, T. (1993). A test–retest study of cerebral blood flow during somatosensory stimulation in depressed patients with schizophrenia and major depression. *Eur Arch Psychiatry Clin Neurosci*, 242(4), 250–254.

Ebert, D., Feistel, H., Barocka, A., and Kaschka, W. (1994). Increased limbic blood flow and total sleep deprivation in major depression with melancholia. *Psychiatry Res*, 55(2), 101–109.

Ebmeier, K.P., Glabus, M.F., Prentice, N., Ryman, A., and Goodwin, G.M. (1998). A voxel-based analysis of cerebral perfusion in dementia and depression of old age. *Neuroimage*, 7(3), 199–208.

Edmonstone, Y., Austin, M.P., Prentice, N., Dougall, N., Freeman, C.P., Ebmeier, K.P., and Goodwin, G.M. (1994). Uptake of ^{99m}Tc-exametazime shown by single photon emission computerized tomography in obsessive-compulsive disorder compared with major depression and normal controls. *Acta Psychiatr Scand*, 90(4), 298–303.

Elizagarate, E., Cortes, J., Gonzalez Pinto, A., Gutierrez, M., Alonso, I., Alcorta, P., Ramirez, M., de Heredia, J.L., Figuerido, J.L. (2001). Study of the influence of electroconvulsive therapy on the regional cerebral blood flow by HMPAO-SPECT. *J Affect Disord*, 65(1), 55–59.

Elkis, H., Friedman, L., Wise, A., Meltzer, H.Y. (1995). Meta-analyses of studies of ventricular enlargement and cortical sulcal prominence in mood disorders. Comparisons with controls or patients with schizophrenia. *Arch Gen Psychiatry*, 52(9), 735–746.

Elliott, R., Baker, S.C., Rogers, R.D., O'Leary, D.A., Paykel, E.S., Frith, C.D., Dolan, R.J., and Sahakian, B.J. (1997). Prefrontal dysfunction in depressed patients performing a complex planning task: A study using positron emission tomography. *Psychol Med*, 27(4), 931–942.

Elliott, R., Sahakian, B.J., Michael, A., Paykel, E.S., and Dolan, R.J. (1998). Abnormal neural response to feedback on planning and guessing tasks in patients with unipolar depression. *Psychol Med*, 28(3), 559–571.

Ende, G., Braus, D.F., Walter, S., Weber-Fahr, W., and Henn, F.A. (2000a). The hippocampus in patients treated with electroconvulsive therapy: A proton magnetic resonance spectroscopic imaging study. *Arch Gen Psychiatry*, 57(10), 937–943.

Ende, G., Braus, D.F., Walter, S., Weber-Fahr, W., Soher, B., Maudsley, A.A., and Henn, F.A. (2000b). Effects of age, medication, and illness duration on the N-acetyl aspartate signal of the anterior cingulate region in schizophrenia. *Schizophr Res*, 41(3), 389–395.

Epperson, C.N., Haga, K., Mason, G.F., Sellers, E., Gueorguieva, R., Zhang, W., Weiss, E., Rothman, D.L., and Krystal, J.H. (2002). Cortical gamma-aminobutyric acid levels across the menstrual cycle in healthy women and those with premenstrual dysphoric disorder: A proton magnetic resonance spectroscopy study. *Arch Gen Psychiatry*, 59(9), 851–858.

Ernst, M., Zametkin, A.J., Phillips, R.L., and Cohen, R.M. (1998). Age-related changes in brain glucose metabolism in adults with attention-deficit/hyperactivity disorder and control subjects. *J Neuropsychiatry Clin Neurosci*, 10(2), 168–177.

Escalona, P.R., Early, B., McDonald, W.M., and Doraiswamy, P.M. (1993). Reduction of cerebellar volume in major depression: A controlled MRI study. *Depression*, 1, 156–158.

Farchione, T.R., Moore, G.J., and Rosenberg, D.R. (2002). Proton magnetic resonance spectroscopic imaging in pediatric major depression. *Biol Psychiatry*, 52(2), 86–92.

Federoff, J.P., Starkstein, S.E., Forrester, A.W., Geisler, F.H., Jorge, R.E., Arndt, S.V., and Robinson, R.G. (1992). Depression in patients with acute traumatic brain injury. *Am J Psychiatry*, 149(7), 918–923.

Felber, S.R., Pycha, R., Hummer, M., Aichner, F.T., and Fleischhacker, W.W. (1993). Localized proton and phosphorus magnetic resonance spectroscopy following electroconvulsive therapy. *Biol Psychiatry*, 33(8-9), 651–654.

Figiel, G.S., Coffey, C.E., and Weiner, R.D. (1989a). Brain magnetic resonance imaging in elderly depressed patients receiving electroconvulsive therapy. *Convulsive Ther*, 5(1), 26–34.

Figiel, G.S., Krishnan, K.R., Breitner, J.C., and Nemeroff, C.B. (1989b). Radiologic correlates of antidepressant-induced delirium: The possible significance of basal-ganglia lesions. *J Neuropsychiatry Clin Neurosci*, 1(2), 188–190.

Figiel, G.S., Coffey, C.E., Djang, W.T., Hoffman, G. Jr., and Doraiswamy, P.M. (1990a). Brain magnetic resonance imaging findings in ECT-induced delirium. *J Neuropsychiatry Clin Neurosci*, 2(1), 53–58.

Figiel, G.S., Krishnan, K.R., and Doraiswamy, P.M. (1990b). Subcortical structural changes in ECT-induced delirium. *J Geriatr Psychiatry Neurol*, 3(3), 172–176.

Figiel, G.S., Krishnan, K.R., Doraiswamy, P.M., Rao, V.P., Nemeroff, C.B., and Boyko, O.B. (1991a). Subcortical hyperintensities on brain magnetic resonance imaging: A comparison between late age onset and early onset elderly depressed subjects. *Neurobiol Aging*, 12(3), 245–247.

Figiel, G.S., Krishnan, K.R., Rao, V.P., Doraiswamy, M., Ellinwood, E.H. Jr., Nemeroff, C.B., Evans, D., and Boyko, O. (1991b). Subcortical hyperintensities on brain magnetic resonance imaging: A comparison of normal and bipolar subjects. *J Neuropsychiatry Clin Neurosci*, 3(1), 18–22.

Folstein, S.E. and Folstein, M.F. (1983). Psychiatric features of Huntington's disease: Recent approaches and findings. *Psychiatr Dev*, 1(2), 193–205.

Fox, P.T. and Raichle, M.E. (1986). Focal physiological uncoupling of cerebral blood flow and oxidative metabolism during somatosensory stimulation in human subjects. *Proc Natl Acad Sci USA*, 83(4), 1140–1144.

Frazier, J.A., Chiu, S., Breeze, J.L., Makris, N., Lange, N., Kennedy, D.N., Herbert, M.R., Bent, E.K., Koneru, V.K., Dieterich, M.E., Hodge, S.M., Rauch, S.L., Grant, P.E., Cohen, B.M., Seidman, L.J., Caviness, V.S., and Biederman, J. (2005). Structural brain magnetic resonance imaging of limbic and thalamic volumes in pediatric bipolar disorder. *Am J Psychiatry*, 162(7), 1256–1265.

Frey, R., Metzler, D., Fischer, P., Heiden, A., Scharfetter, J., Moser, E., and Kasper, S. (1998). Myo-inositol in depressive and healthy subjects determined by frontal 1H-magnetic resonance spectroscopy at 1.5 tesla. *J Psychiatr Res*, 32(6), 411–420.

Friedman, S.D., Dager, S.R., Parow, A., Hirashima, F., Demopulos, C., Stoll, A.L., Lyoo, I.K., Dunner, D.L., and Renshaw, P.F. (2004). Lithium and valproic acid treatment effects on brain chemistry in bipolar disorder. *Biol Psychiatry*, 56(5), 340–348.

Frodl, T., Meisenzahl, E., Zetzsche, T., Bottlender, R., Born, C., Groll, C., Jager, M., Leinsinger, G., Hahn, K., and Moller, H.J. (2002a). Enlargement of the amygdala in patients with a first episode of major depression. *Biol Psychiatry*, 51(9), 708–714.

Frodl, T., Meisenzahl, E.M., Zetzsche, T., Born, C., Groll, C., Jager, M., Leinsinger, G., Bottlender, R., Hahn, K., and Moller, H.J. (2002b). Hippocampal changes in patients with a first episode of major depression. *Am J Psychiatry*, 159(7), 1112–1118.

Frodl, T., Meisenzahl, E.M., Zetzsche, T., Born, C., Jager, M., Groll, C., Bottlender, R., Leinsinger, G., and Moller, H.J. (2003). Larger amygdala volumes in first depressive episode as compared to recurrent major depression and healthy control subjects. *Biol Psychiatry*, 53(4), 338–344.

Frodl, T., Meisenzahl, E.M., Zetzsche, T., Hohne, T., Banac, S., Schorr, C., Jager, M., Leinsinger, G., Bottlender, R., Reiser, M., and Moller, H.J. (2004). Hippocampal and amygdala changes in patients with major depressive disorder and healthy controls during a 1-year follow-up. *J Clin Psychiatry*, 65(4), 492–499.

Frye, M.A., Bertolino, A., et al. (2000). *A 1H-MRSI hippocampal study in bipolar patients with a history of alcohol abuse*. 55th Annual Convention and Scientific Program of the Society of Biological Psychiatry, Chicago, IL, May 11–13.

Frye, M.A., Yue, K., et al. (2001). *Decreased basal ganglia n-acetyl-aspartate in mania*. 40th Annual Meeting of the American College of Neuropsychopharmacology, Waikaloa, Hawaii, December 9–13.

Fujikawa, T., Yamawaki, S., and Touhouda, Y. (1993). Incidence of silent cerebral infarction in patients with major depression. *Stroke*, 24(11), 1631–1634.

Fujikawa, T., Yamawaki, S., and Touhouda, Y. (1995). Silent cerebral infarctions in patients with late-onset mania. *Stroke*, 26(6), 946–949.

Fujikawa, T., Yokota, N., Muraoka, M., and Yamawaki, S. (1996). Response of patients with major depression and silent cerebral infarction to antidepressant drug therapy, with emphasis on central nervous system adverse reactions. *Stroke*, 27(11), 2040–2042.

Fujikawa, T., Yanai, I., and Yamawaki, S. (1997). Psychosocial stressors in patients with major depression and silent cerebral infarction. *Stroke*, 28(6), 1123–1125.

Galynker, I.I., Cai, J., Ongseng, F., Finestone, H., Dutta, E., and Serseni, D. (1998). Hypofrontality and negative symptoms in major depressive disorder. *J Nucl Med*, 39(4), 608–612.

Gemar, M.C., Kapur, S., Segal, Z.V., Brown, G.M., and Houle, S. (1996). Effects of self-generated sad mood on regional cerebral activity: A PET study in normal subjects. *Depression*, 4(2), 81–88.

George, M.S., Ketter, T.A., Gill, D.S., Haxby, J.V., Ungerleider, L.G., Herscovitch, P., and Post, R.M. (1993). Brain regions involved in recognizing facial emotion or identity: An oxygen-15 PET study. *J Neuropsychiatry Clin Neurosci*, 5(4), 384–394.

George, M.S., Kellner, C.H., Bernstein, H., and Goust, J.M. (1994). A magnetic resonance imaging investigation into mood disorders in multiple sclerosis. *J Nerv Ment Dis*, 182(7), 410–412.

George, M.S., Ketter, T.A., Parekh, P.I., Herscovitch, P., and Post, R.M. (1995a). Brain activity during transient sadness and happiness in healthy women. *Am J Psychiatry*, 152(3), 341–351.

George, M.S., Kimbrell, T., et al. (1995b). *Actively depressed subjects have difficulty inducing, and blunted limbic rCBF during, transient sadness*. 148th Annual Meeting of the American Psychiatric Association, Miami, FL, May 20–25.

George, M.S., Wassermann, E.M., Williams, W.A., Callahan, A., Ketter, T.A., Basser, P., Hallett, M., and Post, R.M. (1995c). Daily repetitive transcranial magnetic stimulation (rTMS) improves mood in depression. *Neuroreport*, 6(14), 1853–1856.

George, M.S., Ketter, T.A., Parekh, P.I., Herscovitch, P., and Post, R.M. (1996). Gender differences in regional cerebral blood flow during transient self-induced sadness or happiness. *Biol Psychiatry*, 40(9), 859–871.

George, M.S., Ketter, T.A. Parekh, P.I., and Gill, D.S. (1997a). Depressed subjects have decreased rCBF activation during facial emotion recognition. *CNS Spectrums*, 2(10), 45–55.

George, M.S., Ketter, T.A., Parekh, P.I., Rosinsky, N., Ring, H.A., Pazzaglia, P.J., Marangell, L.B., Callahan, A.M., and Post, R.M. (1997b). Blunted left cingulate activation in mood disorder subjects during a response interference task (the Stroop). *J Neuropsychiatry Clin Neurosci*, 9(1), 55–63.

Giedd, J.N., Blumenthal, J., Jeffries, N.O., Castellanos, F.X., Liu, H., Zijdenbos, A., Paus, T., Evans, A.C., and Rapoport, J.L. (1999). Brain development during childhood and adolescence: A longitudinal MRI study. *Nat Neurosci*, 2(10), 861–863.

Ginsberg, M.D., Chang, J.Y., Kelley, R.E., Yoshii, F., Barker, W.W., Ingenito, G., and Boothe, T.E. (1988). Increases in both cerebral glucose utilization and blood flow during execution of a somatosensory task. *Ann Neurol*, 23(2), 152–160.

Gonzalez, R.G., Guimaraes, A.R., Sachs, G.S., Rosenbaum, J.F., Garwood, M., and Renshaw, P.F. (1993). Measurement of human brain lithium in vivo by MR spectroscopy. *AJNR Am J Neuroradiol*, 14(5), 1027–1037.

Goodwin, G.M., Austin, M.P., Dougall, N., Ross, M., Murray, C., O'Carroll, R.E., Moffoot, A., Prentice, N., and Ebmeier, K.P. (1993). State changes in brain activity shown by the uptake of 99mTc-exametazime with single photon emission tomography in major depression before and after treatment. *J Affect Disord*, 29(4), 243–253.

Goodwin, G.M., Cavanagh, J.T., Glabus, M.F., Kehoe, R.F., O'Carroll, R.E., and Ebmeier, K.P. (1997). Uptake of ^{99m}Tc-exametazime shown by single photon emission computed tomography before and after lithium withdrawal in bipolar patients: Associations with mania. *Br J Psychiatry*, 170, 426–430.

Goyer, P.F., Schulz, P.M., Semple, W.E., Gross, M., Nordahl, T.E., King, A.C., Wehr, T.A., and Cohen, R.M. (1992). Cerebral glucose metabolism in patients with summer seasonal affective disorder. *Neuropsychopharmacology*, 7(3), 233–240.

Grachev, I.D. and Apkarian, A.V. (2000). Chemical heterogeneity of the living human brain: A proton MR spectroscopy study on the effects of sex, age, and brain region. *Neuroimage*, 11(5 Pt. 1), 554–563.

Grachev, I.D., and Apkarian, A.V. (2001). Aging alters regional multichemical profile of the human brain: An in vivo 1H-MRS study of young versus middle-aged subjects. *J Neurochem*, 76(2), 582–593.

Grasso, M.G., Pantano, P., Ricci, M., Intiso, D.F., Pace, A., Padovani, A., Orzi, F., Pozzilli, C., and Lenzi, G.L. (1994). Mesial temporal cortex hypoperfusion is associated with depression in subcortical stroke. *Stroke*, 25(5), 980–985.

Greenwald, B.S., Kramer-Ginsberg, E., Krishnan, R.R., Ashtari, M., Aupperle, P.M., and Patel, M. (1996). MRI signal hyperintensities in geriatric depression. *Am J Psychiatry*, 153(9), 1212–1215.

Greenwald, B.S., Kramer-Ginsberg, E., Bogerts, B., Ashtari, M., Aupperle, P., Wu, H., Allen, L., Zeman, D., and Patel, M. (1997). Qualitative magnetic resonance imaging findings in geriatric depression. Possible link between later-onset depression and Alzheimer's disease? *Psychol Med*, 27(2), 421–431.

Greenwald, B.S., Kramer-Ginsberg, E., Krishnan, K.R., Ashtari, M., Auerbach, C., and Patel, M. (1998). Neuroanatomic localization of magnetic resonance imaging signal hyperintensities in geriatric depression. *Stroke*, 29(3), 613–617.

Grodd, W., Schneider, F., Klose, U., and Nagele, T. (1995). Functional magnetic resonance tomography of psychological functions exemplified by experimentally induced emotions. *Radiologe*, 35(4), 283–289.

Gruber, S., Frey, R., Mlynarik, V., Stadlbauer, A., Heiden, A., Kasper, S., Kemp, G.J., and Moser, E. (2003). Quantification of metabolic differences in the frontal brain of depressive patients and controls obtained by 1H-MRS at 3 Tesla. *Invest Radiol*, 38(7), 403–408.

Gur, R.E., Skolnick, B.E., Gur, R.C., Caroff, S., Rieger, W., Obrist, W.D., Younkin, D., and Reivich, M. (1984). Brain function in psychiatric disorders. II. Regional cerebral blood flow in medicated unipolar depressives. *Arch Gen Psychiatry*, 41(7), 695–699.

Gur, R.C., Mozley, L.H., Mozley, P.D., Resnick, S.M., Karp, J.S., Alavi, A., Arnold, S.E., and Gur, R.E. (1995). Sex differences in regional cerebral glucose metabolism during a resting state. *Science*, 267(5197), 528–531.

Guze, B.H., and Szuba, M.P. (1992). Leukoencephalopathy and major depression: A preliminary report. *Psychiatry Res*, 45(3), 169–175.

Gyulai, L., Bolinger, L., Leigh, J.S. Jr., Barlow, C., and Chance, B. (1984). Phosphorylethanolamine: The major constituent of the phosphomonoester peak observed by 31P-NMR on developing dog brain. *FEBS Lett*, 178(1), 137–142.

Gyulai, L., Wicklund, S.W., Greenstein, R., Bauer, M.S., Ciccione, P., Whybrow, P.C., Zimmerman, J., Kovachich, G., and Alves, W. (1991). Measurement of tissue lithium concentration by lithium magnetic resonance spectroscopy in patients with bipolar disorder. *Biol Psychiatry*, 29(12), 1161–1170.

Gyulai, L., Alavi, A., Broich, K., Reilley, J., Ball, W.B., and Whybrow, P.C. (1997). I-123 iofetamine single-photon computed emission tomography in rapid cycling bipolar disorder: A clinical study. *Biol Psychiatry*, 41(2), 152–161.

Hagman, J.O., Buchsbaum, M.S., Wu, J.C., Rao, S.J., Reynolds, C.A., and Blinder, B.J. (1990). Comparison of regional brain metabolism in bulimia nervosa and affective disorder assessed with positron emission tomography. *J Affect Disord*, 19(3), 153–162.

Hallcher, L.M., and Sherman, W.R. (1980). The effects of lithium ion and other agents on the activity of myo-inositol-1-phosphatase from bovine brain. *J Biol Chem*, 255(22), 10896–10901.

Hallett, M., Dubinsky, R.M., Zeffiro, T., and Bierner, S.M. (1994). Comparison of glucose metabolism and cerebral blood flow during cortical motor activation. *J Neuroimaging*, 4(1), 1–5.

Hamakawa, H., Kato, T., Murashita, J., and Kato, N. (1998). Quantitative proton magnetic resonance spectroscopy of the basal ganglia in patients with affective disorders. *Eur Arch Psychiatry Clin Neurosci*, 248(1), 53–58.

Hamakawa, H., Kato, T., Shioiri, T., Inubushi, T., and Kato, N. (1999). Quantitative proton magnetic resonance spectroscopy of the bilateral frontal lobes in patients with bipolar disorder. *Psychol Med*, 29(3), 639–644.

Hamidi, M., Drevets, W.C., and Price, J.L. (2004). Glial reduction in amygdala in major depressive disorder is due to oligodendrocytes. *Biol Psychiatry*, 55(6), 563–569.

Harvey, I., Persaud, R., Ron, M.A., Baker, G., and Murray, R.M. (1994). Volumetric MRI measurements in bipolars compared with schizophrenics and healthy controls. *Psychol Med*, 24(3), 689–699.

Hauser, P., Altshuler, L.L., Berrettini, W., Dauphinais, I.D., Gelernter, J., and Post, R.M. (1989a). Temporal lobe measurement in primary affective disorder by magnetic resonance imaging. *J Neuropsychiatry Clin Neurosci*, 1(2), 128–134.

Hauser, P., Dauphinais, I.D., Berrettini, W., DeLisi, L.E., Gelernter, J., and Post, R.M. (1989b). Corpus callosum dimensions measured by magnetic resonance imaging in bipolar affective disorder and schizophrenia. *Biol Psychiatry*, 26(7), 659–668.

Hauser, P., Matochik, J., Altshuler, L.L., Denicoff, K.D., Conrad, A., Li, X., and Post, R.M. (2000). MRI-based measurements of temporal lobe and ventricular structures in patients with bipolar I and bipolar II disorders. *J Affect Disord*, 60(1), 25–32.

Heath, R.G., Franklin, D.E., Walker, C.F., and Keating, J.W. Jr. (1982). Cerebellar vermal atrophy in psychiatric patients. *Biol Psychiatry*, 17(5), 569–583.

Hedges, L.V., and Olkin, I. (1985). *Statistical Methods for Meta-analysis*. Orlando, FL: National Academy Press.

Henry, M.E., Schmidt, M.E., Matochik, J.A., Stoddard, E.P., and Potter, W.Z. (2001). The effects of ECT on brain glucose: A pilot FDG PET study. *J ECT*, 17(1), 33–40.

Hickie, I., Scott, E., Mitchell, P., Wilhelm, K., Austin, M.P., and Bennett, B. (1995). Subcortical hyperintensities on magnetic resonance imaging: Clinical correlates and prognostic significance in patients with severe depression. *Biol Psychiatry*, 37(3), 151–160.

Hickie, I., Scott, E., Wilhelm, K., and Brodaty, H. (1997). Subcortical hyperintensities on magnetic resonance imaging in patients with severe depression: A longitudinal evaluation. *Biol Psychiatry*, 42(5), 367–374.

Hirayasu, Y., Shenton, M.E., Salisbury, D.F., Kwon, J.S., Wible, C.G., Fischer, I.A., Yurgelun-Todd, D., Zarate, C., Kikinis, R., Jolesz, F.A., and McCarley, R.W. (1999). Subgenual cingulate cortex volume in first-episode psychosis. *Am J Psychiatry*, 156(7), 1091–1093.

Hirono, N., Mori, E., Ishii, K., Ikejiri, Y., Imamura, T., Shimomura, T., Hashimoto, M., Yamashita, H., and Sasaki, M. (1998). Frontal lobe hypometabolism and depression in Alzheimer's disease. *Neurology*, 50(2), 380–383.

Ho, A.P., Gillin, J.C., Buchsbaum, M.S., Wu, J.C., Abel, L., and Bunney, W.E. Jr. (1996). Brain glucose metabolism during non-rapid eye movement sleep in major depression. A positron emission tomography study. *Arch Gen Psychiatry*, 53(7), 645–652.

Hoge, E.A., Friedman, L., and Schulz, S.C. (1999). Meta-analysis of brain size in bipolar disorder. *Schizophr Res*, 37(2), 177–181.

Holthoff, V.A., Beuthien-Baumann, B., Pietrzyk, U., Pinkert, J., Oehme, L., Franke, W.G., and Bach, O. (1999). Changes in regional cerebral perfusion in depression: SPECT monitoring of response to treatment. *Nervenarzt*, 70(7), 620–626.

Honer, W.G., Hurwitz, T., Li, D.K., Palmer, M., and Paty, D.W. (1987). Temporal lobe involvement in multiple sclerosis patients with psychiatric disorders. *Arch Neurol*, 44(2), 187–190.

Horn, S. (1974). Some psychological factors in Parkinsonism. *J Neurol Neurosurg Psychiatry*, 37(1), 27–31.

Hornig, M., Mozley, P.D., and Amsterdam, J.D. (1997). HMPAO SPECT brain imaging in treatment-resistant depression. *Prog Neuropsychopharmacol Biol Psychiatry*, 21(7), 1097–1114.

Horska, A., Kaufmann, W.E., Brant, L.J., Naidu, S., Harris, J.C., and Barker, P.B. (2002). In vivo quantitative proton MRSI study of brain development from childhood to adolescence. *J Magn Reson Imaging*, 15(2), 137–143.

Howard, R.J., Beats, B., et al. (1993). White matter changes in late onset depression: A magnetic resonance imaging study [letter]. *Int J Geriat Psychiatry*, 8, 183–185.

Howard, R., Cox, T., Almeida, O., Mullen, R., Graves, P., Reveley, A., and Levy, R. (1995). White matter signal hyperintensities in the brains of patients with late paraphrenia and the normal, community-living elderly. *Biol Psychiatry*, 38(2), 86–91.

Hsieh, M.H., McQuoid, D.R., Levy, R.M., Payne, M.E., MacFall, J.R., and Steffens, D.C. (2002). Hippocampal volume and antidepressant response in geriatric depression. *Int J Geriatr Psychiatry*, 17(6), 519–525.

Hurwitz, T.A., Clark, C., Murphy, E., Klonoff, H., Martin, W.R., and Pate, B.D. (1990). Regional cerebral glucose metabolism in major depressive disorder. *Can J Psychiatry*, 35(8), 684–688.

Husain, M.M., McDonald, W.M., Doraiswamy, P.M., Figiel, G.S., Na, C., Escalona, P.R., Boyko, O.B., Nemeroff, C.B., and Krishnan, K.R. (1991). A magnetic resonance imaging study of putamen nuclei in major depression. *Psychiatry Res*, 40(2), 95–99.

Iacono, W.G., Smith, G.N., Moreau, M., Beiser, M., Fleming, J.A., Lin, T.Y., and Flak, B. (1988). Ventricular and sulcal size at the onset of psychosis. *Am J Psychiatry*, 145(7), 820–824.

Iidaka, T., Nakajima, T., Kawamoto, K., Fukuda, H., Suzuki, Y., Maehara, T., and Shiraishi, H. (1996). Signal hyperintensities on brain magnetic resonance imaging in elderly depressed patients. *Eur Neurol*, 36(5), 293–299.

Iidaka, T., Nakajima, T., Suzuki, Y., Okazaki, A., Maehara, T., and Shiraishi, H. (1997). Quantitative regional cerebral flow measured by Tc-99M HMPAO SPECT in mood disorder. *Psychiatry Res*, 68(2-3), 143–154.

Irwin, W., Davidson, R.J., Lowe, M.J., Mock, B.J., Sorenson, J.A., and Turski, P.A. (1996). Human amygdala activation detected with echo-planar functional magnetic resonance imaging. *Neuroreport*, 7(11), 1765–1769.

Ito, H., Kawashima, R., Awata, S., Ono, S., Sato, K., Goto, R., Koyama, M., Sato, M., and Fukuda, H. (1996). Hypoperfusion in the limbic system and prefrontal cortex in depression: SPECT with anatomic standardization technique. *J Nucl Med*, 37(3), 410–414.

Jacoby, R.J., and Levy, R. (1980). Computed tomography in the elderly. 3. Affective disorder. *Br J Psychiatry*, 136, 270–275.

Jacoby, R.J., Levy, R., and Bird, J.M. (1981). Computed tomography and the outcome of affective disorder: A follow-up study of elderly patients. *Br J Psychiatry*, 139, 288–292.

Janowsky, D.S., el-Yousef, M.K., Davis, J.M, and Sekerke, H.J. (1972). A cholinergic-adrenergic hypothesis of mania and depression. *Lancet*, 2(778), 632–635.

Janssen, J., Hulshoff Pol, H.E., Lampe, I.K., Schnack, H.G., de Leeuw, F.E., Kahn, R.S., and Heeren, T.J. (2004). Hippocampal changes and white matter lesions in early-onset depression. *Biol Psychiatry*, 56(11), 825–831.

Jenkins, M., Malloy, P., Salloway, S., Cohen, R., Rogg, J., Tung, G., Kohn, R., Westlake, R., Johnson, E.G., and Richardson, E. (1998). Memory processes in depressed geriatric patients with and without subcortical hyperintensities on MRI. *J Neuroimaging*, 8(1), 20–26.

Jensen, H.V., Plenge, P., Stensgaard, A., Mellerup, E.T., Thomsen, C., Aggernaes, H., and Henriksen, O. (1996). Twelve-hour brain lithium concentration in lithium maintenance treatment of manic-depressive disorder: Daily versus alternate-day dosing schedule. *Psychopharmacology (Berl)*, 124(3), 275–278.

Jernigan, T.L., Press, G.A., and Hesselink, J.R. (1990). Methods for measuring brain morphologic features on magnetic resonance images: Validation and normal aging. *Arch Neurol*, 47(1), 27–32.

Jernigan, T.L., Archibald, S.L., Berhow, M.T., Sowell, E.R., Foster, D.S., and Hesselink, J.R. (1991). Cerebral structure on MRI, Part I: Localization of age-related changes. *Biol Psychiatry*, 29(1), 55–67.

Jeste, D.V., Lohr, J.B., and Goodwin, F.K. (1988). Neuroanatomical studies of major affective disorders. A review and suggestions for further research. *Br J Psychiatry*, 153, 444–459.

Johnstone, E.C., Owens, D.G., Crow, T.J., Colter, N., Lawton, C.A., Jagoe, R., and Kreel, L. (1986). Hypothyroidism as a correlate of lateral ventricular enlargement in manic-depressive and neurotic illness. *Br J Psychiatry*, 148, 317–321.

Johnstone, E.C., Owens, D.G., Crow, T.J., Frith, C.D., Alexandropolis, K., Bydder, G., and Colter, N. (1989). Temporal lobe structure as determined by nuclear magnetic resonance in schizophrenia and bipolar affective disorder. *J Neurol Neurosurg Psychiatry*, 52(6), 736–741.

Jorge, R.E., Robinson, R.G., Starkstein, S.E., Arndt, S.V., Forrester, A.W., and Geisler, F.H. (1993). Secondary mania following traumatic brain injury. *Am J Psychiatry*, 150(6), 916–921.

Jung, R.E., Yeo, R.A., Love, T.M., Petropoulos, H., Sibbitt, W.L. Jr., and Brooks, W.M. (2002). Biochemical markers of mood: A proton magnetic resonance spectroscopy study of normal human brain. *Biol Psychiatry*, 51(3), 224–229.

Kanakaratnam, G., and Direkze, M. (1976). Aspects of primary tumours of the frontal lobe. *Br J Clin Pract*, 30(11–12), 220–221.

Kanaya, T., and Yonekawa, M. (1990). Regional cerebral blood flow in depression. *Jpn J Psychiatry Neurol*, 44(3), 571–576.

Kato, T., Shioiri, T., Takahashi, S., and Inubushi, T. (1991). Measurement of brain phosphoinositide metabolism in bipolar patients using in vivo ³¹P-MRS. *J Affect Disord*, 22(4), 185–190.

Kato, T., Takahashi, S., and Inubushi, T. (1992a). Brain lithium concentration by ⁷Li- and ¹H-magnetic resonance spectroscopy in bipolar disorder. *Psychiatry Res*, 45(1), 53–63.

Kato, T., Takahashi, S., Shioiri, T., and Inubushi T. (1992b). Brain phosphorous metabolism in depressive disorders detected by phosphorus-31 magnetic resonance spectroscopy. *J Affect Disord*, 26(4), 223–230.

Kato, T., Shioiri, T., Inubushi, T., and Takahashi, S. (1993a). Brain lithium concentrations measured with lithium-7 magnetic resonance spectroscopy in patients with affective disorders: Relationship to erythrocyte and serum concentrations. *Biol Psychiatry*, 33(3), 147–152.

Kato, T., Takahashi, S., Shioiri, T., and Inubushi, T. (1993b). Alterations in brain phosphorous metabolism in bipolar disorder detected by in vivo ³¹P and ⁷Li magnetic resonance spectroscopy. *J Affect Disord*, 27(1), 53–59.

Kato, T., Inubushi, T., and Takahashi, S. (1994a). Relationship of lithium concentrations in the brain measured by lithium-7 magnetic resonance spectroscopy to treatment response in mania. *J Clin Psychopharmacol*, 14(5), 330–335.

Kato, T., Shioiri, T., Murashita, J., Hamakawa, H., Inubushi, T., and Takahashi, S. (1994b). Phosphorus-31 magnetic resonance spectroscopy and ventricular enlargement in bipolar disorder. *Psychiatry Res*, 55(1), 41–50.

Kato, T., Takahashi, S., Shioiri, T., Murashita, J., Hamakawa, H., and Inubushi, T. (1994c). Reduction of brain phosphocreatine in bipolar II disorder detected by phosphorus-31 magnetic resonance spectroscopy. *J Affect Disord*, 31(2), 125–133.

Kato, T., Shioiri, T., Murashita, J., Hamakawa, H., Inubushi, T., and Takahashi, S. (1995a). Lateralized abnormality of high-energy phosphate and bilateral reduction of phosphomonoester measured by phosphorus-31 magnetic resonance spectroscopy of the frontal lobes in schizophrenia. *Psychiatry Res*, 61(3), 151–160.

Kato, T., Shioiri, T., Murashita, J., Hamakawa, H., Takahashi, Y., Inubushi, T., and Takahashi, S. (1995b). Lateralized abnormality of high energy phosphate metabolism in the frontal lobes of patients with bipolar disorder detected by phase-encoded ³¹P-MRS. *Psychol Med*, 25(3), 557–566.

Kato, T., Fujii, K., Shioiri, T., Inubushi, T., and Takahashi, S. (1996a). Lithium side effects in relation to brain lithium concentration measured by lithium-7 magnetic resonance spectroscopy. *Prog Neuropsychopharmacol Biol Psychiatry*, 20(1), 87–97.

Kato, T., Hamakawa, H., Shioiri, T., Murashita, J., Takahashi, Y., Takahashi, S., and Inubushi, T. (1996b). Choline-containing compounds detected by proton magnetic resonance spectroscopy in the basal ganglia in bipolar disorder. *J Psychiatry Neurosci*, 21(4), 248–254.

Kato, T., Murashita, J., Kamiya, A., Shioiri, T., Kato, N., and Inubushi, T. (1998). Decreased brain intracellular pH measured by 31P-MRS in bipolar disorder: A confirmation in drug-free patients and correlation with white matter hyperintensity. *Eur Arch Psychiatry Clin Neurosci*, 248(6), 301–306.

Kaufman, M.J., Henry, M.E., Frederick, B.D., Hennen, J., Villafuerte, R.A., Stoddard, E.P., Schmidt, M.E., Cohen, B.M., and Renshaw, P.F. (2003). Selective serotonin reuptake inhibitor discontinuation syndrome is associated with a rostral anterior cingulate choline metabolite decrease: A proton magnetic resonance spectroscopic imaging study. *Biol Psychiatry*, 54(5), 534–553.

Kaur, S., Sassi, R.B., Axelson, D., Nicoletti, M., Brambilla, P., Monkul, E.S., Hatch, J.P., Keshavan, M.S., Ryan, N., Birmaher, B., and Soares, J.C. (2005). Cingulate cortex anatomical abnormalities in children and adolescents with bipolar disorder. *Am J Psychiatry*, 162(9), 1637–1643.

Kegeles, L.S., Malone, K.M., Slifstein, M., Ellis, S.P., Xanthopoulos, E., Keilp, J.G., Campbell, C., Oquendo, M., Van Heertum, R.L., and Mann, J.J. (2003). Response of cortical metabolic deficits to serotonergic challenge in familial mood disorders. *Am J Psychiatry*, 160(1), 76–82.

Kellner, C.H., Rubinow, D.R., Gold, P.W., and Post, R.M. (1983). Relationship of cortisol hypersecretion to brain CT scan alterations in depressed patients. *Psychiatry Res*, 8(3), 191–197.

Kellner, C.H., Rubinow, D.R., and Post, R.M. (1986). Cerebral ventricular size and cognitive impairment in depression. *J Affect Disord*, 10(3), 215–219.

Kemmerer, M., Nasrallah, H.A., et al. (1994). *Increased hippocampal volume in bipolar disorder* [abstract]. 49th Annual Meeting of the Society of Biological Psychiatry, Philadelphia, PA, May 18–22.

Kennedy, S.H., Evans, K.R., Kruger, S., Mayberg, H.S., Meyer, J.H., McCann, S., Arifuzzman, A.I., Houle, S., and Vaccarino, F.J. (2001). Changes in regional brain glucose metabolism measured with positron emission tomography after paroxetine treatment of major depression. *Am J Psychiatry*, 158(6), 899–905.

Keshavan, M.S., Pettegrew, J.W., et al. (1992). Membrane phospholipids and lithium response in schizophrenia: A ³¹P-MRS study. Abstract VIII.B.1. *Schizophr Res*, 6, 134.

Ketter, T.A., and Drevets, W.C. (2002). Neuroimaging studies of bipolar depression: Functional neuropathology, treatment effects, and predictors of clinical response. *Clin Neurosci Res*, 2(3-4), 182–192.

Ketter, T.A., and Wang, P.W. (2002). Predictors of treatment response in bipolar disorders: Evidence from clinical and brain imaging studies. *J Clin Psychiatry*, 63(Suppl. 3), 21–25.

Ketter, T.A., and Wang, P.W. (2003). The emerging differential roles of GABAergic and antiglutamatergic agents in bipolar disorders. *J Clin Psychiatry*, 64(Suppl. 3), 15–20.

Ketter, T.A., Andreason, P.J., et al. (1993). *Blunted CBF response to procaine in mood disorders.* 146th Annual Meeting of the American Psychiatric Association, San Francisco, CA, May 22–27.

Ketter, T.A., Andreason, P.J., George, M.S., Lee, C., Gill, D.S., Parekh, P.I., Willis, M.W., Herscovitch, P., and Post, R.M. (1996a). Anterior paralimbic mediation of procaine-induced emotional and psychosensory experiences. *Arch Gen Psychiatry*, 53(1)59–69.

Ketter, T.A., George, M.S., Kimbrell, T.A., and Benson, B.E. (1996b). Functional brain imaging, limbic function, and affective disorders. *Neuroscientist*, 2(1), 55–65.

Ketter, T.A., Winsberg, M.E., et al. (1997). *Amygdalar metabolism decreases with thirty minute self-induction of depressed mood by recalling sad memories.* 36th Annual Meeting of the American College of Neuropsychopharmacology, Waikoloa, HI, December 8–12.

Ketter, T.A., Kimbrell, T.A., George, M.S., Willis, M.W., Benson, B.E., Danielson, A., Frye, M.A., Herscovitch, P., and Post, R.M. (1999). Baseline cerebral hypermetabolism associated with carbamazepine response, and hypometabolism with nimodipine response in mood disorders. *Biol Psychiatry*, 46(10), 1364–1374.

Ketter, T.A., Wang, P.W., et al. (2000). *Baseline hypofrontality and divalproex response in bipolar disorders.* 55th Annual Convention and Scientific Program of the Society of Biological Psychiatry, Chicago, IL, May 11–13.

Ketter, T.A., Kimbrell, T.A., George, M.S., Dunn, R.T., Speer, A.M., Benson, B.E., Willis, M.W., Danielson, A., Frye, M.A., Herscovitch, P., and Post, R.M. (2001). Effects of mood and subtype on cerebral glucose metabolism in treatment-refractory bipolar disorders. *Biol Psychiatry*, 49(2), 97–109.

Ketter, T.A., Wang, P.W., et al. (2002). Brain anatomic circuits and the pathophysiology of affective disorders. In J.C. Soares (Ed.), *Brain Imaging in Affective Disorders* (pp. 79–118). New York: Marcel Dekker.

Ketter, T.A., Wang, P.W., Becker, O.V., Nowakowska, C., and Yang, Y. (2003). The diverse roles of anticonvulsants in bipolar disorders. *Ann Clin Psychiatry*, 15(2), 95–108.

Ketter, T.A., Wang, P.W., Becker, O.V., Nowakowska, C., and Yang, Y. (2004). Psychotic bipolar disorders: Dimensionally similar to or categorically different from schizophrenia? *J Psychiatry Res*, 38(1), 47–61.

Kimbrell, T.A., Little, J.T., Dunn, R.T., Frye, M.A., Greenberg, B.D., Wassermann, E.M., Repella, J.D., Danielson, A.L., Willis, M.W., Benson, B.E., Speer, A.M., Osuch, E., George, M.S., and Post, R.M. (1999). Frequency dependence of antidepressant response to left prefrontal repetitive transcranial magnetic stimulation (rTMS) as a function of baseline cerebral glucose metabolism. *Biol Psychiatry*, 46(12), 1603–1613.

Kimbrell, T.A., Ketter, T.A., George, M.S., Little, J.T., Benson, B.E., Willis, M.W., Herscovitch, P., and Post, R.M. (2002). Regional cerebral glucose utilization in patients with a range of severities of unipolar depression. *Biol Psychiatry*, 51(3), 237–252.

Kishimoto, H., Takazu, O., Ohno, S., Yamaguchi, T., Fujita, H., Kuwahara, H., Ishii, T., Matsushita, M., Yokoi, S., and Iio, M. (1987). ^{11}C-glucose metabolism in manic and depressed patients. *Psychiatry Res*, 22(1), 81–88.

Kling, A.S., Metter, E.J., Riege, W.H., and Kuhl, D.E. (1986). Comparison of PET measurement of local brain glucose metabolism and CAT measurement of brain atrophy in chronic schizophrenia and depression. *Am J Psychiatry*, 143(2), 175–180.

Kolbeinsson, H., Arnaldsson, O.S., Petursson, H., and Skulason, S. (1986). Computed tomographic scans in ECT-patients. *Acta Psychiatr Scand*, 73(1), 28–32.

Komoroski, R.A., Newton, J.E., Walker, E., Cardwell, D., Jagannathan, N.R., Ramaprasad, S., and Sprigg, J. (1990). In vivo NMR spectroscopy of lithium-7 in humans. *Magn Reson Med*, 15(3), 347–356.

Komoroski, R.A., Newton, J.E., Sprigg, J.R., Cardwell, D., Mohanakrishnan, P., and Karson, C.N. (1993). In vivo ^{7}Li nuclear magnetic resonance study of lithium pharmacokinetics and chemical shift imaging in psychiatric patients. *Psychiatry Res*, 50(2), 67–76.

Kowatch, R.A., Devous, M.D. Sr., Harvey, D.C., Mayes, T.L., Trivedi, M.H., Emslie, G.J., and Weinberg, W.A. (1999). A SPECT HMPAO study of regional cerebral blood flow in depressed adolescents and normal controls. *Prog Neuropsychopharmacol Biol Psychiatry*, 23(4), 643–656.

Krabbendam, L., Honig, A., Wiersma, J., Vuurman, E.F., Hofman, P.A., Derix, M.M., Nolen, W.A., and Jolles, J. (2000). Cognitive dysfunctions and white matter lesions in patients with bipolar disorder in remission. *Acta Psychiatr Scand*, 101(4), 274–280.

Kramer-Ginsberg, E., Greenwald, B.S., Krishnan, K.R., Christiansen, B., Hu, J., Ashtari, M., Patel, M., and Pollack, S. (1999). Neuropsychological functioning and MRI signal hyperintensities in geriatric depression. *Am J Psychiatry*, 156(3), 438–444.

Krishnan, K.R. (1993). Neuroanatomic substrates of depression in the elderly. *J Geriatr Psychiatry Neurol*, 6(1), 39–58.

Krishnan, K.R., Goli, V., Ellinwood, E.H., France, R.D., Blazer, D.G., and Nemeroff, C.B. (1988). Leukoencephalopathy in patients diagnosed as major depressive. *Biol Psychiatry*, 23(5), 519–522.

Krishnan, K.R., Doraiswamy, P.M., Lurie, S.N., Figiel, G.S., Husain, M.M., Boyko, O.B., Ellinwood, E.H. Jr., and Nemeroff, C.B. (1991). Pituitary size in depression. *J Clin Endocrinol Metab*, 72(2), 256–259.

Krishnan, K.R., McDonald, W.M., Escalona, P.R., Doraiswamy, P.M., Na, C., Husain, M.M., Figiel, G.S., Boyko, O.B., Ellinwood, E.H., and Nemeroff, C.B. (1992). Magnetic resonance imaging of the caudate nuclei in depression. Preliminary observations. *Arch Gen Psychiatry*, 49(7), 553–557.

Krishnan, K.R., McDonald, W.M., Doraiswamy, P.M., Tupler, L.A., Husain, M., Boyko, O.B., Figiel, G.S., and Ellinwood, E.H. Jr. (1993). Neuroanatomical substrates of depression in the elderly. *Eur Arch Psychiatry Clin Neurosci*, 243(1), 41–46.

Krishnan, K.R., Hays, J.C., and Blazer, D.G. (1997). MRI-defined vascular depression. *Am J Psychiatry*, 154(4), 497–501.

Kronhaus, D.M., Lawrence, N.S., Williams, A.M., Frangou, S., Brammer, M.J., Williams, S.C.R., Andrew, C.M., and Phillips, M.L. (2006). Stroop performance in bipolar disorder: Further evidence for abnormalities in the ventral prefrontal cortex. *Bipolar Disord*, 8, 28–39.

Krüger, S., Seminowicz, D., Goldapple, K., Kennedy, S.H., and Mayberg, H.S. (2003). State and trait influences on mood regulation in bipolar disorder: Blood flow differences with an acute mood challenge. *Biol Psychiatry*, 54(11), 1274–1283.

Krüger, S., Braunig, P., and Grunze, H. (2006). Official guidelines for the treatment of acute mania. *Psychiatr Prax*, 33(Suppl. 1), S2–S6.

Kuhl, D.E., Metter, E.J., Riege, W.H., and Phelps, M.E. (1982). Effects of human aging on patterns of local cerebral glucose utilization determined by the [18F]fluorodeoxyglucose method. *J Cereb Blood Flow Metab*, 2(2), 163–71.

Kuhl, D.E., Metter, E.J., et al. (1985). Patterns of cerebral glucose utilization in depression, multiple infarct dementia, and Alzheimer's disease. In L. Sokoloff (Ed.), *Brain Imaging and Brain Function* (pp. 211–226). New York: Raven Press.

Kumar, A., Mozley, D., et al. (1991). Semiquantitative I-123 IMP SPECT studies in late onset depression before and after treatment. *Int J Geriatr Psychiatry*, 6, 775–777.

Kumar, A., Newberg, A., Alavi, A., Berlin, J., Smith, R., and Reivich, M. (1993). Regional cerebral glucose metabolism in late-life depression and Alzheimer disease: A preliminary positron emission tomography study. *Proc Natl Acad Sci USA*, 90(15), 7019–7023.

Kumar, A., Miller, D.S., et al. (1996). *Focal anatomic substrates in late-life depression.* 149th Annual Meeting of the American Psychiatric Association, New York, NY, May 4–9.

Kumar, A., Schweizer, E., Jin, Z., Miller, D., Bilker, W., Swan, L.L., and Gottlieb, G. (1997). Neuroanatomical substrates of late-life minor depression. A quantitative magnetic resonance imaging study. *Arch Neurol*, 54(5), 613–617.

Kumar, A., Jin, Z., Bilker, W., Udupa, J., and Gottlieb, G. (1998). Late-onset minor and major depression: Early evidence for common neuroanatomical substrates detected by using MRI. *Proc Natl Acad Sci USA*, 95(13), 7654–7658.

Kumar, A., Bilker, W., Jin, Z., Udupa, J., and Gottlieb, G. (1999). Age of onset of depression and quantitative neuroanatomic measures: Absence of specific correlates. *Psychiatry Res*, 91(2), 101–110.

Kumar, A., Bilker, W., Jin, Z., and Udupa, J. (2000). Atrophy and high intensity lesions: Complementary neurobiological mechanisms in late-life major depression. *Neuropsychopharmacology*, 22(3), 264–274.

Kushner, M., Tobin, M., Alavi, A., Chawluk, J., Rosen, M., Fazekas, F., Alavi, J., and Reivich, M. (1987). Cerebellar glucose consumption in normal and pathologic states using fluorine-FDG and PET. *J Nucl Med*, 28(11), 1667–1670.

Kushnir, T., Itzchak, Y., Valevski, A., Lask, M., Modai, I., and Navon, G. (1993). Relaxation times and concentrations of ^{7}Li in the brain of patients receiving lithium therapy. *NMR Biomed*, 6(1), 39–42.

Kusumakar, V., MacMaster, F.P., Gates, L., Sparkes, S.J., and Khan, S.C. (2001). Left medial temporal cytosolic choline in early onset depression. *Can J Psychiatry*, 46(10), 959–964.

Kwon, A.H., Rogers, L.J., et al. (2002). *Reduced thalamic volumes in recurrent, familial major depressive disorder*. 57th Annual Convention and Scientific Program of the Society of Biological Psychiatry, Philadelphia, PA, May 16–18.

Lacerda, A.L., Nicoletti, M.A., Brambilla, P., Sassi, R.B., Mallinger, A.G., Frank, E., Kupfer, D.J., Keshavan, M.S., and Soares, J.C. (2003). Anatomical MRI study of basal ganglia in major depressive disorder. *Psychiatry Res*, 124(3), 129–140.

Lacerda, A.L., Keshavan, M.S., Hardan, A.Y., Yorbik, O., Brambilla, P., Sassi, R.B., Nicoletti, M., Mallinger, A.G., Frank, E., Kupfer, D.J., and Soares, J.C. (2004). Anatomic evaluation of the orbitofrontal cortex in major depressive disorder. *Biol Psychiatry*, 55(4), 353–358.

Lafer, B., Renshaw, P.F., et al. (1994). *Proton MRS of the basal ganglia in bipolar disorder*. 49th Annual Meeting of the Society of Biological Psychiatry, Philadelphia, PA, May 18–22.

Lai, T., Payne, M.E., Byrum, C.E., Steffens, D.C., and Krishnan, K.R. (2000). Reduction of orbital frontal cortex volume in geriatric depression. *Biol Psychiatry*, 48(10), 971–975.

Lammers, C.S., Doraiswamy, P.M., et al. (1991). MRI of corpus callosum and septum pellucidum in depression [letter]. *Biol Psychiatry*, 29(3), 300–301.

Lane, R.D., Reiman, E.M., Ahern, G.L., Schwartz, G.E., and Davidson, R.J. (1997). Neuroanatomical correlates of happiness, sadness, and disgust. *Am J Psychiatry*, 154(7), 926–933.

Lange, C., and Irle, E. (2004). Enlarged amygdala volume and reduced hippocampal volume in young women with major depression. *Psychol Med*, 34(6), 1059–1064.

Lauer, C.J., Wiegand, M., and Krieg, J.C. (1992). All-night electroencephalographic sleep and cranial computed tomography in depression. A study of unipolar and bipolar patients. *Eur Arch Psychiatry Clin Neurosci*, 242(2-3), 59–68.

Lavretsky, H., Kurbanyan, K., Ballmaier, M., Mintz, J., Toga, A., and Kumar, A. (2004). Sex differences in brain structure in geriatric depression. *Am J Geriatr Psychiatry*, 12(6), 653–657.

Lawrence, N.S., Williams, A.M., Surguladze, S., Giampietro, V., Brammer, M.J., Andrew, C., Frangou, S., Ecker, C., and Phillips, M.L. (2004). Subcortical and ventral prefrontal cortical neural responses to facial expressions distinguish patients with bipolar disorder and major depression. *Biol Psychiatry*, 55(6), 578–587.

Lebrun-Grandie, P., Baron, J.C., Soussaline, F., Loch'h, C., Sastre, J., and Bousser, M.G. (1983). Coupling between regional blood flow and oxygen utilization in the normal human brain. A study with positron tomography and oxygen 15. *Arch Neurol*, 40(4), 230–236.

Lennox, B.R., Park, S.B., Jones, P.B., and Morris, P.G. (1999). Spatial and temporal mapping of neural activity associated with auditory hallucinations [letter]. *Lancet*, 353(9153), 644.

Lenze, E.J., and Sheline, Y.I. (1999). Absence of striatal volume differences between depressed subjects with no comorbid medical illness and matched comparison subjects. *Am J Psychiatry*, 156(12), 1989–1991.

Lenze, E., Cross, D., McKeel, D., Neuman, R.J., and Sheline, Y.I. (1999). White matter hyperintensities and gray matter lesions in physically healthy depressed subjects. *Am J Psychiatry*, 156(10), 1602–1607.

Lesser, I.M., Miller, B.L., Boone, K.B., Hill-Gutierrez, E., Mehringer, C.M., Wong, K., and Mena, I. (1991). Brain injury and cognitive function in late-onset psychotic depression. *J Neuropsychiatry Clin Neurosci*, 3, 33–40.

Lesser, I.M., Mena, I., Boone, K.B., Miller, B.L., Mehringer, C.M., and Wohl, M. (1994). Reduction of cerebral blood flow in older depressed patients. *Arch Gen Psychiatry*, 51(9), 677–686.

Lesser, I.M., Boone, K.B., Mehringer, C.M., Wohl, M.A., Miller, B.L., and Berman, N.G. (1996). Cognition and white matter hyperintensities in older depressed patients. *Am J Psychiatry*, 153(10), 1280–1287.

Levine, J., Barak, Y., Gonzalves, M., Szor, H., Elizur, A., Kofman, O., and Belmaker, R.H. (1995). Double-blind, controlled trial of inositol treatment of depression. *Am J Psychiatry*, 152(5), 792–794.

Lewine, R.R., Risch, S.C., Risby, E., Stipetic, M., Jewart, R.D., Eccard, M., Caudle, J., and Pollard, W. (1991). Lateral ventricle–brain ratio and balance between CSF HVA and 5-HIAA in schizophrenia. *Am J Psychiatry*, 148(9), 1189–1194.

Lewine, R.R., Hudgins, P., Brown, F., Caudle, J., and Risch, S.C. (1995). Differences in qualitative brain morphology findings in schizophrenia, major depression, bipolar disorder, and normal volunteers. *Schizophr Res*, 15(3), 253–259.

Lim, K.O., Rosenbloom, M.J., Faustman, W.O., Sullivan, E.V., and Pfefferbaum, A. (1999). Cortical gray matter deficit in patients with bipolar disorder. *Schizophr Res*, 40(3), 219–227.

Liotti, M., Mayberg, H.S., Brannan, S.K., McGinnis, S., Jerabek, P., and Fox, P.T. (2000). Differential limbic—cortical correlates of sadness and anxiety in healthy subjects: Implications for affective disorders. *Biol Psychiatry*, 48(1), 30–42.

Liotti, M., Mayberg, H.S., McGinnis, S., Brannan, S.L., and Jerabek, P. (2002). Unmasking disease-specific cerebral blood flow abnormalities: Mood challenge in patients with remitted unipolar depression. *Am J Psychiatry*, 159(11), 1830–1840.

Lippmann, S., Manshadi, M., Baldwin, H., Drasin, G., Rice, J., and Alrajeh, S. (1982). Cerebellar vermis dimensions on computerized tomographic scans of schizophrenic and bipolar patients. *Am J Psychiatry*, 139(5), 667–668.

Lippmann, S., Manshadi, M., Baldwin, H., Drasin, G., Wagemaker, H., Rice, J., and Alrajeh, S. (1985). Cerebral CAT scan imaging in schizophrenic and bipolar patients. *J Ky Med Assoc*, 83(1), 13–15.

Lisanby, S.H., McDonald, W.M., Massey, E.W., Doraiswamy, P.M., Rozear, M., Boyko, O.B., Krishnan, K.R., and Nemeroff, C. (1993). Diminished subcortical nuclei volumes in Parkinson's disease by MR imaging. *J Neural Transm Suppl*, 40, 13–21.

Little, J.T., Ketter, T.A., Kimbrell, T.A., Danielson, A., Benson, B., Willis, M.W., and Post, R.M. (1996). Venlafaxine or bupropion responders but not nonresponders show baseline prefrontal and paralimbic hypometabolism compared with controls. *Psychopharmacol Bull*, 32(4), 629–635.

Little, J.T., Ketter, T.A., Kimbrell, T.A., Dunn, R.T., Benson, B.E., Willis, M.W., Luckenbaugh, D.A., and Post, R.M. (2005). Bupropion and venlafaxine responders differ in pretreatment regional cerebral metabolism in unipolar depression. *Biol Psychiatry*, 57(3), 220–228.

Lloyd, A.J., Ferrier, I.N., Barber, R., Gholkar, A., Young, A.H., and O'Brien, J.T. (2004). Hippocampal volume change in depression: Late- and early-onset illness compared. *Br J Psychiatry*, 184, 488–495.

Lochhead, R.A., Parsey, R.V., Oquendo, M.A., and Mann, J.J. (2004). Regional brain gray matter volume differences in patients with bipolar disorder as assessed by optimized voxel-based morphometry. *Biol Psychiatry*, 55(12), 1154–1162.

Loeber, R.T., Sherwood, A.R., Renshaw, P.F., Cohen, B.M., and Yurgelun-Todd, D.A. (1999). Differences in cerebellar blood volume in schizophrenia and bipolar disorder. *Schizophr Res*, 37(1), 81–89.

Loeber, R.T., Gruber, S.A., Cohen, B.M., Renshaw, P.F., Sherwood, A.R., and Yurgelun-Todd, D.A. (2002). Cerebellar blood volume in bipolar patients correlates with medication. *Biol Psychiatry*, 51(5), 370–376.

Lopez-Larson, M.P., DelBello, M.P., Zimmerman, M.E., Schwiers, M.L., and Strakowski, S.M. (2002). Regional prefrontal gray and white matter abnormalities in bipolar disorder. *Biol Psychiatry*, 52(2), 93–100.

Losfescu, D.V., Renshaw, P.F. et al. (2002). *Brain MRI white matter hyperintensities correlate with improved treatment outcome in depression.* 57th Annual Convention and Scientific Program of the Society of Biological Psychiatry, Philadelphia, PA, May 16–18.

Luchins, D.J., Lewine, R.R., and Meltzer, H.Y. (1984). Lateral ventricular size, psychopathology, and medication response in the psychoses. *Biol Psychiatry*, 19(1), 29–44.

Lyoo, I.K., Demopulos, C.M., Hirashima, F., Ahn, K.H., and Renshaw, P.F. (2003). Oral choline decreases brain purine levels in lithium-treated subjects with rapid-cycling bipolar disorder: A double-blind trial using proton and lithium magnetic resonance spectroscopy. *Bipolar Disord*, 5(4), 300–306.

Lyoo, I.K., Kim, M.J., Stoll, A.L., Demopulos, C.M., Parow, A.M., Dager, S.R., Friedman, S.D., Dunner, D.L., and Renshaw, P.F. (2004). Frontal lobe gray matter density decreases in bipolar I disorder. *Biol Psychiatry*, 55(6), 648–651.

Lyoo, I.K., Sung, Y.H., Dager, S.R., Friedman, S.D., Lee, J.Y., Kim, S.J., Kim, N., Dunner, D.L., and Renshaw, P.F. (2006). Regional cerebral cortical thinning in bipolar disorder. *Bipolar Disord*, 8(1), 65–74.

MacFall, J.R., Payne, M.E., Provenzale, J.E., and Krishnan, K.R. (2001). Medial orbital frontal lesions in late-onset depression. *Biol Psychiatry*, 49(9), 803–806.

MacHale, S.M., Lawrie, S.M., Cavanagh, J.T., Glabus, M.F., Murray, C.L., Goodwin, G.M., and Ebmeier, K.P. (2000). Cerebral perfusion in chronic fatigue syndrome and depression. *Br J Psychiatry*, 176, 550–556.

MacLean, P.D. (1952). Some psychiatric implications of physiological studies on the frontotemporal portion of limbic system (visceral brain). *Electroencephalogr Clin Neurophysiol*, 4, 407–418.

MacMaster, F.P., and Kusumakar, V. (2004a). MRI study of the pituitary gland in adolescent depression. *J Psychiatr Res*, 38(3), 231–236.

MacMaster, F.P., and Kusumakar, V. (2004b). Hippocampal volume in early-onset depression. *BMC Med*, 2, 2.

MacQueen, G.M., Campbell, S., McEwen, B.S., Macdonald, K., Amano, S., Joffe, R.T., Nahmias, C., and Young, L.T. (2003). Course of illness, hippocampal function, and hippocampal volume in major depression. *Proc Natl Acad Sci USA*, 100(3), 1387–1392.

Maes, M., Dierckx, R., Meltzer, H.Y., Ingels, M., Schotte, C., Vandewoude, M., Calabrese, J., and Cosyns, P. (1993). Regional cerebral blood flow in unipolar depression measured with Tc-99m-HMPAO single photon emission computed tomography: Negative findings. *Psychiatry Res*, 50(2), 77–88.

Malberg, J.E. (2004). Implications of adult hippocampal neurogenesis in antidepressant action. *J Psychiatry Neurosci*, 29(3), 196–205.

Malhi, G.S., Lagopoulos, J., Sachdev, P., Mitchell, P.B., Ivanovski, B., and Parker, G.B. (2004). Cognitive generation of affect in hypomania: An fMRI study. *Bipolar Disord*, 6(4), 271–285.

Malhi, G.S., Lagopoulos, J., Sachdev, P.S., Ivanovski, B., and Shnier, R. (2005). An emotional stroop functional MRI study of euthymic bipolar disorder. *Bipolar Disord*, 7(Suppl. 5), 58–69.

Manji, H.K., and Lenox, R.H. (2000). Signaling: Cellular insights into the pathophysiology of bipolar disorder. *Biol Psychiatry*, 48(6), 518–530.

Manji, H.K., Drevets, W.C., and Charney, D.S. (2001). The cellular neurobiology of depression. *Nat Med*, 7(5), 541–547.

Mann, J.J., Malone, K.M., Diehl, D.J., Perel, J., Cooper, T.B., and Mintun, M.A. (1996). Demonstration in vivo of reduced serotonin responsivity in the brain of untreated depressed patients. *Am J Psychiatry*, 153(2), 174–182.

Marangell, L.B., Ketter, T.A., George, M.S., Pazzaglia, P.J., Callahan, A.M., Parekh, P., Andreason, P.J., Horwitz, B., Herscovitch, P., and Post, R.M. (1997). Inverse relationship of peripheral thyrotropin-stimulating hormone levels to brain activity in mood disorders. *Am J Psychiatry*, 154(2), 224–230.

Martinot, J.L., Hardy, P., Feline, A., Huret, J.D., Mazoyer, B., Attar-Levy, D., Pappata, S., and Syrota, A. (1990). Left prefrontal glucose hypometabolism in the depressed state: A confirmation. *Am J Psychiatry*, 147(10), 1313–1317.

Mason, G.F., Sanacora, G., et al. (2000). *Cortical GABA reduced in unipolar but not bipolar depression.* 55th Annual Convention and Scientific Program of the Society of Biological Psychiatry, Chicago, IL, May 11–13.

Matsuo, K., Kato, T., Fukuda, M., and Kato, N. (2000). Alteration of hemoglobin oxygenation in the frontal region in elderly depressed patients as measured by near-infrared spectroscopy. *J Neuropsychiatry Clin Neurosci*, 12(4), 465–471.

Matsuo, K., Kato, N., and Kato, T. (2002). Decreased cerebral haemodynamic response to cognitive and physiological tasks in mood disorders as shown by near-infrared spectroscopy. *Psychol Med*, 32(6), 1029–1037.

Mayberg, H.S. (1994). Frontal lobe dysfunction in secondary depression. *J Neuropsychiatry Clin Neurosci*, 6(4), 428–442.

Mayberg, H.S. (1997). Limbic-cortical dysregulation: A proposed model of depression. *J Neuropsychiatry Clin Neurosci*, 9(3), 471–481.

Mayberg, H.S., Starkstein, S.E., Sadzot, B., Preziosi, T., Andrezejewski, P.L., Dannals, R.F., Wagner, H.N. Jr., and Robinson, R.G. (1990). Selective hypometabolism in the inferior frontal lobe in depressed patients with Parkinson's disease. *Ann Neurol*, 28(1), 57–64.

Mayberg, H.S., Starkstein, S.E., and Morris, P.L. (1991). Remote cortical hypometabolism following focal basal ganglia injury: Relationship to secondary changes in mood. Abstract 540S. *Neurology*, 41(Suppl. 1), 266.

Mayberg, H.S., Starkstein, S.E., Peyser, C.E., Brandt, J., Dannals, R.F., and Folstein, S.E. (1992). Paralimbic frontal lobe hypometabolism in depression associated with Huntington's disease. *Neurology*, 42(9), 1791–1797.

Mayberg, H.S., Lewis, P.J., Regenold, W., and Wagner, H.N. Jr. (1994). Paralimbic hypoperfusion in unipolar depression. *J Nucl Med*, 35(6), 929–934.

Mayberg, H.S., Brannan, S.K., Mahurin, R.K., Jerabek, P.A., Brickman, J.S., Tekell, J.L., Silva, J.A., McGinnis, S., Glass, T.G., Martin, C.C., and Fox, P.T. (1997). Cingulate function in depression: A potential predictor of treatment response. *Neuroreport*, 8(4), 1057–1061.

Mayberg, H.S., Liotti, M., Brannan, S.K., McGinnis, S., Mahurin, R.K., Jerabek, P.A., Silva, J.A., Tekell, J.L., Martin, C.C., Lancaster, J.L., and Fox, P.T. (1999). Reciprocal limbic–cortical function and negative mood: Converging PET findings in depression and normal sadness. *Am J Psychiatry*, 156(5), 675–682.

Mayberg, H.S., Brannan, S.K., Tekell, J.L., Silva, J.A., Mahurin, R.K., McGinnis, S., and Jerabek, P.A. (2000). Regional metabolic effects of fluoxetine in major depression: Serial changes and relationship to clinical response. *Biol Psychiatry*, 48(8), 830–843.

Mayberg, H.S., Silva, J.A., Brannan, S.K., Tekell, J.L., Mahurin, R.K., McGinnis, S., and Jerabek, P.A. (2002). The functional neuroanatomy of the placebo effect. *Am J Psychiatry*, 159(5), 728–737.

McDonald, C., Bullmore, E., Sham, P., Chitnis, X., Suckling, J., MacCabe, J., Walshe, M., and Murray, R.M. (2005). Regional volume deviations of brain structure in schizophrenia and psychotic bipolar disorder: Computational morphometry study. *Br J Psychiatry*, 186, 369–377.

McDonald, W.M., Krishnan, K.R., Doraiswamy, P.M., and Blazer, D.G. (1991). Occurrence of subcortical hyperintensities in elderly subjects with mania. *Psychiatry Res*, 40(4), 211–220.

McDonald, W.M., Tupler, L.A., Marsteller, F.A., Figiel, G.S., DiSouza, S., Nemeroff, C.B., and Krishnan, K.R. (1999). Hyperintense lesions on magnetic resonance images in bipolar disorder. *Biol Psychiatry*, 45(8), 965–971.

McDonald, C., Zanelli, J., Rabe-Hesketh, S., Ellison-Wright, I., Sham, P., Kalidindi, S., Murray, R.M., and Kennedy, N. (2004). Meta-analysis of magnetic resonance imaging brain morphometry studies in bipolar disorder. *Biol Psychiatry,* 56(6), 411–417.

McIntosh, A.M., Job, D.E., Moorhead, T.W., Harrison, L.K., Forrester, K., Lawrie, S.M., and Johnstone, E.C. (2004). Voxel-based morphometry of patients with schizophrenia or bipolar disorder and their unaffected relatives. *Biol Psychiatry*, 56(8), 544–552.

McIntosh, A.M., Job, D.E., Moorhead, T.W., Harrison, L.K., Lawrie, S.M., and Johnstone, E.C. (2005). White matter density in patients with schizophrenia, bipolar disorder and their unaffected relatives. *Biol Psychiatry*, 58(3), 254–257.

Mendez, M.F., Adams, N.L., and Lewandowski, K.S. (1989). Neurobehavioral changes associated with caudate lesions. *Neurology*, 39, 349–354.

Mervaala, E., Fohr, J., Kononen, M., Valkonen-Korhonen, M., Vainio, P., Partanen, K., Partanen, J., Tiihonen, J., Viinamaki, H., Karjalainen, A.K., and Lehtonen, J. (2000). Quantitative MRI of the hippocampus and amygdala in severe depression. *Psychol Med*, 30(1), 117–125.

Mervaala, E., Kononen, M., Fohr, J., Husso-Saastamoinen, M., Valkonen-Korhonen, M., Kuikka, J.T., Viinamaki, H., Tammi, A.K., Tiihonen, J., Partanen, J., and Lehtonen, J. (2001). SPECT and neuropsychological performance in severe depression treated with ECT. *J Affect Disord*, 66(1), 47–58.

Michael, N., Erfurth, A., Ohrmann, P., Arolt, V., Heindel, W., and Pfleiderer, B. (2003a). Metabolic changes within the left dorsolateral prefrontal cortex occurring with electroconvulsive therapy in patients with treatment-resistant unipolar depression. *Psychol Med*, 33(7), 1277–1284.

Michael, N., Erfurth, A., Ohrmann, P., Gossling, M., Arolt, V., Heindel, W., and Pfleiderer, B. (2003b). Acute mania is accompanied by elevated glutamate/glutamine levels within the left dorsolateral prefrontal cortex. *Psychopharmacology*, 168(3), 344–346.

Migliorelli, R., Starkstein, S.E., Teson, A., de Quiros, G., Vazquez, S., Leiguarda, R., and Robinson, R.G. (1993). SPECT findings in patients with primary mania. *J Neuropsychiatry Clin Neurosci*, 5(4), 379–383.

Miller, D.S., Kumar, A., et al. (1994). MRI high-intensity signals in depression and Alzheimer's disease. *Am J Geriatr Psychiatry*, 2(4), 332–337.

Mindham, R.H. (1970). Psychiatric symptoms in Parkinsonism. *J Neurol Neurosurg Psychiatry*, 33(2), 188–191.

Mitterschiffthaler, M.T., Kumari, V., Malhi, G.S., Brown, R.G., Giampietro, V.P., Brammer, M.J., Suckling, J., Poon, L., Simmons, A., Andrew, C., and Sharma, T. (2003). Neural response to pleasant stimuli in anhedonia: An fMRI study. *Neuroreport*, 14(2), 177–182.

Miura, S.A., Schapiro, M.B., Grady, C.L., Kumar, A., Salerno, J.A., Kozachuk, W.E., Wagner, E., Rapoport, S.I., and Horwitz, B. (1990). Effect of gender on glucose utilization rates in healthy humans: A positron emission tomography study. *J Neurosci Res*, 27(4), 500–504.

Moeller, J.R., Ishikawa, T., Dhawan, V., Spetsieris, P., Mandel, F., Alexander, G.E., Grady, C., Pietrini, P., and Eidelberg, D. (1996). The metabolic topography of normal aging. *J Cereb Blood Flow Metab*, 16(3), 385–398.

Moller, A., Wiedemann, G., Rohde, U., Backmund, H., and Sonntag, A. (1994). Correlates of cognitive impairment and depressive mood disorder in multiple sclerosis. *Acta Psychiatr Scand*, 89(2), 117–121.

Moore, C.M., Christensen, J.D., Lafer, B., Fava, M., and Renshaw, P.F. (1997). Lower levels of nucleoside triphosphate in the basal ganglia of depressed subjects: A phosphorous-31 magnetic resonance spectroscopy study. *Am J Psychiatry*, 154(1), 116–118.

Moore, C.M., Breeze, J.L., Kukes, T.J., Rose, S.L., Dager, S.R., Cohen, B.M., and Renshaw, P.F. (1999). Effects of myo-inositol ingestion on human brain myo-inositol levels: A proton magnetic resonance spectroscopic imaging study. *Biol Psychiatry*, 45(9), 1197–1202.

Moore, C.M., Breeze, J.L., Gruber, S.A., Babb, S.M., Frederick, B.B., Villafuerte, R.A., Stoll, A.L., Hennen, J., Yurgelun-Todd, D.A., Cohen, B.M., and Renshaw, P.F. (2000). Choline, myo-inositol and mood in bipolar disorder: A proton magnetic resonance spectroscopic imaging study of the anterior cingulate cortex. *Bipolar Disord*, 2(3 Pt. 2), 207–216.

Moore, C.M., Demopulos, C.M., Henry, M.E., Steingard, R.J., Zamvil, L., Katic, A., Breeze, J.L., Moore, J.C., Cohen, B.M., and Renshaw, P.F. (2002). Brain-to-serum lithium ratio and age: An in vivo magnetic resonance spectroscopy study. *Am J Psychiatry*, 159(7), 1240–1242.

Moore, G.J., Bebchuk, J.M., Parrish, J.K., Faulk, M.W., Arfken, C.L., Strahl-Bevacqua, J., and Manji, H.K. (1999). Temporal dissociation between lithium-induced changes in frontal lobe myo-inositol and clinical response in manic-depressive illness. *Am J Psychiatry*, 156(12), 1902–1908.

Moore, G.J., Bebchuk, J.M., Hasanat, K., Chen, G., Seraji-Bozorgzad, N., Wilds, I.B., Faulk, M.W., Koch, S., Glitz, D.A., Jolkovsky, L., and Manji, H.K. (2000a). Lithium increases N-acetyl-aspartate in the human brain: In vivo evidence in support of bcl-2's neurotrophic effects? *Biol Psychiatry*, 48(1), 1–8.

Moore, G.J., Bebchuk, J.M., Wilds, I.B., Chen, G., and Manji, H.K. (2000b). Lithium-induced increase in human brain grey matter. *Lancet*, 356(9237), 1241–1242.

Moore, P.B., Shepherd, D.J., Eccleston, D., Macmillan, I.C., Goswami, U., McAllister, V.L., and Ferrier, I.N. (2001). Cerebral white matter lesions in bipolar affective disorder: Relationship to outcome. *Br J Psychiatry*, 178, 172–176.

Morris, J.S., Frith, C.D., Perrett, D.I., Rowland, D., Young, A.W., Calder, A.J., and Dolan, R.J. (1996). A differential neural response in the human amygdala to fearful and happy facial expressions. *Nature*, 383(6603), 812–815.

Morris, J.S., Friston, K.J., Buchel, C., Frith, C.D., Young, A.W., Calder, A.J., and Dolan, R.J. (1998a). A neuromodulatory role for the human amygdala in processing emotional facial expressions. *Brain*, 121(Pt. 1), 47–57.

Morris, J.S., Ohman, A., and Dolan, R.J. (1998b). Conscious and unconscious emotional learning in the human amygdala. *Nature*, 393(6684), 467–470.

Mozley, P.D., Hornig-Rohan, M., Woda, A.M., Kim, H.J., Alavi, A., Payer, F., and Amsterdam, J.D. (1996). Cerebral HMPAO SPECT in patients with major depression and healthy volunteers. *Prog Neuropsychopharmacol Biol Psychiatry*, 20(3), 443–458.

Mukherjee, S., Schnur, D.B., Lo, E.S., Sackeim, H.A., and Cooper, T.B. (1993). Post-dexamethasone cortisol levels and computerized tomographic findings in manic patients. *Acta Psychiatr Scand*, 88(3), 145–148.

Murashita, J., Kato, T., Shioiri, T., Inubushi, T., and Kato, N. (2000). Altered brain energy metabolism in lithium-resistant bipolar disorder detected by photic stimulated 31P-MR spectroscopy. *Psychol Med*, 30(1), 107–115.

Murata, T., Kimura, H., Omori, M., Kado, H., Kosaka, H., Iidaka, T., Itoh, H., and Wada, Y. (2001). MRI white matter hyperintensities, (1)H-MR spectroscopy and cognitive function in geriatric depression: A comparison of early- and late-onset cases. *Int J Geriatr Psychiatry*, 16(12), 1129–1135.

Murphy, D.G., DeCarli, C., Schapiro, M.B., Rapoport, S.I., and Horwitz, B. (1992). Age-related differences in volumes of subcortical nuclei, brain matter, and cerebrospinal fluid in healthy men as measured with magnetic resonance imaging. *Arch Neurol*, 49(8), 839–845.

Murphy, D.G., Murphy, D.M., Abbas, M., Palazidou, E., Binnie, C., Arendt, J., Campos Costa, D., and Checkley, S.A. (1993). Seasonal affective disorder: Response to light as measured by electroencephalogram, melatonin suppression, and cerebral blood flow. *Br J Psychiatry*, 163, 327–331, 335–337.

Murphy, D.G., DeCarli, C., McIntosh, A.R., Daly, E., Mentis, M.J., Pietrini, P., Szczepanik, J., Schapiro, M.B., Grady, C.L., Horwitz, B., and Rapoport, S.I. (1996). Sex differences in human brain morphometry and metabolism: An in vivo quantitative magnetic resonance imaging and positron emission tomography study on the effect of aging. *Arch Gen Psychiatry*, 53(7), 585–594.

Nasrallah, H.A., Jacoby, C.G., and McCalley-Whitters, M. (1981). Cerebellar atrophy in schizophrenia and mania [letter]. *Lancet*, 1(8229), 1102.

Nasrallah, H.A., McCalley-Whitters, M., and Jacoby, C.G. (1982a). Cerebral ventricular enlargement in young manic males: A controlled CT study. *J Affect Disord*, 4(1), 15–19.

Nasrallah, H.A., McCalley-Whitters, M., and Jacoby, C.G. (1982b). Cortical atrophy in schizophrenia and mania: A comparative CT study. *J Clin Psychiatry*, 43(11), 439–441.

Nasrallah, H.A., McCalley-Whitters, M., and Pfohl, B. (1984). Clinical significance of large cerebral ventricles in manic males. *Psychiatry Res*, 13(2), 151–156.

Navarro, V., Gasto, C., Lomena, F., Mateos, J.J., and Marcos, T. (2001). Frontal cerebral perfusion dysfunction in elderly late-onset major depression assessed by 99MTC-HMPAO SPECT. *Neuroimage*, 14(1 Pt. 1), 202–205.

Nebes, R.D., Vora, I.J., Meltzer, C.C., Fukui, M.B., Williams, R.L., Kamboh, M.I., Saxton, J., Houck, P.R., DeKosky, S.T., and Reynolds, C.F. III. (2001). Relationship of deep white matter hyperintensities and apolipoprotein E genotype to depressive symptoms in older adults without clinical depression. *Am J Psychiatry*, 158(6), 878–884.

Nobler, M.S., Sackeim, H.A., Prohovnik, I., Moeller, J.R., Mukherjee, S., Schnur, D.B., Prudic, J., and Devanand, D.P. (1994). Regional cerebral blood flow in mood disorders, III. Treatment and clinical response. *Arch Gen Psychiatry*, 51(11), 884–897.

Nobler, M.S., Roose, S.P., Prohovnik, I., Moeller, J.R., Louie, J., Van Heertum, R.L., and Sackeim, H.A. (2000). Regional cerebral blood flow in mood disorders V: Effects of antidepressant medication in late-life depression. *Am J Geriatr Psychiatry*, 8(4), 289–296.

Nofzinger, E.A., Nichols, T.E., Meltzer, C.C., Price, J., Steppe, D.A., Miewald, J.M., Kupfer, D.J., and Moore, R.Y. (1999). Changes in forebrain function from waking to REM sleep in depression: Preliminary analyses of [18F]FDG PET studies. *Psychiatry Res*, 91(2), 59–78.

Nofzinger, E.A., Berman, S., Fasiczka, A., Miewald, J.M., Meltzer, C.C., Price, J.C., Sembrat, R.C., Wood, A., and Thase, M.E. (2001). Effects of bupropion SR on anterior paralimbic function during waking and REM sleep in depression: Preliminary findings using [18F]-FDG PET. *Psychiatry Res*, 106(2), 95–111.

Noga, J.T., Vladar, K., and Torrey, E.F. (2001). A volumetric magnetic resonance imaging study of monozygotic twins discordant for bipolar disorder. *Psychiatry Res*, 106(1), 25–34.

Nudmamud, S., Reynolds, L.M., and Reynolds, G.P. (2003). N-acetylaspartate and N-acetylaspartylglutamate deficits in superior temporal cortex in schizophrenia and bipolar disorder: A postmortem study. *Biol Psychiatry*, 53(12), 1138–1141.

Nugent, A.C., Milham, M.P., Bain, E.E., Mah, L., Cannon, D.M., Marrett, S., Zarate, C.A., Pine, D.S., Price, J.L., and Drevets, W.C. (2006). Cortical abnormalities in bipolar disorder investigated with MRI and voxel-based morphometry. *Neuroimage*, 30(2), 485–497.

O'Brien, J., Desmond, P., Ames, D., Schweitzer, I., Harrigan, S., and Tress, B. (1996). A magnetic resonance imaging study of white matter lesions in depression and Alzheimer's disease. *Br J Psychiatry*, 168(4), 477–485.

O'Connell, R.A., Van Heertum, R.L., Billick, S.B., Holt, A.R., Gonzalez, A., Notardonato, H., Luck, D., and King, L.N. (1989). Single photon emission computed tomography (SPECT) with [^{123}I]IMP in the differential diagnosis of psychiatric disorders. *J Neuropsychiatry Clin Neurosci*, 1(2), 145–153.

O'Connell, R.A., Van Heertum, R.L., Luck, D., Yudd, A.P., Cueva, J.E., Billick, S.B., Cordon, D.J., Gersh, R.J., and Masdeu, J.C. (1995). Single-photon emission computed tomography of the brain in acute mania and schizophrenia. *J Neuroimaging*, 5(2), 101–104.

Ohaeri, J.U., Adeyinka, A.O., Enyidah, S.N., and Osuntokun, B.O. (1995). Schizophrenic and manic brains in Nigerians. Computerised tomography findings. *Br J Psychiatry*, 166(4), 496–500.

Ohara, K., Isoda, H., Suzuki, Y., Takehara, Y., Ochiai, M., Takeda, H., Igarashi, Y., and Ohara, K. (1998). Proton magnetic resonance spectroscopy of the lenticular nuclei in bipolar I affective disorder. *Psychiatry Res*, 84(2-3), 55–60.

Öngür, D., Drevets, W.C., and Price, J.L. (1998). Glial reduction in the subgenual prefrontal cortex in mood disorders. *Proc Natl Acad Sci USA*, 95(22), 13290–13295.

Osuch, E.A., Ketter, T.A., Kimbrell, T.A., George, M.S., Benson, B.E., Willis, M.W., Herscovitch, P., and Post, R.M. (2000). Regional cerebral metabolism associated with anxiety symptoms in affective disorder patients. *Biol Psychiatry*, 48(10), 1020–1023.

Pande, A.C., Grunhaus, L.J., Aisen, A.M., and Haskett, R.F. (1990). A preliminary magnetic resonance imaging study of ECT-treated depressed patients. *Biol Psychiatry*, 27(1), 102–104.

Pantel, J., Schroder, J., Essig, M., Popp, D., Dech, H., Knopp, M.V., Schad, L.R., Eysenbach, K., Backenstrass, M., and Friedlinger, M. (1997). Quantitative magnetic resonance imaging in geriatric depression and primary degenerative dementia. *J Affect Disord*, 42(1), 69–83.

Pantel, J., Schroder, J., Essig, M., Schad, L.R., Popp, D., Eysenbach, K., Jauss, M., and Knopp, M.V. (1998). Volumetric brain findings in late depression. A study with quantified magnetic resonance tomography. *Nervenarzt*, 69(11), 968–974.

Papez, J.W. (1937). A proposed mechanism of emotion. *Arch Neurol Psychiatry*, 38, 725–743.

Parashos, I.A., Tupler, L.A., Blitchington, T., and Krishnan, K.R. (1998). Magnetic-resonance morphometry in patients with major depression. *Psychiatry Res*, 84(1), 7–15.

Pardo, J.V., Pardo, P.J., and Raichle, M.E. (1993). Neural correlates of self-induced dysphoria. *Am J Psychiatry*, 150(5), 713–719.

Pascual-Leone, A., and Pallardó, F. (1996). *Beneficial effects of repetitive transcranial magnetic stimulation (rTMS) in depression are associated with normalization of prefrontal hypometabolism*. 8th Congress of the Association of European Psychiatrists, London, England, July 7–12.

Passe, T.J., Rajagopalan, P., Tupler, L.A., Byrum, C.E., MacFall, J.R., and Krishnan, K.R. (1997). Age and sex effects on brain morphology. *Prog Neuropsychopharmacol Biol Psychiatry*, 21(8), 1231–1237.

Pearlson, G.D., and Veroff, A.E. (1981). Computerised tomographic scan changes in manic-depressive illness [letter]. *Lancet*, 2(8244), 470.

Pearlson, G.D., Garbacz, D.J., Breakey, W.R., Ahn, H.S., and DePaulo, J.R. (1984a). Lateral ventricular enlargement associated with persistent unemployment and negative symptoms in both schizophrenia and bipolar disorder. *Psychiatry Res*, 12(1), 1–9.

Pearlson, G.D., Garbacz, D.J., Tompkins, R.H., Ahn, H.S., Gutterman, D.F., Veroff, A.E., and DePaulo, J.R. (1984b). Clinical correlates of lateral ventricular enlargement in bipolar affective disorder. *Am J Psychiatry*, 141(2), 253–256.

Pearlson, G.D., Rabins, P.V., Kim, W.S., Speedie, L.J., Moberg, P.J., Burns, A., and Bascom, M.J. (1989). Structural brain CT changes and cognitive deficits in elderly depressives with and without reversible dementia ('pseudodementia'). *Psychol Med*, 19(3), 573–584.

Pearlson, G.D., Barta, P.E., Powers, R.E., Menon, R.R., Richards, S.S., Aylward, E.H., Federman, E.B., Chase, G.A., Petty, R.G., and Tien, A.Y. (1997). Ziskind-Somerfeld Research Award 1996. Medial and superior temporal gyral volumes and cerebral asymmetry in schizophrenia versus bipolar disorder. *Biol Psychiatry*, 41(1), 1–14.

Persaud, R., Russow, H., Harvey, I., Lewis, S.W., Ron, M., Murray, R.M., and du Boulay, G. (1997). Focal signal hyperintensities in schizophrenia. *Schizophr Res*, 27(1), 55–64.

Petit-Taboue, M.C., Landeau, B., Desson, J.F., Desgranges, B., and Baron, J.C. (1998). Effects of healthy aging on the regional cerebral metabolic rate of glucose assessed with statistical parametric mapping. *Neuroimage*, 7(3), 176–184.

Pettegrew, J.W., Keshavan, M.S., Panchalingam, K., Strychor, S., Kaplan, D.B., Tretta, M.G., and Allen, M. (1991). Alterations in brain high-energy phosphate and membrane phospholipid metabolism in first-episode, drug-naive schizophrenics. A pilot study of the dorsal prefrontal cortex by in vivo phosphorus 31 nuclear magnetic resonance spectroscopy. *Arch Gen Psychiatry*, 48(6), 563–568.

Petty, F., Rush, A.J., Davis, J.M., Calabrese, J.R., Kimmel, S.E., Kramer, G.L., Small, J.G., Miller, M.J., Swann, A.E., Orsulak, P.J., Blake, M.E., and Bowden, C.L. (1996). Plasma GABA predicts acute response to divalproex in mania. *Biol Psychiatry*, 39, 278–284.

Pfefferbaum, A., Mathalon, D.H., Sullivan, E.V., Rawles, J.M., Zipursky, R.B., and Lim, K.O. (1994). A quantitative magnetic resonance imaging study of changes in brain morphology from infancy to late adulthood. *Arch Neurol*, 51(9), 874–887.

Pfleiderer, B., Michael, N., Erfurth, A., Ohrmann, P., Hohmann, U., Wolgast, M., Fiebich, M., Arolt, V., and Heindel, W. (2003). Effective electroconvulsive therapy reverses glutamate/glutamine deficit in the left anterior cingulum of unipolar depressed patients. *Psychiatry Res*, 122(3), 185–192.

Phillips, M.L., Young, A.W., Senior, C., Brammer, M., Andrew, C., Calder, A.J., Bullmore, E.T., Perrett, D.I., Rowland, D., Williams, S.C., Gray, J.A., and David, A.S. (1997). A specific neural substrate for perceiving facial expressions of disgust. *Nature*, 389(6650), 495–498.

Phillips, M.L., Young, A.W., Scott, S.K., Calder, A.J., Andrew, C., Giampietro, V., Williams, S.C., Bullmore, E.T., Brammer, M., and Gray, J.A. (1998). Neural responses to facial and vocal expressions of fear and disgust. *Proc R Soc Lond B Biol Sci*, 265(1408), 1809–1817.

Philpot, M.P., Banerjee, S., Needham-Bennett, H., Costa, D.C., and Ell, P.J. (1993). 99mTc-HMPAO single photon emission tomography in late life depression: A pilot study of regional cerebral blood flow at rest and during a verbal fluency task. *J Affect Disord*, 28(4), 233–240.

Pillai, J.J., Friedman, L., Stuve, T.A., Trinidad, S., Jesberger, J.A., Lewin, J.S., Findling, R.L., Swales, T.P., and Schulz, S.C. (2002). Increased presence of white matter hyperintensities in adolescent patients with bipolar disorder. *Psychiatry Res*, 114(1), 51–56.

Pillay, S.S., Yurgelun-Todd, D.A., Bonello, C.M., Lafer, B., Fava, M., and Renshaw, P.F. (1997). A quantitative magnetic resonance imaging study of cerebral and cerebellar gray matter volume in primary unipolar major depression: Relationship to treatment response and clinical severity. *Biol Psychiatry*, 42, 79–84.

Pillay, S.S., Renshaw, P.F., Bonello, C.M., Lafer, B.C., Fava, M., and Yurgelun-Todd, D. (1998). A quantitative magnetic resonance imaging study of caudate and lenticular nucleus gray matter volume in primary unipolar major depression: Relationship to treatment response and clinical severity. *Psychiatry Res*, 84(2-3), 61–74.

Pizzagalli, D.A., Oakes, T.R., Fox, A.S., Chung, M.K., Larson, C.L., Abercrombie, H.C., Schaefer, S.M., Benca, R.M., and Davidson, R.J. (2004). Functional but not structural subgenual prefrontal cortex abnormalities in melancholia. *Mol Psychiatry*, 9(4), 325, 393–405.

Plenge, P., Stensgaard, A., Jensen, H.V., Thomsen, C., Mellerup, E.T., and Henriksen, O. (1994). 24-hour lithium concentration in human brain studied by Li-7 magnetic resonance spectroscopy. *Biol Psychiatry*, 36(8), 511–516.

Posener, J.A., Wang, L., Price, J.L., Gado, M.H., Province, M.A., Miller, M.I., Babb, C.M., and Csernansky, J.G. (2003). High-dimensional mapping of the hippocampus in depression. *Am J Psychiatry*, 160(1), 83–89.

Post, R.M., DeLisi, L.E., Holcomb, H.H., Uhde, T.W., Cohen, R., and Buchsbaum, M.S. (1987). Glucose utilization in the temporal cortex of affectively ill patients: Positron emission tomography. *Biol Psychiatry*, 22(5), 545–553.

Pouwels, P.J., and Frahm, J. (1998). Regional metabolite concentrations in human brain as determined by quantitative localized proton MRS. *Magn Reson Med*, 39(1), 53–60.

Pujol, J., Cardoner, N., Benlloch, L., Urretavizcaya, M., Deus, J., Losilla, J.M., Capdevila, A., and Vallejo, J. (2002). CSF spaces of the Sylvian fissure region in severe melancholic depression. *Neuroimage*, 15, 103–106.

Rabins, P.V., Pearlson, G.D., Aylward, E., Kumar, A.J., and Dowell, K. (1991). Cortical magnetic resonance imaging changes in elderly inpatients with major depression. *Am J Psychiatry*, 148(5), 617–620.

Raichle, M.E., Grubb, R.L. Jr., Gado, M.H., Eichling, J.O., and Ter-Pogossian, M.M. (1976). Correlation between regional cerebral blood flow and oxidative metabolism. In vivo studies in man. *Arch Neurol*, 33(8), 523–526.

Raichle, M.E., Taylor, J.R., et al. (1985). Brain circulation and metabolism in depression. In T. Greitz, D.H. Ingvar, and L. Widen (Eds.), *The Metabolism of the Human Brain Studied with Positron Emission Tomography* (pp. 453–456). New York: Raven Press.

Rajkowska, G. (1997). *Quantitative histopathology of prefrontal cortex in affective disorders.* 36th Annual Meeting of the American College of Neuropsychopharmacology, Waikoloa, HI, December 8–12.

Rao, V.P., Krishnan, K.R., Goli, V., Saunders, W.B., Ellinwood, E.H. Jr., Blazer, D.G., and Nemeroff, C.B. (1989). Neuroanatomical changes and hypothalamo–pituitary–adrenal axis abnormalities. *Biol Psychiatry*, 26(7), 729–732.

Rasgon, N.L., Thomas, M.A., Guze, B.H., Fairbanks, L.A., Yue, K., Curran, J.G., and Rapkin, A.J. (2001). Menstrual cycle–related brain metabolite changes using 1H magnetic resonance spectroscopy in premenopausal women: A pilot study. *Psychiatry Res*, 106(1), 47–57.

Raz, S. (1993). Structural cerebral pathology in schizophrenia: Regional or diffuse? *J Abnorm Psychol*, 102(3), 445–452.

Raz, S., and Raz, N. (1990). Structural brain abnormalities in the major psychoses: A quantitative review of the evidence from computerized imaging. *Psychol Bull*, 108(1), 93–108.

Reiman, E.M., Armstrong, S.M., Matt, K.S., and Mattox, J.H. (1996). The application of positron emission tomography to the study of the normal menstrual cycle. *Hum Reprod*, 11(12), 2799–2805.

Reischies, F.M., Hedde, J.P., and Drochner, R. (1989). Clinical correlates of cerebral blood flow in depression. *Psychiatry Res*, 29(3), 323–326.

Renshaw, P.F., and Wicklund, S. (1988). In vivo measurement of lithium in humans by nuclear magnetic resonance spectroscopy. *Biol Psychiatry*, 23(5), 465–475.

Renshaw, P.F., Johnson, K.A., et al. (1992). *New onset depression in patients with AIDS dementia complex (ADC) is associated with frontal lobe perfusion defects on HMPAO-SPECT scan.* 31st Annual Meeting of the American College of Neuropsychopharmacology, San Juan, Puerto Rico, December 14–18.

Renshaw, P.F., Yurgelun-Todd, D.A., Tohen, M., Gruber, S., and Cohen, B.M. (1995). Temporal lobe proton magnetic resonance spectroscopy of patients with first-episode psychosis. *Am J Psychiatry*, 152(3), 444–446.

Renshaw, P.F., Stoll, A.L., et al. (1996). *A choline deficit hypothesis for the progression of bipolar disorder with age.* 35th Annual Meeting of the American College of Neuropsychopharmacology, San Juan, Puerto Rico, December 9–13.

Renshaw, P.F., Lafer, B., Babb, S.M., Fava, M., Stoll, A.L., Christensen, J.D., Moore, C.M., Yurgelun-Todd, D.A., Bonello, C.M., Pillay, S.S., Rothschild, A.J., Nierenberg, A.A., Rosenbaum, J.F., and Cohen, B.M. (1997). Basal ganglia choline levels in depression and response to fluoxetine treatment: An in vivo proton magnetic resonance spectroscopy study. *Biol Psychiatry*, 41(8), 837–843.

Rieder, R.O., Mann, L.S., Weinberger, D.R., van Kammen, D.P., and Post, R.M. (1983). Computed tomographic scans in patients with schizophrenia, schizoaffective, and bipolar affective disorder. *Arch Gen Psychiatry*, 40(7), 735–739.

Riedl, U., Barocka, A., Kolem, H., Demling, J., Kaschka, W.P., Schelp, R., Stemmler, M., and Ebert, D. (1997). Duration of lithium treatment and brain lithium concentration in patients with unipolar and schizoaffective disorder: A study with magnetic resonance spectroscopy. *Biol Psychiatry*, 41(8), 844–850.

Ring, H.A., Bench, C.J., Trimble, M.R., Brooks, D.J., Frackowiak, R.S., and Dolan, R.J. (1994). Depression in Parkinson's disease. A positron emission study. *Br J Psychiatry*, 165(3), 333–339.

Risch, S.C., Lewine, R.J., Kalin, N.H., Jewart, R.D., Risby, E.D., Caudle, J.M., Stipetic, M., Turner, J., Eccard, M.B., and Pollard, W.E. (1992). Limbic–hypothalamic–pituitary–adrenal axis activity and ventricular-to-brain ratio studies in affective illness and schizophrenia. *Neuropsychopharmacology*, 6(2), 95–100.

Rosenberg, D.R., Paulson, L.D., et al. (2000). *Brain chemistry in pediatric depression.* 55th Annual Convention and Scientific Program of the Society of Biological Psychiatry, Chicago, IL, May 11–13.

Rossi, A., Stratta, P., Petruzzi, C., De Donatis, M., Nistico, R., and Casacchia, M. (1987). A computerised tomographic study in DSM-III affective disorders. *J Affect Disord*, 12(3), 259–262.

Rossi, A., Stratta, P., di Michele, V., Bolino, F., Nistico, R., de Leonardis, R., Sabatini, M.D., and Casacchia, M. (1989). A computerized tomographic study in patients with depressive disorder: A comparison with schizophrenic patients and controls. *Acta Psychiatr Belg*, 89(1-2), 56–61.

Rothschild, A.J., Benes, F., Hebben, N., Woods, B., Luciana, M., Bakanas, E., Samson, J.A., and Schatzberg, A.F. (1989). Relationships between brain CT scan findings and cortisol in psychotic and nonpsychotic depressed patients. *Biol Psychiatry*, 26(6), 565–575.

Roy, P.D., Zipursky, R.B., Saint-Cyr, J.A., Bury, A., Langevin, R., and Seeman, M.V. (1998). Temporal horn enlargement is present in schizophrenia and bipolar disorder. *Biol Psychiatry*, 44(6), 418–422.

Roy-Byrne, P.P., Post, R.M., Kellner, C.H., Joffe, R.T., and Uhde, T.W. (1988). Ventricular-brain ratio and life course of illness in patients with affective disorder. *Psychiatry Res*, 23(3), 277–284.

Rubin, E., Sackeim, H.A., Prohovnik, I., Moeller, J.R., Schnur, D.B., and Mukherjee, S. (1995). Regional cerebral blood flow in mood disorders: IV. Comparison of mania and depression. *Psychiatry Res*, 61(1), 1–10.

Rusch, B.D., Abercrombie, H.C., Oakes, T.R., Schaefer, S.M., and Davidson, R.J. (2001). Hippocampal morphometry in depressed patients and control subjects: Relations to anxiety symptoms. *Biol Psychiatry*, 50(12), 960–964.

Rush, A.J., Schlessor, M.A., Stokely, E., and Bonte, F.R. (1982). Cerebral blood flow in depression and mania. *Psychopharmacol Bull*, 18, 6–8.

Sachs, G.S., Renshaw, P.F., Lafer, B., Stoll, A.L., Guimaraes, A.R., Rosenbaum, J.F., and Gonzalez, R.G. (1995). Variability of brain lithium levels during maintenance treatment: A magnetic resonance spectroscopy study. *Biol Psychiatry*, 38(7), 422–428.

Sackeim, H.A. (1996). *Physiological perturbations in late-life depression: Implications for neuronal circuitry and effects of treatment.* 35th Annual Meeting of the American College of Neuropsychopharmacology, San Juan, Puerto Rico, December 9–13.

Sackeim, H.A., Prohovnik, I., Moeller, J.R., Brown, R.P., Apter, S., Prudic, J., Devanand, D.P., and Mukherjee, S. (1990). Regional cerebral blood flow in mood disorders. I. Comparison of major depressives and normal controls at rest. *Arch Gen Psychiatry*, 47(1), 60–70.

Sackeim, H.A., Prohovnik, I., Moeller, J.R., Mayeux, R., Stern, Y., and Devanand, D.P. (1993). Regional cerebral blood flow in mood disorders. II. Comparison of major depression and Alzheimer's disease. *J Nucl Med*, 34(7), 1090–1101.

Salloway, S., Malloy, P., Kohn, R., Gillard, E., Duffy, J., Rogg, J., Tung, G., Richardson, E., Thomas, C., and Westlake, R. (1996). MRI and neuropsychological differences in early- and late-life-onset geriatric depression. *Neurology*, 46(6), 1567–1574.

Salmon, E., Maquet, P., Sadzot, B., Degueldre, C., Lemaire, C., and Franck, G. (1991). Decrease of frontal metabolism demonstrated by positron emission tomography in a population of healthy elderly volunteers. *Acta Neurol Belg*, 91(5), 288–295.

Sanacora, G., Mason, G.F., Rothman, D.L., Behar, K.L., Hyder, F., Petroff, O.A., Berman, R.M., Charney, D.S., and Krystal, J.H. (1999). Reduced cortical gamma-aminobutyric acid levels in depressed patients determined by proton magnetic resonance spectroscopy. *Arch Gen Psychiatry*, 56(11), 1043–1047.

Sanacora, G., Mason, G.F., Rothman, D.L., and Krystal, J.H. (2002). Increased occipital cortex GABA concentrations in depressed patients after therapy with selective serotonin reuptake inhibitors. *Am J Psychiatry*, 159(4), 663–665.

Sanacora, G., Mason, G.F., Rothman, D.L., Hyder, F., Ciarcia, J.J., Ostroff, R.B., Berman, R.M., and Krystal, J.H. (2003). Increased cortical GABA concentrations in depressed patients receiving ECT. *Am J Psychiatry*, 160(3), 577–579.

Sanches, M., Sassi, R.B., Axelson, D., Nicoletti, M., Brambilla, P., Hatch, J.P., Keshavan, M.S., Ryan, N.D., Birmaher, B., and Soares, J.C. (2005). Subgenual prefrontal cortex of child and adolescent bipolar patients: A morphometric magnetic resonance imaging study. *Psychiatry Res*, 138(1), 43–49.

Sappey-Marinier, D., Calabrese, G., Hetherington, H.P., Fisher, S.N., Deicken, R., Van Dyke, C., Fein, G., and Weiner, M.W. (1992a). Proton magnetic resonance spectroscopy of human brain: Applications to normal white matter, chronic infarction, and MRI white matter signal hyperintensities. *Magn Reson Med*, 26(2), 313–327.

Sappey-Marinier, D., Deicken, R.F., Fein, G., Calabrese, G., Hubesch, B., Van Dyke, C., Dillon, W.P., Davenport, L., Meyerhoff, D.J., and Weiner, M.W. (1992b). Alterations in brain phosphorus metabolite concentrations associated with areas of high signal intensity in white matter at MR imaging. *Radiology*, 183(1), 247–256.

Sassi, R.B., Nicoletti, M., Brambilla, P., Harenski, K., Mallinger, A.G., Frank, E., Kupfer, D.J., Keshavan, M.S., and Soares, J.C. (2001). Decreased pituitary volume in patients with bipolar disorder. *Biol Psychiatry*, 50(4), 271–280.

Sassi, R.B., Brambilla, P., et al. (2002a). *Lithium influences the volume of the cingulate cortex in bipolar mood disorder patients.* 57th Annual Convention and Scientific Program of the Society of Biological Psychiatry, Philadelphia, PA, May 16–18.

Sassi, R.B., Nicoletti, M., Brambilla, P., Mallinger, A.G., Frank, E., Kupfer, D.J., Keshavan, M.S., and Soares, J.C. (2002b). Increased gray matter volume in lithium-treated bipolar disorder patients. *Neurosci Lett*, 329(2), 243–245.

Sassi, R.B., Brambilla, P., Nicoletti, M., Mallinger, A.G., Frank, E., Kupfer, D.J., Keshavan, M.S., and Soares, J.C. (2003). White matter hyperintensities in bipolar and unipolar patients with relatively mild-to-moderate illness severity. *J Affect Disord*, 77(3), 237–245.

Sassi, R.B., Brambilla, P., Hatch, J.P., Nicoletti, M.A., Mallinger, A.G., Frank, E., Kupfer, D.J., Keshavan, M.S., and Soares, J.C. (2004). Reduced left anterior cingulate volumes in untreated bipolar patients. *Biol Psychiatry*, 56(7), 467–475.

Sassi, R.B., Stanley, J.A., Axelson, D., Brambilla, P., Nicoletti, M.A., Keshavan, M.S., Ramos, R.T., Ryan, N., Birmaher, B., and Soares, J.C. (2005). Reduced NAA levels in the dorsolateral prefrontal cortex of young bipolar patients. *Am J Psychiatry*, 162(11), 2109–2115.

Sax, K.W., Strakowski, S.M., Zimmerman, M.E., DelBello, M.P., Keck, P.E. Jr., and Hawkins, J.M. (1999). Frontosubcortical neuroanatomy and the continuous performance test in mania. *Am J Psychiatry*, 156(1), 139–141.

Saxena, S., Brody, A.L., Ho, M.L., Alborzian, S., Ho, M.K., Maidment, K.M., Huang, S.C., Wu, H.M., Au, S.C., and Baxter, L.R. Jr. (2001). Cerebral metabolism in major depression and obsessive-compulsive disorder occurring separately and concurrently. *Biol Psychiatry*, 50(3), 159–170.

Scarr, E., Pavey, G., Sundram, S., MacKinnon, A., and Dean, B. (2003). Decreased hippocampal NMDA, but not kainite or AMPA receptors in bipolar disorder. *Bipolar Disord*, 5(4), 257–264.

Schlaepfer, T.E., Harris, G.J., Tien, A.Y., Peng, L.W., Lee, S., Federman, E.B., Chase, G.A., Barta, P.E., and Pearlson, G.D. (1994). Decreased regional cortical gray matter volume in schizophrenia. *Am J Psychiatry*, 151(6), 842–848.

Schlageter, N.L., Horwitz, B., Creasey, H., Carson, R., Duara, R., Berg, G.W., and Rapoport, S.I. (1987). Relation of measured brain glucose utilisation and cerebral atrophy in man. *J Neurol Neurosurg Psychiatry*, 50(6), 779–785.

Schlegel, S., and Kretzschmar, V. (1987). Computed tomography in affective disorders. Part I: ventricular and sulcal measurements. *Biol Psychiatry*, 22(1), 4–14.

Schlegel, S., Aldenhoff, J.B., Eissner, D., Lindner, P., and Nickel, O. (1989a). Regional cerebral blood flow in depression: Associations with psychopathology. *J Affect Disord*, 17(3), 211–218.

Schlegel, S., Frommberger, U., and Buller, R. (1989b). Computerized tomography (CT) in affective disorders: Relationship with psychopathology. *Psychiatry Res*, 29(3), 271–272.

Schlegel, S., von Bardeleben, U., Wiedemann, K., Frommberger, U., and Holsboer, F. (1989c). Computerized brain tomography measures compared with spontaneous and suppressed plasma cortisol levels in major depression. *Psychoneuroendocrinology*, 14(3), 209–216.

Schneider, F., Gur, R.E., Mozley, L.H., Smith, R.J., Mozley, P.D., Censits, D.M., Alavi, A., and Gur, R.C. (1995). Mood effects on limbic blood flow correlate with emotional self-rating: A PET study with oxygen-15 labeled water. *Psychiatry Res*, 61(4), 265–283.

Schneider, F., Grodd, W., Weiss, U., Klose, U., Mayer, K.R., Nagele, T., and Gur, R.C. (1997). Functional MRI reveals left amygdala activation during emotion. *Psychiatry Res*, 76(2-3), 75–82.

Schneider, F., Weiss, U., Kessler, C., Salloum, J.B., Posse, S., Grodd, W., and Muller-Gartner, H.W. (1998). Differential amygdala activation in schizophrenia during sadness. *Schizophr Res*, 34(3), 133–142.

Schneider, F., Hatbel, U., Kessler, C., Salloum, J.B., and Posse, S. (2000). Gender differences in regional cerebral activity during sadness. *Hum Brain Mapping*, 9(4), 226–238.

Schwartz, J.M., Baxter, L.R. Jr., Mazziotta, J.C., Gerner, R.H., and Phelps, M.E. (1987). The differential diagnosis of depression. Relevance of positron emission tomography studies of cerebral glucose metabolism to the bipolar–unipolar dichotomy. *JAMA*, 258(10), 1368–1374.

Schwartz, P.J., Loe, J.A., Bash, C.N., Bove, K., Turner, E.H., Frank, J.A., Wehr, T.A., and Rosenthal, N.E. (1997). Seasonality and pituitary volume. *Psychiatry Res*, 74(3), 151–157.

Scott, A.I., Dougall, N., Ross, M., O'Carroll, R.E., Riddle, W., Ebmeier, K.P., and Goodwin, G.M. (1994). Short-term effects of electroconvulsive treatment on the uptake of ^{99m}Tc-exametazime into brain in major depression shown with single photon emission tomography. *J Affect Disord*, 30(1), 27–34.

Scott, M.L., Golden, C.J., Ruedrich, S.L., and Bishop, R.J. (1983). Ventricular enlargement in major depression. *Psychiatry Res*, 8(2), 91–93.

Shah, P.J., Ebmeier, K.P., Glabus, M.F., and Goodwin, G.M. (1998). Cortical grey matter reductions associated with treatment-resistant chronic unipolar depression. Controlled magnetic resonance imaging study. *Br J Psychiatry*, 172, 527–532.

Shah, S.A., Doraiswamy, P.M., Husain, M.M., Escalona, P.R., Na, C., Figiel, G.S., Patterson, L.J., Ellinwood, E.H. Jr., McDonald, W.M., and Boyko, O.B. (1992). Posterior fossa abnormalities in major depression: A controlled magnetic resonance imaging study. *Acta Psychiatr Scand*, 85(6), 474–479.

Sharma, R., Venkatasubramanian, P.N., Barany, M., and Davis, J.M. (1992). Proton magnetic resonance spectroscopy of the brain in schizophrenic and affective patients. *Schizophr Res*, 8(1), 43–49.

Sharma, V., Menon, R., Carr, T.J., Densmore, M., Mazmanian, D., and Williamson, P.C. (2003). An MRI study of subgenual prefrontal cortex in patients with familial and non-familial bipolar I disorder. *J Affect Disord*, 77(2), 167–171.

Sheline, Y.I., Wang, P.W., Gado, M.H., Csernansky, J.G., and Vannier, M.W. (1996). Hippocampal atrophy in recurrent major depression. *Proc Natl Acad Sci USA*, 93(9), 3908–3913.

Sheline, Y.I., Sanghavi, M., Mintun, M.A., and Gado, M.H. (1999). Depression duration but not age predicts hippocampal volume loss in medically healthy women with recurrent major depression. *J Neurosci*, 19(12), 5034–5043.

Sheline, Y.I., Barch, D.M., Barany, M., and Davis, J.M. (2001). Increased amygdala response to masked emotional faces in depressed subjects resolves with antidepressant treatment: An fMRI study. *Biol Psychiatry*, 50(9), 651–658.

Sheline, Y.I., Gado, M.H., and Kraemer, H.C. (2003). Untreated depression and hippocampal volume loss. *Am J Psychiatry*, 160(8), 1516–1518.

Shenton, M.E., Wible, C.G., and McCarley, R.W. (1997). A review of magnetic resonance imaging studies of brain abnormalities in schizophrenia. In K.R.R. Krishnan and P.M. Doriaswamy (Eds.), *Brain Imaging in Clinical Psychiatry* (pp. 297–380). New York: Marcel Dekker.

Shima, S., Shikano, T., Kitamura, T., Masuda, Y., Tsukumo, T., Kanba, S., and Asai, M. (1984). Depression and ventricular enlargement. *Acta Psychiatr Scand*, 70(3), 275–277.

Shiraishi, H., Koizumi, J., Hori, M., Terashima, Y., Suzuki, T., Saito, K., Mizukami, K., Tanaka, Y., and Yamaguchi, N. (1992). A computerized tomographic study in patients with delusional and non-delusional depression. *Jpn J Psychiatry Neurol*, 46(1), 99–105.

Silfverskiöld, P., and Risberg, J. (1989). Regional cerebral blood flow in depression and mania. *Arch Gen Psychiatry*, 46(3), 253–259.

Silverstone, P.H., Hanstock, C.C., Fabian, J., Staab, R., and Allen, P.S. (1996). Chronic lithium does not alter human myo-inositol or phosphomonoester concentrations as measured by 1H and 31P MRS. *Biol Psychiatry*, 40(4), 235–246.

Silverstone, P.H., Rotzinger, S., Pukhovsky, A., and Hanstock, C.C. (1999). Effects of lithium and amphetamine on inositol metabolism in the human brain as measured by 1H and 31P MRS. *Biol Psychiatry*, 46(12), 1634–1641.

Silverstone, P.H., Wu, R.H., O'Donnell, T., Ulrich, M., Asghar, S.J., and Hanstock, C.C. (2002). Chronic treatment with both lithium and sodium valproate may normalize phosphoinositol cycle activity in bipolar patients. *Hum Psychopharmacol*, 17(7), 321–327.

Silverstone, P.H., Wu, R.H., O'Donnell, T., Ulrich, M., Asghar, S.J., and Hanstock, C.C. (2003). Chronic treatment with lithium, but not sodium valproate, increases cortical N-acetylaspartate concentrations in euthymic bipolar patients. *Int Clin Psychopharmacol*, 18(2), 73–79.

Silverstone, P.H., Asghar, S.J., O'Donnell, T., Ulrich, M., and Hanstock, C.C. (2004). Lithium and valproate protect against dextro-amphetamine induced brain choline concentration changes in bipolar disorder patients. *World J Biol Psychiatry*, 5(1), 38–44.

Silverstone, T., McPherson, H., Li, Q., and Doyle, T. (2003). Deep white matter hyperintensities in patients with bipolar depression, unipolar depression and age-matched control subjects. *Bipolar Disord*, 5(1), 53–57.

Simpson, S., Baldwin, R.C., Jackson, A., and Burns, A.S. (1998). Is subcortical disease associated with a poor response to antidepressants? Neurological, neuropsychological and neuroradiological findings in late-life depression. *Psychol Med*, 28(5), 1015–1026.

Simpson, S.W., Baldwin, R.C., Burns, A., and Jackson, A. (2001). Regional cerebral volume measurements in late-life depression: Relationship to clinical correlates, neuropsychological impairment and response to treatment. *Int J Geriatr Psychiatry*, 16(5), 469–476.

Smith, E.A., Russell, A., Lorch, E., Banerjee, S.P., Rose, M., Ivey, J., Bhandari, R., Moore, G.J., and Rosenberg, D.R. (2003). Increased medial thalamic choline found in pediatric patients with obsessive-compulsive disorder versus major depression or healthy control subjects: A magnetic resonance spectroscopy study. *Biol Psychiatry*, 54(12), 1399–1405.

Smith, K.A., Morris, J.S., Friston, K.J., Cowen, P.J., and Dolan, R.J. (1999). Brain mechanisms associated with depressive relapse and associated cognitive impairment following acute tryptophan depletion. *Br J Psychiatry*, 174, 525–529.

Soares, J.C., Boada, F., et al. (1999). *NAA and choline measurements in the anterior cingulate of bipolar disorder patients.* 54th Annual Convention and Scientific Program of the Society of Biological Psychiatry, Washington, DC, May 13–15.

Soares, J.C., Boada, F., Spencer, S., Mallinger, A.G., Dippold, C.S., Wells, K.F., Frank, E., Keshavan, M.S., Gershon, S., and Kupfer, D.J. (2001). Brain lithium concentrations in bipolar disorder patients: Preliminary (7)Li magnetic resonance studies at 3 T. *Biol Psychiatry*, 49(5), 437–443.

Sonawalla, S.B., Renshaw, P.F., Moore, C.M., Alpert, J.E., Nierenberg, A.A., Rosenbaum, J.F., and Fava, M. (1999). Compounds containing cytosolic choline in the basal ganglia: A potential biological marker of true drug response to fluoxetine. *Am J Psychiatry*, 156(10), 1638–1640.

Speer, A.M., Upadhyaya, V.H., et al. (1997). *New windows into bipolar illness: Serial perfusion MRI scanning in rapid-cycling bipolar patients.* 150th Annual Meeting of the American Psychiatric Association, San Diego, CA, May 17–22.

Sprengelmeyer, R., Rausch, M., Eysel, U.T., and Przuntek, H. (1998). Neural structures associated with recognition of facial expressions of basic emotions. *Proc R Soc Lond B Biol Sci*, 265(1409), 1927–1931.

Standish-Barry, H.M., Hale, A.S., Honig, A., Bouras, N., Bridges, P.K., and Bartlett, J.R. (1985). Ventricular size, the dexamethasone suppression test and outcome of severe endogenous depression following psychosurgery. *Acta Psychiatr Scand*, 72(2), 166–171.

Starkstein, S.E., and Robinson, R.G. (1989). Affective disorders and cerebrovascular disease. *Br J Psychiatry*, 154, 170–182.

Starkstein, S.E., Mayberg, H.S., Berthier, M.L., Fedoroff, P., Price, T.R., Dannals, R.F., Wagner, H.N., Leiguarda, R., and Robinson, R.G. (1990). Mania after brain injury: Neuroradiological and metabolic findings. *Ann Neurol*, 7(6), 652–659.

Steffens, D.C., and Krishnan, K.R. (1998). Structural neuroimaging and mood disorders: Recent findings, implications for classification, and future directions. *Biol Psychiatry*, 43(10), 705–712.

Steffens, D.C., Byrum, C.E., McQuoid, D.R., Greenberg, D.L., Payne, M.E., Blitchington, T.F., MacFall, J.R., and Krishnan, K.R. (2000). Hippocampal volume in geriatric depression. *Biol Psychiatry*, 48(4), 301–309.

Steingard, R.J., Yurgelun-Todd, D.A., Hennen, J., Moore, J.C., Moore, C.M., Vakili, K., Young, A.D., Katic, A., Beardslee, W.R., and Renshaw, P.F. (2000). Increased orbitofrontal cortex levels of choline in depressed adolescents as detected by in vivo proton magnetic resonance spectroscopy. *Biol Psychiatry*, 48(11), 1053–1061.

Steingard, R.J., Renshaw, P.F., Hennen, J., Lenox, M., Cintron, C.B., Young, A.D., Connor, D.F., Au, T.H., and Yurgelun-Todd, D.A. (2002). Smaller frontal lobe white matter volumes in depressed adolescents. *Biol Psychiatry*, 52(5), 413–417.

Stern, R.A., and Bachmann, D.L. (1991). Depressive symptoms following stroke. *Am J Psychiatry*, 148, 351–356.

Stoll, A.L., Renshaw, P.F., Sachs, G.S., Guimaraes, A.R., Miller, C., Cohen, B.M., Lafer, B., and Gonzalez, R.G. (1992). The human brain resonance of choline-containing compounds is similar in patients receiving lithium treatment and controls: An in vivo proton magnetic resonance spectroscopy study. *Biol Psychiatry*, 32(10), 944–949.

Stoll, A.L., Renshaw, P.F., De Micheli, E., Wurtman, R., Pillay, S.S., and Cohen, B.M. (1995). Choline ingestion increases the resonance of choline-containing compounds in human brain: An in vivo proton magnetic resonance study. *Biol Psychiatry*, 37(3), 170–174.

Stoll, A.L., Sachs, G.S., Cohen, B.M., Lafer, B., Christensen, J.D., and Renshaw, P.F. (1996). Choline in the treatment of rapid-cycling bipolar disorder: Clinical and neurochemical findings in lithium-treated patients. *Biol Psychiatry*, 40(5), 382–388.

Strakowski, S.M., Wilson, D.R., Tohen, M., Woods, B.T., Douglass, A.W., and Stoll, A.L. (1993a). Structural brain abnormalities in first-episode mania. *Biol Psychiatry*, 33(8-9), 602–609.

Strakowski, S.M., Woods, B.T., Tohen, M., Wilson, D.R., Douglass, A.W., and Stoll, A.L. (1993b). MRI subcortical signal hyperintensities in mania at first hospitalization. *Biol Psychiatry*, 33(3), 204–206.

Strakowski, S.M., DelBello, M.P., Sax, K.W., Zimmerman, M.E., Shear, P.K., Hawkins, J.M., and Larson, E.R. (1999). Brain magnetic resonance imaging of structural abnormalities in bipolar disorder. *Arch Gen Psychiatry*, 56(3), 254–260.

Strakowski, S.M., DelBello, M.P., Zimmerman, M.E., Getz, G.E., Mills, N.P., Ret, J., Shear, P., and Adler, C.M. (2002). Ventricular and periventricular structural volumes in first- versus multiple-episode bipolar disorder. *Am J Psychiatry*, 159(11), 1841–1847.

Strasser, H.C., Honeycutt, N.A., et al. (2002). *Amygdala volumes in psychotic versus nonpsychotic bipolar disorder and schizophrenia.* 57th Annual Convention and Scientific Program of the Society of Biological Psychiatry, Philadelphia, PA, May 16–18.

Swayze, V.W. II, Andreasen, N.C., Alliger, R.J., Ehrhardt, J.C., and Yuh, W.T. (1990). Structural brain abnormalities in bipolar affective disorder. Ventricular enlargement and focal signal hyperintensities. *Arch Gen Psychiatry*, 47(11), 1054–1059.

Swayze, V.W. II, Andreasen, N.C., Alliger, R.J., Yuh, W.T., and Ehrhardt, J.C. (1992). Subcortical and temporal structures in affective disorder and schizophrenia: A magnetic resonance imaging study. *Biol Psychiatry*, 31(3), 221–240.

Tan, J., Bluml, S., Hoang, T., Dubowitz, D., Mevenkamp, G., and Ross, B. (1998). Lack of effect of oral choline supplement on the concentrations of choline metabolites in human brain. *Magn Reson Med*, 39(6), 1005–1010.

Tanaka, Y., Hazama, H., Fukuhara, T., and Tsutsuim T. (1982). Computerized tomography of the brain in manic-depressive patients: A controlled study. *Folia Psychiatr Neurol Jpn*, 36, 137–143.

Targum, S.D., Rosen, L.N., DeLisi, L.E., Weinberger, D.R., and Citrin, C.M. (1983). Cerebral ventricular size in major depressive disorder: Association with delusional symptoms. *Biol Psychiatry*, 18(3), 329–336.

Taylor, W.D., Payne, M.E., Krishnan, K.R., Wagner, H.R., Provenzale, J.M., Steffens, D.C., and MacFall, J.R. (2001). Evidence of white matter tract disruption in MRI hyperintensities. *Biol Psychiatry*, 50(3), 179–183.

Taylor, W.D., Steffens, D.C., MacFall, J.R., McQuoid, D.R., Payne, M.E., Provenzale, J.M., and Krishnan, K.R. (2003). White matter hyperintensity progression and late-life depression outcomes. *Arch Gen Psychiatry*, 60(11), 1090–1096.

Taylor, W.D., MacFall, J.R., Payne, M.E., McQuoid, D.R., Provenzale, J.M., Steffens, D.C., and Krishman, K.R. (2004). Late-life depression and microstructural abnormalities in dorsolateral prefrontal cortex white matter. *Am J Psychiatry*, 161(7), 1293–1296.

Teneback, C.C., Nahas, Z., Speer, A.M., Molloy, M., Stallings, L.E., Spicer, K.M., Risch, S.C., and George, M.S. (1999). Changes in prefrontal cortex and paralimbic activity in depression following two weeks of daily left prefrontal TMS. *J Neuropsychiatry Clin Neurosci*, 11(4), 426–435.

Thomas, K.M., Drevets, W.C., Whalen, P.J., Eccard, C.H., Dahl, R.E., Ryan, N.D., and Casey, B.J. (2001). Amygdala response to facial expressions in children and adults. *Biol Psychiatry*, 49(4), 309–316.

Thomas, P., Vaiva, G., Samaille, E., Maron, M., Alaix, C., Steinling, M., and Goudemand, M. (1993). Cerebral blood flow in major depression and dysthymia. *J Affect Disord*, 29(4), 235–242.

Trivedi, M.H., Blackburn, T., et al. (1995). *Effects of amphetamine in major depressive disorder using functional MRI.* 50th Annual Meeting of the Society of Biological Psychiatry, Miami, FL, May 17–20.

Tsai, L., Nasrallah, H.A., and Jacoby, C.G. (1983). Hemispheric asymmetries on computed tomographic scans in schizophrenia and mania. *Arch Gen Psychiatry*, 39, 1286–1289.

Tutus, A., Kibar, M., Sofuoglu, S., Basturk, M., and Gonul, A.S. (1998a). A technetium-99m hexamethylpropylene amine oxime brain single-photon emission tomography study in adolescent patients with major depressive disorder. *Eur J Nucl Med*, 25(6), 601–606.

Tutus, A., Simsek, A., Sofuoglu, S., Nardali, M., Kugu, N., Karaaslan, F., and Gonul, A.S. (1998b). Changes in regional cerebral blood flow demonstrated by single photon emission computed tomography in depressive disorders: Comparison of unipolar vs. bipolar subtypes. *Psychiatry Res*, 83(3), 169–177.

Upadhyaya, A.K., Abou-Saleh, M.T., Wilson, K., Grime, S.J., and Critchley, M. (1990). A study of depression in old age using single-photon emission computerised tomography. *Br J Psychiatry Suppl*, 157(Suppl. 9), 76–81.

Vakili, K., Pillay, S.S., Lafer, B., Fava, M., Renshaw, P.F., Bonello-Cintron, C.M., and Yurgelun-Todd, D.A. (2000). Hippocampal volume in primary unipolar major depression: A magnetic resonance imaging study. *Biol Psychiatry*, 47(12), 1087–1090.

Van den Bossche, B., Maes, M., Brussaard, C., Schotte, C., Cosyns, P., De Moor, J., and De Schepper, A. (1991). Computed tomography of the brain in unipolar depression. *J Affect Disord*, 21(1), 67–74.

Vasile, R.G., Schwartz, R.B., Garada, B., Holman, B.L., Alpert, M., Davidson, P.B., and Schildkraut, J.J. (1996). Focal cerebral perfusion defects demonstrated by 99mTc-hexamethylpropyleneamine oxime SPECT in elderly depressed patients. *Psychiatry Res*, 67(1), 59–70.

Vasile, R.G., Sachs, G., Anderson, J.L., Lafer, B., Matthews, E., and Hill, T. (1997). Changes in regional cerebral blood flow following light treatment for seasonal affective disorder: Responders versus nonresponders. *Biol Psychiatry*, 42(11), 1000–1005.

Velakoulis, D., Pantelis, C., McGorry, P.D., Dudgeon, P., Brewer, W., Cook, M., Desmond, P., Bridle, N., Tierney, P., Murrie, V., Singh, B., and Copolov, D. (1999). Hippocampal volume in first-episode psychoses and chronic schizophrenia: A high-resolution magnetic resonance imaging study. *Arch Gen Psychiatry*, 56(2), 133–141.

Videbech, P. (1997). MRI findings in patients with affective disorder: A meta-analysis. *Acta Psychiatr Scand*, 96(3), 157–168.

Videbech, P., and Ravnkilde, B. (2004). Hippocampal volume and depression: A meta-analysis of MRI studies. *Am J Psychiatry*, 161(11), 1957–1966.

Videbech, P., Ravnkilde, B., Pedersen, A.R., Egander, A., Landbo, B., Rasmussen, N.A., Andersen, F., Stodkilde-Jorgensen, H., Gjedde, A., and Rosenberg, R. (2001). The Danish PET/depression project: PET findings in patients with major depression. *Psychol Med*, 31(7), 1147–1158.

Videbech, P., Ravnkilde, B., Pedersen, T.H., Hartvig, H., Egander, A., Clemmensen, K., Rasmussen, N.A., Andersen, F., Gjedde, A., and Rosenberg, R. (2002). The Danish PET/depression project: Clinical symptoms and cerebral blood flow. A regions-of-interest analysis. *Acta Psychiatr Scand*, 106(1), 35–44.

Vita, A., Sacchetti, E., and Cazzullo, C.L. (1988). A CT follow-up study of cerebral ventricular size in schizophrenia and major affective disorder. *Schizophr Res*, 1, 165–166.

Volk, S.A., Kaendler, S.H., Hertel, A., Maul, F.D., Manoocheri, R., Weber, R., Georgi, K., Pflug, B., and Hor, G. (1997). Can response to partial sleep deprivation in depressed patients be predicted by regional changes of cerebral blood flow? *Psychiatry Res*, 75, 67–74.

Volkow, N.D., Fowler, J.S., et al. (1991). *Abnormal dopamine brain activity in cocaine abusers.* 30th Annual Meeting of the American College of Neuropsychopharmacology, San Juan, Puerto Rico, December 9–13.

Volkow, N.D., Wang, G.J., Fowler, J.S., Hitzemann, R., Pappas, N., Pascani, K., and Wong, C. (1997). Gender differences in cerebellar metabolism: Test–retest reproducibility. *Am J Psychiatry*, 154(1), 119–121.

Volz, H.P., Rzanny, R., Riehemann, S., May, S., Hegewald, H., Preussler, B., Hubner, G., Kaiser, W.A., and Sauer, H. (1998). 31P magnetic resonance spectroscopy in the frontal lobe of major depressed patients. *Eur Arch Psychiatry Clin Neurosci*, 248(6), 289–295.

von Gunten, A., Fox, N.C., Cipolotti, L., and Ron, M.A. (2000). A volumetric study of hippocampus and amygdala in depressed patients with subjective memory problems. *J Neuropsychiatry Clin Neurosci*, 12(4), 493–498.

Vythilingam, M., Heim, C., Newport, J., Miller, A.H., Anderson, E., Bronen, R., Brummer, M., Staib, L., Vermetten, E., Charney, D.S., Nemeroff, C.B., and Bremner, J.D. (2002). Childhood trauma associated with smaller hippocampal volume in women with major depression. *Am J Psychiatry*, 159(12), 2072–2080.

Vythilingam, M., Charles, H.C., Tupler, L.A., Blitchington, T., Kelly, L., and Krishnan, K.R. (2003). Focal and lateralized subcortical abnormalities in unipolar major depressive disorder: An automated multivoxel proton magnetic resonance spectroscopy study. *Biol Psychiatry*, 54(7), 744–750.

Wang, G.J., Volkow, N.D., et al. (1994). Intersubject variability of brain glucose metabolic measurements in young normal males. *J Nucl Med*, 35(9), 1457–1466.

Wang, P.W., Dieckmann, N., et al. (2002). *3 Tesla ¹H-magnetic resonance spectroscopic measurements of prefrontal cortical gamma-aminobutyric acid (GABA) levels in bipolar disorder patients and healthy volunteers.* 57th Annual Convention and Scientific Program of the Society of Biological Psychiatry, Philadelphia, PA, May 16–18.

Ward, K.E., Friedman, L., Wise, A., and Schulz, S.C. (1996). Meta-analysis of brain and cranial size in schizophrenia. *Schizophr Res*, 22(3), 197–213.

Watanabe, A., Kato, N., and Kato, T. (2002). Effects of creatine on mental fatigue and cerebral hemoglobin oxygenation. *Neurosci Res*, 42(4), 279–285.

Weinberger, D.R., DeLisi, L.E., Perman, G.P., Targum, S., and Wyatt, R.J. (1982). Computed tomography in schizophreniform disorder and other acute psychiatric disorders. *Arch Gen Psychiatry*, 39(7), 778–783.

Whalen, P.J., Rauch, S.L., Etcoff, N.L., McInerney, S.C., Lee, M.B., and Jenike, M.A. (1998). Masked presentations of emotional facial expressions modulate amygdala activity without explicit knowledge. *J Neurosci*, 18(1), 411–418.

Wilke, M., Kowatch, R.A., DelBello, M.P., Mills, N.P., and Holland, S.K. (2004). Voxel-based morphometry in adolescents with bipolar disorder: First results. *Psychiatry Res*, 131(1), 57–69.

Willis, M.W., Ketter, T.A., Kimbrell, T.A., George, M.S., Herscovitch, P., Danielson, A.L., Benson, B.E., and Post, R.M. (2002). Age, sex and laterality effects on cerebral glucose metabolism in healthy adults. *Psychiatry Res*, 114(1), 23–37.

Wilson, J., Kupfer, D.J., et al. (2002). *Ventral striatal metabolism is increased in depression, and decreases with treatment.* 57th Annual Convention and Scientific Program of the Society of Biological Psychiatry, Philadelphia, PA, May 16–18.

Winsberg, M.E., Sachs, N., Tate, D.L., Adalsteinsson, E., Spielman, D., and Ketter, T.A. (2000). Decreased dorsolateral prefrontal N-acetyl aspartate in bipolar disorder. *Biol Psychiatry*, 47(6), 475–481.

Woods, B.T., Yurgelun-Todd, D., Benes, F.M., Frankenburg, F.R., Pope, H.G. Jr., and McSparren, J. (1990). Progressive ventricular enlargement in schizophrenia: Comparison to bipolar affective disorder and correlation with clinical course. *Biol Psychiatry*, 27(3), 341–352.

Woods, B.T., Brennan, S., Yurgelun-Todd, D., Young, T., and Panzarino, P. (1995a). MRI abnormalities in major psychiatric disorders: An exploratory comparative study. *J Neuropsychiatry Clin Neurosci*, 7(1), 49–53.

Woods, B.T., Yurgelun-Todd, D., Mikulis, D., and Pillay, S.S. (1995b). Age-related MRI abnormalities in bipolar illness: A clinical study. *Biol Psychiatry*, 38(12), 846–847.

Wu, J.C., Gillin, J.C., Buchsbaum, M.S., Hershey, T., Johnson, J.C., and Bunney, W.E. Jr. (1992). Effect of sleep deprivation on brain metabolism of depressed patients. *Am J Psychiatry*, 149(4), 538–543.

Wu, J.C., Buchsbaum, M.S., Johnson, J.C., Hershey, T.G., Wagner, E.A., Teng, C., and Lottenberg, S. (1993). Magnetic resonance and positron emission tomography imaging of the corpus callosum: Size, shape and metabolic rate in unipolar depression. *J Affect Disord*, 28(1), 15–25.

Wu, J., Buchsbaum, M.S., Gillin, J.C., Tang, C., Cadwell, S., Wiegand, M., Najafi, A., Klein, E., Hazen, K., Bunney, W.E. Jr., Fallon, J.H., and Keator, D. (1999). Prediction of antidepressant effects of sleep deprivation by metabolic rates in the ventral anterior cingulate and medial prefrontal cortex. *Am J Psychiatry*, 156(8), 1149–1158.

Wu, R.H., O'Donnell, T., Ulrich, M., Asghar, S.J., Hanstock, C.C., and Silverstone, P.H. (2004). Brain choline concentrations may not be altered in euthymic bipolar disorder patients chronically treated with either lithium or sodium valproate. *Ann Gen Hosp Psychiatry*, 3(1), 13.

Wurthmann, C., Bogerts, B., and Falkai, P. (1995). Brain morphology assessed by computed tomography in patients with geriatric depression, patients with degenerative dementia, and normal control subjects. *Psychiatry Res*, 61(2), 103–111.

Yates, W.R., Jacoby, C.G., and Andreasen, N.C. (1987). Cerebellar atrophy in schizophrenia and affective disorder. *Am J Psychiatry*, 144(4), 465–467.

Yazici, K.M., Kapucu, O., Erbas, B., Varoglu, E., Gulec, C., and Bekdik, C.F. (1992). Assessment of changes in regional cerebral blood flow in patients with major depression using the ⁹⁹mTc-HMPAO single photon emission tomography method. *Eur J Nucl Med*, 19(12), 1038–1043.

Yildiz, A., Demopulos, C.M., Moore, C.M., Renshaw, P.F., and Sachs, G.S. (2001a). Effect of lithium on phosphoinositide metabolism in human brain: A proton decoupled (31)P magnetic resonance spectroscopy study. *Biol Psychiatry*, 50(1), 3–7.

Yildiz, A., Sachs, G.S., Dorer, D.J., and Renshaw, P.F. (2001b). 31P Nuclear magnetic resonance spectroscopy findings in bipolar illness: A meta-analysis. *Psychiatry Res*, 106(3), 181–191.

Yoshii, F., Barker, W.W., Chang, J.Y., Loewenstein, D., Apicella, A., Smith, D., Boothe, T., Ginsberg, M.D., Pascal, S., and Duara, R. (1988). Sensitivity of cerebral glucose metabolism to age, gender, brain volume, brain atrophy, and cerebrovascular risk factors. *J Cereb Blood Flow Metab*, 8(5), 654–661.

Young, R.C., Nambudiri, D., et al. (1988). *Ventricular-brain ratio and response to nortriptyline in geriatric depression* [abstract]. 43rd Annual Meeting of the Society of Biological Psychiatry.

Young, R.C., Bocksberger, J.P., et al. (1996). *Putamen volume and age at onset in geriatric mania.* 149th Annual Meeting of the American Psychiatric Association, New York, NY, May 4–9.

Yurgelun-Todd, D.A., Gruber, S.A., Kanayama, G., Killgore, W.D., Baird, A.A., and Young, A.D. (2000). fMRI during affect discrimination in bipolar affective disorder. *Bipolar Disord*, 2(3 Pt. 2), 237–248.

Zipursky, R.B., Seeman, M.V., Bury, A., Langevin, R., Wortzman, G., and Katz, R. (1997). Deficits in gray matter volume are present in schizophrenia but not bipolar disorder. *Schizophr Res*, 26(2-3), 85–92.

Zubenko, G.S., Sullivan, P., Nelson, J.P., Belle, S.H., Huff, F.J., and Wolf, G.L. (1990). Brain imaging abnormalities in mental disorders of late life. *Arch Neurol*, 47(10), 1107–1111.

CHAPTER 16

Abe, M., Herzog, E.D., and Block, G.D. (2000). Lithium lengthens the circadian period of individual suprachiasmatic nucleus neurons. *Neuroreport*, 11(14), 3261–3264.

Achermann, P., and Borbely, A.A. (1998). Coherence analysis of the human sleep electroencephalogram. *Neuroscience*, 85(4), 1195–1208.

Aeschbach, D., and Borbely, A.A. (1993). All-night dynamics of the human sleep EEG. *J Sleep Res*, 2(2), 70–81.

Aeschbach, D., Matthews, J.R., Postolache, T.T., Jackson, M.A., Giesen, H.A., and Wehr, T.A. (1999). Two circadian rhythms in the human electroencephalogram during wakefulness. *Am J Physiol*, 277(6 Pt. 2), R1771–R1779.

Aeschbach, D., Postolache, T. T., Sher, L., Matthews, J.R., Jackson, M.A., and Wehr, T.A. (2001a). Evidence from the waking electroencephalogram that short sleepers live under higher homeostatic sleep pressure than long sleepers. *Neuroscience*, 102(3), 493–502.

Aeschbach, D., Sher, L., Postolache, T.T., Matthews, J.R., Jackson, M.A., and Wehr, T.A. (2001b). A longer biological night in long sleepers than in short sleepers. *Sleep*, 24(Suppl.), 8.

Aeschbach, D., Sher, L., Postolache, T.T., Matthews, J.R., Jackson, M.A., and Wehr, T.A. (2003). A longer biological night in long sleepers than in short sleepers. *J Clin Endocrinol Metab*, 88(1), 26–30.

Albert, R., Merz, A., Schubert, J., and Ebert, D. (1998). Sleep deprivation and subsequent sleep phase advance stabilizes the positive effect of sleep deprivation in depressive episodes. *Nervenarzt*, 69(1), 66–69.

Allada, R., Emery, P., Takahashi, J. S., and Rosbash, M. (2001). Stopping time: The genetics of fly and mouse circadian clocks. *Annu Rev Neurosci*, 24, 1091–1119.

Allen, G., Rappe, J., Earnest, D. J., and Cassone, V. M. (2001). Oscillating on borrowed time: Diffusible signals from immortalized suprachiasmatic nucleus cells regulate circadian rhythmicity in cultured fibroblasts. *J Neurosci*, 21(20), 7937–7943.

Amzica, F., and Steriade, M. (1998). Electrophysiological correlates of sleep delta waves. *Electroencephalogr Clin Neurophysiol*, 107(2), 69–83.

Anand, A., Charney, D.S., Delgado, P.L., McDougle, C.J., Heninger, G.R., and Price, L.H. (1994). Neuroendocrine and behavioral responses to intravenous m-chlorophenylpiperazine (mCPP) in depressed patients and healthy comparison subjects. *Am J Psychiatry*, 151(11), 1626–1630.

Anderson, J.L., Vasile, R.G., Mooney, J.J., Bloomingdale, K.L., Samson, J.A., and Schildkraut, J.J. (1992). Changes in norepi-

nephrine output following light therapy for fall/winter seasonal depression. *Biol Psychiatry*, 32(8), 700–704.

Anderson, J.L., Rosen, L.N., Mendelson, W.B., Jacobsen, F.M., Skwerer, R.G., Joseph-Vanderpool, J.R., Duncan, C.C., Wehr, T.A., and Rosenthal, N.E. (1994). Sleep in fall/winter seasonal affective disorder: Effects of light and changing seasons. *J Psychosom Res*, 38(4), 323–337.

Arbisi, P.A., Depue, R.A., Spoont, M.R., Leon, A., and Ainsworth, B. (1989). Thermoregulatory response to thermal challenge in seasonal affective disorder: A preliminary report. *Psychiatry Res*, 28(3), 323–334.

Arbisi, P.A., Depue, R.A., Krauss, S., Spoont, M.R., Leon, A., Ainsworth, B., and Muir, R. (1994). Heat-loss response to a thermal challenge in seasonal affective disorder. *Psychiatry Res*, 52(2), 199–214.

Archer, S.N., Robilliard, D.L., Skene, D.J., Smits, M., Williams, A., Arendt, J., and von Schantz, M. (2003). A length polymorphism in the circadian clock gene *Per3* is linked to delayed sleep phase syndrome and extreme diurnal preference. *Sleep*, 26(4), 413–415.

Asada, H., Fukuda, Y., Tsunoda, S., Yamaguchi, M., and Tonoike, M. (1999). Frontal midline theta rhythms reflect alternative activation of prefrontal cortex and anterior cingulate cortex in humans. *Neurosci Lett*, 274(1), 29–32.

Aschoff, J.C. (1981a). History and clinical symptoms of brain tumors. *Aktuelle Probl Chir Orthop*, 18, 15–19.

Aschoff, J.C. (1981c). Free running and entrained circadian rhythms. In J. Aschoff (Ed.), *Handbook of Behavorial Neurobiology, Vol. 4 Biological Rhythms* (pp. 81–93). New York: Plenum Press.

Aschoff, J.C., and Wever, R. (1980). On reproducibility of circadian rhythms in man [in German]. *Klin Wochenschr*, 58(7), 323–335.

Aschoff, J.C., and Wever, R. (1981). The circadian system as discussed in psychiatric research. In T.A. Wehr and F.K. Goodwin (Eds.), *Circadian Rhythms in Psychiatry* (pp. 311–331). Pacific Grove, CA: The Boxwood Press.

Aschoff, U. (1981b). Scotopic and photopic parts of light and dark vibrations in the electrooculograph. *Dev Ophthalmol*, 4, 149–166.

Ashman, S.B., Monk, T.H., Kupfer, D.J., Clark, C.H., Myers, F.S., Frank, E., and Leibenluft, E. (1999). Relationship between social rhythms and mood in patients with rapid cycling bipolar disorder. *Psychiatry Res*, 86(1), 1–8.

Asikainen, M., Toppila, J., Alanko, L., Ward, D.J., Stenberg, D., and Porkka-Heiskanen, T. (1997). Sleep deprivation increases brain serotonin turnover in the rat. *Neuroreport*, 8(7), 1577–1582.

Avery, D.H., Bolte, M.A., Dager, S.R., Wilson, L.G., Weyer, M., Cox, G.B., and Dunner, D.L. (1993). Dawn simulation treatment of winter depression: A controlled study. *Am J Psychiatry*, 150(1), 113–117.

Avery, D.H., Bolte, M.A., and Ries, R. (1998). Dawn simulation treatment of abstinent alcoholics with winter depression. *J Clin Psychiatry*, 59(1), 36–42; quiz 43–34.

Baastrup, P.C., and Schou, M. (1967). Lithium as a prophylactic agent: Its effect agains recurrent depression and manic-depressive psychosis. *Arch Gen Psychiatry*, 16, 162–172.

Baillarger, J. (1854). Note sur un genre de folie dont les accés sont caractérisés par deux périodes régulières, l'une de dépression et l'autre d'excitation. *Gazette Hebdomadaire de Medecine et Chirurgie*, 132, 263–265.

Barbini, B., Bertelli, S., Colombo, C., and Smeraldi, E. (1996). Sleep loss, a possible factor in augmenting manic episode. *Psychiatry Res*, 65(2), 121–125.

Barbini, B., Colombo, C., Benedetti, F., Campori, E., Bellodi, L., and Smeraldi, E. (1998). The unipolar–bipolar dichotomy and the response to sleep deprivation. *Psychiatry Res*, 79(1), 43–50.

Barinaga, M. (2002). Circadian clock. How the brain's clock gets daily enlightenment. *Science*, 295(5557), 955–957.

Bauer, M., Grof, P., Rasgon, N., Bschor, T., Glenn, T., and Whybrow, P.C. (2006). Temporal relation between sleep and mood in patients with bipolar disorder. *Bipolar Disord*, 8(2), 160–167.

Beersma, D.G. (1990). Do winter depressives experience summer nights in winter? *Arch Gen Psychiatry*, 47(9), 879–880.

Benca, R.M., Obermeyer, W.H., Thisted, R.A., and Gillin, J.C. (1992). Sleep and psychiatric disorders. A meta-analysis. *Arch Gen Psychiatry*, 49(8), 651–668, discussion 669–670.

Benedetti, F., Barbini, B., Campori, E., Colombo, C., and Smeraldi, E. (1996). Dopamine agonist amineptine prevents the antidepressant effect of sleep deprivation. *Psychiatry Res*, 65(3), 179–184.

Benedetti, F., Barbini, B., Lucca, A., Campori, E., Colombo, C., and Smeraldi, E. (1997). Sleep deprivation hastens the antidepressant action of fluoxetine. *Eur Arch Psychiatry Clin Neurosci*, 247(2), 100–103.

Benedetti, F., Colombo, C., Barbini, B., Campori, E., and Smeraldi, E. (1999a). Ongoing lithium treatment prevents relapse after total sleep deprivation. *J Clin Psychopharmacol*, 19(3), 240–245.

Benedetti, F., Serretti, A., Colombo, C., Campori, E., Barbini, B., di Bella, D., and Smeraldi, E. (1999b). Influence of a functional polymorphism within the promoter of the serotonin transporter gene on the effects of total sleep deprivation in bipolar depression. *Am J Psychiatry*, 156(9), 1450–1452.

Benedetti, F., Barbini, B., Campori, E., Fulgosi, M.C., Pontiggia, A., and Colombo, C. (2001a). Sleep phase advance and lithium to sustain the antidepressant effect of total sleep deprivation in bipolar depression: New findings supporting the internal coincidence model? *J Psychiatr Res*, 35(6), 323–329.

Benedetti, F., Campori, E., Barbini, B., Fulgosi, M.C., and Colombo, C. (2001b). Dopaminergic augmentation of sleep deprivation effects in bipolar depression. *Psychiatry Res*, 104(3), 239–246.

Benna, C., Scannapieco, P., Piccin, A., Sandrelli, F., Zordan, M., Rosato, E., Kyriacou, C.P., Valle, G., and Costa, R. (2000). A second *timeless* gene in *Drosophila* shares greater sequence similarity with mammalian *tim*. *Curr Biol*, 10(14), R512–R513.

Berger, M., Riemann, D., Hochli, D., and Spiegel, R. (1989). The cholinergic rapid eye movement sleep induction test with RS-86. State or trait marker of depression? *Arch Gen Psychiatry*, 46(5), 421–428.

Berger, M., Vollmann, J., Hohagen, F., Konig, A., Lohner, H., Voderholzer, U., and Riemann, D. (1997). Sleep deprivation combined with consecutive sleep phase advance as a fast-acting therapy in depression: An open pilot trial in medicated and unmedicated patients. *Am J Psychiatry*, 154(6), 870–872.

Berger, P.A., Watson, S.J., Akil, H., and Barchas, J.D. (1986). Investigating opioid peptides in schizophrenia and depression. *Res Publ Assoc Res Nerv Ment Dis*, 64, 309–333.

Berson, D.M., Dunn, F.A., and Takao, M. (2002). Phototransduction by retinal ganglion cells that set the circadian clock. *Science*, 295(5557), 1070–1073.

Blacker, C.V., Thomas, J.M., and Thompson, C. (1997). Seasonality prevalence and incidence of depressive disorder in a general practice sample: Identifying differences in timing by caseness. *J Affect Disord*, 43(1), 41–52.

Blacker, D., Faraone, S.V., Rosen, A.E., Guroff, J.J., Adams, P., Weissman, M.M., and Gershon, E.S. (1996). Unipolar relatives in bipolar pedigrees: A search for elusive indicators of underlying bipolarity. *Am J Med Genet*, 67(5), 445–454.

Blazer, D.G., Kessler, R.C., and Swartz, M.S. (1998). Epidemiology of recurrent major and minor depression with a seasonal pattern. The National Comorbidity Survey. *Br J Psychiatry*, 172, 164–167.

Blehar, M.C., and Lewy, A.J. (1990). Seasonal mood disorders: Consensus and controversy. *Psychopharmacol Bull*, 26(4), 465–494.

Booker, J.M., and Hellekson, C.J. (1992). Prevalence of seasonal affective disorder in Alaska. *Am J Psychiatry*, 149(9), 1176–1182.

Borbely, A. (1982). A two process model of sleep regulation. *Hum Neurobiol*, 1(3), 195–204.

Borbely, A.A., and Wirz-Justice, A. (1982). Sleep, sleep deprivation and depression. A hypothesis derived from a model of sleep regulation. *Hum Neurobiol*, 1(3), 205–210.

Borbely, A.A., Steigrad, P., and Tobler, I. (1980). Effect of sleep deprivation on brain serotonin in the rat. *Behav Brain Res*, 1(2), 205–210.

Borbely, A.A., Achermann, P., Trachsel, L., and Tobler, I. (1989). Sleep initiation and initial sleep intensity: Interactions of homeostatic and circadian mechanisms. *J Biol Rhythms*, 4(2), 149–160.

Bouhuys, A.L., van den Burg, W., and van den Hoofdakker, R.H. (1995). The relationship between tiredness prior to sleep deprivation and the antidepressant response to sleep deprivation in depression. *Biol Psychiatry*, 37(7), 457–461.

Braun, A.R., Balkin, T.J., Wesenten, N.J., Carson, R.E., Varga, M., Baldwin, P., Selbie, S., Belenky, G., and Herscovitch, P. (1997). Regional cerebral blood flow throughout the sleep–wake cycle. An H_2(15)O PET study. *Brain*, 120 (Pt. 7), 1173–1197.

Bremner, J.D., Innis, R.B., Salomon, R.M., Staib, L.H., Ng, C.K., Miller, H.L., Bronen, R.A., Krystal, J.H., Duncan, J., Rich, D., Price, L.H., Malison, R., Dey, H., Soufer, R., and Charney, D.S. (1997). Positron emission tomography measurement of cerebral metabolic correlates of tryptophan depletion–induced depressive relapse. *Arch Gen Psychiatry*, 54(4), 364–374.

Breslau, N., Roth, T., Rosenthal, L., and Andreski, P. (1996). Sleep disturbance and psychiatric disorders: A longitudinal epidemiological study of young adults. *Biol Psychiatry*, 39(6), 411–418.

Brewerton, T.D., Berrettini, W.H., Nurnberger, J.I. Jr, and Linnoila, M. (1988). Analysis of seasonal fluctuations of CSF monoamine metabolites and neuropeptides in normal controls: Findings with 5HIAA and HVA. *Psychiatry Res*, 23(3), 257–265.

Brown, L.F., Reynolds, C.F. III, Monk, T.H., Prigerson, H.G., Dew, M.A., Houck, P.R., Mazumdar, S., Buysse, D.J., Hoch, C.C., and Kupfer, D.J. (1996). Social rhythm stability following late-life spousal bereavement: Associations with depression and sleep impairment. *Psychiatry Res*, 62(2), 161–169.

Brown, R.P., Sweeney, J., Loutsch, E., Kocsis, J., and Frances, A. (1984). Involutional melancholia revisited. *Am J Psychiatry*, 141(1), 24–28.

Brunner, D.P., Krauchi, K., Dijk, D.J., Leonhardt, G., Haug, H.J., and Wirz-Justice, A. (1996). Sleep electroencephalogram in seasonal affective disorder and in control women: Effects of midday light treatment and sleep deprivation. *Biol Psychiatry*, 40(6), 485–496.

Buchsbaum, M.S., Hazlett, E.A., Wu, J., and Bunney, W.E. Jr. (2001). Positron emission tomography with deoxyglucose-F18 imaging of sleep. *Neuropsychopharmacology*, 25(5 Suppl.), S50–S56.

Bunney, W.E., and Bunney, B.G. (2000). Molecular clock genes in man and lower animals: Possible implications for circadian abnormalities in depression. *Neuropsychopharmacology*, 22(4), 335–345.

Bunney, W.E., Jr., Murphy, D.L., Goodwin, F.K., and Borge, G.F. (1972a). The "switch process" in manic-depressive illness. I. A systematic study of sequential behavioral changes. *Arch Gen Psychiatry*, 27(3), 295–302.

Bunney, W.E., Jr., Goodwin, F.K., Murphy, D.L., House, K.M., and Gordon, E.K. (1972b). The "switch process" in manic-depressive illness. II. Relationship to catecholamines, REM sleep, and drugs. *Arch Gen Psychiatry*, 27(3), 304–309.

Burgess, H.J., Fogg, L.F., Young, M.A., and Eastman, C.I. (2004). Bright light therapy for winter depression—Is phase advancing beneficial? *Chronobiol Int*, 21(4-5), 759–775.

Burton, R. ([1621] 2001). *The Anatomy of Melancholy*. New York: New York Review of Books.

Buysse, D.J., Frank, E., Lowe, K.K., Cherry, C.R., and Kupfer, D.J. (1997). Electroencephalographic sleep correlates of episode and vulnerability to recurrence in depression. *Biol Psychiatry*, 41(4), 406–418.

Campbell, S.S., and Murphy, P.J. (1998). Extraocular circadian phototransduction in humans. *Science*, 279(5349), 396–399.

Campbell, S.S., Dawson, D., and Zulley, J. (1993). When the human circadian system is caught napping: Evidence for endogenous rhythms close to 24 hours. *Sleep*, 16(7), 638–640.

Cantor, C.H., Hickey, P.A., and De Leo, D. (2000). Seasonal variation in suicide in a predominantly Caucasian tropical/subtropical region of Australia. *Psychopathology*, 33(6), 303–306.

Carlsson, A., Svennerholm, L., and Winblad, B. (1980). Seasonal and circadian monoamine variations in human brains examined post mortem. *Acta Psychiatr Scand Suppl*, 280, 75–85.

Carney, P.A., Fitzgerald, C.T., and Monaghan, C.E. (1988). Influence of climate on the prevalence of mania. *Br J Psychiatry*, 152, 820–823.

Cartwright, R.D. (1983). Rapid eye movement sleep characteristics during and after mood-disturbing events. *Arch Gen Psychiatry*, 40(2), 197–201.

Cassidy, F., and Carroll, B.J. (2002). Seasonal variation of mixed and pure episodes of bipolar disorder. *J Affect Disord*, 68(1), 25–31.

Chang, P.P., Ford, D.E., Mead, L.A., Cooper-Patrick, L., and Klag, M.J. (1997). Insomnia in young men and subsequent depression. The Johns Hopkins Precursors Study. *Am J Epidemiol*, 146(2), 105–114.

Chapman, J., Arlazoroff, A., Goldfarb, L.G., Cervenakova, L., Neufeld, M.Y., Werber, E., Herbert, M., Brown, P., Gajdusek, D.C., and Korczyn, A.D. (1996). Fatal insomnia in a case of familial Creutzfeldt-Jakob disease with the codon 200(Lys) mutation. *Neurology*, 46(3), 758–761.

Chen, D., Buchanan, G.F., Ding, J.M., Hannibal, J., and Gillette, M.U. (1999). Pituitary adenylyl cyclase–activating peptide: A pivotal modulator of glutamatergic regulation of the suprachiasmatic circadian clock. *Proc Natl Acad Sci USA*, 96(23), 13468–13473.

Chouvet, G., Mouret, J., Coindet, J., Siffre, M., and Jouvet, M. (1974). Periodicite bicircadienne du cycle veille-sommeil dans de conditions hors du temps: Etude polygraphique. *Electroencephalogr Clin Neurophysiol*, 37, 367–380.

Cohen, P., and Frame, S. (2001). The renaissance of GSK3. *Nat Rev Mol Cell Biol*, 2(10), 769–776.

Colombo, C., Benedetti, F., Barbini, B., Campori, E., and Smeraldi, E. (1999). Rate of switch from depression into mania after therapeutic sleep deprivation in bipolar depression. *Psychiatry Res*, 86(3), 267–270.

Colombo, C., Lucca, A., Benedetti, F., Barbini, B., Campori, E., and Smeraldi, E. (2000). Total sleep deprivation combined with lithium and light therapy in the treatment of bipolar depression: Replication of main effects and interaction. *Psychiatry Res*, 95(1), 43–53.

Cummings, M.A., Berga, S.L., Cummings, K.L., Kripke, D.F., Haviland, M.G., Golshan, S., and Gillin, J.C. (1989). Light suppression of melatonin in unipolar depressed patients. *Psychiatry Res*, 27(3), 351–355.

Czeisler, C.A., Shanahan, T.L., Klerman, E.B., Martens, H., Brotman, D.J., Emens, J.S., Klein, T., and Rizzo, J.F. III. (1995). Suppression of melatonin secretion in some blind patients by exposure to bright light. *N Engl J Med*, 332(1), 6–11.

Czeisler, C.A., Duffy, J.F., Shanahan, T.L., Brown, E.N., Mitchell, J.F., Rimmer, D.W., Ronda, J.M., Silva, E.J., Allan, J.S., Emens, J.S., Dijk, D.J., and Kronauer, R.E. (1999). Stability, precision, and near-24-hour period of the human circadian pacemaker. *Science*, 284(5423), 2177–2181.

Dahl, K., Avery, D.H., Lewy, A.J., Savage, M.V., Brengelmann, G.L., Larsen, L.H., Vitiello, M.V., and Prinz, P.N. (1993). Dim light melatonin onset and circadian temperature during a constant routine in hypersomnic winter depression. *Acta Psychiatr Scand*, 88(1), 60–66.

Davis, C., and Levitan, R.D. (2005). Seasonality and seasonal affective disorder (SAD): An evolutionary viewpoint tied to energy conservation and reproductive cycles. *J Affect Disord*, 87(1), 3–10.

Demet, E.M., Chicz-Demet, A., Fallon, J.H., and Sokolski, K.N. (1999). Sleep deprivation therapy in depressive illness and Parkinson's disease. *Prog Neuropsychopharmacol Biol Psychiatry*, 23(5), 753–784.

Dement, W., and Kleitman, N. (1957). Cyclic variations in EEG during sleep and their relation to eye movements, body motility, and dreaming. *Electroencephalogr Clin Neurophysiol*, 9, 673–690.

Depue, R.A., Arbisi, P., Spoont, M.R., Krauss, S., Leon, A., and Ainsworth, B. (1989). Seasonal and mood independence of low basal prolactin secretion in premenopausal women with seasonal affective disorder. *Am J Psychiatry*, 146(8), 989–995.

Depue, R.A., Arbisi, P., Krauss, S., Iacono, W.G., Leon, A., Muir, R., and Allen, J. (1990). Seasonal independence of low prolactin concentration and high spontaneous eye blink rates in unipolar and bipolar II seasonal affective disorder. *Arch Gen Psychiatry*, 47(4), 356–364.

Detre, T., Himmelhoch, J., Swartzburg, M., Anderson, C.M., Byck, R., and Kupfer, D.J. (1972). Hypersomnia and manic-depressive disease. *Am J Psychiatry*, 128(10), 1303–1305.

Devinsky, O., Morrell, M.J., and Vogt, B.A. (1995). Contributions of anterior cingulate cortex to behaviour. *Brain*, 118(Pt. 1), 279–306.

Dietzel, D.P., and Ciullo, J.V. (1996). Spontaneous pneumothorax after shoulder arthroscopy: A report of four cases. *Arthroscopy*, 12(1), 99–102.

Dijk, D.J., Duffy, J.F., and Czeisler, C.A. (1992). Circadian and sleep/wake dependent aspects of subjective alertness and cognitive performance. *J Sleep Res*, 1(2), 112–117.

Dijk, D.J., Duffy, J.F., and Czeisler, C.A. (2000). Contribution of circadian physiology and sleep homeostasis to age-related changes in human sleep. *Chronobiol Int*, 17(3), 285–311.

Ding, J.M., Faiman, L.E., Hurst, W.J., Kuriashkina, L.R., and Gillette, M.U. (1997). Resetting the biological clock: mediation of nocturnal CREB phosphorylation via light, glutamate, and nitric oxide. *J Neurosci*, 17(2), 667–675.

Ding, J.M., Buchanan, G.F., Tischkau, S.A., Chen, D., Kuriashkina, L., Faiman, L.E., Alster, J.M., McPherson, P.S., Campbell, K.P., and Gillette, M.U. (1998). A neuronal ryanodine receptor mediates light-induced phase delays of the circadian clock. *Nature*, 394(6691), 381–384.

Drevets, W.C. (1999). Prefrontal cortical–amygdalar metabolism in major depression. *Ann NY Acad Sci*, 877, 614–637.

Drevets, W.C., Price, J.L., Simpson, J.R. Jr., Todd, R.D., Reich, T., Vannier, M., and Raichle, M.E. (1997). Subgenual prefrontal cortex abnormalities in mood disorders. *Nature*, 386(6627), 824–827.

Duffy, J.F., Dijk, D.J., Klerman, E.B., and Czeisler, C.A. (1998). Later endogenous circadian temperature nadir relative to an earlier wake time in older people. *Am J Physiol*, 275(5 Pt. 2), R1478–R1487.

Duffy, J.F., Zeitzer, J.M., Rimmer, D.W., Klerman, E.B., Dijk, D.J., and Czeisler, C.A. (2002). Peak of circadian melatonin rhythm occurs later within the sleep of older subjects. *Am J Physiol Endocrinol Metab*, 282(2), E297–E303.

Duncan, W.C., Jr. (1996). Circadian rhythms and the pharmacology of affective illness. *Pharmacol Ther*, 71(3), 253–312.

Duncan, W.C., Jr., Gillin, J.C., Post, R.M., Gerner, R.H., and Wehr, T.A. (1980). Relationship between EEG sleep patterns and clinical improvement in depressed patients treated with sleep deprivation. *Biol Psychiatry*, 15(6), 879–889.

Eagles, J.M. (1994). The relationship between mood and daily hours of sunlight in rapid cycling bipolar illness. *Biol Psychiatry*, 36(6), 422–424.

Eagles, J.M., Mercer, G., Boshier, A.J., and Jamieson, F. (1996). Seasonal affective disorder among psychiatric nurses in Aberdeen. *J Affect Disord*, 37(2–3), 129–135.

Earnest, D.J., Liang, F.Q., Ratcliff, M., and Cassone, V.M. (1999). Immortal time: Circadian clock properties of rat suprachiasmatic cell lines. *Science*, 283(5402), 693–695.

Eastman, C.I., Gallo, L.C., Lahmeyer, H.W., and Fogg, L.F. (1993). The circadian rhythm of temperature during light treatment for winter depression. *Biol Psychiatry*, 34(4), 210–220.

Eastman, C., Young, M.A., Fogg, L.F., Liu, L., and Meaden. (1998). Bright light treatment of winter depression. *Arch Gen Psychiatry*, 55, 883–889.

Eastwood, M.R., and Peter, A.M. (1988). Epidemiology and seasonal affective disorder. *Psychol Med*, 18(4), 799–806.

Ebert, D., and Berger, M. (1998). Neurobiological similarities in antidepressant sleep deprivation and psychostimulant use: A psychostimulant theory of antidepressant sleep deprivation. *Psychopharmacology (Berl)*, 140(1), 1–10.

Ebert, D., Feistel, H., and Barocka, A. (1991). Effects of sleep deprivation on the limbic system and the frontal lobes in affective disorders: A study with tc-^{99m}-HMPAO SPECT. *Psychiatry Res*, 40(4), 247–251.

Ebert, D., Feistel, H., Kaschka, W., Barocka, A., and Pirner, A. (1994). Single photon emission computerized tomography assessment of cerebral dopamine D2 receptor blockade in depression before and after sleep deprivation—Preliminary results. *Biol Psychiatry*, 35(11), 880–885.

Ebisawa, T., Uchiyama, M., Kajimura, N., Mishima, K., Kamei, Y., Katoh, M., Watanabe, T., Sekimoto, M., Shibui, K., Kim, K., Kudo, Y., Ozeki, Y., Sugishita, M., Toyoshima, R., Inoue, Y., Yamada, N., Nagase, T., Ozaki, N., Ohara, O., Ishida, N., Okawa, M., Takahashi, K., and Yamauchi, T. (2001). Association of structural polymorphisms in the human period3 gene with delayed sleep phase syndrome. *EMBO Rep*, 2(4), 342–346.

Ehlers, C.L., Frank, E., and Kupfer, D.J. (1988). Social zeitgebers and biological rhythms: A unified approach to understanding the etiology of depression. *Arch Gen Psychiatry*, 45, 948–952.

Enoch, M.A., Goldman, D., Barnett, R., Sher, L., Mazzanti, C.M., and Rosenthal, N.E. (1999). Association between seasonal affective disorder and the 5-HT2A promoter polymorphism, –1438G/A. *Mol Psychiatry*, 4(1), 89–92.

Falret, J. (1890). La folie circulaire ou folie a formes alternes. In *Etudes Cliniques sur les Maladies Mentales et Nerveuses*. Paris: Librairie JB Bailliere et Fils.

Feldman-Naim, S., Turner, E.H., and Leibenluft, E. (1997). Diurnal variation in the direction of mood switches in patients with rapid-cycling bipolar disorder. *J Clin Psychiatry*, 58(2), 79–84.

Fernstorm, J.D., and Wurtman, R.J. (1971). Brain serotonin content: Increase following ingestion of carbohydrate diet. *Science*, 174, 1023–1025.

Field, M.D., Maywood, E.S., O'Brien, J.A., Weaver, D.R., Reppert, S.M., and Hastings, M.H. (2000). Analysis of clock proteins in mouse SCN demonstrates phylogenetic divergence of the circadian clockwork and resetting mechanisms. *Neuron*, 25(2), 437–447.

Foster, F.G., Kupfer, D.J., Coble, P., and McPartland, R.J. (1976). Rapid eye movement sleep density. An objective indicator in severe medical-depressive syndromes. *Arch Gen Psychiatry*, 33(9), 1119–1123.

Frank, E., Hlastala, S., Ritenour, A., Houck, P., Tu, X.M., Monk, T.H., Mallinger, A.G., and Kupfer, D.J. (1997). Inducing lifestyle regularity in recovering bipolar disorder patients: Results from the maintenance therapies in bipolar disorder protocol. *Biol Psychiatry*, 41(12), 1165–1173.

Frank, E., Swartz, H.A., and Kupfer, D.J. (2000). Interpersonal and social rhythm therapy: Managing the chaos of bipolar disorder. *Biol Psychiatry*, 48(6), 593–604.

Franken, P., Malafosse, A., and Tafti, M. (1999). Genetic determinants of sleep regulation in inbred mice. *Sleep*, 22(2), 155–169.

Friston, K.J., Sharpley, A.L., Solomon, R.A., and Cowen, P.J. (1989). Lithium increases slow wave sleep: Possible mediation by brain 5-HT2 receptors? *Psychopharmacology (Berl)*, 98(1), 139–140.

Fritzsche, M., Heller, R., Hill, H., and Kick, H. (2001). Sleep deprivation as a predictor of response to light therapy in major depression. *J Affect Disord*, 62(3), 207–215.

Gann, H., Riemann, D., Hohagen, F., Strauss, L.G., Dressing, H., Muller, W.E., and Berger, M. (1993). 48-hour rapid cycling: Results of psychopathometric, polysomnographic, PET imaging and neuro-endocrine longitudinal investigations in a single case. *J Affect Disord*, 28(2), 133–140.

Garcia-Borreguero, D., Jacobsen, F.M., Murphy, D.L., Joseph-Vanderpool, J.R., Chiara, A., and Rosenthal, N.E. (1995). Hormonal responses to the administration of m-chlorophenylpiperazine in patients with seasonal affective disorder and controls. *Biol Psychiatry*, 37(10), 740–749.

Gardner, J.P., Fornal, C.A., and Jacobs, B.L. (1997). Effects of sleep deprivation on serotonergic neuronal activity in the dorsal raphe nucleus of the freely moving cat. *Neuropsychopharmacology*, 17(2), 72–81.

Georgi, F. (1947). Psychophysische Korrelationen: III. Psychiatrische Probleme im Lichte der Rhythmusforschung. *Schweiz Med Wochenschr*, 49, 1276–1280.

Gerner, R.H., Post, R.M., Gillin, J.C., and Bunney, W.E. Jr. (1979). Biological and behavioral effects of one night's sleep deprivation in depressed patients and normals. *J Psychiatr Res*, 15(1), 21–40.

Ghadirian, A.M., Murphy, B.E., and Gendron, M.J. (1998). Efficacy of light versus tryptophan therapy in seasonal affective disorder. *J Affect Disord*, 50(1), 23–27.

Giles, D.E., Jarrett, R.B., Roffwarg, H.P., and Rush, A.J. (1987a). Reduced rapid eye movement latency. A predictor of recurrence in depression. *Neuropsychopharmacology*, 1(1), 33–39.

Giles, D.E., Roffwarg, H.P., and Rush, A.J. (1987b). REM latency concordance in depressed family members. *Biol Psychiatry*, 22(7), 910–914.

Giles, D.E., Biggs, M.M., Rush, A.J., and Roffwarg, H.P. (1988). Risk factors in families of unipolar depression. I. Psychiatric illness and reduced REM latency. *J Affect Disord*, 14(1), 51–59.

Giles, D.E., Jarrett, R.B., Biggs, M.M., Guzick, D.S., and Rush, A.J. (1989). Clinical predictors of recurrence in depression. *Am J Psychiatry*, 146, 764–767.

Gillin, J.C. (1983). The sleep therapies of depression. *Prog Neuropsychopharmacol Biol Psychiatry*, 7(2–3), 351–364.

Gillin, J.C., Wyatt, R.J., Fram, D., and Snyder, F. (1978). The relationship between changes in REM sleep and clinical improvement in depressed patients treated with amitriptyline. *Psychopharmacology (Berl)*, 59(3), 267–272.

Gillin, J.C., Duncan, W., Pettigrew, K.D., Frankel, B.L., and Snyder, F. (1979a). Successful separation of depressed, normal, and insomniac subjects by EEG sleep data. *Arch Gen Psychiatry*, 36(1), 85–90.

Gillin, J.C., Sitaram, N., and Duncan, W.C. (1979b). Muscarinic supersensitivity: A possible model for the sleep disturbance of primary depression? *Psychiatry Res*, 1(1), 17–22.

Gillin, J.C., Sitaram, N., and Mendelson, W.B. (1982). Acetylcholine, sleep, and depression. *Hum Neurobiol*, 1(3), 211–219.

Goldman, B.D. (2001). Mammalian photoperiodic system: Formal properties and neuroendocrine mechanisms of photoperiodic time measurement. *J Biol Rhythms*, 16(4), 283–301.

Goldman, B.D., and Eliott, J.A. (1988). Photoperiodism and seasonality in hamsters. Role of the pineal gland. In M.H. Stetson (Ed.), *Processing of Environmental Information in Vertebrates*. New York: Springer-Verlag.

Gooley, J.J., Lu, J., Chou, T.C., Scammell, T.E., and Saper, C.B. (2001). Melanopsin in cells of origin of the retinohypothalamic tract. *Nat Neurosci*, 4(12), 1165.

Gorman, M.R., and Zucker, I. (1997). Pattern of change in melatonin duration determines testicular responses in siberian hamsters, *Phodopus sungorus*. *Biol Reprod*, 56(3), 668–673.

Gould, T., and Manji, H. (2002a). Signaling networks in the pathophysiology and treatment of mood disorders. *J Psychosom Res*, 53(2), 687.

Gould, T.D., and Manji, H.K. (2002b). The Wnt signaling pathway in bipolar disorder. *Neuroscientist*, 8, 187–201.

Gresham, S.C., Agnew, H.W., and Williams. R.L. (1965). The sleep of depressed patients: An EEG and eye movement study. *Arch Gen Psychiatry*, 13, 503–507.

Griesinger, W. (1867). *Mental Pathology and Therapeutics*. Translated by C.L. Robertson and J. Rutherford. London: New Sydenhem Society.

Grunhaus, L., Shipley, J.E., Eiser, A., Pande, A.C., Tandon, R., Krahn, D.D., Demitrack, M.A., Remen, A., Hirschmann, S., Greden, J.F. (1997). Sleep-onset rapid eye movement after electroconvulsive therapy is more frequent in patients who respond less well to electroconvulsive therapy. *Biol Psychiatry*, 42(3), 191–200.

Guillemette, J., Hebert, M., Paquet, J., and Dumont, M. (1998). Natural bright light exposure in the summer and winter in subjects with and without complaints of seasonal mood variations. *Biol Psychiatry*, 44(7), 622–628.

Hakkarainen, R., Johansson, C., Kieseppa, T., Partonen, T., Koskenvuo, M., Kaprio, J., and Lonnqvist, J. (2003). Seasonal changes, sleep length and circadian preference among twins with bipolar disorder. *BMC Psychiatry*, 3, 6.

Halberg, G. (1968). Physiologic considerations underlying rhythmometry, with special reference to emotional illness. In J. DeAjuriaguerra (Ed.), *Cycles Biologiques et Psychiatrie* (pp. 73–126). Symposium Bel-Air III. Geneva: Masson et Cie.

Hallam, K.T., Olver, J.S., and Norman, T.R. (2005). Effect of sodium valproate on nocturnal melatonin sensitivity to light in healthy volunteers. *Neuropsychopharmacology*, 30(7), 1400–1404.

Hamada, T., Yamanouchi, S., Watanabe, A., Shibata, S., and Watanabe, S. (1999). Involvement of glutamate release in substance P–induced phase delays of suprachiasmatic neuron activity rhythm in vitro. *Brain Res*, 836(1–2), 190–193.

Han, L., Wang, K., Cheng, Y., Du, Z., Rosenthal, N.E., and Primeau, F. (2000a). Summer and winter patterns of seasonality in Chinese college students: A replication. *Compr Psychiatry*, 41(1), 57–62.

Han, L., Wang, K., Cheng, Y., Du, Z., and Rosenthal, N.E. (2000b). Seasonal variations in mood and behavior in Chinese medical students. *Am J Psychiatry*, 157, 133–135.

Hannibal, J., Hindersson, P., Knudsen, S.M., Georg, B., and Fahrenkrug, J. (2002). The photopigment melanopsin is exclusively present in pituitary adenylate cyclase–activating polypeptide-containing retinal ganglion cells of the retinohypothalamic tract. *J Neurosci*, 22(1), RC191.

Harding, G.F., Alford, C.A., and Powell, T.E. (1985). The effect of sodium valproate on sleep, reaction times, and visual evoked potential in normal subjects. *Epilepsia*, 26(6), 597–601.

Harvey, A.G., Schmidt, D.A., Scarna, A., Semier, C.N., and Goodwin, G.M. (2005). Sleep-related functioning in euthymic patients with bipolar disorder, patients with insomnia, and subjects without sleep problems. *Am J Psychiatry*, 162(1), 50–57.

Hattar, S., Liao, H.W., Takao, M., Berson, D.M., and Yau, K.W. (2002). Melanopsin-containing retinal ganglion cells: Architecture, projections, and intrinsic photosensitivity. *Science*, 295(5557), 1065–1070.

Hauri, P., Chernik, D., Hawkins, D., and Mendels, J. (1974). Sleep of depressed patients in remission. *Arch Gen Psychiatry*, 31(3), 386–391.

Healy, D., and Waterhouse, J.M. (1995). The circadian system and the therapeutics of the affective disorders. *Pharmacol Ther*, 65(2), 241–263.

Hebert, M., Dumont, M., and Lachapelle, P. (2002). Electrophysiological evidence suggesting a seasonal modulation of retinal sensitivity in subsyndromal winter depression. *J Affect Disord*, 68(2–3), 191–202.

Herzog, E.D., and Schwartz, W.J. (2002). Invited review: A neural clockwork for encoding circadian time. *J Appl Physiol*, 92(1), 401–408.

Herzog, E.D., Takahashi, J.S., and Block, G.D. (1998). Clock controls circadian period in isolated suprachiasmatic nucleus neurons. *Nat Neurosci*, 1(8), 708–713.

Hobson, J.A., and Steriade, M. (1986). Neuronal basis of behavioral state control. In V.B. Mountcastle, F. Blum, S.R. Geiger (Eds.), *Handbook of Physiology: A Critical, Comprehensive Presentation of Physiological Knowledge and Concepts* (Vol. IV, Section 1, The Nervous System) (pp. 701–823). Bethesda, MD: American Physiological Society.

Huber, R., Deboer, T., and Tobler, I. (2000). Effects of sleep deprivation on sleep and sleep EEG in three mouse strains: Empirical data and simulations. *Brain Res*, 857(1–2), 8–19.

Hudson, J.I., Lipinski, J.F., Frankenburg, F.R., Grochocinski, V.J., and Kupfer, D.J. (1988). Electroencephalographic sleep in mania. *Arch Gen Psychiatry*, 45(3), 267–273.

Hudson, J.I., Lipinski, J.F., Keck, P.E. Jr., Aizley, H.G., Lukas, S.E., Rothschild, A.J., Waternaux, C.M., and Kupfer, D.J. (1992). Polysomnographic characteristics of young manic patients. Comparison with unipolar depressed patients and normal control subjects. *Arch Gen Psychiatry*, 49(5), 378–383.

Hunt, N., Sayer, H., and Silverstone, T. (1992). Season and manic relapse. *Acta Psychiatr Scand*, 85(2), 123–126.

Illnerova, H., and Vanecek, J. (1982). Two-oscillator structure of the pacemaker controlling the circadian-rhythm of N-acetyltransferase in the rat pineal-gland. *J Comp Physiol*, 145(4), 539–548.

Ishii, R., Shinosaki, K., Ukai, S., Inouye, T., Ishihara, T., Yoshimine, T., Hirabuki, N., Asada, H., Kihara, T., Robinson, S.E., and Takeda, M. (1999). Medial prefrontal cortex generates frontal midline theta rhythm. *Neuroreport*, 10(4), 675–679.

Jac, M., Kiss, A., Sumova, A., Illnerova, H., and Jezova, D. (2000a). Daily profiles of arginine vasopressin mRNA in the suprachiasmatic, supraoptic and paraventricular nuclei of the rat hypothalamus under various photoperiods. *Brain Res*, 887(2), 472–476.

Jac, M., Sumova, A., and Illnerova, H. (2000b). c-Fos rhythm in subdivisions of the rat suprachiasmatic nucleus under artificial and natural photoperiods. *Am J Physiol Regul Integr Comp Physiol*, 279(6), R2270–R2276.

Jacobsen, F.M., Mueller, E.A., Rosenthal, N.E., Rogers, S., Hill, J.L., and Murphy, D.L. (1994). Behavioral responses to intravenous meta-chlorophenylpiperazine in patients with seasonal affective disorder and control subjects before and after phototherapy. *Psychiatry Res*, 52(2), 181–197.

Jang, K.L., Lam, R.W., Livesley, W.J., and Vernon, P.A. (1997a). Gender differences in the heritability of seasonal mood change. *Psychiatry Res*, 70(3), 145–154.

Jang, K.L., Lam, R.W., Livesley, W.J., and Vernon, P.A. (1997b). The relationship between seasonal mood change and personality: More apparent than real? *Acta Psychiatr Scand*, 95(6), 539–543.

Janowsky, D.S., el-Yousef, M.K., Davis, J.M., and Sekerke, H.J. (1972). A cholinergic–adrenergic hypothesis of mania and depression. *Lancet*, 2(7778), 632–635.

Johnsson, A., Pflug, B., Engelmann, W., and Klemke, W. (1979). Effect of lithium carbonate on circadian periodicity in humans. *Pharmakopsychiatr Neuropsychopharmakol*, 12(6), 423–425.

Johnsson, A., Engelmann, W., Pflug, B., and Klemke, W. (1980). Influence of lithium ions on human circadian rhythms. *Z Naturforsch [C]*, 35(5–6), 503–507.

Johnsson, A., Engelmann, W., Pflug, B., and Klemke, W. (1983). Period lengthening of human circadian rhythms by lithium carbonate, a prophylactic for depressive disorders. *Int J Chronobiol*, 8(3), 129–147.

Jones, C.R., Campbell, S.S., Zone, S.E., Cooper, F., DeSano, A., Murphy, P.J., Jones, B., Czajkowski, L., and Ptacek, L.J. (1999). Familial advanced sleep-phase syndrome: A short-period circadian rhythm variant in humans. *Nat Med*, 5(9), 1062–1065.

Jones, P.M., and Berney, T.P. (1987). Early onset rapid cycling bipolar affective disorder. *J Child Psychol Psychiatry*, 28, 731–738.

Jones, S.H., Hare, D.J., and Evershed, K. (2005). Actigraphic assessment of circadian activity and sleep patterns in bipolar disorder. *Bipolar Disord*, 7(2), 176–186.

Joseph-Vanderpool, J.R., Jacobsen, F.M., Murphy, D.L., Hill, J.L., and Rosenthal, N.E. (1993). Seasonal variation in behavioral responses to m-CPP in patients with seasonal affective disorder and controls. *Biol Psychiatry*, 33(7), 496–504.

Kafka, M.S., Marangos, P.J., and Moore, R.Y. (1985). Suprachiasmatic nucleus ablation abolishes circadian rhythms in rat brain neurotransmitter receptors. *Brain Res*, 327(1-2), 344–347.

Kalsbeek, A., van Heerikhuize, J.J., Wortel, J., and Buijs, R.M. (1996). A diurnal rhythm of stimulatory input to the hypothalamo-pituitary-adrenal system as revealed by timed intrahypothalamic administration of the vasopressin V1 antagonist. *J Neurosci*, 16(17), 5555–5565.

Kasper, S., Rogers, S.L., Yancey, A., Schulz, P.M., Skwerer, R.G., and Rosenthal, N.E. (1989a). Phototherapy in individuals with and without subsyndromal seasonal affective disorder. *Arch Gen Psychiatry*, 46(9), 837–844.

Kasper, S., Wehr, T.A., Bartko, J.J., Gaist, P.A., and Rosenthal, N.E. (1989b). Epidemiological findings of seasonal changes in mood and behavior. A telephone survey of Montgomery County, Maryland. *Arch Gen Psychiatry*, 46(9), 823–833.

Kavaliers, M., and Ralph, C.L. (1981). Encephalic photoreceptor involvement in the entrainment and control of circadian activity of young American alligators. *Physiol Behav*, 26(3), 413–418.

Klemfuss, H. (1992). Rhythms and the pharmacology of lithium. *Pharmacol Ther*, 56(1), 53–78.

Klemfuss, H., and Kripke, D.F. (1995). Antimanic drugs stabilize hamster circadian rhythms. *Psychiatry Res*, 57(3), 215–222.

Knowles, J.B., Cairns, J., MacLean, A.W., Delva, N., Prowse, A., Waldron, J., and Letemendia, F.J. (1986). The sleep of remitted bipolar depressives: Comparison with sex and age-matched controls. *Can J Psychiatry*, 31(4), 295–298.

Kraepelin, E. (1921). *Manic-Depressive Insanity and Paranoia*. Edinburgh: E & S Livingstone.

Kripke, D.F. (1983). Phase-advance theories for affective illness. In T.A. Wehr and F.K. Goodwin (Eds.), *Circadian Rhythms in Psychiatry* (pp. 41–69). Pacific Grove, CA: Boxwood Press.

Kripke, D.F. (1995). Mortality risk of major depression. *Am J Psychiatry*, 152(6), 962.

Kripke, D.F. (1998). Light treatment for nonseasonal depression: Speed, efficacy, and combined treatment. *J Affect Disord*, 49(2), 109–117.

Kripke, D.F., Mullaney, D.J., Atkinson, M.L., and Wolf, S. (1978). Circadian rhythms disorders in manic depressives. *Biol Psychiatry*, 13, 335–351.

Kripke, D.F., Ancoli-Israel, S., Klauber, M.R., Wingard, D.L., Mason, W.J., and Mullaney, D.J. (1997). Prevalence of sleep-disordered breathing in ages 40–64 years: A population-based survey. *Sleep*, 20(1), 65–76.

Kripke, D.F., Garfinkel, L., Wingard, D.L., Klauber, M.R., and Marler, M.R. (2002). Mortality associated with sleep duration and insomnia. *Arch Gen Psychiatry*, 59(2), 131–136.

Kuhs, H., and Tölle, R. (1991). Sleep deprivation therapy. *Biol Psychiatry*, 29(11), 1129–1148.

Kukopulos, A., and Reginaldi, D. (1973). Does lithium prevent depressions by suppressing manias? *Int Pharmacopsychiatry*, 8(3), 152–158.

Kupfer, D.J. (1976). REM latency: A psychobiologic marker for primary depressive disease. *Biol Psychiatry*, 11(2), 159–174.

Kupfer, D.J., and Foster, F.G. (1972). Interval between onset of sleep and rapid-eye-movement sleep as an indicator of depression. *Lancet*, 2(7779), 684–686.

Kupfer, D.J., Wyatt, R.J., Greenspan, K., Scott, J., and Snyder, F. (1970). Lithium carbonate and sleep in affective illness. *Arch Gen Psychiatry*, 23(1), 35–40.

Kupfer, D.J., Foster, F.G., Reich, L., Thompson, S.K., and Weiss, B. (1976). EEG sleep changes as predictors in depression. *Am J Psychiatry*, 133(6), 622–626.

Kupfer, D.J., Spiker, D.G., Coble, P.A., and Shaw, D.H. (1978). Electroencephalographic sleep recordings and depression in the elderly. *J Am Geriatr Soc*, 26(2), 53–57.

Kupfer, D.J., Spiker, D.G., Coble, P.A., Neil, J.F., Ulrich, R., and Shaw, D.H. (1981). Sleep and treatment prediction in endogenous depression. *Am J Psychiatry*, 138(4), 429–434.

Kupfer, D.J., Ehlers, C.L., Frank, E., Grochocinski, V.J., McEachran, A.B., and Buhari, A. (1994). Persistent effects of antidepressants: EEG sleep studies in depressed patients during maintenance treatment. *Biol Psychiatry*, 35(10), 781–793.

Kusumi, I., Koyama, T., and Yamashita, I. (1994). Serotonin-induced platelet intracellular calcium mobilization in depressed patients. *Psychopharmacology (Berl)*, 113(3–4), 322–327.

Lam, R.W., and Levitan, R.D. (1996). *Tryptophan Augmentation of Light Therapy in Patients with Seasonal Affective Disorder* (Vol. 8). Bethesda, MD: Society for Light Treatment and Biological Rhythms.

Lam, R.W., and Levitan, R.D. (2000). Pathophysiology of seasonal affective disorder: A review. *J Psychiatry Neurosci*, 25(5), 469–480.

Lam, R.V., and Levitt, A.J. (1999). *Canadian Consensus Guidelines for the Treatment of Seasonal Affective Disorder*. Vancouver, WA: Clinical & Academic Publishing.

Lam, R.W., Berkowitz, A.L., Berga, S.L., Clark, C.M., Kripke, D.F., and Gillin, J.C. (1990). Melatonin suppression in bipolar and unipolar mood disorders. *Psychiatry Res*, 33(2), 129–134.

Lam, R.W., Beattie, C.W., Buchanan, A., and Mador, J.A. (1992a). Electroretinography in seasonal affective disorder. *Psychiatry Res*, 43(1), 55–63.

Lam, R.W., Buchanan, A., Mador, J.A., Corral, M.R., and Remick, R.A. (1992b). The effects of ultraviolet-A wavelengths in light therapy for seasonal depression. *J Affect Disord*, 24(4), 237–243.

Lam, R.W., Beattie, C., Mador, J.A., Corral, M.R., Buchanan, A., and Zis, A.P. (1993). *The Effects of Light Therapy on Retinal Electrophysiologic Tests in Winter Depression*. Bethesda, MD: Society for Light Treatment and Biological Rhythms.

Lam, R.W., Gorman, C.P., Michalon, M., Steiner, M., Levitt, A.J., Corral, M.R., Watson, G.D., Morehouse, R.L., Tam, W., and Joffe, R.T. (1995). Multicenter, placebo-controlled study of fluoxetine in seasonal affective disorder. *Am J Psychiatry*, 152(12), 1765–1770.

Lam, R.W., Zis, A.P., Grewal, A., Delgado, P.L., Charney, D.S., and Krystal, J.H. (1996). Effects of rapid tryptophan depletion in patients with seasonal affective disorder in remission after light therapy. *Arch Gen Psychiatry*, 53(1), 41–44.

Lam, R.W., Levitan, R.D., Tam, E.M., Yatham, L.N., Lamoureux, S., and Zis, A.P. (1997). L-tryptophan augmentation of light therapy in patients with seasonal affective disorder. *Can J Psychiatry*, 42(3), 303–306.

Lam, R.W., Bowering, T.A., Tam, E.M., Grewal, A., Yatham, L.N., Shiah, I.S., and Zis, A.P. (2000). Effects of rapid tryptophan depletion in patients with seasonal affective disorder in natural summer remission. *Psychol Med*, 30(1), 79–87.

Lam, R.W., Lee, S.K., Tam, E.M., Grewal, A., and Yatham, L.N. (2001a). An open trial of light therapy for women with seasonal affective disorder and comorbid bulimia nervosa. *J Clin Psychiatry*, 62(3), 164–168.

Lam, R.W., Tam, E.M., Grewal, A., and Yatham, L.N. (2001b). Effects of alpha-methyl-para-tyrosine-induced catecholamine depletion in patients with seasonal affective disorder in summer remission. *Neuropsychopharmacology*, 25(Suppl. 5), S97–S101.

Lam, R.W., Tam, E.M., Yatham, L.N., Shiah, I.S., and Zis, A.P. (2001c). Seasonal depression: The dual vulnerability hypothesis revisited. *J Affect Disord*, 63(1–3), 123–132.

Lambert, G.W., Reid, C., Kaye, D.M., Jennings, G.L., and Esler, M.D. (2002). Effect of sunlight and season on serotonin turnover in the brain. *Lancet*, 360(9348), 1840–1842.

Larkin, J.E., Freeman, D.A., and Zucker, I. (2001). Low ambient temperature accelerates short-day responses in Siberian hamsters by altering responsiveness to melatonin. *J Biol Rhythms*, 16(1), 76–86.

Leibenluft, E., and Wehr, T.A. (1992). Is sleep deprivation useful in the treatment of depression? *Am J Psychiatry*, 149(2), 159–168.

Leibenluft, E., Turner, E.H., Feldman-Naim, S., Schwartz, P.J., Wehr, T.A., and Rosenthal, N.E. (1995). Light therapy in patients with rapid cycling bipolar disorder: Preliminary results. *Psychopharmacol Bull*, 31(4), 705–710.

Leibenluft, E., Albert, P.S., Rosenthal, N.E., and Wehr, T.A. (1996a). Relationship between sleep and mood in patients with rapid-cycling bipolar disorder. *Psychiatry Res*, 63(2–3), 161–168.

Leibenluft, E., Feldman-Naim, S., Turner, E.H., Schwartz, P.J., and Wehr, T.A. (1996b). Salivary and plasma measures of dim light melatonin onset (DLMO) in patients with rapid cycling bipolar disorder. *Biol Psychiatry*, 40(8), 731–735.

Lenox, R.H., Gould, T.D., and Manji, H.K. (2002). Endophenotypes in bipolar disorder. *Am J Med Genet*, 114(4), 391–406.

Leonhardt, G., Wirz-Justice, A., Krauchi, K., Graw, P., Wunder, D., and Haug, H. J. (1994). Long-term follow-up of depression in seasonal affective disorder. *Compr Psychiatry*, 35(6), 457–464.

Leu, S.J., Shiah, I.S., Yatham, L.N., Cheu, Y.M., and Lam, R.W. (2001). Immune-inflammatory markers in patients with seasonal affective disorder: Effects of light therapy. *J Affect Disord*, 63(1–3), 27–34.

Levitan, R.D., Kaplan, A.S., Brown, G.M., Vaccarino, F.J., Kennedy, S.H., Levitt, A.J., and Joffe, R.T. (1998). Hormonal and subjective responses to intravenous m-chlorophenylpiperazine in women with seasonal affective disorder. *Arch Gen Psychiatry*, 55(3), 244–249.

Levitan, R.D., Jain, U.R., and Katzman, M.A. (1999a). Seasonal affective symptoms in adults with residual attention-deficit hyperactivity disorder. *Compr Psychiatry*, 40(4), 261–267.

Levitan, R.D., Masellis, M., Kennedy, J.L., Kennedy, S.H., Kaplan, A.S., and Vaccario, F.J. (1999b). Polymorphism in serotonin genes in seasonal affective disorder and bulimia. *Biol Psychiatry*, 43(Suppl. 8), 271.

Levitt, A.J., Boyle, M.H., Joffe, R.T., and Baumal, Z. (2000). Estimated prevalence of the seasonal subtype of major depression in a Canadian community sample. *Can J Psychiatry*, 45(7), 650–654.

Lewis, P.R., and Lobban, M.C. (1957). Dissociation of diurnal rhythms in human subjects living in abnormal time routines. *Q J Exp Physiol Cognate Med Sci*, 42, 371–386.

Lewy, A.J., and Sack, R.L. (1988). The phase-shift hypothesis of seasonal affective disorder. *Am J Psychiatry*, 145(8), 1041–1043.

Lewy, A.J., and Sack, R.L. (1989). The dim light melatonin onset as a marker for circadian phase position. *Chronobiol Int*, 6(1), 93–102.

Lewy, A.J., Wehr, T.A., Goodwin, F.K., Newsome, D.A., and Markey, S.P. (1980). Light suppresses melatonin secretion in humans. *Science*, 210(4475), 1267–1269.

Lewy, A.J., Wehr, T.A., Goodwin, F.K., Newsome, D.A., and Rosenthal, N.E. (1981). Manic-depressive patients may be supersensitive to light. *Lancet*, 1(8216), 383–384.

Lewy, A.J., Kern, H.A., Rosenthal, N.E., and Wehr, T.A. (1982). Bright artificial light treatment of a manic-depressive patient with a seasonal mood cycle. *Am J Psychiatry*, 139, 1496–1498.

Lewy, A.J., Sack, R.L., and Singer, C.M. (1985). Immediate and delayed effects of bright light on human melatonin production: Shifting "dawn" and "dusk" shifts the dim light melatonin onset (DLMO). *Ann NY Acad Sci*, 453, 253–259.

Lewy, A.J., Nurnberger, J.I., Wehr, T.A., Pack, D., Becker, L.E., Powell, R.-L., and Newsome, D.A. (1985a). Supersensitivity to light: Possible trait marker for manic-depressive illness. *Am J Psychiatry*, 142, 725–727.

Lewy, A.J., Sack, R.L., Miller, L.S., and Hoban, T.M. (1987a). Antidepressant and circadian phase-shifting effects of light. *Science*, 235(4786), 352–354.

Lewy, A.J., Sack, R.L., Singer, C.M., and White, D.M. (1987b). The phase shift hypothesis for bright light's therapeutic mechanism of action: Theoretical considerations and experimental evidence. *Psychopharmacol Bull*, 23(3), 349–353.

Lewy, A.J., Bauer, V.K., Cutler, N.L., Sack, R.L., Ahmed, S., Thomas, K.H., Blood, M.L., and Jackson, J.M. (1998). Morning vs. evening light treatment of patients with winter depression. *Arch Gen Psychiatry*, 55(10), 890–896.

Lewy, A.J., Emens, J., Sack, R.L., Hasler, B.P., and Bernert, R.A. (2003). Zeitgeber hierarchy in humans: Resetting the circadian phase positions of blind people using melatonin. *Chronobiol Int*, 20(5), 837–852.

Lewy, A.J., Emens, J., Jackman, A., and Yuhas, K. (2006). Circadian uses of melatonin in humans. *Chronobiol Int*, 23(1–2), 403–412.

Linkowski, P., Mendlewicz, J., LeClercq, R., Brasseur, M., Hubain, P., Golstein, J., Copinschi, G., and Van Cauter, E. (1985a). The 24-hour profile of adrenocorticotropin and cortisol in major depressive illness. *J Clin Endocrinol Metab*, 61, 429–438.

Linkowski, P., Van Cauter, E., Leclercq, R., Desmedt, D., Brasseur, M., Golstein, J., Copinschi, G., and Mendlewicz, J. (1985b). ACTH, cortisol and growth hormone 24-hour profiles in major depressive illness. *Acta Psychiatr Belg*, 85(5), 615–623.

Linkowski, P., Kerkhofs, M., Rielaert, C., and Mendlewicz, J. (1986). Sleep during mania in manic-depressive males. *Eur Arch Psychiatry Neurol Sci*, 235(6), 339–341.

Linkowski, P., Kerkhofs, M., Van Onderbergen, A., Hubain, P., Copinschi, G., L'Hermite-Baleriaux, M., Leclercq, R., Brasseur, M., Mendlewicz, J., and Van Cauter, E. (1994). The 24-hour profiles of cortisol, prolactin, and growth hormone secretion in mania. *Arch Gen Psychiatry*, 51(8), 616–624.

Liu, C., and Reppert, S.M. (2000). GABA synchronizes clock cells within the suprachiasmatic circadian clock. *Neuron*, 25(1), 123–128.

Liu, C., Weaver, D.R., Jin, X., Shearman, L.P., Pieschl, R.L., Gribkoff, V.K., and Reppert, S.M. (1997a). Molecular dissection of two distinct actions of melatonin on the suprachiasmatic circadian clock. *Neuron*, 19(1), 91–102.

Liu, C., Weaver, D.R., Strogatz, S.H., and Reppert, S.M. (1997b). Cellular construction of a circadian clock: Period determination in the suprachiasmatic nuclei. *Cell*, 91(6), 855–860.

Lobban, M.C., Tredre, B., Elithorn, A., and Bridges, P. (1963). Diurnal rhythms of electrolyte excretion in depressive illness. *Nature*, 199, 667–669.

Lockley, S.W., Skene, D.J., Thapan, K., English, J., Ribeiro, D., Haimov, I., Hampton, S., Middleton, B., von Schantz, M., and Arendt, J. (1998). Extraocular light exposure does not suppress plasma melatonin in humans. *J Clin Endocrinol Metab*, 83(9), 3369–3372.

Loo, H., Hale, A., and D'Haenen, H. (2002). Determination of the dose of agomelatine, a melatoninergic agonist and selective 5-HT(2c) antagonist, in the treatment of major depressive disorder: A placebo-controlled dose range study. *Int Clin Psychopharmacol*, 17(5), 239–247.

Low, K.G., and Feissner, J.M. (1998). Seasonal affective disorder in college students: Prevalence and latitude. *J Am Coll Health*, 47(3), 135–137.

Lowrey, P.L., Shimomura, K., Antoch, M.P., Yamazaki, S., Zemenides, P.D., Ralph, M.R., Menaker, M., and Takahashi, J.S. (2000). Positional syntenic cloning and functional characterization of the mammalian circadian mutation *tau*. *Science*, 288(5465), 483–492.

Madden, P.A., Heath, A.C., Rosenthal, N.E., and Martin, N.G. (1996). Seasonal changes in mood and behavior. The role of genetic factors. *Arch Gen Psychiatry*, 53(1), 47–55.

Magnusson, A. (2000). An overview of epidemiological studies on seasonal affective disorder. *Acta Psychiatr Scand*, 101(3), 176–184.

Magnusson, A., and Axelsson, J. (1993). The prevalence of seasonal affective disorder is low among descendants of Icelandic emigrants in Canada. *Arch Gen Psychiatry*, 50(12), 947–951.

Magnusson, A., and Stefansson, J.G. (1993). Prevalence of seasonal affective disorder in Iceland. *Arch Gen Psychiatry*, 50(12), 941–946.

Malkoff-Schwartz, S., Frank, E., Anderson, B., Sherrill, J. T., Siegel, L., Patterson, D., and Kupfer, D.J. (1998). Stressful life events and social rhythm disruption in the onset of manic and depressive bipolar episodes: A preliminary investigation. *Arch Gen Psychiatry*, 55(8), 702–707.

Malpaux, B., Daveau, A., Maurice-Mandon, F., Duarte, G., and Chemineau, P. (1998). Evidence that melatonin acts in the pre-mammillary hypothalamic area to control reproduction in the ewe: Presence of binding sites and stimulation of luteinizing hormone secretion by in situ microimplant delivery. *Endocrinology*, 139(4), 1508–1516.

Maquet, P., Peters, J., Aerts, J., Delfiore, G., Degueldre, C., Luxen, A., and Franck, G. (1996). Functional neuroanatomy of human rapid-eye-movement sleep and dreaming. *Nature*, 383(6596), 163–166.

Martinek, S., Inonog, S., Manoukian, A.S., and Young, M.W. (2001). A role for the segment polarity gene *shaggy/GSK-3* in the *Drosophila* circadian clock. *Cell*, 105(6), 769–779.

Mayberg, H.S., Brannan, S.K., Mahurin, R.K., Jerabek, P.A., Brickman, J.S., Tekell, J.L., Silva, J.A., McGinnis, S., Glass, T.G., Martin, C.C., and Fox, P.T. (1997). Cingulate function in depression: A potential predictor of treatment response. *Neuroreport*, 8(4), 1057–1061.

McGrath, R.E., Buckwald, B., and Resnick, E.V. (1990). The effect of L-tryptophan on seasonal affective disorder. *J Clin Psychiatry*, 51(4), 162–163.

Mendels, J., and Chernik, D.A. (1973). The effect of lithium carbonate on the sleep of depressed patients. *Int Pharmacopsychiatry*, 8(3), 184–192.

Mendelson, W.B., and Basile, A.S. (2001). The hypnotic actions of the fatty acid amide, oleamide. *Neuropsychopharmacology*, 25(Suppl. 5), S36–S39.

Mendelson, W.B., Gillin, J.C., and Wyatt, R.J. (1997). *Human Sleep and Its Disorders*. New York: Plenum Press.

Meyer, T.D., and Maier, S. (2006). Is there evidence for social rhythm instability in people at risk for affective disorders? *Psychiatry Res*, 141(1), 103–114.

Middleton, B., Arendt, J., and Stone, B.M. (1996). Human circadian rhythms in constant dim light (8 lux) with knowledge of clock time. *J Sleep Res*, 5(2), 69–76.

Millar, A., Espie, C.A., and Scott, J. (2004). The sleep of remitted bipolar outpatients: A controlled naturalistic study using actigraphy. *J Affect Disord*, 80(2-3), 145–153.

Mistlberger, R.E., and Holmes, M.M. (2000). Behavioral feedback regulation of circadian rhythm phase angle in light–dark entrained mice. *Am J Physiol Regul Integr Comp Physiol*, 279(3), R813–R821.

Mizukawa, R., Ishiguro, S., Takada, H., Kishimoto, A., Ogura, C., and Hazama, H. (1991). Long-term observation of a manic-depressive patient with rapid cycles. *Biol Psychiatry*, 29(7), 671–678.

Modell, J.G., Rosenthal, N.E., Harriett, A.E., Krishen, A., Asgharian, A., Foster, V.J., Metz, A., Rockett, C.B., and Wightman, D.S. (2005). Seasonal affective disorder and its prevention by anticipatory treatment with bupropion XL. *Biol Psychiatry*, 58(8), 658–667.

Molin, J., Mellerup, E., Bolwig, T., Scheike, T., and Dam, H. (1996). The influence of climate on development of winter depression. *J Affect Disord*, 37(2–3), 151–155.

Monk, T.H., Flaherty, J.F., Frank, E., Hoskinson, K., and Kupfer, D.J. (1990). The Social Rhythm Metric. An instrument to quantify the daily rhythms of life. *J Nerv Ment Dis*, 178(2), 120–126.

Monk, T.H., Buysse, D.J., Reynolds, C.F. III, Jarrett, D.B., and Kupfer, D.J. (1992). Rhythmic vs. homeostatic influences on mood, activation, and performance in young and old men. *J Gerontol*, 47(4), P221–227.

Montgomery, S.A., Kennedy, S.H., Burrows, G.D., Lejoyeux, M., and Hindmarch, I. (2004). Absence of discontinuation symptoms with agomelatine and occurrence of discontinuation symptoms with paroxetine: A randomized, double-blind, placebo-controlled discontinuation study. *Int Clin Psychopharmacol*, 19(5), 271–280.

Moore, R.Y. (1996a). Entrainment pathways and the functional organization of the circadian system. *Prog Brain Res*, 111, 103–119.

Moore, R.Y. (1996b). Neural control of the pineal gland. *Behav Brain Res*, 73(1–2), 125–130.

Morgan, P.J., Messager, S., Webster, C., Barrett, P., and Ross, A. (1999). How does the melatonin receptor decode a photoperiodic signal in the pars tuberalis? *Adv Exp Med Biol*, 460, 165–174.

Morin, L.P. (1999). Serotonin and the regulation of mammalian circadian rhythmicity. *Ann Med*, 31(1), 12–33.

Morken, G., Lilleeng, S., and Linaker, O.M. (2002). Seasonal variation in suicides and in admissions to hospital for mania and depression. *J Affect Disord*, 69(1–3), 39–45.

Morrissey, S.A., Raggatt, P.T., James, B., and Rogers, J. (1996). Seasonal affective disorder: Some epidemiological findings from a tropical climate. *Aust N Z J Psychiatry*, 30(5), 579–586.

Moscovitch, A., Blashko, C., Wiseman, R., Goldberg, M., and Martindale, J. (1995). *A double-blind, placebo-controlled study of sertaline in patients with seasonal affective disorder.* New Research Abstracts. American Psychiatric Association Annual Meeting.

Mrosovsky, N. (1988). Phase response curves for social entrainment. *J Comp Physiol [A]*, 162, 35–46.

Mrosovsky, N., Salmon, P.A., and Vrang, N. (1998). Revolutionary science: An improved running wheel for hamsters. *Chronobiol Int*, 15(2), 147–158.

Mrugala, M., Zlomanczuk, P., Jagota, A., and Schwartz, W.J. (2000). Rhythmic multiunit neural activity in slices of hamster suprachiasmatic nucleus reflect prior photoperiod. *Am J Physiol Regul Integr Comp Physiol*, 278(4), R987–R994.

Murase, S., Murase, S., Kitabatake, M., Yamauchi, T., and Mathe, A.A. (1995). Seasonal mood variation among Japanese residents of Stockholm. *Acta Psychiatr Scand*, 92(1), 51–55.

Murray, G., Michalak, E.E., Levitt, A.J., Levitan, R.D., Enns, M.W., Morehouse, R., and Lam, R.W. (2006). O sweet spot where art thou? Light treatment of seasonal affective disorder and the circadian time of sleep. *J Affect Disord*, 90(2-3), 227–231.

Myers, D.H., and Davies, P. (1978). The seasonal incidence of mania and its relationship to climatic variables. *Psychol Med*, 8, 433–440.

Nagayama, H., Hasama, N., Tsuchiyama, K., Yamada, K., Ihara, J., and Yanagisawa, T. (1992). Circadian temperature and sleep–wake rhythms in depression. *Jpn J Psychiatry Neurol*, 46(1), 244–245.

Nelson, R.J. (1990). Photoperiodic responsiveness in house mice. *Physiol Behav*, 48, 403–408.

Nelson, R.J. (2004). Seasonal immune function and sickness responses. *Trends Immunol*, 25(4), 187–192.

Nelson, R.J., and Zucker, I. (1981). Photoperiodic control of reproduction in olfactory-bulbectomized rats. *Neuroendocrinology*, 32, 266–271.

Nelson, R.J., Demas, G.E., Klein, S.L., and Kriegsfeld, L.J. (2002). *Seasonal Patterns of Stress, Immune Function and Disease.* New York: Cambridge University Press.

Neumeister, A., Goessler, R., Lucht, M., Kapitany, T., Bamas, C., and Kasper, S. (1996). Bright light therapy stabilizes the antidepressant effect of partial sleep deprivation. *Biol Psychiatry*, 39(1), 16–21.

Neumeister, A., Praschak-Rieder, N., Besselmann, B., Rao, M.L., Gluck, J., and Kasper, S. (1997). Effects of tryptophan depletion on drug-free patients with seasonal affective disorder during a stable response to bright light therapy. *Arch Gen Psychiatry*, 54(2), 133–138.

Neumeister, A., Praschak-Rieder, N., Hesselmann, B., Vitouch, O., Rauh, M., Barocka, A., and Kasper, S. (1998a). Effects of tryptophan depletion in fully remitted patients with seasonal affective disorder during summer. *Psychol Med*, 28(2), 257–264.

Neumeister, A., Praschak-Rieder, N., Hesselmann, B., Vitouch, O., Rauh, M., Barocka, A., Tauscher, J., and Kasper, S. (1998b). Effects of tryptophan depletion in drug-free depressed patients who responded to total sleep deprivation. *Arch Gen Psychiatry*, 55(2), 167–172.

Neumeister, A., Turner, E.H., Matthews, J.R., Postolache, T.T., Barnett, R.L., Rauh, M., Vetticad, R.G., Kasper, S., and Rosenthal, N.E. (1998c). Effects of tryptophan depletion vs. catecholamine depletion in patients with seasonal affective disorder in remission with light therapy. *Arch Gen Psychiatry*, 55(6), 524–530.

Neumeister, A., Konstantinidis, A., Praschak-Rieder, N., Willeit, M., Hilger, E., Stastny, J., and Kasper, S. (2001). Monoaminergic function in the pathogenesis of seasonal affective disorder. *Int J Neuropsychopharmacol*, 4(4), 409–420.

Nievergelt, C.M., Kripke, D.F., Remick, R.A., Sadovnick, A.D., McElroy, S.L., Keck, P.E. Jr., and Kelsoe, J.R. (2005). Examination of the clock gene cryptochrome 1 in bipolar disorder: Mutational analysis and absence of evidence for linkage or association. *Psychiatr Genet*, 15(1), 45–52.

Nofzinger, E.A., Reynolds, C.F. III, Thase, M.E., Frank, E., Jennings, J.R., Fasiczka, A.L., Sullivan, L.R., and Kupfer, D.J. (1995). REM sleep enhancement by bupropion in depressed men. *Am J Psychiatry*, 152(2), 274–276.

Nofzinger, E.A., Mintun, M.A., Wiseman, M., Kupfer, D.J., and Moore, R.Y. (1997). Forebrain activation in REM sleep: An FDG PET study. *Brain Res*, 770(1–2), 192–201.

Nofzinger, E.A., Price, J.C., Meltzer, C.C., Buysse, D.J., Villemagne, V.L., Miewald, J.M., Sembrat, R.C., Steppe, D.A., and Kupfer, D.J. (2000). Towards a neurobiology of dysfunctional arousal in depression: The relationship between beta EEG power and regional cerebral glucose metabolism during NREM sleep. *Psychiatry Res*, 98(2), 71–91.

Norden, M.J., and Avery, D.H. (1993). A controlled study of dawn simulation in subsyndromal winter depression. *Acta Psychiatr Scand*, 88(1), 67–71.

Nurnberger, J.I. Jr., Berrettini, W., Tamarkin, L., Hamovit, J., Norton, J., and Gershon, E. (1988). Supersensitivity to melatonin suppression by light in young people at high risk for affective disorder. A preliminary report. *Neuropsychopharmacology*, 1(3), 217–223.

Nurnberger, J. Jr., Berrettini, W., Mendelson, W., Sack, D., and Gershon, E.S. (1989). Measuring cholinergic sensitivity: I. Arecoline effects in bipolar patients. *Biol Psychiatry*, 25(5), 610–617.

Nurnberger, J.I. Jr., Adkins, S., Lahiri, D.K., Mayeda, A., Hu, K., Lewy, A., Miller, A., Bowman, E.S., Miller, M.J., Rau, L., Smiley, C., and Davis-Singh, D. (2000). Melatonin suppression by light in euthymic bipolar and unipolar patients. *Arch Gen Psychiatry*, 57(6), 572–579.

Okawa, M., Shirakawa, S., Uchiyama, M., Oguri, M., Kohsaka, M., Mishima, K., Sakamoto, K., Inoue, H., Kamei, K., and

Takahashi, K. (1996). Seasonal variation of mood and behaviour in a healthy middle-aged population in Japan. *Acta Psychiatr Scand*, 94(4), 211–216.

Oren, D.A., Moul, D.E., Schwartz, P.J., Brown, C., Yamada, E.M., and Rosenthal, N.E. (1994a). Exposure to ambient light in patients with winter seasonal affective disorder. *Am J Psychiatry*, 151(4), 591–593.

Oren, D.A., Moul, D.E., Schwartz, P.J., Wehr, T.A., and Rosenthal, N.E. (1994b). A controlled trial of levodopa plus carbidopa in the treatment of winter seasonal affective disorder: A test of the dopamine hypothesis. *J Clin Psychopharmacol*, 14(3), 196–200.

Oren, D.A., Schulkin, J., and Rosenthal, N.E. (1994c). 1,25 $(OH)_2$ vitamin D_3 levels in seasonal affective disorder: Effects of light. *Psychopharmacology (Berl)*, 116(4), 515–516.

Oren, D.A., Levendosky, A.A., Kasper, S., Duncan, C.C., and Rosenthal, N.E. (1996). Circadian profiles of cortisol, prolactin, and thyrotropin in seasonal affective disorder. *Biol Psychiatry*, 39(3), 157–170.

O'Rourke, D.A., Wurtman, J.J., Brzezinski, A., Nader, T.A., and Chew, B. (1987). Serotonin implicated in etiology of seasonal affective disorder. *Psychopharmacol Bull*, 23(3), 358–359.

Ostenfeld, I. (1986). Abstinence from night sleep as a treatment for endogenous depressions. The earliest observations in a Danish mental hospital (1954) and an analysis of the causal mechanism. *Dan Med Bull*, 33(1), 45–49.

Ozaki, N., Rosenthal, N.E., Moul, D.E., Schwartz, P.J., and Oren, D.A. (1993). Effects of phototherapy on electrooculographic ratio in winter seasonal affective disorder. *Psychiatry Res*, 49(2), 99–107.

Ozaki, N., Ono, Y., Ito, A., and Rosenthal, N.E. (1995a). Prevalence of seasonal difficulties in mood and behavior among Japanese civil servants. *Am J Psychiatry*, 152(8), 1225–1227.

Ozaki, N., Rosenthal, N.E., Myers, F., Schwartz, P.J., and Oren, D.A. (1995b). Effects of season on electro-oculographic ratio in winter seasonal affective disorder. *Psychiatry Res*, 59(1-2), 151–155.

Palmai, G., and Blackwell, B. (1965). The diurnal pattern of salivary flow in normal and depressed patients. *Br J Psychiatry*, 111, 334–338.

Papoušek, M. (1975). Chronobiologische Aspekte der Zyklothymie. *Fortschritte der Neurologie, Psychiatrie und Ihrer Grenzgebiete*, 43, 381–440.

Partinen, M., Kaprio, J., Koskenvuo, M., Putkonen, P., and Langinvainio, H. (1983). Genetic and environmental determination of human sleep. *Sleep*, 6(3), 179–185.

Partonen, T., and Lonnqvist, J. (1993). Effects of light on mood. *Ann Med*, 25(4), 301–302.

Partonen, T., and Lonnqvist, J. (1996). Seasonal variation in bipolar disorder. *Br J Psychiatry*, 169(5), 641–646.

Partonen, T., Appelberg, B., and Partinen, M. (1993a). Effects of light treatment on sleep structure in seasonal affective disorder. *Eur Arch Psychiatry Clin Neurosci*, 242(5), 310–313.

Partonen, T., Partinen, M., and Lonnqvist, J. (1993b). Frequencies of seasonal major depressive symptoms at high latitudes. *Eur Arch Psychiatry Clin Neurosci*, 243(3–4), 189–192.

Payne, J.L., Quiroz, J.A., Zarate, C.A. Jr., and Manji, H.K. (2002). Timing is everything: Does the robust upregulation of noradrenergically regulated plasticity genes underlie the rapid antidepressant effects of sleep deprivation? *Biol Psychiatry*, 52(10), 921–926.

Peck, D.F. (1990). Climatic variables and admissions for mania: A reanalysis. *J Affect Disord*, 20(4), 249–250.

Penn, J.S., and Williams, T.P. (1986). Photostasis: Regulation of daily photon-catch by rat retinas in response to various cyclic illuminances. *Exp Eye Res*, 43(6), 915–928.

Pereira, D.S., Tufik, S., Louzada, F.M., Benedito-Silva, A.A., Lopez, A.R., Lemos, N.A., Korczak, A.L., D'Almeida, V., and Pedrazzoli, M. (2005). Association of the length of polymorphism in the human *per3* gene with the delayed sleep-phase syndrome: Does latitude have an influence upon it? *Sleep*, 28(1), 29–32.

Perlman, C.A., Johnson, S.L., and Mellman, T.A. (2006). The prospective impact of sleep duration on depression and mania. *Bipolar Disord*, 8(3), 271–274.

Petridou, E., Papadopoulos, F.C., Frangakis, C.E., Skalkidou, A., and Trichopoulos, D. (2002). A role of sunshine in the triggering of suicide. *Epidemiology*, 13(1), 106–109.

Pfaffenberger, B., Hardt, I., Huhnerfuss, H., Konig, W.A., Rimkus, G., Glausch, A., Schurig, V., and Hahn, J. (1994). Enantioselective degradation of alpha-hexachlorocyclohexane and cyclodiene insecticides in roe-deer liver samples from different regions of Germany. *Chemosphere*, 29(7), 1543–1554.

Pflug, B., and Tölle, R. (1971). Disturbance of the 24-hour rhythm in endogenous depression and the treatment of endogenous depression by sleep deprivation. *Int Pharmacopsychiatry*, 6, 187–196.

Pflug, B., Erikson, R., and Johnsson, A. (1976). Depression and daily temperature: A long-term study. *Acta Psychiatr Scand*, 54, 254–266.

Pflug, B., Johnsson, A., and Ekse, A.T. (1981). Manic-depressive states and daily temperature. *Acta Psychiatr Scand*, 63, 277–289.

Pflug, B., Johnsson, A., and Martin, W. (1983). Alterations in the circadian temperature rhythms in depressed patients. In T.A. Weher and F.K. Goodwin (Eds.), *Circadian Rhythms in Psychiatry* (pp. 71–76). Pacific Grove, CA: Boxwood Press.

Phiel, C.J., and Klein, P.S. (2001). Molecular targets of lithium action. *Annu Rev Pharmacol Toxicol*, 41, 789–813.

Pittendrigh, C.S., and Daan, S. (1976). A functional analysis of circadian pacemakers in nocturnal rodents. V. Pacemaker structure: A clock for all seasons. *J Comp Physiol*, 106, 333–355.

Pizzagalli, D., Pascual-Marqui, R.D., Nitschke, J.B., Oakes, T.R., Larson, C.L., Abercrombie, H.C., Schaefer, S.M., Koger, J.V., Benca, R.M., and Davidson, R.J. (2001). Anterior cingulate activity as a predictor of degree of treatment response in major depression: Evidence from brain electrical tomography analysis. *Am J Psychiatry*, 158(3), 405–415.

Placidi, F., Diomedi, M., Scalise, A., Marciani, M. G., Romigi, A., and Gigli, G.L. (2000a). Effect of anticonvulsants on nocturnal sleep in epilepsy. *Neurology*, 54(5 Suppl. 1), S25–S32.

Placidi, F., Marciani, M.G., Diomedi, M., Scalise, A., Pauri, F., Giacomini, P., and Gigli, G.L. (2000b). Effects of lamotrigine on nocturnal sleep, daytime somnolence and cognitive functions in focal epilepsy. *Acta Neurol Scand*, 102(2), 81–86.

Placidi, F., Scalise, A., Marciani, M.G., Romigi, A., Diomedi, M., and Gigli, G.L. (2000c). Effect of antiepileptic drugs on sleep. *Clin Neurophysiol*, 111(Suppl. 2), S115–S119.

Plyte, S.E., Hughes, K., Nikolakaki, E., Pulverer, B.J., and Woodgett, J.R. (1992). Glycogen synthase kinase-3: Functions in oncogenesis and development. *Biochim Biophys Acta*, 1114(2–3), 147–162.

Postolache, T.T., and Oren, D.A. (2005). Circadian phase shifting, alerting, and antidepressant effects of bright light treatment. *Clin Sports Med*, 24(2), 381–413, xii.

Postolache, T.T., Hardin, T.A., Myers, F.S., Turner, E.H., Yi, L.Y., Barnett, R.L., Matthews, J.R., and Rosenthal, N.E. (1998). Greater improvement in summer than with light treatment in winter in patients with seasonal affective disorder. *Am J Psychiatry*, 155(11), 1614–1616.

Postolache, T.T., Benson, B.E., Guzman, A., Mathews, J.R., Turner, E.H., Wehr, T.A., Rosenthal, N.E., and Drevets, W.C. (2002a). Acute effects of light treatment on cerebral blood flow in healthy subjects. *Chronobiol Int*, 19, 984–985.

Postolache, T.T., Benson, B.E., Guzman, A., Mathews, J.R., Turner, E.H., Wehr, T.A., Rosenthal, N.E., and Drevets, W.C. (2002b). *Acute effects of light treatment on cerebral blood flow in healthy subjects and patients with seasonal affective disorder.* Symposium on Healthy Lighting. Eindhoven, The Netherlands: Light & Health Research Foundation.

Postolache, T.T., Matthews, J.R., Turner, E.H., Benson, B.E., Guzman, A., Rosenthal, N.E., and Drevets, W.C. (2002c). Cerebral blood flow in depressed individuals with sad as compared to matched controls. *Chronobiol Int*, 19(5), 986.

Postolache, T.T., Wehr, T.A., Doty, R.L., Sher, L., Turner, E.H., Bartko, J.J., and Rosenthal, N.E. (2002d). Patients with seasonal affective disorder have lower odor detection thresholds than control subjects. *Arch Gen Psychiatry*, 59(12), 1119–1122.

Postolache, T.T., Komarow, H.D., Stiller, J.W., and Tonelli, L.H. (2005a). Allergy, depression, and suicide. *Directions in Psychiatry*, 25(6), 59–70.

Postolache, T.T., Stiller, J.W., Herrell, R., Goldstein, M.A., Shreeram, S.S., Zebrak, R., Thrower, C.M., Volkov, J., No, M.J., Volkov, I., Rohan, K.J., Redditt, J., Parmar, M., Mohyuddin, F., Olsen, C., Moca, M., Tonelli, L.H., Merikangas, K., and Komarow, H.D. (2005b). Tree pollen peaks are associated with increased nonviolent suicide in women. *Mol Psychiatry*, 10, 232–238.

Provencio, I., Jiang, G., De Grip, W.J., Hayes, W.P., and Rollag, M.D. (1998). Melanopsin: An opsin in melanophores, brain, and eye. *Proc Natl Acad Sci USA*, 95(1), 340–345.

Provencio, I., Rodriguez, I.R., Jiang, G., Hayes, W.P., Moreira, E.F., and Rollag, M.D. (2000). A novel human opsin in the inner retina. *J Neurosci*, 20(2), 600–605.

Provencio, I., Rollag, M.D., and Castrucci, A.M. (2002). Photoreceptive net in the mammalian retina. *Nature*, 415(6871), 493.

Puchalski, W., and Lynch, G.R. (1986). Evidence for differences in the circadian organization of hamsters exposed to short day photoperiod. *J Comp Physiol [A]*, 159(1), 7–11.

Rasanen, M., Lehtinen, J.C., Niinikoski, H., Keskinen, S., Ruottinen, S., Salminen, M., Ronnemaa, T., Viikari, J., and Simell, O. (2002a). Dietary patterns and nutrient intakes of 7-year-old children taking part in an atherosclerosis prevention project in Finland. *J Am Diet Assoc*, 102(4), 518–524.

Rasanen, P., Hakko, H., Jokelainen, J., and Tiihonen, J. (2002b). Seasonal variation in specific methods of suicide: A national register study of 20,234 Finnish people. *J Affect Disord*, 71(1–3), 51–59.

Rasanen, T.L., Alhonen, L., Sinervirta, R., Keinanen, T., Herzig, K.H., Suppola, S., Khomutov, A.R., Vepsalainen, J., and Janne, J. (2002c). A polyamine analogue prevents acute pancreatitis and restores early liver regeneration in transgenic rats with activated polyamine catabolism. *J Biol Chem*, 277(42), 39867–39872.

Reinink, E., Bouhuys, N., Wirz-Justice, A., and van den Hoofdakker, R. (1990). Prediction of the antidepressant response to total sleep deprivation by diurnal variation of mood. *Psychiatry Res*, 32(2), 113–124.

Reinink, E., Bouhuys, A.L., Gordijn, M.C., and Van Den Hoof-dakker, R.H. (1993). Prediction of the antidepressant response to total sleep deprivation of depressed patients: Longitudinal versus single day assessment of diurnal mood variation. *Biol Psychiatry*, 34(7), 471–481.

Reme, C., Terman, M., and Wirz-Justice, A. (1990). Are deficient retinal photoreceptor renewal mechanisms involved in the pathogenesis of winter depression? *Arch Gen Psychiatry*, 47(9), 878–879.

Reppert, S.M., and Weaver, D.R. (2000). Comparing clockworks: Mouse versus fly. *J Biol Rhythms*, 15(5), 357–364.

Reppert, S.M., and Weaver, D.R.. (2001). Molecular analysis of mammalian circadian rhythms. *Annu Rev Physiol*, 63, 647–676.

Reynolds, C.F. III, Buysse, D.J., Brunner, D.P., Begley, A.E., Dew, M.A., Hoch, C.C., Hall, M., Houck, P.R., Mazumdar, S., Perel, J.M., and Kupfer, D.J. (1997). Maintenance nortriptyline effects on electroencephalographic sleep in elderly patients with recurrent major depression: Double-blind, placebo- and plasma-level-controlled evaluation. *Biol Psychiatry*, 42(7), 560–567.

Riemann, D., and Berger, M. (1989). EEG sleep in depression and in remission and the REM sleep response to the cholinergic agonist RS 86. *Neuropsychopharmacology*, 2(2), 145–152.

Riemann, D., and Berger, M. (1990). The effects of total sleep deprivation and subsequent treatment with clomipramine on depressive symptoms and sleep electroencephalography in patients with a major depressive disorder. *Acta Psychiatr Scand*, 81(1), 24–31.

Riemann, D., Wiegand, M., and Berger, M. (1991). Are there predictors for sleep deprivation response in depressed patients? *Biol Psychiatry*, 29(7), 707–710.

Riemann, D., Hohagen, F., Konig, A., Schwarz, B., Gomille, J., Voderholzer, U., and Berger, M. (1996). Advanced vs. normal sleep timing: Effects on depressed mood after response to sleep deprivation in patients with a major depressive disorder. *J Affect Disord*, 37(2–3), 121–128.

Riemann, D., Konig, A., Hohagen, F., Kiemen, A., Voderholzer, U., Backhaus, J., Bunz, J., Wesiack, B., Hermle, L., and Berger, M. (1999). How to preserve the antidepressive effect of sleep deprivation: A comparison of sleep phase advance and sleep phase delay. *Eur Arch Psychiatry Clin Neurosci*, 249(5), 231–237.

Riemann, D., Berger, M., and Voderholzer, U. (2001). Sleep and depression—results from psychobiological studies: An overview. *Biol Psychol*, 57(1-3), 67–103.

Rosenthal, N.E., Sack, D.A., Gillin, J.C., Lewy, A.J., Goodwin, F.K., Davenport, Y., Mueller, P.S., Newsome, D.A., and Wehr, T.A. (1984). Seasonal affective disorder. A description of the syndrome and preliminary findings with light therapy. *Arch Gen Psychiatry*, 41(1), 72–80.

Rosenthal, N.E., Sack, D.A., Carpenter, C.J., Parry, B.L., Mendelson, W.B., and Wehr, T.A. (1985). Antidepressant effects of light in seasonal affective disorder. *Am J Psychiatry*, 142(2), 163–170.

Rosenthal, N.E., Jacobsen, F.M., Sack, D.A., Arendt, J., James, S.P., Parry, B.L., and Wehr, T.A. (1988). Atenolol in seasonal affective disorder: A test of the melatonin hypothesis. *Am J Psychiatry*, 145(1), 52–56.

Rosenthal, N.E., Genhart, M.J., Caballero, B., Jacobsen, F.M., Skwerer, R.G., Coursey, R.D., Rogers, S., and Spring, B.J. (1989). Psychobiological effects of carbohydrate- and protein-rich meals in patients with seasonal affective disorder and normal controls. *Biol Psychiatry*, 25(8), 1029–1040.

Rosenthal, N.E., Levendosky, A.A., Skwerer, R.G., Joseph-Vanderpool, J.R., Kelly, K.A., Hardin, T., Kasper, S., Della-Bella, P., and Wehr, T.A. (1990). Effects of light treatment on core body temperature in seasonal affective disorder. *Biol Psychiatry*, 27(1), 39–50.

Rosenthal, N.E., Mazzanti, C.M., Barnett, R.L., Hardin, T.A., Turner, E.H., Lam, G.K., Ozaki, N., and Goldman, D. (1998). Role of serotonin transporter promoter repeat length polymorphism (5-HTTLPR) in seasonality and seasonal affective disorder. *Mol Psychiatry*, 3(2), 175–177.

Rudorfer, M.V., Skwerer, R.G., and Rosenthal, N.E. (1993). Biogenic amines in seasonal affective disorder: Effects of light therapy. *Psychiatry Res*, 46(1), 19–28.

Ruger, M., Gordijn, M.C., Beersma, D.G., de Vries, B., and Daan, S. (2003). Acute and phase-shifting effects of ocular and extraocular light in human circadian physiology. *J Biol Rhythms*, 18(5), 409–419.

Rush, A.J., Erman, M.K., Giles, D.E., Schlesser, M.A., Carpenter, G., Vasavada, N., and Roffwarg, H.P. (1986). Polysomnographic findings in recently drug-free and clinically remitted depressed patients. *Arch Gen Psychiatry*, 43(9), 878–884.

Saanjarvi, S., Lauerma, H., Helenius, S., and Saanlehto, S. (1997). Seasonal affective disorder common in Finland. *Biol Psychiatry*, 42, 255S.

Sack, D.A., Nurnberger, J., Rosenthal, N.E., Ashburn, E., and Wehr, T.A. (1985). Potentiation of antidepressant medications by phase advance of the sleep–wake cycle. *Am J Psychiatry*, 142(5), 606–608.

Sack, D.A., Duncan, W., Rosenthal, N.E., Mendelson, W.E., and Wehr, T.A. (1988). The timing and duration of sleep in partial sleep deprivation therapy of depression. *Acta Psychiatr Scand*, 77, 219–224.

Sack, R.L., Lewy, A.J., Wite, D.M., Singer, C.M., Fireman, M.J., and Vandiver, R. (1990). Morning vs. evening light treatment for winter depression. Evidence that therapeutic effects of light mediated by circadian phase shift. *Arch Gen Psychiatry*, 47, 343–351.

Saper, C.B., Chou, T.C., and Scammell, T.E. (2001). The sleep switch: Hypothalamic control of sleep and wakefulness. *Trends Neurosci*, 24, 726–731.

Sato, T., Bottlender, R., Sievers, M., and Moller, H.J. (2006). Distinct seasonality of depressive episodes differentiates unipolar depressive patients with and without depressive mixed states. *J Affect Disord*, 90(1), 1–5.

Schilgen, B., and Tölle, R. (1980). Partial sleep deprivation as therapy for depression. *Arch Gen Psychiatry*, 37, 267–271.

Schilling, A., and Perret, M. (1993). Removal of the olfactory bulbs modifies the gonadal responses of photoperiod in the lesser mouse lemur (microcebus murinus). *Biol Reprod*, 49, 58–65.

Schlager, D.S. (1994). Early-morning administration of short-acting beta blockers for treatment of winter depression. *Am J Psychiatry*, 151(9), 1383–1385.

Schreiber, W., Lauer, C.J., Krumrey, K., Holsboer, F., and Krieg, J.C. (1992). Cholinergic REM sleep induction test in subjects at high risk for psychiatric disorders. *Biol Psychiatry*, 32(1), 79–90.

Schremser, J.L., and Williams, T.P. (1995a). Rod outer segment (ROS) renewal as a mechanism for adaptation to a new intensity environment. I. Rhodopsin levels and ROS length. *Exp Eye Res*, 61(1), 17–23.

Schremser, J.L., and Williams, T.P. (1995b). Rod outer segment (ROS) renewal as a mechanism for adaptation to a new intensity environment. II. Rhodopsin synthesis and packing density. *Exp Eye Res*, 61(1), 25–32.

Schulz, H., and Lund, R. (1983). Sleep onset REM episodes are associated with circadian parameters of body temperature: A study in depressed patients and normal controls. *Biol Psychiatry*, 18, 1411–1426.

Schulz, H., and Lund, R. (1985). On the origin of early REM episodes in the sleep of depressed patients: A comparison of three hypotheses. *Psychiatry Res*, 16(1), 65–77.

Schulz, H., Lund, R., Cording, C., and Dirlich, G. (1979). Bimodal distribution of REM sleep latencies in depression. *Biol Psychiatry*, 14(4), 595–600.

Schwartz, P.J., Murphy, D.L., Wehr, T.A., Garcia-Borreguero, D., Oren, D.A., Moul, D.E., Ozaki, N., Snelbaker, A.J., and Rosenthal, N.E. (1997). Effects of meta-chlorophenylpiperazine infusions in patients with seasonal affective disorder and healthy control subjects. Diurnal responses and nocturnal regulatory mechanisms. *Arch Gen Psychiatry*, 54(4), 375–385.

Schwartz, P.J., Rosenthal, N.E., Kajimura, N., Han, L., Turner, E.H., Bender, C., and Wehr, T.A. (2000). Ultradian oscillations in cranial thermoregulation and electroencephalographic slow-wave activity during sleep are abnormal in humans with annual winter depression. *Brain Res*, 866(1–2), 152–167.

Schwartz, P.J., Rosenthal, N.E., and Wehr, T.A. (2001a). Band-specific electroencephalogram and brain cooling abnormalities during NREM sleep in patients with winter depression. *Biol Psychiatry*, 50(8), 627–632.

Schwartz, W.J., de la Iglesia, H.O., Zlomanczuk, P., and Illnerova, H. (2001b). Encoding le quattro stagioni within the mammalian brain: Photoperiodic orchestration through the suprachiasmatic nucleus. *J Biol Rhythms*, 16(4), 302–311.

Sharpley, A.L., Walsh, A.E., and Cowen, P.J. (1992). Nefazodone—a novel antidepressant—may increase REM sleep. *Biol Psychiatry*, 31(10), 1070–1073.

Shearman, L.P., Jin, X., Lee, C., Reppert, S.M., and Weaver, D.R. (2000a). Targeted disruption of the *mPer3* gene: Subtle effects on circadian clock function. *Mol Cell Biol*, 20(17), 6269–6275.

Shearman, L.P., Sriram, S., Weaver, D.R., Maywood, E.S., Chaves, I., Zheng, B., Kume, K., Lee, C.C., van der Horst, G.T., Hastings, M.H., and Reppert, S.M. (2000b). Interacting molecular loops in the mammalian circadian clock. *Science*, 288(5468), 1013–1019.

Shen, H., Watanabe, M., Tomasiewicz, H., Rutishauser, U., Magnuson, T., and Glass, J.D. (1997). Role of neural cell adhesion molecule and polysialic acid in mouse circadian clock function. *J Neurosci*, 17(13), 5221–5229.

Sher, L., Matthews, J.R., Turner, E.H., Postolache, T.T., Katz, K.S., and Rosenthal, N.E. (2001). Early response to light therapy partially predicts long-term antidepressant effects in patients with seasonal affective disorder. *J Psychiatry Neurosci*, 26(4), 336–338.

Shin, K., Schaffer, A., Levitt, A.J., and Boyle, M.H. (2005). Seasonality in a community sample of bipolar, unipolar and control subjects. *J Affect Disord*, 86(1), 19–25.

Siegel, J.M., and Rogawski, M.A. (1988). A function for REM sleep: Regulation of noradrenergic receptor sensitivity. *Brain Res*, 472(3), 213–233.

Siffre, M. (1975). Six months alone in a cave. *Natl Geographic*, 147, 426–435.

Silverstone, T., Romans, S., Hunt, N., and McPherson, H. (1995). Is there a seasonal pattern of relapse in bipolar affective disorders? A dual northern and southern hemisphere cohort study. *Br J Psychiatry*, 167(1), 58–60.

Sitaram, N., Wyatt, R.J., Dawson, S., and Gillin, J.C. (1976). REM sleep induction by physostigmine infusion during sleep. *Science*, 191(4233), 1281–1283.

Sitaram, N., Gillin, J.G., and Bunney, W.E. Jr. (1978a). Circadian variation in the time of "switch" of a patient with 48-hour manic-depressive cycles. *Biol Psychiatry*, 13(5), 567–574.

Sitaram, N., Moore, A.M., and Gillin, J.C. (1978b). Experimental acceleration and slowing of REM sleep ultradian rhythm by cholinergic agonist and antagonist. *Nature*, 274(5670), 490–492.

Sitaram, N., Nurnberger, J.I. Jr., Gershon, E.S., and Gillin, J.C. (1980). Faster cholinergic REM sleep induction in euthymic patients with primary affective illness. *Science*, 208(4440), 200–202.

Sitaram, N., Nurnberger, J.I. Jr., Gershon, E.S., and Gillin, J.C. (1982). Cholinergic regulation of mood and REM sleep: Potential model and marker of vulnerability to affective disorder. *Am J Psychiatry*, 139(5), 571–576.

Skene, D.J., Lockley, S.W., Thapan, K., and Arendt, J. (1999). Effects of light on human circadian rhythms. *Reprod Nutr Dev*, 39(3), 295–304.

Skwerer, R.G., Jacobsen, F.M., Duncan, C.C., Kelly, K.A., Sack, D.A., Tamarkin, L., Gaist, P.A., Kasper, S., and Rosenthal, N.E. (1988). Neurobiology of seasonal affective disorder and phototherapy. *J Biol Rhythms*, 3(2), 135–154.

Slater, E. (1938). Zur Periodic des manische-depressiven Irreseins. *Z Neurol Psychiatrie*, 162, 794–801.

Smeraldi, E., Benedetti, F., Barbini, B., Campori, E., and Colombo, C. (1999). Sustained antidepressant effect of sleep deprivation combined with pindolol in bipolar depression. A placebo-controlled trial. *Neuropsychopharmacology*, 20(4), 380–385.

Smith, G.S., Reynolds, C.F. III, Pollock, B., Derbyshire, S., Nofzinger, E., Dew, M.A., Houck, P.R., Milko, D., Meltzer, C.C., and Kupfer, D.J. (1999). Cerebral glucose metabolic response to combined total sleep deprivation and antidepressant treatment in geriatric depression. *Am J Psychiatry*, 156(5), 683–689.

Souêtre, E. (1990). Sleep disorders related to anxiety. *Presse Med*, 19(40), 1839–1841.

Souêtre, E., Pringuey, D., Salvati, E., and Robert, P. (1985). Rythmes circadiens de la température centrale et de la cortisolémie dans les dépressions endogènes. *L'Encéphale*, 11, 185–198.

Souêtre, E., Salvati, E., Wehr, T.A., Sack, D.A., Krebs, B., and Darcourt, G. (1988). Twenty-four-hour profiles of body temperature and plasma TSH in bipolar patients during depression and during remission and in normal control subjects. *Am J Psychiatry*, 145(9), 1133–1137.

Souêtre, E., Salvati, E., Belugou, J.L., Pringuey, D., Candito, M., Krebs, B., Ardisson, J.L., and Darcourt, G. (1989). Circadian rhythms in depression and recovery: Evidence for blunted amplitude as the main chronobiological abnormality. *Psychiatry Res*, 28(3), 263–278.

Spiegel, K., Leproult, R., and Van Cauter, E. (1999). Impact of sleep debt on metabolic and endocrine function. *Lancet*, 354(9188), 1435–1439.

Steiger, A., von Bardeleben, U., Herth, T., and Holsboer, F. (1989). Sleep EEG and nocturnal secretion of cortisol and growth hormone in male patients with endogenous depression before treatment and after recovery. *J Affect Disord*, 16(2-3), 189–195.

Steiger, A., Gerken, A., Benkert, O., and Holsboer, F. (1993a). Differential effects of the enantiomers R(−) and S(+) oxaprotiline on major endogenous depression, the sleep EEG and neuroendocrine secretion: Studies on depressed patients and normal controls. *Eur Neuropsychopharmacol*, 3(2), 117–126.

Steiger, A., Trachsel, L., Guldner, J., Hemmeter, U., Rothe, B., Rupprecht, R., Vedder, H., and Holsboer, F. (1993b). Neurosteroid pregnenolone induces sleep-EEG changes in man compatible with inverse agonistic GABAA-receptor modulation. *Brain Res*, 615(2), 267–274.

Steiger, A., von Bardeleben, U., Guldner, J., Lauer, C., Rothe, B., and Holsboer, F. (1993c). The sleep EEG and nocturnal hormonal secretion studies on changes during the course of depression and on effects of CNS-active drugs. *Prog Neuropsychopharmacol Biol Psychiatry*, 17(1), 125–137.

Stephan, F.K. (1983). Circadian rhythm dissociation induced by periodic feeding in rats with suprachiasmatic lesions. *Behav Brain Res*, 7(1), 81–98.

Steriade, M. (1994). Sleep oscillations and their blockage by activating systems. *J Psychiatry Neurosci*, 19(5), 354–358.

Swade, C., and Coppen, A. (1980). Seasonal variations in biochemical factors related to depressive illness. *J Affect Disord*, 2(4), 249–255.

Tafti, M., Chollet, D., Valatx, J.L., and Franken, P. (1999). Quantitative trait loci approach to the genetics of sleep in recombinant inbred mice. *J Sleep Res*, 8(Suppl. 1), 37–43.

Takano, A., Uchiyama, M., Kajimura, N., Mishima, K., Inoue, Y., Kamei, Y., Kitajima, T., Shibui, K., Katoh, M., Watanabe, T., Hashimotodani, Y., Nakajima, T., Ozeki, Y., Hori, T., Yamada, N., Toyoshima, R., Ozaki, N., Okawa, M., Nagai, K., Takahashi, K., Isojima, Y., Yamauchi, T., and Ebisawa, T. (2004). A missense variation in human casein kinase I epsilon gene that induces functional alteration and shows an inverse association with circadian rhythm sleep disorders. *Neuropsychopharmacology*, 29(10), 1901–1909.

Takei, N., O'Callaghan, E., Sham, P., Glover, G., Tamura, A., and Murray, R. (1992). Seasonality of admissions in the psychoses: Effect of diagnosis, sex, and age at onset. *Br J Psychiatry*, 161, 506–511.

Terman, J.S., and Terman, M. (1999). Photopic and scotopic light detection in patients with seasonal affective disorder and control subjects. *Biol Psychiatry*, 46(12), 1642–1648.

Terman, J.S., Terman, M., Lo, E.S., and Cooper, T.B. (2001). Circadian time of morning light administration and therapeutic response in winter depression. *Arch Gen Psychiatry*, 58(1), 69–75.

Terman, M., Boticelli, S.R., and Link, B.G., et al. (1989a). Seasonal symptom patters in New York: Patients and population. In C. Thomson, and T. Silverstone (Eds.), *Seasonal Affective Disorder* (pp. 77–95). London: CNS Publishers.

Terman, M., Terman J.-S., Quitkin, F., McGrath, P., Stewart, J., and Rafferty, B. (1989b). Light treatment for seasonal affective disorder: A review of efficacy. *Neuropsychopharmacology*, 2, 1–22.

Terman, M., Terman, J.S., and Ross, D.C. (1998). A controlled study of timed bright light and negative air ionization for treatment of winter depression. *Arch Gen Psychiatry*, 55, 875–882.

Thase, M.E., Himmelhoch, J.M., Mallinger, A.G., Jarrett, D.B., and Kupfer, D.J. (1989). Sleep EEG and DST findings in anergic bipolar depression. *Am J Psychiatry*, 146(3), 329–333.

Thase, M.E., Kupfer, D.J., Buysse, D.J., Frank, E., Simons, A.D., McEachran, A.B., Rashid, K.F., and Grochocinski, V.J. (1995). Electroencephalographic sleep profiles in single-episode and recurrent unipolar forms of major depression: I. Comparison during acute depressive states. *Biol Psychiatry*, 38(8), 506–515.

Thase, M.E., Fasiczka, A.L., Berman, S.R., Simons, A.D., and Reynolds, C.F. III. (1998). Electroencephalographic sleep profiles before and after cognitive behavior therapy of depression. *Arch Gen Psychiatry*, 55(2), 138–144.

Thomson, C., Rodin, I., and Birtwhistle, J. (1999). Light therapy for seasonal and nonseasonal affective disorder: A Cochrane meta-analysis, 11.

Thorell, L.H., Kjellman, B., Arned, M., Lindwall-Sundel, K., Walinder, J., and Wetterberg, L. (1999). Light treatment of seasonal affective disorder in combination with citalopram or placebo with 1-year follow-up. *Int Clin Psychopharmacol*, 14(Suppl. 2), S7–S11.

Toh, K.L., Jones, C.R., He, Y., Eide, E.J., Hinz, W.A., Virshup, D.M., Ptacek, L.J., and Fu, Y.H. (2001). An hPer2 phosphorylation site mutation in familial advanced sleep phase syndrome. *Science*, 291(5506), 1040–1043.

Tonelli, L.H., and Postolache, T.T. (2006). *Behavioral, cellular, and molecular responses in the brain induced by allergy to tree pollen*. Presented at the Neuroscience Meeting, Atlanta, GA.

Tonelli, L.H., Rujescu, D., Stiller, J.W., Giegling, I., Schneider, B., Maurer, K., Bratzke, H.J., Schnabel, A., and Postolache, T.T. (2006). Gender-specific cytokine gene expression in the brain of suicide victims. *Biol Psychiatry*, 59, 245S–246S.

Toth, L.A. (2001). Identifying genetic influences on sleep: An approach to discovering the mechanisms of sleep regulation. *Behav Genet*, 31(1), 39–46.

Totterdell, P., Reynolds, S., Parkinson, B., and Briner, R.B. (1994). Associations of sleep with everyday mood, minor symptoms and social interaction experience. *Sleep*, 17(5), 466–475.

Tsai, S.Y., Yang, Y.Y., Kuo, C.J., Chen, C.C., and Leu, S.J. (2001). Effects of symptomatic severity on elevation of plasma soluble interleukin-2 receptor in bipolar mania. *J Affect Disord*, 64(2–3), 185–193.

Tsujimoto, T., Yamada, N., Shimoda, K., Hanada, K., and Takahashi, S. (1990). Circadian rhythms in depression. Part II: Circadian rhythms in inpatients with various mental disorders. *J Affect Disord*, 18(3), 199–210.

Tsuno, N., Besset, A., and Ritchie, K. (1977). Sleep and depression. *J Clin Psychiatry*, 66(10), 1254–1269.

Van Cauter, E., and Turek, F.W. (1986). Depression: A disorder of timekeeping? *Perspect Biol Med*, 29(4), 510–519.

Van Den Burg, W., Beersma, D.G., Bouhuys, A.L., and Van Den Hoofdakker, R.H. (1992). Self-rated arousal concurrent with the antidepressant response to total sleep deprivation of patients with a major depressive disorder: A disinhibition hypothesis. *J Sleep Res*, 1(4), 211–222.

van den Hoofdakker, R.H. (1997). Total sleep deprivation: Clinical and theoretical aspects. In A.V. Honig, and H.M. Praag (Eds.), *Depression: Neurobiological, Psychopathological and Therapeutic Advances* (pp. 564–589). Chichester, England: John Wiley & Sons,

van den Hoofdakker, R.H., and Beersma, D.G. (1985). On the explanation of short REM latencies in depression. *Psychiatry Res*, 16(2), 155–163.

van der Horst, G.T., Muijtjens, M., Kobayashi, K., Takano, R., Kanno, S., Takao, M., de Wit, J., Verkerk, A., Eker, A.P., van

Leenen, D., Buijs, R., Bootsma, D., Hoeijmakers, J.H., and Yasui, A. (1999). Mammalian Cry1 and Cry2 are essential for maintenance of circadian rhythms. *Nature*, 398(6728), 627–630.

van Houwelingen, C.A., and Beersma, D.G. (2001a). Seasonal changes in 24-h patterns of suicide rates: A study on train suicides in The Netherlands. *J Affect Disord*, 66(2–3), 215–223.

van Houwelingen, C.A., and Beersma, D.G. (2001b). Seasonal variation in suicides: Hidden not vanished. *Br J Psychiatry*, 178, 380.

Van Sweden, B. (1986). Disturbed vigilance in mania. *Biol Psychiatry*, 21(3), 311–313.

Vitaterna, M.H., King, D.P., Chang, A.M., Kornhauser, J.M., Lowrey, P.L., McDonald, J.D., Dove, W.F., Pinto, L.H., Turek, F.W., and Takahashi, J.S. (1994). Mutagenesis and mapping of a mouse gene, *Clock*, essential for circadian behavior. *Science*, 264(5159), 719–725.

Vitaterna, M.H., Selby, C.P., Todo, T., Niwa, H., Thompson, C., Fruechte, E.M., Hitomi, K., Thresher, R.J., Ishikawa, T., Miyazaki, J., Takahashi, J.S., and Sancar, A. (1999). Differential regulation of mammalian period genes and circadian rhythmicity by cryptochromes 1 and 2. *Proc Natl Acad Sci USA*, 96(21), 12114–12119.

Vogel, G.W., Vogel, F., McAbee, R.S., and Thurmond, A.J. (1980). Improvement of depression by REM sleep deprivation. New findings and a theory. *Arch Gen Psychiatry*, 37(3), 247–253.

Volk, S.A., Kaendler, S.H., Hertel, A., Maul, F.D., Manoocheri, R., Weber, R., Georgi, K., Pflug, B., and Hor, G. (1997). Can response to partial sleep deprivation in depressed patients be predicted by regional changes of cerebral blood flow? *Psychiatry Res*, 75(2), 67–74.

Vollmann, J., and Berger, M. (1993). Sleep deprivation with consecutive sleep-phase advance therapy in patients with major depression: A pilot study. *Biol Psychiatry*, 33(1), 54–57.

Vollrath, M., Wicki, W., and Angst, J. (1989). The Zurich study. VIII. Insomnia: Association with depression, anxiety, somatic syndromes, and course of insomnia. *Eur Arch Psychiatry Neurol Sci*, 239(2), 113–124.

von Economo, C. (1930). Sleep as a problem of localization. *J Nerv Ment*, 71, 249–259.

von Zerssen, D., Barthelmes, H., Dirlich, G., Doerr, P., Emrich, H.M., von Lindern, L., Lund, R., and Pirke, K.M. (1985). Circadian rhythms in endogenous depression. *Psychiatry Res*, 16(1), 51–63.

Wacker, H.R., Krauchi, K., Wirz-Justice, A., and Battegay, R. (1992). *"Seasonality" is correlated with affective and not with anxiety disorders*. 4th Annual Meeting on Light Treatment and Biological Rhythms, Bethesda, MD.

Wagner, S., Castel, M., Gainer, H., and Yarom, Y. (1997). GABA in the mammalian suprachiasmatic nucleus and its role in diurnal rhythmicity. *Nature*, 387(6633), 598–603.

Webb, W.B., and Campbell, S.S. (1983). Relationships in sleep characteristics of identical and fraternal twins. *Arch Gen Psychiatry*, 40(10), 1093–1095.

Wehr, T.A. (1989). Sleep loss: A preventable cause of mania and other excited states. *J Clin Psychiatry*, 50(Suppl.), 8–16, discussion 45–7.

Wehr, T.A. (1990). Manipulations of sleep and phototherapy: Nonpharmacological alternatives in the treatment of depression. Clin Neuropharmacol, 13(Suppl. 1), S54–S65.

Wehr, T.A. (1991a). The durations of human melatonin secretion and sleep respond to changes in daylength (photoperiod). *J Clin Endocrinol Metab*, 73(6), 1276–1280.

Wehr, T.A. (1991b). Sleep-loss as a possible mediator of diverse causes of mania. *Br J Psychiatry*, 159, 576–578.

Wehr, T.A. (1992a). A brain-warming function for REM sleep. *Neurosci Biobehav Rev*, 16(3), 379–397.

Wehr, T.A. (1992b). Improvement of depression and triggering of mania by sleep deprivation. *JAMA*, 267(4), 548–551.

Wehr, T.A. (1992c). In short photoperiods, human sleep is biphasic. *J Sleep Res*, 1(2), 103–107.

Wehr, T.A. (1996). A "clock for all seasons" in the human brain. *Prog Brain Res*, 111, 321–342.

Wehr, T.A. (2001). Photoperiodism in humans and other primates: Evidence and implications. *J Biol Rhythms*, 16, 348–364.

Wehr, T.A., and Goodwin, F.K. (Eds.). (1981). *Stress, Circadian Rhythms and Affective Disorders. Stress and Coping. Unit I: Psychophysiology*. Philadelphia: SmithKline Corporation.

Wehr, T.A., and Goodwin, F.K. (1983a). *Circadian Rhythms in Psychiatry*. Pacific Grove, CA: Boxwood Press.

Wehr, T.A., and Goodwin, F.K. (1983b). Introduction. In T.A. Wehr and F.K. Goodwin (Eds.), *Circadian Rhythms in Psychiatry* (pp. 1–15). Pacific Grove, CA: Boxwood Press.

Wehr, T.A., and Goodwin, F.K. (1983c). Biological rhythms in manic-depressive illness. In T.A. Wehr and F.K. Goodwin (Eds.), *Circadian Rhythms in Psychiatry* (pp. 129–184). Pacific Grove, CA: Boxwood Press.

Wehr, T.A., and Rosenthal, N.E. (1989). Seasonality and affective illness. *Am J Psychiatry*, 146(7), 829–839.

Wehr, T.A., and Sack, D.A. (1988). The relevance of sleep research to affective illness. In W.P. Koella, F. Obál, H. Schulz, and P. Visser, *Sleep '86* (pp. 207–211). New York: Gustav Fischer Verlag.

Wehr, T.A., and Wirz-Justice, A. (1981). Internal coincidence model for sleep deprivation and depression. In W.P. Koella (Ed.), *Sleep 80* (pp. 26–33). Basel: Karger.

Wehr, T.A., and Wirz-Justice, A. (1982). Circadian rhythm mechanisms in affective illness and in antidepressant drug action. *Pharmacopsychiatria*, 15(1), 31–39.

Wehr, T.A., Wirz-Justice, A., Goodwin, F.K., Duncan, W., and Gillin, J.C. (1979). Phase advance of the circadian sleep–wake cycle as an antidepressant. *Science*, 206(4419), 710–713.

Wehr, T.A., Goodwin, F.K., Wirz-Justice, A., Breitmaier, J., and Craig, C. (1982). 48-hour sleep–wake cycles in manic-depressive illness: Naturalistic observations and sleep deprivation experiments. *Arch Gen Psychiatry*, 39(5), 559–565.

Wehr, T.A., Rosenthal, N.E., Sack, D.A., and Gillin, J.C. (1985a). Antidepressant effects of sleep deprivation in bright and dim light. *Acta Psychiatr Scand*, 72, 161–165.

Wehr, T.A., Sack, D.A., Duncan, W.C., Mendelson, W.B., Rosenthal, N.E., Gillin, J.C., and Goodwin, F.K. (1985b). Sleep and circadian rhythms in affective patients isolated from external time cues. *Psychiatry Res*, 15(4), 327–339.

Wehr, T.A., Jacobsen, F.M., Sack, D.A., Arendt, J., Tamarkin, L., and Rosenthal, N.E. (1986). Phototherapy of seasonal affective disorder. Time of day and suppression of melatonin are not critical for antidepressant effects. *Arch Gen Psychiatry*, 43(9), 870–875.

Wehr, T.A., Sack, D.A., and Rosenthal, N.E. (1987). Sleep reduction as a final common pathway in the genesis of mania. *Am J Psychiatry*, 144(2), 201–204.

Wehr, T.A., Giesen, H.A., Schulz, P.M., Anderson, J.L., Joseph-Vanderpool, J.R., Kelly, K., Kasper, S., and Rosenthal, N.E. (1991). Contrasts between symptoms of summer depression and winter depression. *J Affect Disord*, 23(4), 173–183.

Wehr, T.A., Moul, D.E., Barbato, G., Giesen, H.A., Seidel, J.A., Barker, C., and Bender, C. (1993). Conservation of photoperiod-responsive mechanisms in humans. *Am J Physiol*, 265(4 Pt. 2), R846–R857.

Wehr, T.A., Giesen, H.A., Moul, D.E., Turner, E.H., and Schwartz, P.J. (1995). Suppression of men's responses to seasonal changes in day length by modern artificial lighting. *Am J Physiol*, 269(1 Pt. 2), R173–R178.

Wehr, T.A., Turner, E.H., Shimada, J.M., Lowe, C.H., Barker, C., and Leibenluft, E. (1998). Treatment of rapidly cycling bipolar patient by using extended bed rest and darkness to stabilize the timing and duration of sleep. *Biol Psychiatry*, 43(11), 822–828.

Wehr, T.A., Aeschbach, D., and Duncan, W.C. Jr. (2001a). Evidence for a biological dawn and dusk in the human circadian timing system. *J Physiol*, 535(Pt. 3), 937–951.

Wehr, T.A., Duncan, W.C. Jr., Sher, L., Aeschbach, D., Schwartz, P.J., Turner, E.H., Postolache, T.T., and Rosenthal, N.E. (2001b). A circadian signal of change of season in patients with seasonal affective disorder. *Arch Gen Psychiatry*, 58(12), 1108–1114.

Weissman, M.M., Greenwald, S., Nino-Murcia, G., and Dement, W.C. (1997). The morbidity of insomnia uncomplicated by psychiatric disorders. *Gen Hosp Psychiatry*, 19(4), 245–250.

Weitzman, E.D. (1982). Chronobiology of man. Sleep, temperature and neuroendocrine rhythms. *Hum Neurobiol*, 1(3), 173–183.

Welsh, D.K., and Moore-Ede, M.C. (1990). Lithium lengthens circadian period in a diurnal primate, *Saimiri sciureus*. *Biol Psychiatry*, 28(2), 117–126.

Welsh, D.K., Logothetis, D.E., Meister, M., and Reppert, S.M. (1995). Individual neurons dissociated from rat suprachiasmatic nucleus express independently phased circadian firing rhythms. *Neuron*, 14(4), 697–706.

Wever, R.A. (1979). *The Circadian System of Man: Results of Experiments under Temporal Isolation*. New York: Springer-Verlag.

Wever, R.A. (1980). Phase shifts of human circadian rhythms due to shifts of artificial zeitgebers. *Chronobiologia*, 7, 303–327.

Wever, R.A. (1983). Fractional desynchronization of human circadian rhythms. A method for evaluating entrainment limits and functional interdependencies. *Pflugers Arch*, 396(2), 128–137.

Wiegand, M., Berger, M., Zulley, J., Lauer, C., and von Zerssen, D. (1987). The influence of daytime naps on the therapeutic effect of sleep deprivation. *Biol Psychiatry*, 22(3), 389–392.

Wiegand, M., Riemann, D., Schreiber, W., Lauer, C.J., and Berger, M. (1993). Effect of morning and afternoon naps on mood after total sleep deprivation in patients with major depression. *Biol Psychiatry*, 33(6), 467–476.

Wilamowska, A., Pawlikowski, M., Klencki, M., and Kunert-Radek, J. (1992). Food restriction enhances melatonin effects on the pituitary-gonadal axis in female rats. *J Pineal Res*, 13(1), 1–5.

Williams, R.J., and Schmidt, G.G. (1993). Frequency of seasonal affective disorder among individuals seeking treatment at a northern Canadian mental health center. *Psychiatry Res*, 46(1), 41–45.

Winton, F., Corn, T., Huson, L.W., Franey, C., Arendt, J., and Checkley, S.A. (1989). Effects of light treatment upon mood and melatonin in patients with seasonal affective disorder. *Psychol Med*, 19(3), 585–590.

Wirz-Justice, A., and Richter, R. (1979). Seasonality in biochemical determinations: A source of variance and a clue to the temporal incidence of affective illness. *Psychiatry Res*, 1(1), 53–60.

Wirz-Justice, A., and Van den Hoofdakker, R.H. (1999). Sleep deprivation in depression: What do we know, where do we go? *Biol Psychiatry*, 46(4), 445–453.

Wirz-Justice, A., Pühringer, W., and Hole, G. (1979). Response to sleep deprivation as a predictor of therapeutic results with antidepressant drugs. *Am J Psychiatry*, 136, 1222–1223.

Wirz-Justice, A., Graw, P., Krauchi, K., Gisin, B., Jochum, A., Arendt, J., Fisch, H.U., Buddeberg, C., and Poldinger, W. (1993a). Light therapy in seasonal affective disorder is independent of time of day or circadian phase. *Arch Gen Psychiatry*, 50(12), 929–937.

Wirz-Justice, A., Graw, P., and Pecker, S. (1993b). The seasonal pattern questionnaire (SPAQ): Some comments. *Bull Soc Light Treat Biol Rhythms*, 5, 257–287.

Wirz-Justice, A., Graw, P., Roosli, H., Glauser, G., and Fleischhauer, J. (1999a). An open trial of light therapy in hospitalised major depression. *J Affect Disord*, 52(1–3), 291–292.

Wirz-Justice, A., Krauchi, K., Graw, P., Schulman, J., and Wirz, H. (1999b). *Seasonality in Switzerland: An epidemiological survey.* 4th Annual Meeting on Light Treatment and Biological Rhythms, Bethesda, MD.

Wirz-Justice, A., Quinto, C., Cajochen, C., Werth, E., and Hock, C. (1999c). A rapid-cycling bipolar patient treated with long nights, bedrest, and light. *Biol Psychiatry*, 45(8), 1075–1077.

Wirz-Justice, A., Benedetti, F., Berger, M., Lam, R.W., Martiny, K., Terman, M., and Wu, J.C. (2005). Chronotherapeutics (light and wake therapy) in affective disorders. *Psychol Med*, 35(7), 939–944.

Woodgett, J.R. (2001). Judging a protein by more than its name: GSK-3. *Sci STKE*, 2001(100), RE12.

Wu, J.C., and Bunney, W.E. (1990). The biological basis of an antidepressant response to sleep deprivation and relapse: Review and hypothesis. *Am J Psychiatry*, 147(1), 14–21.

Wu, J.C., Gillin, J.C., Buchsbaum, M.S., Hershey, T., Johnson, J.C., and Bunney, W.E. Jr. (1992). Effect of sleep deprivation on brain metabolism of depressed patients. *Am J Psychiatry*, 149(4), 538–543.

Wu, J., Buchsbaum, M.S., Gillin, J.C., Tang, C., Cadwell, S., Wiegand, M., Najafi, A., Klein, E., Hazen, K., Bunney, W.E. Jr., Fallon, J.H., and Keator, D. (1999). Prediction of antidepressant effects of sleep deprivation by metabolic rates in the ventral anterior cingulate and medial prefrontal cortex. *Am J Psychiatry*, 156(8), 1149–1158.

Wu, J.C., Buchsbaum, M., and Bunney, W.E. Jr. (2001). Clinical neurochemical implications of sleep deprivation's effects on the anterior cingulate of depressed responders. *Neuropsychopharmacology*, 25(Suppl. 5), S74–S78.

Yamada, N., Martin-Iverson, M.T., Daimon, K., Tsujimoto, T., and Takahashi, S. (1995). Clinical and chronobiological effects of light therapy on nonseasonal affective disorders. *Biol Psychiatry*, 37(12), 866–873.

Yamazaki, S., Goto, M., and Menaker, M. (1999). No evidence for extraocular photoreceptors in the circadian system of the Syrian hamster. *J Biol Rhythms*, 14(3), 197–201.

Yang, J.D., Elphick, M., Sharpley, A.L., and Cowen, P.J. (1989). Effects of carbamazepine on sleep in healthy volunteers. *Biol Psychiatry*, 26(3), 324–328.

Young, M.A., Watel, L.G., Lahmeyer, H.W., and Eastman, C.I. (1991). The temporal onset of individual symptoms in winter depression: Differentiating underlying mechanisms. *J Affect Disord*, 22(4), 191–197.

Young, M.A., Meaden, P.M., Fogg, L.F., Cherin, E.A., and Eastman, C.I. (1997). Which environmental variables are related to the onset of seasonal affective disorder? *J Abnorm Psychol*, 106(4), 554–562.

Zheng, B., Larkin, D.W., Albrecht, U., Sun, Z.S., Sage, M., Eichele, G., Lee, C.C., and Bradley, A. (1999). The *mPer2* gene encodes a functional component of the mammalian circadian clock. *Nature*, 400(6740), 169–173.

Zis, A.P., and Goodwin, F.K. (1979). Major affective disorder as a recurrent illness: A critical review. *Arch Gen Psychiatry*, 36, 835–839.

Zylka, M.J., Shearman, L.P., Levine, J.D., Jin, X., Weaver, D.R., and Reppert, S.M. (1998a). Molecular analysis of mammalian *timeless*. *Neuron*, 21(5), 1115–1122.

Zylka, M.J., Shearman, L.P., Weaver, D.R., and Reppert, S.M. (1998b). Three period homologs in mammals: Differential light responses in the suprachiasmatic circadian clock and oscillating transcripts outside of brain. *Neuron*, 20(6), 1103–1110.

Chapter 17

Abou-Saleh, M.T., and Coppen, A. (1986). Who responds to prophylactic lithium? *J Affect Disord*, 10, 115–125.

Almy, G.L., and Taylor, M.A. (1973). Lithium retention in mania. *Arch Gen Psychiatry*, 29, 232–234.

Altshuler, L., Suppes, T., Black, D., Nolen, W.A., Keck, P.E. Jr., Frye, M.A., McElroy, S., Kupka, R., Grunze, H., Walden, J., Leverich, G., Denicoff, K., Luckenbaugh, D., and Post, R. (2003). Impact of antidepressant discontinuation after acute bipolar depression remission on rates of depressive relapse at 1-year follow-up. *Am J Psychiatry*, 160(7), 1252–1262.

Baldessarini, R.J., Tondo, L., Hennen, J., and Floris, G. (1999). Latency and episodes before treatment: Response to lithium maintenance in bipolar I and II disorder. *Bipolar Disord*, 2, 91–97.

Baldessarini, R.J., Tondo, L., Floris, G., and Hennen, J. (2000). Effects of rapid cycling on response to lithium maintenance treatment in 360 bipolar I and II disorder patients. *J Affect Disord*, 61(1-2), 13–22.

Baldessarini, R.J., Pompili, M., and Tondo, L. (2006). Suicidal risk in antidepressant drug trials. *Arch Gen Psychiatry*, 63(3), 246–248.

Bauer, M.S., Kirk, G.F., Gavin, C., and Williford, W.O. (2001). Determinants of functional outcome and healthcare costs in bipolar disorder: A high-intensity follow-up study. *J Affect Disord*, 65, 231–241.

Bauer, M., Grof, P., and Müller-Oerlinghausen, B. (Eds.) (2002). *Lithium in Neuropsychiatry: The Comprehensive Guide.* Abington, England: Informa UK.

Bauer, M.S., McBride, L., Williford, W.O., Glick, H., Kinosian, B., Altshuler, L., Beresford, T., Kilbourne, A.M., Sajatovic, M., and Cooperative Studies Program 430 Study Team. (2006a). Collaborative care for bipolar disorder: Part I. Intervention and implementation in a randomized effectiveness trial. *Psychiatr Serv*, 57(7), 927–936.

Bauer, M.S., McBride, L., Williford, W.O., Glick, H., Kinosian, B., Altshuler, L., Beresford, T., Kilbourne, A.M., Sajatovic, M., and Cooperative Studies Program 430 Study Team. (2006b). Collaborative care for bipolar disorder: Part II. Impact on clinical outcome, function, and costs. *Psychiatr Serv*, 57(7), 937–945.

Begley, C.E., Annegers, J.F., Swann, A.C., Lewis, C., Coan, S., Schnapp, W.B., and Bryant-Comstock, L. (2001). The lifetime cost of bipolar disorder in the U.S.: An estimate for new cases in 1998. *Pharmacoeconomics*, 19(5 Pt. 1), 483–495.

Benson, K., and Hartz, A.J. (2000). A comparison of observational studies and randomized, controlled trials. *N Engl J Med*, 342, 1878–1886.

Blanco, C., Lajc, G., Olfson, M., Marcus, S.C., and Pincus, H.A. (2002). Trends in the treatment of bipolar disorder by outpatient psychiatrists. *Am J Psychiatry*, 159, 1005–1010.

Bowden, C.L., Brugger, A.M., Swann, A.C., Calabrese, J.R., Janicak, P.G., Petty, F., Dilsaver, S.C., Davis, J.M., Rush, A.J., Small, J.G., for the Depakote Mania Study Group. (1994). Efficacy of divalproex vs. lithium and placebo in the treatment of mania. The Depakote Mania Study Group. *JAMA*, 271(12), 918–924.

Calabrese, J.R., and Rapport, D.J. (1999). Mood stabilizers and the evolution of maintenance study designs in bipolar I disorder. *J Clin Psychiatry*, 60 (Suppl. 5), 5–13.

Calabrese, R.J., Hirschfeld, R.M.A., Reed, M., Davies, M.A., Frye, M.A., Keck, P.E., Lewis, L., McElroy, S.L., McNulty, J.P., and Wagner, K.D. (2003). Impact of bipolar disorder on a U.S. community sample. *J Clin Psychiatry*, 64, 425–432.

Chisholm, D., van Ommeren, M., Ayuso-Mateos, J.L., and Saxena, S. (2005). Cost-effectiveness of clinical interventions for reducing the global burden of bipolar disorder. *Br J Psychiatry*, 187, 559–567.

Coate, M. (1964). *Beyond all Reason*. London: Constable & Co.

Conus, P., Cotton, S., Abdel-Baki, A., Lambert, M., Berk, M., and McGorry, P.D. (2006). Symptomatic and functional outcome 12 months after a first episode of psychotic mania: Barriers to recovery in a catchment area sample. *Bipolar Disorders*, 8, 221–231.

Cooper, T.B., and Simpson, G.M. (1976). The 24-hour lithium level as a prognosticator of dosage requirements: A 2-year follow-up study. *Am J Psychiatry*, 133(4), 440–443.

Coryell, W., Scheftner, W., Keller, M., Endicott, J., Maser, J., and Klerman, G.L. (1993). The enduring psychosocial consequences of mania and depression. *Am J Psychiatry*, 150(5), 720–727.

Dardennes, R., Thuile, J., Friedman, S., and Guelfi, J.D. (2006). The costs of bipolar disorder. *Encephale*, 32(1 Pt. 1), 18–25.

Dion, G., Tohen, M., Anthony, W., and Waternaux, C. (1988). Symptoms and functioning of patients with bipolar disorder six months after hospitalization. *Hosp Commun Psychiatry*, 39, 652–657.

Ellenor, G.L., and Dishman, B.R. (1995). Pharmaceutical care role model in psychiatry—pharmacist prescribing. *Hosp Pharm*, 30(5), 377–378.

Fava, G.A., Molnar, G., Block, B., Lee, J.S., and Pereni, G.I. (1984). The lithium loading dose method in a clinical setting. *Am J Psychiatry*, 141, 812–813.

Fenn, H.H., Robinson, D., Luby, V., Dangel, C., Buxton, E., Beattie, M., Kraemer, H., and Yesavage, J.A. (1996). Trends in pharmacotherapy of schizoaffective and bipolar affective disorders: A 5-year naturalistic study. *Am J Psychiatry*, 153(5), 711–713.

Fountoulakis, K.N., Vieta, E., Sanchez-Moreno, J., Kaprinis, S.G., Goikolea, J.M., and Kaprinis, G.S. (2005). Treatment guidelines for bipolar disorder: A critical review. *J Affect Disord*, 86(1), 1–10.

Frances, A., Docherty, J.P., and Kahn, D.A. (1996). The Expert Consensus Guideline Series: Treatment of bipolar disorder. *J Clin Psychiatry*.

Franchini, L., Zanardi, R., Smeraldi, E., and Gasperini, M. (1999). Early onset of lithium prophylaxis as a predictor of good long-term outcome. *Eur Arch Psychiatry Clin Neurosci*, 249, 227–230.

Frangou, S., Raymont, V., and Bettany, D. (2002). The Maudsley bipolar disorder project: A survey of psychotropic prescribing patterns in bipolar I disorder. *Bipolar Disord*, 4, 378–385.

Gardner, H.H., Kleinman, N.L., Brook, R.A., Rajagopalan, K., Brizee, T.J., and Smeeding, J.E. (2006). The economic impact of bipolar disorder in an employed population from an employer perspective. *J Clin Psychiatry*, 67(8), 1209–1218.

Gelenberg, A.J., Kane, J.M., Keller, M.B., Lavori, P., Rosenbaum, J.F., Cole, K., and Lavelle, J. (1989). Comparison of standard and low serum levels of lithium for maintenance treatment of bipolar disorder. *N Engl J Med*, 321, 1489–1493.

Ghaemi, N., Sachs, G.S., and Goodwin, F.K. (2000). What is to be done? Controversies in the diagnosis and treatment of manic-depressive illness. *World J Biol Psychiatry*, 1(2), 65–74.

Ghaemi, S.N., Ko, J.Y., and Goodwin, F.K. (2002). "Cade's disease" and beyond: Misdiagnosis, antidepressant use, and a proposed definition for bipolar spectrum disorder. *Can J Psychiatry*, 47(2), 125–134.

Ghaemi, S.N., Hsu, D.J., Thase, M.E., Wisniewski, S.R., Nierenberg, A.A., Miyahara, S., and Sachs, G. (2006). Pharmacological treatment patterns at study entry for the first 500 STEP-BD participants. *Psychiatr Serv*, 57(5), 660–665.

Gillberg, I.C., Hellgren, L., and Gillberg, C. (1993). Psychotic disorders diagnosed in adolescence. Outcome at age 30 years. *J Child Psychol Psychiatry*, 34(7), 1173–1185.

Giroux, R. (Ed.) (1967). *Robert Lowell: Collected Prose*. New York: Farrar, Straus, Giroux.

Gitlin, M.J., Swendsen, J., Heller, T.L., and Hammen, C. (1995). Relapse and impairment in bipolar disorder. *Am J Psychiatry*, 152(11), 1635–1640.

Goldberg, J.F., and Ernst, C.L. (2002). Features associated with the delayed initiation of mood stabilizers at illness onset in bipolar disorder. *J Clin Psychiatry*, 63(11), 985–991.

Goodwin, F.K. (1999). Anticonvulsant therapy and suicide risk in affective disorders. *J Clin Psychiatry*, 60 (Suppl. 2), 89–93.

Goodwin, F.K. (2003). Impact of formularies of clinical innovation. *J Clin Psychiatry*, 64(Suppl. 17), 11–14.

Goodwin, F.K., and Goldstein, M.A. (2003). Optimizing lithium treatment in bipolar disorder: A review of the literature and clinical recommendations. *J Psychiatr Pract*, 9(5), 333–343.

Goodwin, F.K., Murphy, D.L., and Bunney, W.E. Jr. (1969). Lithium carbonate treatment in depression and mania: A longitudinal double-blind study. *Arch Gen Psychiatry*, 21, 486–496.

Goodwin, F.K., Fireman, B., Simon, G.E., Hunkeler, E.M., Lee, J., and Revicki, D. (2003). Suicide risk in bipolar disorder during treatment with lithium and divalproex. *JAMA*, 290(11), 1467–1473.

Goodwin, G.M. (2003). Evidence-based guidelines for treating bipolar disorder: Recommendations from the British Association for Psychopharmacology. *J Psychopharmacol*, 17, 149–173.

Goodwin, G.M., and Young, A.H. (2003). The British Association for Psychopharmacology guidelines for treatment of bipolar disorder: A summary. *J Psychopharmacol*, 17(4 Suppl.), 3–6.

Gray, G. (2002). Evidence-based medicine: An introduction for psychiatrists. *J Psychiatr Pract*, 8, 5–13.

Greenspan, K., Green, R., and Durrell, J. (1968). Retention and distribution patterns of lithium, a pharmacological tool in studying the pathophysiology of manic-depressive psychosis. *Am J Psychiatry*, 125, 512–519.

Griffith, J.L., and Griffith, M.E. (2002). *Engaging the Sacred in Psychotherapy: How to Talk with People about Their Spiritual Lives*. New York: Guilford Press.

Grunze, H., Kasper, S., Goodwin, G., Bowden, C.L., Baldwin, D., Licht, R.W., Vieta, E., Möller, H.-J., and WFSBP Task Force on Treatment Guidelines for Bipolar Disorders. (2002). The World Federation of Societies of Biological Psychiatry (WFSBP) Guidelines for the Biological Treatment of Bipolar Disorders. Part I: Treatment of bipolar depression. *World J Psychiatry*, 3, 115–124.

Grunze, H., Kasper, S., Goodwin, G., Bowden, C.L., Baldwin, D., Licht, R.W., Vieta, E., Möller, H.-J., and WFSBP Task Force on Treatment Guidelines for Bipolar Disorders. (2003). The World Federation of Societies of Biological Psychiatry (WFSBP) Guidelines for the Biological Treatment of Bipolar Disorders. Part II: Treatment of mania. *World J Psychiatry*, 4, 5–13.

Grunze, H., Kasper, S., Goodwin, G., Bowden, C.L., Möller, H.-J., and WFSBP Task Force on Treatment Guidelines for Bipolar Disorders. (2004). The World Federation of Societies of Biological Psychiatry (WFSBP) Guidelines for the Biological Treatment of Bipolar Disorders. Part III: Maintenance treatment. *World J Psychiatry*, 5, 120–135.

Heres, S., Davis, J., Maino, K., Jetzinger, E., Kissling, W., and Leucht, S. (2006). Why olanzapine beats risperidone, risperidone beats quetiapine, and quetiapine beats olanzapine: An exploratory analysis of head-to-head comparison studies of second-generation antipsychotics. *Am J Psychiatry*, 163(2), 185–194.

Himmelhoch, J.M. (2003). On the usefulness of clinical case studies. *Bipolar Disord*, 5, 69–71.

Hirschfeld, R.M.A., Bowden, C.L., Gitlin, M.J., Keck, P.E., Perlis, R.H., and Suppes, T. (2002). Practice guideline for the treatment of patients with bipolar disorder (revision). *Am J Psychiatry*, 159(Suppl.), 1–50.

Hirschfeld, R.M.A., Calabrese, J.R., Weissman, M.M., Reed, M., Davies, M.A., Frye, M.A., Keck, P.E. Jr., Lewis, L., McElroy, S.L., McNulty, J.P., and Wagner, K.D. (2003). Screening for bipolar disorder in the community. *J Clin Psychiatry*, 64, 53–59.

Hunkeler, E.M., Westphal, J.R., and Williams, M. (1995). Developing a system for automated monitoring of psychiatric outpatients: A first step to improve quality. *HMO Pract*, 9(4), 162–167.

Jackson, A., Cavanagh, J., and Scott, J. (2003). A systematic review of manic and depressive prodromes. *J Affect Disord*, 74(3), 209–217.

Jaffe, S.L., and Yager, J. (1999). A pilot study of a district branch-based educational intervention: Awareness and reactions. *Acad Psychiatry*, 23, 9–13.

Josephson, A., and Peteet, J. (Eds.). (2004). *Handbook of Spirituality and Worldview in Clinical Practice*. Arlington, VA: American Psychiatric Publishing.

Judd, L.L., Akiskal, H.S., Schettler, P.J., Endicott, J., Leon, A.C., Solomon, D.A., Coryell, W., Maser, J.D., and Keller, M.B. (2005). Psychosocial disability in the course of bipolar I and II disorders: A prospective, comparative, longitudinal study. *Arch Gen Psychiatry*, 62(12), 1322–1330.

Keck, P.E., Strakowski, S.M., Hawkins, J.M., Dunayevich, E., Tugrul, K.C., Bennett, J.A., and McElroy, S.L. (2001). A pilot study of rapid lithium administration in the treatment of acute mania. *Bipolar Disord*, 4(4), 68–72.

Keck, P.E., Perlis, R.H., Otto, M.W., Carpenter, D., Ross, R., and Docherty, J.P. (2004). The Expert Consensus Guideline Series: Treatment of bipolar disorder 2004. *Postgrad Med Special Report*, 1, 120.

Kessler, R.C., Akiskal, H.S., Ames, M., Birnbaum, H., Greenberg, M.A., Jin, R., Merikangas, K.R., Simon, G.E., and Wang, P.S. (2006). Prevalence and effects of mood disorders on work performance in a nationally representative sample of U.S. workers. *Am J Psychiatry*, 163(9), 1561–1569.

Ketter, T.A., Frye, M.A., Cora-Locatelli, G., Kimbrell, T.A., and Post, R.M. (1999). Metabolism and excretion of mood stabilizers and new anticonvulsants. *Cell Mol Neurobiol*, 19(4), 511–532.

Kleinman, L., Lowin, A., Flood, E., Gandhi, G., Edgell, E., and Revicki, D. (2003). Costs of bipolar disorder. *Pharmacoeconomics*, 21(9), 601–622.

Kuhn, R. (1957). Über die Behandlung depressiver Zustände mit einem Iminodibenzylderivat (G 22355). [Treatment of depressive states with an iminodibenzyl derivative (G 22355)]. *Schweiz Med Wochenschrift*, 87, 1135–1140.

Kukopulos, A., Minnai, G., and Müller-Oerlinghausen, B. (1985). The influence of mania and depression on the pharmacokinetics of lithium: A longitudinal single-case study. *J Affect Disord*, 8, 159–166.

Levine, J., Chengappa, K.N.R., Brar, J.S., Gershon, S., Yablonsky, E., Stapf, D., and Kupfer, D.J. (2000). Psychotropic drug prescription patterns among patients with bipolar I disorder. *Bipolar Disord*, 2, 120–130.

Li, J., McCombs, J.S., and Stimmel, G.L. (2002). Cost of treating bipolar disorder in the California Medicaid (Medi-Cal) program. *J Affect Disord*, 71(1–3), 131–139.

Licht, R.W. (2002). Limits of the applicability and generalizability of drug trials in mania. *Bipolar Disord*, 4(Suppl. 1), 66–68.

Licht, R.W., Vestergaard, P., Kessing, L.V., Larsen, J.K., Thomsen, P.H., and Danish Psychiatric Association, and the Child and Adolescent Psychiatric Association in Denmark. (2003). Psychopharmacological treatment with lithium and antiepileptic drugs: Suggested guidelines from the Danish Psychiatric Association and the Child and Adolescent Psychiatric Association in Denmark. *Acta Psychiatr Scand*, 108(Suppl. 419), 1–22.

Lieberman, D.Z., Saggese, J.M., and Goodwin, F.K. (2006). Different views on the use of lithium across continents. In M. Bauer, P. Goff, and B. Muller-Oerlinghausen (Eds.), *Lithium and Neuropsychiatry: The Comprehensive Guide*. London: Taylor & Francis.

Lim, P.Z., Tunis, S.L., Edell, W.S., Jensik, S.E., and Tohen, M. (2001). Medication prescribing patterns for patients with bipolar I disorder in hospital settings: Adherence to published practice guidelines. *Bipolar Disord*, 3, 154–173.

Lish, J.D., Dime-Meenan, S., Whybrow, P.C., Price, R.A., and Hirschfeld, R.M. (1994). The National Depressive and Manic-Depressive Association (DMDA) survey of bipolar members. *J Affect Disord*, 31, 281–294.

Lloyd, A.J., Harrison, C.L., Ferrier, I.N., and Young, A.H. (2003). The pharmacological treatment of bipolar affective disorder: Practice is improving but could still be better. *J Psychopharmacol*, 17(2), 230–233.

Matza, L.S., Rajagopalan, K.S., Thompson, C.L., and de Lissovoy, G. (2005). Misdiagnosed patients with bipolar disorder: Comorbidities, treatment patterns, and direct treatment costs. *J Clin Psychiatry*, 66(11), 1432–1440.

McElroy, S.L., Frye, M., Denicoff, K., Altshuler, L., Nolen, W., Kupka, R., Suppes, T., Keck, P.E. Jr., Leverich, G.S., Kmetz, G.F., and Post, R.M. (1998). Olanzapine in treatment-resistant bipolar disorder. *J Affect Disord*, 49(2), 119–122.

McIntyre, R.S., Konarski, J.Z., Soczynska, J.K., Wilkins, K., Panjwani, G., Bouffard, B., Bottas, A., and Kennedy, S.H. (2006). Medical comorbidity in bipolar disorder: Implications for functional outcomes and health service utilization. *Psychiatr Serv*, 57(8), 1140–1144.

Murray, C.J., and Lopez, A.D. (1996). Evidence-based health policy: Lessons from the global burden of disease study. *Science*, 274(5288), 740–743.

O'Connell, R.A., Mayo, J.A., and Flatow, L., Cuthbertson, B., and O'Brien, B.E. (1991). Outcome of bipolar disorder on long-term treatment with lithium. *Br J Psychiatry*, 159, 123–129.

Perlis, R.H. (2005). The role of pharmacologic treatment guidelines for bipolar disorder. *J Clin Psychiatry*, 66(Suppl. 3), 37–47.

Perlis, R.H., Ostacher, M.J., Patel, J.K., Marangell, L.B., Zhang, H., Wisniewski, S.R., Ketter, T.A., Miklowitz, D.J., Otto, M.W., Gyulai, L., Reilly-Harrington, N.A., Nierenberg, A.A., Sachs, G.S., and Thase, M.E. (2006). Predictors of recurrence in bipolar disorder: Primary outcomes from the Systematic Treatment Enhancement Program for Bipolar Disorder (STEP-BD). *Am J Psychiatry*, 163(2), 217–224.

Perry, A., Tarrier, N., Morriss, R., McCarthy, E., and Limb, K. (1999). Randomised controlled trial of efficacy of teaching patients with bipolar disorder to identify early symptoms of relapse and obtain treatment. *BMJ*, 318(7177), 149–153.

Perry, P.J., Alexander, B., Prince, R.A., and Dunner, F.J. (1984). Prospective evaluation of two lithium maintenance dose schedules. *J Clin Psychopharmacol*, 4, 242–246.

Post, R.M. (2005). The impact of bipolar depression. *J Clin Psychiatry*, 66(Suppl. 5), 5–10.

Post, R.M., and Luckenbaugh, D.A. (2003). Unique design issues in clinical trials of patients with bipolar affective disorder. *J Psychiatr Res*, 37(1), 61–73.

Prien, R.F., Caffey, E.M. Jr., and Klett, J. (1974). Factors associated with treatment success in lithium carbonate prophylaxis: Report of the Veterans Administration and National Institute of Mental Health Collaborative Study Group. *Arch Gen Psychiatry*, 31, 189–192.

Pugh, C.B., and Garnett, W.R. (1991). Current issues in the treatment of epilepsy. *Clin Pharmacol*, 10(5), 335–358.

Reinares, M., Vieta, E., Colom, F., Martinez-Aran, A., Torrent, C., Comes, M., Goikolea, J.M., Benabarre, A., Daban, C., and Sanchez-Moreno, J. (2006). What really matters to bipolar patients' caregivers: Sources of family burden. *J Affect Disord*, 94(1-3), 157–163.

Rush, A.J., Post, R.M., Nolen, W.A., Keck, P.E. Jr., Suppes, T., Altshuler, L., and McElroy, S.L. (2000). Methodological issues in developing new acute treatments for patients with bipolar illness. *Biol Psychiatry*, 48(6), 615–624.

Schaffer, A., Cairney, J., Cheung, A.H., Veldhuizen, S., and Levitt, A.J. (2006). Use of treatment services and pharmacotherapy for bipolar disorder in a general population-based mental health survey. *J Clin Psychiatry*, 67(3), 386–393.

Serry, M. (1969). The lithium excretion test I: Clinical application and interpretation. *Aust NZ J Psychiatry*, 3, 390–394.

Simon, G.E., and Unutzer, J. (1999). Health care utilization and costs among patients treated for bipolar disorder in an insured population. *Psychiatr Serv*, 50(10), 1303–1308.

Simon, G.E., Ludman, E.J., Unutzer, J., Bauer, M.S., Operskalski, B., and Rutter, C. (2005). Randomized trial of a population-based care program for people with bipolar disorder. *Psychol Med*, 35(1), 13–24.

Simon, G.E., Ludman, E.J., Bauer, M.S., Unutzer, J., and Operskalski, B. (2006). Long-term effectiveness and cost of a systematic care program for bipolar disorder. *Arch Gen Psychiatry*, 63(5), 500–508.

Soldani, F., Ghaemi, S.N., and Baldessarini, R.J. (2005). Research reports on treatments for bipolar disorder: Preliminary assessment of methodological quality. *Acta Psychiatr Scand*, 112(1), 72–74.

Spiker, D.G., and Pugh, D.D. (1976). Combining tricyclic and monoamine oxidase inhibitor antidepressants. *Arch Gen Psychiatry*, 33, 828–830.

Strakowski, S.M., Sax, K.W., McElroy, S.L., Keck, P.E., Hawkins, J.M., and West, S.A. (1998). Course of psychiatric and substance abuse syndromes co-occurring with bipolar disorder after a first psychiatric hospitalization. *J Clin Psychiatry*, 59(9), 465–471.

Strakowski, S.M., DelBello, M.P., Fleck, D.E., and Arndt, S. (2000). The impact of substance abuse on the course of bipolar disorder. *Biol Psychiatry*, 48(6), 477–485.

Suppes, T., Dennehy, E.B., Hirschfeld, R.M., Altshuler, L.L., Bowden, C.L., Calabrese, J.R., Crismon, M.L., Ketter, T.A., Sachs, G.S., and Swann, A.C. (2005). The Texas implementation of medication algorithms: Update to the algorithms for treatment of bipolar I disorder. *J Clin Psychiatry*, 66(7), 870–886.

Swann, A.C., Bowden, C.L., Calabrese, J.R., Dilsaver, S.C., and Morris, D.D. (1999). Differential effect of number of previous episodes of affective disorder on response to lithium or divalproex in acute mania. *Am J Psychiatry*, 156(8), 1264–1266.

Tohen, M., Waternaux, C.M., and Tsuang, M.T. (1990). Outcome in mania. A 4-year prospective follow-up of 75 patients utilizing survival analysis. *Arch Gen Psychiatry*, 47(12), 1106–1111.

Tohen, M., Tsuang, M.T., and Goodwin, D.C. (1992). Prediction of outcome in mania by mood-congruent or mood-incongruent psychotic features. *Am J Psychiatry*, 149(11), 1580–1584.

Tohen, M., Hennen, J., Zarate, C.M., Jr., Baldessarini, R.J., Strakowski, S.M., Stoll, A.L., Faedda, G.L., Suppes, T., Gebre-Medhin, P., and Cohen, B.M. (2000). Two-year syndromal and functional recovery in 219 cases of first-episode major affective disorder with psychotic features. *Am J Psychiatry*, 157(2), 220–228.

Tohen, M., Baker, R.W., Altshuler, L.L., Zarate, C.A., Suppes, T., Ketter, T.A., Milton, D.R., Risser, R., Gilmore, J.A., Breier, A., and Tollefson, G.A. (2002). Olanzapine versus divalproex in the treatment of acute mania. *Am J Psychiatry*, 159(6), 1011–1017.

Tohen, M., Calabrese, J.R., Sachs, G.S., Banov, M.D., Detke, H.C., Risser, R., Baker, R.W., Chou, J.C., and Bowden, C.L. (2006). Randomized, placebo-controlled trial of olanzapine as maintenance therapy in patients with bipolar I disorder responding to acute treatment with olanzapine. *Am J Psychiatry*, 163(2), 247–256.

Vestergaard, P. (2004). Guidelines for maintenance treatment of bipolar disorder: Are there discrepancies between European and North American recommendations? *Bipolar Disord*, 6(6), 519–522.

Vestergaard, P., and Schou, M. (1987). Does long-term lithium treatment induce diabetes mellitus? *Neuropsychobiology*, 17, 130–132.

Vieta, E., and Carne, X. (2005). The use of placebo in clinical trials on bipolar disorder: A new approach for an old debate. *Psychother Psychosom*, 74(1), 10–16.

Wang, P.S., Lane, M., Olfson, M., Pincus, H.A., Wells, K.B., and Kessler, R.C. (2005). Twelve-month use of mental health services in the United States. *Arch Gen Psychiatry*, 62, 629–640.

Wightman, W.P.D. (1971). *The Emergency of Scientific Medicine*. Edinburgh: Oliver & Boyd.

Winokur, G., Coryell, W., Keller, M., Endicott, J., and Akiskal, H. (1993). A prospective follow-up of patients with bipolar and primary unipolar affective disorder. *Arch Gen Psychiatry*, 50, 457–465.

Wyatt, R.J., and Henter, I. (1995). An economic evaluation of manic-depressive illness—1991. *Soc Psychiatry Psychiatr Epidemiol*, 30(5), 213–219.

Yatham, L.N., Kennedy, S.H., O'Donovan, C., Parikh, S., MacQueen, G., McIntyre, R., Sharma, V., Silverstone, P., Alda, M., Baruch, P., Beaulieu, S., Daigneault, A., Milev, R., Young, L.T., Ravindran, A., Schaffer, A., Connolly, M., and Gorman, C.P. (2005). Canadian Network for Mood and Anxiety Treatments (CANMAT) guidelines for the management of patients with bipolar disorder: Consensus and controversies. *Bipolar Disord*, 7(Suppl. 3), 5–69.

Zajecka, J.M., Weisler, R., Sachs, G., Swann, A.C., Wozniak, P., and Sommerville, K.W. (2002). A comparison of the efficacy, safety, and tolerability of divalproex sodium and olanzapine in the treatment of bipolar disorder. *J Clin Psychiatry*, 63(12), 1148–1155.

Ziegler, V.E., Wylie, L.T., and Biggs, J.T. (1978). Intrapatient variability of serial steady-state plasma tricyclic antidepressant concentrations. *J Pharm Sci*, 67(4), 554–555.

Chapter 18

Abbott Laboratories. (2005). *Abbott's Depakote® ER (Divalproex Sodium Extended-Release Tablets) approved for acute mania or mixed episodes associated with bipolar disorder*. Available: http://abbott.com/news/press_release.cfm?id=1034 [January 27, 2006].

Altshuler, L.L., Keck, P.E. Jr., McElroy, S.L., Suppes, T., Brown, E.S., Denicoff, K., Frye, M., Gitlin, M., Hwang, S., Goodman, R., Leverich, G., Nolen, W., Kupka, R., and Post, R. (1999). Gabapentin in the acute treatment of refractory bipolar disorder. *Bipolar Disord*, 1(1), 61–65.

Amann, B., and Grunze, H. (2005). Neurochemical underpinnings in bipolar disorder and epilepsy. *Epilepsia*, 46(Suppl. 4), 26–30.

Anand, A., Oren, D.A., Berman, R.M., Cappiello, A., and Charney, D.S. (1999). Lamotrigine treatment of lithium failure outpatient mania: A double-blind placebo-controlled trial. *Bipolar Disord*, S1(1), 23.

Aronson, T.A., Shukla, S., and Hirschowitz, J. (1989). Clonazepam treatment of five lithium-refractory patients with bipolar disorder. *Am J Psychiatry*, 146(1), 77–80.

Baker, R.W., Goldberg, J.F., Tohen, M., Milton, D.R., Stauffer, V.L., and Schuh, L.M. (2002). The impact of response to previous mood stabilizer therapy on response to olanzapine versus placebo for acute mania. *Bipolar Disord*, 4(1), 43–49.

Baker, R.W., Milton, D.R., Stauffer, V.L., Gelenberg, A., and Tohen, M. (2003a). Placebo-controlled trials do not find association of olanzapine with exacerbation of bipolar mania. *J Affect Disord*, 73(1-2), 147–153.

Baker, R.W., Tohen, M., Fawcett, J., Risser, R.C., Schuh, L.M., Brown, E., Stauffer, V.L., Shao, L., and Tollefson, G.D. (2003b). Acute dysphoric mania: Treatment response to olanzapine compared to placebo. *J Clin Psychopharmacol*, 23(2), 132–137.

Baker, R.W., Brown, E., Akiskal, H.S., Calabrese, J.R., Ketter, T.A., Schuh, L.M., Trzepacz, P.T., Watkin, J.G., and Tohen, M. (2004). Efficacy of olanzapine combined with valproate or lithium in the treatment of dysphoric mania. *Br J Psychiatry*, 185, 472–478.

Baldessarini, R.J., Tondo, L., Floris, G., and Hennen, J. (2000). Effects of rapid cycling on response to lithium maintenance treatment in 360 bipolar I and II disorder patients. *J Affect Disord*, 61(1-2), 13–22.

Baldessarini, R.J., Hennen, J., Wilson, M., Calabrese, J., Chengappa, R., Keck, P.E. Jr., McElroy, S.L., Sachs, G., Vieta, E., Welge, J.A., Yatham, L.N., Zarate, C.A. Jr., Baker, R.W., and Tohen, M. (2003). Olanzapine versus placebo in acute mania: Treatment responses in subgroups. *J Clin Psychopharmacol*, 23(4), 370–376.

Ballenger, J.C., and Post, R.M. (1980). Carbamazepine in manic-depressive illness: A new treatment. *Am J Psychiatry*, 137(7), 782–790.

Barbini, B., Scherillo, P., Benedetti, F., Crespi, G., Colombo, C., and Smeraldi, E. (1997). Response to clozapine in acute mania is more rapid than that of chlorpromazine. *Int Clin Psychopharmacol*, 12(2), 109–112.

Barton, B.M., and Gitlin, M.J. (1987). Verapamil in treatment-resistant mania: An open trial. *J Clin Psychopharmacol*, 7(2), 101–103.

Benabarre, A., Vieta, E., Colom, F., Martinez, A., Reinares, M., and Corbella, B. (2001). Treatment of mixed mania with risperidone and mood stabilizers. *Can J Psychiatry*, 46(9), 866–867.

Benazzi, F. (1998). Mania associated with donepezil. *Int J Geriatr Psychiatry*, 13(11), 814–815.

Benedetti, A., Lattanzi, L., Pini, S., Musetti, L., Dell'Osso, L., and Cassano, G.B. (2004). Oxcarbazepine as add-on treatment in patients with bipolar manic, mixed or depressive episode. *J Affect Disord*, 79(1-3), 273–277.

Bennett, J., Goldman, W.T., and Suppes, T. (1997). Gabapentin for treatment of bipolar and schizoaffective disorders. *J Clin Psychopharmacol*, 17(2), 141–142.

Berigan, T.R. (2002). Zonisamide treatment of bipolar disorder: A case report. *Can J Psychiatry*, 47(9), 887.

Berk, M., Ichim, L., and Brook, S. (1999). Olanzapine compared to lithium in mania: A double-blind randomized controlled trial. *Int Clin Psychopharmacol*, 14(6), 339–343.

Bersani, G. (2004). Levetiracetam in bipolar spectrum disorders: First evidence of efficacy in an open add-on study. *Hum Psycholpharmacol*, 19, 355–356.

Black, D.W., Winokur, G., and Nasrallah, A. (1987). Treatment of mania: A naturalistic study of electroconvulsive therapy versus lithium in 438 patients. *J Clin Psychiatry*, 48, 132–139.

Bowden, C.L. (1995). Predictors of response to divalproex and lithium. *J Clin Psychiatry*, 56(Suppl. 3), 25–30.

Bowden, C.L., Brugger, A.M., Swann, A.C., Calabrese, J.R., Janicak, P.G., Petty, F., Dilsaver, S.C., Davis, J.M., Rush, A.J., Small, J.G., Garza-Treviño, E.S., Risch, S.C., Goodnick, P.J., and Morris, D.D. (1994). Efficacy of divalproex vs. lithium and

placebo in the treatment of mania. The Depakote Mania Study Group. *JAMA*, 271(12), 918–924.

Bowden, C.L., Janicak, P.G., Orsulak, P., Swann, A.C., Davis, J.M., Calabrese, J.R., Goodnick, P., Small, J.G., Rush, A.J., Kimmel, S.E., Risch, S.C., and Morris, D.D. (1996). Relation of serum valproate concentration to response in mania. *Am J Psychiatry*, 153(6), 765–770.

Bowden, C.L., Calabrese, J.R., McElroy, S.L., Rhodes, L.J., Keck, P.E. Jr., Cookson, J., Anderson, J., Bolden-Watson, C., Ascher, J., Monaghan, E., and Zhou, J. (1999). The efficacy of lamotrigine in rapid cycling and non-rapid cycling patients with bipolar disorder. *Biol Psychiatry*, 45(8), 953–958.

Bowden, C.L., Grunze, H., Mullen, J., Brecher, M., Paulsson, B., Jones, M., Vagero, M., and Svensson, K. (2005). A randomized, double-blind, placebo-controlled efficacy and safety study of quetiapine or lithium as monotherapy for mania in bipolar disorder. *J Clin Psychiatry*, 66(1), 111–121.

Bowden, C.L., Calabrese, J.R., Wallin, B.A., Swann, A.C., McElroy, S.L., Risch, S.C., and Hirschfeld, M.A. (1995). Illness characteristics of patients in clinical drug studies of mania. *Psychopharmacol Bull*, 31(1), 103–109.

Bowden, C.L., Swann, A.C., Calabrese, J.R., Rubenfaer, L.M., Wozniak, P.J., Collins, M.A., Abi-Saab, W., Saltarelli, M., for the Depakote ER Mania Study Group. (2006). A randomized, placebo-controlled, multicenter study of divalproex sodium extended release in the treatment of acute mania. *J Clin Psychiatry*, 67(10), 1501–1510.

Bozikas, V.P., Petrikis, P., Kourtis, A., Youlis, P., and Karavatos, A. (2002). Treatment of acute mania with topiramate in hospitalized patients. *Prog Neuropsychopharmacol Biol Psychiatry*, 26(6), 1203–1206.

Bradwejn, J., Shriqui, C., Koszycki, D., and Meterissian, G. (1990). Double-blind comparison of the effects of clonazepam and lorazepam in acute mania. *J Clin Psychopharmacol*, 10(6), 403–408.

Braunig, P., and Kruger, S. (2003). Levetiracetam in the treatment of rapid cycling bipolar disorder. *J Psychopharmacol*, 17, 239–241.

Brook, S., Lucey, J.V., and Gunn, K.P. (2000). Intramuscular ziprasidone compared with intramuscular haloperidol in the treatment of acute psychosis. Ziprasidone I.M. Study Group. *J Clin Psychiatry*, 61(12), 933–941.

Burt, T., Sachs, G.S., and Demopulos, C. (1999). Donepezil in treatment-resistant bipolar disorder. *Biol Psychiatry*, 45(8), 959–964.

Cabras, P.L., Hardoy, M.J., Hardoy, M.C., and Carta, M.G. (1999). Clinical experience with gabapentin in patients with bipolar or schizoaffective disorder: Results of an open-label study. *J Clin Psychiatry*, 60(4), 245–248.

Calabrese, J.R., and Delucchi, G.A. (1990). Spectrum of efficacy of valproate in 55 patients with rapid-cycling bipolar disorder. *Am J Psychiatry*, 147(4), 431–434.

Calabrese, J.R., Markovitz, P.J., Kimmel, S.E., and Wagner, S.C. (1992). Spectrum of efficacy of valproate in 78 rapid-cycling bipolar patients. *J Clin Psychopharmacol*, 12(Suppl. 1), 53S–56S.

Calabrese, J.R., Kimmel, S.E., Woyshville, M.J., Rapport, D.J., Faust, C.J., Thompson, P.A., and Meltzer, H.Y. (1996). Clozapine for treatment-refractory mania. *Am J Psychiatry*, 153(6), 759–764.

Calabrese, J.R., Bowden, C.L., McElroy, S.L., Cookson, J., Andersen, J., Keck, P.E. Jr., Rhodes, L., Bolden-Watson, C., Zhou, J., and Ascher, J.A. (1999). Spectrum of activity of lamotrigine in treatment-refractory bipolar disorder. *Am J Psychiatry*, 156(7), 1019–1023.

Calabrese, J.R., Suppes, T., Bowden, C.L., Sachs, G.S., Swann, A.C., McElroy, S.L., Kusumakar, V., Ascher, J.A., Earl, N.L., Greene, P.L., and Monaghan, E.T. (2000). A double-blind, placebo-controlled, prophylaxis study of lamotrigine in rapid-cycling bipolar disorder. Lamictal 614 Study Group. *J Clin Psychiatry*, 61(11), 841–850.

Calabrese, J.R., Keck, P.E. Jr., McElroy, S.L., and Shelton, M.D. (2001). A pilot study of topiramate as monotherapy in the treatment of acute mania. *J Clin Psychopharmacol*, 21(3), 340–342.

Calabrese, J.R., Shelton, M.D., Rapport, D.J., Youngstrom, E.A., Jackson, K., Bilali, S., Ganocy, S.J., and Findling, R.L. (2005). A 20-month, double-blind, maintenance trial of lithium versus divalproex in rapid-cycling bipolar disorder. *Am J Psychiatry*, 162(11), 2152–2161.

Chase, P.B., and Biros, M.H. (2002). A retrospective review of the use and safety of droperidol in a large, high-risk, inner-city emergency department patient population. *Acad Emerg Med*, 9(12), 1402–1410.

Chen, S.T., Altshuler, L.L., Melnyk, K.A., Erhart, S.M., Miller, E., and Mintz, J. (1999). Efficacy of lithium vs. valproate in the treatment of mania in the elderly: A retrospective study. *J Clin Psychiatry*, 60(3), 181–186.

Chengappa, K.N., Rathore, D., Levine, J., Atzert, R., Solai, L., Parepally, H., Levin, H., Moffa, N., Delaney, J., and Brar, J.S. (1999). Topiramate as add-on treatment for patients with bipolar mania. *Bipolar Disord*, 1(1), 42–53.

Chengappa, K.N., Baker, R.W., Shao, L., Yatham, L.N., Tohen, M., Gershon, S., and Kupfer, D.J. (2003). Rates of response, euthymia and remission in two placebo-controlled olanzapine trials for bipolar mania. *Bipolar Disord*, 5(1), 1–5.

Chengappa, K.N.R., Schwarzman, L.K., Hulihan, J.F., Xiang, J., and Rosenthal, N.R., for the Clinical Affairs Product Support Study-168 Investigators. (2006). Adjunctive topiramate therapy in patients receiving a mood stabilizer for bipolar disorder: A randomized, placebo-controlled trial. *J Clin Psychiatry*, 67, 1698–1706.

Chisholm, K.A., Dennehy, E.B., and Suppes, T. (2001). *Clinical responses to quetiapine add-on for the treatment of refractory bipolar disorder.* 8th International Conference on Bipolar Disorder, Pittsburgh, PA.

Chou, J.C., Zito, J.M., Vitrai, J., Craig, T.J., Allingham, B.H., and Czobor, P. (1996). Neuroleptics in acute mania: A pharmacoepidemiologic study. *Ann Pharmacother*, 30(12), 1396–1398.

Chou, J.C., Czobor, P., Charles, O., Tuma, I., Winsberg, B., Allen, M.H., Trujillo, M., and Volavka, J. (1999). Acute mania: Haloperidol dose and augmentation with lithium or lorazepam. *J Clin Psychopharmacol*, 19(6), 500–505.

Chouinard, G., Young, S.N., and Annable, L. (1983). Antimanic effect of clonazepam. *Biol Psychiatry*, 18(4), 451–466.

Chouinard, G., Annable, L., Turnier, L., Holobow, N., and Szkrumelak, N. (1993). A double-blind randomized clinical trial of rapid tranquilization with I.M. clonazepam and I.M. haloperidol in agitated psychotic patients with manic symptoms. *Can J Psychiatry*, 38(Suppl. 4), S114–S121.

Ciapparelli, A., Dell'Osso, L., Tundo, A., Pini, S., Chiavacci, M.C., Di Sacco, I., and Cassano, G.B. (2001). Electroconvulsive therapy in medication-nonresponsive patients with mixed mania and bipolar depression. *J Clin Psychiatry*, 62(7), 552–555.

Cipriani, A., Rendell, J.M., and Geddes, J.R. (2006). Haloperidol alone or in combination for acute mania. *Cochrane Database Syst Rev*, 19, 3:CD004362.

Curtin, F., and Schultz, P. (2004). Clonazepam and larazepam in acute mania: A Bayesian meta-analysis. *J Affect Disord*, 78, 201–208.

Dalkilic, A., Diaz, E., Baker, C.B., Pearsall, H.R., and Woods, S.W. (2000). Effects of divalproex versus lithium on length of hospital stay among patients with bipolar disorder. *Psychiatr Serv*, 51(9), 1184–1186.

Dam, M. (1994). Practical aspects of oxcarbazepine treatment. *Epilepsia*, 35(Suppl. 3), S23–S25.

Daniel, D.G., Zimbroff, D.L., Swift, R.H., and Harrigan, E.P. (2004). The tolerability of intramuscular ziprasidone and haloperidol treatment and the transition to oral therapy. *Int Clin Psychopharmacol*, 19(1), 9–15.

Dean, C.E. (2000). Prasterone (DHEA) and mania. *Ann Pharmacother*, 34(12), 1419–1422.

DelBello, M.P., Findling, R.L., Kushner, S., Wang, D., Olson, W.H., Capece, J.A., Fazzio, L., and Rosenthal, N.R. (2005). A pilot controlled trial of topiramate for mania in children and adolescents with bipolar disorder. *J Am Acad Child Adolesc Psychiatry*, 44(6), 539–547.

Denicoff, K.D., Smith-Jackson, E.E., Disney, E.R., Ali, S.O., Leverich, G.S., and Post, R.M. (1997). Comparative prophylactic efficacy of lithium, carbamazepine, and the combination in bipolar disorder. *J Clin Psychiatry*, 58(11), 470–478.

Desai, N.G., Gangahar, B.N., Channabasavanna, S.M., and Shetty, K.T. (1987). Carbamazepine hastens therapeutic action of lithium in mania. *Proceedings of the International Conference on New Directions in Affective Disorders*, 97.

Dose, M., Emrich, H.M., Cording-Tommel, C., and von Zerssen, D. (1986). Use of calcium antagonists in mania. *Psychoneuroendocrinology*, 11(2), 241–243.

Dubovsky, S.L., Franks, R.D., Allen, S., and Murphy, J. (1986). Calcium antagonists in mania: A double-blind study of verapamil. *Psychiatry Res*, 18(4), 309–320.

Dunayevich, E., and Strakowski, S.M. (2000). Quetiapine for treatment-resistant mania. *Am J Psychiatry*, 157(8), 1341.

Dunner, D.L. (2000). Optimizing lithium treatment. *J Clin Psychiatry*, 61(Suppl. 9), 76–81.

Dunner, D.L., and Fieve, R.R. (1974). Clinical factors in lithium carbonate prophylaxis failure. *Arch Gen Psychiatry*, (2), 229–233.

Dwight, M.M., Keck, P.E. Jr., Stanton, S.P., Strakowski, S.M., and McElroy, S.L. (1994). Antidepressant activity and mania associated with risperidone treatment of schizoaffective disorder. *Lancet*, 344(8921), 554–555.

Eden Evins, A., Demopulos, C., Nierenberg, A., Culhane, M.A., Eisner, L., and Sachs, G. (2006). A double-blind, placebo-controlled trial of adjunctive donepezil in treatment-resistant mania. *Bipolar Disord*, 8(1), 75–80.

Edwards, R., Stephenson, U., and Flewett, T. (1991). Clonazepam in acute mania: A double-blind trial. *Aust N Z J Psychiatry*, 25(2), 238–242.

Emilien, G., Maloteaux, J.M., Seghers, A., and Charles, G. (1996). Lithium compared to valproic acid and carbamazepine in the treatment of mania: A statistical meta-analysis. *Eur Neuropsychopharmacol*, 6(3), 245–252.

Emrich, H.M. (1990). Studies with oxcarbazepine in acute mania. *Int Clin Psychopharmacol*, 5(Suppl.), 83–88.

Emrich, H.M., Dose, M., and von Zerssen, D. (1985). The use of sodium valproate, carbamazepine and oxcarbazepine in patients with affective disorders. *J Affect Disord*, 8(3), 243–250.

Erfurth, A., Kammerer, C., Grunze, H., Normann, C., and Walden. J. (1998). An open label study of gabapentin in the treatment of acute mania. *J Psychiatr Res*, 32(5), 261–264.

Fink, M. (1999). Delirious mania. *Bipolar Disord*, 1(1), 54–60.

Fink, M., (2006). ECT in therapy-resistant mania: Does it have a place? *Bipolar Disord*, 8(3), 307–309.

Freeman, T.W., Clothier, J.L., Pazzaglia, P., Lesem, M.D., and Swann, A.C. (1992). A double-blind comparison of valproate and lithium in the treatment of acute mania. *Am J Psychiatry*, 149(1), 108–111.

Frye, M.A., Altshuler, L.L., Szuba, M.P., Finch, N.N., and Mintz, J. (1996). The relationship between antimanic agent for treatment of classic or dysphoric mania and length of hospital stay. *J Clin Psychiatry*, 57(1), 17–21.

Frye, M.A., Ketter, T.A., Kimbrell, T.A., Dunn, R.T., Speer, A.M., Osuch, E.A., Luckenbaugh, D.A., Cora-Ocatelli, G., Leverich, G.S., and Post, R.M. (2000). A placebo-controlled study of lamotrigine and gabapentin monotherapy in refractory mood disorders. *J Clin Psychopharmacol*, 20(6), 607–612.

Garfinkel, P.E., Stancer, H.C., and Persad, E. (1980). A comparison of haloperidol, lithium carbonate and their combination in the treatment of mania. *J Affect Disord*, 2(4), 279–288.

Garza-Trevino, E.S., Overall, J.E., and Hollister, L.E. (1992). Verapamil versus lithium in acute mania. *Am J Psychiatry*, 149(1), 121–122.

Ghaemi, S.N., and Goodwin, F.K. (2001). Gabapentin treatment of the non-refractory bipolar spectrum: An open case series. *J Affect Disord*, 65(2), 167–171.

Ghaemi, S.N., and Katzow, J.J. (1999). The use of quetiapine for treatment-resistant bipolar disorder: A case series. *Ann Clin Psychiatry*, 11(3), 137–140.

Ghaemi, S.N., and Sachs, G.S. (1997). Long-term risperidone treatment in bipolar disorder: 6-month follow up. *Int Clin Psychopharmacol*, 12(6), 333–338.

Ghaemi, S.N., Katzow, J.J., Desai, S.P., and Goodwin, F.K. (1998). Gabapentin treatment of mood disorders: A preliminary study. *J Clin Psychiatry*, 59(8), 426–429.

Giannini, A.J., Houser, W.L. Jr., Loiselle, R.H., Giannini, M.C., and Price, W.A. (1984). Antimanic effects of verapamil. *Am J Psychiatry*, 141(12), 1602–1603.

Goldberg, J.F., and Burdick, K.E. (2002). Levetiracetam for acute mania. *Am J Psychiatry*, 159(1), 148.

Gonzalez-Pinto, Lalaguna, B., Mosquera, F., Perez de Heredia, J.L., Gutierrez, M., Ezcurra, J., Gilaberte, I., and Tohen, M. (2001). Use of olanzapine in dysphoric mania. *J Affect Disord*, 66(2–3), 247–253.

Goodnick, P.J., and Meltzer, H.Y. (1984). Treatment of schizoaffective disorders. *Schizophr Bull*, 10, 30–48.

Goodwin, F.K., and Ebert, M. (1973). Lithium in mania: Clinical trials and controlled trials. In S. Gershon and B. Shopsin (Eds.), *Lithium: Its Role in Psychiatric Research* (pp. 237–252). New York: Plenum Press.

Goodwin, F.K., Murphy, D.L., and Bunney, W.E. Jr. (1969). Lithium-carbonate treatment in depression and mania. A longitudinal double-blind study. *Arch Gen Psychiatry*, 21(4), 486–496.

Gouliaev, G., Licht, R.W., Vestergaard, P., Merinder, L., Lund, H., and Bjerre, L. (1996). Treatment of manic episodes: Zuclopenthixol and clonazepam versus lithium and clonazepam. *Acta Psychiatr Scand*, 93(2), 119–124.

Green, A.I., Tohen, M., Patel, J.K., Banov, M., DuRand, C., Berman, I., Chang, H., Zarate, C., Jr., Posener, J., Lee, H., Dawson, R., Richards, C., Cole, J.O., and Schatzberg, A.F. (2000). Clozapine in the treatment of refractory psychotic mania. *Am J Psychiatry*, 157(6), 982–986.

Grisaru, N., Chudakov, B., Yaroslavsky, Y., and Belmaker, R.H. (1998). Transcranial magnetic stimulation in mania: A controlled study. *Am J Psychiatry*, 155(11), 1608–1610.

Grunze, H.C., Erfurth, A., Amann, B., Giupponi, G., Kammerer, C., and Walden, J. (1999a). Intravenous valproate loading in acutely manic and depressed bipolar I patients. *J Clin Psychopharmacol*, 19(4), 303–309.

Grunze, H.C., Erfurth, A., Marcuse, A., Amann, B., Normann, C., and Walden, J. (1999b). Tiagabine appears not to be efficacious in the treatment of acute mania. *J Clin Psychiatry*, 60(11), 759–762.

Grunze, H.C., Normann, C., Langosch, J., Schaefer, M., Amann, B., Sterr, A., Schloesser, S., Kleindienst, N., and Walden, J. (2001). Antimanic efficacy of topiramate in 11 patients in an open trial with an on-off-on design. *J Clin Psychiatry*, 62(6), 464–468.

Grunze, H.C., Kasper, S., Goodwin, G., Bowden, C., Baldwin, D., Licht, R.W., Vieta, E., Moller, H.J., and WFSBP Task Force on Treatment Guidelines for Bipolar Disorders. (2003). The World Federation of Societies of Biological Psychiatry (WFSBP) guidelines for the biological treatment of bipolar disorders, Part II: Treatment of mania. *World J Biol Psychiatry*, 4(1), 5–13.

Guille, C., Sachs, G.S., and Ghaemi, S.N. (2000). A naturalistic comparison of clozapine, risperidone, and olanzapine in the treatment of bipolar disorder. *J Clin Psychiatry*, 61(9), 638–642.

Hamilton, I. (1982). *Robert Lowell: A Biography*. New York: Random House.

Harada, T., and Otsuki, S. (1986). Antimanic effect of zotepine. *Clin Ther*, 8(4), 406–414.

Hatzimanolis, J., Lykouras, L., Oulis, P., and Christodoulou, G.N. (1999). Gabapentin as monotherapy in the treatment of acute mania. *Eur Neuropsychopharmacol*, 9(3), 257–258.

Heiden, A., Frey, R., Presslich, O., Blasbichler, T., Smetana, R., and Kasper, S. (1999). Treatment of severe mania with intravenous magnesium sulphate as a supplementary therapy. *Psychiatry Res*, 89, 239–246.

Hellewell, J.S. (2002). Oxcarbazepine (Trileptal) in the treatment of bipolar disorders: A review of efficacy and tolerability. *J Affect Disord*, 72(Suppl.), S23–S34.

Hillert, A., Maier, W., Wetzel, H., and Benkert, O. (1992). Risperidone in the treatment of disorders with a combined psychotic and depressive syndrome: A functional approach. *Pharmacopsychiatry*, 25(5), 213–217.

Hirschfeld, R.M., Allen, M.H., McEvoy, J.P., Keck, P.E. Jr., and Russell, J.M. (1999). Safety and tolerability of oral loading divalproex sodium in acutely manic bipolar patients. *J Clin Psychiatry*, 60(12), 815–818.

Hirschfeld, R.M., Baker, J.D., Wozniak, P., Tracy, K., and Sommerville, K.W. (2003). The safety and early efficacy of oral-loaded divalproex versus standard-titration divalproex, lithium, olanzapine, and placebo in the treatment of acute mania associated with bipolar disorder. *J Clin Psychiatry*, 64(7), 841–846.

Hirschfeld, R.M., Keck, P.E. Jr., Kramer, M., Karcher, K., Canuso, C., Eerdekens, M., and Grossman, F. (2004). Rapid antimanic effect of risperidone monotherapy: A 3-week multicenter, double-blind, placebo-controlled trial. *Am J Psychiatry*, 161(6), 1057–1065.

Hummel, B., Walden, J., Stampfer, R., Dittmann, S., Amann, B., Sterr, A., Schaefer, M., Frye, M.A., and Grunze, H. (2002). Acute antimanic efficacy and safety of oxcarbazepine in an open trial with an on-off-on design. *Bipolar Disord*, 4(6), 412–417.

Ichim, L., Berk, M., and Brook, S. (2000). Lamotrigine compared with lithium in mania: A double-blind randomized controlled trial. *Ann Clin Psychiatry*, 12(1), 5–10.

Isometsa, E.T., Henriksson, M.M., Aro, H.M., and Lonnqvist, J.K. (1994). Suicide in bipolar disorder in Finland. *Am J Psychiatry*, 151(7), 1020–1024.

Janicak, P.G., Sharma, R.P., Pandey, G., and Davis, J.M. (1998). Verapamil for the treatment of acute mania: A double-blind, placebo-controlled trial. *Am J Psychiatry*, 155(7), 972–973.

Jochum, T., Bar, K.J., and Sauer, H. (2002). Topiramate induced manic episode. *J Neurol Neurosurg Psychiatry*, 73(2), 208–209.

Juckel, G., Hegerl, U., Mavrogiorgou, P., Gallinat, J., Mager, T., Tigges, P., Dresel, S., Schroter, A., Stotz, G., Meller, I., Greil, W., and Moller, H.J. (2000). Clinical and biological findings in a case with 48-hour bipolar ultrarapid cycling before and during valproate treatment. *J Clin Psychiatry*, 61(8), 585–593.

Kanba, S., Yagi, G., Kamijima, K., Suzuki, T., Tajima, O., Otaki, J., Arata, E., Koshikawa, H., Nibuya, M., Kinoshita, N., and Asai, M. (1994). The first open study of zonisamide, a novel anticonvulsant, shows efficacy in mania. *Prog Neuropsychopharmacol Biol Psychiatry*, 18(4), 707–715.

Keck, P.E. Jr. (2005). Bipolar depression: A new role for atypical antipsychotics? *Bipolar Disord*, 7(Suppl. 4), 34–40.

Keck, P.E. Jr., Wilson, D.R., Strakowski, S.M., McElroy, S.L., Kizer, D.L., Balistreri, T.M., Holtman, H.M., and DePriest, M. (1995). Clinical predictors of acute risperidone response in schizophrenia, schizoaffective disorder, and psychotic mood disorders. *J Clin Psychiatry*, 56(10), 466–470.

Keck, P.E. Jr., Nabulsi, A.A., Taylor, J.L., Henke, C.J., Chmiel, J.J., Stanton, S.P., and Bennett, J.A. (1996). A pharmacoeconomic model of divalproex vs. lithium in the acute and prophylactic treatment of bipolar I disorder. *J Clin Psychiatry*, 57(5), 213–222.

Keck, P.E. Jr., Reeves, K.R., and Harrigan, E.P. (2001). Ziprasidone in the short-term treatment of patients with schizoaffective disorder: Results from two double-blind, placebo-controlled, multicenter studies. *J Clin Psychopharmacol*, 21(1), 27–35.

Keck, P.E. Jr., Marcus, R., Tourkodimitris, S., Ali, M., Liebeskind, A., Saha, A., Ingenito, G., and Aripiprazole Study Group. (2003a). A placebo-controlled, double-blind study of the efficacy and safety of aripiprazole in patients with acute bipolar mania. *Am J Psychiatry*, 160(9), 1651–1658.

Keck, P.E. Jr., Versiani, M., Potkin, S., West, S.A., Giller, E., Ice, K., and Ziprasidone in Mania Study Group. (2003b). Ziprasidone in the treatment of acute bipolar mania: A three-week, placebo-controlled, double-blind, randomized trial. *Am J Psychiatry*, 160(4), 741.

Ketter, T.A. (2005). *Advances in Treatment of Bipolar Disorder* (Review of Psychiatry). Arlington, VA: American Psychiatric Association.

Ketter, T.A., Kalali, A.H., Weisler, R.H., and SPD417 Study Group. (2004). A 6-month, multicenter, open-label evaluation of beaded, extended-release carbamazepine capsule monotherapy in bipolar disorder patients with manic or mixed episodes. *J Clin Psychiatry*, 65(5), 668–673.

Khanna, S., Vieta, E., Lyons, B., Grossman, F., Eerdekens, M., and Kramer, M. (2005). Risperidone in the treatment of acute bipolar mania: A double-blind, placebo-controlled study of 290 patients. *Br J Psychiatry*, 187, 229–234.

Kinrys, G. (2000). Hypomania associated with omega3 fatty acids. *Arch Gen Psychiatry*, 57(7), 715–716.

Kushner, S.F., Khan, A., Lane, R., and Olson, W.H. (2006). Topiramate monotherapy in the management of acute mania: Results of four double-blind placebo-controlled trials. *Bipolar Disord*, 8(1), 15–27.

Lambert, P.A., Cavaz, G., Borselli, S., and Carrel, S. (1966). Action neuro-psychotrope d'un nouvel anti-épileptique: Le dépamide. *Ann Med Psychol*, 1, 707–710.

Lenox, R.H., Newhouse, P.A., Creelman, W.L., and Whitaker, T.M. (1992). Adjunctive treatment of manic agitation with lorazepam versus haloperidol: A double-blind study. *J Clin Psychiatry*, 53(2), 47–52.

Lerer, B., Moore, N., Meyendorff, E., Cho, S.R., and Gershon, S. (1987). Carbamazepine versus lithium in mania: A double-blind study. *J Clin Psychiatry*, 48(3), 89–93.

Lessig, M.C., Shapira, N.A., and Murphy, T.K. (2001). Topiramate for reversing atypical antipsychotic weight gain. *J Am Acad Child Adolesc Psychiatry*, 40(12), 1364.

Letmaier, M., Schreinzer, D., Wolf, R., and Kasper, S. (2001). Topiramate as a mood stabilizer. *Int Clin Psychopharmacol*, 16(5), 295–298.

Letmaier, M., Schreinzer, D., Thierry, N., Wolf, R., and Kasper, S. (2004). Drug therapy of acute manias: A retrospective data analysis of inpatients from 1997 to 1999. *Nervenarzt*, 75(3), 249–257.

Letmaier, M., Schreinzer, D., Reinfried, L., Glauninger, G., Thierry, N., Kapitany, T., and Kasper, S. (2006). Typical neuroleptics vs. atypical antipsychotics in the treatment of acute mania in a natural setting. *Int J Neuropsychopharmacol*, 9(5), 529–537.

Levy, N.A., and Janicak, P.G. (2000). Calcium channel antagonists for the treatment of bipolar disorder. *Bipolar Disord*, 2, 108–119.

Licht, R.W., Gouliaev, G., Vestergaard, P., and Frydenberg, M. (1997). Generalisability of results from randomised drug trials: A trial on antimanic treatment. *Br J Psychiatry*, 170, 264–267.

Maggs, R. (1963). Treatment of manic illness with lithium carbonate. *Br J Psychiatry*, 109, 56–65.

Manji, H.K., and Chen, G. (2002). PKC, MAP kinases and the bcl-2 family of proteins as long-term targets for mood stabilizers. *Mol Psychiatry*, 7(Suppl. 1), S46–S56.

Marcotte, D. (1998). Use of topiramate, a new anti-epileptic as a mood stabilizer. *J Affect Disord*, 50(2), 245–251.

Margolese, H.C., Beauclair, L., Szkrumelak, N., and Chouinard, G. (2003). Hypomania induced by adjunctive lamotrigine. *Am J Psychiatry*, 160(1), 183–188.

McElroy, S.L., and Keck, P.E. Jr. (2000). Pharmacologic agents for the treatment of acute bipolar mania. *Biol Psychiatry*, 48(6), 539–557.

McElroy, S.L., Keck, P.E. Jr., Pope, H.G. Jr., and Hudson, J.I. (1988). Valproate in the treatment of rapid-cycling bipolar disorder. *J Clin Psychopharmacol*, 8(4), 275–279.

McElroy, S.L., Keck, P.E. Jr., Pope, H.G. Jr., Hudson, J.I., Faedda, G.L., and Swann, A.C. (1992) Clinical and research implications of the diagnosis of dysphoric or mixed mania or hypomania. *Am J Psychiatry*, 149(12), 1633–1644.

McElroy, S.L., Keck, P.E., Stanton, S.P., Tugrul, K.C., Bennett, J.A., and Strakowski, S.M. (1996). A randomized comparison of divalproex oral loading versus haloperidol in the initial treatment of acute psychotic mania. *J Clin Psychiatry*, 57(4), 142–146.

McElroy, S.L., Soutullo, C.A., Keck, P.E. Jr., and Kmetz, G.F. (1997). A pilot trial of adjunctive gabapentin in the treatment of bipolar disorder. *Ann Clin Psychiatry*, 9(2), 99–103.

McElroy, S.L., Suppes, T., Keck, P.E., Frye, M.A., Denicoff, K.D., Altshuler, L.L., Brown, E.S., Nolen, W.A., Kupka, R.W., Rochussen, J., Leverich, G.S., and Post, R.M. (2000). Open-label adjunctive topiramate in the treatment of bipolar disorders. *Biol Psychiatry*, 47(12), 1025–1033.

McElroy, S.L., Suppes, T., Keck, P.E. Jr., Black, D., Frye, M.A., Altshuler, L.L., Nolen, W.A., Kupka, R.W., Leverich, G.S., Walden, J., Grunze, H., and Post, R.M. (2005). Open-label adjunctive zonisamide in the treatment of bipolar disorders: A prospective trial. *J Clin Psychiatry*, 66(5), 617–624.

McIntyre, R.S., Brecher, M., Paulsson, B., Huizar, K., and Mullen, J. (2005). Quetiapine or haloperidol as monotherapy for bipolar mania: A 12-week, double-blind, randomised, parallel-group, placebo-controlled trial. *Eur Neuropsychopharmacol*, 15(5), 573–585.

Meehan, K., Zhang, F., David, S., Tohen, M., Janicak, P., Small, J., Koch, M., Rizk, R., Walker, D., Tran, P., and Breier, A. (2001). A double-blind, randomized comparison of the efficacy and safety of intramuscular injections of olanzapine, lorazepam, or placebo in treating acutely agitated patients diagnosed with bipolar mania. *J Clin Psychopharmacol*, 21(4), 389–397.

Michael, N., and Erfurth, A. (2004). Treatment of bipolar mania with right prefrontal rapid transcranial magnetic stimulation. *J Affect Disord*, 78, 253–257.

Miller, D.S., Yatham, L.N., and Lam, R.W. (2001). Comparative efficacy of typical and atypical antipsychotics as add-on therapy to mood stabilizers in the treatment of mania. *J Clin Psychiatry*, 62(12), 9750–9980.

Milstein, V., Small, J.G., Klapper, M.H., Small, I.F., Miller, M.J., and Kellams, J.J. (1987). Uni- versus bilateral ECT in the treatment of mania. *Convuls Ther*, 3(1), 1–9.

Mishory, A., Yaroslavsky, Y., Bersudsky, Y., and Belmaker, R.H. (2000). Phenytoin as an antimanic anticonvulsant: A controlled study. *Am J Psychiatry*, 157(3), 463–465.

Modell, J.G., Lenox, R.H., and Weiner, S. (1985). Inpatient clinical trial of lorazepam for the management of manic agitation. *J Clin Psychopharmacol*, 5(2), 109–113.

Mukherjee, S., Sackeim, H.A., and Schnur, D.B. (1994). Electroconvulsive therapy of acute manic episodes: A review of 50 years' experience. *Am J Psychiatry*, 151(2), 169–176.

Muller, P., and Heipertz, R. (1977). Treatment of manic psychosis with clozapine [in German]. *Fortschr Neurol Psychiatr Grenzgeb*, 45(7), 420–424.

Muller-Oerlinghausen, B., Retzow, A., Henn, F.A., Giedke, H., and Walden, J. (2000). Valproate as an adjunct to neuroleptic medication for the treatment of acute episodes of mania: A prospective, randomized, double-blind, placebo-controlled, multicenter study. European Valproate Mania Study Group. *J Clin Psychopharmacol*, 20(2), 195–203.

Nierenberg, A.A., Burt, T., Matthews, J., and Weiss, A.P. (1999). Mania associated with St. John's Wort. *Biol Psychiatry*, 46(12), 1707–1708.

Normann, C., Langosch, J., Schaerer, L.O., Grunze, H., and Walden, J. (1999). Treatment of acute mania with topiramate. *Am J Psychiatry*, 156(12), 2014.

Okuma, T., Inanaga, K., Otsuki, S., Sarai, K., Takahashi, R., Hazama, H., Mori, A., and Watanabe, S. (1981). A preliminary double-blind study on the efficacy of carbamazepine in prophylaxis of manic-depressive illness. *Psychopharmacology (Berl)*, 73(1), 95–96.

Okuma, T., Yamashita, I., Takahashi, R., Itoh, H., Otsuki, S., Watanabe, S., Sarai, K., Hazama, H., and Inanaga, K. (1990). Comparison of the antimanic efficacy of carbamazepine and lithium carbonate by double-blind controlled study. *Pharmacopsychiatry*, 23(3), 143–150.

Pande, A.C., Crockatt, J.G., Janney, C.A., Werth, J.L., and Tsaroucha, G. (2000). Gabapentin in bipolar disorder: A placebo-controlled trial of adjunctive therapy. Gabapentin Bipolar Disorder Study Group. *Bipolar Disord*, 2 (3 Pt. 2), 249–255.

Pascual-Leone, A., and Catala, M.D. (1996). Lateralized effect of rapid-rate transcranial magnetic stimulation on the prefrontal contex on mood. *Neurology*, 46, 499–502.

Pazzaglia, P.J., Post, R.M., Ketter, T.A., Callahan, A.M., Marangell, L.B., Frye, M.A., George, M.S., Kimbrell, T.A., Leverich, G.S., Cora-Locatelli, G., and Luckenbaugh, D. (1998). Nimodipine monotherapy and carbamazepine augmentation in patients with refractory recurrent affective illness. *J Clin Psychopharmacol*, 18(5), 404–413.

Pecuch, P.W., and Erfurth, A. (2001). Topiramate in the treatment of acute mania. *J Clin Psychopharmacol*, 21(2), 243–244.

Perlis, R.H., Baker, R.W., Zarate, C.A. Jr., Brown, E.B., Schuh, L.M., Jamal, H.H., and Tohen, M. (2006a). Olanzapine versus risperidone in the treatment of manic or mixed states in bipolar disorder: A randomized, double-blind trial. *J Clin Psychiatry*, 67, 1747–1753.

Perlis, R.H., Welge, J.A., Vornik, L.A., Hirschfeld, R.M., and Keck, P.E. Jr. (2006b). Atypical antipsychotics in the treatment of mania: A meta-analysis of randomized, placebo-controlled trials. *J Clin Psychiatry*, 67(4), 509–516.

Perugi, G., Toni, C., Ruffolo, G., Sartini, S., Simonini, E., and Akiskal, H. (1999). Clinical experience using adjunctive gabapentin in treatment-resistant bipolar mixed states. *Pharmacopsychiatry*, 32(4), 136–141.

Peuskens, J., Moller, H.J., and Puech, A. (2002). Amisulpride improves depressive symptoms in acute exacerbations of schizophrenia: Comparison with haloperidol and risperidone. *Eur Neuropsychopharmacol*, 12(4), 305–310.

Phrolov, K., Applebaum, J., Levine, J., Miodovnick, H., and Belmaker, R.H. (2004). Single-dose intravenous valproate in acute mania. *J Clin Psychiatry*, 65(1), 68–70.

Pope, H.G., Jr., McElroy, S.L., Keck, P.E., and Hudson, J.I. (1991). Valproate in the treatment of acute mania. A placebo-controlled study. *Arch Gen Psychiatry*, 48(1), 62–68.

Post, R.M., Uhde, T.W., and Kramlinger, K.G. (1986a). Carbamazepine treatment of mania: Clinical and biochemical aspects. *Clin Neuropharmacol*, 9, 547–549.

Post, R.M., Uhde, T.W., Roy-Byrne, P.P., and Joffe, R.T. (1986b). Antidepressant effects of carbamazepine. *Am J Psychiatry*, 143(1), 29–34.

Post, R.M., Uhde, T.W., Roy-Byrne, P.P., and Joffe, R.T. (1987). Correlates of antimanic response to carbamazepine. *Psychiatry Research*, 21(1), 71–83.

Post, R.M., Frye, M.A., Denicoff, K.D., Leverich, G.S., Dunn, R.T., Osuch, E.A., Speer, A.M., Obrocea, G., and Jajodia, K. (2000). Emerging trends in the treatment of rapid cycling bipolar disorder: A selected review. *Bipolar Disord*, 2(4), 305–315.

Potkin, S.G., Keck, P.E. Jr., Segal, S., Ice, K., and English, P. (2005). Ziprasidone in acute bipolar mania: A 21-day randomized, double-blind, placebo-controlled replication trial. *J Clin Psychopharmacol*, 25(4), 301–310.

Powers, P., Sachs, G.S., Kushner, S.F., Wang, D., Olson, W., Capece, J., Fazzio, L., and Rosenthal, N. (2004). Topiramate in adults with acute bipolar I mania: Pooled results. In 157th Annual Meeting of the American Psychiatric Association. New York, NY: American Psychiatric Association.

Prien, R.F., and Caffey, E.M. Jr. (1976). Relationship between dosage and response to lithium prophylaxis in recurrent depression. *Am J Psychiatry*, 133(5), 567–570.

Prien, R.F., Caffey, E.M. Jr., and Klett, C.J. (1972). Comparison of lithium carbonate and chlorpromazine in the treatment of mania. Report of the Veterans Administration and National Institute of Mental Health Collaborative Study Group. *Arch Gen Psychiatry*, 26(2), 146–153.

Rifkin, A., Doddi, S., Karajgi, B., Borenstein, M., and Munne, R. (1994). Dosage of haloperidol for mania. *Br J Psychiatry*, 165, 113–116.

Rucci, P., Frank, E., Kostelnik, B., Fagiolini, A., Mallinger, A.G., Swartz, H.A., Thase, M.E., Siegel, L., Wilson, D., and Kupfer, D.J. (2002). Suicide attempts in patients with bipolar I disorder during acute and maintenance phases of intensive treatment with pharmacotherapy and adjunctive psychotherapy. *Am J Psychiatry*, 159(7), 1160–1164.

Rudorfer, M.V., Linnoila, M., and Potter, W.Z. (1987). Combined lithium and electroconvulsive therapy: Pharmacokinetic and pharmacodynamic interactions. *Convuls Ther*, 3(1), 40–45.

Sachs, G.S., Printz, D.J., Kahn, D.A., Carpenter, D., and Docherty, J.P. (2000). The expert consensus guideline series: Medication treatment of bipolar disorder 2000. *Postgrad Med*, Spec. No. 1–104.

Sachs, G.S., Grossman, F., Ghaemi, S.N., Okamoto, A., and Bowden, C.L. (2002). Combination of a mood stabilizer with risperidone or haloperidol for treatment of acute mania: A double-blind, placebo-controlled comparison of efficacy and safety. *Am J Psychiatry*, 159(7), 1146–1154.

Sachs, G., Chengappa, K.N., Suppes, T., Mullen, J.A., Brecher, M., Devine, N.A., and Sweitzer, D.E. (2004). Quetiapine with lithium or divalproex for the treatment of bipolar mania: A randomized, double-blind, placebo-controlled study. *Bipolar Disord*, 6(3), 213–223.

Sajatovic, M., Brescan, D.W., Perez, D.E., DiGiovanni, S.K., Hattab, H., Ray, J.B., and Bingham, C.R. (2001). Quetiapine alone and added to a mood stabilizer for serious mood disorders. *J Clin Psychiatry*, 62(9), 728–732.

Sanger, T.M., Tohen, M., Vieta, E., Dunner, D.L., Bowden, C.L., Calabrese, J.R., Feldman, P.D., Jacobs, T.G., and Breier, A. (2003). Olanzapine in the acute treatment of bipolar I disorder with a history of rapid cycling. *J Affect Disord*, 73(1–2), 155–161.

Schaffer, A., and Levitt, A.J. (2005). Double-blind, placebo-controlled pilot study of mexiletine for acute mania or hypomania. *J Clin Psychopharmacol*, 25(5), 507–508.

Schaffer, L.C., Schaffer, C.B., and Howe, J. (2002). An open case series on the utility of tiagabine as an augmentation in refractory bipolar outpatients. *J Affect Disord*, 71(1-3), 259–263.

Schatzberg, A.F., and Nemeroff, C.B. (Eds.). (1998). *The American Psychiatric Publishing Textbook of Psychopharmacology* (2nd Edition). Arlington, VA: American Psychiatric Association.

Schou, M., Juel-Nielsen, N, Strömgren, E., and Voldby, H. (1954). The treatment of manic psychoses by the administration of lithium salts. *J Neurol Neurosurg Psychiatry*, 17, 250–260.

Segal, J., Berk, M., and Brook, S. (1998). Risperidone compared with both lithium and haloperidol in mania: A double-blind randomized controlled trial. *Clin Neuropharmacol*, 21(3), 176–180.

Shaldubina, A., Stahl, Z., Furszpan, M., Regenold, W.T., Shapiro, J., Belmaker, R.H., and Bersudsky, Y. (2006). Inositol deficiency diet and lithium effects. *Bipolar Disord*, 8(2), 152–159.

Shi, L., Namjoshi, M.A., Zhang, F., Gandhi, G., Edgell, E.T., Tohen, M., Breier, A., and Haro, J.M. (2002). Olanzapine versus haloperidol in the treatment of acute mania: Clinical outcomes, health-related quality of life and work status. *Int Clin Psychopharmacol*, 17(5), 227–237.

Shopsin, B., Gershon, S., Thompson, H., and Collins, P. (1975). Psychoactive drugs in mania. A controlled comparison of lithium carbonate, chlorpromazine, and haloperidol. *Arch Gen Psychiatry*, 32(1), 34–42.

Short, C., and Cooke, L. (1995). Hypomania induced by gabapentin. *Br J Psychiatry*, 166(5), 679–680.

Small, J.G., Klapper, M.H., Kellams, J.J., Miller, M.J., Milstein, V., Sharpley, P.H., and Small, I.F. (1988). Electroconvulsive treatment compared with lithium in the management of manic states. *Arch Gen Psychiatry*, 45(8), 727–732.

Small, J.G., Klapper, M.H., Milstein, V., Kellams, J.J., Miller, M.J., Marhenke, J.D., and Small, I.F. (1991). Carbamazepine compared with lithium in the treatment of mania. *Arch Gen Psychiatry*, 48(10), 915–921.

Small, J.G., Klapper, M.H., Marhenke, J.D., Milstein, V., Woodham, G.C., and Kellams, J.J. (1995). Lithium combined with carbamazepine or haloperidol in the treatment of mania. *Psychopharmacol Bull*, 31(2), 265–272.

Smulevich, A.B., Khanna, S., Eerdekens, M., Karcher, K., Kramer, M., and Grossman, F. (2005). Acute and continuation risperidone monotherapy in bipolar mania: A 3-week placebo-controlled trial followed by a 9-week double-blind trial of risperidone and haloperidol. *Eur Neuropsychopharmacol*, 15(1), 75–84.

Sokolski, K.N., Green, C., Maris, D.E., and DeMet, E.M. (1999). Gabapentin as an adjunct to standard mood stabilizers in outpatients with mixed bipolar symptomatology. *Ann Clin Psychiatry*, 11(4), 217–222.

Stanton, S.P., Keck, P.E. Jr., and McElroy, S.L. (1997). Treatment of acute mania with gabapentin. *Am J Psychiatry*, 154(2), 287.

Stokes, P.E., Shamoian, C.A., Stoll, P.M., and Patton, M.J. (1971). Efficacy of lithium as acute treatment of manic-depressive illness. *Lancet*, 1(7713), 1319–1325.

Suppes, T., McElroy, S.L., Gilbert, J., Dessain, E.C., and Cole, J.O. (1992). Clozapine in the treatment of dysphoric mania. *Biol Psychiatry*, 32(3), 270–280.

Suppes, T., Webb, A., Paul, B., Carmody, T., Kraemer, H., and Rush, A.J. (1999). Clinical outcome in a randomized 1-year trial of clozapine versus treatment as usual for patients with treatment-resistant illness and a history of mania. *Am J Psychiatry*, 156(8), 1164–1169.

Suppes, T., Chisholm, K.A., Dhavale, D., Frye, M.A., Altshuler, L.L., McElroy, S.L., Keck, P.E., Nolen, W.A., Kupka, R., Denicoff, K.D., Leverich, G.S., Rush, A.J., and Post, R.M. (2002).

Tiagabine in treatment refractory bipolar disorder: A clinical case series. *Bipolar Disord*, 4(5), 283–289.

Swann, A.C., Bowden, C.L., Morris, D., Calabrese, J.R., Petty, F., Small, J., Dilsaver, S.C., and Davis, J.M. (1997). Depression during mania. Treatment response to lithium or divalproex. *Arch Gen Psychiatry*, 54(1), 37–42.

Swann, A.C., Bowden, C.L., Calabrese, J.R., Dilsaver, S.C., and Morris, D.D. (1999). Differential effect of number of previous episodes of affective disorder on response to lithium or divalproex in acute mania. *Am J Psychiatry*, 156(8), 1264.

Swann, A.C., Bowden, C.L., Calabrese, J.R., Dilsaver, S.C., and Morris, D.D. (2002). Pattern of response to divalproex, lithium, or placebo in four naturalistic subtypes of mania. *Neuropsychopharmacology*, 26(4), 530–536.

Tohen, M., Castillo, J., Pope, H.G. Jr., and Herbstein, J. (1994). Concomitant use of valproate and carbamazepine in bipolar and schizoaffective disorders. *J Clin Psychopharmacol*, 14(1), 67–70.

Tohen, M., Zarate, C.A. Jr., Centorrino, F., Hegarty, J.I., Froeschl, M., and Zarate, S.B. (1996). Risperidone in the treatment of mania. *J Clin Psychiatry*, 57(6), 249–253.

Tohen, M., Sanger, T.M., McElroy, S.L., Tollefson, G.D., Chengappa, K.N., Daniel, D.G., Petty, F., Centorrino, F., Wang, R., Grundy, S.L., Greaney, M.G., Jacobs, T.G., David, S.R., and Toma, V. (1999). Olanzapine versus placebo in the treatment of acute mania. Olanzapine HGEH Study Group. *Am J Psychiatry*, 156(5), 702–709.

Tohen, M., Jacobs, T.G., Grundy, S.L., McElroy, S.L., Banov, M.C., Janicak, P.G., Sanger, T., Risser, R., Zhang, F., Toma, V., Francis, J., Tollefson, G.D., and Breier, A. (2000). Efficacy of olanzapine in acute bipolar mania: A double-blind, placebo-controlled study. The Olanzipine HGGW Study Group. *Arch Gen Psychiatry*, 57(9), 841–849.

Tohen, M., Zhang, F., Taylor, C.C., Burns, P., Zarate, C., Sanger, T., and Tollefson, G. (2001). A meta-analysis of the use of typical antipsychotic agents in bipolar disorder. *J Affect Disord*, 65(1), 85–93.

Tohen, M., Baker, R.W., Altshuler, L.L., Zarate, C.A., Suppes, T., Ketter, T.A., Milton, D.R., Risser, R., Gilmore, J.A., Breier, A., and Tollefson, G.D. (2002). Olanzapine versus divalproex sodium for the treatment of acute mania. *Am J Psychiatry*, 159(6), 1011–1017.

Tohen, M., Ketter, T.A., Zarate, C.A., Suppes, T., Frye, M., Altshuler, L., Zajecka, J., Schuh, L.M., Risser, R.C., Brown, E., and Baker, R.W. (2003a). Olanzapine versus divalproex sodium for the treatment of acute mania and maintenance of remission: A 47-week study. *Am J Psychiatry*, 160(7), 1263–1271.

Tohen, M., Goldberg, J.F., Gonzalez-Pinto, Arrillaga, A.M., Azorin, J.M., Vieta, E., Hardy-Bayle, M.C., Lawson, W.B., Emsley, R.A., Zhang, F., Baker, R.W., Risser, R.C., Namjoshi, M.A., Evans, A.R., and Breier, A. (2003b). A 12-week, double-blind comparison of olanzapine vs. haloperidol in the treatment of acute mania. *Arch Gen Psychiatry*, 60(12), 1218–1226.

Tohen, M., Chengappa, K.N., Suppes, T., Baker, R.W., Zarate, C.A., Bowden, C.L., Sachs, G.S., Kupfer, D.J., Ghaemi, S.N., Feldman, P.D., Risser, R.C., Evans, A.R., and Calabrese, J.R. (2004). Relapse prevention in bipolar I disorder: 18-month comparison of olanzapine plus mood stabiliser vs. mood stabiliser alone. *Br J Psychiatry*, 184, 337–345.

Vieta, E., Gasto, C., Colom, F., Reinares, M., Martinez-Aran, A., Benabarre, A., and Akiskal, H.S. (2001). Role of risperidone in bipolar II: An open 6-month study. *J Affect Disord*, 67(1–3), 213–219.

Vieta, E., Brugue, E., Goikolea, J.M., Sanchez-Moreno, J., Reinares, M., Comes, M., Colom, F., Martinez-Aran, A., Benabarre, A., and Torrent, C. (2003). *Risperidone monotherapy in acute bipolar mania*. Poster, Meeting of the American College of Neuropsychopharmacology, Puerto Rico, 222.

Vieta, E., Bourin, M., Sanchez, R., Marcus, R., Stock, E., McQuade, R., Carson, W., Abou-Gharbia, N., Swanink, R., Iwamoto, T., and Aripoprazole Study Group. (2005). Effectiveness of aripiprazole vs. haloperidol in acute bipolar mania: Double-blind, randomised, comparative 12-week trial. *Br J Psychiatry*, 187, 235–242.

Walton, S.A., Berk, M., and Brook, S. (1996). Superiority of lithium over verapamil in mania: A randomized, controlled, single-blind trial. *J Clin Psychiatry*, 57(11), 543–546.

Weisler, R.H., Kalali, A.H., Ketter, T.A., and SPD417 Study Group. (2004). A multicenter, randomized, double-blind, placebo-controlled trial of extended-release carbamazepine capsules as monotherapy for bipolar disorder patients with manic or mixed episodes. *J Clin Psychiatry*, 65(4), 478–484.

Weisler, R.H., Keck, P.E. Jr., Swann, A.C., Cutler, A.J., Ketter, T.A., Kalali, A.H., and SPD417 Study Group. (2005). Extended-release carbamazepine capsules as monotherapy for acute mania in bipolar disorder: A multicenter, randomized, double-blind, placebo-controlled trial. *J Clin Psychiatry*, 66(3), 323–330.

Winokur, G., and Kadrmas, A. (1989). A polyepisodic course in bipolar illness: Possible clinical relationships. *Compr Psychiatry*, 30(2), 121–127.

Winokur, G., Coryell, W., Keller, M., and Scheftner, W.A. (1990). Relationship of electroconvulsive therapy to course in affective illness: A collaborative study. *Eur Arch Psychiatry Clin Neurosci*, 240(1), 54–59.

Yatham, L.N., Grossman, F., Augustyns, I., Vieta, E., and Ravindran, A. (2003). Mood stabilisers plus risperidone or placebo in the treatment of acute mania. International, double-blind, randomised controlled trial. *Br J Psychiatry*, 182, 141–147.

Yatham, L.N., Binder, C., Kusumakar, V., and Riccardelli, R. (2004). Risperidone plus lithium versus risperidone plus valproate in acute and continuation treatment of mania. *Int Clin Psychopharmacol*, 19(2), 103–109.

Zajecka, J.M., Weisler, R., Sachs, G., Swann, A.C., Wozniak, P., and Sommerville, K.W. (2002). A comparison of the efficacy, safety, and tolerability of divalproex sodium and olanzapine in the treatment of bipolar disorder. *J Clin Psychiatry*, 63(12), 1148–1155.

Zarate, C.A. Jr., Tohen, M., and Baldessarini, R.J. (1995). Clozapine in severe mood disorders. *J Clin Psychiatry*, 56(9), 411–417.

Zarate, C.A. Jr., Tohen, M., and Baraibar, G. (1997). Combined valproate or carbamazepine and electroconvulsive therapy. *Ann Clin Psychiatry*, 9(1), 19–25.

Zarate, C.A. Jr., Rothschild, A., Fletcher, K.E., Madrid, A., and Zapatel, J. (2000). Clinical predictors of acute response with quetiapine in psychotic mood disorders. *J Clin Psychiatry*, 61(3), 185–189.

CHAPTER 19

Abraham, G., Milev, R., and Stuart Lawson, J. (2006). T3 augmentation of SSRI resistant depression. *J Affect Disord*, 91(2-3), 211–215.

Abrams, R. (Ed.). (1997). *Electroconvulsive Therapy* (third edition). New York: Oxford University Press.

Ahokas, A., Aito, M., and Rimon, R. (2000). Positive treatment effect of estradiol in postpartum psychosis: A pilot study. *J Clin Psychiatry*, 61(3), 166–169.

Ahokas, A., Kaukoranta, J., Wahlbeck, K., and Aito, M. (2001). Estrogen deficiency in severe postpartum depression: Successful treatment with sublingual physiologic 17 beta-estradiol: A preliminary study. *J Clin Psychiatry*, 62(5), 332–336.

Akiskal, H.S. (1995). Switching from "unipolar" to bipolar II: An 11-year prospective study of clinical and temperamental predictors in 559 patients. *Arch Gen Psychiatry*, 52, 114–123.

Akiskal, H.S., Maser, J.D., Zeller, P.J., Endicott, J., Coryell, W., Keller, M., Warshaw, M., Clayton, P., and Goodwin, F. (1995). Switching from 'unipolar' to bipolar II. An 11-year prospective study of clinical and temperamental predictors in 559 patients. *Arch Gen Psychiatry*, 52(2), 114–123.

Akiskal, H.S., Hantouche, E.G., Allilaire, J.F., Sechter, D., Bourgeois, M.L., Azorin, J.M., Chatenet-Duchene, L., and Lancrenon, S. (2003). Validating antidepressant-associated hypomania (bipolar III): A systematic comparison with spontaneous hypomania (bipolar II). *J Affect Disord*, 73(1-2), 65–74.

Alpert, J.E., Papakostas, G., Mischoulon, D., Worthington, J.J. III, Petersen, T., Mahal, Y., Burns, A., Bottiglieri, T., Nierenberg, A.A., and Fava, M. (2004). S-Adenosyl-L-methionine (SAMe) as an adjunct for resistant major depressive disorder: An open trial following partial or nonresponse to selective serotonin reuptake inhibitors or venlafaxine. *J Clin Psychopharmacol*, 24(6), 661–664.

Altshuler, L.L., Post, R.M., Leverich, G.S., Mikalauskas, K., Rosoff, A., and Ackerman, L. (1995). Antidepressant-induced mania and cycle acceleration: A controversy revisited. *Am J Psychiatry*, 152(8), 1130–1138.

Altshuler, L.L., Keck, P.E. Jr., McElroy, S.L., Suppes, T., Brown, E.S., Denicoff, K., Frye, M., Gitlin, M., Hwang, S., Goodman, R., Leverich, G., Nolen, W., Kupka, R., and Post, R. (1999). Gabapentin in the acute treatment of refractory bipolar disorder. *Bipolar Disord*, 1(1), 61–65.

Altshuler, L., Kiriakos, L., Calcagno, J., Goodman, R., Gitlin, M., Frye, M., and Mintz, J. (2001a). The impact of antidepressant discontinuation versus antidepressant continuation on 1-year risk for relapse of bipolar depression: A retrospective chart review. *J Clin Psychiatry*, 62(8), 612–616.

Altshuler, L.L., Bauer, M., Frye, M.A., Gitlin, M.J., Mintz, J., Szuba, M.P., Leight, K.L., and Whybrow, P.C. (2001b). Does thyroid supplementation accelerate tricyclic antidepressant response? A review and meta-analysis of the literature. *Am J Psychiatry*, 158(10), 1617–1622.

Altshuler, L., Suppes, T., Black, D., Nolen, W.A., Keck, P.E. Jr., Frye, M.A., McElroy, S., Kupka, R., Grunze, H., Walden, J., Leverich, G., Denicoff, K., Luckenbaugh, D., and Post, R. (2003). Impact of antidepressant discontinuation after acute bipolar depression remission on rates of depressive relapse at 1-year follow-up. *Am J Psychiatry*, 160(7), 1252–1262.

Altshuler, L.L., Suppes, T., Black, D.O., Nolen, W.A., Leverich, G., Keck, P.E., Frye, M.A., Kupka, R., McElroy, S.L., Grunze, H., Kitchen, C.M., and Post, R. (2006). Lower switch rate in depressed patients with bipolar II than bipolar I disorder treated adjunctively with second-generation antidepressants. *Am J Psychiatry*, 163(2), 313–315.

American Psychiatric Association. (2002). Practice guidelines for the treatment of patients with bipolar depression (revision). *Am J Psychiatry*, 159(Suppl. 4), 1–50.

Amsterdam, J. (1998). Efficacy and safety of venlafaxine in the treatment of bipolar II major depressive episode. *J Clin Psychopharmacol*, 18(5), 414–417.

Amsterdam, J.D., and Garcia-Espana, F. (2000). Venlafaxine monotherapy in women with bipolar II and unipolar major depression. *J Affect Disord*, 59(3), 225–229.

Amsterdam, J.D., Garcia-Espana, F., Fawcett, J., Quitkin, F.M., Reimherr, F.W., Rosenbaum, J.F., Schweizer, E., and Beasley, C. (1998). Efficacy and safety of fluoxetine in treating bipolar II major depressive episode. *J Clin Psychopharmacol*, 18(6), 435–440.

Anand, A., Bukhari, L., Jennings, S.A., Lee, C., Kamat, M., Shekhar, A., Nurnberger, J.I. Jr., and Lightfoot, J. (2005). A preliminary open-label study of zonisamide treatment for bipolar depression in 10 patients. *J Clin Psychiatry*, 66(2), 195–198.

Angst, J. (1985). Switch from depression to mania: A record study over decades between 1920 and 1982. *Psychopathology*, 18(2-3), 140–154.

Angst, J., Angst, K., Baruffol, I., and Meinherz-Surbeck, R. (1992). ECT-induced and drug-induced hypomania. *Convuls Ther*, 8(3), 179–185.

Arieli, A., and Lepkifker, E. (1981). The antidepressant effect of lithium. *Curr Dev Psychopharmacol*, 6, 165–190.

Arnold, O.H., and Kryspin-Exner, K. (1965). Zur Frage der Beeinflussung des Verlaufes des manisch-depressiven Krankheitsgeschehens durch Antidepressiva. [The problem of control of manic-depressive processes by antidepressants]. *Wien Med Wochenschr*, 115, 929–934.

Aronson, R., Offman, H.J., Joffe, R.T., and Naylor, C.D. (1996). Triiodothyronine augmentation in the treatment of refractory depression. A meta-analysis. *Arch Gen Psychiatry*, 53(9), 842–848.

Artaud, A. (1965). *Artaud Anthology*. Edited by J. Hirschman. San Francisco: City Lights Press.

Aubry, J.M., Simon, A.E., and Bertschy, G. (2000). Possible induction of mania and hypomania by olanzapine or risperidone: A critical review of reported cases. *J Clin Psychiatry*, 61(9), 649–655.

Austin, M.P., Souza, F.G., and Goodwin, G.M. (1991). Lithium augmentation in antidepressant-resistant patients. A quantitative analysis. *Br J Psychiatry*, 159, 510–514.

Baastrup, P.C., and Schou, M. (1967). Lithium as a prophylactic agent. Its effect against recurrent depressions and manic-depressive psychosis. *Arch Gen Psychiatry*, 16(2), 162–172.

Baastrup, P.C., Poulsen, J.C., Schou, M., Thomsen, K., and Amdisen, A. (1970). Prophylactic lithium: Double-blind discontinuation in manic-depressive and recurrent-depressive disorders. *Lancet*, 2(7668), 326–330.

Baker, R.W., Milton, D.R., Stauffer, V.L., Gelenberg, A., and Tohen, M. (2003). Placebo-controlled trials do not find association of olanzapine with exacerbation of bipolar mania. *J Affect Disord*, 73(1-2), 147–153.

Baldassano, C.F., Sachs, G., and Stoll, A.L. (1995). Paroxetine for bipolar depression: Outcome in patients failing prior to antidepressant trials. *Depression*, 3182–3186.

Baldassano, C.F., Ghaemi, S.N., Chang, A., Lyman, A., and Lipari, M. (2004). Acute treatment of bipolar depression with adjunctive zonisamide: A retrospective chart review. *Bipolar Disord*, 6(5), 432–434.

Baldessarini, R.J., Tondo, L., Hennen, J., and Viguera, A.C. (2002). Is lithium still worth using? An update of selected recent research. *Harv Rev Psychiatry*, 10(2), 59–75.

Baldessarini, R.J., Pompili, M., and Tondo, L. (2006). Suicide in bipolar disorder: Risks and management. *CNS Spectr*, 11(6), 465–471.

Balon, R., Mufti, R., and Arfken, C.L. (1999). A survey of prescribing practices for monoamine oxidase inhibitors. *Psychiatr Serv*, 50(7), 945–947.

Barbini, B., Colombo, C., Benedetti, F., Campori, E., Bellodi, L., and Smeraldi, E. (1998). The unipolar–bipolar dichotomy and the response to sleep deprivation. *Psychiatry Res*, 79(1), 43–50.

Baron, M., Gershon, E.S., Rudy, V., Jonas, W.Z., and Buchsbaum, M. (1975). Lithium carbonate response in depression. Prediction by unipolar/bipolar illness, average-evoked response, catechol-O-methyl transferase, and family history. *Arch Gen Psychiatry*, 32(9), 1107–1111.

Bauer, M., and Döpfmer, S. (1999). Lithium augmentation in treatment-resistant depression: Meta-analysis of placebo-controlled studies. *J Clin Psychopharmacol*, 19(5), 427–434.

Bauer, M., and Döpfmer, S. (2000). Lithium augmentation in treatment-resistant depression: Meta-analysis of placebo-controlled studies. *J Clin.Psychopharmacol*, 20(2), 287.

Bauer, M.D., Hellweg, R., Graf, K.J., and Baumgartner, A. (1998). Treatment of refractory depression with high-dose thyroxine. *Neuropsychopharmacology*, 18(6), 444–455.

Bauer, M., Heinz, A., and Whybrow, P.C. (2002). Thyroid hormones, serotonin and mood: Of synergy and significance in the adult brain. *Mol Psychiatry*, 7(2), 140–156.

Bauer, M., London, E.D., Silverman, D.H., Rasgon, N., Kirchheiner, J., and Whybrow, P.C. (2003). Thyroid, brain and mood modulation in affective disorder: Insights from molecular research and functional brain imaging. *Pharmacopsychiatry*, 36(Suppl. 3), S215–S221.

Bauer, M., Rasgon, N., Grof, P., Altshuler, L., Gyulai, L., Lapp, M., Glenn, T., and Whybrow, P.C. (2005). Mood changes related to antidepressants: A longitudinal study of patients with bipolar disorder in a naturalistic setting. *Psychiatry Res*, 133(1), 73–80.

Bauer, M., Grof, P., and Muller-Oelingausen, B. (2006). The acute antidepressive effects of lithium: From monotherapy to augmentation therapy in major depression. In *Lithium in Neuropsychiatry: The Comprehensive Guide*. London: Taylor & Francis Book Ltd.

Bauer, M.S., and Whybrow, P.C. (1986). The effect of changing thyroid function on cyclic affective illness in a human subject. *Am J Psychiatry*, 142(5), 633–636.

Bauer, M.S., and Whybrow, P.C. (1990). Rapid cycling bipolar affective disorder. II. Treatment of refractory rapid cycling with high-dose levothyroxine: A preliminary study. *Arch Gen Psychiatry*, 47(5), 435–440.

Baumann, P., Nil, R., Souche, A., Montaldi, S., Baettig, D., Lambert, S., Uehlinger, C., Kasas, A., Amey, M., and Jonzier-Perey, M. (1996). A double-blind, placebo-controlled study of citalopram with and without lithium in the treatment of therapy-resistant depressive patients: A clinical, pharmacokinetic, and pharmacogenetic investigation. *J Clin Psychopharmacol*, 16(4), 307–314.

Benazzi, F. (1997). Antidepressant-associated hypomania in outpatient depression: A 203-case study in private practice. *J Affect Disord*, 46(1), 73–77.

Benazzi, F. (2001). Prevalence and clinical correlates of residual depressive symptoms in bipolar II disorder. *Psychother Psychosom*, 70(5), 232–238.

Benedetti, F., Barbini, B., Campori, E., Colombo, C., and Smeraldi, E. (1996). Dopamine agonist amineptine prevents the antidepressant effect of sleep deprivation. *Psychiatry Res*, 65(3), 179–184.

Benedetti, F., Colombo, C., Barbini, B., Campori, E., and Smeraldi, E. (1999). Ongoing lithium treatment prevents relapse after total sleep deprivation. *J Clin Psychopharmacol*, 19(3), 240–245.

Benedetti, F., Barbini, B., Campori, E., Fulgosi, M.C., Pontiggia, A., and Colombo, C. (2001a). Sleep phase advance and lithium to sustain the antidepressant effect of total sleep deprivation in bipolar depression: New findings supporting the internal coincidence model? *J Psychiatr Res*, 35(6), 323–329.

Benedetti, F., Campori, E., Barbini, B., Fulgosi, M.C., and Colombo, C. (2001b). Dopaminergic augmentation of sleep deprivation effects in bipolar depression. *Psychiatry Res*, 104(3), 239–246.

Benedetti, F., Colombo, C., Serretti, A., Lorenzi, C., Pontiggia, A., Barbini, B., and Smeraldi. E. (2003). Antidepressant effects of light therapy combined with sleep deprivation are influenced by a functional polymorphism within the promoter of the serotonin transporter gene. *Biol Psychiatry*, 154(7), 687–692.

Benedetti, F., Barbini, B., Fulgosi, M.C., Colombo, C., Dallaspezia, S., Pontiggia, A., and Smeraldi, E. (2005). Combined total sleep deprivation and light therapy in the treatment of drug-resistant bipolar depression: Acute response and long-term remission rates. *J Clin Psychiatry*, 66(12), 1535–1540.

Berger, M., Vollmann, J., Hohagen, F., Konig, A., Lohner, H., Voderholzer, U., and Riemann, D. (1997). Sleep deprivation combined with consecutive sleep phase advance as a fast-acting therapy in depression: An open pilot trial in medicated and unmedicated patients. *Am J Psychiatry*, 154(6), 870–872.

Berv, D., Klugman, J., Rosenquist, K.J., Hsu, D.J., and Ghaemi, S.N. (2002). *Oxcarbazepine treatment of refractory bipolar depression* [abstract]. 15th Congess of the European College of Neuropsychopharmacology, Barcelona, Spain.

Berzewski, H., Van Moffaert, M., and Gagiano, C.A. (1997). Efficacy and tolerability of reboxetine compared with imipramine in a double-blind study in patients suffering from major depressive offsodes. *Eur Neuropsychopharmacol*, 7(Suppl. 1), S37–S47.

Bhagwagar, Z., and Goodwin, G.M. (2002). The role of lithium in the treatment of bipolar depression. *Clin Neurosci Res*, 2(3-4), 222–227.

Black, D.W., Winokur, G., and Nasrallah, A. (1986). ECT in unipolar and bipolar disorders: A naturalistic evaluation of 460 patients. *Convuls Ther*, 2(4), 231–237.

Blanco, C., Laje, G., Olfson, M., Marcus, S.C., and Pincus, H.A. (2002). Trends in the treatment of bipolar disorder by outpatient psychiatrists. *Am J Psychiatry*, 159(6), 1005–1010.

Bodkin, J.A., and Amsterdam, J.D. (2002). Transdermal selegiline in major depression: A double-blind, placebo-controlled, parallel-group study in outpatients. *Am J Psychiatry*, 159(11), 1869–1875.

Boerlin, H.L., Gitlin, M.J., Zoellner, L.A., and Hammen, C.L. (1998). Bipolar depression and antidepressant-induced mania: A naturalistic study. *J Clin Psychiatry*, 59(7), 374–379.

Bottlender, R., Rudolf, D., Strauss, A., and Moller, H.J. (1998). Antidepressant-associated maniform states in acute treatment of patient with bipolar I depression. *Eur Arch Psychiatry Clin Neurosci*, 248, 296–300.

Bouckoms, A., and Mangini, L. (1993). Pergolide: An antidepressant adjuvant for mood disorders? *Psychopharmacol Bull*, 29(2), 207–211.

Bowden, C.L. (2001). Clinical correlates of therapeutic response in bipolar disorder. *J Affect Disord*, 67(1-3), 257–265.

Bowden, C.L., Brugger, A.M., Swann, A.C., Calabrese, J.R., Janicak, P.G., Petty, F., Dilsaver, S.C., Davis, J.M., Rush, A.J., and Small, J.G. (1994). Efficacy of divalproex vs. lithium and placebo in the treatment of mania. The Depakote Mania Study Group. *JAMA*, 271(12), 918–924.

Bowden, C.L., Calabrese, J.R., Sachs, G., Yatham, L.N., Asghar, S.A., Hompland, M., Montgomery, P., Earl, N., Smoot, T.M., DeVeaugh-Geiss, J., and Lamictal 606 Study Group. (2003). A placebo-controlled 18-month trial of lamotrigine and lithium maintenance treatment in recently manic or hypomanic patients with bipolar I disorder. *Arch Gen Psychiatry*, 60(4), 392–400.

Bowden, C.L., Collins, M.A., McElroy, S.L., Calabrese, J.R., Swann, A.C., Weisler, R.H., and Wozniak, P.J. (2005). Relationship of mania symptomatology to maintenance treatment response with divalproex, lithium, or placebo. *Neuropsychopharmacology*, 30(10), 1932–1939.

Bressa, G.M. (1994). S-adenosyl-l-methionine (SAMe) as antidepressant: Meta-analysis of clinical studies. *Acta Neurol Scand Suppl*, 154, 7–14.

Brown, E.S., Bobadilla, L., and Rush, A.J. (2001). Ketoconazole in bipolar patients with depressive symptoms: A case series and literature review. *Bipolar Disord*, 3(1), 23–29.

Bruijn, J.A., Moleman, P., Mulder, P.G., and van den Broek, W.W. (1998). Comparison of 2 treatment strategies for depressed inpatients: Imipramine and lithium addition or mirtazapine and lithium addition. *J Clin Psychiatry*, 59(12), 657–663.

Burt, T., Lisanby, S.H., and Sackeim, H.A. (2002). Neuropsychiatric applications of transcranial magnetic stimulation: A meta-analysis. *Int J Neuropsychopharmacol*, 5(1), 73–103.

Cade, J.F. (2000). Lithium salts in the treatment of psychotic excitement. 1949. *Bull World Health Organ*, 78(4), 518–520.

Calabrese J. (2005). One-year outcome with antidepressant treatment of bipolar depression: Is the glass half empty or half full? *Acta Psychiatr Scand*, 112(2), 85–87.

Calabrese, J.R., Bowden, C.L., McElroy, S.L., Cookson, J., Andersen, J., Keck, P.E. Jr., Rhodes, L., Bolden-Watson, C., Zhou, J., and Ascher, J.A. (1999a). Spectrum of activity of lamotrigine in treatment-refractory bipolar disorder. *Am J Psychiatry*, 156(7), 1019–1023.

Calabrese, J.R., Bowden, C.L., Sachs, G.S., Ascher, J.A., Monaghan, E., and Rudd, G.D. (1999b). A double-blind placebo-controlled study of lamotrigine monotherapy in outpatients with bipolar I depression. Lamictal 602 Study Group. *J Clin Psychiatry*, 60(2), 79–88.

Calabrese, J.R., Bowden, C.L., Sachs, G., Yatham, L.N., Behnke, K., Mehtonen, O.P., Montgomery, P., Ascher, J., Paska, W., Earl, N., DeVeaugh-Geiss, J., and Lamictal 605 Study Group. (2003). A placebo-controlled 18-month trial of lamotrigine and lithium maintenance treatment in recently depressed patients with bipolar I disorder. *J Clin Psychiatry*, 64(9), 1013–1024.

Calabrese, J.R., Keck, P.E. Jr., Macfadden, W., Minkwitz, M., Ketter, T.A., Weisler, R.G., Cutler, A.J., McCoy, R., Wilson, E., Mullen, J., and the Bolder Study Group. (2005). A randomized, double-blind, placebo-controlled trial of quetiapine in the treatment of bipolar I or II depression. *Am J Psychiatry*, 162(7), 1351–1360.

Carlson, P.J., Merlock, M.C., and Suppes, T. (2004). Adjunctive stimulant use in patients with bipolar disorder: Treatment of residual depression and sedation. *Bipolar Disord*, 6(5), 416–420.

Chengappa, K.N., Levine, J., Gershon, S., Mallinger, A.G., Hardan, A., Vagnucci, A., Pollock, B., Luther, J., Buttenfield, J., Verfaille, S., and Kupfer, D.J. (2000). Inositol as an add-on treatment for bipolar depression. *Bipolar Disord*, 21(1), 47–55.

Cohn, J.B., Collins, G., Ashbrook, E., and Wernicke, J.F. (1989). A comparison of fluoxetine imipramine and placebo in patients with bipolar depressive disorder. *Int Clin Psychopharmacol*, 4(4), 313–322.

Cole, D.P., Thase, M.E., Mallinger, A.G., Soares, J.C., Luther, J.F., Kupfer, D.J., and Frank, E. (2002). Slower treatment response in bipolar depression predicted by lower pretreatment thyroid function. *Am J Psychiatry*, 159(1), 116–121.

Colombo, C., Benedetti, F., Barbini, B., Campori, E., and Smeraldi, E. (1999). Rate of switch from depression into mania after therapeutic sleep deprivation in bipolar depression. *Psychiatry Res*, 86(3), 267–270.

Colombo, C., Lucca, A., Benedetti, F., Barbini, B., Campori, E., and Smeraldi, E. (2000). Total sleep deprivation combined with lithium and light therapy in the treatment of bipolar depression: Replication of main effects and interaction. *Psychiatry Res*, 95(1), 43–53.

Corya, S.A., Perlis, R.H., Keck, P.E. Jr., Lin, D.Y., Case, M.G., Williamson, D.J., and Tohen, M.F. (2006). A 24-week open-label extension study of olanzapine-fluoxetine combination and olanzapine monotherapy in the treatment of bipolar depression. *J Clin Psychiatry*, 67(5), 798–806.

Coryell, W., Endicott, J., and Keller, M. (1992). Rapidly cycling affective disorder. Demographics, diagnosis, family history, and course. *Arch Gen Psychiatry*, 49(2), 126–131.

Coryell, W., Endicott, J., Maser, J.D., Keller, M.B., Leon, A.C., and Akiskal, H.S. (1995). Long-term stability of polarity distinctions in the affective disorders. *Am J Psychiatry*, 152, 385–390.

Coryell, W., Winokur, G., Solomon, D., Shea, T., Leon, A., and Keller, M. (1997). Lithium and recurrence in a long-term follow-up of bipolar affective disorder. *Psychol Med*, 27(2), 281–189.

Coupland, N.J., Ogilvie, C.J., Hegadoren, K.M., Seres, P., Hanstock, C.C., and Allen, P.S. (2005). Decreased prefrontal myo-inositol in major depressive disorder. *Biol Psychiatry*, 57(12), 1526–1534.

Crane, G.E. (1956). The psychiatric side effects of iproniazid. *Am J Psychiatry*, 112, 494–501.

Daly, J.J., Prudic, J., Devanand, D.P., Nobler, M.S., Lisanby, S.H., Peyser, S., Roose, S.P., and Sackeim, H.A. (2001). ECT in bipolar and unipolar depression: Differences in speed of response. *Bipolar Disord*, 3(2), 95–104.

Daskalakis, Z.J., Christensen, B.K., Fitzgerald, P.B., and Chen, R. (2002). Transcranial magnetic stimulation: A new investigational and treatment tool in psychiatry. *J Neuropsychiatry*, 14(4), 406–415.

Davidson, J.R., Abraham, K., Connor, K.M., and McLeod, M.N. (2003). Effectiveness of chromium in atypical depression: A placebo-controlled trial. *Biol Psychiatry*, 53(3), 261–264.

Davis, J.M., Janicak, P.G., and Hogan, D.M. (1999). Mood stabilizers in the prevention of recurrent affective disorders: A meta-analysis. *Acta Psychiatr Scand*, 100(6), 406–417.

Davis, L.L., Kabel, D., Patel, D., Choate, A.D., Foslien-Nash, C., Gurguis, G.N., Kramer, G.L., and Petty, F. (1996). Valproate as an antidepressant in major depressive disorder. *Psychopharmacol Bull*, 32(4), 647–652.

Davis, L.L., Bartolucci, A., and Petty, F. (2005). Divalproex in the treatment of bipolar depression: A placebo-controlled study. *J Affect Disord*, 85(3), 259–266.

Dean, C.E. (2000). Prasterone (DHEA) and mania. *Ann Pharmacother*, 34(12), 1419–1422.

DeBattista, C., Lembke, A., Solvason, H.B., Ghebremichael, R., and Poirier, J. (2004). A prospective trial of modafinil as an adjunctive treatment of major depression. *J Clin Psychopharmacol*, 24(1), 87–90.

DelBello, M.P., Schwiers, M.L., Rosenberg, H.L., and Strakowski, S.M. (2002). A double-blind, randomized, placebo-controlled study of quetiapine as adjunctive treatment for adolescent mania. *J Am Acad Child Adolesc Psychiatry*, 41(10), 1216–1223.

Delle Chiaie, R., Pancheri, P., and Scapicchio, P. (2002). Efficacy and tolerability of oral and intramuscular S-adenosyl-L-methionine 1,4-butanedisulfonate (SAMe) in the treatment of major depression: Comparison with imipramine in 2 multicenter studies. *Am J Clin Nutr*, 76(5), 1172S–1176S.

De Montigny, C., Grunberg, F., Mayer, A., and Deschenes, J.P. (1981). Lithium induces rapid relief of depression in tricyclic antidepressant drug non-responders. *Br J Psychiatry*, 138, 252–256.

Desai, A.K., and Grossberg, G.T. (2003). Herbals and botanicals in geriatric psychiatry. *Am J Geriatr Psychiatry*, 11(5), 498–506.

Detke, M.J., Lu, Y., Goldstein, D.J., McNamara, R.K., and Demitrack, M.A. (2002). Duloxetine 60 mg once daily dosing versus placebo in the acute treatment of major depression. *J Psychiatr Res*, 36(6), 383–390.

Dilsaver, S.C., Swann, S.C., Chen, Y.W., Shoaib, A., Joe, B., Krajewski, K.J., Gruber, N., and Tsai, Y. (1996). Treatment of bipolar depression with carbamazepine: Results of an open study. *Biol Psychiatry*, 40(9), 935–937.

Djousse, L., Pankow, J.S., Eckfeldt, J.H., Folsom, A.R., Hopkins, P.N., Province, M.A., Hong, Y., and Ellison, R.C. (2001). Relation between dietary linolenic acid and coronary artery disease in the National Heart, Lung, and Blood Institute Family Heart Study. *Am J Clin Nutr*, 74(5), 612–661.

Dolberg, O.T., Dannon, P.N., Schreiber, S., and Grunhaus, L. (2002). Transcranial magnetic stimulation in patients with bipolar depression: A double-blind, controlled study. *Bipolar Disord*, 4(Suppl. 1), 94–95.

Dube, S., Corya, S.A., and Andersen, S.W. (2002). Olanzapine-fluoxetine combination for treatment of psychotic depression. *Eur Psychiatry*, 17(Suppl. 1), 130.

Dunn, R.T., Gilmer, W., and Fleck, J. (2006). *Divalproex monotherapy for acute bipolar depression: A double-blind, randomized placebo-controlled trial.* Presented at the 159th Annual Meeting of the American Psychiatric Association, Toronto, Canada, May 20–25.

Eastman, C.I., Young, M.A., Fogg, L.F., Liu, L., and Meaden, P.M. (1998). Bright light treatment of winter depression: A placebo-controlled trial. *Arch Gen Psychiatry*, 55(10), 883–889.

Eden Evins, A., Demopulos, C., Yovel, I., Culhane, M., Ogutha, J., Grandin, L.D., Nierenberg, A.A., and Sachs, G.S. (2006). Inositol augmentation of lithium or valproate for bipolar depression. *Bipolar Disord*, 8 (2), 168–174.

El-Mallakh, R.S. (1999). Rapid fade of antidepressant effect of nefazodone in bipolar depression. *J Clin Psychiatry*, 60, 559.

El-Mallakh, R.S. (2000). An open study of methylphenidate in bipolar depression. *Bipolar Disord*, 2(1), 56–59.

Erfurth, A., Michael, N., Stadtland, C., and Arolt, V. (2002). Bupropion as add-on strategy in difficult-to-treat bipolar depressive patients. *Neuropsychobiology*, 45(Suppl. 1), 33–36.

Ernst, C.L., and Goldberg, J.F. (2002). The reproductive safety profile of mood stabilizers, atypical antipsychotics, and broad-spectrum psychotropics. *J Clin Psychiatry*, 63(Suppl. 4), 42–55.

Faedda, G.L., Tondo, L., Teicher, M.H., Baldessarini, R.J., Gelbard, H.A., and Floris, G.F. (1993). Seasonal mood disorders. Patterns of seasonal recurrence in mania and depression. *Arch Gen Psychiatry*, 50(1), 17–23.

Fagiolini, A., Kupfer, D.J., Scott, J., Swartz, H.A., Cook, D., Novick, D.M., and Frank E. (2006). Hypothyroidism in patients with bipolar I disorder treated primarily with lithium. *Epidemiol Psychiatr Soc*, 15(2), 123–127.

Fava, M. (2000). Management of nonresponse and intolerance: Switching strategies. *J Clin Psychiatry*, 61(Suppl. 2), 10–12.

Fava, M., Rosenbaum, J.F., McGrath, P.J., Stewart, J.W., Amsterdam, J.D., and Quitkin, F.M. (1994). Lithium and tricyclic augmentation of fluoxetine treatment for resistant major depression: A double-blind, controlled study. *Am J Psychiatry*, 151(9), 1372–1374.

Fava, M., Thase, M.E., and DeBattista, C. (2005). A multicenter, placebo-controlled study of modafinil augmentation in partial responders to selective serotonin reuptake inhibitors with persistent fatigue and sleepiness. *J Clin Psychiatry*, 66(1), 85–93.

Fieve, R.R., Platman, S.R., and Plutchik, R.R. (1968). The use of lithium on affective disorders. I: Acute endogenous depression. *Am J Psychiiatry*, 125, 487–491.

Fink, M. (2001). Convulsive therapy: A review of the first 55 years. *J Affect Disord*, 63(1-3), 1–15.

Fogelson, D.L., Bystritsky, A., and Pasnau, R. (1992). Bupropion in the treatment of bipolar disorders: The same old story? *J Clin Psychiatry*, 53(12), 443–446.

Frangou, S., and Lewis, M. (2002). The Maudsley Bipolar Disorder Project: A double-blind, randomized, placebo controlled trial of Ethyl-EPA as an adjunct treatment of depression in bipolar disorder. *Bipolar Disord*, 4, 123.

Frangou, S., Lewis, M., and McCrone, P. (2006). Efficacy of ethyl-eicosapentaenoic acid in bipolar depression: Randomised double-blind placebo-controlled study. *Br J Psychiatry*, 188, 46–50.

Frankenburg, F.R., and Zanarini, M.C. (2002). Divalproex sodium treatment of women with borderline personality disorder and bipolar II disorder: A double-blind placebo-controlled pilot study. *J Clin Psychiatry*, 63(5), 442–446.

Frankle, W.G., Perlis, R.H., Deckersbach, T., Grandin, L.D., Gray, S.M., Sachs, G.S., and Nierenberg, A.A. (2002). Bipolar depression: Relationship between episode length and antidepressant treatment. *Psychol Med*, 32(8), 1417–1423.

Freeman, M.P., Hibbeln, J.R., Wisner, K.L., Davis, J.M., Mischoulon, D., Peet, M., Keck, P.E., Jr., Marangell, L.B., Richardson, A.J., Lake, J., and Stoll, A.L. (2006). Omega-3 fatty acids: Evidence basis for treatment and future research in psychiatry. *J Clin Psychiatry*, 67, 1954–1967.

Frye, M.A., Denicoff, K.D., Bryan, A.L., Smith-Jackson, E.E., Ali, S.O., Luckenbaugh, D., Leverich, G.S., and Post, R.M. (1999). Association between lower serum free T4 and greater mood instability and depression in lithium-maintained bipolar patients. *Am J Psychiatry*, 156(12), 1909–1914.

Frye, M., Ketter, T.A., Kimbrell, T.A., Dunn, R.T., Speer, A.M., Osuch, E.A., Luckenbaugh, D.A., Cora-Ocatelli, G., Leverich, G.S., and Post, R.M. (2000). A placebo-controlled sudy of lamotrigine and gabapentin monotherapy in refractory mood disorders. *J Clin Psychopharmacol*, 20(6), 607–612.

Frye, M.A., Calabrese, J.R., Reed, M.L., Wagner, K.D., Lewis, L., McNulty, J., and Hirschfeld, R.M. (2005). Use of health care services among persons who screen positive for bipolar disorder. *Psychiatr Serv*, 56(12), 1529–1533.

Frye, M.A., Yatham, L.N., Calabrese, J.R., Bowden, C.L., Ketter, T.A., Suppes, T., Adams, B.E., and Thompson, T.R. (2006). Incidence and time course of subsyndromal symptoms in patients with bipolar I disorder: An evaluation of 2 placebo-controlled trials. *J Clin Psychiatry*, 67(11), 1721–1728.

Gao, K., and Calabrese, J.R. (2005). New treatment studies for bipolar depression. *Bipolar Disord*, 7(Suppl. 5), 13–23.

Gelenberg, A.J., Kane, J.M., Keller, M.B., Lavori, P., Rosenbaum, J.F., Cole, K., and Lavelle, J. (1989). Comparison of standard and low serum levels of lithium for maintenance treatment of bipolar disorder. *N Engl J Med*, 321(22), 1489–1493.

Geller, B., Zimerman, B., Williams, M., Bolhofner, K., and Craney, J.L. (2001). Bipolar disorder at prospective follow-up of adults who had prepubertal major depressive disorder. *Am J Psychiatry*, 158(1), 125–127.

George, M.S., Sackeim, H.A., Rush, A.J., Marangell, L.B., Nahas, Z., Husain, M.M., Lisanby, S., Burt, T., Goldman, J., and Ballenger, J.C. (2000). Vagus nerve stimulation: A new tool for brain research and therapy. *Biol Psychiatry*, 47(4), 287–295.

George, M.S., Rush, A.J., Marangell, L.B., Sackeim, H.A., Brannan, S.K., Davis, S.M., Howland, R., Kling, M.A., Moreno, F., Rittberg, B., Dunner, D., Schwartz, T., Carpenter, L., Burke, M., Ninan, P., and Goodnick, P. (2005). A one-year comparison of vagus nerve stimulation with treatment as usual for treatment-resistant depression. *Biol Psychiatry*, 58(5), 364–373.

Ghaemi, S.N., and Goodwin, F.K. (2001a). Gabapentin treatment of the non-refractory bipolar spectrum: An open case series. *J Affect Disord*, 65, 167–171.

Ghaemi, S.N., and Goodwin, F.K. (2001b). Long-term naturalistic treatment of depressive symptoms in bipolar illness with divalproex vs. lithium in the setting of minimal antidepressant use. *J Affect Disord*, 65(3), 281–287.

Ghaemi, S.N., and Goodwin, F.K. (2005). Antidepressants for bipolar depression. *Am J Psychiatry*, 162(8), 1545–1546.

Ghaemi, S.N., and Hsu, D.J. (2005). Evidence-based treatment of bipolar disorder. In D.J. Stein, B. Lerer, and S. Stahl (Eds.), *Evidence-Based Psychopharmacology* (pp. 22–55). Cambridge, UK: Cambridge University Press.

Ghaemi, S.N., Katzow, J.J., Desai, S.P., and Goodwin, F.K. (1998). Gabapentin treatment of mood disorders: A preliminary study. *J Clin Psychiatry*, 59(8), 426–429.

Ghaemi, S.N., Boiman, E.E., and Goodwin, F.K. (2000). Diagnosing bipolar disorder and the effect of antidepressants: A naturalistic study. *J Clin Psychiatry*, 61(10), 804–808.

Ghaemi, S.N., Lenox, M.S., and Baldessarini, R.J. (2001). Effectiveness and safety of long-term antidepressant treatment in bipolar disorder. *J Clin Psychiatry*, 62, 565–569.

Ghaemi, S., Ko, J.Y., and Katzow, J.J. (2002). Oxcarbazepine treatment of refractory bipolar disorder: A retrospective chart review. *Bipolar Disord*, (1), 70–74.

Ghaemi, S.N., Berv, D.A., Klugman, J., Rosenquist, K.J., and Hsu, D.J. (2003a). Oxcarbazepine treatment of bipolar disorder. *J Clin Psychiatry*, 64(8), 943–945.

Ghaemi, S.N., Soldani, F., and Hsu, D. (2003b). Evidenced-based pharmacotherpy of bipolar disorder. *Int J Neuropsychopharmacol*, 6(3), 303–308.

Ghaemi, S.N., Hsu, D.J., Soldani, F., and Goodwin, F.K. (2003c). Antidepressants in bipolar disorder: The case for caution. *Bipolar Disord*, (6), 421–433.

Ghaemi, S.N., Rosenquist, K.J., Ko, J.Y., Baldassano, C.F., Kontos, N.J., and Baldessarini, R.J. (2004). Antidepressant treatment in bipolar versus unipolar depression. *Am J Psychiatry*, 161(1), 163–165.

Ghaemi, S.N., Hsu, D.J., Thase, M.E., Wisniewski, S.R., Nierenberg, A.A., Miyahara, S., and Sachs, G. (2006). Pharmacological treatment patterns at study entry for the first 500 STEP-BD participants. *Psychiatr Serv*, 57(5), 660–665.

Giedke, H., Klingberg, S., Schwarzler, F., and Schweinsberg, M. (2003). Direct comparison of total sleep deprivation and late partial sleep deprivation in the treatment of major depression. *J Affect Disord*, 85–93.

Gijsman, H.J., Geddes, J.R., Rendell, J.M., Nolen, W.A., and Goodwin, G.M. (2004). Antidepressants for bipolar depression: A systematic review of randomized, controlled trials. *Am J Psychiatry*, 161(9), 1537–1547.

Gjessing, R. (1938). Disturbances of somatic functions in catatonia with periodic course, and their compensation. *J Mental Sci*, 84, 608–621.

Goldberg, J.F., and Truman, C.J. (2003). Antidepressant-induced mania: An overview of current controversies. *Bipolar Disord*, 5, 407–420.

Goldberg, J.F., and Whiteside, J.E. (2002). The association between substance abuse and antidepressant-induced mania in bipolar disorder: A preliminary study. *J Clin Psychiatry*, 63(9), 791–795.

Goldberg, J.F., Singer, T.M., and Garno, J.L. (2001). Suicidality and substance abuse in affective disorders. *J Clin Psychiatry*, 62(Suppl. 25), 35–43.

Goldberg, J.F., Burdick, K.E., and Endick, C.J. (2004). Preliminary randomized, double-blind, placebo-controlled trial of pramipexole added to mood stabilizers for treatment-resistant bipolar depression. *Am J Psychiatry*, 161(3), 564–566.

Goldberg, J.F., and Nassir Ghaemi, S. (2005). Benefits and limitations of antidepressants and traditional mood stabilizers for treatment of bipolar depression. *Bipolar Disord*, 7(Suppl. 5), 3–12.

Golden, R.N., Gaynes, B.N., Ekstrom, R.D., Hamer, R.M., Jacobsen, F.M., Suppes, T., Wisner, K.L., and Nemeroff, C.B. (2005). The efficacy of light therapy in the treatment of mood disorders: A review and meta-analysis of the evidence. *Am J Psychiatry*, 162(4), 656–662.

Goldstein, D.J., Mallinckrodt, C., Lu, Y., and Demitrack, M.A. (2002). Duloxetine in the treatment of major depressive disorder: A double-blind clinical trial. *J Clin Psychiatry*, 63(3), 225–231.

Gonzalez-Pinto, A., Lalaguna, B., Mosquera, F., Perez de Heredia, J.L., Gutierrez, M., Ezcurra, J., Gilaberte, I., and Tohen, M. (2001). Use of olanzapine in dysphoric mania. *J Affect Disord*, 66(2–3), 247–253.

Goodwin, F.K., Murphy, D.L., and Bunney, W.F. Jr. (1969). Lithium carbonate treatment in depression and mania: A longitudinal double blind study. *Arch Gen Psychiatry*, 21, 486–496.

Goodwin, F.K., Murphy, D.L., Dunner, D.L., and Bunney, W.E. (1972). Lithium response in unipolar vs. bipolar depression. *Am J Psychiaty*, 129, 44–47.

Goodwin, F.K., Prange, A.J. Jr., Post, R.M., Muscettola, G., and Lipton, M.A. (1982). Potentiation of antidepressant effects by L-triiodothyronine in tricyclic nonresponders. *Am J Psychiatry*, 139, 34–38.

Goodwin, G.M., Bowden, C.L., Calabrese, J.R., Grunze, H., Kasper, S., White, R., Greene, P., and Leadbetter, R. (2004). A pooled analysis of 2 placebo-controlled 18-month trials of lamotrigine and lithium maintenance in bipolar I disorder. *J Clin Psychiatry*, 65(3), 432–441.

Goren, J.L., and Levin, J.M. (2000). Mania with bupropion: A dose-related phenomenon? *Ann Pharmacother*, 34(5), 619–621.

Grunebaum, M.F., Ellis, S.P., Li, S., Oquendo, M.A., and Mann, J.J. (2004). Antidepressants and suicide risk in the United States, 1985–1999. *J Clin Psychiatry*, 65(11), 1456–1462.

Grunhaus, L., Schreiber, S., Dolberg, O.T., Hirshman, S., and Dannon, P.N. (2002). Response to ECT in major depression: Are there differences between unipolar and bipolar depression? *Bipolar Disord*, 4(Suppl. 1), 91–93.

Grunze, H., Kasper, S., Goodwin, G., Bowden, C., Baldwin, D., Licht, R., Vieta, E., Moller, H.J., and World Federation of Societies of Biological Psychiatry Task Force on Treatment Guidelines for Bipolar Disorders. (2002). World Federation of Societies of Biological Psychiatry (WFSBP) guidelines for biological treatment of bipolar disorders. Part I: Treatment of bipolar depression. *World J Biol Psychiatry*, 3(3), 115–124.

Hantouche, E.G., Akiskal, H.S., Lancrenon, S., Allilaire, J.F., Sechter, D., Azorin, J.M., Bourgeois, M., Fraud, J.P., and Chatenet-Duchene, L. (1998). Systematic clinical methodology for validating bipolar-II disorder: Data in mid-stream from a French national multi-site study (EPIDEP). *J Affect Disord*, 50(2-3), 163–173.

Hantouche, E.G., Akiskal, H.S., Lancrenon, S., and Chatenet-Duchene, L. (2005). Mood stabilizer augmentation in apparently "unipolar" MDD: Predictors of response in the naturalistic French national EPIDEP study. *J Affect Disord*, 84(2-3), 243–249.

Henderson, L., Yue, Q.Y., Bergquist, C., Gerden, B., and Arlett, P. (2002). St. John's wort (*Hypericum perforatum*): Drug interactions and clinical outcomes. *Br J Clin Pharmacol*, 54(4), 349–356.

Hendrick, V., Altshuler, L.L., and Szuba, M.P. (1994). Is there a role for neuroleptics in bipolar depression? *J Clin Psychiatry*, 55(12), 533–535.

Henry, C., and Demotes-Mainard, J. (2003). Avoiding drug-induced switching in patients with bipolar depression. *Drug Safety*, 26(5), 337–351.

Henry, C., Sorbara, F., Lacoste, J., Gindre, C., and Leboyer, M. (2001). Antidepressant-induced mania in bipolar patients: Identification of risk factors. *J Clin Psychiatry*, 62(4), 249–255.

Hibbeln, J.R. (2002). Seafood consumption, the DHA content of mothers' milk and prevalence rates of postpartum depression: A cross-national, ecological analysis. *J Affect Disord*, 69(1-3), 15–29.

Hibbeln, J.R., Umhau, J.C., Linnoila, M., George, D.T., Ragan, P.W., Shoaf, S.E., Vaughan, M.R., Rawlings, R., and Salem, N. (1998). A replication study of violent and nonviolent subjects: CSF metabolites of serotonin and dopamine are predicted by plasma essential fatty acids. *Biol Psychiatry*, 44, 243–249.

Himmelhoch, J.M., Thase, M.E., Mallinger, A.G., and Houck, P. (1991). Tranylcypromine versus imipramine in anergic bipolar depression. *Am J Psychiatry*, 148(7), 910–916.

Hirschfeld, R.M., Fochtmann, L.J., and McIntyre, J.S. (2005). Antidepressants for bipolar depression. *Am J Psychiatry*, 162(8), 1546–1547.

Hirschfeld, R.M., Weisler, R.H., Raines, S.R., Macfadden, W. for the BOLDER Study Group. (2006). Quetiapine in the treatment of anxiety in patients with bipolar I or II depression: A secondary analysis from a randomized, double-blind, placebo-controlled study. *J Clin Psychiatry*, 67(3), 355–362.

Hlastala, S.A., Frank, E., Mallinger, A.G., Thase, M.E., Ritenour, A.M., and Kupfer, D.J. (1997). Bipolar depression: An underestimated treatment challenge. *Depress Anxiety*, 5(2), 73–83.

Hoencamp, E., Haffmans, J., Dijken, W.A., and Huijbrechts, I.P. (2000). Lithium augmentation of venlafaxine: An open-label trial. *J Clin Psychopharmacol*, 20(5), 538–543.

Holsboer, F. (2001). Prospects for antidepressant drug discovery. *Biol Psychol*, 57(1-3), 47–65.

Holtzheimer, P.E. III, Russo, J., and Avery, D.H. (2001). A meta-analysis of repetitive transcranial magnetic stimulation in the treatment of depression. *Psychopharmacol Bull*, 35(4), 149–169.

Hussain, M.Z., and Chaudhry, Z. (1999). Treatment of bipolar depression with topiramate. *Eur Neuropsychopharmacol*, 9(Suppl. 5), S222.

Hypericum Depression Trial Study Group. (2002). Effect of *Hypericum perforatum* (St. John's wort) in major depressive disorder: A randomized controlled trial. *JAMA*, 287(14), 1807–1814.

Isometsa, E.T., Henriksson, M.M., Aro, H.M., and Lonnqvist, J.K. (1994). Suicide in bipolar disorder in Finland. *Am J Psychiatry*, 151(7), 1020–1024.

Jackson, A., Cavanagh, J., and Scott, J. (2003). A systematic review of manic and depressive prodromes. *J Affect Disord*, 74(3), 209–217.

Janicak, P.G., Davis, J.M., Gibbons, R.D., Ericksen, S., Chang, S., and Gallagher, P. (1985). Efficacy of ECT: A meta-analysis. *Am J Psychiatry*, 142(3), 297–302.

Joffe, R.T. (1988). Triiodothyronine potentiation of the antidepressant effect of phenelzine. *J Clin Psychiatry*, 49, 409–410.

Joffe, R.T. (1992). Triiodothyronine potentiation of fluoxetine in depressed patients. *Can J Psychiatry*, 37(1), 48–50.

Joffe, R.T. (1998). The use of thyroid supplements to augment antidepressant medication. *J Clin Psychiatry*, 59(Suppl. 5), 26–29.

Joffe, R.T., Singer, W., Levitt, A.J., and MacDonald, C. (1993). A placebo-controlled comparison of lithium and triiodothyronine augmentation of tricyclic antidepressants in unipolar refractory depression. *Arch Gen Psychiatry*, 50(5), 387–393.

Joffe, R.T., MacQueen, G.M., Marriott, M., Robb, J., Begin, H., and Young, L.T. (2002). Induction of mania and cycle acceleration in bipolar disorder: Effect of different classes of antidepressant. *Acta Psychiatr Scand*, 105(6), 427–430.

Joffe, R.T., MacQueen, G.M., Marriott, M., and Young, L.T. (2005). One-year outcome with antidepressant—treatment of bipolar depression. *Acta Psychiatr Scand*, 112(2), 105–109.

Johnson, G. (1974). Antidepressant effect of lithium. *Compr Psychiatry*, 15(1), 43–47.

Judd, L.L., Schettler, P.J., Akiskal, H.S., Maser, J., Coryell, W., Solomon, D., Endicott, J., and Keller, M. (2003). Long-term symptomatic status of bipolar I vs. bipolar II disorders. *Int J Neuropsychopharmacol*, 6(2), 127–137.

Kanba, S., Yagi, G., Kamijima, K., Suzuki, T., Tajima, O., Otaki, J., Arata, E., Koshikawa, H., Nibuya, M., and Kinoshita, N. (1994). The first open study of zonisamide, a novel anticonvulsant, shows efficacy in mania. *Prog Neuropsychopharmacol Biol Psychiatry*, 18(4), 707–715.

Kaplan, B.J., Simpson, J.S., Ferre, R.C., Gorman, C.P., McMullen, D.M., and Crawford, S.G. (2001). Effective mood stabilization with a chelated mineral supplement: An open-label trial in bipolar disorder. *J Clin Psychiatry*, 62(12), 936–944.

Kasper, S., and Dienel, A. (2002). Cluster analysis of symptoms during antidepressant treatment with Hypericum extract in mildly to moderately depressed out-patients. A meta-analysis of data from three randomized, placebo-controlled trials. *Psychopharmacology (Berl)*, 164(3), 301–308.

Katona, C.L., Abou-Saleh, M.T., Harrison, D.A., Nairac, B.A., Edwards, D.R., Lock, T., Burns, R.A., and Robertson, M.M. (1995). Placebo-controlled trial of lithium augmentation of fluoxetine and lofepramine. *Br J Psychiatry*, 166(1), 80–86.

Kaufman, K.R. (1998). Adjunctive tiagabine treatment of psychiatric disorders: Three cases. *Ann Clin Psychiatry*, 10(4), 181–184.

Keck, P.E., Mintz, J., McElroy, S., Freeman, M., Suppes, T., Frye, M., Altshuler, L., Kupka, R., Nolen, W., Leverich, G., Denicoff, D., Grunze, H., Duan, N., and Post, R. (2006). Double-blind, randomized, placebo-controlled trials of ethyl-eicosapentanoate in the treatment of bipolar depression and rapid cycling bipolar disorder. *Biol Psychiatry*, 60(9), 1020–1022.

Keitner, G.I., Solomon, D.A., Ryan, C.E., Miller, I.W., Mallinger, A., Kupfer, D.J., and Frank, E. (1996). Prodromal and residual symptoms in bipolar I disorder. *Compr Psychiatry*, 37(5), 362–367.

Kennedy, S.H. (1997). Continuation and maintenance treatments in major depression: The neglected role of monoamine oxidase inhibitors. *J Psychiatry Neurosci*, 22(2), 127–131.

Khan, A.U. (1981). A comparison of the therapeutic and cardiovascular effects of a single nightly dose of Prothiaden (dothiepin, dosulepin) and Lentizol (sustained-release amitriptyline) in depressed elderly patients. *J Int Med Res*, 9(2), 108–112.

Kielholz, P., Terzani, S., and Poldinger, W. (1979). The long-term treatment of periodical and cyclic depressions with flupenthixol decanoate. *Int Pharmacopsychiatry*, 14(6), 305–309.

Klein, E., Kreinin, I., Chistyakov, A., Koren, D., Mecz, L., Marmur, S., Ben-Shachar, D., and Feinsod, M. (1999). Therapeutic efficacy of right prefrontal slow repetitive transcranial magnetic stimulation in major depression: A double-blind controlled study. *Arch Gen Psychiatry*, 56(4), 315–320.

Kline, M.D., and Jaggers, E.D. (1999). Mania onset while using dehydroepiandrosterone. *Am J Psychiatry*, 156(6), 971.

Klufas, A., and Thompson, D. (2001). Topiramate-induced depression. *Am J Psychiatry*, 158(10), 1736.

Koukopoulos, A., Reginaldi, D., Laddomada, P., Floris, G., Serra, G., and Tondo, L. (1980). Course of the manic-depressive cycle and changes caused by treatment. *Pharmakopsychiatr Neuropsychopharmakol*, 13(4), 156–167.

Koukopoulos, A., Faedda, G., Proietti, R., D'Amico, S., de Pisa, E., and Simonetto, C. (1992). Mixed depressive syndrome. *Encephale*, 18(1), 19–21.

Kovacs, M. (1996). Presentation and course of major depressive disorder during childhood and later years of the life span. *J Am Acad Child Adolesc Psychiatry*, 35(6), 705–715.

Krahl, S.E., Senanayake, S.S., Pekary, A.E., and Sattin, A. (2004). Vagus nerve stimulation (VNS) is effective in a rat model of antidepressant action. *J Psychiatr Res*, 38(3), 237–240.

Kripke, D.F. (1998). Light treatment for nonseasonal depression: Speed, efficacy, and combined treatment. *J Affect Disord*, 49(2), 109–117.

Kuhn, R. (1958). The treatment of depressive states with G22355 (imipramine hydrochloride). *Am J Psychiatry*, 115, 459–464.

Kupfer, D.J., and Spiker, D.G. (1981). Refractory depression: Prediction of non-response by clinical indicators. *J Clin Psychiatry*, 42(8), 307–312.

Kupfer, D.J., Chengappa, K.N., Gelenberg, A.J., Hirschfeld, R.M., Goldberg, J.F., Sachs, G.S., Grochocinski, V.J., Houck, P.R., and Kolar, A.B. (2001). Citalopram as adjunctive therapy in bipolar depression. *J Clin Psychiatry*, 62(12), 985–990.

Kusumakar, V., and Yatham, L.N. (1997). An open study of lamotrigine in refractory bipolar depression. *Psychiatry Res*, 72(2), 145–148.

Lake, C.R., Tenglin, R., Chernow, B., and Holloway, H.C. (1983). Psychomotor stimulant-induced mania in a genetically predisposed patient: A review of the literature and report of a case. *J Clin Psychopharmacol*, 3(2), 97–100.

Lecrubier, Y., Boyer, P., Turjanski, S., and Rein, W. (1997). Amisulpride versus imipramine and placebo in dysthymia and major depression. Amisulpride Study Group. *J Affect Disord*, 43(2), 95–103.

Levine, J., Barak, Y., Gonzalves, M., Szor, I.I., Elizur, A., Kofman, O., and Belmaker, R.H. (1995). Double-blind, controlled trial of inositol treatment of depression. *Am J Psychiatry*, 152(5), 792–794.

Lewis, J.L., and Winokur, G. (1982). The induction of mania: A natural history study with controls. *Arch Gen Psychiatry*, 39, 303–306.

Lewy, A.J., Bauer, V.K., Cutler, N.L., Sack, R.L., Ahmed, S., Thomas, K.H., Blood, M.L., and Jackson, J.M. (1998). Morning vs. evening light treatment of patients with winter depression. *Arch Gen Psychiatry*, 55(10), 890–896.

Lieber, C.S., and Packer, L. (2002). S-adenosylmethionine: Molecular, biological, and clinical aspects: An introduction. *Am J Clin Nutr*, 76(5), 1148S–1150S.

Linder, J., Fyro, B., Pettersson, U., and Werner, S. (1989). Acute antidepressant effect of lithium is associated with fluctuation of calcium and magnesium in plasma. A double-blind study on the antidepressant effect of lithium and clomipramine. *Acta Psychiatr Scand*, 80(1), 27–36.

Lipinski, J.F., Cohen, B.M., Frankenburg, F., Tohen, M., Waternaux, C., Altesman, R., Jones, B., and Harris, P. (1984). Open trial of S-adenosylmethionine for treatment of depression. *Am J Psychiatry*, 141(3), 448–450.

Lisanby, S.H., Schlaepfer, T.E., Fisch, H.U., and Sackeim, H.A. (2001a). Magnetic seizure therapy of major depression. *Arch Gen Psychiatry*, 58(3), 303–305.

Lisanby, S.H., Gutman, D., Luber, B., Schroeder, C., and Sackeim, H.A. (2001b). Sham TMS: Intracerebral measurement of the induced electrical field and the induction of motor-evoked potentials. *Biol Psychiatry*, 49(5), 460–463.

MacQueen, G.M., and Trevor Young, L. (2001). Bipolar II disorder: Symptoms, course, and response to treatment. *Psychiatr Serv*, 52(3), 358–361.

MacQueen, G.M., Trevor Young, L., Marriott, M., Robb, J., Begin, H., and Joffe, R.T. (2002). Previous mood state predicts response and switch rates in patients with bipolar depression. *Acta Psychiatr Scand*, 105(6), 414–418.

Malison, R.T., Anand, A., Pelton, G.H., Kirwin, P., Carpenter, L., McDougle, C.J., Heninger, G.R., and Price, L.H. (1999). Limited efficacy of ketoconazole in treatment-refractory major depression. *J Clin Psychopharmacol*, 19(5), 466–470.

Manji, H., Moore, G., and Chen, G. (2001). Bipolar disorder: Leads from the molecular and cellular mechanisms of action of mood stabilizers. *Br J Psychiatry*, 178(41), 107s–119s.

Manwani, S., Pardo, T.B., and Ghaemi, S.N. (2004). *Bipolar disorder, substance-abuse, and antidepressant-induced mania* [abstract]. 157th Annual Meeting of the American Psychiatric Association, New York City, NY.

Manwani, S.G., Pardo, T.B., Albanese, M.J., Zablotsky, B., Goodwin, F.K., Ghaemi, S.N. (2006). Substance use disorder and other predictors of antidepressant-induced mania: A retrospective chart review. *J Clin Psychiatry*, 67(9), 1341–1345.

Marangell, L.B. (2004). The importance of subsyndromal symptoms in bipolar disorder. *J Clin Psychiatry*, 65(Suppl. 10), 24–27.

Marangell, L.B., Rush, A.J., George, M.S., Sackeim, H.A., Johnson, C.R., Husain, M.M., Nahas, Z., and Lisanby, S.H. (2002). Vagus nerve stimulation (VNS) for major depressive episodes: One-year outcomes. *Biol Psychiatry*, 51(4), 280–287.

Marangell, L.B., Martinez, J.M., Zboyan, H.A., Kertz, B., Kim, H.F., and Puryear, L.J. (2003). A double-blind, placebo-controlled study of the omega-3 fatty acid docosahexaenoic acid in the treatment of major depression. *Am J Psychiatry*, 160(5), 996–998.

Marcotte, D. (1998). Use of topiramate, a new anti-epileptic as a mood stabilzer. *J Affect Disord*, 50, 245–251.

McAskill, R., Mir, S., and Taylor, D. (1998). Pindolol augmentation of antidepressant therapy. *Br J Psychiatry*, 173, 203–208.

McElroy, S.L., and Keck, P.E. Jr. (1993). Treatment guidelines for valproate in bipolar and schizoaffective disorders. *Can J Psychiatry*, 38(3 Suppl. 2), S62–S66.

McElroy, S.L., Suppes, T., Keck, P.E. Jr., Black, D., Frye, M.A., Altshuler, L.L., Nolen, W.A., Kupka, R.W., Leverich, G.S., Walden, J., Grunze, H., and Post, R.M. (2005). Open-label adjunctive zonisamide in the treatment of bipolar disorders: A prospective trial. *J Clin Psychiatry*, 66(5), 617–624.

McIntyre, R.S., Mancini, D.A., McCann, S., Srinivasan, J., Sagman, D., and Kennedy, S.H. (2002). Topiramate versus bupropion SR when added to mood stabilizer therapy for the depressive phase of bipolar disorder: A preliminary single-blind study. *Bipolar Disord*, 4, 207–213.

McLeod, M.N., and Golden, R.N. (2000). Chromium treatment of depression. *Int J Neuropsychopharmacol*, 3(4), 311–314.

McQuade, R., and Young, A.H. (2000). Future therapeutic targets in mood disorders: The glucocorticoid receptor. *Br J Psychiatry*, 177, 390–395.

Mendels, J., Sedcunda, S.K., and Dyson, W.L. (1972). A controlled study of the antidepressant effects of lithium carbonate. *Arch Gen Psychiatry*, 26, 154–157.

Menza, M.A., Kaufman, K.R., and Castellanos, A. (2000). Modafinil augmentation of antidepressant treatment in depression. *J Clin Psychiatry*, 61(5), 378–381.

Miller, L.J. (1994). Use of electroconvulsive therapy during pregnancy. *Hosp Community Psychiatry*, 45(5), 444–450.

Mischoulon, D., and Fava, M. (2000). Docosahexanoic acid and omega-3 fatty acids in depression. *Psychiatr Clin North Am*, 23(4), 785–794.

Moller, H.J., and Grunze, H. (2000). Have some guidelines for the treatment of acute bipolar depression gone too far in the restriction of antidepressants? *Eur Arch Psychiatry Clin Neurosci*, 250(2), 57–68.

Moller, H.J., Bottlender, R., Grunze, H., Strauss, A., and Wittmann, J. (2001). Are antidepressants less effective in the acute treatment of bipolar I compared to unipolar depression? *J Affect Disord*, 67(1–3), 141–146.

Montgomery, S.A., and Asberg, M. (1979). A new depression scale designed to be sensitive to change. *Br J Psychiatry*, 134, 382–389.

Moustgaard, G. (2000). Treatment-refractory depression successfully treated with the combination of mirtazapine and lithium. *J Clin Psychopharmacol*, 20(2), 268.

Mundo, E., Walker, M., Cate, T., Macciardi, F., and Kennedy, J.L. (2001). The role of serotonin transporter protein gene in antidepressant-induced mania in bipolar disorder: Preliminary findings. *Arch Gen Psychiatry*, 58, 539–544.

Mundo, E., Cattaneo, E., Russo, M., and Altamura, A.C. (2006). Clinical variables related to antidepressant-induced mania in bipolar disorder. *J Affect Disord*, 92(2–3), 227–230.

Nahas, Z., Kozel, F.A., Li, X., Anderson, B., and George, M.S. (2003). Left prefrontal transcranial magnetic stimulation (TMS) treatment of depression in bipolar affective disorder: A pilot study of acute safety and efficacy. *Bipolar Disord*, 5(1), 40–47.

Nahas, Z., Marangell, L.B., Husain, M.M., Rush, A.J., Sackeim, H.A., Lisanby, S.H., Martinez, J.M., and George, M.S. (2005). Two-year outcome of vagus nerve stimulation (VNS) for treatment of major depressive episodes. *J Clin Psychiatry*, 66(9), 1097–1104.

Nasr, S., Wendt, B., and Steiner, K. (2006). Absence of mood switch with and tolerance to modafinil: A replication study from a large private practice. *J Affect Disord*, 95(1-3), 111–114.

Nemeroff, C.B., Evans, D.L., Gyulai, L., Sachs, G.S., Bowden, C.L., Gergel, I.P., Oakes, R., and Pitts, C.D. (2001). Double-blind, placebo-controlled comparison of imipramine and paroxetine in the treatment of bipolar depression. *Am J Psychiatry*, 158(6), 906–912.

Nemeroff, C.B., Schatzberg, A.F., Goldstein, D.J., Detke, M.J., Mallinckrodt, C., Lu, Y., and Tran, P.V. (2002). Duloxetine for the treatment of major depressive disorder. *Psychopharmacol Bull*, 36(4), 106–132.

Nemets, B., Stahl, Z., and Belmaker, R.H. (2002). Addition of omega-3 fatty acid to maintenance medication treatment for recurrent unipolar depressive disorder. *Am J Psychiatry*, 159(3), 477–479.

Nierenberg, A.A., Burt, T., Matthews, J., and Weiss, A.P. (1999). Mania associated with St. John's wort. *Biol Psychiatry*, 46(12), 1707–1708.

Nierenberg, A.A., Trivedi, M.H., Fava, M., Biggs, M.M., Shores-Wilson, K., Wisniewski, S.R., Balasubramani, G.K., and Rush, A.J. (2006). Family history of mood disorder and characteristics of major depressive disorder: A STAR(*)D (sequenced treatment alternatives to relieve depression) study. *J Psychiatr Res*, 41(3-4), 214–221.

Normann, C., Hummel, B., Scharer, L.O., Horn, M., Grunze, H., and Walden, J. (2002). Lamotrigine as adjunct to paroxetine in acute depression: A placebo-controlled, double-blind study. *J Clin Psychiatry*, 63(4), 337–344.

Noyes, R. Jr., Dempsey, G.M., Blum, A., and Cavanaugh, G.L. (1974). Lithium treatment of depression. *Compr Psychiatry*, 15, 187–193.

Obrocea, G.V., Dunn, R.M., Frye, M.A., Ketter, T.A., Luckenbaugh, D.A., Leverich, G.S., Speer, A.M., Osuch, E.A., Jajodia, K., and Post, R.M. (2002). Clinical predictors of response to lamotrigine and gabapentin monotherapy in refractory affective disorders. *Biol Psychiatry*, 51(3), 253–260.

Osher, Y., Bersudsky, Y., and Belmaker, R.H. (2005). Omega-3 eicosapentaenoic acid in bipolar depression: Report of a small open-label study. *J Clin Psychiatry*, 66(6), 726–729.

Osser, D.N., Najarian, D.M., and Dufresne, R.L. (1999). Olanzapine increases weight and serum triglyceride levels. *J Clin Psychiatry*, 60(11), 767–770.

Parker, G., Gibson, N.A., Brotchie, H., Heruc, G., Rees, A.M., and Hadzi-Pavlovic, D. (2006). Omega-3 fatty acids and mood disorders. *Am J Psychiatry*, 163(6), 969–978.

Peet, M. (1994). Induction of mania with selective serotonin reuptake inhibitors and tricyclic antidepressants. *Br J Psychiatry*, 164(4), 549–550.

Peet, M. (2004). Nutrition and schizophrenia: Beyond omega-3 fatty acids. *Prostaglandins Leukot Essent Fatty Acids*, 70(4), 417–422.

Peet, M., and Horrobin, D.F. (2002). A dose-ranging study of the effects of ethyl-eicosapentaenoate in patients with ongoing depression despite apparently adequete treatment with standard drugs. *Arch Gen Psychiatry*, 59(10), 913–919.

Penland, H.R., and Ostroff, R.B. (2006). Combined use of lamotrigine and electroconvulsive therapy in bipolar depression: A case series. *J ECT*, 22(2), 142–147.

Perlis, R.H., Brown, E., Baker, R.W., and Nierenberg, A.A. (2006). Clinical features of bipolar depression versus major depressive disorder in large multicenter trials. *Am J Psychiatry*, 163(2), 225–231.

Perugi, G., Toni, C., Ruffolo, G., Frare, F., and Akiskal, H. (2001). Adjunctive dopamine agonists in treatment-resistant bipolar II depression: An open case series. *Pharmacopsychiatry*, 34(4), 137–141.

Physicians' Desk Reference. (2006). *2006 Physicians' Desk Reference (PDR): Your Complete Print and Electronic Drug Information Solution.* Montvale, NJ: Thomson Healthcare.

Post, R.M., Uhde, T.W., Roy-Byrne, P.P., and Joffe, R.T. (1986). Antidepressant effects of carbamazepine. *Am J Psychiatry*, 143(1), 29–34.

Post, R.M., Ketter, T.A., Denicoff, K., Pazzaglia, P.J., Leverich, G.S., Marangell, L.B., Callahan, A.M., George, M.S., and Frye, M.A. (1996). The place of anticonvulsant therapy in bipolar illness. *Psychopharmacology*, 128(2), 115–129.

Post, R.M., Leverich, G.S., Nolen, W.A., Kupka, R.W., Altshuler, L.L., Frye, M.A., Suppes, T., McElroy, S., Keck, P., Grunze, H., Walden, J., and Stanley Foundation Bipolar Network. (2003). A re-evaluation of the role of antidepressants in the treatment of bipolar depression: Data from the Stanley Foundation Bipolar Network. *Bipolar Disord*, 5(6), 396–406.

Post, R.M., Altshuler, L.L., Leverich, G.S., Frye, M.A., Nolen, W.A., Kupka, R.W., Suppes, T., McElroy, S., Keck, P.E. Jr., Denicoff, K.D., Grunze, H., Walden, J., Kitchen, C.M., and Mintz, J. (2006). Mood switch in bipolar depression: Comparison of adjunctive venlafaxine, bupropion, and sertraline. *Br J Psychiatry*, 189, 124–131.

Price, L.H., Charney, D.S., and Heninger, G.R. (1985). Efficacy of lithium-tranylcypromine treatment in refractory depression. *Am J Psychiatry*, 142(5), 619–623.

Prien, R.F. (1984). NIMH report. Five-center study clarifies use of lithium, imipramine for recurrent affective disorders. *Hosp Community Psychiatry*, 35(11), 1097–1098.

Prien, R.F., Kupfer, D.J., Mansky, P.A., Small, J.G., Tuason, V.B., Voss, C.B., and Johnson, W.E. (1984). Drug therapy in the prevention of recurrences in unipolar and bipolar affective diorders: A report of the NIMH Collaborative Study Group comparing lithium carbonate, imipramine, and a lithium carbonate-imipramine combination. *Arch Gen Psychiatry*, 41, 1096–1104.

Prien, R.F., Himmelhoch, J.M., and Kupfer, D.J. (1988). Treatment of mixed mania. *J Affect Disord*, 15, 9–15.

Quitkin, F.M., Kane, J., Rifkin, A., Ramos-Lorenzi, J.R., and Nayak, D.V. (1981). Prophylactic lithium carbonate with and without imipramine for bipolar 1 patients. A double-blind study. *Arch Gen Psychiatry*, 38(8), 902–907.

Rachid, F., Bertschy, G., Bondolfi, G., and Aubry, J.M. (2004). Possible induction of mania or hypomania by atypical antipsychotics: An updated review of reported cases. *J Clin Psychiatry*, 65(11), 1537–1545.

Ranjan, S., and Chandra, P.S. (2005). Modafinil-induced irritability and aggression: A report of 2 bipolar patients. *J Clin Psychopharmacol*, 25(6), 628–629.

Rao, A.V., and Nammalvar, N. (1977). The course and outcome in depressive illness: A follow-up study of 122 cases in Madurai, India. *Br J Psychiatry*, 130, 392–396.

Raskin, S., Teitelbaum, A., Zislin, J., and Durst, R. (2006). Adjunctive lamotrigine as a possible mania inducer in bipolar patients, *Am J Psychiatry*, 163(1), 159–160.

Riemann, D., Voderholzer, U., and Berger, M. (2002). Sleep and sleep–wake manipulations in bipolar depression. *Neuropsychobiology*, 45(Suppl. 1), 7–12.

Rocca, P., Fonzo, V., Ravizza, L., Rocca, G., Scotta, M., Zanalda, E., and Bogetto, F. (2002). A comparison of paroxetine and amisulpride in the treatment of dysthymic disorder. *J Affect Disord*, 70(3), 313–317.

Rohan, M., Parow, A., Stoll, A.L., Demopulos, C., Friedman, S., Dager, S., Hennen, J., Cohen, B.M., and Renshaw, P.F. (2004). Low-field magnetic stimulation in bipolar depression using an MRI-based stimulator. *Am J Psychiatry*, 161(1), 93–98.

Rosenthal, N.E., Sack, D.A., Gillin, J.C., Lewy, A.J., Goodwin, F.K., Davenport, Y., Mueller, P.S., Newsome, D.A., and Wehr, T.A. (1984). Seasonal affective disorder. A description of the syndrome and preliminary findings with light therapy. *Arch Gen Psychiatry*, 41(1), 72–80.

Rozans, M., Dreisbach, A., Lertora, J.J., and Kahn, M.J. (2002). Palliative uses of methylphenidate in patients with cancer: A review. *J Clin Oncol*, 20(1), 335–339.

Rudas, S., Schmitz, M., Pichler, P., and Baumgartner, A. (1999). Treatment of refractory chronic depression and dysthymia with high-dose thyroxine. *Biol Psychiatry*, 45(2), 229–233.

Rush, A.J., George, M.S., Sackeim, H.A., Marangell, L.B., Husain, M.M., Giller, C., Nahas, Z., Haines, S., Simpson, R.K. Jr., and Goodman, R. (2000). Vagus nerve stimulation (VNS) for treatment-resistant depressions: A multicenter study. *Biol Psychiatry*, 47(4), 276–286.

Rush, A.J., Marangell, L.B., Sackeim, H.A., George, M.S., Brannan, S.K., Davis, S.M., Howland, R., Kling, M.A., Rittberg,

B.R., Burke, W.J., Rapaport, M.H., Zajecka, J., Nierenberg, A.A., Husain, M.M., Ginsberg, D., and Cooke, R.G. (2005). Vagus nerve stimulation for treatment-resistant depression: A randomized, controlled acute phase trial. *Biol Psychiatry*, 58(5), 347–354.

Rybakowski, J.K., Suwalska, A., Lojko, D., Rymaszewska, J., and Kiejna, A. (2005). Bipolar mood disorder among Polish psychiatric outpatients treated for major depression. *J Affect Disord*, 84(2-3), 141–147.

Sachs, G. (2004). Strategies for improving treatment of bipolar disorder: Intergration of measurement and management. *Acta Psychiatr Scand*, 422(Suppl.), 7–17.

Sachs, G. (2005). *Advances in the treatment of acute bipolar depression. Advances in the treatment of bipolar disorders.* Washington, DC: American Psychiatric Association.

Sachs, G.S., Thase, M.E., Otto, M.W., Bauer, M., Miklowitz, D., Wisniewski, S.R., Lavori, P., Lebowitz, B., Rudorfer, M., Frank, E., Nierenberg, A.A., Fava, M., Bowden, C., Ketter, T., Marangell, L., Calabrese, J., Kupfer, D., and Rosenbaum, J.F. (1994). A double-blind trial of bupropion versus desipramine for bipolar depression. *J Clin Psychiatry*, 55(9), 391–393.

Sachs, G.S., Printz, D.J., Kahn, D.A., Carpenter, D., and Docherty, J.P. (2000). The expert consensus guideline series: Medication treatment of bipolar disorder 2000. *Postgrad Med*, 1–104.

Sachs, G.S., Altshuler, L.L., and Ketter, T.A. (2001). *Divalproex versus placebo for the treatment of bipolar depression* [abstract]. Annual Meeting of the American College of Neuropsychopharmacology, Puerto Rico.

Sachs, G.S., Thase, M.E., Otto, M.W., Bauer, M., Miklowitz, D., Wisniewski, S.R., Lavori, P., Lebowitz, B., Rudorfer, M., Frank, E., Nierenberg, A.A., Fava, M., Bowden, C., Ketter, T., Marangell, L., Calabrese, J., Kupfer, D., and Rosenbaum, J.F. (2003). Rationale, design, and methods of the systematic treatment enhancement program for bipolar disorder (STEP-BD). *Biol Psychiatry*, 53(11), 1028–1042.

Sachs, G., Chengappa, K.N., Suppes, T., Mullen, J.A., Brecher, M., Devine, N.A., and Sweitzer, D.E. (2004). Quetiapine with lithium or divalproex for the treatment of bipolar mania: A randomized, double-blind, placebo-controlled study. *Bipolar Disord*, 6(3), 213–223.

Sackeim, H.A., Rush, A.J., George, M.S., Marangell, L.B., Husain, M.M., Nahas, Z., Johnson, C.R., Seidman, S., Giller, C., Haines, S., Simpson, R.K. Jr., and Goodman, R.R. (2001). Vagus nerve stimulation (VNS) for treatment-resistant depression: Efficacy, side effects, and predictors of outcome. *Neuropsychopharmacology*, 25(5), 713–728.

Sajatovic, M., Brescan, D.W., Perez, D.E., DiGiovanni, S.K., Hattab, H., Ray, J.B., and Bingham, C.R. (2001). Quetiapine alone and added to a mood stabilizer for serious mood disorders. *J Clin Psychiatry*, 62(9), 728–732.

Sajatovic, M., Mullen, J.A., and Sweitzer, D.E. (2002). Efficacy of quetiapine and risperidone against depressive symptoms in outpatients with psychosis. *J Clin Psychiatry*, 63(12), 1156–1163.

Salzman, C., Wong, E., and Wright, B. (2002). Drug and ECT treatment of depression in the elderly, 1996–2001: A literature review. *Biol Psychiatry*, 52(3), 265.

Satel, S.L., and Nelson, J.C. (1989). Stimulants in the treatment of depression: A critical overview. *J Clin Psychiatry*, 50(7), 241–249.

Sato, T., Bottlender, R., Sievers, M., Schroter, A., Kleindienst, N., and Moller, H.J. (2004). Evaluating the inter-episode stability of depressive mixed states. *J Affect Disord*, 81(2), 103–113.

Schaffer, A., Zuker, P., and Levitt, A. (2006). Randomized, double-blind pilot trial comparing lamotrigene versus citalopram for the treatment of bipolar depression. *J Affect Disord*, 96, 95–99.

Schatzberg, A.F. (2000). Clinical efficacy of reboxetine in major depression. *J Clin Psychiatry*, 61(Suppl. 10), 31–38.

Schlatter, F.J., Soutullo, C.A., and Cervera-Enguix, S. (2001). First break of mania associated with topiramate treatment. *J Clin Psychopharmacol*, 21(4), 464–466.

Schweiger, U., Deuschle, M., Weber, B., Korner, A., Lammers, C.H., Schmider, J., Gotthardt, U., and Heuser, I. (1999). Testosterone, gonadotropin, and cortisol secretion in male patients with major depression. *Psychosom Med*, 61(3), 292–296.

Seidman, S.N., and Rabkin, J.G. (1998). Testosterone replacement therapy for hypogonadal men with SSRI-refractory depression. *J Affect Disord*, 48(2-3), 157–161.

Serby, M. (2001). Manic reactions to ECT. *Am J Geriatr Psychiatry*, 9(2), 180.

Serretti, A., Artioli, P., Zanardi, R., and Rossini, D. (2003). Clinical features of antidepressant associated manic and hypomanic switches in bipolar disorder. *Progr Neuropsychopharmacol Biol Psychiatry*, 27, 751–757.

Shapira, B., Oppenheim, G., Zohar, J., Segal, M., Malach, D., and Belmaker, R.H. (1985). Lack of efficacy of estrogen supplementation to imipramine in resistant female depressives. *Biol Psychiatry*, 20(5), 576–579.

Sharma, B., Khan, M., and Smith, A. (2005). A closer look at treatment resistant depression: Is it due to a bipolar diathesis? *J Affect Disord*, 84(2-3), 251–257.

Shelton, R.C., Keller, M.B., Gelenberg, A., Dunner, D.L., Hirschfeld, R., Thase, M.E., Russell, J., Lydiard, R.B., Crits-Cristoph, P., Gallop, R., Todd, L., Hellerstein, D., Goodnick, P., Keitner, G., Stahl, S.M., and Halbreich, U. (2001). Effectiveness of St. John's wort in major depression: A randomized controlled trial, *JAMA*, 285(15), 1978–1986.

Shergill, S.S., and Katona, C.L. (1997). Pharmacological choices after one antidepressant fails: A survey of UK psychiatrists. *J Affect Disord*, 43(1), 19–25.

Shimon, H., Agam, G., Belmaker, R.H., Hyde, T.M., and Kleinman, J.E. (1997). Reduced frontal cortex inositol levels in postmortem brain of suicide victims and patients with bipolar disorder. *Am J Psychiatry*, 154(8), 1148–1150.

Silverstone, T. (2001). Moclobemide vs. imipramine in bipolar depression: A multicentre double-blind clinical trial. *Acta Psychiatr Scand*, 104(2), 104–109.

Simpson, S.G., and DePaulo, J.R. (1991). Fluoxetine treatment of bipolar II depression. *J Clin Psychopharmacol*, 11(1), 52–54.

Smeraldi, E. (1998). Amisulpride versus fluoxetine in patients with dysthymia or major depression in partial remission: A double-blind, comparative study. *J Affect Disord*, 48(1), 47–56.

Smeraldi, E., Benedetti, F., Barbini, B., Campori, E., and Colombo, C. (1999). Sustained antidepressant effect of sleep deprivation combined with pindolol in bipolar depression. A placebo-controlled trial. *Neuropsychopharmacology*, 20(4), 380–385.

Smeraldi, E., Benedetti, F., Barbini, B., Campori, E., and Colombo, C. (2003). Sustained antidepressant effect of sleep deprivation combined with pindolol in bipolar depression: A placebo controlled trial. *Neuropsychopharmacology*, 20(4), 380–383.

Soares, C.N., Almeida, O.P., Joffe, H., and Cohen, L.S. (2001). Efficacy of estradiol for the treatment of depressive disorders in perimenopausal women: A double-blind, randomized, placebo-controlled trial. *Arch Gen Psychiatry*, (6), 529–534.

Sporn, J., and Sachs, G. (1997). The anticonvulsant lamotrigine in treatment-resistant manic-depressive illness. *J Clin Psychopharmacol*, 17(3), 185–189.

Sporn, J., Ghaemi, S.N., Sambur, M.R., Rankin, M.A., Recht, J., Sachs, G.S., Rosenbaum, J.F., and Fava, M. (2000). Pramipexole augmentation in the treatment of unipolar and bipolar depression: A retrospective chart review. *Ann Clin Psychiatry*, 12(3), 137–140.

Stokes, P.E., Shamoian, C.A., Stoll, P.M., and Patton, M.J. (1971). Efficacy of lithium as acute treatment of manic-depressive illness. *Lancet*, 1, 1319–1325.

Stoll, A.L., Mayer, P.V., Kolbrener, M., Goldstein, E., Suplit, B., Lucier, J., Cohen, B.M., and Tohen, M. (1994). Antidepressant-associated mania: A controlled comparison with spontaneous mania. *Am J Psychiatry*, 151(11), 1642–1650.

Stoll, A.L., Pillay, S.S., Diamond, L., Workum, S.B., and Cole, J.O. (1996). Methylphenidate augmentation of serotonin selective reuptake inhibitors: A case series. *J Clin Psychiatry*, 57(2), 72–76.

Stoll, A.L., Severus, W.E., Freeman, M.P., Rueter, S., Zboyan, H.A., Diamond, E., Cress, K.K., and Marangell, L.B. (1999). Omega 3 fatty acids in bipolar disorder: A preliminary double-blind, placebo-controlled trial. *Arch Gen Psychiatry*, 56(5), 407–412.

Su, K.P., Huang, S.Y., Chiu, C.C., and Shen, W.W. (2003). Omega-3 fatty acids in major depressive disorder. A preliminary double-blind, placebo-controlled trial. *Eur Neuropsychopharmacol*, 13(4), 267–271.

Suppes, T., Brown, E.S., McElroy, S.L., Keck, P.E. Jr., Nolen, W., Kupka, R., Frye, M., Denicoff, K.D., Altshuler, L., Leverich, G.S., and Post, R.M. (1999). Lamotrigine for the treatment of bipolar disorder: A clinical case series. *J Affect Disord*, 53(1), 95–98.

Suppes, T., McElroy, S.L., Keck, P.E., Altshuler, L., Frye, M.A., Grunze, H., Leverich, G.S., Nolen, W.A., Chisholm, K., Dennehy, E.B., and Post, R.M. (2004). Use of quetiapine in bipolar disorder: A case series with prospective evaluation. *Int Clin Psychopharmacol*, 19(3), 173–174.

Suppes, T., Mintz, J., McElroy, S.L., Altshuler, L.L., Kupka, R.W., Frye, M.A., Keck, P.E. Jr., Nolen, W.A., Leverich, G.S., Grunze, H., Rush, A.J., and Post, R.M. (2005). Mixed hypomania in 908 patients with bipolar disorder evaluated prospectively in the Stanley Foundation Bipolar Treatment Network: A sex-specific phenomenon. *Arch Gen Psychiatry*, 62(10), 1089–1096.

Szuba, M.P., Baxter, L.R. Jr., Altshuler, L.L., Allen, E.M., Guze, B.H., Schwartz, J.M., and Liston, E.H. (1994). Lithium sustains the acute antidepressant effects of sleep deprivation: Preliminary findings from a controlled study. *Psychiatry Res*, 51(3), 283–295.

Tamada, R.S., Issler, C.K., Amaral, J.A., Sachs, G.S., and Lafer, B. (2004). Treatment emergent affective switch: A controlled study. *Bipolar Disord*, 6(4), 333–337.

Taylor, D.M., and McAskill, R. (2000). Atypical antipsychotics and weight gain—a systematic review. *Acta Psychiatr Scand*, 101(6), 416–432.

Terman, M., and Terman, J.S. (1999). Bright light therapy: Side effects and benefits across the symptom spectrum. *J Clin Psychiatry*, 60(11), 799–808.

Terman, M., Terman, J.S., Quitkin, F.M., McGrath, P.J., Stewart, J.W., and Rafferty, B. (1989). Light therapy for seasonal affective disorder. A review of efficacy. *Neuropsychopharmacology*, 2(1), 1–22.

Terman, M., Terman, J.S., and Ross, D.C. (1998). A controlled trial of timed bright light and negative air ionization for treatment of winter depression. *Arch Gen Psychiatry*, 55(10), 875–882.

Tevar, R., Jho, D.H., Babcock, T., Helton, W.S., and Espat, N.J. (2002). Omega-3 fatty acid supplementation reduces tumor growth and vascular endothelial growth factor expression in a model of progressive non-metastasizing malignancy. *JPEN J Parenter Enteral Nutr*, 26(5), 285–289.

Thase, M.E. (2002). What role do atypical antipsychotic drugs have in treatment-resistant depression? *J Clin Psychiatry*, 63(2), 95–103.

Thase, M.E., Mallinger, A.G., McKnight, D., and Himmelhoch, J.M. (1992). Treatment of imipramine-resistant recurrent depression, IV: A double-blind crossover study of tranylcypromine for anergic bipolar depression. *Am J Psychiatry*, 149(2), 195–198.

Thase, M.E., Blomgren, S.L., Birkett, M.A., Apter, J.T., and Tepner, R.G. (1997). Fluoxetine treatment of patients with major depressive disorder who failed initial treatment with sertraline. *J Clin Psychiatry*, 58(1), 16–21.

Thase, M.E., Entsuah, A.R., and Rudolph, R.L. (2001). Remission rates during treatment with venlafaxine or selective serotonin reuptake inhibitors. *Br J Psychiatry*, 178, 234–241.

Thase, M.E., Bhargava, M., and Sachs, G.S. (2003). Treatment of bipolar depression: Current status, continued challenges, and the STEP-BD approach. *Psychiatr Clin North Am*, 26(2), 495–518.

Till, E., and Vuckovic, S. (1970). Uber den Einfluss der thymoleptischen Behandlung auf den Verlauf endogener Depressionen. *Int Pharmacopsychiatry*, 4, 210–219.

Tohen, M., Risser, R.C., Baker, R.W., Evans, A.R., Tollefson, G., and Breier, A. (2002). *Olanzapine in the treatment of bipolar depression*. Poster presented at 155th Annual Meeting. Philadelphia: American Psychiatric Association.

Tohen, M., Vieta, E., Calabrese, J., Ketter, T.A., Sachs, G., Bowden, C., Mitchell, P.B., Centorrino, F., Risser, R., Baker, R.W., Evans, A.R., Beymer, K., Dube, S., Tollefson, G.D., and Breier, A. (2003a). Efficacy of olanzapine and olanzapine-fluoxetine combination in the treatment of bipolar I depression. *Arch Gen Psychiatry*, 61(2), 176.

Tohen, M., Zarate, C.A. Jr., Hennen, J., Khalsa, H.M., Strakowski, S.M., Gebre-Medhin, P., Salvatore, P., and Baldessarini, R.J. (2003b). The McLean-Harvard First-Episode Mania Study: Prediction of recovery and first recurrence. *Am J Psychiatry*, 160(12), 2099–2107.

Trivedi, M.H., Rush, A.J., Wisniewski, S.R., Nierenberg, A.A., Warden, D., Ritz, L., Norquist, G., Howland, R.H., Lebowitz, B., McGrath, P.J., Shores-Wilson, K., Biggs, M.M., Balasubramani, G.K., and Fava, M., for the STAR*D Study Team. (2006). Evaluation of outcomes with citalopram for depression using measurement-based care in STAR*D: Implications for clinical practice. *Am J Psychiatry*, 163(1), 28–40.

Tuuainen, A., Kripke, D.F., and Endo, T. (2004). Light therapy for non-seasonal depression. *Cochrane Database Syst Rev*, (2), CD004050.

UK ECT Review Group. (2003). Efficacy and safety of electroconvulsive therapy in depressive disorders: A systematic review and meta-analysis. *Lancet*, 361(9360), 799–808.

Versiani, M., Mehilane, L., Gaszner, P., and Arnaud-Castiglioni, R. (1999). Reboxetine, a unique selective NRI, prevents relapse and recurrence in long-term treatment of major depressive disorder. *J Clin Psychiatry*, 60(6), 400–406.

Vieta, E., Colom, F., Martinez-Aran, A., Reinares, M., Benabarre, A., Corbella, B., and Gasto, C. (2001). Reboxetine-induced hypomania. *J Clin Psychiatry*, 62(8), 655–656.

Vieta, E., Martinez-Aran, A., Goikolea, J.M., Torrent, C., Colom, F., Benabarre, A., and Reinares, M. (2002). A randomized trial comparing paroxetine and venlafaxine in the treatment of bipolar depressed patients taking mood stabilizers. *J Clin Psychiatry*, 63(6), 508–512.

Visser, H., and Van der Mast, R. (2005). Bipolar disorder, antidepressants, and induction of hypomania or mania: A systemic review. *World J Biol Psychiatry*, 6, 231–241.

Wagner, G.J., and Rabkin, R. (2000). Effects of dextroamphetamine on depression and fatigue in men with HIV: A double-blind, placebo-controlled trial. *J Clin Psychiatry*, 61(6), 436–440.

Waldmeier, P.C. (1993). Newer aspects of the reversible inhibitor of MAOA and serotonin reuptake, brofaromine. *Prog Neuropsychopharmacol Biol Psychiatry*, 17(2), 183–198.

Walker, S.E., Shulman, K.I., Tailor, S.A., and Gardner, D. (1996). Tyramine content of previously restricted foods in monoamine oxidase inhibitor diets. *J Clin Psychopharmacol*, 16(5), 383–388.

Walter, G., Lyndon, B., and Kubb, R. (1998). Lithium augmentation of venlafaxine in adolescent major depression. *Aust NZ J Psychiatry*, 32(3), 457–459.

Watanabe, S., Ishino, H., and Otsuki, S. (1975). Double-blind comparison of lithium carbonate and imipramine in treatment of depression. *Arch Gen Psychiatry*, 32(5), 659–668.

Wehr, T., and Goodwin, F.K. (1979a). Tricyclics modulate frequency of mood cycles. *Chronobiologia*, 6(4), 377–385.

Wehr, T., and Goodwin, F.K. (1979b). Rapid cycling in manic-depressives induced by tricyclic antidepressants. *Arch Gen Psychiatry*, 36(5), 555–559.

Wehr, T.A., Goodwin, F.K., Wirz-Justice, A., Breitmaier, J., and Craig, C. (1982). 48-hour sleep–wake cycles in manic-depressive illness: Naturalistic observations and sleep deprivation experiments. *Arch Gen Psychiatry*, 39(5), 559–565.

Wehr, T.A., Sacks, D.A., Rosenthal, N.E., and Cowdry, R.W. (1988). Rapid cycling affective disorder: Contributing factors and treatment responses in 51 patients. *Am J Psychiatry*, 145(2), 179–184.

Whybrow, P.C. (1994). The therapeutic use of triiodothyronine and high-dose thyroxine in psychiatric disorder. *Acta Med Austriaca*, 21(2), 47–52.

Wiegand, M., Riemann, D., Schreiber, W., Lauer, C.J., and Berger, M. (1993). Effect of morning and afternoon naps on mood after total sleep deprivation in patients with major depression. *Biol Psychiatry*, 33(6), 467–476.

Williamson, D., Brown, E., Perlis, R.H., Ahl, J., Baker, R.W., and Tohen, M. (2006). Clinical relevance of depressive symptom improvement in bipolar I depressed patients. *J Affect Disord*, 92(2-3), 261–266.

Winsberg, M.E., DeGolia, S.G., Strong, C.M., and Ketter, T.A. (2001). Divalproex therapy in medication-naive and mood-stabilizer-naive bipolar II depression. *J Affect Disord*, 67(1-3), 207–212.

Wirshing, D.A., Spellberg, B.J., Erhart, S.M., Marder, S.R., and Wirshing, W.C. (1998). Novel antipsychotics and new-onset diabetes. *Biol Psychiatry*, 44(8), 778–783.

Wirz-Justice, A., and van den Hoofdakker, R.H. (1999). Sleep deprivation in depression: What do we know, where do we go? *Biol.Psychiatry*, 46(4), 445–453.

Wolkowitz, O.M., and Reus, V.I. (1999). Treatment of depression with antiglucocorticoid drugs. *Psychosom Med*, 61(5), 698–711.

Wolkowitz, O.M., Reus, V.I., Chan, T., Manfredi, F., Raum, W., Johnson, R., and Canick, J. (1999a). Antiglucocorticoid treatment of depression: Double-blind ketoconazole. *Biol Psychiatry*, 45(8), 1070–1074.

Wolkowitz, O.M., Reus, V.I., Keebler, A., Nelson, N., Friedland, M., Brizendine, L., and Roberts, E. (1999b). Double-blind treatment of major depression with dehydroepiandrosterone. *Am J Psychiatry*, 156(4), 646–649.

Wong, A.H., Smith, M., and Boon, H.S. (1998a). Herbal remedies in psychiatric practice. *Arch Gen Psychiatry*, 55(11), 1033–1044.

Wong, A.H., Smith, M., and Boon, H.S. (1998b). Herbal remedies in psychiatric practice. *Arch Gen Psychiatry*, 55(11), 1033–1044.

Wong, E.H., Sonders, M.S., Amara, S.G., Tinholt, P.M., Piercey, M.F., Hoffmann, W.P., Hyslop, D.K., Franklin, S., Porsolt, R.D., Bonsignori, A., Carfagna, N., and McArthur, R.A. (2000). Reboxetine: A pharmacologically potent, selective, and specific norepinephrine reuptake inhibitor. *Biol Psychiatry*, 47(9), 818–829.

Worrall, E.P., Moody, J.P., Peet, M., Dick, P., Smith, A., Chambers, C., Adams, M., and Naylor, G.J. (1979). Controlled studies of the acute antidepressant effects of lithium. *Br J Psychiatry*, 135, 255–262.

Wu, J.C., and Bunney, W.E. (1990). The biological basis of an antidepressant response to sleep deprivation and relapse: Review and hypothesis. *Am J Psychiatry*, 147(1), 14–21.

Yatham, L.N., Calabrese, J.R., and Kusumakar, V. (2003). Bipolar depression: Criteria for treatment selection, definition of refractoriness, and treatment options. *Bipolar Disord*, 5(2), 85–97.

Yildiz, A., and Sachs, G.S. (2003). Do antidepressants induce rapid cycling? A gender-specific association. *J Clin Psychiatry*, 64(7), 814–818.

Young, A.H., Gallagher, P., and Porter, R.J. (2002). Elevation of the cortisol-dehydroepiandrosterone ratio in drug-free depressed patients. *Am J Psychiatry*, 159(7), 1237–1239.

Young, E.A., and Korszun, A. (2002). The hypothalamic-pituitary-gonadal axis in mood disorders. *Endocrinol Metab Clin North Am*, 31(1), 63–78.

Young, L., Robb, J.C., Patelis-Siotis, I., MacDonald, C., and Joffe, R.T. (1997). Acute treatment of bipolar depression with gabapentin. *Biol Psychiatry*, 42(9), 851–853.

Young, L.T., Joffe, R.T., Robb, J.C., MacQueen, G.M., Marriott M., and Patelis-Siotis, I. (2000). Double-blind comparison of addition of a second mood stabilizer versus an antidepressant to an initial mood stabilizer for treatment of patients with bipolar depression. *Am J Psychiatry*, 1, 124–126.

Zabara, J. (1988). Neuroinhibition of xylazine induced emesis. *Pharmacol Toxicol*, 63(2), 70–74.

Zanarini, M.C., and Frankenburg, F.R. (2003). Omega-3 fatty acid treatment of women with borderline personality disorder: A double-blind, placebo-controlled pilot study. *Am J Psychiatry*, 160(1), 167–169.

Zarate, C.A. Jr., Rothschild, A., Fletcher, K.E., Madrid, A., and Zapatel, J. (2000). Clinical predictors of acute response with quetiapine in psychotic mood disorders. *J Clin Psychiatry*, 61(3), 185–189.

Zarate, C.A. Jr., Payne, J.L., Singh, J., Quiroz, J.A., Luckenbaugh, D.A., Denicoff, K.D., Charney, D.S., and Manji, H.K. (2004). Pramipexole for bipolar II depression: A placebo-controlled proof of concept study. *Biol Psychiatry*, 56(1), 54–60.

Zarate, C.A. Jr., Quiroz, J.A., Singh, J.B., Denicoff, K.D., De Jesus, G., Luckenbaugh, D.A., Charney, D.S., and Manji, H.K. (2005). An open-label trial of the glutamate-modulating agent riluzole in combination with lithium for the treatment of bipolar depression. *Biol Psychiatry*, 57(4), 430–432.

Zornberg, G.L., and Pope, H.G. Jr. (1993). Treatment of depression in bipolar disorder: New directions for research. *J Clin Psychopharmacol*, 13(6), 397–408.

Zwil, A.S., Bowring, M.A., Price, T.R., Goetz, K.L., Greenbarg, J.B., and Kane-Wanger, G. (1990). Prospective electroconvulsive therapy in the presence of intracranial tumor. *Convuls Ther*, 6(4), 299–307.

CHAPTER 20

Aagaard, J., and Vestergaard, P. (1990). Predictors of outcome in prophylactic lithium treatment: A 2-year prospective study. *J Affect Disord*, 18(4), 259–266.

Abrams, R. (1990). ECT as prophylactic treatment for bipolar disorder. *Am J Psychiatry*, 147(3), 373–374.

Ahlfors, U.G. Baastrup, P.C., Dencker, S.J., Elgen, K., Lingjaerde, O., Pedersen, V., Schou, M., and Aaskoven, O. (1981). Flupenthixol decanoate in recurrent manic-depressive illness: A comparison with lithium. *Acta Psychiatr Scand*, 64(3), 226–237.

Ahmed, Z., and Anderson, I.M. (2001). Treatment of bipolar affective disorder in clinical practice. *J Psychopharmacol*, 15(1), 55–57.

Ahrens, B., Grof, P., Moller, H.J., Muller-Oerlinghausen, B., and Wolf, T. (1995). Extended survival of patients on long-term lithium treatment. *Can J Psychiatry*, 241–246.

Akiskal, H. 2000. Mood disorders. In M.H. Beers, R. Berkow (Eds.), *The Merck Manual of Diagnosis and Therapy* (17th edition). Rahway, NJ: Merck Research Laboratories.

Allan, S.J., Kavanagh, G.M., Herd, R.M., and Savin, J.A. (2004). The effect of inositol supplements on the psoriasis of patients taking lithium: A randomized, placebo-controlled trial. *Br J Dermatol*, 150(5), 966–969.

Allen, M.H., Hirschfeld, R.M., Wozniak, P.J., Baker, J.D., and Bowden, C.L. (2006). Linear relationship of valproate serum concentration to response and optimal serum levels for acute mania. *Am J Psychiatry*, 163(2), 272–275.

Allison, D.B. (2001). Antipsychotic-induced weight gain: A review of the literature. *J Clin Psychiatry*, 62(Suppl. 7), 22–31.

Altshuler, L.L., Cohen, L., Szuba, M.P., Burt, V.K., Gitlin, M., and Mintz, J. (1996). Pharmacologic management of psychiatric illness during pregnancy: Dilemmas and guidelines. *Am J Psychiatry*, 153(5), 592–606.

Altshuler, L.L., Keck, P.E. Jr., McElroy, S.L., Suppes, T., Brown, E.S., Denicoff, K., Frye, M., Gitlin, M., Hwang, S., Goodman, R., Leverich, G., Nolen, W., Kupka, R., and Post, R. (1999). Gabapentin in the acute treatment of refractory bipolar disorder. *Bipolar Disord*, 1(1), 61–65.

American Psychiatric Association. (2002). Practice guideline for the treatment of patients with bipolar disorder (revision). *Am J Psychiatry*, 159(Suppl. 4), 1–50.

Amsterdam, J.D., Garcia-Espana, F., Fawcett, J., Quitkin, F.M., Reimherr, F.W., Rosenbaum, J.F., Schweizer, E., and Beasley, C. (1998). Efficacy and safety of fluoxetine in treating bipolar II major depressive episode. *J Clin Psychopharmacol*, 18(6), 435–440.

Andrade, C., and Kurinji, S. (2002). Continuation and maintenance ECT: A review of recent research. *J ECT*, 18(3), 149–158.

Angst, J., Weis, P., Grof, P., Baastrup, P.C., and Schou, M. (1970). Lithium prophylaxis in recurrent affective disorders. *Br J Psychiatry*, 116, 604–614.

Appleby, L., Mortensen, P.B., Faragher, E.B. (1998). Suicide and other causes of mortality after post-partum psychiatric admission. *Br J Psychiatry*, 173, 209–211.

Atmaca, M. (2002). Weight gain and serum leptin levels in patients on lithium treatment. *Neuropsychobiology*, 46(2), 67–69.

Austin, M.P. (1992). Puerperal affective psychosis: Is there a case for lithium prophylaxis? *Br J Psychiatry*, 161, 692–694.

Baastrup, P.C., and Schou, M. (1967). Lithium as a prophylactic agent: Its effect against recurrent depressions and manic-depressive psychosis. *Arch Gen Psychiatry*, 16(2), 162–172.

Baastrup, P.C., Poulsen, J.C., Schou, M., Thomsen, K., and Amdisen, A. (1970). Prophylactic lithium: Double blind discontinuation in manic-depressive and recurrent-depressive disorders. *Lancet*, 2(7668), 326–330.

Baethge C., Smolka, M.N., Gruschka, P., Berghofer, A., Schlattmann, P., Bauer, M., Altshuler, L., Grof, P., and Muller-Oerlinghausen, B. (2003). Does prophylaxis-delay in bipolar disorder influence outcome? Results for a long-term study of 147 patients. *Acta Psychiatr Scand*, 107, 260–267.

Baethge, C., Baldessarini, R.J., Mathiske-Schmidt, K., Hennen, J., Berghofer, A., Muller-Oerlinghausen, B. (2005). Long-term combination therapy versus monotherapy with lithium and carbamazepine in 46 bipolar I patients. *J Clin Psychiatry*, 66(2), 174–182.

Baldessarini, R.J. (1988). A summary of current knowledge of tardive dyskinesia. *Encephale*, 14, 263–268.

Baldessarini, R.J., and Tondo, L. (2000). Does lithium treatment still work? Evidence of stable responses over three decades. *Arch Gen Psychiatry*, 57(2), 187–190.

Baldessarini, R.J., Tondo, L., Faedda, G., Floris, G., Suppes, T., and Rudas, N. (1996). Effects of the rate of discontinuing lithium maintenance treatment in bipolar disorders. *J Clin Psychiatry*, 57, 441–448.

Baldessarini, R.J., Tondo, L., Floris, G., and Rudas, N. (1997). Reduced morbidity after gradually discontinuing lithium in bipolar I and II disorders: A replication study. *Am J Psychiatry*, 154, 551–553.

Baldessarini, R.J., Tondo, L., Hennen, J., and Floris, G. (1999a). Latency and episodes before treatment: Response to lithium maintenance in bipolar I and II disorders. *Bipolar Disord*, 1(2), 91–97.

Baldessarini, R.J., Tondo, L., and Viguera, A.C. (1999b). Discontinuing lithium maintenance treatment in bipolar disorders: Risks and implications. *Bipolar Disord*, 1(1), 17–24.

Baldessarini, R.J., Tondo, L., Floris, G., and Hennen, J. (2000). Effects of rapid cycling on response to lithium maintenance treatment in 360 bipolar I and II disorder patients. *J Affect Disord*, 61(1-2), 13–22.

Baldessarini, R.J., Tondo, L., Hennen, J., and Viguera, A.C. (2002). Is lithium still worth using? An update of selected recent research. *Harv Rev Psychiatry*, 10(2), 59–75.

Baldessarini, R.J., Tondo, L., and Hennen, J. (2003). Treatment-latency and previous episodes: Relationships to pretreatment morbidity and response to maintenance treatment in bipolar I and II disorders. *Bipolar Disord*, 5(3), 169–179.

Baldessarini, R.J., Pompili, M., and Tondo, L. (2006). Suicidal risk in antidepressant drug trials. *Arch Gen Psychiatry*, 63(3), 246–248.

Ballenger, J.C., and Post, R.M. (1978). Therapeutic effects of carbamazepine in affective illness: A preliminary report. *Commun Psychopharmacol*, 2, 159–175.

Ballenger, J.C., and Post, R.M. (1980). Carbamazepine in manic-depressive illness: A new treatment. *Am J Psychiatry*, 137(7), 782–790.

Banov, M.D., Zarate, C.A. Jr., Tohen, M., Scialabba, D., Wines, J.D. Jr., Kolbrener, M., Kim, J.W., and Cole, J.O. (1994). Clozapine therapy in refractory affective disorders: Polarity predicts response in long-term follow-up. *J Clin Psychiatry*, 55(7), 295–300.

Baptista, T., Lacruz, A., de Mendoza, S., Guillen, M.M., Burguera, J.L., de Burguera, M., and Hernandez, L. (2000). Endocrine effects of lithium carbonate in healthy premenopausal women: Relationship with body weight regulation. *Prog Neuropsychopharmacol Biol Psychiatry*, 24(1), 1–16.

Baptista, T., Kin, N.M., Beaulieu, S., and de Baptista, E.A. (2002). Obesity and related metabolic abnormalities during antipsychotic drug administration: Mechanisms, management and research perspectives. *Pharmacopsychiatry*, 35(6), 205–219.

Barton, C.D. Jr., Dufer, D., Monderer, R., Cohen, M.J., Fuller, H.J., Clark, M.R., and DePaulo, J.R. Jr. (1993). Mood variability in normal subjects on lithium. *Biol Psychiatry*, 34(12), 878–884.

Bauer, J., Jarre, A., Klingmuller, D., and Elger, C.E. (2000). Polycystic ovary syndrome in patients with focal epilepsy: A study in 93 women. *Epilepsy Res*, 41(2), 163–167.

Bauer, M.S., and Mitchner, L. (2004). What is a "mood stabilizer"? An evidence-based response. *Am J Psychiatry*, 161(1), 3–18.

Bauer, M.S., and Whybrow, P.C. (1990). Rapid cycling bipolar affective disorder: II. Treatment of refractory rapid cycling with high-dose levothyroxine: A preliminary study. *Arch Gen Psychiatry*, 47(5), 435–440.

Bauer, M., and Whybrow, P.C. (2001). Thyroid hormones, neural tissue, and mood modulation. *World J Biol Psychiatry*, 2, 59–69.

Bauer, M., Berghofer, A., Bschor, T., Baumgartner, A., Kiesslinger, U., Hellweg, R., Adli, M., Baethge, C., and Muller-Oerlinghausen, B. (2002). Supraphysiological doses of L-thyroxine in the maintenance treatment of prophylaxis-resistant affective disorders. *Neuropsychopharmacology*, 27(4), 620–628.

Baumgartner, A. (2000). Thyroxine and the treatment of affective disorders: An overview of the results of basic and clinical research. *Int J Neuropsychopharmacol*, 3(2), 149–165.

Bech, P. (2006). The full story of lithium: A tribute to Mogens Schou (1918–2005). *Psychother Psychosom* 75(5), 265–269.

Berghofer, A., Kossmann, B., and Muller-Oerlinghausen, B. (1996). Course of illness and pattern of recurrences in patients with affective disorders during long-term lithium prophylaxis: A retrospective analysis over 15 years. *Acta Psychiatr Scand*, 93(5), 349–354.

Bendz, H., Aurell, M., and Lanke, J. (2001). A historical cohort study of kidney damage in long-term lithium patients: Continued surveillance needed. *Eur Psychiatry*, 16(4), 199–206.

Birt, J. (2003). Management of weight gain associated with antipsychotics. *Ann Clin Psychiatry*, 15(1), 49–58.

Blackwell, B., and Shepherd, M. (1968). Prophylactic lithium: Another therapeutic myth? *Lancet*, 968–971.

Bocchetta, A., Chillotti, C., Severino, G., Ardau, R., and Del Zompo, M. (1997). Carbamazepine augmentation in lithium-refractory bipolar patients: A prospective study on long-term prophlyactic effectiveness. *J Clin Psychopharmacol*, 17(2), 92–96.

Bocchetta, A., Mossa, P., Velluzzi, F., Mariotti, S., Zompo, M.D., and Loviselli, A. (2001). Ten-year follow-up of thyroid function in lithium patients. *J Clin Psychopharmacol*, 21(6), 594–598.

Bollini, P., Pampallona, S., Orza, M.J., Adams, M.E., and Chalmers, T.C. (1994). Antipsychotic drugs: Is more worse? A meta-analysis of the published randomized control trials. *Psychol Med*, 24(2), 307–316.

Bonari, L., Pinto, N., Ahn, E., Einarson, A., Steiner, M., and Koren, G. (2004). Perinatal risks of untreated depression during pregnancy. *Can J Psychiatry*, 49(11), 726–735.

Bowden, C.L. (1998). Key treatment studies of lithium in manic-depressive illness: Efficacy and side effects. *J Clin Psychiatry*, 59(Suppl. 6), 13–19; discussion 20.

Bowden, C.L., Brugger, A.M., Swann, A.C., Calabrese, J.R., Janicak, P.G., Petty, F., Dilsaver, S.C., Davis, J.M., Rush, A.J., and Small, J.G. (1994). Efficacy of divalproex vs lithium and placebo in the treatment of mania. The Depakote Mania Study Group. *JAMA*, 271(12), 918–924.

Bowden, C.L., Calabrese, J.R., McElroy, S.L., Rhodes, L.J., Keck, P.E. Jr., Cookson, J., Anderson, J., Bolden-Watson. C., Ascher, J., Monaghan, E., and Zhou, J. (1999). The efficacy of lamotrigine in rapid cycling and non-rapid cycling patients with bipolar disorder. *Biol Psychiatry*, 45(8), 953–958.

Bowden, C.L., Calabrese, J.R., McElroy, S.L., Gyulai, L., Wassef, A., Petty, F., Pope, H.G. Jr., Chou, J.C., Keck, P.E. Jr., Rhodes, L.J., Swann, A.C., Hirschfeld, R.M., and Wozniak, P.J. (2000a). A randomized, placebo-controlled 12-month trial of divalproex and lithium in treatment of outpatients with bipolar I disorder. Divalproex Maintenance Study Group. *Arch Gen Psychiatry*, 57(5), 481–489.

Bowden, C.L., Lecrubier, Y., Bauer, M., Goodwin, G., Greil, W., Sachs, G., and von Knorring, L. (2000b). Maintenance therapies for classic and other forms of bipolar disorder. *J Affect Disord*, 59(Suppl. 1), S57–S67.

Bowden, C.L., Calabrese, J.R., Sachs, G., Yatham, L.N., Asghar, S.A., Hompland, M., Montgomery, P., Earl, N., Smoot, T.M., DeVeaugh-Geiss, J., and Lamictal 606 Study Group. (2003a). A placebo-controlled 18-month trial of lamotrigine and lithium maintenance treatment in recently manic or hypomanic patients with bipolar I disorder. *Arch Gen Psychiatry*, 60(4), 392.

Bowden, C.L., Calabrese, J.R., Sachs, G., Yatham, L.N., Asghar, S.A., Hompland, M., Montgomery, P., Earl, N., Smoot, T.M., DeVeaugh-Geiss, J., for Lamictal 606 Study Group. (2003b). A placebo-controlled 18-month trial of lamotrigine and lithium maintenance treatment in recently manic or hypomanic patients with bipolar I disorder. *Arch Gen Psychiatry*, 60(4), 392–400.

Bowden, C.L., Myers, J.E., Grossman, F., and Xie, Y. (2004). Risperidone in combination with mood stabilizers: A 10-week continuation phase study in bipolar I disorder. *J Clin Psychiatry*, 65(5), 707–714.

Bowden, C.L., Collins, M.A., McElroy, S.L., Calabrese, J.R., Swann, A.C., Weisler, R.H. (2005). Relationship of mania symptomatology to maintenance treatment response with divalproex, lithium, or placebo. *Neuropsychopharmacology*, 30(10), 1932–1939.

Bowden, C.L., Calabrese, J.R., Ketter, T.A., Sachs, G.S., White, R.L., and Thompson, T.R. (2006). Impact of lamotrigine and lithium on weight in obese and nonobese patients with bipolar I disorder. *Am J Psychiatry*, 163(7), 1199–1201.

Bowden, R.C., Grof, P., and Grof, E. (1991). Less frequent lithium administration and lower urine volume. *Am J Psychiatry*, 148(2), 189–192.

Burt, T., Sachs, G.S., and Demopulos, C. (1999). Donepezil in treatment-resistant bipolar disorder. *Biol Psychiatry*, 45(8), 959–964.

Byrne, S.E., and Rothschild, A.J. (1998). Loss of antidepressant efficacy during maintenance therapy: Possible mechanisms and treatments. *J Clin Psychiatry*, 59(6), 279–288.

Cade, J.F.J. (1949). Lithium salts in the treatment of psychotic excitement. *Med J Aust*, 36, 349–352.

Calabrese, J.R., and Delucchi, G.A. (1990). Spectrum of efficacy of valproate in 55 patients with rapid-cycling bipolar disorder. *Am J Psychiatry*, 147(4), 431–434.

Calabrese, J.R., and Rapport, D.J. (1999). Mood stabilizers and the evolution of maintenance study designs in bipolar I disorder. *J Clin Psychiatry*, 60(Suppl. 5), 5–13; discussion 14–15.

Calabrese, J.R., Rapport, D.J., Kimmel, S.E., Reece, B., and Woyshville, M.J. (1993). Rapid cycling bipolar disorder and its treatment with valproate. *Can J Psychiatry*, 38(3 Suppl. 2), S57–S61.

Calabrese, J.R., Bowden, C.L., McElroy, S.L., Cookson, J., Andersen, J., Keck, P.E. Jr., Rhodes, L., Bolden-Watson, C., Zhou, J., and Ascher, J.A. (1999a). Spectrum of activity of lamotrigine in treatment-refractory bipolar disorder. *Am J Psychiatry*, 156(7), 1019–1023.

Calabrese, J.R., Bowden, C.L., Sachs, G.S., Ascher, J.A., Monaghan, E., and Rudd, G.D. (1999b). A double-blind placebo-controlled study of lamotrigine monotherapy in outpatients with bipolar I depression. Lamictal 602 Study Group. *J Clin Psychiatry*, 60(2), 79–88.

Calabrese, J.R., Suppes, T., Bowden, C.L., Sachs, G.S., Swann, A.C., McElroy, S.L., Kusumakar, V., Ascher, J.A., Earl, N.L., Greene, P.L., and Monaghan, E.T. (2000). A double-blind, placebo-controlled, prophylaxis study of lamotrigine in rapid-cycling bipolar disorder. Lamictal 614 Study Group. *J Clin Psychiatry*, 61(11), 841–850.

Calabrese, J.R., Shelton, M.D., Rapport, D.J., Kujawa, M., Kimmel, S.E., and Caban, S. (2001). Current research on rapid cycling bipolar disorder and its treatment. *J Affect Disord*, 67(1–3), 241–255.

Calabrese, J.R., Sullivan, J.R., Bowden, C.L., Suppes, T., Goldberg, J.F., Sachs, G.S., Shelton, M.D., Goodwin, F.K., Frye, M.A., and Kusumakar, V. (2002). Rash in multicenter trials of lamotrigine in mood disorders: Clinical relevance and management. *J Clin Psychiatry*, 63(11), 1012–1019.

Calabrese, J.R., Bowden, C.L., Sachs, G., Yatham, L.N., Behnke, K., Mehtonen, O.P., Montgomery, P., Ascher, J., Paska, W., Earl, N., DeVeaugh-Geiss, J., and Lamictal 605 Study Group. (2003). A placebo-controlled 18-month trial of lamotrigine and lithium maintenance treatment in recently depressed patients with bipolar I disorder. *J Clin Psychiatry*, 64(9), 1013–1024.

Calabrese, J.R., Shelton, M.D., Rapport, D.J., Youngstrom, E.A., Jackson, K., Bilali, S., Ganocy, S.J., and Findling, R.L. (2005). A 20-month, double-blind, maintenance trial of lithium versus divalproex in rapid-cycling bipolar disorder. *Am J Psychiatry*, 162(11), 2152–2161.

Calabrese, J.R., Goldberg, J.F., Ketter, T.A., Suppes, T., Frye, M., White, R., DeVeaugh-Geiss, A., and Thompson, T.R. (2006). Recurrence in bipolar I disorder: A post hoc analysis excluding relapses in two double-blind maintenance studies. *Biol Psychiatry*, 59(11), 1061–1064.

Calil, H.M., Zwicker, A.P., and Klepacz, S. (1990). The effects of lithium carbonate on healthy volunteers: Mood stabilization? *Biol Psychiatry*, 27(7), 711–722.

Carta, M.G. Hardoy, M.C., Grunze, H., and Carpiniello, B. (2002). The use of tiagabine in affective disorders. *Pharmacopsychiatry*, 35(1), 33–34.

Cavanagh, J., Smyth, R., and Goodwin, G.M. (2004). Relapse into mania or depression following lithium discontinuation: A 7-year follow-up. *Acta Psychiatr Scand*, 109(2), 91–95.

Champion, L.M., Nem, J.Y., Culver, J.L., Wong, P.W., Marsh, W.K., Bonner, J.C., and Ketter, T.C. (2006). *Effectiveness of lamotrigine in a clinical setting*. APA New Research Poster. Presented at American Psychiatric Association Meeting, Toronto, Canada.

Chang, J.S., Ha, K-S., Lee, K.Y., Kim, Y.S., and Ahn, Y.M. (2006). The effects of long-term clozapine add-on therapy on the rehospitalization rate and the mood polarity patterns in bipolar disorders. *J Clin Psychiatry*, 67(3), 461–467.

Chaudron, L.H., and Jefferson, J.W. (2000). Mood stabilizers during breastfeeding: A review. *J Clin Psychiatry*, 61(2), 79–90.

Chaudron, L.H., and Pies, R.W. (2003). The relationship between postpartum psychosis and bipolar disorder: A review. *J Clin Psychiatry*, 64(11), 1284–1292.

Chen, S.T., Altshuler, L.L., Melnyk, K.A., Erhart, S.M., Miller, E., and Mintz, J. (1999). Efficacy of lithium vs. valproate in the treatment of mania in the elderly: A retrospective study. *J Clin Psychiatry*, 60(3), 181–186.

Chengappa, K.N., Chalasani, L., Brar, J.S., Parepally, H., Houck, P., and Levine, J. (2002). Changes in body weight and body mass index among psychiatric patients receiving lithium, valproate, or topiramate: An open-label, nonrandomized chart review. *Clin Ther*, 24(10), 1576–1584.

Ciapparelli, A., Dell'Osso, L., Pini, S., Chiavacci, M.C., Fenzi, M., and Cassano, G.B. (2000). Clozapine for treatment-refractory schizophrenia, schizoaffective disorder, and psychotic bipolar disorder: A 24-month naturalistic study. *J Clin Psychiatry*, 61(5), 329–334.

Cohen, L.S., Friedman, J.M., Jefferson, J.W., Johnson, E.M., and Weiner, M.L. (1994). A reevaluation of risk of in utero exposure to lithium. *JAMA*, 271(2), 146–150.

Cole, D.P., Thase, M.E., Mallinger, A.G., Soares, J.C., Luther, J.F., Kupfer, D.J., and Frank, E. (2002). Slower treatment response in bipolar depression predicted by lower pretreatment thyroid function. *Am J Psychiatry*, 159(1), 116–121.

Conney, J., and Kaston, B. (1999). Pharmacoeconomic and health outcome comparison of lithium and divalproex in a VA geriatric nursing home population: Influence of drug-related morbidity on total cost of treatment. *Am J Manag Care*, 5(2), 197–204.

Coppen, A., Noguera, R., Bailey, J., Burns, B.H., Swani, M.S., Hare, E.H., Gardner, R., and Maggs, R. (1971). Prophylactic lithium in affective disorders: Controlled trial. *Lancet*, 2(7719), 275–279.

Coppen, A., Peet, M., Bailey, J., Noguera, R., Burns, B.H., Swani, M.S., Maggs, R., and Gardner, R. (1973). Double-blind and open prospective studies on lithium prophylaxis in affective disorders. *Psychiatr Neurol Neurochir*, 76(6), 501–510.

Correll, C.U., Frederickson, A.M., Kane, J.M., and Manu, P. (2006). Metabolic syndrome and the risk of coronary disease in 367 patients treated with second-generation antipsychotic drugs. *J Clin Psychiatry*, 67(4), 575–583.

Coryell, W., Winokur, G., Solomon, D., Shea, T., Leon, A., and Keller, M. (1997). Lithium and recurrence in a long-term follow-up of bipolar affective disorder. *Psychol Med*, 27(2), 281–289.

Coryell, W., Solomon, D., Leon, A.C., Akiskal, H.S., Keller, M.B., Scheftner, W.A., and Mueller, T. (1998). Lithium discontinuation and subsequent effectiveness. *Am J Psychiatry*, 155(7), 895.

Coxhead, N., Silverstone, T., and Cookson, J. (1992). Carbamazepine versus lithium in the prophylaxis of bipolar affective disorder. *Acta Psychiatr Scand*, 85(2), 114–118.

Crawford, P. (2002). Interactions between antiepileptic drugs and hormonal contraception. *CNS Drugs*, 16(4), 263–272.

Cundall, R.L., Brooks, P.W., and Murray, L.G. (1972). A controlled evaluation of lithium prophylaxis in affective disorders. *Psychol Med*, 2(3), 308–311.

Cunnington, M., and Tennis, P. (2005). Lamotrigine and the risk of malformations in pregnancy. *Neurology*, 64(6), 955–960.

Davis, J.M., Janicak, P.G., and Hogan, D.M. (1999). Mood stabilizers in the prevention of recurrent affective disorders: A meta-analysis. *Acta Psychiatr Scand*, 100(6), 406–417.

Dean, C., Williams, R.J., and Brockington, I.F. (1989). Is puerperal psychosis the same as bipolar manic-depressive disorder? A family study. *Psychol Med*, 19(3), 637–647.

de Camargo, O.A., and Bode, H. (1999). Agranulocytosis associated with lamotrigine. *BMJ*, 318(7192), 1179.

Denicoff, K.D., Smith-Jackson, E.E., Bryan, A.L., Ali, S.O., and Post, R.M. (1997a). Valproate prophylaxis in a prospective clinical trial of refractory bipolar disorder. *Am J Psychiatry*, 154(10), 1456–1458.

Denicoff, K.D., Smith-Jackson, E.E., Disney, E.R., Ali, S.O., Leverich, G.S., and Post, R.M. (1997b). Comparative prophylactic efficacy of lithium, carbamazepine, and the combination in bipolar disorder. *J Clin Psychiatry*, 58(11), 470–478.

DePaulo, J.R. Jr., Folstein, M.F., and Correa, E.I. (1982). The course of delirium due to lithium intoxication. *J Clin Psychiatry*, 43(11), 447–449.

Deshauer, D., Fergusson, D., Duffy, A., Albuquerque, J., and Grof, P. (2005). Re-evaluation of randomized control trials of lithium monotherapy: A cohort effect. *Bipolar Disord*, 7(4), 382–387.

Dettling, M., and Anghelescu, I.G. (2006). Antipsychotic drugs and schizophrenia. *N Engl J Med*, 354(3), 298–300.

Dickson, W.E., and Kendell, R.E. (1986). Does maintenance lithium therapy prevent recurrences of mania under ordinary clinical conditions? *Psychol Med*, 16(3), 521–530.

Duffy, A., Alda, M., Kutcher, S., Cavazzoni, P., Robertson, C., Grof, E., and Grof, P. (2002). A prospective study of the offspring of bipolar parents responsive and nonresponsive to lithium treatment. *J Clin Psychiatry*, 63(12), 1171–1178.

Dunner, D.L., and Fieve, R.R. (1974). Clinical factors in lithium carbonate prophylaxis failure. *Arch Gen Psychiatry*, 30(2), 229–233.

Dunner, D.L., Dwyer, T., and Fieve, R.R. (1976). Depressive symptoms in patients with unipolar and bipolar affective disorder. *Compr Psychiatry*, 17(3), 447–451.

Dunner, D.L., Patrick, V., and Fieve, R.R. (1977). Rapid cycling manic depressive patients. *Compr Psychiatry*, 18(6), 561–566.

Eberhard-Gran, M., Eskild, A., and Opjordsmoen, S. (2005). Treating mood disorders during pregnancy: Safety considerations. *Drug Saf*, 28(8), 695–706.

Ernst, C.L., and Goldberg, J.F. (2002). The reproductive safety profile of mood stabilizers, atypical antipsychotics, and broad-spectrum psychotropics. *J Clin Psychiatry*, 63(Suppl. 4), 42–55.

Esparon, J., Kolloori, J., Naylor, G.J., McHarg, A.M., Smith, A.H., and Hopwood, S.E. (1986). Comparison of the prophylactic action of flupenthixol with placebo in lithium treated manic-depressive patients. *Br J Psychiatry*, 148, 723–725.

Eyer, F., Pfab, R., Felgenhauer, N., Lutz, J., Heemann, U., Steimer, W., Zondler, S., Fichtl, B., and Zilker, T. (2006). Lithium poisoning: pharmacokinetics and clearance during different therapeutic measures. *J Clin Psychopharmacol*, 26(3), 325–330.

Faedda, G.L., Tondo, L., Baldessarini, R.J., Suppes, T., and Tohen, M. (1993). Outcome after rapid vs. gradual discontinuation of lithium treatment in bipolar mood disorders. *Arch Gen Psychiatry*, 50, 448–455.

Fagiolini, A., Frank, E., Houck, P.R., Mallinger, A.G., Swartz, H.A., Buysse, D.J., Ombao, H., and Kupfer, D.J. (2002). Prevalence of obesity and weight change during treatment in patients with bipolar I disorder. *J Clin Psychiatry*, 63(6), 528–533.

Fagiolini, A., Frank, E., Scott, J.A., Turkin, S., and Kupfer, D.J. (2005). Metabolic syndrome in bipolar disorder: Findings from the Bipolar Disorder Center for Pennsylvanians. *Bipolar Disord*, 7(5), 424–430.

Fava, G.A. (2003). Can long-term treatment with antidepressant drugs worsen the course of depression? *J Clin Psychiatry*, 64(2), 123–133.

Fieve, R.R., Kumbaraci, T., and Dunner, D.L. (1976). Lithium prophylaxis of depression in bipolar I, bipolar II, and unipolar patients. *Am J Psychiatry*, 133(8), 925–929.

Folstein, M.F., DePaulo, J.R. Jr., and Trepp, K. (1982). Unusual mood stability in patients taking lithium. *Br J Psychiatry*, 140, 188–191.

Forty, L., Jones, L., Macgregor, S., Caesar, S., Cooper, C., Hough, A., Dean, L., Dave, S., Farmer, A., McGuffin, P., Brewster, S., Craddock, N., and Jones, I. (2006). Familiality of postpartum depression in unipolar disorder: Results of a family study. *Am J Psychiatry*, 163(9), 1549–1553.

Frangou, S., Raymont, V., and Bettany, D. (2002). The Maudsley bipolar disorder project: A survey of psychotropic prescribing patterns in bipolar I disorder. *Bipolar Disord*, 4(6), 378–385.

Frank, E., Kupfer, D.J., Wagner, E.F., McEachran, A.B., and Cornes, C. (1991). Efficacy of interpersonal psychotherapy as a maintenance treatment of recurrent depression: Contributing factors. *Arch Gen Psychiatry*, 48(12), 1053–1059.

Frankenburg, F.R., and Zanarini, M.C. (2002). Divalproex sodium treatment of women with borderline personality disorder and bipolar II disorder: A double-blind placebo-controlled pilot study. *J Clin Psychiatry*, 63(5), 442–446.

Freeman, M.P., and Stoll, A.L. (1998). Mood stabilizer combinations: A review of safety and efficacy. *Am J Psychiatry*, 155(1), 12–21.

Frye, M.A., Denicoff, K.D., Bryan, A.L., Smith-Jackson, E.E., Ali, S.O., Luckenbaugh, D., Leverich, G.S., and Post, R.M. (1999).

Association between lower serum free T4 and greater mood instability and depression in lithium-maintained bipolar patients. *Am J Psychiatry*, 156(12), 1909–1914.

Frye, M., Ketter, T.A., Kimbrell, T.A., Dunn, R.T., Speer, A.M., Osuch, E.A., Luckenbaugh, D.A., Cora-Ocatelli, G., Leverich, G.S., and Post, R.M. (2000). A placebo-controlled study of lamotrigine and gabapentin monotherapy in refractory mood disorders. *J Clin Psychopharmacol*, 20(6), 607–612.

Garza-Trevino, E.S., Overall, J.E., and Hollister, L.E. (1992). Verapamil versus lithium in acute mania. *Am J Psychiatry*, 149(1), 121–122.

Geddes, J.R., Rendell, J.M., and Goodwin, G. (2002). BALANCE: A large simple trial of maintenance treatment for bipolar disorder. *World Psychiatry*, 1(1), 48–51.

Geddes, J.R., Burgess, S., Hawton, K., Jamison, K., and Goodwin, G.M. (2004). Long-term lithium therapy for bipolar disorder: Systematic review and meta-analysis of randomized controlled trials. *Am J Psychiatry*, 161(2), 217–222.

Gelenberg, A.J., Kane, J.M., Keller, M.B., Lavori, P., Rosenbaum, J.F., Cole, K., and Lavelle, J. (1989). Comparison of standard and low serum levels of lithium for maintenance treatment of bipolar disorder. *N Engl J Med*, 321(22), 1489–1493.

Gentile, S. (2004). Clinical utilization of atypical antipsychotics in pregnancy and lactation. *Ann Pharmacother*, 38(7–8), 1265–1271.

Gentile, S. (2006). Prophylactic treatment of bipolar disorder in pregnancy and breastfeeding: Focus on emerging mood stabilizers. *Bipolar Disord*, 8(3), 207–220.

Ghaemi, S.N. (2001). On defining "mood stabilizer." *Bipolar Disord*, 3(3), 154–158.

Ghaemi, S.N., and Goodwin, F.K. (2001). Long-term naturalistic treatment of depressive symptoms in bipolar illness with divalproex vs. lithium in the setting of minimal antidepressant use. *J Affect Disord*, 65(3), 281–287.

Ghaemi, S.N., and Goodwin, F.K. (2005). Antidepressants for bipolar depression. *Am J Psychiatry*, 162(8), 1545–1546.

Ghaemi, S.N., and Sachs, G.S. (1997). Long-term risperidone treatment in bipolar disorder: 6-Month follow up. *Int Clin Psychopharmacol*, 12(6), 333–338.

Ghaemi, S.N., Boiman, E.E., and Goodwin, F.K. (2000). Diagnosing bipolar disorder and the effect of antidepressants: A naturalistic study. *J Clin Psychiatry*, 804–808.

Ghaemi, S.N., Lenox, M.S., and Baldessarini, R.J. (2001a). Effectiveness and safety of long-term antidepressant treatment in bipolar disorder. *J Clin Psychiatry*, 62(7), 565–569.

Ghaemi, S.N., Manwani, S.G., Katzow, J.J., Ko, J.Y., and Goodwin, F.K. (2001b). Topiramate treatment of bipolar spectrum disorders: A retrospective chart review. *Ann Clin Psychiatry*, 13(4), 185–189.

Ghaemi, S.N., Ko, J.Y., and Katzow, J.J. (2002). Oxcarbazepine treatment of refractory bipolar disorder: A retrospective chart review. *Bipolar Disord*, 4, 70–74.

Ghaemi, S.N., Hsu, D.J., Rosenquist, K.J., Pardo, T.B., and Goodwin, F.K. (2000). Extrapyramidal side effects with atypical neuroleptics in bipolar disorder. *Prog Neuropsychopharmacol Biol Psychiatry*, 30(2), 209–213.

Gitlin, M. (1999). Lithium and the kidney: An updated review. *Drug Saf*, 20(3), 231–243.

Glazer, W.M., Sonnenberg, J.G., Reinstein, M.J., and Akers, R.F. (2004). A novel, point-of-care test for lithium levels: Description and reliability. *J Clin Psychiatry*, 65(5), 652–655.

Goldberg, J.F., Garno, J.L., Leon, A.C., Kocsis, J.H., and Portera, L. (1998). Rapid titration of mood stabilizers predicts remission from mixed or pure mania in bipolar patients. *J Clin Psychiatry*, 59(4), 151–158.

Goodnick, P.J. (1993). Verapamil prophylaxis in pregnant women with bipolar disorder. *Am J Psychiatry*, 150(10), 1560.

Goodwin, F.K. (1989). The biology of recurrence: New directions for the pharmacologic bridge. *J Clin Psychiatry*, 50(Suppl.), 40–44; discussion 45–47.

Goodwin, F.K. (2003). Rationale for using lithium in combination with other mood stabilizers in the management of bipolar disorder. *J Clin Psychiatry*, 64(Suppl. 5), 18–24.

Goodwin, F.K., and Goldstein, M. (2003). Optimizing lithium treatment in bipolar disorder: A review of the literature and clinical recommendations. *J Psychiatr Pract*, 9(5), 1–11.

Goodwin, F.K., and Jamison, K.R. (1990). *Manic-Depressive Illness*. New York: Oxford University Press.

Goodwin, G.M. (1994). Recurrence of mania after lithium withdrawal: Implications for the use of lithium in the treatment of bipolar affective disorder. *Br J Psychiatry*, 164(2), 149–152.

Goodwin, G.M., and Geddes, J.R. (2003). Latest maintenance data on lithium in bipolar disorder. *Eur Neuropsychopharmacol*, 13(Suppl. 2), S51–S55.

Goodwin, G.M., Cavanagh, J.T., Glabus, M.F., Kehoe, R.F., O'Carroll, R.E., and Ebmeier, K.P. (1997). Uptake of ^{99m}Tc-exametazime shown by single photon emission computed tomography before and after lithium withdrawal in bipolar patients: Associations with mania. *Br J Psychiatry*, 170, 426–430.

Goodwin, G.M., Bowden, C.L., Calabrese, J.R., Grunze, H., Kasper, S., White, R., Greene, P., and Leadbetter, R. (2004). A pooled analysis of 2 placebo-controlled 18-month trials of lamotrigine and lithium maintenance in bipolar I disorder. *J Clin Psychiatry*, 65(3), 432–441.

Graham, K.A., Gu, H., Lieberman, J.A., Harp, J.B., and Perkins, D.O. (2005). Double-blind, placebo-controlled investigation of amantadine for weight loss in subjects who gained weight with olanzapine. *Am J Psychiatry*, 162(9), 1744–1746.

Greil, W., and Kleindienst, N. (1999). Lithium versus carbamazepine in the maintenance treatment of bipolar II disorder and bipolar disorder not otherwise specified. *Int Clin Psychopharmacol*, 14(5), 283–285.

Greil, W., Ludwig-Mayerhofer, W., Erazo, N., Engel, R.R., Czernik, A., Giedke, H., Muller-Oerlinghausen, B., Osterheider, M., Rudolf, G.A., Sauer, H., Tegeler, J., and Wetterling, T. (1997). Lithium vs. carbamazepine in the maintenance treatment of schizoaffective disorder: A randomised study. *Eur Arch Psychiatry Clin Neurosci*, 247(1), 42–50.

Grof, P., and Alda, M. (2000). Discrepancies in the efficacy of lithium. *Arch Gen Psychiatry*, 57(2), 191.

Grof, P., Cakulis, P., and Dostal, T. (1970). Lithium dropouts: A follow-up study of patients who discontinued prophylactic treatment. *Int Pharmacopsychiatry*, 5, 162–169.

Grof, P., Alda, M., Grof, E., Zvolsky, P., and Walsh, M. (1994). Lithium response and genetics of affective disorders. *J Affect Disord*, 32(2), 85–95.

Grof, P., Robbins, W., Alda, M., Berghoefer, A., Vojtechovsky, M., Nilsson, A. (2000). Protective effect of pregnancy in women with lithium-responsive bipolar disorder. *J Affect Disord*, 61(1–2), 31–39.

Gruenwald J., The Medical Economics Team, and PDR Physicians Desk Reference Team (Eds.). (2004). *PDR for Herbal Medicines* (3rd edition). Montvale, NJ: Thompson PDR.

Grunze, H., Erfurth, A., Marcuse, A., Amann, B., Normann, C., and Walden, J. (1999). Tiagabine appears not to be efficacious in the treatment of acute mania. *J Clin Psychiatry*, 60(11), 759–762.

Grunze, H., Kasper, S., Goodwin, G., Bowden, C., Baldwin, D., Licht, R. (2002). World Federation of Societies of Biological Psychiatry (WFSBP) guidelines for biological treatment of bipolar disorders. Part I: Treatment of bipolar depression. *World J Biol Psychiatry*, 3(3), 115–124.

Grunze, H., Kasper, S., Goodwin, G., Bowden, C., Moller, H.J., WFSBP Task Force on Treatment Guidelines for Bipolar Disorders. (2004). The World Federation of Societies of Biological Psychiatry (WFSBP) guidelines for the biological treatment of bipolar disorders, part III: Maintenance treatment. *World J Biol Psychiatry*, 5(3), 120–135.

Guo, J.J., Keck, P.E., Corey-Lisle, P.K., Li, H., Jiang, D., Jang, R., and L'italien, G.J. (2006). Risk of diabetes mellitus associated with atypical antipsychotic use among patients with bipolar disorder: A retrospective, population-based, case-control study. *J Clin Psychiatry*, 67(7), 1055–1061.

Gyulai, L., Bowden, C.L., McElroy, S.L., Calabrese, J.R., Petty, F., Swann, A.C., Chou, J.C., Wassef, A., Risch, C.S., Hirschfeld, R.M., Nemeroff, C.B., Keck, P.E. Jr., Evans, D.L., and Wozniak, P.J. (2003). Maintenance efficacy of divalproex in the prevention of bipolar depression. *Neuropsychopharmacology*, 28(7), 1374–1382.

Harrow, M., Goldberg, J.F., Grossman, L.S., and Meltzer, H.Y. (1990). Outcome in manic disorders: A naturalistic follow-up study. *Arch Gen Psychiatry*, 47(7), 665–671.

Hartong, E.G., Moleman, P., Hoogduin, C.A., Broekman, T.G., Nolen, W.A., and LitCar Group. (2003). Prophylactic efficacy of lithium versus carbamazepine in treatment-naive bipolar patients. *J Clin Psychiatry*, 64(2), 144–151.

Henderson, D.C., Cagliero, E., Gray, C., Nasrallah, R.A., Hayden, D.L., Schoenfeld, D.A., and Goff, D.C. (2000). Clozapine, diabetes mellitus, weight gain, and lipid abnormalities: A five-year naturalistic study. *Am J Psychiatry*, 157(6), 975–981.

Hendrick, V., Altshuler, L., and Whybrow, P. (1998). Psychoneuroendocrinology of mood disorders: The hypothalamic-pituitary-thyroid axis. *Psychiatr Clin North Am*, 21(2), 277–292.

Holinger, P.C., and Wolpert, E.A. (1979). A ten year follow-up of lithium use. *IMJ Ill Med J*, 156(2), 99–104.

Hopkins, H.S., and Gelenberg, A.J. (2000). Serum lithium levels and the outcome of maintenance therapy of bipolar disorder. *Bipolar Disord*, 3(5), 174–179.

Isaksson, A., Ottosson, J.O., and Perris, C. (1969). Methologische aspekte der Forschung über prophylaktische Behandlung bei affektiven Psychosen. In H. Hippius and H. Selbach (Eds.), *Das Depressive Syndrom* (pp. 561–574). Munich: Urban and Schwarzenberg.

Isojarvi, J.I., Laatikainen, T.J., Pakarinen, A.J., Juntunen, K.T., and Myllyla, V.V. (1993). Polycystic ovaries and hyperandrogenism in women taking valproate for epilepsy. *N Engl J Med*, 329(19), 1383–1388.

Jacobsen, F.M., and Comas-Diaz, L. (1999). Donepezil for psychotropic-induced memory loss. *J Clin Psychiatry*, 60(10), 698–704.

Jacobson, S.J., Jones, K., Johnson, K., Ceolin, L., Kaur, P., Sahn, D., Donnenfeld, A.E., Rieder, M., Santelli, R., Smythe, J. (1992). Prospective multicentre study of pregnancy outcome after lithium exposure during first trimester. *Lancet*, 339(8792), 530–533.

Jamison, K.R., Gerner, R.H., and Goodwin, F.K. (1979). Patient and physician attitudes toward lithium: Relationship to compliance. *Arch Gen Psychiatry*, 36(Spec. No. 8), 866–869.

Joffe, H., Hall, J.E., Cohen, L.S., Taylor, A.E., and Baldessarini, R.J. (2003). A putative relationship between valproic acid and polycystic ovarian syndrome: Implications for treatment of women with seizure and bipolar disorders. *Harv Rev Psychiatry*, 11(2), 99–108.

Joffe, H., Cohen, L.S., Suppes, T., McLaughlin, W.L., Lavori, P., and Adams, J.M. (2006). Valproate is associated with new-onset oligoamenorrhea with hyperandrogenism in women with bipolar disorder. *Biol Psychiatry*, 59(11), 1078–1086.

Johnston, A.M., and Eagles, J.M. (1999). Lithium-associated clinical hypothyroidism: Prevalence and risk factors. *Br J Psychiatry*, 175, 336–339.

Jones, I., and Craddock, N. (2001). Familiality of the puerperal trigger in bipolar disorder: Results of a family study. *Am J Psychiatry*, 158(6), 913–917.

Jones, I., and Craddock, N. (2005). Bipolar disorder and childbirth: The importance of recognising risk. *Br J Psychiatry*, 186, 453–454.

Judd, L.L., Akiskal, H.S., Schettler, P.J., Endicott, J., Leon, A.C., and Solomon, D.A. (2005). Psychosocial disability in the course of bipolar I and II disorders: A prospective, comparative, longitudinal study. *Arch Gen Psychiatry*, 62(12), 1322–1330.

Kahn, D.A., Sachs, G.S., Printz, D.J., Carpenter, D., Docherty, J.P., and Ross, R. (2000). Medication treatment of bipolar disorder 2000: A summary of the expert consensus guidelines. *J Psychiatr Pract*, 6(4), 197–211.

Kallen, A.J. (1994). Maternal carbamazepine and infant spina bifida. *Reprod Toxicol*, 8(3), 203–205.

Kallner, G., Lindelius, R., Petterson, U., Stockman, O., and Tham, A. (2000). Mortality in 497 patients with affective disorders attending a lithium clinic or after having left it. *Pharmacopsychiatry*, 33(1), 8–13.

Kane, J.M., Quitkin, R.A., Ramos-Lorenzi, J.R., Nayak, D.D., and Howard, A. (1982). Lithium carbonate and imipramine in the prophylaxis of unipolar and bipolar II illness: A prospective, placebo-controlled comparison. *Arch Gen Psychiatry*, 39, 1065–1069.

Kanner, A.M., and Frey, M. (2000). Adding valproate to lamotrigine: A study of their pharmacokinetic interaction. *Neurology*, 55(4), 588–591.

Kaplan, B.J., Simpson, J.S., Ferre, R.C., Gorman, C.P., McMullen, D.M., and Crawford, S.G. (2001). Effective mood stabilization with a chelated mineral supplement: An open-label trial in bipolar disorder. *J Clin Psychiatry*, 62(12), 936–944.

Kaplan, B.J., Fisher, J.E., Crawford, S.G., Field, C.J., and Kolb, B. (2004). Improved mood and behavior during treatment with a mineral-vitamin supplement: A open-label case series of children. *J Child Adolesc Psychopharmacol*, 14(1), 115–122.

Keck, P.E. Jr., and McElroy, S.L. (2003). Redefining mood stabilization. *J Affect Disord*, 73(1–2), 163–169.

Keck, P.E., McElroy, S.L., Strakowski, S.M., Balistreri, T.M., Kizer, D.I., and West, S.A. (1996). Factors associated with maintenance antipsychotic treatment of patients with bipolar disorder. *J Clin Psychiatry*, 57(4), 147–151.

Keck, P.E. Jr., Mendlwicz, J., Calabrese, J.R., Fawcett, J., Suppes, T., Vestergaard, P.A., and Carbonell, C. (2000). A review of randomized, controlled clinical trials in acute mania. *J Affect Disord*, 59(Suppl. 1), S31–S37.

Keck, P.E. Jr., Calabrese, J.R., McQuade, R.D., Carson, W.H., Carlson, B.X., Rollin, L.M., Marcus, R.N., Sanchez, R., and Aripiprazole Study Group. (2006). A randomized, double-blind, placebo-controlled 26-week trial of aripiprazole in recently manic patients with bipolar I disorder. *J Clin Psychiatry*, 67(4), 626–637.

Keller, M.B., Lavori, P.W., Mueller, T.I., Endicott, J., Coryell, W., Hirschfeld, R.M., and Shea, T. (1992). Time to recovery, chronicity, and levels of psychopathology in major depression: A 5-year prospective follow-up of 431 subjects. *Arch Gen Psychiatry*, 49(10), 809–816.

Keller, M.B., Lavori, P.W., Coryell, W., Endicott, J., and Mueller, T.I. (1993). Bipolar I: A five-year prospective follow-up. *J Nerv Ment Dis*, 181(4), 238–245.

Ketter, T.A., and Calabrese, J.R. (2002). Stabilization of mood from below versus above baseline in bipolar disorder: A new nomenclature. *J Clin Psychiatry*, 63(2), 146–151.

Ketter, T.A., Wang, P.W., Chandler, R.A., Alarcon, A.M., Becker, O.V., Nowakowska, C., O'Keeffe, C.M., and Schumacher, M.R. (2005). Dermatology precautions and slower titration yield low incidence of lamotrigine treatment-emergent rash. *J Clin Psychiatry*, 66(5), 642–645.

Ketter, T.A., Houston, J. P., Adams, D.H., Risser, R.C., Meyers, A.L., Williamson, D.J., and Tohen, M. (2006). Differential efficacy of olanzapine and lithium in preventing manic or mixed recurrence in patients with bipolar I disorder based on number of previous manic or mixed episodes. *J Clin Psychiatry*, 67(1), 95–101.

King, J.R., and Hullin, R.P. (1983). Withdrawal symptoms from lithium: Four case reports and a questionnaire study. *Br J Psychiatry*, 143, 30–35.

Kirov, G., Tredget, J., John R., Owen, M.J., and Lazarus, J.H. (2005). A cross-sectional and a prospective study of thyroid disorders in lithium-treated patients. *J Affect Disord*, 87(2-3), 313–317.

Kishimoto, A. (1992). The treatment of affective disorder with carbamazepine: Prophylactic synergism of lithium and carbamazepine combination. *Prog Neuropsychopharmacol Biol Psychiatry*, 16(4), 483–493.

Kishimoto, A., Ogura, C., Hazama, H., and Inoue, K. (1983). Long-term prophylactic effects of carbamazepine in affective disorder. *Br J Psychiatry*, 143, 327–331.

Kleindienst, N., and Greil, W. (2002). Inter-episodic morbidity and drop-out under carbamazepine and lithium in the maintenance treatment of bipolar disorder. *Psychol Med*, 32(3), 493–501.

Kleindienst, N., Greil, W., Ruger, B., and Moller, H.J. (1999). The prophylactic efficacy of lithium—transient or persistent? *Eur Arch Psychiatry Clin Neurosci*, 249(3), 144–149.

Kleindienst, N., Engel, R., and Greil, W. (2005). Which clinical factors predict response to prophylactic lithium? A systematic review for bipolar disorders. *Bipolar Disord*, 7(5), 404–417.

Kleiner, J., Altshuler, L., Hendrick, V., and Hershman, J.M. (1999). Lithium-induced subclinical hypothyroidism: Review of the literature and guidelines for treatment. *J Clin Psychiatry*, 60(4), 249–255.

Knoll, J., Stegman, K., and Suppes, T. (1998). Clinical experience using gabapentin adjunctively in patients with a history of mania or hypomania. *J Affect Disord*, 49(3), 229–233.

Kukopulos, A., Reginaldi, D., Laddomada, P., Floris, G., Serra, G., and Tondo, L. (1980). Course of the manic-depressive cycle and changes caused by treatment. *Pharmakopsychiatr Neuropsychopharmakol*, 13(4), 156–167.

Kupka, R.W., Nolen, W.A., Post, R.M., McElroy, S.L., Altshuler, L.L., Denicoff, K.D., Frye, M.A., Keck, P.E. Jr., Leverich, G.S., Rush, A.J., Suppes, T., Pollio, C., Drexhage, H.A. (2002). High rate of autoimmune thyroiditis in bipolar disorder: Lack of association with lithium exposure. *Biol Psychiatry*, 51(4), 305–311.

Kupka, R.W., Luckenbaugh, D.A., Post, R.M., Leverich, G.S., and Nolen, W.A. (2003). Rapid and non-rapid cycling bipolar disorder: A meta-analysis of clinical studies. *J Clin Psychiatry*, 64(12), 1483–1494.

Kusalic, M. (1992). Grade II and grade III hypothyroidism in rapid-cycling bipolar patients. *Neuropsychobiology*, 25(4), 177–181.

Lambert, P.A., Borselli, S., Marcou, G., Bouchardy, M., and Cabrol, G. (1971). Long-term thymoregulative action of Depamide in manic-depressive psychoses. *Ann Med Psychol (Paris)*, 2(3), 442–448.

Laurell, B., and Ottosson, J.O. (1968). Prophylactic lithium? *Lancet*, 2(7580), 1245–1246.

Lepkifker, E., Sverdlik, A., Iancu, I., Ziv, R., Segev, S., and Kotler, M. (2004). Renal insufficiency in long-term lithium treatment. *J Clin Psychiatry*, 65(6), 850–856.

Leucht, S., Wahlbeck, K., Hamann, J., and Kissling, W. (2003). New generation antipsychotics versus low-potency conventional antipsychotics: A systematic review and meta-analysis. *Lancet*, 361(9369), 1581–1589.

Levy, E., Margolese, H.C., and Chouinard, G. (2002). Topiramate produced weight loss following olanzapine-induced weight gain in schizophrenia. *J Clin Psychiatry*, 63(11), 1045.

Licht, R.W., Vestergaard, P., Rasmussen, N.A., Jepsen, K., Brodersen, A., and Hansen, P.E. (2001). A lithium clinic for bipolar patients: 2-Year outcome of the first 148 patients. *Acta Psychiatr Scand*, 104(5), 387–390.

Lieberman, D.Z., and Goodwin, F.K. (2004). Separate and concomitant use of lamotrigine, lithium, and divalproex in bipolar disorders. *Curr Psychiatry Rep*, 6(6), 459–465.

Lipkovich, I., Citrome, L., Perlis, R., Deberdt, W., Houston, J.P., Ahl, J., and Hardy, T. (2006). Early predictors of substantial weight gain in bipolar patients treated with olanzapine. *J Clin Psychopharmacol*, 26(3), 316–320.

Littlejohn, R., Leslie, F., and Cookson, J. (1994). Depot antipsychotics in the prophylaxis of bipolar affective disorder. *Br J Psychiatry*, 165(6), 827–829.

Luby, E.D., and Singareddy, R.K. (2003). Long-term therapy with lithium in a private practice clinic: A naturalistic study. *Bipolar Disord*, 5(1), 62–68.

Luznat, R.M., Murphy, D.P., and Nunn, C.M.H. (1988). Carbamazepine vs. lithium treatment and prophylaxis of mania. *Br J Psychiatry*, 153, 198–204.

Lydon, E., and El-Mallakh, R.S. (2006). Naturalistic long-term use of methylphenidate in bipolar disorder. *J Clin Psychopharmacol*, 26(5), 516–518.

Macritchie, K.A., Geddes, J.R., Scott, J., Haslam, D.R., and Goodwin, G.M. (2001). Valproic acid, valproate and divalproex in the maintenance treatment of bipolar disorder. *Cochrane Database Syst Rev*, (3):CD003196.

Macritchie, K.A.N., Geddes, J.R., Scott, J., Haslam, D.R.S., and Goodwin, G.M. (2002). Valproic acid, valproate and divalproex in the maintenance treatment of bipolar disorder. *Cochrane Database Syst Rev*, (3), CD003196.

Maj, M., Starace, F., Nolfe, G., and Kemali, D. (1986). Minimum plasma lithium levels required for effective prophylaxis in DSM III bipolar disorder: A prospective study. *Pharmacopsychiatry*, 19, 420–423.

Maj, M., Pirozzi, R., and Magliano, L. (1995). Nonresponse to reinstituted lithium prophylaxis in previously responsive bipolar patients: prevalence and predictors. *Am J Psychiatry*, 152(12), 1810–1811.

Maj, M., Pirozzi, R., and Magliano, L. (1996). Late non-response to lithium prophylaxis in bipolar patients: Prevalence and predictors. *J Affect Disord*, 39(1), 39–42.

Maj, M., Pirozzi, R., Magliano, L., and Bartoli, L. (1998). Long-term outcome of lithium prophylaxis in bipolar disorder: A 5-year prospective study of 402 patients at a lithium clinic. *Am J Psychiatry*, 155(1), 30–35.

Maj, M., Pirozzi, R., Bartoli, L., and Magliano, L. (2002). Long-term outcome of lithium prophylaxis in bipolar disorder with mood-incongruent psychotic features: A prospective study. *J Affect Disord*, 71(1–3), 195–198.

Malone, K., Papagni, K., Ramini, S., and Keltner, N.L. (2004). Antidepressants, antipsychotics, benzodiazepines, and the breast-feeding dyad. *Perspect Psychiatr Care*, 40(2), 73–85.

Marcotte, D. (1998). Use of topiramate, a new anti-epileptic as a mood stabilizer. *J Affect Disord*, 50(2–3), 245–251.

Markar, H.R., and Mander, A.J. (1989). Efficacy of lithium prophylaxis in clinical practice. *Br J Psychiatry*, 155, 496–500.

Markowitz, G.S., Radhakrishnan, J., Kambham, N., Valeri, A.M., Hines, W.H., D'Agati, V.D. (2000). Lithium nephrotoxicity: A progressive combined glomerular and tubulointerstitial nephropathy. *J Am Soc Nephrol*, 11(8), 1439–1448.

McElroy, S.L., Suppes, T., Keck, P.E., Frye, M.A., Denicoff, K.D., Altshuler, L.L., Brown, E.S., Nolen, W.A., Kupka, R.W., Rochussen, J., Leverich, G.S., and Post, R.M. (2000). Open-label adjunctive topiramate in the treatment of bipolar disorders. *Biol Psychiatry*, 47(12), 1025–1033.

McIntyre, R.S., Girgla, S., Binder, C., Riccardelli, R., and Kennedy, S.H. (2002). *Efficacy of topiramate as adjunctive therapy to mood stabilizers in patients with bipolar I or II disorder.* Poster presented at the Meeting of the American College of Neurosychopharmacology, Puerto Rico.

McIntyre, R.S., Mancini, D.A., McCann, S., Srinivasan, J., and Kennedy, S.H. (2003). Valproate, bipolar disorder and polycystic ovarian syndrome. *Bipolar Disord*, 5(1), 28–35.

McKenna, K., Koren, G., Tetelbaum, M., Wilton, L., Shakir, S., Diav-Citrin, O., Levinson, A., Zipursky, R.B., and Einarson, A. (2005). Pregnancy outcome of women using atypical antipsychotic drugs: A prospective comparative study. *J Clin Psychiatry*, 66(4), 444–449; quiz 546.

McQuade, R.D., Stock, E., Marcus, R., Jody, D., Gharbia, N.A., Vanveggel, S., Archibald, D., Carson, W.H. (2004). A comparison of weight change during treatment with olanzapine or aripiprazole: Results from a randomized, double-blind study. *J Clin Psychiatry*, 65(Suppl. 18), 47–56.

Melia, P.I. (1970). Prophylactic lithium: A double-blind trial in recurrent affective disorders. *Br J Psychiatry*, 115, 621–624.

Miller, A.L., Bowden, C.L., and Plewes, J. (1985). Lithium and impairment of renal concentrating ability. *J Affect Disord*, 9(2), 115–119.

Mishory, A., Winokur, M., and Bersudsky, Y. (2003). Prophylactic effect of phenytoin in bipolar disorder: A controlled study. *Bipolar Disord*, 5, 464–467.

Mockenhaupt, M., Messenheimer, J., Tennis, P., and Schlingmann, J. (2005). Risk of Stevens-Johnson syndrome and toxic epidermal necrolysis in new users of antiepileptics. *Neurology*, 64, 1134–1138.

Moretti, M.E., Koren, G., Verjee, Z., and Ito, S. (2003). Monitoring lithium in breast milk: An individualized approach for breast-feeding mothers. *Ther Drug Monit*, 25(3), 364–366.

Movig, K.L., Leufkens, H.G., Belitser, S.V., Lenderink, A.W., and Egberts, A.C. (2002). Selective serotonin reuptake inhibitor-induced urinary incontinence. *Pharmacoepidemiol Drug Saf*, 11(4), 271–279.

Movig, K.L., Baumgarten, R., Leufkens, H.G., van Laarhoven, J.H., and Egberts, A.C. (2003). Risk factors for the development of lithium-induced polyuria. *Br J Psychiatry*, 182, 319–323.

Munoz, R. (2002). *Oxcarbazepine for the treatment of bipolar disorder.* Poster presented to the Meeting of the American Psychiatric Association, Philadelphia, PA.

Murray, M., Hopwood S., Balfour, D.J.K., Ogston, S., and Hewick, D.S. (1983). The influence of age on lithium efficacy and side effects in out-patients. *Pscychol Med*, 13, 53–60.

Narendran, R., Young, C.M., Valenti, A.M., Pristach, C.A., Pato, M.T., and Grace, J.J. (2001). Olanzapine therapy in treatment-resistant psychotic mood disorders: A long-term follow-up study. *J Clin Psychiatry*, 62(7), 509–516.

Nascimento, A.L., Appolinario, J.C., Segenreich, D., Cavalcanti, M.T., and Brasil, M.A. (2006). Maintenance electroconvulsive therapy for recurrent refractory mania. *Bipolar Disord*, 8(3), 301–303.

Nasr, S., and Caspar, M. (2002). *Oxcarbazepine for the treatment of bipolar disorder.* Poster presented to the Meeting of the American Psychiatric Association, Philadelphia, PA.

Nemeroff, C.B. (2003). Advancing the treatment of mood and anxiety disorders: The first 10 years' experience with paroxetine. *Psychopharmacol Bull*, 37(Suppl. 1), 6–7.

Newcomer, J.W. (2006). Medical risk in patients with bipolar disorder and schizophrenia. *J Clin Psychiatry*, 67(Suppl. 9), 25–30.

Newcomer, J.W., Haupt, D.W., Fucetola, R., Melson, A.K., Schweiger, J.A., Cooper, B.P., and Selke, G. (2002). Abnormalities in glucose regulation during antipsychotic treatment of schizophrenia. *Arch Gen Psychiatry*, 59(4), 337–345.

Newport, D.J., Viguera, A.C., Beach, A.J., Ritchie, J.C., Cohen, L.S., and Stowe, Z.N. (2005). Lithium placental passage and obstetrical outcome: Implications for clinical management during late pregnancy. *Am J Psychiatry*, 162(11), 2162–2170.

Noack, C.H., and Trautner, E.M. (1951). The lithium treatment of maniacal psychosis. *Med J Aust*, 2(7), 219–222.

Nonacs, R., and Cohen, L.S. (2003). Assessment and treatment of depression during pregnancy: An update. *Psychiatr Clin North Am*, 26, 547–562.

Nulman, I., Rovet, J., Stewart, D.E., Wolpin, J., Pace-Asciak, P., Shuhaiber, S., and Koren, G. (2002). Child development following exposure to tricyclic antidepressants or fluoxetine throughout fetal life: A prospective, controlled study. *Am J Psychiatry*, 159(11), 1889–1895.

O'Donovan, C., Kusumakar, V., Graves, G.R., and Bird, D.C. (2002). Menstrual abnormalities and polycystic ovary syndrome in women taking valproate for bipolar mood disorder. *J Clin Psychiatry*, 63(4), 322–330.

Okuma, T. (1993). Effects of carbamazepine and lithium on affective disorders. *Neuropsychobiology*, 27(3), 138–145.

Okuma, T., Kishimoto, A., Inoue, K., Matsumoto, H., and Ogura, A. (1973). Anti-manic and prophylactic effects of carbamazepine (Tegretol) on manic depressive psychosis: A preliminary report. *Folia Psychiatr Neurol Jpn*, 27(4), 283–297.

Okuma, T., Koga, I., and Uchida, Y. (1976). Sensitivity to chlorpromazine effects on brain function of schizophrenics and normals: A preliminary report. *Psychopharmacology (Berl)*, 51(1), 101–105.

Okuma, T., Inanaga, K., Otsuki, S., Sarai, K., Takahashi, R., Hazama, H., Mori, A., and Watanabe, S. (1981). A preliminary double-blind study on the efficacy of carbamazepine in prophylaxis of manic-depressive illness. *Psychopharmacology (Berl)*, 73(1), 95–96.

Pande, A.C., Crockatt, J.G., Janney, C.A., Werth, J.L., and Tsaroucha, G. (2000). Gabapentin in bipolar disorder: A placebo-controlled trial of adjunctive therapy. Gabapentin Bipolar Disorder Study Group. *Bipolar Disord*, 2 (3 Pt. 2), 249–255.

Parker, G., Tully, L., Olley, A., and Hadzi-Pavlovic, D. (2006). SSRIs as mood stabilizers for bipolar II disorder? A proof of concept study. *J Affect Disord*, 92(2-3), 205–214.

Passmore, M.J., Garnham, J., Duffy, A., MacDougall, M., Munro, A., Slaney, C., Teehan, A., and Alda, M. (2003). Phenotypic spectra of bipolar disorder in responders to lithium versus lamotrigine. *Bipolar Disord*, 5(2), 110–114.

Pazzaglia, P.J., Post, R.M., Ketter, T.A., George, M.S., and Marangell, L.B. (1993). Preliminary controlled trial of nimodipine in ultra-rapid cycling affective dysregulation. *Psychiatry Res*, 49(3), 257–272.

Pazzaglia, P.J., Post, R.M., Ketter, T.A., Callahan, A.M., Marangell, L.B., Frye, M.A., George, M.S., Kimbrell, T.A., Leverich, G.S., Cora-Locatelli, G., and Luckenbaugh, D. (1998). Nimodipine monotherapy and carbamazepine augmentation in patients with refractory recurrent affective illness. *J Clin Psychopharmacol*, 18(5), 404–413.

Perlis, R.H., Sachs, G.S., Lafer, B., Otto, M.W., Faraone, S.V., Kane, J.M., and Rosenbaum, J.F. (2002). Effect of abrupt change from standard to low serum levels of lithium: A reanalysis of double-blind lithium maintenance data. *Am J Psychiatry*, 159(7), 1155.

Perlis, R.H., Ostacher, M.J., Patel, J.K., Marangell, L.B., Zhang, H., Wisniewski, S.R., Ketter, T.A., Miklowitz, D.J., Otto, M.W., Gyulai, L., Reilly-Harrington, N.A., Nierenberg, A.A., Sachs, G.S., and Thase, M.E. (2006). Predictors of recurrence in bipolar disorder: Primary outcomes from the Systematic Treatment Enhancement Program for Bipolar Disorder (STEP-BD). *Am J Psychiatry*, 163(2), 217–224.

Perselow, E.D., Dunner, D.L., Fieve, R.R., and Lautin A. (1980). Lithium carbonate and weight gain. *J Affect Disord*, 2, 303–310.

Petrides, G., Dhossche, D., Fink, M., and Francis, A. (1994). Continuation ECT: Relapse prevention in affective disorders. *Convuls Ther*, 10(3), 189–194.

Pies, R. (2000). Free drug fraction versus free drug concentration. *J Clin Psychiatry*, 61(6), 449.

Placidi, G.F., Lenzi, A., Lazzerini, F., Cassano, G.B., and Akiskal, H.S. (1986). The comparative efficacy and safety of carbamazepine versus lithium: A randomized, double blind three year trial in 83 patients. *J Clin Psychiatry*, 47, 490–494.

Plenge, P., Mellerup, E.T., and Bolwig, T.G. (1982). Lithium treatment: Does the kidney prefer one daily dose instead of two? *Acta Psychiatr Scand*, 66, 121–128.

Poole, A.J., James, H.D., and Hughes, W.C. (1978). Treatment experiences in the lithium clinic at St. Thomas Hospital. *J R Soc Med*, 71(12), 890–894.

Popper, C.W. (2001). Do vitamins or minerals (apart from lithium) have mood stabilizing effects? *J Clin Psychiatry*, 62(12), 933–935.

Post, R.M., Uhde, T.W., Roy-Byrne, P.P., and Joffe, R.T. (1986). Antidepressant effects of carbamazepine. *Am J Psychiatry*, 143(1), 29–34.

Post, R.M., Uhde, T.W., Roy-Byrne, P.P., and Joffe, R.T. (1987). Correlates of antimanic response to carbamazepine. *Psychiatry Res*, 21(1), 71–83.

Post, R.M., Leverich, G.S., Altshuler, L., and Mikalauskas, K. (1992). Lithium-discontinuation-induced refractoriness: Preliminary observations. *Am J Psychiatry*, 149(12), 1727–1729.

Post, R.M., Altshuler, L.L., Frye, M.A., Suppes, T., Rush, A.J., Keck, P.E. Jr., McElroy, S.L., Denicoff, K.D., Leverich, G.S., Kupka, R., and Nolen, W.A. (2001). Rate of switch in bipolar patients prospectively treated with second-generation antidepressants as augmentation to mood stabilizers. *Bipolar Disord*, 3(5), 259–265.

Presne, C., Fakhouri, F., Noel, L.H., Stengel, B., Even, C., Kreis, H., Mignon, F., and Grunfeld, J.P. (2003). Lithium-induced nephropathy: Rate of progression and prognostic factors. *Kidney Int*, 64(2), 585–592.

Prien, R.F., Caffey, E.M. Jr., and Klett, C.J. (1973a). Prophylactic efficacy of lithium carbonate in manic-depressive illness: Report of the Veterans Administration and National Institute of Mental Health collaborative study group. *Arch Gen Psychiatry*, 28(3), 337–341.

Prien, R.F., Klett, C.J., and Caffey, E.M. Jr. (1973b). Lithium carbonate and imipramine in prevention of affective episodes: A comparison in recurrent affective illness. *Arch Gen Psychiatry*, 29(3), 420–425.

Prien, R.F., Klett, C.J., and Caffey, E.M. Jr. (1974). Lithium prophylaxis in recurrent affective illness. *Am J Psychiatry*, 131(2), 198–203.

Prien, R.F., Kupfer, D.J., Mansky, P.A., Small, J.G., Tuason, V.B., Voss, C.B., and Johnson, W.E. (1984). Drug therapy in the prevention of recurrences in unipolar and bipolar affective disorders: Report of NIMH Collaborative study group comparing lithium carbonate, imipramine, and a lithium carbonate-imipramine combination. *Arch Gen Psychiatry*, 41, 1096–1104.

Quitkin, F.M., Kane, J.M., Rifkin, A., Ramos-Lorenzi, J.R., Saraf, K., Howard, A., and Klein, D.F. (1981). Lithium and imipramine in the prophylaxis of unipolar and bipolar II depression: A prospective, placebo-controlled comparison [proceedings]. *Psychopharmacol Bull*, 17(1), 142–144.

Revicki, D.A., Hirschfeld, R.M., Ahearn, E.P., Weisler, R.H., Palmer, C., and Keck, P.E. Jr. (2005). Effectiveness and medical costs of divalproex versus lithium in the treatment of bipolar disorder: Results of a naturalistic clinical trial. *J Affect Disord*, 86(2-3), 183–193.

Rhodes, L.J. (2000). Maintenance ECT replaced with lamotrigine. *Am J Psychiatry*, 157(12), 2058.

Rybakowski, J., Chlopocka-Wozniak, M., Kapelski, Z., and Strzyzewski, W. (1980). The relative prophylactic efficacy of lithium against manic and depressive recurrences in bipolar patients. *Int Pharmacopsychiatry*, 15(2), 86–90.

Rzany, B., Correia, O., Kelly, J.P., Naldi, L., Auquier, A., and Stern, R. (1999). Risk of Stevens-Johnson syndrome and toxic epidermal necrolysis during first weeks of antiepileptic therapy: A case-control study. Study Group of the International Case Control Study on Severe Cutaneous Adverse Reactions. *Lancet*, (353), 2190–2194.

Sachs, G.S. (1996). Bipolar mood disorder: practical strategies for acute and maintenance phase treatment. *J Clin Psychopharmacol*, 16(2 Suppl. 1), 32S–47S.

Sachs, G.S., Lafer, B., Stoll, A.L., Banov, M., Thibault, A.B., Tohen, M., and Rosenbaum, J.F. (1994). A double-blind trial of bupropion versus desipramine for bipolar depression. *J Clin Psychiatry*, 55(9), 391–393.

Sachs, G., Bowden, C., Calabrese, J.R., Ketter, T., Thompson, T., White, R., and Bentley, B. (2006). Effects of lamotrigine and lithium on body weight during maintenance treatment of bipolar I disorder. *Bipolar Disord*, 8(2), 175–181.

Sajatovic, M., Gyulai, L., Calabrese, J.R., Thompson, T.R., Wilson, B.G., White, R., and Evoniuk, G. (2005). Maintenance treatment outcomes in older patients with bipolar I disorder. *Am J Geriatr Psychiatry*, 13(4), 305–311.

Sanger, T.M., Grundy, S.L., Gibson, P.J., Namjoshi, M.A., Greaney, M.G., and Tohen, M.F. (2001). Long-term olanzapine therapy in the treatment of bipolar I disorder: An open-label continuation phase study. *J Clin Psychiatry*, 62(4), 273–281.

Sashidharan, S.P., and McGuire, R.J. (1983). Recurrence of affective illness after withdrawal of long-term lithium treatment. *Acta Psychiatr Scand*, 68, 126–133.

Schaffer, L.C., and Schaffer, C.B. (1999). Tiagabine and the treatment of refractory bipolar disorder. *Am J Psychiatry*, 156(12), 2014–2015.

Schaffer, L.C., Schaffer, C.B., and Howe, J. (2002). An open case series on the utility of tiagabine as an augmentation in refractory bipolar outpatients. *J Affect Disord*, 71(1-3), 259–263.

Schou, M. (1963). Normothymics, "mood-normalizer." *Br J Psychiatry*, 109, 803–809.

Schou, M. (1968). Lithium in psychiatric therapy and prophylaxis. *J Psychiatr Res*, 6(1), 67–95.

Schou, M. (2001). Lithium treatment at 52. *J Affect Disord*, 67(1-3), 21–32.

Schou, M., Juel-Nielsen, N., Stromgren, E., and Voldby, H. (1954). The treatment of manic psychoses by the administration of lithium salts. *J Neurochem*, 17(4), 250–260.

Schou, M., Amidsen, A., Eskjer, J.S., and Olsen, T. (1968). Occurrence of goitre during lithium treatment. *BMJ*, 3, 710–713.

Schou, M., Baastrup, P.C., Grof, P., Weis, P., and Angst, J. (1970). Pharmacological and clinical problems of lithium prophylaxis. *Br J Psychiatry*, 116(535), 615–619.

Schrauwen, E., and Ghaemi, S.N. (2006). Galantamine treatment of cognitive impairment in bipolar disorder: Four cases. *Bipolar Disord*, 8(2), 196–199.

Schumann, C., Lenz, G., Berghofer, A., and Muller-Oerlinghausen, B. (1999). Non-adherence with long-term prophylaxis: A 6-year naturalistic follow-up study of affectively ill patients. *Psychiatry Res*, 89(3), 247–257.

Severus, W.E., Grunze, H., Kleindienst, N., Frangou, S., and Moeller, H.J. (2005). Is the prophylactic antidepressant efficacy of lithium in bipolar I disorder dependent on study design and lithium level? *J Clin Psychopharmacol*, 25(5), 457–462.

Sharma, V., Smith, A., and Mazmanian, D. (2006). Olanzapine in the prevention of postpartum psychosis and mood episodes in bipolar disorder. *Bipolar Disord*, 8(4), 400–404.

Shulman, K.I., Sykora, K., Gill, S., Mamdani, M., Bronskill, S., Wodchis, W.P., Anderson, G., and Rochon, P. (2005). Incidence of delirium in older adults newly prescribed lithium or valproate: A population-based cohort study. *J Clin Psychiatry*, 66(4), 424–427.

Sienaert, P., and Peuskens, J. (2006). Electroconvulsive therapy: An effective therapy of medication-resistant bipolar disorder. *Bipolar Disord*, 8(3), 304–306.

Silverstone, T., McPherson, H., Hunt, N., and Romans, S. (1998). How effective is lithium in the prevention of relapse in bipolar disorder? A prospective naturalistic follow-up study. *Aust NZ J Psychiatry*, 32(1), 61–66.

Sobotka, J.L., Alexander, B., and Cook, B.L. (1990). A review of carbamazepine's hematologic reactions and monitoring recommendations. *DICP*, 24(12), 1214–1219.

Solomon, D.A., Ryan, C.E., Keitner, G.I., Miller, I.W., Shea, M.T., Kazim, A., and Keller, M.B. (1997). A pilot study of lithium carbonate plus divalproex sodium for the continuation and maintenance treatment of patients with bipolar I disorder. *J Clin Psychiatry*, 58(3), 95–99.

Solomon, D.A., Leon, A.C., Mueller, T.I., Coryell, W., Teres, J.J., Posternak, M.A., Judd, L.L., Endicott, J., and Keller, M.B. (2005). Tachyphylaxis in unipolar major depressive disorder. *J Clin Psychiatry*, 66(3), 283–290.

Solvason, H.B. (2000). Agranulocytosis associated with lamotrigine. *Am J Psychiatry*, 157(10), 1704.

Souza, F.G., Mander, A.J., and Goodwin, G.M. (1990). The efficacy of lithium in prophylaxis of unipolar depression: Evidence from its discontinuation. *Br J Psychiatry*, 157, 718–722.

Spinelli, M.G. (2004). Maternal infanticide associated with mental illness: Prevention and promise of saved lives. *Am J Psychiatry*, 161(9), 1548–1557.

Sporn, J., and Sachs, G. (1997). The anticonvulsant lamotrigine in treatment-resistant manic-depressive illness. *J Clin Psychopharmacol*, 17(3), 185–189.

Stallone, F., Shelley, E., Mendlewicz, J., and Fieve, R.R. (1973). The use of lithium in affective disorders: 3. A double-blind study of prophylaxis in bipolar illness. *Am J Psychiatry*, 130(9), 1006–1010.

Steckler, T.L. (1994). Lithium- and carbamazepine-associated sinus node dysfunction: Nine-year experience in a psychiatric hospital. *J Clin Psychopharmacol*, 14(5), 336–339.

Stewart, D.E. (2000). Antidepressant drugs during pregnancy and lactation. *Int Clin Psychopharmacol*, 15(Suppl. 3), S19–S24.

Stewart, D.E., Klompenhouwer, J.L., Kendell, R.E., and van Hulst, A.M. (1991). Prophylactic lithium in puerperal psychosis: The experience of three centres. *Br J Psychiatry*, 158, 393–397.

Suppes, T., and Dennehy, E.B. (2002). Evidence-based long-term treatment of bipolar II disorder. *J Clin Psychiatry*, 63(Suppl. 10), 29–33.

Suppes, T., Baldessarini, R.J., Faedda, G.L., and Tohen, M. (1991). Risk of recurrence following discontinuation of lithium treatment in bipolar disorder. *Arch Gen Psychiatry*, 48(12), 1082–1088.

Suppes, T., Brown, E.S., McElroy, S.L., Keck, P.E. Jr., Nolen, W., Kupka, R., Frye, M., Denicoff, K.D., Altshuler, L., Leverich,

G.S., and Post, R.M. (1999a). Lamotrigine for the treatment of bipolar disorder: A clinical case series. *J Affect Disord*, 53(1), 95–98.

Suppes, T., Webb, A., Paul, B., Carmody, T., Kraemer, H., and Rush, A.J. (1999b). Clinical outcome in a randomized 1-year trial of clozapine versus treatment as usual for patients with treatment-resistant illness and a history of mania. *Am J Psychiatry*, 156(8), 1164–1169.

Suppes, T., Ozcan, M.E., and Carmody, T. (2004). Response to clozapine of rapid cycling versus non-cycling patients with a history of mania. *Bipolar Disord*, 6(4), 329–332.

Suppes, T., Brown, E., Schuh, L.M., Baker, R.W., and Tohen, M. (2005). Rapid versus non-rapid cycling as a predictor of response to olanzapine and divalproex sodium for bipolar mania and maintenance of remission: Post hoc analyses of 47-week data. *J Affect Disord*, 89(1–3), 69–77.

Swann, A.C., Bowden, C.L., Calabrese, J.R., Dilsaver, S.C., and Morris, D.D. (1999). Differential effect of number of previous episodes of affective disorder on response to lithium or divalproex in acute mania. *Am J Psychiatry*, 156(8), 1264–1266.

Swann, A.C., Bowden, C.L., Calabrese, J.R., Dilsaver, S.C., and Morris, D.D. (2000). Mania: Differential effects of previous depressive and manic episodes on response to treatment. *Acta Psychiatr Scand*, 101(6), 444–451.

Thisted, E., and Ebbesen, F. (1993). Malformations, withdrawal manifestations, and hypoglycaemia after exposure to valproate in utero. *Arch Dis Child*, 69(Spec. No. 3), 288–291.

Tohen, M., Castillo, J., Baldessarini, R.J., Zarate, C. Jr., and Kando, J.C. (1995). Blood dyscrasias with carbamazepine and valproate: A pharmacoepidemiological study of 2,228 patients at risk. *Am J Psychiatry*, 152(3), 413–418.

Tohen, M., Bowden, C., Greil, W., Jacobs, T.G., Baker, R.W., Evans, A.R., and Cassano, G. (2002). *Olanzapine in relapse prevention of bipolar disorder.* Poster presented to the Meeting of the American College of Neurosychopharmacology, Puerto Rico.

Tohen, M., Ketter, T.A., Zarate, C.A., Suppes, T., Frye, M., Altshuler, L., Zajecka, J., Schuh, L.M., Risser, R.C., Brown, E., and Baker, R.W. (2003). Olanzapine versus divalproex sodium for the treatment of acute mania and maintenance of remission: A 47-week study. *Am J Psychiatry*, 160(7), 1263–1271.

Tohen, M., Chengappa, K.N., Suppes, T., Baker, R.W., Zarate, C.A., Bowden, C.L., Sachs, G.S., Kupfer, D.J., Ghaemi, S.N., Feldman, P.D., Risser, R.C., Evans, A.R., and Calabrese, J.R. (2004). Relapse prevention in bipolar I disorder: 18-Month comparison of olanzapine plus mood stabilizer v. mood stabilizer alone. *Br J Psychiatry*, 184, 337–345.

Tohen, M., Calabrese, J.R., Sachs, G.S., Banov, M.D., Detke, H.C., Risser, R., Baker, R.W., Chou, J.C., and Bowden, C.L. (2006). Randomized, placebo-controlled trial of olanzapine as maintenance therapy in patients with bipolar I disorder responding to acute treatment with olanzapine. *Am J Psychiatry*, 163(2), 247–256.

Tondo, L., Baldessarini, R.J., Floris, G., and Rudas, N. (1997). Effectiveness of restarting lithium treatment after its discontinuation in bipolar I and bipolar II disorders. *Am J Psychiatry*, 154(4), 548–550.

Tondo, L., Baldessarini, R.J., Hennen, J., and Floris, G. (1998). Lithium maintenance treatment of depression and mania in bipolar I and bipolar II disorders. *Am J Psychiatry*, 155(5), 638–645.

Tondo, L., Baldessarini, R.J., and Floris, G. (2001). Long-term clinical effectiveness of lithium maintenance treatment in types I and II bipolar disorders. *Br J Psychiatry*, 41, S184–S190.

Tondo, L., Hennen, J., and Baldessarini, R.J. (2003). Rapid-cycling bipolar disorder: Effects of long term treatments. *Acta Psychiatr Scand*, 108, 4–14.

Trivedi, M.H., Rush, A.J., Wisniewski, S.R., Nierenberg, A.A., Warden, D., Ritz, L., Norquist, G., Howland, R.H., Lebowitz, B., McGrath, P.J., Shores-Wilson, K., Biggs, M.M., Balasubramani, G.K., Fava, M., and STAR*D Study Team. (2006). Evaluation of outcomes with citalopram for depression using measurement-based care in STAR*D: Implications for clinical practice. *Am J Psychiatry*, 163(1), 28–40.

Tsankov, N., Angelova, I., and Kazandjieva, J. (2000). Drug-induced psoriasis: Recognition and management. *Am J Clin Dermatol*, 1(3), 159–165.

Vaidya, N.A., Mahableshwarkar, A.R., and Shahid, R. (2003). Continuation and maintenance ECT in treatment-resistant bipolar disorder. *J ECT*, 19(1), 10–16.

Van Gerpen, M.W., Johnson, J.E., and Winstead, D.K. (1999). Mania in the geriatric patient population: A review of the literature. *Am J Geriatr Psychiatry*, 7(3), 188–202.

Vanelle, J.M., Loo, H., Galinowski, A., de Carvalho, W., Bourdel, M.C., Brochier, P., Bouvet, O., Brochier, T., and Olie, J.P. (1994). Maintenance ECT in intractable manic-depressive disorders. *Convuls Ther*, 10(3), 195–205.

Vestergaard, P. (2004). Guidelines for maintenance treatment of bipolar disorder: Are there discrepancies between European and North American recommendations? *Bipolar Disord*, 6(6), 519–522.

Vestergaard, P., and Schou, M. (1987). Does long-term lithium treatment induce diabetes mellitus? *Neuropsychobiology*, 17(3), 130–132.

Vestergaard, P., Licht, R. W., Brodersen, A., Rasmussen, N.A., Christensen, H., Arngrim, T., Gronvall, B., Kristensen, E., and Poulstrup, I. (1998). Outcome of lithium prophylaxis: A prospective follow-up of affective disorder patients assigned to high and low serum lithium levels. *Acta Psychiatr Scand*, 98(4), 310–315.

Vieta, E., Goikolea, J.M., Corbella, B., Benabarre, A., Reinares, M., Martinez, G., Fernandez, A., Colom, F., Martinez-Aran, A., Torrent, C., and Group for the Study of Risperidone in Affective Disorders (GSRAD). (2001a). Risperidone safety and efficacy in the treatment of bipolar and schizoaffective disorders: Results from a 6-month, multicenter, open study. *J Clin Psychiatry*, 62(10), 818–825.

Vieta, E., Reinares, M., Corbella, B., Benabarre, A., Gilaberte, I., Colom, F., Martinez-Aran, A., Gasto, C., and Tohen, M. (2001b). Olanzapine as long-term adjunctive therapy in treatment-resistant bipolar disorder. *J Clin Psychopharmacol*, 21(5), 469–473.

Vieta, E., Torrent, C., Garcia-Ribas, G., Gilabert, A., Garcia-Pares, G., Rodriguez, A., Cadevall, J., Garcia-Castrillon, J., Lusilla, P., and Arrufat, F. (2002). Use of topiramate in treatment-resistant bipolar spectrum disorders *J Clin Psychopharmacol*, 22(4), 431–435.

Vieta, E., Sanchez-Moreno, J., Goikolea, J.M., Torrent, C., Benabarre, A., Colom, F., Martinez, A., Reinares, M., Comes, M., and Corbella, B. (2003). Adjunctive topiramate in bipolar I disorder. *World J Biol Psychiatry*, 4(4), 172–176.

Vieta, E., Sanchez-Moreno, J., Goikolea, J. M., Colom, F., Martinez-Aran, A., Benabarre, A., Corbella, B., Torrent, C.,

Comes, M., Reinares, M., and Brugue, E. (2004). Effects on weight and outcome of long-term olanzapine-topiramate combination treatment in bipolar disorder. *J Clin Psychopharmacol*, 24(4), 374–378.

Vieta, E., Goikolea, J.M., Martinez-Aran, A., Comes, M., Verger, K., Masramon, X., Sanchez-Moreno, J., and Colom, F. (2006). A double-blind, randomized, placebo-controlled, prophylaxis study of adjunctive gabapentin for bipolar disorder. *J Clin Psychiatry*, 67(3), 473–477.

Viguera, A.C., Nonacs, R., Cohen, L.S., Tondo, L., Murray, A., and Baldessarini, R.J. (2000). Risk of recurrence of bipolar disorder in pregnant and nonpregnant women after discontinuing lithium maintenance. *Am J Psychiatry*, 157(2), 179–184.

Viguera, A.C., Cohen, L.S., Baldessarini, R.J., and Nonacs, R. (2002). Managing bipolar disorder during pregnancy: Weighing the risks and benefits. *Can J Psychiatry*, 47(5), 426–436.

Walden, J., Hesslinger, B., van Calker, D., and Berger, M. (1996). Addition of lamotrigine to valproate may enhance efficacy in the treatment of bipolar affective disorder. *Pharmacopsychiatry*, 29(5), 193–195.

Walden, J., Schaerer, L., Schloesser, S., and Grunze, H. (2000). An open longitudinal study of patients with bipolar rapid cycling treated with lithium or lamotrigine for mood stabilization. *Bipolar Disord*, 2(4), 336–339.

Warner, J.P. (2000). Evidence-based psychopharmacology: 3. Assessing evidence of harm: What are the teratogenic effects of lithium carbonate? *J Psychopharmacol*, 14(1), 77–80.

Watkins, S.E., Callender, K., Thomas, D.R., Tidmarsh, S.F., and Shaw, D.M. (1987). The effect of carbamazepine and lithium on remission from affective illness. *Br J Psychiatry*, 150, 180–182.

Wehr, T.A., and Goodwin, F.K. (1979). Rapid cycling in manic-depressives induced by tricyclic antidepressants. *Arch Gen Psychiatry*, 36(5), 555–559.

Wehr, T.A., Sack, D.A., Rosenthal, N.E., and Cowdry, R.W. (1988). Rapid cycling affective disorder: Contributing factors and treatment responses in 51 patients. *Am J Psychiatry*, 145(2), 179–184.

Wehr, T.A., Turner, E.H., Shimada, J.M., Lowe, C.H., Barker, C., and Leibenluft, E. (1998). Treatment of rapidly cycling bipolar patient by using extended bed rest and darkness to stabilize the timing and duration of sleep. *Biol Psychiatry*, 43(11), 822–828.

Whitwell, J.R. (1936). *Historical Notes on Psychiatry: Early Times—End of 16th Century*. London: H.K. Lewis & Co.

Wisner, K.L., Peindl, K.S., Perel, J.M., Hanusa, B.H., Piontek, C.M., and Baab, S. (2002). Verapamil treatment for women with bipolar disorder. *Biol Psychiatry*, 51(9), 745–752.

Wisner, K.L., Hanusa, B.H., Peindl, K.S., and Perel, J.M. (2004). Prevention of postpartum episodes in women with bipolar disorder. *Biol Psychiatry*, 56(8), 592–596.

Wong, I.C., Mawer, G.E., and Sander, J.W. (1999). Factors influencing the incidence of lamotrigine-related skin rash. *Ann Pharmacother*, 33(10), 1037–1042.

Yonkers, K.A., Wisner, K.L., Stowe, Z., Leibenluft, E., Cohen, L., Miller, L., Manber, R., Viguera, A., Suppes, T., and Altshuler, L. (2004). Management of bipolar disorder during pregnancy and the postpartum period. *Am J Psychiatry*, 161(4), 608–620.

Young, A., Geddes, J., Macritchie, K., Rao, S., and Vasudev, A. (2006). Tiagabine in the maintenance treatment of bipolar disorders. *Cochrane Database Syst Rev*, 19(3), CD005173.

Zarate, C.A. Jr., and Quiroz, J.A. (2003). Combination treatment in bipolar disorder: A review of controlled trials. *Bipolar Disord*, 5(3), 217–225.

Zarate, C.A. Jr., Tohen, M., and Baldessarini, R.J. (1995). Clozapine in severe mood disorders. *J Clin Psychiatry*, 56(9), 411–417.

CHAPTER 21

Aagaard, J., and Vestergaard, P. (1990). Predictors of outcome in prophylactic lithium treatment: A 2-year prospective study. *J Affect Disord*, 18, 259–266.

Abou-Saleh, M.T., and Coppen, A. (1983). Subjective side-effects of amitriptyline and lithium in affective disorders. *Br J Psychiatry*, 142, 391–397.

Adams, J., and Scott, J. (2000). Predicting medication adherence in severe mental disorders. *Acta Psychiatr Scand*, 101(2), 119–124.

Amador, X.F., Flaum, M., Andreasen, N.C., Strauss, D.H., Yale, S.A., Clark, S.C., and Gorman, J.M. (1994). Awareness of illness in schizophrenia, schizoaffective and mood disorders. *Arch Gen Psychiatry*, 51, 826–836.

Angst, J., Weis, P., Grof, P., Baastrup, P.C., and Schou, M. (1970). Lithium prophylaxis in recurrent affective disorders. *Br J Psychiatry*, 116, 604–614.

Ball, J.R., Mitchell, P.B., Corry, J.C., Skillecorn, A., Smith, M., and Malhi, G.S. (2006). A randomized controlled trial of cognitive therapy for bipolar disorder: Focus on long-term change. *J Clin Psychiatry*, 67, 277–286.

Bech, P. (1981). Rating scales for affective disorders: Their validity and consistency. *Acta Psychiatr Scand*, 295, 1–101.

Bech P., Vendsborg, P.B., and Rafaelsen, O.J. (1976). Lithium maintenance treatment of manic-melancholic patients: Its role in the daily routine. *Acta Psychiatr Scand*, 53, 70–81.

Becker, M.H., and Maiman, L.A. (1980). Strategies for enhancing compliance. *J Community Health*, 6, 113–135.

Blackwell, B. (1973). Patient adherence. *N Engl J Med*, 289, 249–252.

Blackwell, B. (1976). Treatment adherence. *Br J Psychiatry*, 129, 513–531.

Blackwell, B. (1980, January). *Why don't patients take their medicines?* Paper presented at the annual meeting of the American Association for the Advancement of Science, Toronto, Canada.

Blackwell, B. (1982). Treatment adherence. In J.H. Greist, J.W. Jefferson, and R.L. Spitzer (Eds.), *Treatment of Mental Disorders* (pp. 501–516). New York: Oxford University Press.

Bonin, J.P. (1999). Psychosocial determinants of lithium compliance in patients with bipolar disorder. *Can J Nurs Res*, 31, 24–40.

Bowskill, R., Clatworthy, J., Parham, R., Rank, T., and Horner, R. (2006). Patient dissatisfaction with information provided about medicines prescribed for bipolar disorder. *J Affect Disord*, Dec. 14 [epub ahead of print].

Boyd, J.R., Covington, T.R., Stanaszek, W.F., and Coussons, R.T. (1974a). Drug defaulting: Part I. Determinants of adherence. *Am J Hosp Pharm*, 31, 362–367.

Boyd, J.R., Covington, T.R., Stanaszek, W.F., and Coussons, R.T. (1974b). Drug defaulting: Part II. Analysis of non-adherence patterns. *Am J Hosp Pharm*, 31, 485–491.

Brookmeyer, R., Johnson, E., and Bollinger, R. (2003). Modeling the optimum duration of antibiotic prophylaxis in an anthrax outbreak. *Proc Natl Acad Sci USA*, 100(17), 10129–10132.

Cade, J.F.J. (1978). Past, present and future. In F.N. Johnson, and S. Johnson (Eds.), *Lithium in Medical Practice* (pp. 5–16). Baltimore: University Park Press.

Cassidy, F., Ahearn, E., and Carroll, B.J. (2001). A prospective study of inter-episode consistency of manic and mixed subtypes of bipolar disorder. *J Affect Disord*, 67(1-3), 181–185.

Clarkin, J.F., Carpenter, D., Hull, J., Wilner, P., and Glick, I. (1998). Effects of psychoeducational intervention for married patients with bipolar disorder and their spouses. *Psychiatr Serv*, 49(4), 531–533.

Cochran, S.D. (1982). *Strategies for Preventing Lithium Non-Adherence in Bipolar Affective Illness*. Unpublished doctoral dissertation, University of California, Los Angeles, CA.

Cochran, S.D. (1984). Preventing medical noncompliance in the outpatient treatment of bipolar affective disorders. *J Consult Clin Psychol*, 52, 873–878.

Cochran, S.D., and Gitlin, M.J. (1988). Attitudinal correlates of lithium adherence in bipolar affective disorders. *J Nerv Ment Dis*, 176, 457–464.

Colom, F., and Vieta, E. (2002). Treatment adherence in bipolar patients. *Clin Approaches Bipolar Disord*, 1, 49–56.

Colom, F., Vieta, E., Martínez-Arán, A., Reinares, M., Benabarre, A., and Gasto, C. (2000). Clinical factors associated with treatment noncompliance in euthymic bipolar patients. *J Clin Psychiatry*, 61, 549–555.

Colom, F., Vieta, E., Martínez-Arán, A., Reinares, M., Goikolea, J.M., Benabarre, A., Torrent, C., Comes, M., Corbella, B., Parramon, G., and Corominas, J. (2003). A randomized trial on the efficacy of group psychoeducation in the prophylaxis in bipolar patients whose disease is in remission. *Arch Gen Psychiatry*, 60, 402–407.

Connelly, C.E., Davenport, Y.B., and Nurnberger, J.I. (1982). Adherence to treatment regimen in a lithium carbonate clinic. *Arch Gen Psychiatry*, 39, 585–588.

Dailey, L.F., Townsend, S.W., Dysken, M.W., and Kuskowski, M.A. (2005). Recidivism in medication-noncompliant serious juvenile offenders with bipolar disorder. *J Clin Psychiatry*, 66, 477–484.

Danion, J.M., Neunreuther, C., Krieger-Finance, F., Imbs, J.L., and Singer, L. (1987). Compliance with long-term lithium treatment in major affective disorders. *Pharmacopsychiatry*, 20, 230–231.

Day, J.C., Bertall, R.P., Roberts, C., Randall, F., Rogers, A., Cattell, D., Healy D., Rae, P., and Power, C. (2005). Attitudes toward antipsychotic medication: The impact of clinical variables and relationships with health professionals. *Arch Gen Psychiatry*, 62, 717–724.

Dell'Osso, L., Pini, S., Tundo, A., Sarno, N., Musetti, L., and Cassano, G.B. (2000). Clinical characteristics of mania, mixed mania, and bipolar depression with psychotic features. *Compr Psychiatry*, 41(4), 242–247.

Dell'Osso, L., Pini, S., Cassano, G.B., Mastrocinque, C., Seckinger, R.A., Saettoni, M., Papasogli, A., Yale, S.A., and Amador, X.F. (2002). Insight into illness in patients with mania, mixed mania, bipolar depression and major depression with psychotic features. *Bipolar Disord*, 4(5), 315–322.

DiMatteo, M.R. (2004). Variations in patients' adherence to medical recommendations: A quantitative review of 50 years of research. *Med Care*, 42(3), 200–209.

Docherty, J.P., and Fiester, S.J. (1985). The therapeutic alliance and compliance with psychopharmacology. In R.E. Hales and A.J. Frances (Eds.), *American Psychiatric Association Annual Review, Vol. 4* (pp. 607–632). Washington, DC: American Psychiatric Press.

Dolder, C., Lacro, J., Dunn, L., and Jeste, D. (2002). Antipsychotic medication adherence: Is there a difference between typical and atypical agents? *Am J Psychiatry*, 159, 103–108.

Fennig, S., Bromet, E.G., Jandorf, L., Schwartz, J., Lavelle, J., and Ram, R. (1995). Eliciting psychotic symptoms using a semistructured interview. *J Nerv Ment Dis*, 181, 20–26.

Fenton, W.S., Blyer, C.R., and Heinssen, R.K. (1997). Determinants of medication adherence in schizophrenia: Empirical and clinical findings. *Schizophrenia Bull*, 23, 637–651.

Fitzgerald, R.G. (1972). Mania as a message: Treatment with family therapy and lithium carbonate. *Am J Psychotherapy*, 26, 547–553.

Frank, E., Prien, R.F., Kupfer, D.J., and Alberts, L. (1985). Implications of nonadherence on research in affective disorders. *Psychopharmacol Bull*, 21, 37–42.

Frank, J.D., and Frank, J.B. (1991). *Persuasion and Healing: A Comparative Study of Psychotherapy*, 3rd ed. Baltimore: Johns Hopkins University Press.

Ghaemi, S.N. (1997). Insight and psychiatric disorder: A review of the literature, with a focus on its clinical relevance for bipolar disorder. *Psychiatr Ann*, 27, 782–790.

Ghaemi, S.N., Stoll, A.L., and Pope, H.G. Jr. (1995). Lack of insight in bipolar disorder: The acute manic episode. *J Nerv Ment Dis*, 183(7), 464–467.

Gianfrancesco, F.D., Rajagopalan, K., Sajatovic M., Wang, R.H. (2006). Treatment adherence among patients with bipolar or manic disorder taking atypical and typical antipsychotics. *J Clin Psychiatry*, 67(2), 222–232.

Gitlin, M.J., and Jamison, K.R. (1984). Lithium clinics: Theory and practice. *Hosp Community Psychiatry*, 35(4), 363–368.

Gitlin, M.J., Cochran, S.D., and Jamison, K.R. (1989). Maintenance lithium treatment: Side effects and adherence. *J Clin Psychiatry*, 50, 127–131.

Glazer, W.M., Sonnenberg, J.G., Reinstein, M.J., and Akers, R.F. (2004). A novel, point-of-case test for lithium levels: Description and reliability. *J Clin Psychiatry*, 65, 652–656.

Goldberg, J.F., Harrow, M., and Leon, A.C. (1996). Lithium treatment of bipolar affective disorders under naturalistic followup conditions. *Psychopharmacol Bull*, 32, 47–54.

Gonzalez-Pinto, A., Mosquera, F., Alonso, M., Lopez, P., Ramirez, F., Vieta, E., and Baldessarini, R.J. (2006). Suicidal risk in bipolar I disorder patients and adolescence to long-term lithium treatment. *Bipolar Disord*, 8, 618–624.

Greenhouse, W.J., Meyer, B., and Johnson, S.L. (2000). Coping and medication adherence in bipolar disorder. *J Affect Disord*, 59, 237–241.

Grof, P., Cakulis, P., and Dostal, T. (1970). Lithium dropouts: A follow-up study of patients who discontinued prophylactic treatment. *Int Pharmacopsychiatry*, 5, 162–169.

Harvey, N.S., and Peet, M. (1991). Lithium maintenance: 2. Effects of personality and attitude on health information acquisition and compliance. *Br J Psychiatry*, 158, 200–204.

Haynes, R.B., Taylor, D.W., and Sackett, D.L. (Eds.). (1979). *Compliance in Health Care*. Baltimore: The Johns Hopkins University Press.

Haynes, R.B., McDonald, H., Garg, A.X., and Montague, P. (2002). Interventions for helping patients to follow prescriptions for medications. *Cochrane Database Syst Rev*, (2):CD000011.

Horne, R., Clatworthy, J., Parham, R., Rank, T., Bowskill, R. (2006). Medication prescribed for bipolar disorder: The role of patients' treatment perceptions in predicting nonadherence. *J Affect Disord*, 915, 566.

Jamison, K.R. (1995). *An Unquiet Mind: A Memoir of Moods and Madness*. New York: Alfred A. Knopf.

Jamison, K.R., Gerner, R.H., and Goodwin, F.K. (1979). Patient and physician attitudes toward lithium: Relationship to adherence. *Arch Gen Psychiatry*, 36, 866–869.

Johnson, R.E., and McFarland, B.H. (1996). Lithium use and discontinuation in a health maintenance organization. *Am J Psychiatry*, 153, 993–1000.

Johnson, S., Winett, C., Miller, I., Bauer, M., Solomon, D., Keitner, G., and Ryan, C. (1998). Life events, medications and bipolar-I disorder. *J Bipolar Disord*, 1, 37–39.

Keck, P.E., McElroy, S.L., Strakowski, S.M., Bourne, M.L., and West, S.A. (1997). Compliance with maintenance treatment in bipolar disorder. *Psychopharmacol Bull*, 33, 87–91.

Keck, P.E., McElroy, S.L., Strakowski, S.M., West, S.A., Sax, K.W., Hawkins, J.M., Bourne, M.L., and Haggard, P. (1998). 12-month outcome of patients with bipolar disorder following hospitalization for a manic or mixed episode. *Am J Psychiatry*, 155, 646–652.

Kerry, J. (1978). Recent developments in patient management. In F.N. Johnson and S. Johnson (Eds.), *Lithium in Medical Practice* (pp. 337–353). Baltimore: University Park Press.

Kleindienst, N., and Greil, W. (2004). Are illness concepts a powerful predictor of adherence to prophylactic treatment in bipolar disorder? *J Clin Psychiatry*, 65, 966–974.

Kucera-Bozarth, K., Beck, N.C., and Lyss, L. (1982). Compliance with lithium regimens. *J Psychosoc Nurs Ment Health Serv*, 20, 11–15.

Kulhara, P., Basu, D., Matoo, S.K., Sharan, P., and Chopra, R. (1999). Lithium prophylaxis of recurrent bipolar affective disorder: Long-term outcome and its psychosocial correlates. *J Affect Disord*, 54, 87–96.

Lam, D., Bright, J., Jones, S., Hayward, P., Schuck, N., Chisholm, D., and Sham, P. (2000). Cognitive therapy for bipolar illness: A pilot study of relapse prevention. *Cognitive Ther Res*, 24, 503–520.

Lam, D.H., Watkins, E.R., Hayward, P., Bright, J., Wright, K., Kerr, N., Parr-Davis, G., and Sham, P. (2003). A randomized controlled study of cognitive therapy for relapse prevention for bipolar affective disorder: Outcome of the first year. *Arch Gen Psychiatry*, 60, 145–152.

Lam, D.H., Hayward, P., Watkins, E.R., Wright, K., and Sham, P. (2005). Relapse prevention in patients with bipolar disorder: Cognitive therapy outcome after 2 years. *Am J Psychiatry*, 162, 324–329.

Lenzi, A., Lazzerini, F., Placidi, G.F., Cassano, G.B., and Akiskal, H.S. (1989). Predictors of adherence with lithium and carbamazepine regimens in the long-term treatment of recurrent mood and related psychotic disorders. *Pharmacopsychiatry*, 22, 34–37.

Maarbjerg, K., Aagaard, J., and Vestergaard, P. (1988). Adherence to lithium prophylaxis: I. Clinical predictors and patient's reasons for non adherence. *Pharmacopsychiatry*, 21, 121–125.

Marken, P.A., Stanislac, W.S., Lacombe, S., Pierce, C., Hornstra, R., and Sommi, R.W. (1992). Profile of a sample of subjects admitted to an acute care psychiatric facility with manic symptoms. *Psychopharmacol Bull*, 28, 201–205.

Mazullo, J.M., and Lasagna, L. (1972). Take thou . . . But is your patient really taking what you prescribed? *Drug Ther*, 2, 11–15.

McDonald, H.P., Garg, A.X., and Haynes, R.B. (2002). Interventions to enhance patient adherence to medication prescriptions: Scientific review. *JAMA*, 288, 2868–2879.

Michalakeas, A., Skoutas, C., Charalambous, A., Peristeris, A., Marinos, V., and Keramari, E. (1994). Insight in schizophrenia and mood disorders and its relation to psychopathology. *Acta Psychiatr Scand*, 90, 46–49.

Miklowitz, D.J. (1992). Longitudinal outcome and medication nonadherence among manic patients with and without mood-incongruent psychotic features. *J Nerv Ment Di*, 180, 703–711.

Miklowitz, D.J., Simoneau, T.L., George, E.L., Richards, J.A., Kalbag, A., Sachs-Ericsson, N., and Suddath, R. (2000). Family-focused treatment of bipolar disorder: 1-Year effects of a psychoeducational program in conjunction with pharmacotherapy. *Biol Psychiatry*, 48(6), 582–592.

Miklowitz, D.J., Richard, J.A., George, E.L., Frank, E., Suddath, R.L., Powell, K.B., and Sacher, J.A. (2003). Integrated family and individual therapy for bipolar disorder: Results of a treatment development study. *J Clin Psychiatry*, 64, 182–191.

Morselli, P.L., Elgie, R., GAMIAN-Europe. (2003). GAMIAN-Europe/BEAM Survey I-global analysis of a patient questionnaire circulated to 3450 members of 12 European advocacy groups operating in the field of mood disorders. *Bipolar Disord* 5, 265–278.

Mukherjee, S., Rosen, A.M., and Skukla, S. (1993). Acceptance by patients of maintenance lithium treatment. *Lithium*, 2, 63–69.

Osterberg, L., and Blaschke, T. (2005). Adherence to medication. *N Engl J Med*, 353, 487–497.

Pallanti, S., Quercioli, L., Pazzagli, A., Rossi, A., Dell'Osso, L., Pini, S., Cassano, G.B. (1999). Awareness of illness and subjective experience of cognitive complaints in patients with bipolar I and bipolar II disorder. *Am J Psychiatry*, 156(7), 1094–1096.

Pampallona, S., Bollini, P., Tibaldi, G., Kupelnick, B., and Munizza, C. (2002). Patient adherence in the treatment of depression. *Br J Psychiatry*, 180, 104–109.

Peralta, V., and Cuetsa, M.J. (1998). Lack of insight in mood disorders. *J Affect Disord*, 49, 55–58.

Perkins, D.O., Johnson, J.L., Hamer, R.M., Zipursky, R.B., Keefe, R.S., Centorrhino, F., Green, A.I., Glick, I.B., Kahn, R.S., Sharma, T., Tohen, M., McEvoy, J.P., Weiden, P.J., and Lieberman, J.A. (2006). Predictors of antipsychotic medication adherence in patients recovering from a first psychotic episode. *Schizophr Res*, 83, 53–63.

Perlick, D.A., Rosenheck, R.A., Clarkin, J.F., Maciejewski, P.K., Sirey, J., Struening, E., and Link, B.G. (2004a). Impact of family burden and affective response on clinical outcome among patients with bipolar disorder. *Psychiatr Serv*, 55, 1029–1035.

Perlick, D.A., Rosenheck, R.A., Kaczynski, R., and Kozma, L. (2004b). Medication non-adherence in bipolar disorder: A patient-centered review of research findings. *Clin Approaches Bipolar Disord* 3, 56–64.

Perry, A., Tarrier, N., Morriss, R., McCarthy, E., and Limb, K. (1999). Randomised controlled trial of efficacy of teaching patients with bipolar disorder to identify early symptoms of relapse and obtain treatment. *BMJ*, 318(7177), 149–153.

Pini, S., Cassano, G.B., Dell'Osso, L., and Amador, X.F. (2001). Insight into illness in schizophrenia, schizoaffective disorder, and mood disorders with psychotic features. *Am J Psychiatry*, 158(1), 122–125.

Polatin, P., and Fieve, R.R. (1971). Patient rejection of lithium carbonate prophylaxis. *JAMA, 218*, 864–866.

Pope, M., and Scott, J. (2003). Do clinicians understand why individuals stop taking lithium? *J Affect Disord, 74*, 287–291.

Sajatovic, M., Davies, M., and Hrouda, D.R. (2004). Enhancement of treatment adherence among patients with bipolar disorder. *Psychiatr Serv, 55*, 264–269.

Sajatovic, M., Bauer, M.S., Kilbourne, A.M., Vertrees, J.E., and Williford, W. (2006a). Self-reported medication treatment adherence among veterans with bipolar disorder. *Psychiatr Serv, 57*, 56–62.

Sajatovic, M., Valenstein, M., Blow, F.C., Ganoczy, D., and Ignacio, R.V. (2006b). Treatment adherence with antipsychotic medications in bipolar disorder. *Bipolar Disord, 8*, 232–241.

Schou, M. (1997). The combat of non-adherence during prophylactic lithium treatment. *Acta Psychiatr Scand, 95*, 361–363.

Schou, M., and Baastrup, P.C. (1973). Personal and social implications of lithium maintenance treatment. In T.A. Ban, J.R. Boissier, G.H. Gessa, H. Heimann, L. Hollister, H.E. Lehmann, I. Munkvad, H. Steinberg, F. Sulser, A Sundwall, and O. Vinar (Eds.), *Psychopharmacology, Sexual Disorders and Drug Abuse* (pp. 65–68). Amsterdam and London: North-Holland Publishing Co.

Schou, M., Baastrup, P. C., Grof, P., Weis, P., and Angst, J. (1970). Pharmacological and clinical problems of lithium prophylaxis. *Br J Psychiatry, 116*, 615–619.

Schumann, C., Lenz, G., Berghofer, A., and Muller-Oerlinghausen, B. (1999). Non-adherence with long-term prophylaxis: A 6-year naturalistic follow-up study of affectively ill patients. *Psychiatry Res, 89*, 247–257.

Scott, J., and Pope, M. (2002a). Nonadherence with mood stabilizers: Prevalence and predictors. *J Clin Psychiatry, 63*, 384–390.

Scott, J., and Pope, M. (2002b). Self-reported adherence to treatment with mood stabilizers, plasma levels, and psychiatric hospitalization. *Am J Psychiatry, 159*, 1927–1929.

Scott, J., Paykel, E., Morriss, R., Bentall, R., Kinderman, P., Johnson, T., Abbott, R., and Hayhurst, H. (2006). Cognitive-behavioural therapy for severe and recurrent bipolar disorders: Randomised controlled trial. *Br J Psychiatry, 188*, 313–320.

Shakir, S.A., Volkmar, F.R., Bacon, S., and Pfefferbaum, A. (1979). Group psychotherapy as an adjunct to lithium maintenance. *Am J Psychiatry, 136*, 455–456.

Silverstone, T., McPherson, H., Hunt, N., and Romans, S. (1998). How effective is lithium in the prevention of relapse in bipolar disorder? A prospective naturalistic follow-up study. *Aust NZ J Psychiatry, 32*, 61–66.

Slavney, P.R. (2005). *Psychotherapy: An Introduction for Psychiatry Residents and Other Mental Health Trainees.* Baltimore: Johns Hopkins University Press.

Stratigos, K., Peselowe, L., Sobel, M., Fieve, R., and Laje, G. (2002, October). *Non-Adherence with Long-Term Mood Stabilizers in Patients with Bipolar Disorder.* Poster presented at the Institute on Psychiatric Services Meeting, Chicago, IL.

Suppes, T., Baldessarini, R.J., Faedda, G.L., and Tohen, M. (1991). Risk of recurrence following discontinuation of lithium treatment in bipolar disorder. *Arch Gen Psychiatry, 48*, 1082–1088.

Svarstad, B.L., Shireman, T., and Sweeney, J.K. (2001). Using drug claims data to assess the relationship of medication adherence with hospitalization costs. *Psychiatr Serv, 52*, 805–811.

Tohen, M., Chengappa, K.N., Suppes, T., Baker, R.W., Zarate, C.A., Bowden, C.L., Sachs, G.S., Kupfer, D.J., Ghaemi, S.N.,

Feldman, P.D., Risser, R.C., Evans, A.R., and Calabrese, J.R. (2004). Relapse prevention in bipolar I disorder: 18-Month comparison of olanzapine plus mood stabilizer vs. mood stabilizer alone. *Br J Psychiatry, 184*, 337–345.

Tsai, S.M., Chen, C., Kuo, C., Lee, J., Lee, H., and Strakowski, S.M. (2001). 15-year outcome of treated bipolar disorder. *J Affect Disord, 63*(1-3), 215–220.

van Gent, E.M., and Zwart, F.M. (1991). Psychoeducation of partners of bipolar-manic patients. *J Affect Disord, 21*(1), 15–18.

Van Putten, T. (1975). Why do patients with manic-depressive illness stop their lithium? *Compr Psychiatry, 16*, 179–183.

Van Putten, T., and Jamison, K.R. (1980). Rejecting of lithium maintenance therapy by the patient. In Johnson, F.N. (ed.), *Handbook of Lithium Therapy* (pp. 103–108). Lancaster, England: NTP Press.

Vestergaard, P., and Amdisen, A. (1983). Patient attitudes toward lithium. *Acta Psychiatr Scand, 67*, 8–12.

Weiss, R.D., Greenfield, S.F., Najavits, L.M., Soto, J.A., Wyner, D., Tohen, M., and Griffin, M.L. (1998). Medication adherence among patients with bipolar disorder and substance use disorder. *J Clin Psychiatry, 59*, 172–174.

Weiss, R.D., Kolodziej, M.E., Najavits, L.M., Greenfield, S.F., and Fucito, L.M. (2000). Utilization of psychosocial treatments by patients diagnosed with bipolar disorder and substance dependence. *Am J Addict, 9*(4), 314–320.

World Health Organization. (2003). *Adherence to Long-Term Therapies: Evidence for Action.* Geneva: World Health Organization.

Yen, C.-F., Chen, C.-S., Yeh, M.-L., Yang, S.-J., Ke, J.-H., and Yen, J.-Y. (2003). Changes of insight in manic episodes and influencing factors. *Compr Psychiatry, 44*, 404–408.

Yen, C.-F., Chen, C.-S., Yeh, M.-L., Ker, J.-H., Yang, S.-J., and Yen, J.-Y. (2004). Correlates of insight among patients with bipolar I disorder in remission. *J Affect Dis, 78*, 57–60.

Young, J.L., Spitz, R.T., Hillbrand, M., and Daneri, G. (1999). Medication adherence failure in schizophrenia: A forensic review of rates, reasons, treatments, and prospects. *J Am Acad Psychiatry Law, 27*, 426–444.

CHAPTER 22

Abraham, K. (1911). Notes on the psycho-analytical investigation and treatment of manic-depressive insanity and allied conditions. In *Selected Papers of Karl Abraham, M.D.* (pp. 137–156). Translated by D. Bryan and A. Strachey. London: Hogarth Press.

Abraham, K. (1927). Notes on the psycho-analytical investigation and treatment of manic-depressive insanity and allied conditions, 1911. In D. Bryan and A. Strachey (Eds.), *Selected Papers of Karl Abraham, M.D.* (pp. 137–156). London: Hogarth Press.

Aleman, A., Agrawal, N., Morgan, K.D., and David, A.S. (2006). Insight in psychosis and neuropsychological function: Meta-analysis. *Br J Psychiatry, 189*, 204–212.

Alloy, L.B., Reilly-Harrington, N., Fresco, D.M., Whitehouse, W.G., and Zechmeister, J.S. (1999). Cognitive styles and life events in subsyndromal unipolar and bipolar disorders: Stability and prospective prediction of depressive and hypomanic mood swings. *J Cogn Psychotherapy, 13*, 21–40.

American Psychiatric Association (APA). (2002). Practice guideline for the treatment of patients with bipolar disorder. *Am J Psychiatry, 159*(Suppl.), 4–50.

Anonymous. (1984). Manic depressive illness. *Lancet*, 2(8414), 1268.

Anthony, E.J. (1975). The influence of a manic-depressive environment on the developing child. In E.J. Anthony and T. Benedek (Eds.), *Depression and Human Existence* (pp. 279–315). Boston: Little, Brown.

Baastrup, P.C., and Schou, M. (1967). Lithium as a prophylactic agent: Its effect against recurrent depression and manic-depressive psychosis. *Arch Gen Psychiatry*, 16, 162–172.

Basco, M.R., and Rush, A.J. (1996). *Cognitive Behavioral Therapy for Bipolar Disorder*. New York: The Guilford Press.

Bauer, M.S., Crits-Christoph, P., Ball, W.A., Dewees, E., McAllister, T., Alahi, P., Cacciola, J., and Whybrow, P.C. (1991). Independent assessment of manic and depressive symptoms by self-rating: Scale characteristics and implications for the study of mania. *Arch Gen Psychiatry*, 48, 807–812.

Beck, A.T., Rush, A.J., Shaw, B.F., and Emery, G. (1979). *Cognitive Therapy of Depression*. New York: The Guilford Press.

Benson, R. (1976). Psychological stress as a cause of lithium prophylaxis failure: A report of three cases. *Dis Nerv Syst*, 37(12), 699–700.

Berk, M., Berk, L., and Castle, D. (2004). A collaborative approach to the treatment alliance in bipolar disorder. *Bipolar Disord*, 6, 504–518.

Callahan, A.M., and Bauer, M.S. (1999). Psychosocial interventions for bipolar disorder. *Psychtr Clin North Am*, 22, 675–688.

Cassidy, F., Murry, E., Forest, K., and Carroll, B.J. (1998). Signs and symptoms of mania in pure and mixed episodes. *J Affect Disord*, 50(2-3), 187–201.

Cassidy, F., McEvoy, J.P., Yang, Y.K., and Wilson, W.H. (2001). Insight is greater in mixed than in pure manic episodes of bipolar I disorder. *J Nerv Ment Dis*, 189(6), 398–399.

Clarkin, J.F., Carpenter, D., Hull, J., Wilner, P., and Glick, I. (1998). Effects of psychoeducational intervention for married patients with bipolar disorder and their spouses. *Psychiatr Serv*, 49, 531–533.

Cochran, S.D. (1984). Preventing medical nonadherence in the outpatient treatment of bipolar affective disorders. *J Consult Clin Psychol*, 52, 873–878.

Cohen, M.B., Baker, G., Cohen, R.A., Fromm-Reichmann, F., and Weighert, E.V. (1954). An intensive study of twelve cases of manic-depressive psychosis. *Psychiatry*, 17, 103–137.

Colom, F., and Vieta, E. (2006). The pivotal note of psychoeducation with long-term treatment of bipolar disorder. In H.S. Akiskal and M. Tohen (Eds.), *Bipolar Psychopharmacotherapy: Caring for the Patient* (pp. 333–345). New York: John Wiley & Sons.

Colom, F., Vieta, E., Martinez-Avan, A., Reinares, M., Goikolea, J.M., Benabarre, A., Torrent, C., Comes, M., Corbella, B., Parramon, G., and Corominas, J. (2003a). A randomized trial on the efficacy of group psychoeducation in the prophylaxis of recurrences in remitted bipolar patients. *Arch Gen Psychiatry*, 60, 402–407.

Colom, F., Vieta, E., Reinares, M., Martinez-Aran, A., Torrent, C., Goikolea, J.M., and Gasto, C. (2003b). Psychoeducation efficacy in bipolar disorders beyond compliance enhancement. *J Clin Psychiatry*, 64, 1101–1105.

Colom, F., Vieta, E., Sánchez-Moreno, J., Martinez-Arán, A., Reinares, M., Goikolea, J.M., and Scott, J. (2005). Stabilizing the stabilizer: Group psychoeducation enhances the stability of serum lithium levels. *Bipolar Disord*, 7(Suppl. 5), 32–36.

Coryell, W., Scheftner, W., Keller, M., Endicott, J., Maser, J., and Klerman, G.L. (1993). The enduring psychosocial consequences of mania and depression. *Am J Psychiatry*, 150, 720–727.

Culver, J.L., Nam, J.Y., Ullal, A., Wang, P.W., Marsh, W., and Ketter, T.A. (2006). *Finding a silver lining: Benefit-finding in bipolar disorder.* Poster presented at the annual meeting of the American Psychiatric Association, Toronto, Canada.

Custance, J. (1952). *Wisdom, Madness, and Folly: The Philosophy of a Lunatic.* New York: Farrar, Strauss, & Cudahy.

Davenport, Y.B., Aldland, M.L., Gold, P.W., and Goodwin, F.K. (1979). Manic-depressive illness: Psychodynamic features of multigenerational families. *Am J Orthopsychiatry*, 49, 24–35.

de Andrés, R.D., Aillon, N., Bardiot, M.C., Bourgeois, P., Mertel, S., Nerfin, F., Romailler, G., Gex-Fabry, M., and Aubry, J.M. (2006). Impact of the life goals group therapy program for bipolar patients: an open study. *J Affect Disord*, 93, 253–257.

Dell'Osso, L., Pini, S., Tundo, A., Sarno, N., Musetti, L., and Cassano, G.B. (2000). Clinical characteristics of mania, mixed mania, and bipolar depression with psychotic features. *Conpr Psychiatry*, 41(4), 242–247.

Dell'Osso, L., Pini, S., Cassano, G.B., Mastrocinque, C., Seckinger, R.A., Saettoni, M., Papasogli, A., Yale, S.A., and Amador, X.F. (2002). Insight into illness in patients with mania, mixed mania, bipolar depression and major depression with psychotic features. *Bipol Disord*, 4(5), 315–322.

Denicoff, K.D., Smith-Jackson, E.E., Disney, E.R., Suddath, R.L., Leverich, G.S., and Post, R.M. (1997). Preliminary evidence of the reliability and validity of the prospective life-chart methodology (LCM-p). *J Psychiatr Res*, 31, 593–603.

Depression and Bipolar Support Alliance (DBSA). http://www.dbsalliance.org/site/PageServer?pagename=home&printer_friendly=1.

Depression and Bipolar Support Alliance (DBSA). http://www.dsballiance.org/site/PageServer?pagename=empower_advance_advancedirectives2. Page created 5/8/2006.

Ehlers, C.L., Frank, E., and Kupfer, D.J. (1988). Social zeitgebers and biological rhythms: A unified approach to understanding the etiology of depression. *Arch Gen Psychiatry*, 45, 948–952.

Endler, A.T., and Gabi, F. (1982). The role of drug level determination in therapy control [in German]. *Med Lab (Stuttg)*, 35(5), 133–136.

English, O.S. (1949). Observations of trends in manic-depressive psychosis. *Psychiatry*, 12, 125–133.

Fallon, I.R.H., Boyd, J.L., and McGill, C.W. (1984). *Family Care of Schizophrenia*. New York: The Guilford Press.

Frank, E., Kupfer, D.J., Ehlers, C.L., Monk, T.H., and Cornes, C. (1994). Interpersonal and social rhythm therapy for bipolar disorder: Integrating interpersonal and behavior approaches. *The Behavior Therapist*, 17, 143–149.

Frank, E., Kupfer, D.J., and Siegel, L.R. (1995). Alliance not adherence: A philosophy of outpatient care. *J Clin Psychiatry*, 56(Suppl.), 11–16.

Frank, E., Swartz, H.A., Mallinger, A.G., Thase, M.E., Weaver, E.V., and Kupfer, D.J. (1999). Adjunctive psychotherapy for bipolar disorder: Effects of changing treatment modality. *J Abnorm Psychol*, 108, 579–587.

Frank, E., Swartz, H.A., and Kupfer, D.J. (2000). Interpersonal and social rhythm therapy: Managing the chaos of bipolar disorder. *Biol Psychiatry*, 48, 593–604.

Frank, E., Kupfer, D.J., Thase, M.E., Mallinger, A.G., Swartz, H.A., Faglioni, A.M., Grochocinski, V., Houck, P., Scott, J.,

Thompson, W., and Monk, T. (2005). Two-year outcomes for interpersonal and social rhythm therapy in individuals with bipolar IV. *Arch Gen Psychiatry*, 62, 996–1004.

Frank, J.D. (1961). *Persuasion and Healing*. New York: Oxford University Press.

Fristad, M.A., Teare, M., Weller, E.B., Weller, R.A., and Salmon, P. (1998). Study III: Development and concurrent validity of the Children's Interview for Psychiatric Syndromes–parent version (P-ChIPS). *J Child Adolesc Psychopharmacol*, 8(4), 221–226.

Fristad, M.A., Goldberg-Arnold, J.S., and Gavazzi, S.M. (2002). Multifamily psychoeducation groups (MFPG) for families of children with bipolar disorder. *Bipolar Disord*, 4(4), 254–262.

Fromm-Reichman, F. (1949). Intensive psychotherapy of manic-depressives: A preliminary report. *Confina Neurologica*, 9, 158–165.

Ghaemi, S.N., Stoll, A.L., and Pope H.R. (1995). Lack of insight in bipolar disorder. The acute manic episode. *J Nerv Ment Dis*, 183(7), 464–467.

Gitlin, M.J., Cochran, S.D., and Jamison, K.R. (1989). Maintenance lithium treatment: Side effects and compliance. *J Clin Psychiatry*, 50(4), 127–131.

Goldberg, J.F., and Harrow, M. (1999). Poor-outcome bipolar disorders. In J.F. Goldberg and M. Harrow (Eds.), *Bipolar Disorders: Clinical Course and Outcome* (pp. 1–19). Washington, DC: American Psychiatric Press.

Goldberg, J.F., Harrow, M., and Grossman, L.S. (1995). Course and outcome in bipolar affective disorder: A longitudinal follow-up study. *Am J Psychiatry*, 152, 379–384.

Goodale, L.C., and Lewis, L. (1999). The effects of support group participation on treatment adherence. In J.C. Soares, S. Gershon (Eds.), Bipolar Disorders. Poster presented at the Third International Conference on Bipolar Disorder, Pittsburgh, PA, June 17–19. *Int J Psychiatry Neurosci*, 1(Suppl. 1), 32.

Goodwin, G. (2002). Hypomania: What's in a name? *Br J Psychiatry*, 181, 94–95.

Graves, A. (1942). *The Eclipse of a Mind*. New York: The Medical Journal Press.

Greene, J. (2001). Benchmarking. Guidelines on kids. *Hosp Health Netw*, 75(7), 26, 28.

Greenson, R.R. (1967). *The Technique and Practice of Psychoanalysis*. New York: International Universities Press.

Haas, G.L., Glick, I.D., Clarkin, J.F., Spencer, J.H., Lewis, A.B., Peyser, J., DeMane, N., Good-Ellis, M., Harris, E., and Lestelle, V. (1988). Inpatient family intervention: A randomized clinical trial: II: Results at hospital discharge. *Arch Gen Psychiatry*, 45, 217–224.

Hamilton, I. (1982). *Robert Lowell: A Biography*. New York: Random House.

Hibbs, E.D., Clarke, G., Hechtman, L., Abikoff, H.B., Greenhill, L.L., and Jensen, P.S. (1997). Manual development for the treatment of child and adolescent disorders. *Psychopharmacol Bull*, 33, 619–629.

Highet, N., Thompson, M., and McNair, B. (2005). Identifying depression in a family member: The carers' experience. *J Affect Disord*, 87, 25–33.

Hirschfeld-Becker, D.R., Gould, R.A., Reilly-Harrington, N., Morabito, C., Cosgrove, V., Guille, C., Fredman, S., and Sachs, G. (1998). *Short-Term Adjunctive Cognitive-Behavioral Group Therapy for Bipolar Disorder: Preliminary Results from a Controlled Trial*. Poster presented at the 32nd Annual Convention of the Association for the Advancement of Behavior Therapy, Washington, DC, November 5–8.

Hollon, S.D., Kendall, P.C., and Lamry, A. (1986). Specificity of depressogenic cognitions in clinical depression. *J Abnorm Psychol*, 95, 52–59.

Honig, A., Hofman, A., Rozendaal, N., and Dingemans, P. (1997). Psycho-education in bipolar disorder: Effect on expressed emotion. *Psychiatry Res*, 72(1), 17–22.

Jackson, A., Cavanagh, J., and Scott, J. (2003). A systematic review of manic and depressive prodromes. *J Affect Disord*, 74, 209–217.

Jamison, K.R. (1991). Manic-depressive illness: The overlooked need for psychotherapy. In B.D. Beitman and G. Klerman (Eds.), *Integrating Pharmacotherapy and Psychotherapy* (pp. 409–420). Washington, DC: American Psychiatric Press.

Jamison, K.R. (1995). *An Unquiet Mind: A Memoir of Moods and Madness*. New York: Alfred A. Knopf.

Jamison, K.R. (2004). *Exuberance: The Passion for Life*. New York: Alfred A. Knopf.

Jamison, K.R. (2006). The many stigmas of mental illness. *Lancet*, 367(9520), 1396–1397.

Jamison, K.R., and Goodwin, F.K. (1983). Psychotherapeutic treatment of manic-depressive patients on lithium. In M. Greenhill and A. Gralnick (Eds.), *The Interrelationship of Psychopharmacology and Psychotherapy* (pp. 53–74). New York: Macmillan.

Jamison, K.R., Gerner, R.H., and Goodwin, F.K. (1979). Patient and physician attitudes toward lithium: Relationship to adherence. *Arch Gen Psychiatry*, 36, 866–869.

Jamison, K.R., Gerner, R.H., Hammen, C., and Padesky, C. (1980). Clouds and silver linings: Positive experiences associated with primary affective disorders. *Am J Psychiatry*, 137, 198–202.

Janowsky, D.S., Leff, M., and Epstein, R.S. (1970). Playing the manic game: Interpersonal maneuvers of the acutely manic patient. *Arch Gen Psychiatry*, 22, 252–261.

Jones, I., Scourfield, J., McCandless, F., and Craddock, N. (2002). Attitudes towards future testing for bipolar disorder susceptibility genes: A preliminary investigation. *J Affect Disord*, 71, 189–193.

Jones, L., Scott, J., Hague, S., Gordon-Smith, K., Heron, J., Caesar, S., Cooper, C., Forty, L., Hyde, S., Lyon, L., Greening, J., Sham, P., Farmer, A., McGuffin, P., Jones, I., and Craddock, N. (2005). Cognitive style in bipolar disorder. *Br J Psychiatry*, 187, 431–437.

Joshi, K.G. (2003). Psychiatric advance directives. *J Psychiatr Prac*, 9, 303–306.

Keck, P.E. Jr., McElroy, S.L., Strakowski, S.M., Bourne, M.L., and West, S.A. (1997). Adherence with maintenance treatment in bipolar disorder. *Psychopharmacol Bull*, 33, 87–91.

Keck, P.E. Jr., McElroy, S.L., and Strakowski, S.M. (1998). Anticonvulsants and antipsychotics in the treatment of bipolar disorder. *J Clin Psychiatry*, 59(Suppl. 6), 74–81.

Kim, E.Y., and Miklowitz, D.J. (2004). Expressed emotion as a predictor of outcome among bipolar patients undergoing family therapy. *J Affect Disord*, 82, 343–352.

Klerman, G.L., Weissman, M.M., Rounsaville, B.J., and Chevron, E.S. (1984). *Interpersonal Psychotherapy of Depression*. New York: Basic Books.

Kraepelin, E. (1904). *Lectures on Clinical Psychiatry*. London: Ballière, Tindall & Cox.

Lam, D.H. (2006). What can we conclude from studies on psychotherapy in bipolar disorder? Invited commentary on . . . Cognitive-behavioral therapy for severe and recurrent bipolar disorders. *Br J Psychiatry*, 188, 321–322.

Lam, D.H., and Wong, G. (1997). Prodromes, coping strategies, insight and social functioning in bipolar affective disorder. *Psychol Med*, 27, 1091–1100.

Lam, D.H., Bright, J., Jones, S., Hayward, P., Schuck, N., Chisholm, D., and Sham, P. (2000). Cognitive therapy of bipolar illness: A pilot study. *Cogn Ther Res*, 24, 503–520.

Lam, D.H., Watkins, E.R., Hayward, P., Bright, J., Wright, K., Kerr, N., Parr-Davis, G., and Sham P. (2003). A randomized controlled study of cognitive therapy for relapse prevention for bipolar affective disorder: Outcome of the first year. *Arch Gen Psychiatry*, 60(2), 145–152.

Lam, D.H., McCrone, P., Wright, K., and Kerr, N. (2005a). Cost-effectiveness of relapse-prevention cognitive therapy for bipolar disorder: 30-month study. *Br J Psychiatry*, 186, 500–506.

Lam, D.H., Hayward, P., Watkins, E.R., Wright, K., and Sham, P. (2005b). Relapse prevention in patients with bipolar disorder: Cognitive therapy outcome after 2 years. *Am J Psychiatry*, 162, 324–329.

Leverich, G.S., and Post, R.M. (1993). *The NIMH Life Chart Manual for Recurrent Affective Illness: The LCM*. Bethesda, MD: Monograph.

Lish, J.D., Dime-Meenan, S., Whybrow, P.C., Price, R.A., and Hirschfeld, R.M.A. (1994). The National Depressive and Manic-depressive Association (DMDA) survey of bipolar members. *J Affect Disord*, 31, 281–294.

Logan, J. (1976). *Josh: My Up and Down, In and Out Life*. New York: Delacorte Press.

Lowell, R. (1959). Home after three months away. In *Life Studies*. New York: Farrar, Strauss, and Cudahy.

Lowell, R. (1977). Since 1939. In *Day by Day*. New York: Farrar, Straus & Giroux.

Marlatt, G.A., and Gordon, J.R. (1985). *Relapse Prevention*. New York: The Guilford Press.

McAlpin, R.N., Goodnick, P.J. (1998). Psychotherapy, in mania: Clinical and research perspectives (pp. 363–381). P.J. Goodnick (Ed.). Washington, DC: American Psychiatric Press.

Miklowitz, D.J., and Goldstein, M.J. (1990). Behavioral family treatment for patients with bipolar affective disorder. *Behav Modif*, 14, 457–489.

Miklowitz, D.J., and Goldstein, M.J. (1997). *Bipolar Disorder: A Family Focused Treatment Approach*. New York: The Guilford Press.

Miklowitz, D.J., Frank, E., and George, E.L. (1996). New psychosocial treatments for the outpatient management of bipolar disorder. *Psychopharm Bull*, 32, 613–621.

Miklowitz, D.J., Simoneau, T.L., George, E.L., Richards, J.A., Kalbag, A., Sachs-Ericsson, N., and Suddath, R. (2000). Family-focused treatment of bipolar disorder: One-year effects of a psychoeducational program in conjunction with pharmacotherapy. *Biol Psychiatry*, 48, 582–592.

Miklowitz, D.J., George, E.L., Axelson, D.A., Kim, E.Y., Birmaher, B., Schneck, C., Beresford, C., Craighead, W.E., and Brent, D.A. (2004). Family-focused treatment for adolescents with bipolar disorder. *J Affect Disord*, 825, S113–S128.

Miklowitz, D.J., Wisniewski, S.R., Miyahara, S., Otto, M.W., and Sachs, G.S. (2005). Perceived criticism from family members as a predictor of the one-year course of bipolar disorder. *Psychiatry Res*, 136, 101–111.

Miklowitz, D.J., Otto, M.W., Wisniewski, S.R., Araga, M., Frank, E., Reilly-Harrington, N.A., Lembke, A., and Sachs, G.S. (2006). Psychotherapy, symptom outcomes, and role functioning over one year among patients with bipolar disorder. *Psychiatr Serv*, 57, 959–969.

Miller, I.W., Keitner, G.I., Bishop, D.S., and Ryan, C.I. (1991). *Families of Bipolar Patients: Dysfunction, Course of Illness, and Pilot Treatment Study*. Presented at the annual meeting of the Association for Advancement of Behavior Therapy, New York.

Miller, I.W., Solomon, D.A., Ryan, C.E., and Keitner, G.I. (2004). Does adjunctive family therapy enhance recovery from bipolar I mood episodes? *J Affect Disord*, 82(3), 431–436.

Molnar, G., Feeney, M.G., and Fava, G.A. (1988). Duration and symptoms of bipolar prodromes. *Am J Psychiatry*, 145, 1576–1578.

Monk, T.H., Kupfer, D.J., Frank, E., and Ritenour, A.M. (1991). The Social Rhythm Metric (SRM): Measuring daily social rhythms over 12 weeks. *Psychiatry Res*, 36, 195–207.

Pallanti, S., Quercioli, L., Pazzagli, A., Rossi, A., Dell'Osso, L., Pini, S., and Cassano, G.B. (1999). Awareness of illness and subjective experience of cognitive complaints in patients with bipolar I and bipolar II disorder. *Am J Psychiatry*, 156(7), 1094–1096.

Pavuluri, M.N., Naylor, M., and Janicak, P. (2002). Recognition and treatment of pediatric bipolar disorder. *Contemp Psychiatry*, 1, 1–10.

Pavuluri, M.N., Graczyk, P.A., Henry, D.B., Carbray, J.A., Heidenreich, J., and Miklowitz, D.J. (2004). Child- and family-focused cognitive-behavioral therapy for pediatric bipolar disorder: Development and preliminary results. *J Am Acad Child Adolesc Psychiatry*, 43, 528–537.

Peet, M., and Harvey, N.S. (1991). Lithium maintenance: 1. A standard education programme for patients. *Br J Psychiatry*, 158, 197–200.

Peralta, V., and Cuesta, M.J. (1998). Lack of insight in mood disorders. *J Affect Disord*, 49(1), 55–58.

Perlick, D.A., Rosenheck, R.A., Clarkin, J.F., Maciejewski, P.K., Sirey, J., Struening, E., and Link, B.G. (2004). Impact of family burden and affective response on clinical outcome among patients with bipolar disorder. *Psychiatr Serv*, 55(9), 1029–1035.

Perry, A., Tarrier, N., Morriss, R., McCarthy, E., and Limb, K. (1999). Randomised controlled trial of efficacy of teaching patients with bipolar disorder to identify early symptoms of relapse and obtain treatment. *BMJ*, 318, 149–153.

Pini, S., Cassano, G.B., Dell'Osso, L., and Amador, X.F. (2001). Insight into illness in schizophrenia, schizoaffective disorder, and mood disorders with psychotic features. *Am J Psychiatry*, 158(1), 122–125.

Post, R.M., Rubinow, D.R., and Ballenger, J.C. (1986). Conditioning and sensitization in the longitudinal course of affective illness. *Br J Psychiatry*, 149, 191–201.

Prien, R.F., and Potter, W.Z. (1990). *Report from the NIMH Workshop on the Treatment of Bipolar Disorder*. Rockville, MD: NIMH Division of Clinical Research.

Rado, S. (1928). The problem of melancholia. *Int J Psychoanal*, 9, 420–438.

Rea, M., Tompson, M., Miklowitz, D., Goldstein, M., Hwang, S., and Mintz, J. (2003). Family-focused treatment versus individual treatment for bipolar disorder: Results of a randomized clinical trial. *J Consult Clin Psychol*, 71, 482–492.

Reiss, E. (1910). *Konstitutionelle Verstimmung und manisch-depressives Irresein: Klinische Untersuchungen über den Zusammenhang von Veranlagung und Psychose.* Berlin: J. Springer.

Rosenfeld, H. (1963). Notes on the psychopathology and psychoanalytic treatment of depressive and manic depressive patients. In H. Azima and B.C. Glueck (Eds.), *Psychiatric Research Report 17* (pp. 73–83). Washington, DC: American Psychiatric Association.

Roy, C.K., and Williams, P. (2005). Barriers to the effective management of bipolar disorder: A survey of psychiatrists based on the UK and USA. *Bipolar Disord*, 7(Suppl. 1), 38–42.

Schou, M. (1980). Social and psychological implications of lithium therapy. In F.N. Johnson (Ed.), *Handbook of Lithium Therapy* (pp. 378–381). Baltimore: University Park Press.

Schou, M., and Baastrup, P.C. (1973). Personal and social implications of lithium maintenance treatment. In T.A. Ban, J.R. Boissier, G.J. Gessa, H. Heimann, L. Hollister, H.E. Lehmann, I. Munkvad, H. Steinberg, F. Sulser, A. Sundwall, and O. Vinar (Eds.), *Psychopharmacology, Sexual Disorders and Drug Abuse.* Amsterdam and London: North-Holland Publishing Company.

Scott, J. (1996). Cognitive therapy of affective disorders: A review. *J Affect Disord*, 37, 1–11.

Scott, J., and Gutierrez, M.J. (2004). The current status of psychological treatments in bipolar disorders: A systematic review of relapse prevention. *Bipolar Disord*, 6, 498–503.

Scott, J., and Pope, M. (2003). Cognitive styles in individuals with bipolar disorders. *Psychol Med*, 33, 1082–1088.

Scott, J., Stanton, B., Garland A., and Ferrier, I.N. (2000). Cognitive vulnerability in patients with bipolar disorder. *Psychol Med*, 30, 467–472.

Scott, J., Garland, A., and Moorhead, S. (2001). A pilot study of cognitive therapy in bipolar disorder. *Psychol Med*, 31(3), 459–467.

Simon, G.E., Ludman, E.J., Unützer, J., Bauer, M.S., Operskalski, B., and Rutter, C. (2005). Randomized trial of a population-based care program for people with bipolar disorder. *Psychol Med*, 35, 13–24.

Slavney, P.R. (2005). *Psychotherapy: An Introduction for Psychiatry Residents and Other Mental Health Trainees.* Baltimore: Johns Hopkins University Press.

Smith, J.A., and Tarrier, N. (1992). Prodromal symptoms in manic depressive psychosis. *Soc Psychiatry Psychiatr Epidemiol*, 27, 245–248.

Smith, L.B., Sapers, B., Reus, V.I., and Freimer, N.B. (1996). Attitudes towards bipolar disorder and predictive genetic testing among patients and providers. *J Med Genet*, 33, 544–559.

Squillace, K., Post, R.M., Savard, R., and Erwin-Gorman, M. (1984). Life charting of the longitudinal course of recurrent affective illness. In: R.M. Post, J.C. Ballenger (Eds.), *Neurobiology of Mood Disorders* (pp. 38–59). Baltimore: Williams & Wilkins.

Srebnik, D.S., Rutherford, L.T., Peto, T., Russo, J., Zick, E., Jaffe, C., and Holtzheimer, P. (2005). The content and clinical utility of psychiatric advance directives. *Psychiatr Serv*, 56, 592–598.

Suppes, T., Swann, A.C., Dennehy, E.B., Habermacher, E.D., Mason, M., Crismon, M.L., Toprac, M.G., Rush, A.J., Shon, S.P., and Altshuler, K.Z, (2001). Texas Medication Algorithm Project: Development and feasability testing of a treatment algorithm for patients with bipolar disorder. *J Clin Psychiatry*, 62, 439–447.

Suppes, T., Dennehy, E.B., Swann, A.C., Bowden, C.L., Calabrese, J.R., Hirschfeld, R.M., Keck, P.E., Sachs, G.S., Crismon, M.L., Toprac, M.G., Shon, S.P., Texas Consensus Conference Panel on Medication Treatment of Bipolar Disorder. (2002). Report of the Texas Consensus Conference Panel on medication treatment of bipolar disorder 2000. *J Clin Psychiatry*, 63(4), 288–299.

Swanson, J.W., Swartz, M.S., Elbogen, E.G., Van Dorn, R.A., Ferron, J., Wagner, H.R., McCauley, B.J., and Kim, M. (2006). Facilitated psychiatric advance directives: A randomized trial of an intervention to foster advance treatment planning among persons with severe mental illness. *Am J Psychiatry*, 163, 1943–1951.

Szmukler, G.I., and Bloch, S. (1997). Family involvement in the care of people with psychoses: An ethical argument. *Br J Psychiatry*, 171, 401–405.

Toprac, M.G., Hopkins, C., Conner, T., Rush, A.J., Crismon, M.L., Dees, M., Rowe, V., and Shon, S.P. (1998). *Texas Medication Algorithm Project (TMAP) Patient Education Plan Guidebook.* Austin, TX: Texas Department of Mental Health and Mental Retardation (TDMHMR).

Toprac, M.G., Rush, J.A., Conner, T.M., Crismon, M.L., Dees, M., Hopkins, C., Rowe, V., and Shon, S.P. (2000). The Texas Medication Algorithm Project Patient and Family Education Program: A consumer-guided initiative. *J Clin Psychiatry*, 61, 477–486.

Trippitelli, C.L., Jamison, K.R., Folstein, M.F., Bartko, J.J., and DePaulo, J.R. (1998). Pilot study on patients' and spouses' attitudes toward potential genetic testing for bipolar disorder. *Am J Psychiatry*, 155, 899–904.

van Gent, E.M., and Zwart, F.M. (1991). Psychoeducation of partners of bipolar-manic patients. *J Affect Disord*, 21(1), 15–18.

Varga, M., Magnusson, A., Flekkøy, K., Rønnerg, U., and Opjordsmoen, S. (2006). Insight, symptoms and neurocognition in bipolar I patients. *J Affect Disord*, 91, 1–9.

Vasile, R.G., Samson, J.A., Bemporad, J., Bloomingdale, K.L., Creasey, D., Fenton, B.T., Gudeman, J.E., and Schildkraut, J.J. (1987). A biopsychosocial approach to treating patients with affective disorders. *Am J Psychiatry*, 144, 341–344.

Verdeli, H. (2004, October). *Modifying IPT for Prevention for Symptomatic Offspring of Bipolar Parents.* Presented at the Symposium, "New Developments in IPT with Adolescents" (L. Mufson Chair). Washington, DC: American Academy of Child and Adolescent Psychiatry.

Wehr, T.A., and Goodwin, F.K. (1987). Can antidepressants cause mania and worsen the course of affective illness? *Am J Psychiatry*, 144, 1403–1411.

Wehr, T.A., Sach, D.A., and Rosenthal, N.E. (1987a). Sleep reduction as a final common pathway in the genesis of mania. *Am J Psychiatry*, 144, 201–204.

Wehr, T.A., Sach, D.A., and Rosenthal, N.E. (1987b). Seasonal affective disorder with summer depression and winter hypomania. *Am J Psychiatry*, 144, 1602–1603.

Weiss, R.D., Griffin, M.L., Greenfield, S.F., Najavits, L.M., Wyner, D., Soto, J.A., and Hennen, J.A. (2000). Group therapy for patients with bipolar disorder and substance dependence: Results of a pilot study. *J Clin Psychiatry*, 61, 361–365.

Weissman, M.M., Markowitz, J.C., and Klerman, G.L. (2000). *Comprehensive Guide to Interpersonal Psychotherapy.* New York: Basic Books.

Wilson, S. (1976). *What Shall We Wear to This Party? The Man in the Gray Flannel Suit: Twenty Years Before and After.* New York: Arbor House.

Wodehouse, P.G. (1975). *The Code of the Woosters.* New York: Random House.

Yen, C.F., Chen, C.S., Yeh, M.L., Yang, S.J., Ke, J.H., and Yen, J.Y. (2003). Changes of insight in manic episodes and influencing factors. *Compr Psychiatry,* 44(5), 404–408.

Zaretsky, A.E., Zindel, V.S., and Gemar, M. (1999). Cognitive therapy for bipolar depression: A pilot study. *Can J Psychiatry,* 44, 491–494.

Chapter 23

Akiskal, H.S., Downs, J., Jordan, P., Watson, S., Daugherty, D., and Pruitt, D.B. (1985). Affective disorders in referred children and younger siblings of manic depressives. *Arch Gen Psychiatry,* 42, 996–1004.

Allison, D.B., Mentore, J.L., Heo, M., Chandler, L.P., Cappelleri, J.C., Infante, M.C., and Weiden, P.J. (1999). Antipsychotic-induced weight gain: A comprehensive research synthesis. *Am J Psychiatry,* 156(11), 1686–1696.

Altshuler, L., Suppes, T., Black, D., Nolen, W.A., Keck, P.E. Jr., Frye, M.A., McElroy, S., Kupka, R., Grunze, H., Walden, J., Leverich, G., Denicoff, K., Luckenbaugh, D., and Post, R. (2003). Impact of antidepressant discontinuation after acute bipolar depression remission on rates of depressive relapse at 1-year follow-up. *Am J Psychiatry,* 160(7), 1252–1262.

Aman, M.G., Singh, N.N., Stewart, A.W., and Field, C.J. (1985). The aberrant behavior checklist: A behavior rating scale for the assessment of treatment effects. *Am J Ment Defic,* 89(5), 485–491.

Aman, M.G., Tasse, M.J., Rojahn, J., and Hammer, D. (1996). The Nisonger CBRF: A child behavior rating form for children with developmental disabilities. *Res Dev Disabil,* 17(1), 41–57.

Aman, M.G., De Smedt, G., Derivan, A., Lyons, B., Findling, R.L., and Risperidone Disruptive Behavior Study Group. (2002). Double-blind, placebo-controlled study of risperidone for the treatment of disruptive behaviors in children with subaverage intelligence. *Am J Psychiatry,* 159(8), 1337–1346.

American Diabetes Association. (2004). Consensus Development Conference on Antipsychotic Drugs and Obesity and Diabetes. http://www.diabetes.org/for=media/2004=press=releases/jan=27-04.jsp.

Annell, A.L. (1969). Lithium in the treatment of children and adolescents. *Acta Psychiatr Scand Suppl,* 207, 19.

Anthony, E.J., and Scott, P. (1960). Manic-depressive psychosis in childhood. *J Child Psychol Psychiatry,* 1, 53–72.

Baldessarini, R.J., Tondo, L., and Viguera, A.C. (1999). Discontinuing lithium maintenance treatment in bipolar disorders: Risks and implications. *Bipolar Disord,* 1(1), 17–24.

Barnett, M.S. (2004). Ziprasidone monotherapy in pediatric bipolar disorder. *J Child Adolesc Psychopharmacol,* 14(3), 471–477.

Barzman, D.H., DelBello, M.P., Kowatch, R.A., Gernert, B., Fleck, D.E., Pathak, S., Rappaport, K., Delgado, S.V., Campbell, P., and Strakowski, S.M. (2004). The effectiveness and tolerability of aripiprazole for pediatric bipolar disorders: A retrospective chart review. *J Child Adolesc Psychopharmacol,* 14(4), 593–600.

Barzman, D.H., Adler, C.M., DelBello, M.P., Stanford, K.E., Kowatch, R.A., and Strakowski, S.M. (2006). Quetiapine efficacy in bipolar adolescents with depressive symptoms. *New Research Abstract,* May 22, 2006. American Psychiatric Association.

Baumer, F.M., Howe, M., Gallelli, K., Simeonova, D.I., Hallmayer, J., and Chang, K.D. (2006). A pilot study of antidepressant-induced mania in pediatric bipolar disorder: Characteristics, risk factors, and the serotonin transporter gene. *Biol Psychiatry,* 60(9), 1005–1012.

Biederman, J., Wozniak, J., Kiely, K., Ablon, S., Faraone, S., Mick, E., Mundy, E., and Kraus, I. (1995). CBCL Clinical Scales discriminate prepubertal children with structured-interview-derived diagnosis of mania from those with ADHD. *J Am Acad Child Adolesc Psychiatry,* 34, 133–140.

Biederman, J., Faraone, S., Mick, E., Wozniak, J., Chen, L., Ouellette, C., Marrs, A., Moore, P., Garcia, J., Mennin, D., and Lelon, E. (1996). Attention-deficit hyperactivity disorder and juvenile mania: An overlooked comorbidity? *J Am Acad Child Adolesc Psychiatry,* 35(8), 997–1008.

Biederman, J., Klein, R.G., Pine, D.S., and Klein, D.F. (1998). Resolved: Mania is mistaken for ADHD in prepubertal children. *J Am Acad Child Adolesc Psychiatry,* 37(10), 1091–1096; discussion 1096–1099.

Biederman, J., Mick, E., Spencer, T.J., Wilens, T.E., and Faraone, S.V. (2000a). Therapeutic dilemmas in the pharmacotherapy of bipolar depression in the young. *J Child Adolesc Psychopharmacol,* 10(3), 185–192.

Biederman, J., Faraone, S.V., Wozniak, J., and Monuteaux, M.C. (2000b). Parsing the associations between bipolar, conduct, and substance use disorders: A familial risk analysis. *Biol Psychiatry,* 48, 1037–1044.

Biederman, J., Mick, E., Wozniak, J., Aleardi, M., Spencer, T., and Faraone, S.V. (2005a). An open-label trial of risperidone in children and adolescents with bipolar disorder. *J Child Adolesc Psychopharmacol,* 15(2), 311–317.

Biederman, J., McDonnell, M.A., Wozniak, J., Spencer, T., Aleardi, M., Falzone, R., Mick, E. (2005b). Aripiprazole in the treatment of pediatric bipolar disorder: A systematic chart review. *CNS Spectr,* 10(2), 141–148.

Buitelaar, J.K., van der Gaag, R.J., Cohen-Kettenis, P., and Melman, C.T. (2001). A randomized controlled trial of risperidone in the treatment of aggression in hospitalized adolescents with subaverage cognitive abilities. *J Clin Psychiatry,* 62(4), 239–248.

Calabrese, J.R., Shelton, M.D., Rapport, D.J., Youngstrom, E.A., Jackson, K., Bilali, S., Ganocy. S.J., and Findling, R.L. (2005). A 20-month, double-blind, maintenance trial of lithium versus divalproex in rapid-cycling bipolar disorder. *Am J Psychiatry,* 162(11), 2152–2161.

Campbell, M., Fish, B., Korein, J., Shapiro, T., Collins, P., and Koh, C. (1972). Lithium and chlorpromazine: A controlled crossover study of hyperactive severely disturbed young children. *J Autism Child Schizophr,* 2(3), 234–263.

Campbell, M., Small, A.M., Green, W.H., Jennings, S.J., Perry, R., Bennett, W.G., and Anderson, L. (1984). Behavioral efficacy of haloperidol and lithium carbonate: A comparison in hospitalized aggressive children with conduct disorder. *Arch Gen Psychiatry,* 41(7), 650–656.

Campbell, M., Adams, P.B., Small, A.M., Kafantaris, V., Silva, R.R., Shell, J., Perry, R., and Overall, J.E. (1995). Lithium in hospitalized aggressive children with conduct disorder: A double-blind and placebo-controlled study. *J Am Acad Child Adolesc Psychiatry,* 34(4), 445–453.

Carandang, C.G., Maxwell, D.J., Robbins, D.R., and Oesterheld, J.R. (2003). Lamotrigine in adolescent mood disorders. *J Am Acad Child Adolesc Psychiatry*, 42(7), 750–751.

Carlson, G.A. (2005a). Early onset bipolar disorder: Clinical and research considerations. *J Clin Child Adolesc Psychol*, 34(2), 333–343.

Carlson, G.A. (2005b). Medication-induced activation in children and adolescents. *Psychiatr Times*, Vol. XXII, issue 10.

Carlson, G.A., and Kelly, K.L. (1998). Manic symptoms in psychiatrically hospitalized children: What do they mean? *J Affect Disord*, 51(2), 123–135.

Carlson, G.A., and Kelly, K.L. (2003). Stimulant rebound: How common is it and what does it mean? *J Child Adolesc Psychopharmacol*, 13(2), 137–142.

Carlson, G.A., and Meyer, S.E. (2006). Phenomenology and diagnosis of bipolar disorder in children, adolescents, and adults: Complexities and developmental issues. *Dev Psychopathol*, 18, 939–969.

Carlson, G.A., and Mick, E. (2003). Drug-induced disinhibition in psychiatrically hospitalized children. *J Child Adolesc Psychopharmacol*, 13, 153–164.

Carlson, G.A., and Strober, M. (1978). Affective disorder in adolescence: Issues in misdiagnosis. *J Clin Psychiatry*, 39, 59–66.

Carlson, G.A., Rapport, M.D., Pataki, C., and Kelly, K.K. (1992a). Lithium in hospitalized children at 4 and 8 weeks: Mood, behavior and cognitive effects. *J Child Psychol Psychiatry*, 33, 411–425.

Carlson, G.A., Rapport, M.D., Pataki, C., and Kelly, K.K. (1992b). The effects of methylphenidate and lithium on attention and activity level. *Am Acad Child Adolesc Psychiatry*, 31, 262–270.

Carlson, G.A., Loney, J., Salisbury, H., and Volpe, R.J. (1998). Young referred boys with DICA-P manic symptoms versus two comparison groups. *J Affect Disord*, 51, 113–121.

Carlson, G.A., Bromet, E.J., and Lavelle, J. (1999). Medication treatment in adolescents versus adults with psychotic mania. *J Child Adolesc Psychopharmacol*, 9, 221–231.

Carlson, G.A., Loney, J., Salisbury, H., Kramer, J.R., and Arthur, C. (2000). Stimulant treatment in young boys with symptoms suggesting childhood mania: A report from a longitudinal study. *J Child Adolesc Psychopharmacol*, 10, 175–184.

Carlson, G.A., Bromet, E.J., Driessens, C., Mojtabai, R., and Schwartz, J.E. (2002). Age at onset, childhood psychopathology, and 2-year outcome in psychotic bipolar disorder. *Am J Psychiatry*, 159, 307–309.

Carlson, G.A., Jensen, P.S., Findling, R.L., Meyer, R.E., Calabrese, J., DelBello, M.P., Emslie, G., Flynn, L., Goodwin, F., Hellander, M., Kowatch, R., Kusumakar, B., Laughren, T., Leibenluft, E., McCracken, J., Nottelmann, E., Pine, D., Sachs, G., Shaffer, D., Simar, R., Strober, M., Weller, E.B., Wozniak, J., and Youngstrom, E.A. (2003). Methodological issues and controversies in clinical trials with child and adolescent patients with bipolar disorder: Report of a consensus conference. *J Child Adolesc Psychopharmacol*, 13(1), 13–27.

Carlson, G.A., Finch, S., Kang, S., Ye, Q., and Bromet, E. (in press). Conversion from depression to mania in 1st admission patients with psychotic bipolar disorder. *J Affect Disord*.

Casey, D.E. (2004). Dyslipidemia and atypical antipsychotic drugs. *J Clin Psychiatry*, 65(Suppl. 18), 27–35.

Chang, K.D., and Ketter, T.A. (2000). Mood stabilizer augmentation with olanzapine in acutely manic children. *J Child Adolesc Psychopharmacol*, 10(1), 45–49.

Chang, K.D., Dienes, K., Blasey, C., Adleman, N., Ketter, T., and Steiner, H. (2003). Divalproex monotherapy in the treatment of bipolar offspring with mood and behavioral disorders and at least mild affective symptoms. *J Clin Psychiatry*, 64(8), 936–942.

Chang, K., Saxena, K., and Howe M. (2006). An open-label study of lamotrigine adjunct or monotherapy for the treatment of adolescents with bipolar depression. *J Am Acad Child Adolesc Psychiatry*, 45(3), 298–304.

Cheung, A.H., Emslie, G.J., and Mayes, T.L. (2005). Review of the efficacy and safety of antidepressants in youth depression. *J Child Psychol Psychiatry*, 46(7), 735–754.

Correll, C.U., and Carlson, H.E.C. (2006). Endocrine and metabolic adverse effects of psychotropic medications in children and adolescents. *J Am Acad Child Adolesc Psychiatry*, 45(7), 771–791.

Correll, C.U., Parikh, U.H., Mughal, T., Olshanskiy, V., Moroff, M., Pleak, R.R., Foley, C., Shah, M., Gutkovich, Z., Kane, J.M., and Malhotra, A.K. (2005). Body composition changes associated with second-generation antipsychotics. *Biol Psychiatry*, 57(Suppl. 8), 36.

Craney, J., and Geller, B. (2003). Clinical implications of antidepressant and stimulant use on switching from depression to mania in children. *J Child Adolesc Psychopharmacol*, 13(2), 201–204.

Craven, C., and Murphy, M. (2000) Carbamazepine treatment of bipolar disorder in an adolescent with cerebral palsy. *J Am Acad Child Adolesc Psychiatry*, 39(6), 680–681.

Davanzo, P.A., Krah, N., Kleiner, J., and McCracken, J. (1999). Nimodipine treatment of an adolescent with ultradian cycling bipolar affective illness. *J Child Adolesc Psychopharmacol*, 9(1), 51–61.

DelBello, M.P., Soutullo, C.A., Hendricks, W., Niemeier, R.T., McElroy, S.L., and Strakowski, S.M. (2001). Prior stimulant treatment in adolescents with bipolar disorder: Association with age at onset. *Bipolar Disord*, 3(2), 53–57.

DelBello, M.P., Schwiers, M.L., Rosenberg, H.L., and Strakowski, S.M. (2002). A double-blind, randomized, placebo-controlled study of quetiapine as adjunctive treatment for adolescent mania. *J Am Acad Child Adolesc Psychiatry*, 41(10), 1216–1223.

DelBello, M.P., Carlson, G.A., Tohen, M., Bromet, E.J., Schwiers, M., and Strakowski, S.M. (2003). Rates and predictors of developing a manic or hypomanic episode 1 to 2 years following a first hospitalization for major depression with psychotic features. *J Child Adolesc Psychopharmacol*, 13, 173–186.

DelBello, M.P., Findling, R.L., Kushner, S., Wang, D., Olson, W.H., Capece, J.A., Fazzio, L., and Rosenthal, N.R. (2005). A pilot controlled trial of topiramate for mania in children and adolescents with bipolar disorder. *J Am Acad Child Adolesc Psychiatry*, 44(6), 539–547.

DelBello, M.P., Kowatch, R.A., Adler, C.M., Stanford, K.E., Welge, J.A., Barzman, D.H., Nelson, E., and Strakowski, S.M. (2006). A double-blind randomized pilot study comparing quetiapine and divalproex for adolescent mania. *J Am Acad Child Adolesc Psychiatry*, 45(3), 305–313.

DeLong, G.R. (1978). Lithium carbonate treatment of select behavior disorders in children suggesting manic depressive illness. *J Pediatr*, 93, 689–694.

DeLong, G.R., and Aldershof, A.L. (1987). Long-term experience with lithium treatment in childhood: Correlation with clinical diagnosis. *Am Acad Child Adolesc Psychiatry*, 26, 389–394.

Deltito, A.J., Levitan, J., Damore, J., Hajal, F., and Zambenedetti, M. (1998). Naturalistic experience with the use of divalproex sodium on an in-patient unit for adolescent psychiatric patients. *Acta Psychiatr Scand*, 97, 236–240.

Donovan, S.J., Stewart, J.W., Nunes, E.V., Quitkin, F.M., Parides, M., Daniel, W., Susser, E., and Klein, D.F. (2000). Divalproex treatment for youth with explosive temper and mood lability: A double-blind, placebo-controlled crossover design. *Am J Psychiatry*, 157(5), 818–820.

Duffy, A., Alda, M., Kutcher, S., Fusee, C., and Grof, P. (1998). Psychiatric symptoms and syndromes among adolescent children of parents with lithium-responsive or lithium-nonresponsive bipolar disorder. *Am J Psychiatry*, 155(3), 431–433.

Dyson, W.L., and Barcai, A. (1970). Treatment of children of lithium-responding parents. *Curr Ther Res Clin Exp*, 12(5), 286–290.

Egeland, J.A., Hostetter, A.M., Pauls, D.L., and Sussex, J.N. (2000). Prodromal symptoms before onset of manic-depressive disorder suggested by first hospital admission histories. *J Am Acad Child Adolesc Psychiatry*, 39(10), 1245–1252.

Egeland, J.A., Shaw, J.A., Endicott, J., Pauls, D.L., Allen, C.R., Hostetter, A.M., and Sussex, J.N. (2003). Prospective study of prodromal features for bipolarity in well Amish children. *J Am Acad Child Adolesc Psychiatry*, 42(7), 786–796.

Endicott, J., and Spitzer, R.L. (1978). A diagnostic interview: The Schedule for Affective Disorders and Schizophrenia. *Arch Gen Psychiatry*, 35(7), 837–844.

Faedda, G.L., Baldessarini, R.J., Glovinsky, I.P., and Austin, N.B. (2004). Treatment-emergent mania in pediatric bipolar disorder: A retrospective case review. *J Affect Disord*, 82(1), 149–158.

Faraone, S.V., Biederman, J., Wozniak, J., Mundy, E., Mennin, D., and O'Donnell, D. (1997). Is comorbidity a marker for juvenile-onset mania? *J Am Acad Child Adolesc Psychiatry*, 36, 1046–1055.

Findling, R.L., and McNamara, N.K. (2004). Atypical antipsychotics in the treatment of children and adolescents: Clinical applications. *J Clin Psychiatry*, 65(Suppl. 6), 30–44.

Findling, R.L., McNamara, N.K., Branicky, L.A., Schluchter, M.D., Lemon, E., and Blumer, J.L. (2000). A double-blind pilot study of risperidone in the treatment of conduct disorder. *J Am Acad Child Adolesc Psychiatry*, 39(4), 509–516.

Findling, R.L., Gracious, B.L., McNamara, N.K., Youngstrom, E.A., Demeter, C.A., Branicky, L.A., and Calabrese, J.R. (2001). Rapid, continuous cycling and psychiatric co-morbidity in pediatric bipolar I disorder. *Bipolar Disord*, 3(4), 202–210.

Findling, R.L., McNamara, N.K., Gracious, B.L., Youngstrom, E.A., Stansbrey, R.J., Reed, M.D., Demeter, C.A., Branicky, L.A., Fisher, K.E., and Calabrese, J.R. (2003). Combination lithium and divalproex sodium in pediatric bipolarity. *J Am Acad Child Adolesc Psychiatry*, 42(8), 895–901.

Findling, R.L., McNamara, N.K., Youngstrom, E.A., Stansbrey, R., Gracious, B.L., Reed, M.D., and Calabrese, J.R. (2005). Double-blind 18-month trial of lithium versus divalproex maintenance treatment in pediatric bipolar disorder. *J Am Acad Child Adolesc Psychiatry*, 44(5), 409–417.

Frazier, J.A., Meyer, M.C., Biederman, J., Wozniak, J., Wilens, T.E., Spencer, T.J., Kim, G.S., and Shapiro, S. (1999). Risperidone treatment for juvenile bipolar disorder: A retrospective chart review. *J Am Acad Child Adolesc Psychiatry*, 38(8), 960–965.

Frazier, J.A., Biederman, J., Tohen, M., Feldman, P.D., Jacobs, T.G., Toma, V., Rater, M.A., Tarazi, R.A., Kim, G.S., Garfield, S.B., Sohma, M., Gonzalez-Heydrich, J., Risser, R.C., and Nowlin, Z.M. (2001). A prospective open-label treatment trial of olanzapine monotherapy in children and adolescents with bipolar disorder. *J Child Adolesc Psychopharmacol*, 11(3), 239–250.

Fristad, M.A., Cummins, J., Verducci, J.S., Teare, M., Weller, E.B., and Weller, R.A. (1998). Study IV: Concurrent validity of the DSM-IV revised Children's Interview for Psychiatric Syndromes (ChIPS). *J Child Adolesc Psychopharmacol*, 8(4), 227–236.

Fristad, M.A., Goldberg-Arnold, J.S., Gavazzi, S.M. (2002). Multifamily psychoeducation groups (MFPG) for families of children with bipolar disorder. *Bipolar Disord*, 4(4), 254–262.

Fristad, M.A., Gavazzi, S.M., and Mackinaw-Koons, B. (2003). Family psychoeducation: An adjunctive intervention for children with bipolar disorder. *Biol Psychiatry*, 53(11), 1000–1008.

Fuchs, D.C. (1994). Clozapine treatment of bipolar disorder in a young adolescent. *J Am Acad Child Adolesc Psychiatry*, 33(9), 1299–1302.

Galanter, C.A., Carlson, G.A., Jensen, P.S., Greenhill, L., Davies, M., Li, W., Chuang, S.Z., Glen Elliott, G.R., Arnold, L.E., March, J.S., Hechtman, L., Pelham, W.E., and Swanson, J.M. (2003). Response to methylphenidate in children with ADHD and manic symptoms in the MTA titration trial. *J Child Adolesc Psychopharmacol*, 13, 123–137.

Geller, B., Cooper, T.B., Sun, K., Zimerman, B., Frazier, J., Williams, M., and Heath, J. (1998a). Double-blind and placebo-controlled study of lithium for adolescent bipolar disorders with secondary substance dependency. *J Am Acad Child Adolesc Psychiatry*, 37(2), 171–178.

Geller, B., Zimerman, B., Williams, M., Bolhofner, K., and Craney, J.L. (2001). Bipolar disorder at prospective follow-up of adults who had prepubertal major depressive disorder. *Am J Psychiatry*, 158(1), 125–127.

Geller, B., Zimerman, B., Williams, M., DelBello, M.P., Frazier, J., and Beringer, L. (2002). Phenomenology of prepubertal and early adolescent bipolar disorder: Examples of elated mood, grandiose behaviors, decreased need for sleep, racing thoughts and hypersexuality. *J Child Adolesc Psychopharmacol*, 12(1), 3–9.

Geller, B., Tillman, R., Craney, J.L., and Bolhofner, K. (2004). Four-year prospective outcome and natural history of mania in children with a prepubertal and early adolescent bipolar disorder phenotype. *Arch Gen Psychiatry*, 61(5), 459–467.

Ghaemi, S.N., Hsu, D.J., Soldani, F., and Goodwin, F.K. (2003). Antidepressants in bipolar disorder: The case for caution. *Bipolar Disord*, 5(6), 421–433.

Ghaziuddin, N., Kutcher, S.P., Knapp, P., and American Academy of Child and Adolescent Psychiatry Work Group on Quality Issues. (2004). Summary of the practice parameter for the use of electroconvulsive therapy with adolescents. *J Am Acad Child Adolesc Psychiatry*, 43(1), 119–122.

Gijsman, H.J., Geddes, J.R., Rendell, J.M., Nolen, W.A., and Goodwin, G.M. (2004). Antidepressants for bipolar depression: A systematic review of randomized, controlled trials. *Am J Psychiatry*, 161(9), 1537–1547.

Glovinsky, I. (2002). A brief history of childhood-onset bipolar disorder through 1980. *Child Adolesc Psychiatr Clin North Am*, 11(3), 443–460.

Gracious, B.L., Findling, R.L., Seman, C., Youngstrom, E.A., Demeter, C.A., and Calabrese, J.R. (2004). Elevated thyrotropin in bipolar youths prescribed both lithium and divalproex sodium. *J Am Acad Child Adolesc Psychiatry*, 43(2), 215–220.

Gram, L.F., and Rafaelsen, O.J. (1972). Lithium treatment of psychotic children and adolescents: A controlled clinical trial. *Acta Psychiatr Scand*, 48(3), 253.

Greene, R.W., and Ablon, J.S. (2005). *Treating Explosive Kids: The Collaborative Problem-Solving Approach*. New York: Guilford Press.

Greene, R.W., Ablon, J.S., and Goring, J.C. (2003). A transactional model of oppositional behavior: Underpinnings of the collaborative problem solving approach. *J Psychosom Res*, 55(1), 67–75.

Greenhill, L.L., Rieder, R.O., Wender, P.H., Buchsbaum, M., and Zhan, T.P. (1973). Lithium carbonate in the treatment of hyperactive children. *Arch Gen Psychiatry*, 28(5), 636.

Harrington, R., and Myatt, T. (2003). Is preadolescent mania the same condition as adult mania? A British perspective. *Biol Psychiatry*, 53, 961–969.

Hazell, P., O'Connell, D., Heathcote, D., and Henry, D. (2002). Tricyclic drugs for depression in children and adolescents. *Cochrane Database Syst Rev*, 2, CD002317.

Hazell, P.L., Carr, V., Lewin, T.J., and Sly, K. (2003). Manic symptoms in young males with ADHD predict functioning but not diagnosis after 6 years. *J Am Acad Child Adolesc Psychiatry*, 42(5), 552–560.

Hill, M.A., Courvoisie, H., Dawkins, K., Nofal, P., and Thomas, B. (1997). ECT for the treatment of intractable mania in two prepubertal male children. *Convuls Ther*, 13(2), 74–82.

Hsu, L.K.G., and Starzynski, J.M. (1986). Mania in adolescence. *J Clin Psychiatry*, 47(12), 596–599.

Humphrey, L.L. (1982). Children's and teachers' perspectives on children's self-control: The development of two rating scales. *J Consult Clin Psychol*, 50(5), 624–633.

Joffe, R.T., MacQueen, G.M., Marriott, M., and Young, L.T. (2005). One-year outcome with antidepressant treatment of bipolar depression. *Acta Psychiatr Scand*, 112(2), 105–109.

Johnson, S.L., Winett, C.A., Meyer, B., Greenhouse, W.J., and Miller, I. (1999). Social support and the course of bipolar disorder. *J Abnorm Psychol*, 108(4), 558–566.

Kafantaris, V., Coletti, D.J., Dicker, R., Padula, G., and Pollack, S. (1998). Are childhood psychiatric histories of bipolar adolescents associated with family history, psychosis, and response to lithium treatment? *J Affect Disord*, 51, 153–164.

Kafantaris, V., Coletti, D.J., Dicker, R., Padula, G., and Kane, J.M. (2001). Adjunctive antipsychotic treatment of adolescents with bipolar psychosis. *J Am Acad Child Adolesc Psychiatry*, 40(12), 1448–1456.

Kafantaris, V., Coletti, D.J., Dicker, R., Padula, G., and Kane, J.M. (2003). Lithium treatment of acute mania in adolescents: A large open trial. *J Am Acad Child Adolesc Psychiatry*, 42(9), 1038–1045.

Kafantaris, V., Coletti, D.J., Dicker, R., Padula, G., Pleak, R.R., and Alvir, J.M. (2004). Lithium treatment of acute mania in adolescents: A placebo-controlled discontinuation study. *J Am Acad Child Adolesc Psychiatry*, 43(8), 984–993.

Kant, R., Chalansani, R., Chengappa, K.N., and Dieringer, M.F. (2004). The off-label use of clozapine in adolescents with bipolar disorder, intermittent explosive disorder, or posttraumatic stress disorder. *J Child Adolesc Psychopharmacol*, 14(1), 57–63.

Kastner, T., and Friedman D.L. (1992). Verapamil and valproic acid treatment of prolonged mania. *J Am Acad Child Adolesc Psychiatry*, 31(2), 271–275.

Kowatch, R.A., Suppes, T., Carmody, T.J., Bucci, J.P., Hume, J.H., Kromelis, M., Emslie, G.J., Weinberg, A., and Rush, A.J. (2000). Effect size of lithium, divalproex sodium, and carbamazepine in children and adolescents with bipolar disorder. *J Am Acad Child Adolesc Psychiatry*, 39(6), 713–720.

Kowatch, R.A., Sethuraman, G., Hume, J.H., Kromelis, M., and Weinberg, W.A. (2003). Combination pharmacotherapy in children and adolescents with bipolar disorder. *Biol Psychiatry*, 53(11), 978–984.

Kowatch, R.A., Fristad, M., Birmaher, B., Wagner, K.D., and Findling, R. (2005). Treatment guidelines for children and adolescents with bipolar disorder. *J Am Acad Child Adolesc Psychiatry*, 44(3), 213–235.

Kusumakar, V., and Yatham, L.N. (1997). An open study of lamotrigine in refractory bipolar depression. *Psychiatry Res*, 72, 145–148.

Lapalme, M., Hodgins, S., and LaRoche, C. (1997). Children of parents with bipolar disorder: A metaanalysis of risk for mental disorders. *Can J Psychiatry*, 42(6), 623–631.

Leibenluft, E., Blair, R.J., Charney, D.S., and Pine, D.S. (2003). Irritability in pediatric mania and other childhood psychopathology. *Ann N Y Acad Sci*, 1008, 201–218.

Lewinsohn, P.M., Klein, D.N., and Seeley, J.R. (2000). Bipolar disorder during adolescence and young adulthood in a community sample. *Bipolar Disord*, 2(3 Pt. 2), 281–293.

Maj, M., Pirozzi, R., Magliano, L., and Bartoli, L. (2002). The prognostic significance of "switching" in patients with bipolar disorder: A 10-year prospective follow-up study. *Am J Psychiatry*, 159(10), 1711–1717. Erratum in *Am J Psychiatry*, 159(12), 2132.

Malone, R.P., Delaney, M.A., Luebbert, J.F., Cater, J., and Campbell, M. (2000). A double-blind placebo-controlled study of lithium in hospitalized aggressive children and adolescents with conduct disorder. *Arch Gen Psychiatry*, 57(7), 649–654.

Mannuzza, S., Klein, R.G., Bessler, A., Malloy, P., and LaPadula, M. (1998). Adult psychiatric status of hyperactive boys grown up. *Am J Psychiatry*, 155(4), 493–498.

Martin, A., Young, C., Leckman, J.F., Mukonoweshuro, C., Rosenheck, R., and Leslie, D. (2004). Age effects on antidepressant-induced manic conversion. *Arch Pediatr Adolesc Med*, 158(8), 773–780.

Masi, G., Mucci, M., and Millepiedi, S. (2002). Clozapine in adolescent inpatients with acute mania. *J Child Adolesc Psychopharmacol*, 12(2), 93–99.

McClellan, J. (2005). Commentary: Treatment guidelines for child and adolescent bipolar disorder. *J Am Acad Child Adolesc Psychiatry*, 44(3), 236–239.

McClellan, J., and Werry, J. (1997). Practice parameters for the assessment and treatment of children and adolescents with bipolar disorder. American Academy of Child and Adolescent Psychiatry. *J Am Acad Child Adolesc Psychiatry*, 36(10 Suppl.), 157S–176S.

McConville, B.J., Arvanitis, L.A., Thyrum, P.T., Yeh, C., Wilkinson, L.A., Chaney, R.O., Foster, K.D., Sorter, M.T., Friedman, L.M., Brown, K.L., and Heubi, J.E. (2000). Pharmacokinetics, tolerability, and clinical effectiveness of quetiapine fumarate: An open-label trial in adolescents with psychotic disorders. *J Clin Psychiatry*, 61(4), 252–260.

McCracken, J.T., McGough, J., Shah, B., Cronin, P., Hong, D., Aman, M.G., Arnold, L.E., Lindsay, R., Nash, P., Hollway, J., McDougle, C.J., Posey, D., Swiezy, N., Kohn, A., Scahill, L.,

Martin, A., Koenig, K., Volkmar, F., Carroll, D., Lancor, A., Tierney, E., Ghuman, J., Gonzalez, N.M., Grados, M., Vitiello, B., Ritz, L., Davies, M., Robinson, J., McMahon, D., and Research Units on Pediatric Psychopharmacology Autism Network. (2002). Risperidone in children with autism and serious behavioral problems. *N Engl J Med*, 347(5), 314–321.

McKnew, D.H., Cytryn, L., Buchsbaum, M.S., Hamovit, J., Lamour, M., Rapoport, J.L., and Gershon, E.S. (1981). Lithium in children of lithium-responding parents. *Psychiatry Res*, 4(2), 171–180.

Meyer, S.E., Carlson, G.A., Wiggs, E.A., Martinez, P.E., Ronsaville, D.S., Klimes-Dougan, B., Gold, P.W., and Radke-Yarrow, M. (2004). A prospective study of the association among impaired executive functioning, childhood attentional problems, and the development of bipolar disorder. *Dev Psychopathol*, 16(2), 461–476.

Mick, E., Biederman, J., Pandina, G., and Faraone, S.V. (2003). A preliminary meta-analysis of the child behavior checklist in pediatric bipolar disorder. *Biol Psychiatry*, 53(11), 1021–1027.

Miklowitz, D.J., Simoneau, T.L., George, E.L., Richards, J.A., Kalbag, A., Sachs-Ericsson, N., and Suddath, R. (2000). Family-focused treatment of bipolar disorder: 1-Year effects of a psychoeducational program in conjunction with pharmacotherapy. *Biol Psychiatry*, 48(6), 582–592.

Miklowitz, D.J., George, E.L., Axelson, D.A., Kim, E.Y., Birmaher, B., Schneck, C., Beresford, C., Craighead, W.E., and Brent, D.A. (2004). Family-focused treatment for adolescents with bipolar disorder. *J Affect Disord*, 82(Suppl. 1), S113–S128.

Papatheodorou, G., Kutcher, S.P., Katic, M., and Szalai, J.P. (1995). The efficacy and safety of divalproex sodium in the treatment of acute mania in adolescents and young adults: An open clinical trial. *J Clin Psychopharmacol*, 15, 110–116.

Pappadopulos, E., Macintyre, J.C. II, Crismon, M.L., Findling, R.L., Malone, R.P., Derivan, A., Schooler, N., Sikich, L., Greenhill, L., Schur, S.B., Felton, C.J., Kranzler, H., Rube, D.M., Sverd, J., Finnerty, M., Ketner, S., Siennick, S.E., and Jensen, P.S. (2003). Treatment Recommendations for the Use of Antipsychotics for Aggressive Youth (TRAAY): Part II. *J Am Acad Child Adolesc Psychiatry*, 42(2), 145–161.

Patel, N.C., DelBello, M.P., Bryan, H.S., Adler, C.M., Kowatch, R.A., Stanford, K., Strakowski, S.M. (2006). Open-label lithium for the treatment of adolescents with bipolar depression. *J Am Acad Child Adolesc Psychiatry*, 45(3), 289–297.

Pavuluri, M.N., Graczyk, P.A., Henry, D.B., Carbray, J.A., Heidenreich, J., and Miklowitz, D.J. (2004a). Child- and family-focused cognitive-behavioral therapy for pediatric bipolar disorder: Development and preliminary results. *J Am Acad Child Adolesc Psychiatry*, 43(5), 528–537.

Pavuluri, M.N., Henry, D.B., Carbray, J.A., Sampson, G., Naylor, M.W., and Janicak, P.G. (2004b). Open-label prospective trial of risperidone in combination with lithium or divalproex sodium in pediatric mania. *J Affect Disord*, 82(Suppl. 1), S103–S111.

Pavuluri, M.N., Henry, D.B., Carbray, J.A., Naylor, M.W., and Janicak, P.G. (2005). Divalproex sodium for pediatric mixed mania: A 6-month prospective trial. *Bipolar Disord*, 7(3), 266–273.

Post, R.M., and Kowatch, R.A. (2006). The health care crisis of childhood-onset bipolar illness: Some recommendations for its amelioration. *J Clin Psychiatry*, 67(1), 115–125.

Post, R.M., Leverich, G.S., Fergus, E., Miller, R., and Luckenbaugh, D. (2002). Parental attitudes towards early intervention in children at high risk for affective disorders. *J Affect Disord*, 70(2), 117–124.

Post, R.M., Leverich, G.S., Nolen, W.A., Kupka, R.W., Altshuler, L.L., Frye, M.A., Suppes, T., McElroy, S., Keck, P., Grunze, H., and Walden, J. (2003). A re-evaluation of the role of antidepressants in the treatment of bipolar depression: Data from the Stanley Foundation Bipolar Network. *Bipolar Disord*, 5(6), 396–406.

Poznanski, E.O., Israel, M.G., and Grossman, J. (1984). Hypomania in a four-year-old. *J Am Acad Child Psychiatry*, 23, 105–110.

Reinblatt, S.P., and Walkup, J.T. (2005). Psychopharmacologic treatment of pediatric anxiety disorders. *Child Adolesc Psychiatr Clin North Am*, 14(4), 877–908.

Rey, J.M., and Walter, G. (1997). Half a century of ECT use in young people. *Am J Psychiatry*, 154(5), 595–602.

Robertson, J.M., and Tanguay, P.E. (1997). Case study: The use of melatonin in a boy with refractory bipolar disorder. *J Am Acad Child Adolesc Psychiatry*, 36(6), 822–825.

Russell, P.S., Tharyan, P., Arun Kumar, K., and Cherian, A. (2002). Electro convulsive therapy in a pre-pubertal child with severe depression. *J Postgrad Med*, 48(4), 290–291.

Schaller, J.L., and Behar, D. (1999). Quetiapine for refractory mania in a child. *J Am Acad Child Adolesc Psychiatry*, 38(5), 498–499.

Scheffer, R.E., Kowatch, R.A., Carmody, T., and Rush, A.J. (2005). Randomized, placebo-controlled trial of mixed amphetamine salts for symptoms of comorbid ADHD in pediatric bipolar disorder after mood stabilization with divalproex sodium. *Am J Psychiatry*, 162(1), 58–64.

Schreier, H.A. (1982). Mania responsive to lecithin in a 13-year-old girl. *Am J Psychiatry*, 139(1), 108–110.

Schur, S.B., Sikich, L., Findling, R.L., Malone, R.P., Crismon, M.L., Derivan, A., Macintyre, J.C. II, Pappadopulos, E., Greenhill, L., Schooler, N., Van Orden, K., and Jensen, P.S. (2003). Treatment Recommendations for the Use of Antipsychotics for Aggressive Youth (TRAAY). Part I: A review. *J Am Acad Child Adolesc Psychiatry*, 42(2), 132–144.

Shaffer, D., Gould, M.S., Brasic, J., Ambrosini, P., Fisher, P., Bird, H., and Aluwahlia, S. (1983). A Children's Global Assessment Scale (CGAS). *Arch Gen Psychiatry*, 40(11), 1228–1231.

Shaw, J.A., Egeland, J.A., Endicott, J., Allen, C.R., and Hostetter, A.M. (2005). A 10-year prospective study of prodromal patterns for bipolar disorder among Amish youth. *J Am Acad Child Adolesc Psychiatry*, 44(11), 1104–1111.

Silva, R.R., Campbell, M., Golden, R.R., Small, A.M., Pataki, C.S., and Rosenberg, C.R. (1992). Side effects associated with lithium and placebo administration in aggressive children. *Psychopharmacol Bull*, 28(3), 319–326.

Snyder, R., Turgay, A., Aman, M., Binder, C., Fisman, S., Carroll, A., and Risperidone Conduct Study Group. (2002). Effects of risperidone on conduct and disruptive behavior disorders in children with subaverage IQs. *J Am Acad Child Adolesc Psychiatry*, 41(9), 1026–1036.

Soutullo, C.A., Casuto, L.S., and Keck, P.E. Jr. (1998). Gabapentin in the treatment of adolescent mania: A case report. *J Child Adolesc Psychopharmacol*, 8, 81–85.

Soutullo, C.A., Sorter, M.T., Foster, K.D., McElroy, S.L., and Keck, P.E. (1999). Olanzapine in the treatment of adolescent acute mania: A report of seven cases. *J Affect Disord*, 53(3), 279–283.

Soutullo, C.A., DelBello, M.P., Ochsner, J.E., McElroy, S.L., Taylor, S.A., Strakowski, S.M., Keck, P.E. Jr. (2002). Severity of bipolarity in hospitalized manic adolescents with history of stimulant or antidepressant treatment. *J Affect Disord*, 70(3), 323–327.

Steiner, H., Petersen, M.L., Saxena, K., Ford, S., and Matthews, Z. (2003). Divalproex sodium for the treatment of conduct disorder: A randomized controlled clinical trial. *J Clin Psychiatry*, 64(10), 1183–1191.

Strakowski, S.M., DelBello, M.P., Kowatch, R., Whitsel, R., and Adler, C. (2006). A single-blind prospective study of quetiapine for the treatment of mood disorders in adolescents who are at high risk for developing bipolar disorder. *New Research Abstract*, May 22, 2006. American Psychiatric Association.

Strober, M., and Carlson, G. (1982). Bipolar illness in adolescents with major depression: Clinical, genetic, and psychopharmacologic predictors in a three- to four-year prospective follow-up investigation. *Arch Gen Psychiatry*, 39(5), 549–555.

Strober, M., Morrell, W., Burroughs, J., Lampert, C., Danforth, H., and Freeman, R. (1988). A family study of bipolar I disorder in adolescence: Early onset of symptoms linked to increased familial loading and lithium resistance. *J Affect Disord*, 15(3), 255–268.

Strober, M., Morrell, W., Lampert, C., and Burroughs, J. (1990). Relapse following discontinuation of lithium maintenance therapy in adolescents with bipolar I illness: A naturalistic study. *Am J Psychiatry*, 147, 457–461.

Strober, M., DeAntonio, M., Schmidt-Lackner, S., Freeman, R., Lampert, C., and Diamond, J. (1998). Early childhood attention deficit hyperactivity disorder predicts poorer response to acute lithium therapy in adolescent mania. *J Affect Disord*, 51, 145–151.

Suppes, T., Baldessarini, R.J., and Faedda, G.L. (1991). Risk of recurrence following discontinuation of lithium in bipolar disorder. *Arch Gen Psychiatry*, 48, 1082–1088.

Taieb, O., Flament, M.F., Chevret, S., Jeammet, P., Allilaire, J.F., Mazet, P., and Cohen, D. (2002). Clinical relevance of electroconvulsive therapy (ECT) in adolescents with severe mood disorder: Evidence from a follow-up study. *Eur Psychiatry*, 17(4), 206–212.

Tillman, R., Geller, B., Craney, J.L., Bolhofner, K., Williams, M., Zimerman, B., Frazier, J., and Beringer, L. (2003). Temperament and character factors in a prepubertal and early adolescent bipolar disorder phenotype compared to attention deficit hyperactive and normal controls. *J Child Adolesc Psychopharmacol*, 13(4), 531–543.

Tohen, M., Kryzhanovskay, L., Carlson, G., DelBello, M., Wozniak, J., Kowatch, R., Wagner, K., Findling, R., Lin, D., Robertson-Plouch, C., Xu, W., Huang, X., Dittman, R., and Biederman, J. (2006). Olanzapine in the treatment of acute mania in adolescents with bipolar I disorder: A 3-week randomized double-blind placebo-controlled study. *New Research Abstract*, May 22, 2006. American Psychiatric Association.

Towbin, K.E., Pradella, A., Gorrindo, T., Pine, D.S., and Leibenluft, E. (2005). Autism spectrum traits in children with mood and anxiety disorders. *J Child Adolesc Psychopharmacol*, 15(3), 452–464.

Tuke, D.H. (1892). *A Dictionary of Psychological Medicine*. Philadelphia: P. Blaikston, Son & Co.

Turgay, A., Binder, C., Snyder, R., and Fisman, S. (2002). Long-term safety and efficacy of risperidone for the treatment of disruptive behavior disorders in children with subaverage IQs. *Pediatrics*, 110(3), e34.

U.S. Food and Drug Administration (FDA). (2004). T.A. Hammad (Ed.), *Relationship between Psychotropic Drugs and Pediatric Suicidality: Review and Evaluation of Clinical Data*. Available: http://www.fda.gov/ohrms/dockets/ac/04/briefing/2004–4065b1-10-TAB08-Hammads-Review.pdf [November 2004].

Varanka, T.M., Weller, R.A., and Weller, E.B. (1988). Fristad, M.A. (Ed.), Lithium treatment of manic episodes with psychotic features in prepubertal children. *Am J Psychiatry*, 145(12), 1557–1559.

Wagner, K.D., Weller, E.B., Carlson, G.A., Sachs, G., Biederman, J., Frazier, J.A., Wozniak, P., Tracy, K., Weller, R.A., and Bowden, C. (2002). An open-label trial of divalproex in children and adolescents with bipolar disorder. *J Am Acad Child Adolesc Psychiatry*, 41(10), 1224–1230.

Wagner, K.D., Jonas, J., Findling, R.L., Ventura, D., and Saikali, K. (2006a). A double-blind, randomized, placebo-controlled trial of escitalopram in the treatment of pediatric depression. *J Am Acad Child Adolesc Psychiatry*, 45(3), 280–288.

Wagner, K.D., Kowatch, R.A., Emslie, G.J., Findling, R.L., Wilens, T.E., McCague, K., D'Souza, J., Wamil, A., Lehman, R.B., Berv, D., and Linden, D. (2006b). A double-blind, randomized, placebo-controlled trial of oxcarbazepine in the treatment of bipolar disorder in children and adolescents. *Am J Psychiatry*, 163(7), 1179–1186.

Walter, G., and Rey, J.M. (2003). Has the practice and outcome of ECT in adolescents changed? Findings from a whole-population study. *J ECT*, 19(2), 84–87.

Walter, G., Rey, J.M., and Mitchell, P.B. (1999). Practitioner review: Electroconvulsive therapy in adolescents. *J Child Psychol Psychiatry*, 40(3), 325–334.

Weissman, M.M., Wolk, S., Goldstein, R.B., Moreau, D., Adams, P., Greenwald, S., Klier, C.M., Ryan, N.D., Dahl, R.E., and Wickramaratne, P. (1999a). Depressed adolescents grown up. *JAMA*, 281(18), 1707–1713.

West, S.A., Keck, P.E., Jr., McElroy, S.L., Strakowski, S.M., Minnery, K.L., McConville, B.J., and Sorter, M.T. (1994). Open trial of valproate in the treatment of adolescent mania. *J Child Adolesc Psychopharmacol*, 4, 263–267.

Woolston, J.L. (1999). Case study: Carbamazepine treatment of juvenile-onset bipolar disorder. *J Am Acad Child Adolesc Psychiatry*, 38(3), 335–338.

Wudarsky, M., Nicolson, R., Hamburger, S.D., Spechler, L., Gochman, P., Bedwell, J., Lenane, M.C., and Rapoport, J.L. (1999). Elevated prolactin in pediatric patients on typical and atypical antipsychotics. *J Child Adolesc Psychopharmacol*, 9(4), 239–245.

Youngerman, J., and Canino, I.A. (1978). Lithium carbonate use in children and adolescents. A survey of the literature. *Arch Gen Psychiatry*, 35(2), 216–224.

Youngstrom, E.A., Findling, R.L., Calabrese, J.R., Gracious, B.L., Demeter, C., Bedoya, D.D., and Price, M. (2004). Comparing diagnostic accuracy of six potential screening instruments for bipolar disorder in youths aged 5 to 17 years. *J Am Acad Child Adolesc Psychiatry*, 43(7), 847–858.

CHAPTER 24

Ahrens, B., Grof, P., Moller, H.J., Muller-Oerlinghausen, B., and Wolf, T. (1995). Extended survival of patients on long-term lithium treatment. *Can J Psychiatry*, 40, 241–246.

Alevizos, B., Lykouras, L., Zervas, I.M., and Christodoulou, G.N. (2002). Risperidone-induced obsessive-compulsive symptoms: A series of six cases. *J Clin Psychopharmacol*, 22(5), 461–467.

Anderson, J.W., Greenway, F.L., Fujioka, K., Gadde, K.M., McKenney, J., and O'Neil, P.M. (2002). Bupropion SR enhances weight loss: A 48-week double-blind, placebo-controlled trial. *Obes Res*, 10, 633–641.

Appolinario, J.C., Bacaltchuk, J., Sichieri, R., Claudino, A.M., Godoy-Matos, A., Morgan, C., Zanella, M.T., and Coutinho, W. (2003). A randomized, double-blind, placebo-controlled study of sibutramine in the treatment of binge-eating disorder. *Arch Gen Psychiatry*, 60, 1109–1116.

Aronson, R., Offman, H.J., Joffe, R.T., and Naylor, C.D. (1996). Triiodothyronine augmentation in the treatment of refractory depression: A meta-analysis. *Arch Gen Psychiatry*, 53, 842–848.

Ballenger, J.C., Davidson, J.R., Lecrubier, Y., Nutt, D.J., Marshall, R.D., Nemeroff, C.B., Shalev, A.Y., and Yehuda, R. (2004). Consensus statement update on posttraumatic stress disorder from the international consensus group on depression and anxiety. *J Clin Psychiatry*, 65(Suppl. 1), 55–62.

Barbarich, N.C., McConaha, C.W., Gaskill, J., La Via, M., Frank, G.K., Achenbach, S., Plotnicov, K.H., and Kaye, W.H. (2004). An open trial of olanzapine in anorexia nervosa. *J Clin Psychiatry*, 65, 1480–1482.

Bauer, M.S., and Whybrow, P.C. (1990). Rapid cycling bipolar affective disorder: II. Treatment of refractory rapid cycling with high-dose levothyroxine: A preliminary study. *Arch Gen Psychiatry*, 47, 435–440.

Bauer, M.S., Berghofer, A., Bschor, T., Baumgartner, A., Kiesslinger, U., Hellweg, R., Adli, M., Baethge, C., and Muller-Oerlinghausen, B. (2002). Supraphysiological doses of L-thyroxine in the maintenance treatment of prophylaxis-resistant affective disorders. *Neuropsychopharmacology*, 27, 620–628.

Bellack, A.S., Bennett, M.E., Gearon, J.S., Brown, C.H., and Yang, Y. (2006). A randomized clinical trial of a new behavioral treatment for drug abuse in people with severe and persistent mental illness. *Arch Gen Psychiatry*, 63, 426–432.

Berton, F., Francesconi, W.G., Madamba, S.G., Zieglgansberger, W., and Siggins, G.R. (1998). Acamprosate enhances N-methyl-D-apartate receptor-mediated neurotransmission but inhibits presynaptic GABA(B) receptors in nucleus accumbens neurons. *Alcohol Clin Exp Res*, 22, 183–191.

Bjorkqvist, S.E., Isohanni, M., Makela, R., and Malinen, L. (1976). Ambulant treatment of alcohol withdrawal symptoms with carbamazepine: A formal multicentre double-blind comparison with placebo. *Acta Psychiatr Scand*, 53, 333–342.

Brady, K.T., Sonne, S.C., Anton, R., and Ballenger, J.C. (1995). Valproate in the treatment of acute bipolar affective episodes complicated by substance abuse: A pilot study. *J Clin Psychiatry*, 56(3), 118–121.

Brady, K.T., Sonne, S.C., Malcolm, R.J., Randall, C.L., Dansky, B.S., Simpson, K., Roberts, J.S., and Brondino, M. (2002). Carbamazepine in the treatment of cocaine dependence: Subtyping by affective disorder. *Exp Clin Psychopharmacol*, 10, 276–285.

Bray, G.A., Hollander, P., Klein, S., Kushner, R., Levy, B., Fitchet, M., and Perry, B.H. (2003). A 6-month randomized, placebo-controlled, dose-ranging trial of topiramate for weight loss in obesity. *Obes Res*, 11, 722–733.

Brown, E.S. (2006). Management of comorbid bipolar disorder and substance abuse. *J Clin Psychiatry*, 67(8), e05.

Brown, E.S., Nejtek, V.A., Perantie, D.C., and Bobadilla, L. (2002). Quetiapine in bipolar disorder and cocaine dependence. *Bipolar Disord*, 4(6), 406–411.

Brown, E.S., Nejtek, V.A., Perantie, D.C., Orsulak, P.J., and Bobadilla, L. (2003). Lamotrigine in patients with bipolar disorder and cocaine dependence. *J Clin Psychiatry*, 64(2), 197–201.

Brown, E.S., Beard, L., Dobbs, L., and Rush, A.J. (2006). Naltrexone in patients with bipolar disorder and alcohol dependence. *Depress Anxiety*, 23(8), 492–495.

Brown, J., Kranzler, H.R., and Del Boca, F.K. (1992). Self-reports by alcohol and drug abuse inpatients: Factors affecting reliability and validity. *Br J Addict*, 87, 1013–1024.

Calabrese, J.R., Shelton, M.D., Bowden, C.L., Rapport, D.J., Suppes, T., Shirley, E.R., Kimmel, S.E., and Caban, S.J. (2001). Bipolar rapid cycling: Focus on depression as its hallmark. *J Clin Psychiatry*, 62(Suppl. 14), 34–41.

Chick, J., Anton, R., Checinski, K., Croop, R., Drummond, D.C., Farmer, R., Labriola, D., Marshall, J., Moncrieff, J., Morgan, M.Y., Peters, T., and Ritson, B. (2000). A multicentre, randomized, double-blind, placebo-controlled trial of naltrexone in the treatment of alcohol dependence or abuse. *Alcohol Alcohol*, 35, 587–593.

Denys, D., de Geus, F., van Meger, H.J., and Westenberg, H.G. (2004). A double blind, randomized, placebo controlled trial of quetiapine addition in patients with obsessive-compulsive disorder refractory to serotonin reuptake inhibitors. *J Clin Psychiatry*, 1040–1048.

Drake, R.E., Xie, H., McHugo, G.J., and Shumway, M. (2004). Three-year outcomes of long-term patients with co-occurring bipolar and substance use disorders. *Biol Psychiatry*, 56(10), 749–756.

Driessen, M., Veltrup, C., Wetterling, T., John, U., and Dilling, H. (1998). Axis I and Axis II comorbidity in alcohol dependence and the two types of alcoholism. *Alcohol Clin Exp Res*, 22, 77–86.

Driessen, M., Meier, S., Hill, A., Wetterling, T., Lange, W., and Junghanns, K. (2001). The course of anxiety, depression and drinking behaviours after completed detoxification in alcoholics with and without comorbid anxiety and depressive disorders. *Alcohol Alcohol*, 36, 249–255.

Dymek, M.P., le Grange, D., Neven, K., and Alverdy, J. (2001). Quality of life and psychosocial adjustment in patients after Roux-en-Y gastric bypass: A brief report. *Obes Surg*, 11, 32–39.

Estroff, T.W., Dackis, C.A., Gold, M.S., and Pottash, A.L. (1985). Drug abuse and bipolar disorders. *Int J Psychiatry Med*, 15, 37–40.

Famularo, R., Stone, K., and Popper, C. (1985). Preadolescent alcohol abuse and dependence. *Am J Psychiatry*, 142, 1187–1189.

Feltner, D.E., Crockatt, J.G., Dubovsky, S.J., Cohn, C.K., Shrivastava, R.K., Targum, S.D., Liu-Dumaw, M., Carter, C.M., and Pande, A.C. (2003). A randomized, double-blind, placebo-controlled, fixed-dose, multicenter study of pregabalin in patients with generalized anxiety disorder. *J Clin Psychopharmacol*, 23(3), 240–249.

Fesler, F.A. (1991). Valproate in combat-related posttraumatic stress disorder. *J Clin Psychiatry*, 52, 361–364.

Foa, E.B., Zoellner, L.A., Feeny, N.C., Hembree, E.A., and Alvarez-Conrad, J. (2002). Does imaginal exposure exacerbate PTSD symptoms? *J Consult Clin Psychol*, 70, 1022–1028.

Forster, P.L., Schoenfeld, F.B., Marmar, C.R., and Lang, A.J. (1995). Lithium for irritability in post-traumatic stress disorder. *J Trauma Stress*, 8, 143–149.

Friedman, M.A., Schwartz, M.B., and Brownell, K.D. (1998). Differential relation of psychological functioning with the history and experience of weight cycling. *J Consult Clin Psychol*, 66, 646–650.

Gadde, K.M., Parker, C.B., Maner, L.G., Wagner, H.R. II, Logue, E.J., Drezner, M.K., and Krishnan, K.R. (2001). Bupropion for weight loss: An investigation of efficacy and tolerability in overweight and obese women. *Obes Res*, 9(9), 544–551.

Gadde, K.M., Franciscy, D.M., Wagner, H.R. II, and Krishnan, K.R. (2003). Zonisamide for weight loss in obese adults: A randomized controlled trial. *JAMA*, 289, 1820–1825.

Gawin, F.H., and Kleber, H.D. (1984). Cocaine abuse treatment: Open pilot trial with deipramine and lithium carbonate. *Arch Gen Psychiatry*, 41, 903–909.

Geller, B., Cooper, T.B., Sun, K., Zimerman, B., Frazier, J., Williams, M., and Heath, J. (1998). Double-blind and placebo-controlled study of lithium for adolescent bipolar disorders with secondary substance dependency. *J Am Acad Child Adolesc Psychiatry*, 37(2), 171–178.

Goldberg, J.F., and Whiteside, J.E. (2002). The association between substance abuse and antidepressant-induced mania in bipolar disorder: A preliminary study. *J Clin Psychiatry*, 63, 791–795.

Goldberg, J.F., Garno, J.L., Leon, A.C., Kocsis, J.H., and Portera, L. (1999). A history of substance abuse complicates remission from acute mania in bipolar disorder. *J Clin Psychiatry*, 60, 733–740.

Goodman, W.K., and Charney, D.S. (1987). A case of alprazolam, but not lorazepam, inducing manic symptoms. *J Clin Psychiatry*, 48, 117–118.

Goodwin, F.K., Prange, A.J. Jr., Post, R.M., Muscettola, G., and Lipton, M.A. (1982). Potentiation of antidepressant effects by L-triiodothyronine in tricyclic nonresponders. *Am J Psychiatry*, 139, 34–38.

Gross, H.A., Ebert, M.H., Faden, V.B., Goldberg, S.C., Nee, L.E., and Kaye, W.H. (1981). A double-blind controlled trial of lithium carbonate primary anorexia nervosa. *J Clin Psychopharmacol*, 1, 376–381.

Haffenden, J. (1982). *The Life of John Berryman*. Boston: Routledge & Kegan Paul.

Hamner, M., Deitsch, S., Brodrick, P., Ulmer, H., and Lorberbaum, J. (2003). Quetiapine treatment in patients with post-traumatic stress disorder: An open trial of adjunctive therapy. *J Clin Psychopharmacol*, 23, 15–20.

Henderson, D.C., Cagliero, E., Copeland, P.M., Borba, C.P., Evins, E., Hayden, D., Weber, M.T., Anderson, E.J., Allison, D.B., Daley, T.B., Schoenfeld, D., and Goff D.C. (2005). Glucose metabolism in patients with schizophrenia treated with atypical antipsychotic agents: A frequently sampled intravenous glucose tolerance test and minimal model analysis. *Arch Gen Psychiatry*, 62, 19–28.

Hertzberg, M.A., Butterfield, M.I., Feldman, M.E., Beckham, J.C., Sutherland, S.M., Connor, K.M., and Davidson, J.R. (1999). A preliminary study of lamotrigine for the treatment of post-traumatic stress disorder. *Biol Psychiatry*, 45, 1226–1229.

Hirschfeld, R.M., Weisler, R.H., Raines, S.R., Macfadden, W., and the BOLDER Study Group. (2006). Quetiapine in the treatment of anxiety in patients with bipolar I or II depression: A secondary analysis from a randomized, double-blind, placebo-controlled study. *J Clin Psychiatry*, 67(3), 355–362.

Hollander, E., Kaplan, A., and Stahl, S.M. (2003). A double-blind, placebo-controlled trial of clonazepam in obsessive-compulsive disorder. *World J Biol Psychiatry*, 4, 30–34.

Hollister, L.E., Johnson, K., Boukhabza, D., and Gillespie, H.K. (1981). Aversive effects of naltrexone in subjects not dependent on opiates. *Drug Alcohol Depend*, 8, 37–41.

Hoopes, S.P., Reimherr, F.W., Hedges, D.W., Rosenthal, N.R., Kamin, M., Karim, R., Capece, J.A., and Karvois, D. (2003). Treatment of bulimia nervosa with topiramate in a randomized, double-blind, placebo-controlled trial: Part 1. Improvement in binge and purge measures. *J Clin Psychiatry*, 64, 1335–1341.

Hsu, L.K., Clement, L., Santhouse, R., and Ju, E.S. (1991). Treatment of bulimia nervosa with lithium carbonate: A controlled study. *J Nerv Ment Dis*, 179, 351–355.

Hutterfield, M., Becker, M., and Conner, K. (2001). Olanzapine in the treatment of post-traumatic stress disorder: A pilot study. *Int Clin Psychopharmacol*, 16, 197–203.

Jain, A.K., Kaplan, R.A., Gadde, K.M., Wadden, T.A., Allison, D.B., Brewer, E.R., Leadbetter, R.A., Richard, N., Haight, B., Jamerson, B.D., Buaron, K.S., and Metz, A. (2002). Bupropion SR vs. placebo for weight loss in obese patients with depressive symptoms. *Obes Res*, 10(10), 1049–1056.

Johnson, B.A., Ait-Daoud, N., Bowden, C.L., DiClemente, C.C., Roache, J.D., Lawson, K., Javors, M.A., and Ma, J.Z. (2003). Oral topiramate for treatment of alcohol dependence: A randomised controlled trial. *Lancet*, 361, 1677–1685.

Kanba, S., Yagi, G., Kamijima, K., Suzuki, T., Tajima, O., Otaki, J., Arata, E., Koshikawa, H., Nibuya, M., and Kinoshita, N. (1994). The first open study of zonisamide, a novel anticonvulsant, shows efficacy in mania. *Prog Neuropsychopharmacol Biol Psychiatry*, 18, 707–715.

Keck, P.E., Jr., McElroy, S.L., and Friedman, L.M. (1992). Valproate and carbamazepine in the treatment of panic and posttraumatic stress disorders, withdrawal states, and behavioral dyscontrol syndromes. *J Clin Psychopharmacol*, 12, 36S–41S.

Keck, P.E., Jr., Taylor, V.E., Tugrul, K.C., McElroy, S.L., and Bennett, J.A. (1993). Valproate treatment of panic disorder and lactate-induced panic attacks. *Biol Psychiatry*, 33, 542–546.

Latt, N.C., Jurd, S., Houseman, J., and Wutzke, S.E. (2002). Naltrexone in alcohol dependence: A randomised controlled trial of effectiveness in a standard clinical setting. *Med J Aust*, 176, 530–534.

Leibow, D. (1983). L-thyroxine for rapid-cycling bipolar illness. *Am J Psychiatry*, 140, 1255.

Lensi, P., Cassano, G.B., Correddu, G., Ravagli, S., Kunovac, J.L., and Akiskal, H.S. (1996). Obsessive-compulsive disorder: Familial-developmental history, symptomatology, comorbidity and course with special reference to gender-related differences. *Br J Psychiatry*, 169, 101–107.

Leverich, G.S., Altshuler, L.L., Frye, M.A., Suppes, T., McElroy, S.L., Keck, P.E. Jr., Kupka, R.W., Denicoff, K.D., Nolen, W.A., Grunze, H., Martinez, M.I., and Post, R.M. (2006). Risk of switch in mood polarity to hypomania or mania in patients with bipolar depression during acute and continuation trials of venlafaxine, sertraline, and bupropion as adjuncts to mood stabilizers. *Am J Psychiatry*, 163(2), 232–239.

Levin, F.R., and Hennessy, G. (2004). Bipolar disorder and substance abuse. *Biol Psychiatry*, 56, 738–748.

Longo, L.P., Campbell, T., and Hubatch, S. (2002). Divalproex sodium (Depakote) for alcohol withdrawal and relapse prevention. *J Addict Dis*, 21, 55–64.

Magura, S., Laudet, A.B., Mahmood, D., Rosenblum, A., and Knight, E. (2002). Adherence to medication regimens and participation in dual-focus self-help groups. *Psychiatr Serv*, 53, 310–316.

Malcolm, R., Ballenger, J.C., Sturgis, E.T., and Anton, R. (1989). Double-blind controlled trial comparing carbamazepine to oxazepam treatment of alcohol withdrawal. *Am J Psychiatry*, 146, 617–621.

Malcolm, R., Myrick, H., and Roberts., J. (2002). The effects of carbamazepine and lorazepam on single versus multitude previous alcohol withdrawals in an outpatient randomized trial. *J Gen Intern Med*, 17, 349–355.

McDougle, C.J., Price, L.H., Goodman, W.K., Charney, D.S., and Heninger, G.R. (1991). A controlled trial of lithium augmentation in fluvoxamine-refractory obsessive-compulsive disorder: Lack of efficacy. *J Clin Psychopharmacol*, 11(3), 175–184.

McDougle, C.J., Epperson, C., Peltion, G., Wasylink, S., and Price, L. (2000). A double blind placebo controlled study of risperidone addition in serotonin reuptake inhibitor-refractory obsessive compulsive disorder. *Arch Gen Psychiatry*, 57, 794–801.

McElroy, S.L., Arnold, L.M., Shapira, N.A., Keck, P.E. Jr., Rosenthal, N.R., Karim, M.R., Kamin, M., and Hudson, J.I. (2003). Topiramate in the treatment of binge eating disorder associated with obesity: A randomized, placebo-controlled trial. *Am J Psychiatry*, 160, 255–261.

McElroy, S.L., Kotwal, R., Hudson, J.I., Nelson, E.B., and Keck, P.E. (2004). Zonisamide in the treatment of binge-eating disorder: An open-label, prospective trial. *J Clin Psychiatry*, 65, 50–56.

Monnelly, E., Ciraulo, D., Knapp, C., and Keane, T. (2003). Low-dose risperidone as adjunctive therapy for irritable aggression in post-traumatic stress disorder. *J Clin Psychopharmacol*, 23, 193–196.

Montgomery, S.A., Tobias, K., Zornberg, G.L., Kasper, S., and Pande, A.C. (2006). Efficacy and safety of pregabalin in the treatment of generalized anxiety disorder: A 6-week, multicenter, randomized, double-blind, placebo-controlled comparison of pregabalin and venlafaxine. *J Clin Psychiatry*, 67(5), 771–782.

Morrison, J.R. (1975). The family histories of manic-depressive patients with and without alcoholism. *J Nerv Ment Dis*, 160, 227–229.

Mueller, T.I., Stout, R.L., Rudden, S., Brown, R.A., Gordon, A., Solomon, D.A., and Recupero, P.R. (1997). A double-blind, placebo-controlled pilot study of carbamazepine for the treatment of alcohol dependence. *Alcohol Clin Exp Res*, 21, 86–92.

Muller-Oerlinghausen, B., Wolf, T., Ahrens, B., Glaenz, T., Schou, M., Grof, E., Grof, P., Lenz, G., Simhandl, C., Thau, K., Vestergaard, P., and Wolf, R. (1996). Mortality of patients who dropped out from regular lithium prophylaxis: A collaborative study by the International Group for the Study of Lithium-treated Patients (IGSLI). *Acta Psychiatr Scand*, 94, 344–347.

Najavits, L.M., Weiss, R.D., Shaw, S.R., and Muenz, L.R. (1998). "Seeking safety": Outcome of a new cognitive-behavioral psychotherapy for women with posttraumatic stress disorder and substance dependence. *J Trauma Stress*, 11, 437–456.

Nunes, E.V., McGrath, P.J., Wager, S., and Quitkin, F.M. (1990). Lithium treatment for cocaine abusers with bipolar spectrum disorders. *Am J Psychiatry*, 147(5), 655–657.

Nuzzo, V., Lupoli, G., Esposito Del Puente, A., Rampone, E., Carpinelli, A., Del Puente, A.E., and Oriente, P. (1998). Bone mineral density in premenopausal women receiving levothyroxine suppressive therapy. *Gynecol Endocrinol*, 12, 333–337.

Ogborne, A.C., and Glaser, F.B. (1985). Evaluating Alcoholics Anonymous. In T.E. Bratter (Ed.), *Alcoholism and Substance Abuse* (pp. 176–192). New York: Free Press.

Olson, G.A., Olson, R.D., and Kastin, A.J. (1996). Endogenous opiates: 1995. *Peptides*, 17, 1421–1466.

Pande, A.C., Davidson, J.R., Jefferson, J.W., Janney, C.A., Katzelnick, D.J., Weisler, R.H., Greist, J.H., and Sutherland, S.M. (1999). Treatment of social phobia with gabapentin: A placebo-controlled study. *J Clin Psychopharmacol*, 19(4), 341–348.

Pande, A.C., Pollack, M.H., Crockatt, J., Greiner, M., Chouinard, G., Lydiard, R.B., Taylor, C.B., Dager, S.R., and Shiovitz, T. (2000). Placebo-controlled study of gabapentin treatment of panic disorder. *J Clin Psychopharmacol*, 20, 467–471.

Pande, A.C., Crockatt, J.G., Feltner, D.E., Janney, C.A., Smith, W.T., Weisler, R., Londborg, P.D., Bielski, R.J., Zimbroff, D.L., Davidson, J.R., and Liu-Dumaw, M. (2003). Pregabalin in generalized anxiety disorder: A placebo-controlled trial. *Am J Psychiatry*, 160(3), 533–540.

Perugi, G., Akiskal, H.S., Pfanner, C., Presta, S., Gemignani, A., Milanfranchi, A., Lensi, P., Ravagli, S., and Cassano, G.B. (1997). The clinical impact of bipolar and unipolar affective comorbidity on obsessive-compulsive disorder. *J Affect Disord*, 46, 15–23.

Perugi, G., Toni, C., Frare, F., Travierso, M.C., Hantouche, E., and Akiskal, H.S. (2002). Obsessive-compulsive-bipolar comorbidity: A systematic exploration of clinical features and treatment outcome. *J Clin Psychiatry*, 63, 1129–1134.

Pigott, T.A., Pato, M.T., L'Heureux, F., Hill, J.L., Grover, G.N., Bernstein, S.E., and Murphy, D.L. (1991). A controlled comparison of adjuvant lithium carbonate or thyroid hormone in clomipramine-treated patients with obsessive-compulsive disorder. *J Clin Psychopharmacol*, 11(4), 242–248.

Pohl, R.B., Feltner, D.E., Fieve, R.R., and Pande, A.C. (2005). Efficacy of pregabalin in the treatment of generalized anxiety disorder: Double-blind, placebo-controlled comparison of BID versus TID dosing. *J Clin Psychopharmacol*, 25(2), 151–158.

Post, R.M., Kramlinger, K.G., Joffe, R.T., Roy-Byrne, P.P., Rosoff, A., Frye, M.A., and Huggins, T. (1997). Rapid cycling bipolar affective disorder: Lack of relation to hypothyroidism. *Psychiatry Res*, 72, 1–7.

Powers, P.S., Santana, C.A., and Bannon, Y.S. (2002). Olanzapine in the treatment of anorexia nervosa: An open label trial. *Int J Eat Disord*, 32, 146–154.

Prange, A.J., Jr., Wilson, I.C., Rabon, A.M., and Lipton, M.A. (1969). Enhancement of imipramine antidepressant activity by thyroid hormone. *Am J Psychiatry*, 126, 457–469.

Reinhold, R.B. (1994). Late results of gastric bypass surgery for morbid obesity. *J Am Coll Nutr*, 13, 326–331.

Rickels, K., Pollack, M.H., Feltner, D.E., Lydiard, R.B., Zimbroff, D.L., Bielski, R.J., Tobias, K., Brock, J.D., Zornberg, G.L., and Pande, A.C. (2005). Pregabalin for treatment of generalized anxiety disorder: A 4-week, multicenter, double-blind, placebo-controlled trial of pregabalin and alprazolam. *Arch Gen Psychiatry*, 62(9), 1022–1030.

Rubio G., Lopez-Munoz. F., and Alamo, C. (2006). Effects of lamotrigine in patients with bipolar disorder and alcohol dependence. *Bipolar Disord*, 8, 289–293.

Rychtarik, R.G., Connors, G.J., Dermen, K.H., and Stasiewicz, P.R. (2000). Alcoholics Anonymous and the use of medications to prevent relapse: An anonymous survey of member attitudes. *J Stud Alcohol*, 61, 134–138.

Salloum, I.M., Cornelius, J.R., Daley, D.C., Kirisci, L., Himmelhoch, J.M., and Thase, M.E. (2005). Efficacy of valproate maintenance in patients with bipolar disorder and alcoholism: A double-blind placebo-controlled study. *Arch Gen Psychiatry*, 62, 37–45.

Sass, H., Soyka, M., Mann, K., and Zieglgansberger, W. (1996). Relapse prevention by acamprosate: Results from a placebo-controlled study on alcohol dependence. *Arch Gen Psychiatry*, 53, 673–680.

Saxena, S., Wang, D., Bystritsky, A., and Baxter, L.R. Jr. (1996). Risperidone augmentation of SRI treatment for refractory obsessive-compulsive disorder. *J Clin Psychiatry*, 57(7), 303–306.

Schuckit, M. (1983). Alcoholic patients with secondary depression. *Am J Psychiatry*, 140, 711–714.

Shapira, N.A., Ward, H.E., Mandoki, M., Murphy, T.K., Yang, M.C., Blier, P., and Goodman, W.K. (2004). A double-blind, placebo-controlled trial of olanzapine addition in fluoxetine-refractory obsessive-compulsive disorder. *Biol Psychiatry*, 55, 553–555.

Solyom, L., DiNicola, V.F., Phil, M., Sookman, D., and Luchins, D. (1985). Is there an obsessive psychosis? Aetiological and prognostic factors of an atypical form of obsessive-compulsive neurosis. *Can J Psychiatry*, 30(5), 372–380.

Sonne, S.C., and Brady, K.T. (2000). Naltrexone for individuals with comorbid bipolar disorder and alcohol dependence. *J Clin Psychopharmacol*, 20, 114–115.

Stancer, H.C., and Persad, E. (1982). Treatment of intractable rapid-cycling manic-depressive disorder with levothyroxine: Clinical observations. *Arch Gen Psychiatry*, 39, 311–312.

Strakowski, S.M., Sax, K.W., McElroy, S.L., Keck, P.E. Jr., Hawkins, J.M., and West, S.A. (1998). Course of psychiatric and substance abuse syndromes co-occurring with bipolar disorder after a first psychiatric hospitalization. *J Clin Psychiatry*, 59(9), 465–471.

Swartz, H.A., Pilkonis, P.A., Frank, E., Proietti, J.M., and Scott, J. (2005). Acute treatment outcomes in patients with bipolar I disorder and comorbid borderline personality disorder receiving medication and psychotherapy. *Bipolar Disord*, 7(2), 192–197.

Tarrier, N., Pilgrim, H., Sommerfield, C., Faragher, B., Reynolds, M., Graham, E., and Barrowclough, C. (1999a). A randomized trial of cognitive therapy and imaginal exposure in the treatment of chronic posttraumatic stress disorder. *J Consult Clin Psychol*, 67, 13–18.

Tarrier, N., Sommerfield, C., Pilgrim, H., and Humphreys, L. (1999b). Cognitive therapy or imaginal exposure in the treatment of post-traumatic stress disorder: Twelve-month follow-up. *Br J Psychiatry*, 175, 571–575.

Taylor, C.B., Youngblood, M.E., Catellier, D., Veith, R.C., Carney, R.M., Burg, M.M., Kaufmann, P.G., Shuster, J., Mellman, T., Blumenthal, J.A., Krishnan, R., Jaffe, A.S., and ENRICHD Investigators (2005). Effects of antidepressant medication on morbidity and mortality in depressed patients after myocardial infarction. *Arch Gen Psychiatry*, 62, 792–798.

Tiihonen, J., Lönnqvist, J., Wahlbeck, K., Klaukka, T., Tanskanen, A., and Haukka, J. (2006). Antidepressants and the risk of suicide, attempted suicide, and overall mortality in a nationwide cohort. *Arch Gen Psychiatry*, 63, 1368–1367.

Tonigan, J.S., Toscova, R., and Miller, W.R. (1996). Meta-analysis of the literature on Alcoholics Anonymous: Sample and study characteristics moderate findings. *J Stud Alcohol*, 57, 65–72.

Uhde, T.W., Stein, M.B., and Post, R.M. (1988). Lack of efficacy of carbamazepine in the treatment of panic disorder. *Am J Psychiatry*, 145, 1104–1109.

Vaillant, G.E. (1978). Alcoholism and drug dependence. In A.M. Nicholi (Ed.), *The Harvard Guide to Modern Psychiatry* (pp. 567–577). Cambridge, MA: Belknap Press.

Vulink, N.C., Denys, D., and Westenberg, H.G. (2005). Bupropion for patients with obsessive-compulsive disorder: An open-label, fixed-dose study. *J Clin Psychiatry*, 66, 228–230.

Weiss, R.D., Greenfield, S.F., Najavits, L.M., Soto, J.A., Wyner, D., Tohen, M., and Griffin, M.L. (1998). Medication compliance among patients with bipolar disorder and substance use disorder. *J Clin Psychiatry*, 59, 172–174.

Weiss, R.D., Najavits, L.M., and Greenfield, S.F. (1999). A relapse prevention group for patients with bipolar and substance use disorders. *J Subst Abuse Treat*, 16, 47–54.

Weiss, R.D., Kolodziej, M.E., Najavits, L.M., Greenfield, S.F., and Fucito, L.M. (2000). Utilization of psychosocial treatments by patients diagnosed with bipolar disorder and substance dependence. *Am J Addict*, 9, 314–320.

Weiss, R.D., Griffin, M.L., Kolodziej, M.E., Greenfield, S.F., Najavits, L.M., Daley, D.C., Doreau, H.R., and Hennen, J.A. (2007). A randomized trial of integrated group therapy versus group drug counseling for patients with bipolar disorder and substance dependence. *Am J Psychiatry*, 164, 100–107.

Whitworth, A.B., Fischer, F., Lesch, O.M., Nimmerrichter, A., Oberbauer, H., Platz, T., Potgieter, A., Walter, H., and Fleischhacker, W.W. (1996). Comparison of acamprosate and placebo in long-term treatment of alcohol dependence. *Lancet*, 347, 1438–1442.

Wilner, K.D., Anziano, R.J., Johnson, A.C., Miceli, J.J., Fricke, J.R., and Titus, C.K. (2002). The anxiolytic effect of the novel antipsychotic ziprasidone compared with diazepam in subjects anxious before dental surgery. *J Clin Psychopharmacol*, 22, 206–210.

CHAPTER 25

Advisory Committee to U.S. Food and Drug Administration. (2004). Center for Drug Evaluation and Research, Psychopharmacologic Drugs Advisory Committee with the Pediatric Subcommittee of the Anti-Infective Drugs Advisory Committee. *February 2 Transcript*. Available: http://www.fda.gov/ohrms/dockets/ac/04/transcripts/4006t1.htm (accessed September 19, 2006).

Akiskal, H.S., Benazzi, F., Perugi, G., and Rihmer, Z. (2005). Agitated "unipolar" depression re-conceptualized as a depressive mixed state: Implications for the antidepressant-suicide controversy. *J Affect Disord*, 85(3), 245–258.

Allen, M.H., and Currier, G.W. (2004). Use of restraints and pharmacotherapy in academic psychiatric emergency services. *Gen Hosp Psychiatry*, 26, 42–49.

American Psychiatric Association. (2003). Practice guidelines for the assessment and treatment of patients with suicidal behaviors. *Am J Psychiatry,* 117 pp. Available at: http://www.psych.org/psych_pract/treatg/pg/pg_suicidalbehaviors.pdf.

Angst, F., Stassen, H.H., Clayton, P.J., and Angst, J. (2002). Mortality of patients with mood disorders: Follow-up over 34–38 years. *J Affect Disord,* 68(2), 167–181.

Angst, J., Angst, F., Gerber-Werder, R., and Gamma, A. (2005b). Suicide in 406 mood-disorder patients with and without long-term medication: A 40 to 44 years' follow-up. *Arch Suicide Res,* 9(3), 279–300.

Appleby, L., Shaw, J., Amos, T., McDonnell, R., Harris, C., McCann, K., Kiernan, K., Davies, S., Bickley, H., and Parsons, R. (1999). Suicide within 12 months of contact with mental health services: National clinical survey. *BMJ,* 318(7193), 1235–1239.

Baldessarini, R.J., and Goodwin, F.K. (2003). *Psychiatric treatments versus suicidal risk.* Submitted to ACNP Task Force on Treatment Effects and Suicide, by invitation.

Baldessarini, R.J., and Goodwin, F.K. (2005). Citizens Petition to the United States Food and Drug Administration: Lithium and Suicide Prevention.

Baldessarini, R.J., and Jamison, K. (1999). Effects of medical interventions on suicidal behavior. *J Clin Psychiatry,* 60(Suppl. 2), 117–122.

Baldessarini, R.J., Tondo, L., and Hennen, J. (1999). Effects of lithium treatment and its discontinuation on suicidal behavior in bipolar manic-depressive disorder. *J Clin Psychiatry,* 60(Suppl. 2), 77–84.

Baldessarini, R.J., Tondo, L., and Hennen, J. (2001). Treating the suicidal patient with bipolar disorder: Reducing suicide risk with lithium. *Ann N Y Acad Sci,* 932:24–38; discussion 39–43.

Baldessarini, R.J., Tondo, L., and Hennen, J. (2003). Lithium treatment and suicide risk in major affective disorders: Update and new findings. *J Clin Psychiatry,* 64(Suppl. 5), 44–52.

Baldessarini, R.J., Pompili, M., and Tondo, L. (2006a). Suicide in bipolar disorder: Risks and management. *CNS Spectr,* 11(6), 465–471.

Baldessarini, R.J., Tondo, L., Davis, P., Pompili, M., Goodwin, F.K., and Hennen, J. (2006b). Decreased risks of suicides and suicide attempts during long-term lithium treatment: A meta-analytic review. *Bipolar Disord,* 8, 625–639.

Barraclough, B., Bunch, J., Nelson, B., and Sainsbury, P. (1974). A hundred cases of suicide: Clinical aspects. *Br J Psychiatry,* 125, 355–373.

Battaglia, J. (2005). Pharmacologic management of acute agitation. *Drugs,* 65, 1207–1222.

Bauer, M.S., Wisniewski, S.R., Marangell, L.B., Chessick, C.A., Allen, M.H., Dennehy, E.B., Miklowitz, D.J., Thase, M.E., and Sachs, G.S. (2006). Are antidepressants associated with new-onset suicidality in bipolar disorder? A prospective study of participants in the Systematic Treatment Enhancement Program for Bipolar Disorder (STEP-BD). *J Clin Psychiatry,* 67, 48–55.

Bradvik, L., and Berglund, M. (2000). Treatment and suicide in severe depression: A case-control study of antidepressant therapy at last contact before suicide. *J ECT,* 16(4), 399–408.

Brent, D.A., Moritz, G., Bridge, J., Perper, J., and Canobbio, R. (1996). Long-term impact of exposure to suicide: A three-year controlled follow-up. *J Am Acad Child Adolesc Psychiatry,* 35(5), 646–653.

Brodersen, A., Licht, R.W., Vestergaard, P., Olesen, A.V., and Morensen, P.B. (2000). Sixteen-year mortality in patients with affective disorder commenced on lithium. *Br J Psychiatry,* 176, 429–433.

Brown, G.K., Ten Have, T., Henriques, G.R., Xie, S.X., Hollander, J.E., and Beck, A.T. (2005). Cognitive therapy for the prevention of suicide attempts: A randomized controlled trial. *JAMA,* 294, 563–570.

Bruce, M.L., Ten Have, T.R., Reynolds, C.F. III, Katz, I.I., Schulberg, H.C., Mulsant, B.H., Brown, G.K., McAvay, G.J., Pearson, J.L., and Alexopoulos, G.S. (2004). Reducing suicidal ideation and depressive symptoms in depressed older primary care patients: A randomized controlled trial. *JAMA,* 291(9), 1081–1091.

Busch, K.A., Fawcett, J., and Jacobs, D.G. (2003). Clinical correlates of inpatient suicide. *J Clin Psychiatry,* 64(1), 14–19.

Cassem, N.H. (1978). Treating the person confronting death. In A.M. Nicholi (Ed.), *Harvard Guide to Modern Psychiatry* (pp. 579–606). Cambridge, MA: Belknap Press of Harvard University Press.

Cerel, J., Fristad, M.A., Weller, E.B., and Weller, R.A. (1999). Suicide-bereaved children and adolescents: A controlled longitudinal examination. *J Am Acad Child Adolesc Psychiatry,* 38(6), 672–679.

Chemtob, C.M., Hamada, R.S., Bauer, G., Kinney, B., and Torigoe, R.Y. (1988a). Patients' suicides: Frequency and impact on psychiatrists. *Am J Psychiatry,* 145(2), 224–228.

Chemtob, C.M., Hamada, R.S., Bauer, G., Torigoe, R.Y., and Kinney, B. (1988b). Patients' suicides: Frequency and impact on psychologists. *Prof Psychol,* 19, 416–420.

Ciapparelli, A., Dell'Osso, L., Pini, S., Chiavacci, M.C., Fenzi, M., and Cassano, G.B. (2000). Clozapine for treatment-refractory schizophrenia, schizoaffective disorder, and psychotic bipolar disorder: A 24-month naturalistic study. *J Clin Psychiatry,* 61(5), 329–334.

Cipriani, A., Wilder, H., Hawton, K., and Geddes, J.R. (2005). Lithium in the prevention of suicidal behavior and all-cause mortality in patients with mood disorders: A systematic review of randomized trials. *Am J Psychiatry,* 162(10), 1805–1819.

Coate, M. (1964). *Beyond All Reason.* London: Constable & Co.

Coppen, A., Standish-Barry, H., Bailey, J., Houston, G., Silicocks, P., and Hermon, C. (1990). Long-term lithium and mortality. *Lancet,* 335, 1347.

Coppen, A., Standish-Barry, H., Bailey, J., Houston, G., Silicocks, P., and Hermon, C. (1991). Does lithium reduce the mortality of recurrent mood disorders? *J Affect Disord,* 23, 1–7.

Coryell, W. (1988). Panic disorder and mortality. *Psychiatr Clin North Am,* 11(2), 433–440.

Dixon, J.F., and Hokin, L.E. (1998). Lithium acutely inhibits and chronically up-regulates and stabilizes glutamate uptake by presynaptic nerve endings in mouse cerebral cortex. *Proc Natl Acad Sci USA,* 95(14), 8363–8368.

Dubicka, B., Hadley, S., and Roberts, C. (2006). Suicidal behavior in youths with depression treated with new-generation antidepressants. *Br J Psychiatry,* 189, 393–398.

Duke University. (2005). *Duke University program on psychiatric advance directives.* Available: http://pad.duhs.duke.edu/index.html [accessed September 19, 2006].

Emslie, G.J., Heiligenstein, J.H., Wagner, K.D., Hoog, S.L., Ernest, D.E., Brown, E., Nilsson, M., and Jacobson, J.G. (2002). Fluoxetine for acute treatment of depression in children and adolescents: A placebo-controlled randomized clinical trial. *J Am Acad Child Adolesc Psychiatr*, 41, 1205–1215.

Faedda, G., Tondo, L., Baldessarini, R.J., Suppes, T., and Tohen, M. (1993). Outcome after rapid vs. gradual discontinuation of lithium treatment in bipolar mood disorders. *Arch Gen Psychiatry*, 50, 448–455.

Fawcett, J., and Barkin, R.L. (1998). Review of the results from clinical studies on the efficacy, safety and tolerability of mirtazapine for the treatment of patients with major depression. *J Affect Disord*, 51(3), 267–285.

Fawcett, J., Scheftner, W., Clark, D., Hedeker, D., Gibbons, R., and Coryell, W. (1987). Clinical predictors of suicide in patients with major affective disorders: A controlled prospective study. *Am J Psychiatry*, 144(1), 35–40.

Fawcett, J., Scheftner, W.A., Fogg, L., Clark, D.C., Young, M.A., Hedeker, D., and Gibbons, R. (1990). Time-related predictors of suicide in major affective disorder. *Am J Psychiatry*, 147(9), 1189–1194.

Fergusson, D., Doucette, S., Glass, K.C., Shapiro, S., Healy, D., Hebert, P., and Hutton, B. (2005). Association between suicide attempts and selective serotonin in reuptake inhibitors: Systematic review of randomized controlled trials. *BMJ*, 330, 396.

Fieve, R.R. (1975). The lithium clinic: A new model for the delivery of psychiatric services. *Am J Psychiatry*, 132, 1018–1022.

Gibbons, R.D., Hur, K., Bhaumik, D.K., and Mann, J.J. (2005). The relationship between antidepressant medication use and rate of suicide. *Arch Gen Psychiatry*, 62(2), 165–172.

Gibbons, R.D., Hur, K., Bhaumik, D.K., and Mann, J.J. (2006). The relationship between antidepressant prescription rates and rate yearly adolescent suicide. *Am J Psychiatry*, 163, 1898–1904.

Gitlin, M.J. (1999). A psychiatrist's reaction to a patient's suicide. *Am J Psychiatry*, 156(10), 1630–1634.

Gitlin, M.J., and Jamison, K.R. (1984). Lithium clinics: Theory and practice. *Hosp Community Psychiatry*, 35, 363–368.

Glazer, W.M. (1997). Olanzapine and the new generation of antipsychotic agents: Patterns of use. *J Clin Psychiatry*, 58(Suppl. 10), 18–21.

Goldstein, R.B., Black, D.W., Nasrallah, A., and Winokur, G. (1991). The prediction of suicide: Sensitivity, specificity and predictive value of a multivariate model applied to suicide among 1906 patients with affective disorders. *Arch Gen Psychiatry*, 48(5), 418–422.

Goodwin, F.K., and Jamison, K.R. (1984). The natural course of manic-depressive illness. In R.M. Post and J.C. Ballenger (Eds.), *Neurobiology of Mood Disorders* (pp. 20–37). Baltimore: Williams & Wilkins.

Goodwin, F.K., Fireman, B., Simon, G.E., Hunkeler, E.M., Lee, J., and Revicki, D. (2003). Suicide risk in bipolar disorder during treatment with lithium and divalproex. *JAMA*, 290(11), 1467–1473.

Grunebaum, M.F., Oquendo, M.A., Burke, A.K., Ellis, S.P., Echavarria, G., Brodsky, B.S., Malone, K.M., and Mann, J.J. (2003). Clinical impact of a 2-week psychotropic medication washout in unipolar depressed inpatients. *J Affect Disord*, 75(3), 291–296.

Hankoff, L.D. (1982). Suicide and attempted suicide. In E.S. Paykel (Ed.), *Handbook of Affective Disorders* (pp. 416–428). New York: Guildford Press.

Hartigan, G.P. (1959). *Experiences with Treatment with Lithium Salts*. Paper read to the Southeastern branch of the Royal Medicopsychological Society, London, UK.

Hawton, K., and Catalan, J. (1982). *Attempted Suicide: A Practical Guide to Its Nature and Management*. New York: Oxford University Press.

Hawton, K., Arensman, E., Townsend, E., Bremner, S., Feldman, E., Goldney, R., Gunnell, D., Hazell, P., van Heeringen, K., House, A., Owens, D., Sakinofsky, I., and Traskman-Bendz, L. (1998). Deliberate self harm: Systematic review of efficacy of psychosocial and pharmacological treatments in preventing repetition. *BMJ*, 317(7156), 441–447.

Hawton, K., Townsend, E., Arensman, E., Gunnell, D., Hazell, P., House, A., and van Heeringen, K. (2000). Psychosocial versus pharmacological treatments for deliberate self harm. *Cochrane Database Syst Rev*, (2), CD001764.

Hendin, H., Lipschitz, A., Maltsberger, J.T., Haas, A.P., and Wynecoop, S. (2000). Therapists' reactions to patients' suicides. *Am J Psychiatry*, 157(12), 2022–2027.

Hendin, H., Haas, A.P., Maltsberger, J.T., Szanto, K., and Rabinowicz, H. (2004). Factors contributing to therapists' distress after the suicide of a patient. *Am J Psychiatry*, 161(8), 1442–1446.

Hepp, U., Wittmann, L., Schnyder, U., and Michel, K. (2004). Psychological and psychosocial interventions after attempted suicide: An overview of treatment studies. *Crisis*, 25(3), 108–117.

Institute of Medicine (IOM). (2002). *Reducing Suicide: A National Imperative*. Washington, DC: National Academy Press.

Isacsson, G. (2000). Suicide prevention: A medical breakthrough? *Acta Psychiatr Scand*, 102(2), 113–117.

Isacsson, G., Redfors, I., Wasserman, D., and Bergman, U. (1994). Choice of antidepressants: Questionnaire survey of psychiatrists and general practitioners in two areas of Sweden. *BMJ*, 309(6968), 1546–1549.

Isacsson, G., Holmgren, P., Druid, H., and Bergman, U. (1997). The utilization of antidepressants—A key issue in the prevention of suicide: An analysis of 5281 suicides in Sweden during the period 1992–1994. *Acta Psychiatr Scand*, 96(2), 94–100.

Isometsa, E.T., Henriksson, M.M., Aro, H.M., Heikkinen, M.E., Kuoppasalmi, K.I., and Lonnqvist, J.K. (1994). Suicide in major depression. *Am J Psychiatry*, 151(4), 530–536.

Isometsa, E.T., Heikkinen, M.E., Marttunen, M.J., Henriksson, M.M., Aro, H.M., and Lonnqvist, J.K. (1995). The last appointment before suicide: Is suicide intent communicated? *Am J Psychiatry*, 152(6), 919–922.

Jacobs, D.G., Baldessarini, R.J., Conwell, Y., Fawcett, J., Horton, L., Meltzer, H., Pfeffer, C.R., and Simon, R.L. (2003). *Practice Guideline for the Assessment and Treatment of Patients with Suicide Behaviors*. Available: http://www.psych.org/psych_pract/treatg/quick_ref_guide/Suibehavs_QRG.pdf (accessed September 19, 2006).

Jamison, K.R. (1995). *An Unquiet Mind*. New York: Knopf.

Jamison, K.R. (1999). *Night Falls Fast: Understanding Suicide*. New York: Random House.

Khan, A., Shad, M.U., and Preskorn, S.H. (2000). Lack of sertraline efficacy probably due to an interaction with carbamazepine. *J Clin Psychiatry*, 61(7), 526–527.

Khan, A., Khan, S., Kolts, R., and Brown, W.A. (2003). Suicide rates in clinical trials of SSRIs, other antidepressants, and placebo: Analysis of FDA reports. *Am J Psychiatry*, 160(4), 790–792.

Kessing, L.V., Sondergard, L., Kvist, K., and Andersen, P.K. (2005). Suicide risk in patients treated with lithium. *Arch Gen Psychiatry*, 62(8), 860–866.

King, R.A., Riddle, M.A., Chappell, P.B., Hardin, M.T., and Anderson, G.M. (1991). Emergence of self-destructive phenomena in children and adolescents during fluoxetine treatment. *J Am Acad Child Adolesc Psychiatry*, 30(2), 179–186.

Knox, K.L., Litts, D.A., Talcott, G.W., Feig, J.C., and Caine, E.D. (2003). Risk of suicide and related adverse outcomes after exposure to a suicide prevention programme in the U.S. Air Force: Cohort study. *BMJ*, 327(7428), 1376.

Knox, K.L., Conwell, Y., and Caine, E.D. (2004). If suicide is a public health problem, what are we doing to prevent it? *Am J Public Health*, 94(1), 37–45.

Leon, A.C. (2005). Fluoxetine plus cognitive behavioural therapy improves symptoms of major depressive disorder in adolescents. *Evid Based Ment Health*, 8, 10.

Londborg, P.D., Smith, W.T., Glaudin, V., and Painter, J.R. (2000). Short-term cotherapy with clonazepam and fluoxetine: Anxiety, sleep disturbance and core symptoms of depression. *J Affect Disord*, 61(1–2), 73–79.

Ludwig, J., and Marcotte, D.E. (2005). Anti-depressants, suicide, and drug regulation. *J Policy Anal Manage*, 24, 249–272.

Luoma, J.B., Martin, C.E., and Pearson, J.L. (2002). Contact with mental health and primary care providers before suicide: A review of the evidence. *Am J Psychiatry*, 159(6), 909–916.

MacKinnon, D.R., and Farberow, N.L. (1976). An assessment of the utility of suicide prediction. *Suicide Life Threat Behav*, 6(2), 86–91.

Malone, K.M., Oquendo, M.A., Haas, G.L., Ellis, S.P., Li, S., and Mann, J.J. (2000). Protective factors against suicidal acts in major depression: Reasons for living. *Am J Psychiatry*, 157(7), 1084–1088.

Marco, C.A., and Vaughan, J. (2005). Emergency management of agitation in schizophrenia. *Am J Emerg Med*, 23, 767–776.

Marder, S.R., (2006). A review of agitation in mental illness: Treatment guidelines and current therapies. *J Clin Psychiatry*, 67(Suppl. 10), 13–21.

McElroy, S.L., Kotwal, R., Kaneria, R., and Keck, P.E. (2006). Antidepressants and suicidal behavior in bipolar disorder. *Bipolar Disord*, 8, 596–617.

Meltzer, H.Y., and Okayli, G. (1995). Reduction of suicidality during clozapine treatment of neuroleptic-resistant schizophrenia: Impact on risk-benefit assessment. *Am J Psychiatry*, 152(2), 183–190.

Meltzer, H.Y., Alphs, L., Green, A.I., Altamura, A.C., Anand, R., Bertoldi, A., Bourgeois, M., Chouinard, G., Islam, M.Z., Kane, J., Krishnan, R., Lindenmayer, J.P., Potkin, S., and International Suicide Prevention Trial Study Group. (2003). Clozapine treatment for suicidality in schizophrenia: International Suicide Prevention Trial (InterSePT). *Arch Gen Psychiatry*, 60(1), 82–91.

Middlebrook, D.W. (1991). *Anne Sexton: A Biography* (p. 36). Boston: Houghton Mifflin.

Miklowitz, D.J., and Taylor, D.O. (2006). Family-focused treatment of the suicidal bipolar patient. *Bipolar Disord*, 8, 640–651.

Modestin, J., Pian, D.D., and Agarwall, P. (2005). Clozapine diminishes suicidal behavior: A retrospective evaluation of clinical record. *J Clin Psychiatry*, 66, 534–538.

Motto, J.A. (1975). The recognition and management of the suicidal patient. In F.F. Flach and S.C. Draghi (Eds.), *The Nature and Treatment of Depression* (pp. 229–254). New York: John Wiley & Sons.

Muller-Oerlinghausen, B., Muser-Causemann, B., and Volk, J. (1992a). Suicides and parasuicides in a high-risk patient group on and off lithium long-term medication. *J Affect Disord*, 25, 261–269.

Muller-Oerlinghausen, B., Berghofer, A., and Ahrens, B. (2003). The antisuicidal and mortality-reducing effect of lithium prophylaxis: Consequences for guidelines in clinical psychiatry. *Can J Psychiatry*, 48(7), 433–439.

Murphy, G.E. (1975). The physician's responsibility for suicide: II. Errors of omission. *Ann Intern Med*, 82(3), 305–309.

Murphy, G.E., Simons, A.D., Wetzel, R.D., and Lustman, P.J. (1984). Cognitive therapy and pharmacotherapy: Singly and together in the treatment of depression. *Arch Gen Psychiatry*, 41, 33–41.

Norton, B., and Whalley, L.J. (1984). Mortality of a lithium-treated population. *Br J Psychiatry*, 145, 277–282.

Nutt, D.J. (1999). Care of depressed patients with anxiety symptoms. *J Clin Psychiatry*, 60(Suppl. 17), 23–27; discussion, 46–48.

Olfson, M., Shaffer, D., Marcus, S.C., and Greenberg, T. (2003). Relationship between antidepressant medication treatment and suicide in adolescents. *Arch Gen Psychiatry*, 60(10), 978–982.

Olfson, M., Marcus, S.C., and Shaffer, D. (2006). Antidepressant drug therapy and suicide in severely depressed children and adults. *Arch Gen Psychiatry*, 63, 865–872.

Oquendo, M.A., Malone, K.M., Ellis, S.P., Sackeim, H.A., and Mann, J.J. (1999). Inadequacy of antidepressant treatment for patients with major depression who are at risk for suicidal behavior. *Am J Psychiatry*, 156(2), 190–194.

Oquendo, M.A., Galfalvy, H., Russo, S., Ellis, S.P., Grunebaum, M.F., Burke, A., and Mann, J.J. (2004). Prospective study of clinical predictors of suicidal acts after a major depressive episode in patients with major depressive disorder or bipolar disorder. *Am J Psychiatry*, 161(8), 1433–1441.

Osman, A., Gutierrez, P.M., Muehlenkamp, J.J., Dix-Richardson, F., Barrios, F.X., and Kopper, B.A. (2004). Suicide Resilience Inventory-25: Development and preliminary psychometric properties. *Psychol Rep*, 94(3 Pt. 2), 1349–1360.

Pirraglia, P.A., Stafford, R.S., and Singer, D.E. (2003). Trends in prescribing of selective serotonin reuptake inhibitors and other newer antidepressant agents in adult primary care. *Prim Care Companion J Clin Psychiatry*, 5(4), 153–157.

Pokorny, A.D. (1983). Prediction of suicide in psychiatric patients: Reports of a prospective study. *Arch Gen Psychiatry*, 40(3), 249–257.

Pokorny, L.J. (1991). A summary measure of client level of functioning: Progress and challenges for use within mental health agencies. *J Ment Health Adm*, 18(2), 80–87.

Prudic, J., and Sackeim, H.A. (1999). Electroconvulsive therapy and suicide risk. *J Clin Psychiatry*, 60(Suppl. 2), 104–110; discussion, 111–116.

Reid, W.H., Mason, M., and Hogan, T. (1998). Suicide prevention effects associated with clozapine therapy in schizophrenia and schizoaffective disorder. *Psychiatr Serv*, 49(8), 1029–1033.

Rihmer, Z. (2004). Decreasing national suicide rates—fact or fiction? *World J Biol Psychiatry*, 5, 55–56.

Rihmer, Z., Rutz, W., and Pihlgren, H. (1995). Depression and suicide on Gotland. An intensive study of all suicides before and after a depression-training programme. *J Affect Disord*, 35, 147–152.

Robins, E., Murphy, G.E., Wilkinson, R.H., Gassner, S., and Kayes, J. (1959). Some clinical considerations in the prevention of suicide based on a study of 134 successful suicides. *Am J Public Health*, 49, 888–899.

Robins, L.N., Helzer, J.E., Croughan, J., and Ratcliff, K.S. (1981). National Institute of Mental Health Diagnostic Interview Schedule: Its history, characteristics, and validity. *Arch Gen Psychiatry*, 38, 381–389.

Roose, S.P., Glassman, A.H., Walsh, B.T., Woodring, S., and Vital-Herne, J. (1983). Depression, delusions, and suicide. *Am J Psychiatry*, 140, 1159–1162.

Rothschild, A.J., and Locke, C.A. (1991). Reexposure to fluoxetine after serious suicide attempts by three patients: The role of akathisia. *J Clin Psychiatry*, 52(12), 491–493.

Roy, A. (1982). Risk factors for suicide in psychiatric patients. *Arch Gen Psychiatry*, 39, 1089–1095.

Rucci, P., Frank, E., Kostelnik, B., Fagiolini, A., Mallinger, A.G., Swartz, H.A., Thase, M.E., Siegel, L., Wilson, D., and Kupfer, D.J. (2002). Suicide attempts in patients with bipolar I disorder during acute and maintenance phases of intensive treatment with pharmacotherapy and adjunctive psychotherapy. *Am J Psychiatry*, 159(7), 1160–1164.

Rush, B. (1812). *Medical Inquiries and Observations upon the Diseases of the Mind*. Philadelphia: Kimber and Richardson.

Sachs, G.S. (2006). A review of agitation in mental illness: Burden of illness and underlying pathology. *J Clin Psychiatry*, 67(Suppl. 10), 5–12.

Schatzberg, A.F. (1998). Noradrenergic versus serotonergic antidepressants: Predictors of treatment response. *J Clin Psychiatry*, 59(Suppl. 14), 15–18.

Sernyak, M.J., Desai, R., Stolar, M., and Rosenheck, R. (2001). Impact of clozapine on completed suicide. *Am J Psychiatry*, 158(6), 931–937.

Sharma, V. (1999). Retrospective controlled study of inpatient ECT: Does it prevent suicide? *J Affect Disord*, 56(2–3), 183–187.

Sharma, V. (2001). Loss of response to antidepressants and subsequent refractoriness: Diagnostic issues in a retrospective case series. *J Affect Disord*, 64(1), 99–106.

Sheard, M.H. (1975). Effect of lithium on human aggression. *Nature*, 230, 113–114.

Shi, L., Thieband, P., and McCombs, J.S. (2004). The impact of unrecognized bipolar disorders for patients treated with depression with antidepressants in the fee-for-services California Medicaid (Medi-Cal) programme. *J Affect Disord*, 82, 373–383.

Simon, G.E., Savarino, J., Operskalski, B., and Wang, P.S. (2006). Suicide risk during antidepressant treatment. *Am J Psychiatry*, 163, 41–47.

Smith, W.T., Londborg, P.D., Glaudin, V., and Painter, J.R. (2002). Summit research: Is extended clonazepam cotherapy of fluoxetine effective for outpatients with major depression? *J Affect Disord*, 70(3), 251–259.

Soomro, G.M. (2004). Deliberate self harm. *Clin Evid*, (12), 1348–1360.

Storosum, J.G., Elferink, A.J., van Zwieten, B.J., van Strik, R., Hoogendijk, W.J., and Broekmans, A.W. (2002). Amisulpride: Is there a treatment for negative symptoms in schizophrenia patients? *Schizophr Bull*, 28(2), 193–201.

Teicher, M.H., Glod, C.A., and Cole, J.O. (1990). Emergence of intense suicidal preoccupation during fluoxetine treatment. *Am J Psychiatry*, 147(2), 207–210.

Teicher, M.H., Glod, C.A., and Cole, J.O. (1993). Antidepressant drugs and the emergence of suicidal tendencies. *Drug Saf*, 8(3), 186–212.

Tiihonen, J., Lönnqvist, J., Wahlbeck, K., Klaukka, T., Tanskanen, A., and Haukka, J. (2006). Antidepressants and the risk of suicide, attempted suicide, and overall mortality in a nationwide cohort. *Arch Gen Psychiatry*, 63, 1358–1367.

Tondo, L., and Baldessarini, R.J. (2000). Reduced suicide risk during lithium maintenance treatment. *J Clin Psychiatry*, 61(Suppl. 9), 97–104.

Tran, P.V., Dellva, M.A., Tollefson, G.D., Wentley, A.L., and Beasley, C.M. (1998). Oral olanzapine versus oral haloperidol in the maintenance treatment of schizophrenia and related psychoses. *Br J Psychiatry*, 172, 499–505.

Treiser, S.L., Cascio, C.S., O'Donohue, T.L., Thoa, N.B., Jacobowitz, D.M., and Kellar, K.J. (1981). Lithium increases serotonin release and decreases serotonin receptors in the hippocampus. *Science*, 213, 1529–1531.

U.S. Food and Drug Administration (FDA). (2004). T.A. Hammad (Ed.), *Relationship between Psychotropic Drugs and Pediatric Suicidality: Review and Evaluation of Clinical Data*. Available: http://www.fda.gov/ohrms/dockets/ac/04/briefing/2004-4065b1-10-TAB08-Hammads-Review.pdf (accessed September 19, 2006).

U.S. Public Health Service. (1999). *The Surgeon General's Call to Action to Prevent Suicide*. Washington, DC: Department of Health and Human Services.

Vestergaard, P., and Aagaard, J. (1991). Five-year mortality in lithium-treated manic-depressive patients. *J Affect Disord*, 21, 33–38.

Wagner, K.D., Robb, A.S., Findling, R.L., Jin, J., Gutierrez, M.M., and Heydorn, W.E. (2004). A randomized, placebo-controlled trial of citalopram for the treatment of major depression in children and adolescents. *Am J Psychiatry*, 161, 1079–1083.

Walker, A.M., Lanza, L.L., Arellano, F., and Rothman, K.J. (1997). Mortality in current and former users of clozapine. *Epidemiology*, 8(6), 671–677.

Weeke, A. (1979). Causes of death in manic-depressives. In M. Schou and E. Strömgren (Eds.), *Origin, Prevention and Treatment of Affective Disorders* (pp. 289–299). London: Academic Press.

West, L.J. (1975). Integrative psychotherapy of depressive illness. In F.F. Flach and S.C. Draghi (Eds.), *The Nature and Treatment of Depression*. New York: John Wiley & Sons.

Winokur, G., Clayton, P.J., and Reich, T. (1969). *Manic Depressive Illness*. St. Louis: CV Mosby.

Wolf, T., Muller-Oerlinghausen, B., Ahrens, B., Grof, P., Schou, M., Feiber, W., Grof, E., Lenz, G., Nilsson, A., Simhandl, C., Thau, K., Vestergaard, P., and Wolf, R. (1996). How to interpret findings on mortality of long-term lithium treated manic-depressive patients? Critique of different methodological approaches. *J Affect Disord*, 39, 127–132.

Yerevanian, B.I., Koek, R.J., and Mintz, J. (2003). Lithium, anticonvulsants and suicidal behavior in bipolar disorder. *J Affect Disord*, 73, 223–228.

Zito, J.M., Safer, D.J., dosReis, S., Gardner, J.F., Magder, L., Soeken, K., Boles, M., Lynch, F., and Riddle, M.A. (2003). Psychotropic practice patterns for youth: A 10-year perspective. *Arch Pediatr Adolesc Med*, 157(1), 17–25.

INDEX

Note: Page numbers followed by the letter b refer to boxes, those followed by f refer to figures, and those followed
by t refer to tables.

Learned helplessness, 467–68
Learning deficits, 291–98. *See also* Memory deficits
Lecithin, for acute mania, in children and
    adolescents, 928
Leucopenia, from carbamazepine, 810
Leukocytes, gene expression in, 451
Level I randomized controlled trials, challenges
    in interpreting, 707–12, 707b, 708t
Levels of evidence, 706–7, 707b
Levels of processing, memory and, 296–98
Levetiracetam, for acute mania, 724, 736,
    746nn23–24
Liability threshold model, 421
Life Chart Method (LCM), 373–74, 881–82
Life events, in triggering episodes, 135–38,
    136t–137t
Life Goals Program, 903–4
Lifestyle changes, 705
Light
    phase response curve, 661, 690n14
    sensitivity to, 671–72
        seasonal affective disorder and, 687–88
    suicide and, 254
Light therapy. *See* Phototherapy
Limbic basal ganglia–thalamocortical circuits,
    610, 610f
Limbic regional cerebral blood flow (rCBF),
    628–29, 629f
Limit setting, 745n7
Linguistic patterns
    in mania versus depression, 52–53, 53t
    in mania versus schizophrenia, 51–52, 52f
Linkage disequilibrium studies, 445
Linkage studies, 423–30, 459
    affected sibling pair method, 426
    complex disorders, 430, 462nn11–12
    findings, 426, 427f
    future directions, 455
    LOD score approach, 425–26, 461–62n9
    meta-analyses, 426–27, 428t
    method, 423–25, 425f
    promising chromosomal regions, 427–30, 427f
Lithium
    for acute hypomania, 728
    for acute mania, 723, 725, 725f, 726, 740
        plus carbamazepine, 733
        in children and adolescents, 912, 917–23,
            918t, 920t–922t, 934n2
        versus clonazepam, 742
        combination therapy, 928
        dosages, 726
        efficacy, 729–33, 730f, 730t, 731t, 732f
        plus haloperidol, 733, 736
        versus lamotrigine, 735
        versus olanzapine, 739
        versus oxcarbazepine, 735
        plus quetiapine, 740
        plus risperidone, 740
        versus risperidone, 740
        versus valproate, 734
        versus verapamil, 743
        plus ziprasidone, 741
    adenyl cyclase and, 543–44, 604n60
    adherence to, 849–68. *See also* Medications,
        adherence
    for aggression, 913, 914t, 929
    Bcl-2 overexpression, 572–74, 573f, 581, 583f

for bipolar depression, 751, 753, 759, 759t, 760t,
    761–62
    versus antidepressants, 759, 760t, 761, 761t
    augmentation of antidepressants, 761–62,
        762t, 793nn16–19
    plus carbamazepine, 763
    in children and adolescents, 911, 929
    plus topiramate, 765
    plus valproate, 763, 794n22
blood levels
    in acute mania, 726
    instant test, 804
    in maintenance, 802, 804, 844n7
cardiovascular mortality and, 949
cholinergic system and, 502–3
chronobiological effects, 672–73
circadian rhythms and, 557, 562f
cognitive impairment from, 275, 306–8, 306f,
    307f, 807
in comorbid conditions
    anxiety disorders, 948
    cardiovascular disease, 949
    eating disorders, 949
    substance abuse, 939, 940t, 941t, 943
creativity and, 403–5, 405f, 405t
CREB and, 543
dermatologic problems from, 807, 844n14
diabetes and, 243–44
discontinuation
    relapse after, 824–25
    suicide risk after, 971
dopaminergic system and, 486–87
effects on normal mood, 824
efficacy, strength of evidence, 838t
G protein signaling and, 543, 604n59
GABAergic system and, 506–7
glucocorticoids and, 494
glutamate and, 512–13
hippocampal neurogenesis with, 576, 578, 578f
historical perspective, 798
for hyperkinesis in children of bipolar parents,
    930
hypothyroidism from, 487, 518, 804, 806, 808,
    842, 845nn20–21, 932
inositol-deficient diet and, 732–33
intoxication, 808–9
intrinsic qualities, adherence and, 865
magnetic resonance spectroscopy, 651–52, 652f
maintenance. *See* Lithium maintenance
marital functioning and, 349–50
for mixed mania, 725, 725f
monitoring, 716, 720nn15–16, 726
as "mood normalizer," 798
neuroprotective effects, 557, 574–75, 574b, 575f,
    581, 606–7n82
neurotrophic effects, 580, 580f–582f, 586b,
    587–89
norepinephrine and, 480
opiates and, 532, 603n49
personality and, 333–34
pharmacogenetics, 453
pharmacology, 715–16
phosphoinositide cycle and, 550–53, 553f,
    604nn62–66
precautions/medical issues, 753
productivity and, 404, 405t
prophylaxis. *See* Lithium maintenance

protein kinase C and, 554, 554f
psychopharmacological revolution initiated
    by, 699, 719n1
REM sleep and, 667
renal effects, 807–8, 844nn15–19
responsiveness to
    as endophenotype, 435
    offspring studies, 215, 219
retinal ganglion cell axon regeneration with,
    576, 577f
serotonergic system and, 496–97
sexual behavior and, 349
side effects, adherence and, 862–63
plus sleep deprivation therapy, 677
suicide and, 254, 762
teratogenicity, 815, 816t
vasopressin and, 533
weight gain from, 806, 844nn11–12, 932
Lithium maintenance, 802, 804, 806–9
    plus anticonvulsants, 839, 848nn87–88
    plus antidepressants, 839, 840t, 841
    plus antipsychotics, 841
    blood levels, 802, 804, 844n7
    breakthrough depression on, 750
    in breast-feeding women, 817–18, 846n45
    versus carbamazepine, 830–31, 831f
    in children and adolescents, 911, 916, 929–30
    differential response, clinical characteristics
        associated with, 828t
    efficacy, 819–29, 832t, 833t
        in bipolar-II disorder, 828, 829t
        contemporary studies using lithium as
            comparator, 821–23, 846nn49–52
        placebo-controlled studies prior to 1980,
            820–21, 821f
        predictors, 825, 827–28, 828t, 846nn56–59
        in rapid cycling, 825–27, 826t–827t
        in recurrent unipolar depression, 800,
            828–29
        renewed controversies, 821–23
        in treating mania versus depression,
            823–24
    in elderly person, 814–15
    versus lamotrigine, 831–34, 834f
    versus olanzapine, 837
    perceived losses associated with, 877–78
    in pregnancy, 815, 816t
    pretreatment evaluation and ongoing
        monitoring, 803t
    recurrence rate bias, 126, 128
    side effects, 804, 806–8, 807t
    before sleep deprivation, 789
    for suicide prevention, 960, 967–71, 968f, 969f,
        970t, 972–73, 976n5
    toxicity treatment, 808–9
    versus valproate, 829–30
Living alone, medication adherence and, 864
Localization of mood systems, brain functional
    asymmetry and, 318–20
Locomotor activity, baseline, 469
LOD score approach, linkage studies, 425–26,
    461–62n9
Lofepramine, for bipolar depression, 762
Logan, Joshua, 875, 879
Lombroso, C., 383
Longitudinal Interval Follow-Up Evaluation
    (LIFE), 373